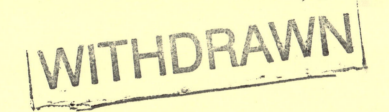

Wiley Encyclopedia of

FORENSIC SCIENCE

Wiley Encyclopedia of
FORENSIC SCIENCE

Volume 4

M–Q

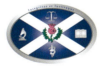

Editors-in-Chief

Allan Jamieson
The Forensic Institute, Glasgow, UK

Andre Moenssens
Forensics and Law Center, Columbia City, IN, USA

WILEY

This edition first published 2009
© 2009 John Wiley & Sons Ltd

Registered office

John Wiley & Sons Ltd, The Atrium, Southern Gate, Chichester, West Sussex, PO19 8SQ, United Kingdom

For details of our global editorial offices, for customer services and for information about how to apply for permission to reuse the copyright material in this book please see our website at www.wiley.com.

Bomb-Pulse Dating, pp. 418–422; Radiocarbon Dating, pp. 2231–2233; Dissociative Disorders, pp. 784–792; Footwear and Foot Impressions: Foot Impressions and Linking Foot to Shoe, pp. 1244–1248; Footwear and Foot Impressions: Overview, pp. 1252–1255; Forged and Counterfeit Documents, pp. 1255–1276, are all US Government works in the public domain and not subject to copyright.

Accreditation: Laboratory, pp. 1–10, is copyright of The American Society of Crime Laboratory Directors/Laboratory Accreditation Board (ASCLD/LAB) and is used here with their consent.

Juvenile Justice: Adolescent Development, pp. 1608–1612, and Juvenile Justice: Transfer to Adult, pp. 1612–1618, are copyright of the John D. and Catherine T. MacArthur Foundation and are used here with their consent.

Bloodstain Pattern Interpretation, pp. 359–396, is copyright of the author and is used here with his consent.

Library of Congress Cataloging-in-Publication Data

Wiley encyclopedia of forensic science / editors in chief, Allan Jamieson, Andre Moenssens.
    p. ; cm.
    Includes bibliographical references and index.
    ISBN 978-0-470-01826-2 (set : cloth)
  1. Forensic sciences–Encyclopedias. I. Jamieson, Allan. II. Moenssens, Andre A. III. Title: Encyclopedia of forensic science.
    [DNLM: 1. Forensic Medicine–Encyclopedias–English. 2. Forensic Sciences–Encyclopedias–English. W 613 W714 2009]
    HV8073.W55 2009
    363.2503–dc22

                                                                2009001881

A catalogue record for this book is available from the British Library.

Set in $9\frac{1}{2}$ / $11\frac{1}{2}$ pt Times by Laserwords Private Limited, Chennai, India
Printed and bound by Grafos S.A., Barcelona, Spain

Contents

viii   *Contents*

x   *Contents*

Contributors

ABBONDANTE, SERENA F. *Australian Federal Police, Weston and Australian Chemical, Biological Radiological and Nuclear Data Centre, Canberra, ACT, Australia*

ABDEL-MONEM, TARIK *University of Nebraska Public Policy Center, Lincoln, NE, USA*

ABOU-KHALIL, BASSEL *Vanderbilt University School of Medicine, Nashville, TN, USA*

ABRAM, KAREN M. *Northwestern University Feinberg School of Medicine, Chicago, IL, USA*

ADAMS, HOLLY A. *Automotive Data Consultants, Centreville, VA, USA*

AITKEN, COLIN G. G. *University of Edinburgh, Edinburgh, UK*

ALBERINK, IVO *Netherlands Forensic Institute, Den Haag, The Netherlands*

ALEKSANDER, ADAM K. *Aleksander & Associates P.A., Boise, ID, USA*

ALLEN, REBECCA S. *Center for Mental Health and Aging, Tuscaloosa, AL, USA*

ALMOG, JOSEPH *The Hebrew University of Jerusalem, Jerusalem, Israel*

ANDERSON, ROBERT N. *RNA Consulting, Inc., Losaltos Hills, CA, USA*

ANDREWS, PAUL *Tyler, TX, USA*

ANETZBERGER, GEORGIA J. *Cleveland State University, Cleveland, OH, USA*

AUMEER-DONOVAN, SHAHEEN *University of Technology, Sydney, New South Wales, Australia*

BADEN, MICHAEL M. *New York State Police, Albany, NY, USA*

BADER, SCOTT *The Forensic Institute, Glasgow, UK*

BAKER, DAVID W. *The MITRE Corporation, McLean, VA, USA*

BALDING, DAVID *Imperial College, London, UK*

BALDWIN, DAVID *London Laboratory, London, UK*

BALLANTYNE, JACK *University of Central Florida and National Center for Forensic Science, Orlando, FL, USA*

BARNES, SEAN *Binghamton University, Binghamton, NY, USA*

BARNI, FILIPPO *Carabinieri Scientific Investigation Department of Rome, Rome, Italy*

BENBOW, M. ERIC *Michigan State University, East Lansing, MI, USA*

BERKOWITZ, SHARI R. *University of California, Irvine, CA, USA*

BERNET, WILLIAM *Vanderbilt University School of Medicine, Nashville, TN, USA*

BEYER, JOCHEN *Monash University, Southbank and Victorian Institute of Forensic Medicine, Melbourne, Victoria, Australia*

BICKNELL, DANNA E. *United States Secret Service, Washington, DC, USA*

BLACK, SUE *University of Dundee, Dundee, Scotland, UK*

BLOCK, STEPHANIE *University of California, Davis, CA*

BOHNERT, MICHAEL *University of Freiburg, Freiburg, Germany*

BOTLUK, DIANA *Stetson University College of Law, Gulfport, FL, USA*

BOTTOMS, BETTE L. *University of Illinois at Chicago, Chicago, IL, USA*

BOWMAN-FOWLER, NICCI *University of California, Irvine, CA, USA*

BRAUN, MICHELLE *Wheaton Franciscan Healthcare, Racine, WI, USA*

BRESLER, SCOTT A. *University of Cincinnati, Cincinnati, OH, USA*

BRICK, JOHN *Intoxikon International, Yardley, PA, USA*

BRIGHT, JO-ANNE *Institute of Environmental Science and Research Limited, Auckland, New Zealand*

BRYANT, VAUGHN M. *Texas A&M University, College Station, TX, USA*

BUCHHOLZ, BRUCE A. *Lawrence Livermore National Laboratory, Livermore, CA, USA*

BUCKLETON, JOHN S. *Institute of Environmental Science and Research, Ltd., Auckland, New Zealand*

BULLING, DENISE *University of Nebraska Public Policy Center, Lincoln, NE, USA*

BURGESS, ANN W. *Boston College, Chestnut Hill, MA, USA*

CANTU, ANTONIO A. *Seven Oaks Place, Falls Church, VA, USA*

CARPENTER, DOUGLAS J. *Combustion Science & Engineering, Inc., Columbia, MD, USA*

CATTANEO, CRISTINA *Universitá degli Studi, Milan, Italy*

CHAMPOD, CHRISTOPHE *Institut de Police Scientifique, University of Lausanne, Lausanne, Switzerland*

CHENG, WING-CHI *Government Laboratory, Hong Kong Special Administrative Region, China*

CHOI, HYEYOUNG *National Institute of Scientific Investigation, Seoul, South Korea*

CHOI, SANGKIL *National Institute of Scientific Investigation, Seoul, South Korea*

CHRISTENSEN, THOMAS C. *San Ramon, CA, USA*

CHUNG, HEESUN *National Institute of Scientific Investigation, Seoul, South Korea*

CLEGG, CARL *West Virginia University, Morgantown, WV, USA*

COBLE, MICHAEL D. *The Armed Forces DNA Identification Laboratory, Rockville, MD, USA*

CONNOR, MELISSA *Nebraska Wesleyan University, Lincoln, NE, USA*

CORNELL, DEWEY G. *University of Virginia, Charlottesville, VA, USA*

COSTANZO, MARK *Claremont McKenna College, Claremont, CA, USA*

COSTELLO, JAN *Loyola Law School, Los Angeles, CA, USA*

COURT, DENISE S. *Barts and The London School of Medicine and Dentistry, London, UK*

COWELL, ANTHONY M. *University of Lincoln, Lincoln, UK*

CROSS, DOUGLAS W. *Lowick Bridge, Ulverston, UK*

CURRAN, JAMES M. *University of Auckland, Auckland, New Zealand*

DAVIS, MALCOLM *Vashaw Scientific, Inc., Norcross, GA, USA*

DAY, STEPHEN P. *Huntingdon Forensic Science Laboratory, Cambridgeshire, UK*

DE ANGELIS, DANILO *Università degli Studi, Milan, Italy*

DE BOECK, GERT *National Institute of Criminalistics and Criminology, Brussels, Belgium*

DE LA TORRE, RAFAEL *Neuropsychopharmacology Program IMIM-Hospital del Mar PRBB, Barcelona, Spain*

DEN DUNNEN, M. *Amsterdam-Amstelland Police, Amsterdam, The Netherlands*

DICKSON, STUART *Institute of Environmental Science and Research Limited, Porirua, New Zealand*

DIETZ, PARK *Threat Assessment Group, Inc., and Park Dietz & Associates, Inc., Newport Beach and University of California, Los Angeles, CA, USA*

DOUGLAS, KEVIN S. *Simon Fraser University, Burnaby, British Columbia, Canada*

DRUMMER, OLAF H. *Monash University, Southbank, Victoria, Australia*

DUTTON, GERARD *Tasmania Police, Hobart, Tasmania, Australia*

DUVINAGE, NICOLAS *Gendarmerie National Forensic Sciences Institute (IRCGN), Rosny-sous-Bios, France*

DU PREEZ, CHARL *University of Technology, Sydney, New South Wales, Australia*

EASTEAL, PATRICIA *University of Canberra, Canberra, ACT, Australia*

EDELMAN, GERDA *Netherlands Forensic Institute, Den Haag, The Netherlands*

EDELSTEIN, BARRY A. *West Virginia University, Morgantown, WV, USA*

EDWARDS, CARL N. *Four Oaks Institute, Dover, MA, USA*

ELKINGTON, KATE S. *Columbia University and New York State Psychiatric Institute, New York, NY, USA*

ERICKSON, STEVEN K. *University of Pennsylvania Law School, Philadelphia, PA, USA*

ERIKSSON, ANDERS F. *Umeå University, Umeå, Sweden*

ERVIN, THOMAS *The MITRE Corporation, McLean, VA, USA*

ESSEIVA, PIERRE *University of Lausanne, Lausanne, Switzerland*

EVETT, IAN W. *London Laboratory, London, UK*

FAGAN, JEFFREY *Columbia Law School, New York, NY, USA*

FELGATE, PETER *Forensic Science South Australia, Adelaide, South Australia, Australia*

FIDDIAN, SUSAN *Victoria Police Forensic Services Department, McLeod, Victoria, Australia*

FINCH, INDRA A. *Center for Forensic Services – Western State Hospital, Tacoma, WA, USA*

FINESCHI, VITTORIO *University of Foggia, Foggia, Italy*

FINKENBINE, RYAN *West Virginia University, Morgantown, WV, USA*

FITTERMAN, ELIZABETH *Stetson University College of Law, Gulfport, FL, USA*

FITZPATRICK, ROBERT W. *Centre for Australian Forensic Soil Science/CSIRO Land and Water, Adelaide, South Australia, Australia*

FLANAGAN, ROBERT J. *King's College Hospital NHS Foundation Trust, London, UK*

FOUND, BRYAN *Latrobe University, Bundoora and Victoria Police Forensic Services Department, Macleod, Victoria, Australia*

FOWLER, NICCI B. *University of California, Irvine, CA, USA*

FRAZIER, LEEANNE *Stetson University College of Law, Gulfport, FL, USA*

FREMOUW, WILLIAM J. *West Virginia University, Morgantown, WV, USA*

FRUDAKIS, TONY *DNAPrint Genomics, Inc., Sarasota, FL, USA*

FRUMKIN, BRUCE *Forensic and Clinical Psychology Associates, South Miami, FL, USA*

GALLO, FRANK J. *Western New England College, Springfield, MA, USA*

GANIS, GIORGIO *Harvard Medical School, Boston, and Atinoulas Martinos Center, Charlestown, and Harvard University, Cambridge, MA, USA*

GARDNER, ROSS M. *Bevel, Gardner and Associates, Inc., Lake City, GA, USA*

GELLER, JEFFREY L. *University of Massachusetts Medical School, Worcester, MA, USA*

GERADTS, ZENO *Netherlands Forensic Institute, Den Haag, The Netherlands*

GERAERTS, ELKE *Harvard University, Cambridge, MA, USA and Maastricht University, Maastricht, The Netherlands*

GEROSTAMOULOS, DIMITRI *Monash University, Southbank, Victoria, Australia*

GIBELLI, DANIELE *Universitá degli Studi, Milan, Italy*

GIBLIN, MARY *Garda Headquarters, Dublin, Ireland*

GILDER, JASON R. *Forensic Bioinformatics, Fairborn, OH, USA*

GILLMAN, VICTORIA C. *Australian Federal Police, Weston and Australian Chemical, Biological Radiological and Nuclear Data Centre, Canberra, ACT, Australia*

GITLOW, STUART *Mount Sinai School of Medicine, New York, NY, USA*

GODDARD, KEN *National Fish and Wildlife Forensics Laboratory, Ashland, OR, USA*

GOODMAN, GAIL S. *University of California, Davis, CA, USA*

GOODWIN, KERRI A. *Towson University, Towson, MD, USA*

GOULD, CHRISTINE E. *West Virginia University, Morgantown, WV, USA*

GRAHAM, ELEANOR A.M. *University of Leicester, Leicester, UK*

GREAVES, CAROLINE *BC Mental Health & Addiction Services, Port Coquitlam and Simon Fraser University, Burnaby, British Columbia, Canada*

GREENBERG, MARTIN S. *University of Pittsburgh, Pittsburgh, PA, USA*

GREENE, EDIE *University of Colorado at Colorado Spring, Colorado Spring, CO, USA*

HACKMAN, LUCINA *University of Dundee, Dundee, UK*

HAMILTON, WARREN D. *Rapidtox Pty. Ltd., Brisbane, Queensland, Australia*

HAMMER, LESLEY *State of Alaska Crime Laboratory, Anchorage, AK, USA*

HANSON, ERIN K. *University of Central Florida and National Center for Forensic Science, Orlando, FL, USA*

HAN, EUNYOUNG *National Institute of Scientific Investigation, Seoul, South Korea*

HARBISON, SALLY-ANN *Institute of Environmental Science and Research Ltd., Auckland, New Zealand*

HART, STEPHEN D. *Simon Fraser University, Burnaby, British Columbia, Canada*

HASEL, LISA E. *Iowa State University, Ames, IA, USA*

HATTERS-FRIEDMAN, SUSAN *University Hospital – Case Medical Center, Cleveland, OH, USA*

HAYNE, HARLENE *University of Otago, Dunedin, New Zealand*

HAZELWOOD, ROBERT R. *Academy Group, Inc., Manassas, VA, USA*

HENDERSON, CAROL *Stetson University College of Law, Gulfport, FL, USA*

HICKS, TACHA N. *Institut de Police Scientifique, University of Lausanne, Lausanne, Switzerland*

HILL, CHERYL A. *West Virginia University, Morgantown, WV, USA*

HONTS, CHARLES ROBERT *Boise State University, Boise, ID, USA*

HOPEN, THOMAS J. *The Bureau of Alcohol, Tobacco, Firearms and Explosives, Atlanta, GA, USA*

HUNTER, JOHN *University of Birmingham, Birmingham, UK*

IKEGAYA, HIROSHI *Kyoto Prefectural University of Medicine, Kyoto, Japan*

ISENSCHMID, DANIEL S. *Wayne County Medical Examiner's Office, Detroit, MI, USA*

JACKSON, GRAHAM *Advance Forensic Science, and University of Abertay Dundee, Dundee, UK*

JACKSON, MICHAEL *New South Wales Police Force, Sydney, New South Wales, Australia*

JAMIESON, ALLAN *The Forensic Institute, Glasgow, UK*

JONES, ALAN W. *National Board of Forensic Medicine, Linköping, Sweden*

JONES, GRAHAM R. *Office of the Chief Medical Examiner, Edmonton, Alberta, Canada*

JONES, PHILIP J. *York, North Yorkshire, UK*

JUST, REBECCA S. *The Armed Forces DNA Identification Laboratory, Rockville, MD, USA*

KARCH, STEVEN B. *Berkeley, CA, USA*

KASSIN, SAUL *John Jay College of Criminal Justice, New York, NY, USA*

KATSUMATA, YOSHINAO *National Research Institute of Police Science, Chiba, Japan*

KATTERWE, HORST *Bundeskriminalamt, Wiesbaden, Germany*

KAYE, DAVID H. *Arizona State University, Tempe, AZ, USA*

KAYE, NEIL S. *Widener University School of Law, Wilmington, DE, USA*

KEATON, RALPH *American Society of Crime Laboratory Directors/ Laboratory Accreditation Board (ASCLD/LAB), Garner, NC, USA*

KEEREWEER, ISAÄC *Netherlands Forensic Institute, The Hague, The Netherlands*

KEHN, ANDRE *University of Wyoming, Laramie, WY, USA*

KENAN, JOSEPH *University of California Los Angeles School of Medicine, Beverly Hills, CA, USA*

KENNEDY, ROBERT *Royal Canadian Mounted Police (Retired), Ottawa, Ontario, Canada*

KERNBACH-WIGHTON, GERHARD *University of Edinburgh, Edinburgh, UK*

KHANMY-VITAL, AITA *University of Lausanne, Lausanne, Switzerland*

KIM, EUNMI *National Institute of Scientific Investigation, Seoul, South Korea*

KINTZ, PASCAL *Laboratoire ChemTox, Illkirch, France*

KIRKBRIDE, K. PAUL *Australian Federal Police, Canberra, ACT, Australia*

KNOLL, IV, JAMES L. *SUNY Upstate Medical University, Syracuse, NY, USA*

KOEHLER, JONATHAN J. *Arizona State University, Tempe, AZ, USA*

KOPERSKI, J. GEORGE *Australian Federal Police, Weston and Australian Chemical, Biological Radiological and Nuclear Data Centre, Canberra, ACT, Australia*

KOSSLYN, STEPHEN M. *Harvard University, Cambridge and Massachusetts General Hospital, Boston, MA, USA*

KRANE, DAN E. *Wright State University, Dayton, OH, USA*

LAMENDOLA, GRETCHEN M. *Nova Southeastern University, Fort Lauderdale, FL, USA*

LANCASTER, SARAH L. *Defence Science and Technology Laboratories, Sevenoaks, UK*

LANGENBURG, GLENN *Minnesota Bureau of Criminal Apprehension, St. Paul, MN, USA*

LAPORTE, GERALD M. *United States Secret Service, Washington, DC, USA*

LAUX, DALE L. *Attorney General's Office, Richfield, OH, USA*

LEBEAU, MARC A. *FBI Laboratory, Quantico, VA, USA*

LEE, JUSEON *National Institute of Scientific Investigation, Seoul, South Korea*

LEE, LI-WEN G. *New York University School of Medicine, New York, NY, USA*

LEE, SOOYEUN *National Institute of Scientific Investigation, Seoul, South Korea*

LENNARD, CHRIS *University of Canberra, Canberra, ACT, Australia*

LENTINI, JOHN J. *Scientific Fire Analysis, LLC, Big Pine Key, FL, USA*

LENZ, KURT W. *Stetson University College of Law, Gulfport, FL, USA*

LEONG, GREGORY B. *University of Washington, Seattle, WA, USA*

LEO, RICHARD A. *University of San Francisco, San Francisco, CA, USA*

LEWIS, SIMON W. *Curtin University of Technology, Perth, Western Australia, Australia*

LIM, MIAE *National Institute of Scientific Investigation, Seoul, South Korea*

LIPTAI, LAURA L. *Biomedical Forensics, Moraga, CA and Orlando, FL, USA*

LOFTUS, ELIZABETH F. *University of California, Irvine, CA, USA*

LOVELL, ROBERT W. *Mercer Island, WA, USA*

LOVELOCK, TINA J. *LGC Forensics, Abingdon, UK*

LUONG, SUSAN *University of Technology, Sydney, New South Wales, Australia*

LYNN, STEVEN JAY *Binghamton University, Binghamton, NY, USA*

MAAT, G.J.R. *Netherlands Forensic Institute, The Hague and Leiden University Medical Center, Leiden, The Netherlands*

MACDONELL, HERBERT L. *Bloodstain Evidence Institute, Corning, NY, USA*

MACEO, ALICE V. *Las Vegas Metropolitan Police Department Forensic Laboratory, Las Vegas, NV, USA*

MACVAUGH III, GILBERT S. *Mississippi State Hospital, Whitfield, MS, USA*

MADEA, BURKHARD *University of Bonn, Bonn, Germany*

MAIDEN, NICHOLAS R. *South Australia Police, Adelaide, South Australiaa, Australia*

MALLETT, XANTHÉ *University of Dundee, Dundee, UK*

MARGOT, PIERRE *University of Lausanne, Lausanne, Switzerland*

MARLEEN, LALOUP *National Institute of Criminalistics and Criminology, Brussels, Belgium*

MARSHALL, MAURICE *Defence Science and Technology Laboratories, Sevenoaks, UK*

MARTELL, DANIEL A. *UCLA, Los Angeles, CA, USA*

MASSONNET, GENEVIÈVE *University of Lausanne, Lausanne, Switzerland*

MASTRUKO, VOJIN *Court Expert Witness, Zagreb, Croatia*

MATTHEWS, ABIGAIL *Binghamton University, Binghamton, NY, USA*

MAZZELLA, W.D. *University of Lausanne, Lausanne, Switzerland*

McCOY, KATRINA *West Virginia University, Morgantown, WV, USA*

McCULLOUGH, JOHN *Garda HQ, Dublin, Ireland*

McDERMOTT, SEAN D. *Forensic Science Laboratory, Dublin, Ireland*

McKENNA, LOUISE *Garda Headquarters, Dublin, Ireland*

McNALLY, RICHARD J. *Harvard University, Cambridge, MA, USA*

MEIJERMAN, L. *Netherlands Forensic Institute, The Hague, and Leiden University Medical Center, Leiden, The Netherlands*

MELOY, J. REID *University of California, San Diego, California, USA*

MELSON, KENNETH E. *American Society of Crime Laboratory Directors/ Laboratory Accreditation Board (ASCLD/LAB), Garner, NC, USA*

MELTON, TERRY *Mitotyping Technologies, LLC, State College, LA, USA*

MERRITT, RICHARD W. *Michigan State University, East Lansing, MI, USA*

MEUWLY, DIDIER *Netherlands Forensic Institute, The Hague, The Netherlands*

MICHEALS, ANASTASIA D. *San Jose State University, San Jose, CA, USA*

MILES, SAMUEL I. *Geffen School of Medicine UCLA, Los Angeles and Cedars-Sinai Medical Center, Los Angeles, CA, USA*

MOENSSENS, ANDRE *Forensics and Law Center, Columbia City, IN, USA*

MOHAMMED, LINTON A. *San Diego Sheriff's Regional Crime Laboratory, San Diego, CA, USA*

MONNARD, FLORENCE *University of Lausanne, Lausanne, Switzerland*

MORETTI, MARLENE M. *Simon Fraser University, Burnaby, British Columbia, Canada*

MORRISH, BRONWYN C. *Australian Federal Police, Weston and Australian Chemical, Biological Radiological and Nuclear Data Centre, Canberra, ACT, Australia*

MUELLER-JOHNSON, KATRIN *University of Cambridge, Cambridge, UK*

MURPHY, JOHN P. *CSIRO Forest Biosciences, Clayton, Victoria, Australia*

NEHSE, KORNELIA *Forensic Science Institute, Berlin, Germany*

NELE, SAMYN *National Institute of Criminalistics and Criminology, Brussels, Belgium*

NELSON, KALLY J. *University of California, Irvine, CA, USA*

NERENBERG, LISA *Private Consultant, Redwood City, CA, USA*

NEUMANN, CEDRIC *The Forensic Science Service Ltd, Birmingham, UK and University of Lausanne, Lausanne, Switzerland*

NEUNER, JOHN K. *American Society of Crime Laboratory Directors/ Laboratory Accreditation Board (ASCLD/LAB), Garner, NC, USA*

NEUSCHATZ, JEFFREY S. *University of Alabama in Huntsville, Huntsville, AL, USA*

NICHOLLS, TONIA L. *BC Mental Health & Addiction Services, Port Coquitlam and University of British Columbia, Vancouver, British Columbia, Canada*

NIKOLOVA, NATALIA L. *Simon Fraser University, Burnaby, British Columbia, Canada*

NORMAN, KEITH W. *Australian Federal Police, Weston, ACT, Australia*

NUNEZ, NARINA L. *University of Wyoming, Laramie, WY, USA*

OJANPERÄ, ILKKA *University of Helsinki, Helsinki, Finland*

OLLEY, J. GREGORY *University of North Carolina, Chapel Hill, NC, USA*

ÖSTRÖM, MATS G. *Umeå University, Umeå, Sweden*

OXLEY, JIMMIE C. *University of Rhode Island, Kingston, RI, USA*

PARK, YONGHOON *National Institute of Scientific Investigation, Seoul, South Korea*

PAYNE-JAMES, JASON *Forensic Healthcare Services, Leigh-on-Sea and Royal College of Physicians and Barts & the Royal London Hospitals, London, UK*

PERRY, SYLVIA *University of Illinois at Chicago, Chicago, IL, USA*

PETERSON, TIAMOYO *University of California, Irvine, CA, USA*

PICHINI, SIMONA *Istituto Superiore di Sanità, Rome, Italy*

PINALS, DEBRA A. *University of California, Sacramento, CA, USA*

PIPER, AUGUST *Seattle, WA, USA*

POLLAK, STEFAN *University of Freiburg, Freiburg, Germany*

POLLANEN, MICHAEL S. *University of Toronto, Toronto, Ontario, Canada*

PORTA, DAVIDE *Università degli Studi, Milan, Italy*

PORTER, GLENN *University of Western Sydney, Penrith South DC, New South Wales, Australia*

POULSEN, HELEN *Institute of Environmental Science and Research Limited, Porirua, New Zealand*

QUINN, MARY J. *San Francisco Probate Court, San Francisco, CA, USA*

RAES, ELKE *Ghent University, Ghent, Belgium*

RAFF, ADAM N. *New York University Medical Center, New York, NY, USA*

RANDOLPH-QUINNEY, PATRICK *University of Dundee, Dundee, UK*

RAYMOND, JENNIFER J. *NSW Police Force, Pemulwuy, New South Wales, Australia*

RAY, NEELANJAN *New York University School of Medicine, New York, NY, USA*

REED, TOM *Widener University School of Law, Wilmington, DE, USA*

RESNICK, PHILLIP J. *Case Western Reserve University Medical School, Cleveland, OH, USA*

RESOR, MICHELLE R. *University of North Carolina at Charlotte, Charlotte, NC, USA*

RESSLER, ROBERT K. *Forensic Behavioral Services, Fredericksburg, VA, USA*

RIEZZO, IRENE *University of Foggia, Foggia, Italy*

ROBERTSON, JAMES *Australian Federal Police, Canberra, ACT, Australia*

ROFFEY, PAUL E. *Australian Federal Police, Weston and University of Canberra, Canberra, ACT, Australia*

ROMERO, ERIN G. *Northwestern University, Chicago, IL, USA*

ROUX, CLAUDE *University of Technology (UTS), Sydney, New South Wales, Australia*

ROYDS, DAVID *Australian Federal Police, Canberra, Australia*

RUIFROK, ARNOUT C. C. *Netherlands Forensic Institute, The Hague, The Netherlands*

SALEKIN, KAREN L. *University of Alabama, Tuscaloosa, AL, USA*

SALSAROLA, DOMINIC *Universitá degli Studi, Milan, Italy*

SAUKKO, PEKKA J. *University of Turku, Kiinamyllynkatu, Turku, Finland*

SAUVAGNAT, FRANÇOIS *Université de Rennes-II, Rennes, France*

SCHIFFER, BEATRICE *University of Lausanne, Lausanne, Switzerland*

SCHNECK, WILLIAM M. *Microvision Northwest-Forensic Consulting, Inc. Spokane, WA, USA*

SCHNEIDER, RICHARD D. *The Ontario Court of Justice and University of Toronto, Toronto, Ontario, Canada*

SCOTT, ALLAN MATHIESON *University of Central Lancashire (UCLAN), Preston, UK*

SCOTT, CHARLES L. *University of California, Sacramento, CA, USA*

SEGOVIA, DAISY A. *University of California, Davis, CA, USA*

SHARFE, GORDON A.I. *Wellington Central Police Station, Wellington, New Zealand*

SHEFCHICK, THOMAS P. *Shefchick Engineering, Sunnyvale, CA, USA*

SHIVER, FARRELL C. *Shiver & Nelson Document Investigation Laboratory, Inc., Woodstock, GA, USA*

SIEGEL, JAY A. *Indiana University Purdue University Indianapolis, Indianapolis, IN, USA*

SILVA, J. ARTURO *Private Practice of Forensic Psychiatry, San Jose, CA, USA*

SINGH, RAJVINDER *Punjabi University, Patiala, India*

SKOPP, GISELA *Ruprecht-Karls University, Heidelberg, Germany*

SMARTY, SYLVESTER *Case Western University/University Hospitals of Cleveland, Cleveland, OH, USA*

SMITH, ANN C. *Columbia City, Indiana, IN, USA*

SMITH, DELANEY M. *Twin Valley Behavioral Healthcare, Columbus, OH, USA*

SMYTH, LARRY D. *Red Toad Road Company, Havre de Grace, MD, USA*

SORRENTINO, RENEE *Institute for Sexual Wellness, Quincy, MA, USA*

SPIEGEL, DAVID *Stanford University School of Medicine, Stanford, CA, USA*

SQUIER, WANEY *John Radcliffe Hospital, Oxford, UK*

STANKOWSKI, JOY E. *Case Western Reserve University, Cleveland, OH, USA*

STAUFFER, ERIC *University of Lausanne, Lausanne, Switzerland*

STEINBERG, LAURENCE *Temple University, Philadelphia, PA, USA*

STRUB, DIANE S. *Simon Fraser University, Burnaby, British Columbia, Canada*

STUDEBAKER, CHRISTINA *ThemeVision LLC, Indianapolis, IN, USA*

TAKATORI, TAKEHIKO *National Research Institute of Police Science, Chiba, Japan*

TARONI, FRANCO *The University of Lausanne, Lausanne, Switzerland*

TEPLIN, LINDA A. *Northwestern University Feinberg School of Medicine, Chicago, IL, USA*

THAKAR, MUKESH KUMAR *Punjabi University, Patiala, India*

THEAN, A. *Netherlands Organisation for Applied Scientific Research (TNO), Delft, The Netherlands*

THOMAS, TRACY A. *West Virginia University, Morgantown, WV, USA*

THOMPSON, CHRISTOPHER *University of California Los Angeles School of Medicine, Los Angeles, CA, USA*

THOMPSON, WILLIAM C. *University of California, Irvine, CA, USA*

THURMAN, JAMES T. *Eastern Kentucky University, Richmond, KY, USA*

TOGLIA, MICHAEL P. *University of North Florida, Jacksonville, FL, USA*

TRAMONTANA, MICHAEL G. *Vanderbilt University Medical Center, Nashville, TN, USA*

TRIDICO, SILVANA R. *Australian Federal Police, Canberra, ACT, Australia*

TULLY, GILLIAN *Forensic Science Service, Birmingham, UK*

TURILLAZZI, EMANUELA *University of Foggia, Foggia, Italy*

TURNER, BARRY *University of Lincoln, Lincoln, UK*

VAN WAALWIJK VAN DOORN, K. *Amsterdam-Amstelland Police, Amsterdam, The Netherlands*

VERSTRAETE, ALAIN G. *Ghent University Hospital, Ghent, Belgium*

VINER, MARK D. *Cranfield Forensic Institute, Defence Academy of the United Kingdom, Shrivenham and St Bartholomew's and the Royal London Hospitals, London, UK*

VITACCO, MICHAEL J. *Mendota Mental Health Institute, Madison, WI, USA*

VUORI, ERKKI *University of Helsinki, Helsinki, Finland*

WALKER, JAMES S. *Vanderbilt University School of Medicine, Nashville, TN, USA*

WALSH, SIMON J. *Australian Federal Police, Canberra, ACT, Australia*

WASHBURN, JASON J. *Northwestern University Feinberg School of Medicine, Chicago, IL, USA*

WEINSTOCK, ROBERT *University of California, Los Angeles, CA, USA*

WEIR, BRUCE S. *University of Washington, Seattle, WA, USA*

WELLS, GARY L. *Iowa State University, Ames, IA, USA*

WENGER, ERIC *Australian Federal Police, Weston and Australian Chemical, Biological Radiological and Nuclear Data Centre, Canberra, ACT, Australia*

WEST, SARA G. *University Hospital Case Medical Center, Cleveland, OH, USA*

WETTON, JON *Forensic Science Service, Birmingham, UK*

WEYERMANN, CÉLINE *University of Lausanne, Lausanne, Switzerland*

WHEATE, RHONDA M. *The Forensic Institute, Glasgow, UK*

WHELPTON, ROBIN *University of London, London, UK*

WILSON, CATHERINE M. *Simon Fraser University, Burnaby, British Columbia, Canada*

WONG, STEVEN H.Y. *Medical College of Wisconsin and Milwaukee County Medical Examiner's Office, Milwaukee, WI, USA*

YANG, SUZANNE *University of Pittsburgh School of Medicine, Pittsburgh, PA, USA*

YORK, CATHERINE *The University of Illinois at Chicago, Chicago, IL, USA*

ZAJAC, RACHEL *University of Otago, Dunedin, New Zealand*

ZEICHNER, ARIE *Hebrew University of Jerusalem, Jerusalem, Israel*

ZOUN, RIKKERT *Netherlands Forensic Institute, The Hague, The Netherlands*

Foreword

Forensic scientists who are attempting to provide guidance that assists investigators and solves crimes are well aware of the capabilities of the various disciplines in which they toil. Even more importantly, they are also cognizant of what their chosen specialty cannot (yet) accomplish. With a carefully nurtured and expanded knowledge base of the strengths and weaknesses of science, experts are often key to solving perplexing and high-profile cases. Their accomplishments on those occasions draw widespread attention from the media but, even more importantly, these experts also labor quietly on a daily basis to solve the more common cases that represent the bulk of their laboratory efforts and analyses. The consumers of forensic science – be they courts, legislative bodies, or regulatory agencies – rely on the solutions and ideas which these dedicated researchers strive to supply.

In the past few decades, there have been many new discoveries and advances in scientific disciplines, enabling forensic science specialists to apply an ever increasing depth of expertise in carrying out their tasks. Cases are being solved today using techniques that were unheard of twenty, ten, five, or even one year ago. It seems as if every issue of a scientific or technical journal that is published reports new innovations that are progressing from the experimental to the practical. In that environment, the *Wiley Encyclopedia of Forensic Science* is no doubt destined to be recognized as the premiere compendium of knowledge. After all, the entries in its volumes have been compiled by recognized, internationally known, and respected experts in every field.

There is no denying the popularity of television programs such as *CSI*, *Cold Case*, *Forensic Files*, and others. Indeed, there is perhaps no topic of greater interest in today's cyber world than the use of forensics to solve crimes. The small (and not-so-small) screen of the home theater also allows people to view a plethora of movies dealing with scientific ways to demystify complex scenarios. Prominent actors are cast in the white coats of laboratory examiners and interact with other participants in an effort to convince us of their prowess.

Through television, the movies, and an ever growing number of Internet sites, the public receives an abundance of information about how crime laboratory science assists in solving mysteries. The so-called "CSI effect" influences jurors, and even some judges, who have come to expect real life to mirror what they see on television, the movies, or what they read in other media. Unfortunately, not all of the information purveyed via these mediums comports with reality. Expectations are inflated beyond the possible. Even the most accomplished expert cannot solve cases in one hour or less as their television counterparts suggest *they* can!

Expectations in the legal profession, the courts, those who serve on juries, and the public at large demand that those who deal with the judicial system be familiar and are knowledgeable about what is possible and what is perhaps coming in the future. Experts, and anyone else who seeks knowledge about forensics, must not only be familiar with the well-established foundations of scientific proof, but must also stay reliably informed about new developments in the various forensic science disciplines. Here again, the *Wiley Encyclopedia of Forensic Science* serves as a complete, accurate, realistic, and up-to-date resource that will sate the knowledge thirst of experts as well as that of consumers of forensic science.

The framework for this five-volume Wiley encyclopedia was designed and compiled by its two Editors-in-Chief, Allan Jamieson of the United Kingdom and Andre Moenssens of the United States, both pre-eminent authorities in forensic science and its practical and legal applications. They are intimately familiar with the formidable strengths of forensic evidence as well as its perhaps less-known weaknesses. In their daunting task to seek a balance reporting on topics from A to Z, all of which straddle different levels of achievement, the Editors-in-Chief were ably assisted by a selection of knowledgeable subject-specialist topic editors and hundreds of contributors from all over the world. The cooperation and efforts of these many leaders in the scientific enterprise ensures that information dispensed in each discipline is reliable, relevant to real-life problems, and useful to a broad audience.

There are over 370 articles written by more than 330 contributors. These articles reference the myriad subjects of forensic science and embrace the physical, biological, behavioral, as well as comparative sciences. Laboratory management and case investigative techniques, laboratory support mechanisms, quality control programs, and discussions on the modern trends in interpreting the confidence level accorded test results by reference to statistical likelihood ratios are also dealt with.

Concerns about the desired exactness of science, and the inexactness of the law, also required that precedent-setting court decisions and discussions of legal principles that impact on a forensic expert's performance be explained and analyzed in these volumes. Issues of examiner education, training, and accreditation in various disciplines, as well as the ethical requirements governing scientists' professional behavior and the problem of expert witness malpractice have not been neglected.

For the layperson, the Encyclopedia provides authoritative answers to most questions about specific forensic problems. For the practitioners in specific fields, it reminds them of the basic fundamentals in their own discipline while it also informs them of the totality of knowledge in other fields so as to better understand the system as a whole and its interrelated complexities. References to published data and source materials appended to most articles allow interested persons to study areas of special concern in greater depth. Truly a collection of useful information on most of what is known as "forensic science", the Encyclopedia provides ready answers for everyone who is either involved or simply interested in forensic science.

In assessing how well John Wiley & Sons and all those associated with the production and publication of these volumes have achieved their objectives, there is no doubt the verdict and judgment will be favorable.

The Honorable Haskell M. Pitluck
Past President, American Academy of Forensic Science
Retired Circuit Judge, State of Illinois
April 2009

Preface

Forensic science is a broad label. It covers the entire complement of human industry and experience at the point where they interface with legal and legislative processes. This interaction may involve civil as well as criminal concerns and often takes the form of expert testimony offered to answer questions posed by a variety of human institutions. In the exercise of that function, the opinions of experts may vary widely in probative value, weight, and persuasiveness. But forensic science also serves therapeutic and human aspects apart from problem solving, and is often a crucial component in the formulation of policy and the passage of regulatory endeavors destined to insure the health and safety of populations.

The advent of DNA profiling has heralded a revolution in forensic science that goes well beyond forensic biology. The techniques and principles used in evaluating forensic scientific evidence are being closely examined at this moment in the light of the work in DNA as an individualization process – considered somewhat as a Holy Grail for forensic science. The ability to develop population databases, based on the easy numerical nature of DNA profiles, enabled the introduction of other approaches to the evaluation of evidence. The scientific rigor of some aspects of this process has posed difficult-to-answer questions for those forensic disciplines that emerged primarily from experience-based endeavors but which, through use, had become accepted in criminal justice systems. The debate as to the response within many of these specialties is ongoing.

This state of events has brought us to an era of unprecedented development and debate, as well as a measure of uncertainty, in some forensic science functions. Several disciplines are now broadly divided into "old school" and "new school" practitioners. It is not easy to predict which school will emerge as the dominant thinking in these disciplines, but it is almost certain that the future will see more scientifically robust techniques of evidence evaluation gaining widespread acceptance.

Many of the entries in this work may represent the seeds of that future. The existence of these competing schools inevitably creates differences of opinion regarding the science. The constant and varied evolution of science means that the state of the art in one discipline (in instrumentation, analytical accuracy, or evaluation) may be very different from the state of the art in another.

Although science may be regarded as international, law is not. Jurisdictional differences also inevitably create differences in the practice of forensic science. We have encouraged authors to be candid, but to represent those differences in their writing, and occasionally different authors will discuss the same or similar topics while offering a slightly different approach. We regard this as healthy and a natural part of the scientific discourse. As such, the debate is encouraged. However, the consequence is that the views expressed within articles are not necessarily the definitive or final word on any topic, nor do they necessarily represent the view of any other author or of the Editors-in-Chief.

In bringing together such a large and varied selection of experts in one major work, we were cognizant that imposing a "house style" would be close to impossible. Our limit seemed to be the adoption of American-English spelling and a single reference style. Inevitably, our workload and a variety of deeply ingrained localized or national approaches will have allowed some departures from the standard to slip through the editorial net. We hope that this does not detract from the content. We did not enforce any particular writing style and the varied entries reflect that.

One thing that all of our authors had to be aware of was that this is a very unusual major technical reference work in that we aimed to inform an audience that includes people who are not forensic science professionals and who may simply be interested in selected topics discussed in these volumes, such as writers, reporters, educators, but who may have only a sketchy knowledge of the core principles or language of science. The work also purports to inform the legal profession, the judiciary, and paralegals. With these different audiences in mind, we have attempted to maintain sufficient depth to provide a valuable reference source for practitioners and academics as well. Only use will establish the degree to which we have been successful in achieving those disparate aims.

The complexity of providing information to a wide potential readership, composed of such a variety of interested parties, placed important choices on the editors in terms of its coverage. No one source can serve all of humanity, and thus the editors sometimes had to make painful judgments on what to include and what to pass over. Sometimes the choices on what to include were dictated in part by the availability of experts willing to share their professional experience with our readers. At other times, choices related simply to the fact that the dividing line between science and pseudoscience required a decision as to whether conclusions reached in a particular field provided sufficient guarantees of trustworthiness and reliability. This in no way can be taken to mean that the lack of appearance here invalidates any particular discipline, nor for that matter that inclusion validates it! Whatever the choice, the editors acted in their best judgment and will remain vigilant so as to select, for later inclusions, those emerging fields currently perhaps on the fringes of forensic science that increase their underlying knowledge-based data and gain a modicum of acceptance in the broader forensic science profession.

No work of this nature is perfect. This will not prevent us from striving to improve it on-line and in subsequent editions. We welcome feedback on any aspect of this work, including topics that, almost certainly, we have missed in our attempts to be all-inclusive.

We are only part of a very large and skilled team including our Editorial Board and the team at Wiley. Our heartfelt thanks go to all of them and in advance to you, the reader, for your feedback which will assist us to provide better resources for your future work.

Allan Jamieson and Andre Moenssens
April 2009

Abbreviations and Acronyms

1,4-BD	1,4-butanediol
16 PF	16 Personality Factor
2,4-DNT	2,4-dinitrotoluene
2,6-DNT	2,6-dinitrotoluene
5-HT	5-Hydroxytryptamine
5HIAA	5-Hydroxyindole Acetic Acid
5HTOL	5-hydroxytryptophol
6-AM	Δ^9-Tetrahydrocannabinol
6-AM	6-Acetylmorphine
AA	Greatest Angular Apertures
AACC	American Association of Clinical Chemists
AAFS	American Academy of Forensic Sciences
AAIDD	American Association on Intellectual and Developmental Disabilities
AAMR	American Association on Mental Retardation
AAPA	American Association of Physical Anthropology
AAPI	Adult–Adolescent Parenting Inventory
AAS	Atomic Absorption Spectrophotometry
AAS	Atomic Absorption Spectroscopy
ABAS-II	Adaptive Behavior Assessment System – Second Edition
ABC	American Board of Criminalistics
ABFDE	American Board of Forensic Document Examiners
ABFE	American Board of Forensic Entomology
ABFM	American Board of Forensic Medicine
ABFO	American Board of Forensic Odontology
ABFP	American Board of Forensic Psychology
ABFT	American Board of Forensic Toxicology
ABI	Applied Biosystems
ABO	ABO Blood Groups
ABPN	American Board of Psychiatry and Neurology
ABPP	American Board of Professional Psychology
ABTS	2, 2′-azino-di-(3-Ethyl-Benzthiazolinesulfonate)
ACE-V	Analysis, Comparison, Evaluation and Verification
ACFE	American College of Forensic Examiners
ACh	Acetylcholine
ACP1	Acid Phosphatase 1
ACPO	Association of Chief Police Officers
ADA	Adenosine Deaminase
ADD	Accumulated Degree-Days

ADH	Accumulated Degree-Hours
ADH	Alcohol Dehydrogenase
ADHD	Attention Deficit Hyperactive Disorder
ADM	Alcohol, Drug, and Mental
ADP	Adenosine Diphosphate
AEDs	Antiepileptic Drugs
AEME	Anhydroecgonine Methylester
AES	Auger Electron Spectroscopy
AF	Acid Fuchsin
AFE	Amniotic Fluid Embolism
AFIS	Automated Fingerprint Identification System
AFM	Atomic Force Microscopy
AFR	Association of Forensic Radiographers
AFTE	Association of Firearm and Tool Mark Examiners
AHG	Antihuman Globulin
AIDS	Acquired Immunodeficiency Syndrome
AIMs	Ancestry Informative Markers
AIP	Acute Interstitial Pneumonitis
AK	Adenylate Kinase
AKA	Alcoholic Ketoacidosis
AKD	Alkyl Ketene Dimer
ALDH	Aldehyde Dehydrogenase
ALFPs	Amplified Fragment Length Polymorphisms
ALI	American Law Institute
ALS	Alternate Light Sources
ALT	Alanine Aminotransaminases
ALTEs	Acute Life-Threatening Events
AM	Antemortem
AMDIS	Automated Mass Spectral Deconvolution and Identification System
AMI	Acute Myocardial Infarction
AMP	Adenosine Monophosphate
AmpFLPs	Amplified Fragment Length Polymorphisms
AMPS	Advanced Mobile Phone System
AMS	Accelerator Mass Spectrometry
AN	Ammonium Nitrate
ANFO	Ammonium Nitrate and Fuel Oil
ANN	Artificial Neural Network
ANSI	American National Standards Institute
AP	Acid Phosphatase
AP	Ammonium Perchlorate
APA	American Psychological Association
APA	American Psychiatric Association
APCI	Atmospheric Pressure Chemical Ionization
APD	Antisocial Personality Disorder
APDS	Autonomous Pathogen Detection System
APHL	Association of Public Health Laboratories
API	Application Programming Interface
API	Atmospheric Pressure Ionization
AP-LS	American Psychology-Law Society

APPITA	Australian Pulp and Paper Industry Technical Association
APS	Adult Protective Services
ARDS	Acute Respiratory Distress Syndrome
ARIs	Actuarial Risk Assessment Instruments
ARVD	Arrhythmogenic Right Ventricular Disease
AS	Autonomous System
ASA	Acetylsalicylic Acid
ASA	Alkenyl Succinyl Anhydride
ASCH	American Society of Clinical Hypnosis
ASCLD	American Society of Crime Laboratory Directors
ASCLD/LAB	American Society of Crime Laboratory Directors/Laboratory Accreditation Board
ASD	Acute Stress Disorder
ASM	American Society of Metals
ASME	American Society of Mechanical Engineer
ASQDE	American Society of Questioned Document Examiners
ASRIS	Australian Soil Resources Information System
AST	Aspartate Aminotransaminases
ASTM	American Society for Testing and Materials
ATF	Alcohol, Tobacco, and Firearms
ATP	Adenosine Triphosphate
ATR	Attenuated Total Reflection
ATR-FTIR	Attenuated Total Reflectance-Fourier Transform Infrared
ATSA	Association for the Treatment of Sexual Abusers
ATV	Atmospheric Pressure Chemical Ionization
AUC	Area Under Curve
BAC	Blood Alcohol Concentration
BAPP	Beta Amyloid Precursor Protein
BARTS	Biological Agent Real-Time Sensor
BAWS	Biological Agent Warning Sensor
BCCH	Broadcast Control Channel
BCTMP	Bleached Chemi-Thermomechanical Hardwood Pulps
BE	Benzoylecgonine
BEECS	Benign Enlargement of the Extracerebral Spaces
BFRL	Building Fire and Research Laboratory
BGA	Ball Grid Array
BHT	Butylated Hydroxytoluene
BISFA	The International Bureau for the Standardization of Man-Made Fibres
BKV	BK Virus
BLEVE	Boiling Liquid and Expanding Vapor Explosion
BMI	Body Mass Index
BNs	Bayesian Networks
BP	Bandpass
bp	Base Pair
BPIF	Bandpass Interference Filters
BPS	Bricklin Perceptual Scales
BrAC	Breath-Alcohol Concentration
BS	Beam Splitter

BSA	Bovine Sera Albumin
BSDL	Boundary-Scan Description Language
BSE	Back-Scattered Electrons
BSE	Black Sheep Effect
BTB	Sickle Cell Anemia
BTEX	Benzene, Toluene, Ethylbenzene, and Xylene
BTU	British Thermal Unit
BWC	Biological and Toxins Weapons Convention
BWS	Battered Woman Syndrome
CA	Carbonic Anhydrase
CA	Cytosine-Adenine
CABs	Conformity Assessment Bodies
CABL	Compositional Analysis of Bullet Lead
CAC	California Association of Criminalistics
CAC	Child Advocacy Center
CAD	Computer-Aided Design
CAD	Coronary Artery Disease
CAF	Cyanoacrylate Fuming
CAFSS	Centre for Australian Forensic Soil Science
CAGE	Computer Aided Glass Evaluation
CAI	Case Assessment and Interpretation
CAI	Competence Assessment Instrument for Standing Trial
CAM	Computer-Aided Modeling
CAN	Cardiovascular Autonomic Neuropathy
CAP	College of American Pathologists
CAPI	Child Abuse Potential Inventory
CAPTA	Child Abuse Prevention and Treatment Act
carboxy-THC	11-Nor-9-carboxytetrahydrocannabinol
CAST/MR	Competence Assessment for Standing Trial for Defendants with Mental Retardation
CAT	Computed Axial Tomography
CBD	Cannabidiol
CBN	Cannabinol
CBRN	Chemical, Biological, Radiological, and Nuclear
CCBEMWG	Common Criteria Biometric Evaluation Methodology Working Group
CCD	Charge Coupled Device
CCSA	Certified Crime Scene Analyst
CCSI	Certified Crime Scene Investigator
CCTV	Closed Circuit Television
CD	Conduct Disorder
CD	Cyclodextrin
CDC	Centers for Disease Control
CDER	Center for Drug Evaluation and Research
CDMA	Frequency Division Multiple Access
CDR	Cartridge Discharge Residues
CDR	Crash Data Recorders
CDT	Carbohydrate Deficient Transferrin
CE	Capillary Electrophoresis

CEDIA	Cloned Enzyme Donor Immunoassay
CEIR	Central Equipment Identify Register
CESB	Council of Engineering and Scientific Specialty Boards
CF	Compact Flash
CF	Corrective Factors
CFA	Confirmatory Factor Analysis
CFAST	Consolidated Model of Fire Growth and Smoke Transport
CFC	Chlorofluorocarbon
CFD	Computational Fluid Dynamics
CGS	Crow–Glassman Scale
CHD	Coronary Heart Disease
CHF	Congestive Heart Failure
CHINS	Children in Need of Supervision
CI	Chemical Ionization
CI	Cognitive Interview
CI-MS	Chemical Ionization Mass Spectrometry
CIFA	Centre for International Forensic Assistance
CIL	Central Identification Laboratory
CIP	Commission Internationale Permanente
CIS	Canadian Information Society
CITES	The Convention on International Trade in Endangered Species Fauna and Flora
CIT	Concealed Information Test
CJA	Criminal Justice Act
CJP	Capital Jury Project
CL	Cathodoluminescence
CMOS	Complementary Metal-Oxide Semiconductor
CMR-R	Comprehension of Miranda Rights-Recognition
CMS	Consecutive Matching Striae
CMYK	Cyan, Magenta, Yellow, and Black
CN	Cyanide
CNS	Central Nervous System
CO	Carbon Monoxide
CO-Hb	Carbon Monoxide Hemoglobin
CODIS	Combined Offender DNA Index System
COHb	Carboxyhemoglobin
COPFS	Crown Office Procurator Fiscal Service
COVR	Classification of Violence Risk
CPA	Cyproterone Acetate
CPD	Continuing Professional Development
CPE	Combined Power of Exclusion
CPF	Cardiac Fibroelastoma
CPGR	Chlorophenolred-β-Galactoside
CPI	Combined Probability of Inclusion
CPIA	Criminal Procedure and Investigations Act
CPK	Creatine Phosphokinase
CPLE	Certified Latent-Print Examiner
CPR	Cardiopulmonary Rescuscitation
CPR	Chlorophenolred
CPR	Civil Procedure Rules

CPS	Child Protective Services
CPSC	Consumer Product Safety Commission
CPVT	Catecholaminergic Polymorphic Ventricular Tachycardia
CQT	Comparison Question Test
CR	Conditioned Response
CRFP	Council for Registration of Forensic Practitioners
CRT	Cathode-Ray Tube
CS	Conditioned Stimuli
CSA	Child Sexual Abuse
CSA	Crime Scene Analyst
CSAAS	Child Sexual Abuse Accommodation Syndrome
CSC	Crime Scene Coordinator
CSCSA	Certified Senior Crime Scene Analyst
CSD	Circuit Switched Data
CSE	Crime Scene Examiner
CSF	Cerebrospinal Fluid
CSFS	Canadian Society of Forensic Science
CSI	Consensual Sexual Intercourse
CSI	Crime Scene Investigators
CSM	Crime Scene Manager
CT	Computed Tomography
CTAB	Hexadecyltrimethlyammonium Bromide
CTS	Collaborative Testing Services
CV	Coefficient of Variation
CV	Curriculum Vita
CVD	Cardiovascular Disease
CVFI	Candidate for the Vehicle Fire Investigator
CW	Chemical Warfare
CWAs	Chemical Warfare Agents
CWC	Chemical Weapons Convention
CYP	Cytochrome P
CYP 2B6	Cytochrome P450 2B6
CYP 2D6	Cytochrome P450 2D6
CYP 3A5	Cytochrome P450 3A5
CYP3A	Cytochrome P450 3A
CZE	Capillary Zone Electrophoresis
D1T2	Direct Thermal Transfer
D2T2	Dye Diffusion Thermal Transfer
D-AMPS	Digital Advanced Mobile Phone System
DA	Dopamine
DAB	Diaminobenzidine
DAB	DNA Advisory Board
DAD	Diffuse Alveolar Damage
DAD	Diode-Array Detector
DAD	Drowning-Associated Diatoms
DAD	Photodiode Array Detection
DADP	Diacetone Diperoxide
DAG	Directed Acyclic Graph
DAI	Diffuse Axonal Injury

DART	Direct Analysis in Real Time
DEA	Drug Enforcement Agency
DECT	Digital Enhanced Cordless Telecommunication
DEM	Digital Elevation Model
DESNOS	Disorder of Extreme Stress not Otherwise Specified
DF	Dedicated File
DFC	Drug-Facilitated Crime
DFO	1,8-diaza-9-fluorenone
DFSA	Drug-Facilitated Sexual Assault
DHCP	Dynamic Host Configuration Protocol
DIC	Differential Interference Contrast
DID	Dissociative Identity Disorder
DIN	Deutsches Institut Für Normung
DIS-IV	Diagnostic Interview Schedule, Version IV
DLC	Diagnostic Link Connector
DM	Diabetes Mellitus
DM	Dichroic Mirror
DMA	Dimethoxyamphetamine
DNA	Deoxyribonucleic Acid
DNS	Domain Name System
DO	Dangerous Offender
DOB	4-Bromo-2,5-dimethoxyamphetamine
DOET	Dimethoxyethylamphetamine
DOM	4-Methyl-2,5-dimethoxyamphetamine
DOP	Degenerate Oligonucleotide Primed
DOS	Denial-of-Service
DOT	Department of Transportation
DPA	Diphenylamine
DPI	Dots Per Inch
DPS	Department of Public Safety
DRE	Drug Recognition Evaluation
DRIFT	Diffuse Reflectance Infrared Fourier Transform
DRM	Deese–Roediger–McDermott
DSC	Differential Scanning Calorimeter
DSM	Diagnostic and Statistical Manual of Mental Disorders
DSM-III	Diagnostic and Statistical Manual of Mental Disorders, Third Edition
DSM-IV	Diagnostic and Statistical Manual of Mental Disorders, Fourth Edition
DSM-IV-TR	Diagnostic and Statistical Manual, Fourth Edition, Text Revision
DSPD	Dangerous Severe Personality Disorder
DTA	Differential Thermal Analysis
DTCs	Diagnostic Trouble Codes
DTGS	Deuterated Triglycine Sulfate
DTO	Dithiooxamide
DTT	Dithiothreitol
DUID	Driving Under the Influence of Drugs
DVI	Disaster Victim Identification
DVT	Deep Venous/Vein Thrombosis
DWI	Driving While Intoxicated

EA	Enzyme Acceptor
EA	European Co-Operation for Accreditation
EAAF	Equipo Argentino De Antropología Forense
EAFE	European Association for Forensic Entomology
EAP	Erythrocyte Acid Phosphatase
EBV	Epstein Barr Virus
EC	Ethyl Centralite
ECA	Epidemiologic Catchment Area
ECD	Electron Capture Detector
ECDS	Empirical Criteria for the Determination of Suicide
ECF	Elemental Chlorine Free
ECHR	European Court of Human Rights
ECLM	European Council of Legal Medicine
ECT	Electroconvulsive Therapy
ED	Enzyme Donor
EDD	Electrostatic Detection Device
EDDP	2-Ethylidene-1,5-Dimethyl-3,3-Diphenylpyrrolidine
EDM	Electrical Discharge Machining
EDMI	Electromyography
EDNAP	European DNA Profiling Group
EDS	Energy-Dispersive Spectrometer
EDS or EDX	Energy-Dispersive X-Ray
EDTA	Ethylene Diamine Tetraacetic Acid
EDX	Energy Dispersive X-Ray
EDXA	Energy Dispersive X-Ray Analysis
EEG	Electro-Encephalogram
EER	Equal Error Rate
EF	Elementary File
EFA	Exploratory Factor Analysis
EFG	European Fibres Group
EGA	Estimated Gestational Age
EGDN	Ethylene Glycol Dinitrate
E-HMM	Ergodic Hidden Markov Models
EI	Electron Impact
EI-MS	Electron Impact Positive Ion Mass Spectrometry
EIA	Environmental Impact Assessment
EIA	Enzyme Immunoassay
EIC	Extracted Ion Chromatogram
EIP	Extracted Ion Profiles
ELISA	Enzyme Linked Immunosorbent Assay
EME	Ecgonine Methyl Ester
EMG	Electromyography
EMIT	Enzyme Multiplied Immunoassay Technique
EMPOP	European DNA Profiling Group MtDNA Population Database
EMS	Enhanced Messaging Service
ENAA	Epithermal Neutron Activation Analysis
ENFSI	European Network of Forensic Science Institutes
EPA	Environmental Protection Agency
EPG	Electropherogram
EPI	Enhanced Product Ion

EPO	Erythropoetin
EPS	Extra-Pyramidal Symptoms
EQA	External Quality Assessment
ERPs	Event-Related Potentials
ESD	Environmental Secondary Detector
EsD	Esterase D
ESDA	Electrostatic Detection Apparatus
ESEM	Environmental SEM
ESI	Electronically Stored Information
ESI	Electrospray Ionization
ESLA	Electrostatic Lifting Apparatus
ESR	Environmental Science Research Limited
EtG	Ethyl Glucuronide
ETK	Explosive Test Kit
EtS	Ethyl Sulfate
EU	European Union
EUCAP	European Collection of Automotive Paint
EWG	Expert Working Group
EX	Exciter Filter
FAAS	Flameless Atomic Absorption Spectroscopy
FABMS	Fast Atom Bombardment Mass Spectrometry
FAEE	Fatty Acid Ethyl Esters
FAME	Fatty Acid Methyl Esters
FAR	False Acceptance Rate
FASE	Forensic Anthropology Society of Europe
FBI	Federal Bureau of Investigation
FDA	Food and Drug Administration
FDE	Forensic Document Examiner
FDR	Firearm Discharge Residue
FDS	Fire Dynamics Simulator
FDS	Fragment Data System
FE	Field Emission
FEC	Forensic Engineering Curriculum
FEPAC	Forensic Science Education Programs Accreditation Commission
FFT	Fast Fourier Transform
FGH	S-Formylglutathione Hydrolase
FHE	Forensic Handwriting Examiner
FIB	Focused Ion Beam
FID	Flame Ionization Detector
FINEX	Forensic International Network of Explosive Examiners
FIRS	Forensic Information Retrieval System
FISH	Fluorescent In Situ Hybridization
FLE	Filtered Light Examination
FLIM	Fluorescence Lifetime Imaging
FLO	Family Liaison Officer
FLS	Forensic Light Source
FMEA	Failure Modes and Effects Analysis
FMJ	Full Metal Jacket

fMRI	Functional Magnetic Resonance Imaging
FMSF	False Memory Syndrome Foundation
FNAA	Fast Neutron Activation Analysis
FOMA	Freedom of Mobile Multimedia Access
FPAC	Forensic Pathology Advisory Commitee
fpc	Finite Population Correction
FPD	Flame Photometric Detection
FPIA	Fluorescence Polarization Immunoassay
FPM	First-Pass Metabolism
FQS-I	Forensic Quality Services-International
FRE	Federal Rules of Evidence
FRI	Function of Rights in Interrogation
FRR	False Rejection Rate
FSAB	Forensic Specialties Accreditation Board
FSF	Forensic Sciences Foundation
FSH	Follicle-Stimulating Hormone
FSS	Forensic Science Society
FSS	Forensic Science Service Ltd
FSSoc	Forensic Science Society (UK)
FTA	Fault Tree Analysis
FTD	Flame Thermoionic Detector
FTIR	Frustrated Total Internal Reflection
FTL	Flash Translation Layer
FTP	File Transfer Protocol
FUT	Fucosyltransferase
FWA	Fluorescent Whitening Agent
G6PDH	Glucose-6-phosphate Dehydrogenase
GABA	Gamma Amino-Butyric Acid
GBL	Gamma Butyrolactone
GC	Gas Chromatography
GC-ECD	Gas Chromatography Electron Capture Detector
GC-FID	Gas Chromatography Flame Ionization Detector
GC-MS	Gas Chromatography-Mass Spectrometry
GC-MS/DFPD	Gas Chromatography-Mass Spectroscopy/Dual Flame Photometric Detection
GCS	Glascow Coma Scale
GD–MS	Glow Discharge–Mass Spectrometry
GERD	Gastroesophageal Reflux Disease
GFAAS	Graphite Furnace Atomic Absorption Spectrophotometry
GGT	Gamma-Glutamyltransferase
GH	Growth Hormone
GHB	γ-Hydroxybutyrate
GIS	Geographic Information System
GKT	Guilty Knowledge Test
GLO	Glyoxylase I
GMM	Gaussian Mixture Models
GMSC	Gateway Mobile Switching Center
GNDS	General Neuropsychological Deficit Scale
GnRH	Gonadotropin-Releasing Hormone

GPA	Grade Point Average
GPB	Glycophorin B
GPR	Ground-Penetrating Radar
GPRS	General Packet Radio Service
GPS	Global Positioning System
GPT	Glutamate-Pyruvate Transaminase
GRC	General Rifling Characteristics
GSM	Global System for Mobile
gsm	Grams Per Square Meter
GSR	Gunshot Residue
GSS	Gudjonsson Suggestibility Scales
GUI	Graphical User Interface
GuSCN	Guanidinium Thiocyanate
GUS	General Unknown Screening
Hb	Heterozygosity Balance
HBFP	Haematoxylin-Basic Fuchsin-Picric Acid
HCM	Hypertrophic Cardiomyopathy
HCN	Hydrogen Cyanide
HCR	Historical Clinical Risk
HELIN	Higher Education Library Information Network
HERG	Human Ether-a-go-go-Related Gene
HF	Human Factor
HFC	Hydrofluorocarbon
HFE	Human Factors Engineering
HFE	Hydrofluoroether
HGN	Horizontal Gaze Nystagmus
HHV-1	Human Herpes Virus Type 1
HIC	Head Injury Criterion
HIV AIDS	Human Immunodeficiency Virus Acquired Immune Deficiency Syndrome
HLA	Human Leucocyte Antigen
HLoQ	Higher Limit of Quantitation
HMTD	Hexamethylene Triperoxide Diamine
HMW	High-Molecular-Weight
HMX	Octogen
HPD	Heavy Petroleum Distillates
HPD	Highest Posterior Density
HPLC	High Performance Liquid Chromatography
HPLC-DAD	High Performance Liquid Chromatography Diode-Array Detector
HPLC-MS	High Performance Liquid Chromatography Mass Spectrometry
HPLC/PMDE	High Performance Liquid Chromatography with a Pendant Mercury Drop Electrode Detector
HPV	Human Papillomavirus
HRGS	High-Resolution Gamma Spectrometry
HRNB	Halstead–Reitan Neuropsychological Battery
HRNTB	Halstead–Reitan Neuropsychological Test Battery
HRR	Heat Release Rate
HSE	Health and Safety Executive

HTTP	Hypertext Transfer Protocol
HWE	Hardy–Weinberg Equilibrium
i.d.	Internal Diameter
I/IS	Insulin or Insulin Secretagogs
IAAC	Inter-American Accreditation Cooperation
IAAI	International Association of Arson Investigators
IABPA	International Association of Bloodstain Pattern Analysts
IACI	International Association for Craniofacial Identification
IAEA	International Atomic Energy Agency
IAFIS	Integrated Automated Fingerprint Identification System
IAFS	International Association of Forensic Scientists
IAI	International Association for Identification
ibd	Identical by Descent
IBG	International Biometrics Group
IBIS	Integrated Ballistics Identification System
IBS	Identical by State
IC	Ion Chromatography
ICC	International Criminal Court
ICC1	Intraclass Correlation Coefficient
ICCID	Integrated Circuit Card Identifier
ICD	International Classification of Diseases
ICDD	International Centre for Diffraction Data
ICF/DIC	Intravascular Coagulation and Fibrinolysis/Disseminated Intravascular Coagulation
ICN	Increased Cycle Number
ICP	Inductively Coupled Plasma
ICP-MS	Inductively Coupled Plasma Mass Spectrometry
ICP-OES	Inductively Coupled Plasma-Optical Emission Spectrometry
ICP/AES	Inductively Coupled Plasma Atomic Emission Spectroscopy
ICP/MS	Inductively Coupled Plasma Mass Spectrometry
ICTR	International Criminal Tribunal for Rwanda
ICTY	International Criminal Tribunal for the Former Yugoslavia
IDA	International Development Agencies
IDEIA	Individuals with Disabilities Education Improvement Act
iDEN	Integrated Digital-Enhanced Network
IDS	Intrusion Detection System
IEC	International Electrotechnical Commission
IED	Improvised Explosive Device
IEEE	Institute of Electrical and Electronic Engineers
IEEGFI	Interpol European Expert Group on Fingerprint Identification
IEF	Isoelectric Focusing
IFSTA	International Fire Service Training Association
IHL	International Humanitarian Law
IIFES	International Institute of Forensic Engineering Sciences
ILAC	International Laboratory Accreditation Cooperation
ILAE	International League against Epilepsy
ILR	Ignitable Liquid Residues
IMED	Indentation Materializer

IMEI/IMSI	International Mobile Equipment Identity/International Mobile Equipment Identity
IMMORTAL	Impaired Motorists, Methods of Roadside Testing and Assessment for Licensing
IMS	Ion Mobility Spectrometry
IMSI	International Mobile Equipment Identity
IMT-2000	International Mobile Telecommunications-2000
INAA	Instrumental Nuclear Activation Analysis
IND	1,2-Indanedione
IND	Improvised Nuclear Device
IND-Zn	Indanedione-Zinc
INFL	International Nuclear Forensic Laboratories
INH	Isoniazid
INS	International Neuropsychological Society
IOFOS	International Organisation for Forensic Odontostomotology
IP	Internet Protocol
IPEP	Improved Primer Extension Preamplification
IQ	Intelligence Quotient
IQC	Internal Quality Control
IR	Infrared
IRA	Irish Republican Army
IRC	Internet Relay Chat
IrDA	Infrared Data Association
IRL	Infrared Luminescence
IRMS	Isotope Ratio Mass Spectrometry
IRR	Infrared Reflectance
IS	Internal Standard
ISFG	International Society of Forensic Genetics
ISO	International Standards Organization
ISP	Internet Service Provider
ITU	International Telecommunication Union
ITWG	International Technical Working Group
JCAH	Joint Commission on Accreditation of Hospitals
JFFS2	Journalized Flash File System
JINS	Juveniles in Need of Supervision
JPAC	Joint Pow/MIA Accounting Command
JPEG2000	Joint Photographic Expert Group 2000
JTAG	Joint Test Action Group
KAAIT	Kaufman Adolescent and Adult Intelligence Test
KBS	Knowledge-Based System
KEBQ	Knowledge of Eyewitness Behavior Questionnaire
KIMS	Kinetic Interaction of Microparticles in Solution
KIPS	Keys to Interactive Parenting Scale
KM	Kastle Meyer test
KSA	Knowledge, Skills, and Abilities
LAB	Laboratory Accreditation Board
LAC	Location Area Code

LAMMA	Laser Microprobe Mass Analysis
LAMPA	Lysergic Acid Methyl Propyl Amide
LAN	Local Area Network
LBA	Logical Block Addressing
LC	Liquid Chromatography
LC/ESI/MS	Liquid Chromatography Electrospray Ionization Mass Spectrometry
LC-MS/MS	Liquid Chromatography Tandem Mass Spectrometry
LC/MS	Liquid Chromatography Mass Spectrometry
LCN	Low Copy Number
LCP	Life-Course Persistent
LCV	Leucocrystal Violet
LD	Lethal Dose
LDA	Linear Discriminant Analysis
LEAA	Law Enforcement Assistance Administration
LED	Light-Emitting Diode
LEL	Lower Explosive Limit
LH	Luteinizing Hormone
LHRH	Luteinizing Hormone-Releasing Hormone
LIBS	Laser-Induced Breakdown Spectroscopy
LLE	Liquid–Liquid Extraction
LLoQ	Lower Limit of Quantification
LMG	Leucomalachite Green
LNNB-CR	Luria–Nebraska Neuropsychological Battery-Children's Revision
LOC	Loss of Consciousness
LOD	Limit of Detection
LOQ	Limit of Quantification
LP	Liquefied Petroleum
LPC	Linear Predictive Coding
LPCC	Linear Prediction Cepstrum Coefficients
LPDs	Light Petroleum Distillates
LQTS	Long QT Syndrome
LR	Likelihood Ratio
LRs	Long Rifles
LSD	Lysergic Acid Diethylamide
LTDNA	Low Template DNA
LTO	Long-Term Offender
LVH	Left Ventricular Hypertrophy
M-FAST	Miller Forensic Assessment of Symptoms Test
M3G	Morphine-3-glucuronide
M6G	Morphine-6-glucuronide
MAC	Media Access Control
MacCAT-CA	MacArthur Competence Assessment Tool-Criminal Adjudication
MacCAT-T	MacArthur Competence and Assessment Tool-Treatment
MacSAC-CD	MacArthur Structured Assessment of the Competencies of Criminal Defendants
MALDI/TOF	Matrix-Assisted Laser Desorption/Ionization Time-of-Flight
MAM	Mechanical, Analytical, and Medical

MAM	Mono acetyl Morphine
MAO	Monoamine Oxidase
MB	Myocardial Bridging
MBD	4-(4-Methoxybenzylamino-7-Nitrobenzofurazan)
MBDB	*N*-Methyl-Benzodioxazoylbutanamine
MC-ICP/MS	Multicollector Inductively Coupled Plasma Mass Spectrometry
MC1R	Melanocortin 1 Receptor
MCMC	Monte Carlo Markov Chain
MCMI	Millon Clinical Multiaxial Inventory
MCQ	Multiple-Choice Questions
MCT	Mercury Cadmium Telluride
MCV	Mean Corpuscular Volume
MDA	3,4-Methylenedioxyamphetamine
MDA	Multiple Displacement Amplification
MDCT	Multislice Computed Tomography
MDE	3,4-Methylenedioxyamphetamine
MDEA	3,4-Methylenedioxy-*N*-Amphetamine
MDMA	3,4 Methylenedioxymethamphetamine
MDMA	Liquid Chromatography Coupled to Mass Spectrometry
MDMA	Methylenedioxymethamphetamine
MDMA	Methylenedioxymeth(yl)amphetamine
MDT	Multidisciplinary Team
ME	Medical Examiner
MECA	Methodology for Epidemiology of Mental Disorders in Children and Adolescents
MECC	Micellar Electrokinetic Chromatography
MECE	Micellar Electrokinetic Capillary Electrophoresis
MEOS	Microsomal Oxidizing System
MERMER	Memory and Encoding Related Multifaceted Electroencephalographic Response
MERS	Medical Error Reporting System
met-Hb	Methemoglobin
MFCC	Mel Frequency Cepstral Coefficients
MGT	Modified Griess Test
MHC	Major Histocompatibility Complex
MHL	Minimal Haplotype Loci
MI	Medullary Index
mIPEP	Modified Improved Primer Extension Preamplification
MIR	Mid-Infrared
MLE	Most Likely Estimate
MLP	Multilocus Profiling
MMC	Multi Media Card
MMDA	Methoxymethylenedioxyamphetamine
MMD	Multimetal Deposition
MMPI-2	Minnesota Multiphasic Personality Inventory 2
MMSD	Mass Memory Storage Device
MMSE	Mini Mental State Examination
MND	Malingering Neurocognitive Dysfunction
MO	Modus Operandi
MPA	Medroxyprogesterone

MPD	Medium Petroleum Distillate
MPD	Modified Physical Developer
MPD	Multiple Personality Disorder
MPS	Metropolitan Police Service
MP	Match Probability
MR	Metabolic Ratios
MRI	Magnetic Resonance Imagery
MRM	Multiple Reaction Monitoring
mRNA	Messenger Ribonucleic Acid
MRS	Magnetic Resonance Spectroscopy
MS	Mass Selective
MS	Mass Spectrometer
MSC	Mobile Switching Center
MSCT	Multislice Computed Tomography
MSD	Mass Selective Detector
MSE	Mental Status Examination
MSP	Microspectrophotometers
mtDNA	Mitochondrial Deoxyribonucleic Acid
MTPA	α-Methoxy-α-(Trifluoromethyl)Phenylacetic Acid
(S)-(+)-MTPACl	(S)-(+)-α-Methoxy-(Trifluoromethyl)Phenylacetyl Chloride
MTT	Dimethylthiazol 2 yl Diphenyltetrazolium Bromide
MVD	Multiwavelength Detection
MVN	Multivariate Normality
MW	Molecular Weight
NA	Numerical Aperture
NAA	Neutron Activation Analysis
NACB	National Academy of Clinical Biochemistry
NAD	Nicotine Adenine Dinucleotide
NADP	Nicontinamide Adenine Dinucleotide Phosphate
NADPH	Reduced Nicontinamide Adenine Dinucleotide Phosphate
NAE	Negligent Adverse Event
NAFE	National Academy of Forensic Engineers
NAFEA	North American Forensic Entomological Association
NAFI	National Association of Fire Investigators
NAGPRA	Native American Graves Protection and Repatriation Act
NAHI	Non-accidental Head Injury
NAME	National Association of Medical Examiners
NAPQI	N-Acetyl-p-benzoquinone Imine
NAS	National Academy of Sciences
NAS	Network Attached Storage
NATA	National Association of Testing Authorities
Native PAGE	Native Gel Electrophoresis
NBS	National Bureau of Standards
NC	Nitrocellulose
NCA	No Cause Apparent
NCANDS	National Child Abuse and Neglect Data System
NCIDD	National Criminal Identification DNA Database
NCIGC-MS	Negative Chemical Ionisation Gas Chromatograph with Mass Spectral Analyser

NCIS	National Coroners Information Service
NCJRS	National Criminal Justice Reference Service
NCNM	Noncorrosive and Nonmercuric
NCS	National Comorbidity Survey
NCSI	Nonconsensual Sexual Intercourse
NCSTL	National Clearinghouse for Science, Technology and the Law
NCVS	National Crime Victimization Survey
NDIS	National DNA Identification System
NDNAD	National DNA Database
nDNA	Nuclear DNA
NE	Norepinephrine
NEISS	National Electronic Injury Surveillance System
NEO-PI	Neo-Personality Inventory
NEO-PI-R	Neo-Personality Inventory-Revised
NFA	National Forensics Association
NFI	Netherlands Forensic Institute
NFIRS	National Fire Incident Reporting System
NFPA	National Fire Protection Association
NFSTC	National Forensic Science Technology Center
NFWFL	National Fish and Wildlife Forensics Laboratory
NG	Nitroglycerine
NGOs	Nongovernmental Organizations
NGRI	Not-Guilty-by-Reason-of-Insanity
NHTSA	National Highway Traffic Safety Administration
NIBIN	National Integrated Ballistic Information Network
NICHD	National Institute of Child Health and Human Development
NIFS	National Institute of Forensic Science
NIJ	National Institute of Justice
NIR	Near Infrared
NIST	National Institute of Standards and Technology
NLQ	Near Letter Quality
NMDA	N-Methyl-D-Aspartic Acid
NMR	Nuclear Magnetic Resonance
NMT	Nordic Mobile Telephones
NP	Neuropsychological
NPD	Nitrogen Phosphorus Detector
NPIA	National Policing Improvements Agency
NRC	National Research Council
NRY	Nonrecombining Region of the Y Chromosomes
NSAID	Nonsteroidal Anti-Inflammatory Drug
NSTC	National Science and Technology Council
NTT	Nippon Telegraph and Telephones
nuDNA	Nuclear Deoxyribonucleic Acid
NVFS	Nonvolatile File System
NY-OCME	New York Office of the Chief Medical Examiner
OBAs	Optical Brightening Agents
OCD	Obsessive Compulsive Disorder
OCDS	Operational Criteria for the Determination of Suicide
OD	Overdose

OEM	Original Equipment Manufacturer
OHS&W	Occupational Health Safety and Wellbeing
OLA	Oligonucleotide Ligation Assay
OOBNs	Object-Oriented Bayesian Networks
OPC	Organic Photoconductor
OPCW	Organization for the Prohibition of Chemical Weapons
OPGs	Orthopantomographs
ORO	Oil Red O
OSHA	Occupational Safety and Health Administration
OS	Operating Systems
OTA	Over the Air
OTC	Over-the-Counter
OVD	Optical Variable Device
P2P	Peer-to-Peer
PAC	Plasma Alcohol Concentration
PACE	Police and Evidence Act
PAE	Preventable Adverse Event
PAI	Personality Assessment Inventory
PAP	Prostatic Acid Phosphatase
PAR	Pseudoautosomal Region
PAS	Preliminary Alcohol Screening
PCA	Principal Component Analysis
PCB	Polychlorinated Biphenyl
PCB	Printed Circuit Board
PCC	Pyridinium Chlorochromate
PCDF	Polychlorinated Dibenzofurans
PCL	Psychopathy Checklist
PCL-R	Psychopathy Checklist-Revised
PCL:SV	Screening Version of the Hare Psychopathy Checklist-Revised
PCP	Phencyclidine
PCP	Primary Care Physician
PCPP	Phenyl Cyclopentyl Piperidine
PCR	Polymerase Chain Reaction
PCRI	Parent–Child Relationship Inventory
PCT	Procalcitonin Concentration
PD	Physical Developer
PDA	Personal Digital Assistant
PDC	Personal Digital Cellular
PDD	Psychophysiological Detection of Deception
PDM	Psychodynamic Diagnostic Manual
PDQ	Paint Data Query
PE	Pulmonary Embolism
Pep A	Peptidase A
PEP	Primer Extension Preamplification
PEP-PCR	Primer Extension Preamplification Polymerase Chain Reaction
PET	Positron Emission Tomography
PETN	Pentaerythritol Tetranitrate
PFA	Psychological First Aid
PGC–MS	Pyrolysis Gas Chromatography–Mass Spectrometry

PGD	6-Phosphogluconate Dehydrogenase
PGM	Phosphoglucomutase
PHA	Preliminary Hazard Analysis
PHA	Public Health Agency
PHP	Phenyl Cyclohexylpyrrolidine
PHT	Pulmonary Hypertension
PID	Photoionization Detector
PIN	Personal Identifying Number
PINS	Persons in Need of Supervision
PLM	Polarized Light Microscope
PLMN	Public Land Mobile Network
PLS	Partial Least-Squares
PM	Postmortem
PMA	*p*-Methoxy-Amphetamine
PMDD	Premenstrual Dysphoric Disorder
PMI	Postmortem Interval
PML	Progressive Multifocal Leukoencephalopathy
PMR	Postmortem Redistribution
PMS	Phenazine Methosulphate
PMS	Premenstrual Syndrome
PMT	Photo Multiplier Tube
PMT	Premenstrual Tension
PNE	Pediatric Neurological Exam
PNES	Psychogenic Nonepileptic Seizures
POCT	Point-of-Care Testing
PORT	Perception-of-Relationships Test
POW	Prisoners of War
ppb	Parts Per Billion
PPD	Postpartum Depression
PPE	Personal Protective Equipment
ppi	Pixels Per Inch
PPI	Proton Pump Inhibitor
PPP	Postpartum Psychosis
pRIA	Protein Radioimmunoassays
PRNU	Photo Response Nonuniformity
PSA	Prostate-Specific Antigen
PSI	Parenting Stress Inventory
PSTN	Public Switched Telephone Network
PTAH	Phosphotungstic Acid-hematoxylin
PTE	Pulmonary ThromboEmbolism
PTFE	Polytetrafluoroethylene
PTSD	PostTraumatic Stress Disorder
PT	Proficiency Testing
PUK	Pin Unlocking Key
PVC	Polyvinyl Chloride
Py-GC-MS	Pyrolysis Gas Chromatography Mass Spectrometry
QA	Quality Assurance
QC	Quality Control
QDE	Questioned Document Examiner

QM	Quality Management
QPN	Qualitative Probabilistic Network
RAID	Redundant Array of Independent Disks
RAM	Random Access Memory
RAPID	Ruggedized Advanced Pathogen Identification Device
RCMP	Royal Canadian Mounted Police
RC	Restructured Clinical
rCRS	Revised Cambridge Reference Sequence
RDC	Research Diagnostic Criteria
RDCT	Rey Dot Counting Test
RDD	Radiological Dispersion Device
RDX	Hexogen
RED	Radiological Emission Device
RF	Renal Failure
RFC	Request for Comment
RFID	Radio Frequency Identification Device
RFLP	Restriction Fragment Length Polymorphism
RFS	Robust File System
RFU	Relative Fluorescence Intensity
RFUs	Relative Fluorescent Units
RGB	Red, Green, and Blue
RH	Retinal Hemorrhage
RI	Refractive Index
RIA	Radio-Immunoassay
RIM	Research in Motion
RMNE	Random Man Not Excluded
RMP	Random Match Probability
ROC	Receiver Operating Characteristic
ROSITA	Roadside Testing Assessment
RP	Readiness Potential
RRT	Relative Retention Time
RSD	Relative Standard Deviation
RT	Retention Time
RT-PCR	Real-Time Polymerase Chain Reaction
RTS	Rape Trauma Syndrome
RUVIS	Reflected Ultraviolet Imaging System
Ry	Ryanodyine Receptor
S/N	Signal-to-Noise Ratio
S/P	Saliva-to-Plasma
SAAMI	Sporting Arms and Ammunition Manufacturers' Institute
SAC	Serum Alcohol Concentration
SADS-C	Schedule of Affective Disorders and Schizophrenia-Change
SAMHSA	Substance Abuse and Mental Health Service Administration
SARS	Severe Acute Respiratory Syndrome
SB-5	Stanford-Binet Intelligence Scale – Fifth Edition
SBP	Sellier Bellot, Prague
SBS	Shaken Baby Syndrome
SCAN	Scandinavian Pulp and Paper Association

SCC	Standards Council of Canada
SCID	Structured Clinical Interview for Diagnostic and Statistical Manual of Mental Disorders, 4th ed.-Text Revision
SDH	Subdural Hemorrhage
SDIS	State DNA Identification System
SDS-PAGE	Sodium Dodecyl Sulphate Polyacrylamide Gel Electrophoresis
SD	Secure Digital
SD	Standard Deviation
SE	Secondary Electron
SEA	Strategic Environmental Assessment
SEIR	Surface-Enhanced Irregular Reflection
SEM/EDS	Scanning Electron Microanalysis with Energy Dispersive Sensor
SEM/EDX	Scanning Electron Microscopy/Energy Dispersive X-Ray
SEM/WDS	Scanning Electron Microanalysis with Wavelength Dispersive Sensor
SEM/WDX	Scanning Electron Microscopy/Wavelength Dispersive X-Ray Spectroscopy
SEM	Scanning Election Microscope
SF-ICP/MS	Sector Field-Inductively Coupled Plasma Mass Spectrometry
SFPE	Society of Fire Protection Engineers
SFST	Standardized Field Sobriety Test
SGAs	Second Generation Antipsychotics
SGM	Second-Generation Multiplex
SIB-R	Scales of Independent Behavior – Revised
SIDS	Sudden Infant Death Syndrome
SIM	Selected Ion Monitoring
SIM	Senior Identification Manager
SIM	Subscriber Identity Module
SIMCA	Soft Independent Modeling of Class Analogy
SIMS	Secondary Ion Mass Spectrometry
SIMS	Structured Inventory of Malingered Symptomatology
SIO	Senior Investigating Officer
SIPRI	Stockholm International Peace Research Institute
SIRS	Structured Interview of Reported Symptoms
SLA	Symbionese Liberation Army
SLP	Single Locus Probes
SLP	Single Locus Profiling
SLR	Single Lens Reflex
SMANZFL	Senior Managers of Australian and New Zealand Forensic Laboratories
SMD	Single-Metal Deposition
SMI	Severe Mental Illness
SMM	Stepwise Mutation Model
SMS	Short Message Service
SMTP	Simple Mail Transfer Protocol
SNAP-IV	Swanson, Nolan, and Pelham
SNP	Single Nucleotide Polymorphism
SNRI	Serotonin and Norepinephrine Reuptake Inhibitor
SOCO	Scenes of Crime Officer
SOFT	Society of Forensic Toxicologists

SOHO	Small and Home Office
SoHT	Society of Hair Testing
SOP	Standard Operating Procedure
SP	Shortpass
SPECT	Single Proton Emission Computed Tomography
SPE	Solid-Phase Extraction
SPIN	Service Planning Instrument
SPJ	Structured Professional Judgment
SPM	Scanning Probe Microscope
SPME	Solid Phase Micro Extraction
SPR	Small Particle Reagent
SRT	Sodium Rhodizonate Test
SSD	Scientific Support Department
SSM	Scientific Support Manager
SSM	Slipped Strand Mispairing
SSO	Sequence Specific Oligonucleotide
SSRI	Selective Serotonin Reuptake Inhibitor
SSSQ	Street Survival Skills Questionnaire
STA	Systematic Toxicology Analysis
STAG	Statistical Analysis of Glass
START	Short-Term Assessment of Risk and Treatability
STD	Sexually Transmitted Diseases
STEM	Scanning Transmission Microscope
STI	Sexually Transmitted Infections
StPO	Criminal Procedure Code
STR	Short Tandem Repeat
SUDEP	Sudden Unexplained Death in Epilepsy
SUDNIC	Sudden Unexpected Death Due to Neoplastic Disease in Infancy and Childhood
SVM	Support-Vector Machines
SVP	Sexually Violent Predator
SWAT	Special Weapons and Tactics
SWGDAM	Scientific Working Group on DNA Analysis Methods
SWEDOC	Science Working Group on Documents
SWGDRUG	Scientific Working Group for the Analysis of Drugs
SWGFAST	Scientific Working Group for Friction Ridge Analysis, Study, and Technology
SWGFEX	Scientific Working Group for Fire and Explosives
SWGGUN	Science Working Group on Guns
SWGhair	Scientific Working Group for Hairs
SWGIT	Scientific Working Group IT
SWGMAT	Scientific Working Group on Materials Analysis
TACS	Total Access Communication System
TAPPI	Technical Association of the Pulp and Paper Industry
TAT	Thematic Apperception Test
TATP	Triacetone Triperoxide
TBI	Traumatic Brain Injury
TBW	Total Body Water
TCD	Thermal Conductivity Detector

TCF	Totally Chlorine Free
TCP	Thienyl Cyclohexyl Piperidine
TCP	Transmission Control Protocol
TDMA	Time Division Multiple Access
TDx	Fluorescent Polarization Assay
TETRA	Terrestrial Trunked Radio
TDM	Target Disk Mode
TDM	Therapeutic Drug Monitoring
TdP	Torsades Des Pointes
TDx	Fluorescent Polarization Assay
TEA	Thermal Energy Analyzer
TEM	Transmission Electron Microscope
TEMED	Tetramethylethylenediamine
TETRA	Terrestrial Trunked Radio
TFPCl	N-(Trifluoroacetyl) Prolyl Chloride
TFS4	Transactional File System
TGA	Thermogravimetric Analysis
THC	Δ^9-Tetrahydrocannabinol
THC-COOH	11-Nor-9-Carboxy-Δ^9-Tetrahydrocannabinol
TIAs	Transient Ischemic Attacks
TIC	Toxic Industrial Chemical
TIC	Total Ion Chromatogram
TIM	Toxic Industrial Material
TIMS	Thermal Ionization Mass Spectrometry
TLC	Thin Layer Chromatography
TMA	Trimethoxyamphetamine
TMOT	Trace Metal Detection Test
TMJ	Total Metal Jacket
TMP	Thermomechanical Pulps
TMS	Trimethylsilyl
TNAZ	1,3,3-Trinitroazetidine
TNT	Trinitrotoluene
TOF	Time-of-Flight
TOF-SIMS	Time-of-Flight Secondary Ion Mass Spectrometry
TOMM	Test of Memory Malingering
TOR	The Onion Routing
TPMT	Thiopurine S-Methyltransferase
TPP	Thermal Protective Performance
TSH	Thyroid-Stimulating Hormone
TSOP	Thin Small-Outline Packages
TSWG	Technical Support Working Group
TTI	Transmit Terminal Identifier
TWGDAM	Technical Working Group on DNA Analysis and Methods
TWGED	Technical Working Group on Education and Training in Forensic Science
TWGFEX	Technical Working Group for Fire and Explosive Analysis
UAC	Urine–Alcohol Concentration
UCS	Unconditioned Stimuli
UDP	User Datagram Protocol

UEL	Upper Explosive Limit
UGPPA	Uniform Guardianship and Protective Proceedings Act
UHP	Ultra High Purity
UKAS/NAMAS	United Kingdom Accreditation Service/National Accreditation of Measurements and Sampling
UKNEQAS	United Kingdom National External Quality Assessment Scheme
UL	Underwriters Laboratories
UM	Ultrarapid Metabolizers
UMTS	Universal Mobile Telecommunication System
UN	United Nations
UNODC	United Nations Office on Drug Control
URN	Unique Reference Number
USDA	United States Department of Agriculture
USSC	United States Supreme Court
UV	Ultraviolet
UV-MSP	Microspectrophotometry Using Visible Light and Ultraviolet Light
UV/Vis	Ultraviolet/Visible
VA	Veterans Administration
VABS II	Vineland Adaptive Behavior Scales II
VCA	Vacuum Cyanoacrylate
VDAG	Vitamin D Binding Alpha Globulin
VIP	Validity Indicator Profile
VMD	Vacuum Metal Deposition
VNTR	Variable Number of Tandem Repeat
VoIP	Voice over Internet Protocol
VoIP/ToIP	Voice over Internet Protocol/Telephone over Internet Protocol
VQ	Vector Quantization
VRAG	Violence Risk Appraisal Guide
VRML	Virtual Reality Modeling Language
VSA	Video Spectral Analysis
VSA	Voice Stress Analyzers
VSA	Volatile Substance Abuse
VSC	Video Spectral Comparator
WADA	World Anti-Doping Agency
WAIS III	Wechsler Adult Intelligence Scale, Third Edition
WAIS-R	Wechsler Adult Intelligence Scale-Revised
WAN	Wide Area Network
WAP	Wireless Access Point
WAP	Wireless Application Protocol
WDX	Wavelength Dispersive X-Ray
WGA	Whole Genome Amplification
WHO	World Health Organization
WIRA	Wool Industries Research Association
WMD	Weapons of Mass Destruction
WMH-CIDI	World Mental Health – Composite International Diagnostic Interview
WMS	Wechsler Memory Scale

WRB	World Reference Base
WSQ	Wavelet Scalar Quantization
WTC	World Trade Center
WWI	World War I
WWII	World War II
XBO	Xenon Short Arc Lamp
XRD	X-Ray Diffraction
XRF	X-Ray Fluorescence Spectroscopy
XSR	eXtended Sector Remapper
Y-STRs	Y-Chromosome Short Tandem Repeats
YAFFS	Yet Another Flash File System
ZD	Z Direction
ZPO	Zivilprozessordnung(Civil Procedure Code)

The International System of Units (SI)

There are many different units of measure for most physical parameters such as length, mass, and temperature. The scientific community have agreed on a single system called the SI (Systeme Internationale) as the accepted international system of such units. SI units are either base or derived. Base units are fundamental and not reducible. Table 1 lists the main base units of interest in the discipline of materials science and engineering.

Derived units are expressed in terms of the base units, using mathematical signs for multiplication and division. For example, the SI units for density are kilogram per cubic meter (kg/m^3). For some derived units, special names and symbols exist; for example, N is used to denote the Newton, the unit of force, which is equivalent to $1\,kg\text{-}m/s^2$. Although many use the '/' notation (e.g. m/s) the system uses a superscript or exponent (to the power of) notation where a negative symbol replaces the '/'. For example, m/s becomes ms^{-1}, and m/s^2 becomes ms^{-2}. Table 2 contains a number of important derived units.

It is sometimes necessary, or convenient, to form names and symbols that are decimal multiples of SI units. Only one prefix is used when a multiple of an SI unit is formed, which should be in the numerator. These prefixes and their approved symbols are given in Table 3. Symbols for the main units are used in this book, SI or otherwise. Some disciplines retain other nomenclatures by practice or convention, although these are departures from the main scientific recommendations.

Table 1 The SI base units

Quantity	SI unit	Symbol
Length	meter	m
Mass	kilogram	kg
Time	second	s
Electric current	ampere	A
Thermodynamic temperature	kelvin	K
Amount of substance	mole	mol

Table 2   Some of the SI derived units (including examples of the superscript notation)

Quantity	Name	Formula	Special symbol
Area	square meter	m^2	–
Volume	cubic meter	m^3	–
Velocity	meter per second	$m/s\ (ms^{-1})$	–
Density	kilogram per cubic meter	kg/m^3	–
Concentration	moles per cubic meter	mol/m^3	–
Force	newton	$kg\cdot m/s^2\ (kg\cdot ms^{-2})$	N
Energy	joule	$kg\cdot m^2/s^2$, Nm	J
Pressure/Stress	pascal	kg/ms^2, N/m^2	Pa
Strain	–	m/m	–
Power, radiant flux	watt	$kg\cdot m^2/s^3$, J/s	W
Viscosity	pascal-second	kg/ms	Pa-s
Frequency (a periodic phenomenon)	hertz	$1/s\ (s^{-1})$	Hz
Electric charge	coulomb	A·s	C
Electric potential	volt	$kg\cdot m^2/s^2 C$	V
Capacitance	farad	$s^2 C/kg\cdot m^2$	F
Electric resistance	ohm	$kg\cdot m^2/sC^2$	Ω
Magnetic flux	weber	$kg\cdot m^2/sC$	Wb
Magnetic flux density	tesla	kg/sC, Wb/m^2	(T)

Table 3   SI multiple and submultiple prefixes

Factors by which multiplied	Prefix	Symbol
10^{12}	tera	T
10^{9}	giga	G
10^{6}	mega	M
10^{3}	kilo	k
10^{-2}	centi[a]	c
10^{-3}	milli	m
10^{-6}	micro	μ
10^{-9}	nano	n
10^{-12}	pico	p

[a] Avoided when possible.

Guide to Legal Citations

What is the Correct Form?

There are many systems for citing sources

When a publication such as this Encyclopedia is to accommodate technical contributions from authorities across the world, there is benefit in uniformity in the form that source references are printed. Thus, for scientific publications, we decided that the Vancouver style would be adopted. For the most part, that format is followed throughout these volumes.

It was more difficult to decide on the format for legal authorities and sources, because there is no single system of citing court cases, statutes, and other law publications. What exists is a conglomeration of conventions that are not always followed by various courts even within the same country. Local custom of reporting legal sources often supersedes what was prescribed as the "official" system in a jurisdiction.

Of course, that is only of limited help. In the United Kingdom, for instance, with no less than a dozen different courts that, at one time or another, publish or have published case reports (e.g., Appeal Cases (second and third series), Chancery Division, Criminal Appeal Reports, Queen's Bench, House of Lords, and other specialty courts), whatever convention exists is not always enlightening when one is confronted with a citation of a court. It is not easy for individuals who are not solicitors, barristers, or trained in law to locate where a particular case report may be found.

The confusion is even greater in the United States where there are 50 different states, each printing their case reports in official and/or unofficial reporter systems. In addition, the federal court system publishes cases decided by the United States Supreme Court (in three different reporter systems), by eleven Circuit Courts of Appeal and the District of Columbia (in two different publication forms), and by numerous United States District Court opinions. Then there is also a multitude of reports for specialized courts or federal agencies.

To seek to impart uniformity in citation form, editors from the Universities of Harvard, Columbia, Yale, and Pennsylvania Law Reviews have devised what is known as *The Bluebook – A Uniform System of Citation*. It is referred to as the *Bluebook*. The latest edition of the tome is the Eighteenth Edition, published in 2007. It comprises 415 pages. Unfortunately, the *Bluebook* has not imparted uniformity in citation form.

First, each of the *Bluebook's* editions advocated using conventions that were later partially modified in successive editions. Furthermore, the *Bluebook* is used essentially by law review journals published by law schools, but courts and other legal writers as well as publishers pay only scant attention to it and report cases in varying ways that they deem rational.

Clearly, then, some leeway must be accorded to authors in these volumes in the way they report case law, statutes, and other legal collections, since there is no one accepted way that might be said to be generally accepted as the "correct" format. In the face of these considerations we decided, as a matter of convenience, that legal sources would be cited in the form that was customary in the jurisdiction where the source originated.

It is more important, then, to understand the purpose that references serve. The purpose of a citation is so that the complete opinion of the court or other legal authority can be readily retrieved. Sadly, the convention whereby decisions of courts are cited makes sense only to legally trained individuals or to persons who work within a relatively closed environment.

Basic requirement of an informative citation form

An adequate citation of a reported opinion of a court is supposed to contain the following: (i) the name (or "style") of the case, (ii) the reporter system wherein the opinion has been published, (iii) the court that decided the case, and (iv) the year of decision. This is the preferred order in which court cases are cited in the United States and in many other countries, though the four elements of an informative citation are not always listed in the same order.

In the United Kingdom, for instance, the preferred form is to start with (i) the case name, (ii) the year of decision in parentheses, and thereafter (iii) the volume number (if available), (iv) the reporting system, (v) the page, (vi) the deciding court if that information is not otherwise clearly indicated by the reporting system, and (vii) the jurisdiction where the case was decided, if that information is not evident from the context or the citation. It is also preferred that cases be cited from official Law Reports rather than from ancillary sources. The Official Reports consist of the Appeal Courts (A.C.), Queen's Bench (Q.B.), Chancery (Ch.), Family (Fam.), and Probate (P) Reports. When citing decisions of the House of Lords, the Privy Council, or other sources that may report appeals from more than one jurisdiction, the jurisdiction from which the appeal was taken should be indicated parenthetically.

Most forensic scientists may be familiar with the way court opinions are published in their own country, but may not understand where and how foreign legal sources may be found. If, for research purposes, it becomes necessary for them to retrieve a complete court opinion or a statute for which the researcher possesses a citation, help in locating the full text referenced may be obtained from law-trained individuals. Major court systems also maintain libraries staffed by knowledgeable librarians. Legal libraries staffed with helpful librarians are further maintained in most law colleges and by many large legal firms.

Because a single uniform system for referencing legal authorities is lacking, some variations may be noted in the citation form used by authors of contributions. With the guidance offered here, the individual who is not legally trained will hopefully be able to decipher the meaning of legal references encountered throughout this Encyclopedia.

Andre Moenssens

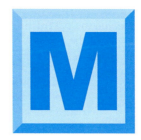

Malingering *see* Delusions, Hallucinations, Posttraumatic Stress Disorder

Malingering: Assessment of *see* Neuropsychological Assessment

Malingering: Forensic Evaluations

Malingering in Forensic Evaluations

The essential feature of malingering, as defined by the *Diagnostic and Statistical Manual of Mental Disorders* (*DSM*), is the "intentional production of false or grossly exaggerated physical or psychological symptoms, motivated by external incentives such as avoiding military duty, avoiding work, obtaining financial compensation, evading criminal prosecution, or obtaining drugs ..." [1] (p. 739). Malingering for the purposes of evading criminal prosecution or obtaining drugs are commonly seen in forensic settings and forensic mental health clinicians often

face difficult decisions when evaluating and treating these individuals. In civil settings, malingering is often related to obtaining potentially large financial settlements.

In order to appropriately assess and manage malingering, clinicians must have in-depth knowledge of the following: (i) prevalence rates of malingering and how the *Diagnostic and Statistical Manual of Mental Disorders* Fourth Edition, Text Revision (*DSM-IV-R*) inadvertently encourages misdiagnosis and mismanagement of malingering-related issues, (ii) common reasons for countertransference toward malingering patients and strategies to avoid it, (iii) empirically validated measures of malingering, and (iv) clinical issues related with the evaluation of malingering.

Malingering and the DSM

Recent evidence [2–4] indicates that malingering is common in forensic settings with prevalence rates ranging from 10 to 29%. Even with the most conservative estimate of malingering, one thing is clear that forensic mental health practitioners cannot rely on the veracity of their patient's self-reports to establish diagnoses or effectively manage their patient's symptoms. Self-report distortion is especially salient in pretrial forensic evaluations where the stakes can be quite high.

For instance, individuals undergoing an evaluation of their mental status (i.e., insanity) at the time of offense, will, at times, embellish pre-existing psychopathology or fabricate mental health symptoms in order to avoid prison sentence[5]. Likewise, competency to stand trial evaluees may feign psychopathology in an attempt to avoid trial altogether [6]. Others malinger for some reasons apart from trying to avoid prosecution. Such reasons include moving to a mental health unit where the environment is often viewed as calmer and safer [7] or to acquire psychotropic medications [8].

How clinicians view the issue of malingering can have significant influence on their treatment of bona fide patients and individuals who are feigning. Unfortunately, countertransference (see next section) often accompanies malingering and staff members frequently make assumptions about other aspects of the patient's presentation based on a malingering diagnosis. Current diagnostic nomenclature does little to disabuse professionals of this potential conflict.

The DSM [1] criteria indicate that malingering should be suspected if any of the following are present: (i) medicolegal context of presentation, (ii) marked discrepancy between the person's claimed stress or disability and the objective findings, (iii) lack of cooperation during the diagnostic evaluation and in complying with the diagnostic evaluation, and (iv) the presence of Antisocial Personality Disorder. In forensic settings, either one or several of these criteria are routinely present for reasons wholly unrelated to malingering. Reliance on these criteria can lead to the misclassification of patients with bona fide mental illnesses as feigning cases. In fact, exclusive reliance on DSM-IV TR criteria can result in up to 80% misclassification rate [9]. If a test for a medical disorder, such as human immunodeficiency virus (HIV), resulted in high false positive rate, the test would be discontinued forthwith.

Avoiding false positives with malingering cases must be the primary responsibility of the forensic examiner. Evaluators must be cognizant that certain evaluees are more at risk to be misdiagnosed as **malingerers**. Research has shown that bona fide patients with lower educational attainment and absence of previous mental health treatment are much more likely to be misclassified as **malingerers** [10]. Clinicians can avoid false positives by conducting comprehensive evaluations that include multiple data sources, continuing to evaluate for psychopathology or cognitive deficits in the presence of malingering, and not making facile assumptions based on incomplete data.

Malingering and Countertransference

An issue that frequently goes unchecked in malingering evaluations is the misuse and conveyance of diagnostic information. One prime example is the use of emotionally laden words by clinicians to describe a malingerer; a clear sign of countertransference [11]. I have overhead staff using terms like "liar", "fraud", or "fake" when describing an individual found to be malingering. These descriptors are clinically useless and result in untoward feelings toward the patient.

Even more distressing is that longitudinally, a malingering diagnosis can follow the patient and subsequent complaints may be dismissed as bogus and misattributed to malingering. As such, clinicians conducting forensic evaluations have an ethical responsibility to minimize harm by accurately reporting their findings [12]. When malingering is identified, discussing situational-specific aspects of the diagnosis would be the first step toward minimizing future consequences.

One way to avoid countertransference with malingering cases is through the use of explanatory models. Rogers [9, 13] introduced explanatory models as a counterperspective to the unitary perspective provided by the DSM. Rogers proposed three explanatory models: (i) criminological, (ii) adaptational, and (iii) pathogenic.

Criminological

The DSM is focused on the criminological model, which closely aligns malingering with antisocial behavior. The criminological model accounts for only a minority of malingering cases, which explains the high rate of false positives associated with the DSM criteria.

Adaptational

A prototypical analysis of the responses of forensic experts [14] reinforced that the majority of individuals who malinger in psycholegal evaluations do so as an adaptive response to adversarial circumstances. The adaptational model allows for the possibility that people facing difficult circumstances engage in deception designed to decrease the likelihood of a bad outcome (e.g., lengthy prison term).

Pathogenic

The pathogenic model posits that feigning can occur as a result of underlying psychopathology. Although this model is infrequently used and has mainly fallen into disfavor, there is some support for this model derived from both a historical perspective and surveys of forensic practitioners [15].

Explanatory models are especially useful if clinicians consider alternative explanations for malingering. Using models to understand malingering can provide objectivity to the assessment process and eliminate emotionally laden statements regarding patients who are engaging in deception.

Measures that Detect Malingering of Psychopathology

The use of extant measures for evaluating feigning is necessary for accurate assessment. In reviewing measures used to systematically assess for the malingering of psychopathology, it is clear that clinicians have several available options. Given space constraints, I primarily focus on measures specifically designed to assess malingering, with the exception of the *Minnesota Multiphasic Personality Inventory Second Edition (MMPI-2)* [16]. Other multiscale inventories with malingering or response style scales such as the Personality Assessment Inventory (PAI) [17] and the Millon Clinical Multiaxial Inventory (MCMI) [18] are not discussed. It should be noted that both the PAI and MCMI-III possess significant psychometric limitations for detecting feigning, although recent research suggests that the PAI does possess utility for screening feigned presentations [3, 19].

- The Structured Interview of Reported Symptoms (SIRS), [16] is an interview designed to comprehensively assess malingering and related response styles. The SIRS is often employed as the criterion measure in feigning research due to its very strong psychometric properties and exceedingly low false positive rate [16]. Its eight primary scales focus on measuring symptom patterns consistent with malingering include rare, combinations, improbable and absurd, blatant, subtle, severity, selectivity, and reported versus observed. Rogers *et al.* [20] performed a confirmatory factor analysis (CFA) of the SIRS with a large sample of forensic referrals. The results obtained strongly support for a two-factor dimensional model: Spurious Presentation and Plausible Presentation. "Spurious Presentation" was consistent with "classic" malingering made up of atypical and rare symptoms. "Plausible Presentation"

was defined by over-reporting actual symptoms of mental illness and issues related to psychological maladjustment. Considering these two factors, Spurious Presentation was focused on the overall content of the report while Plausible Presentation was focused on the magnitude of report.

- The Miller Forensic Assessment of Symptoms Test (M-FAST, [21]) is a 25-item structured interview that consists of seven scales designed to be used to screen for malingering. The M-FAST is closely modeled after the SIRS and consists of seven scales and a total score; the total score is especially effective for identifying patients who are potentially malingering and in need of a more thorough assessment [3]. The M-FAST was subjected to a CFA in order to assess if the two-factor structure found in the SIRS was applicable. Vitacco *et al.* [22] tested models of the M-FAST with 244 forensic patients and cross-validated those findings with 210 forensic patients. Results demonstrated that a single, parsimonious factor emerged that was closely aligned with the SIRS' Spurious Presentation ($r = 0.75$) and moderately related to Plausible Presentation ($r = 0.64$). The clear implication is that the M-FAST is most effective for identifying patients with atypical and rare symptoms.

- The Structured Inventory of Malingered Symptomatology [SIMS, [23]] is a 75-item true/false test composed of five scales: low intelligence, affective disorders, neurological impairment, psychosis, and amnesia. The SIMS evaluates a wide range of feigning aspects, including aspects of cognitive feigning. With the SIRS as a criterion for known-groups design, the SIMS effectively differentiated malingerers from nonmalingerers (M Cohen's $d = 2.25$) with excellent reliability estimates [3]. However, the use of self-report measure has inherent limitations in that aspects of interpersonal presentation are not evaluated. Given that interpersonal interactions are important in evaluating malingering, this limitation is noteworthy.

- The MMPI-2 [16] is a 567-item multiscale inventory designed to assess psychopathology. In addition to its clinical scales, the MMPI-2 contains specialized scales designed to evaluate issues related to response styles. These scales use validated strategies for assessing response styles including (i) rare symptoms, (ii) erroneous stereotypes, (iii) symptom severity, or (iv) obvious and subtle symptoms. Rogers *et al.* completed a large meta-analysis of malingering on the MMPI-2 [24] and generally found robust effect sizes for many malingering scales. However, clinicians should be cautious in using the MMPI-2 to assess malingering for a wide range of cut scores that dramatically vary by disorder and study [24]. Research [25, 26] evaluating the Infrequency (F) and Infrequency Psychopathology [F(p)] scales with large groups of mental health and criminal-forensic patients found the presence of an underlying taxon for both scales.

Clinical Issues Related to Evaluating Malingering

A key consideration in the accurate assessment of malingering is the realization that mentally ill individuals can engage in deception. This is referred to as *partial malingering* [18], which is defined as the exaggeration of current symptomatology or reporting symptoms from a previous episode of mental illness. Partial malingering is common in forensic settings and can contribute to error when clinicians fail to recognize the presence of underlying mental disorder(s). Obtaining a thorough psychosocial history from the patient, interviewing collateral sources, and reviewing available records are useful tools in disentangling bona fide illness from feigned symptoms.

One potentially useful strategy to disentangle pathology and response styles is to employ a structured interview such as the schedule of affective disorders and schizophrenia-change version [(SADS-C), [27]]. The SADS-C provides an extensive evaluation of psychopathology [28], it has two scales (symptom combinations and symptom selectivity) that act as an effective screen for malingering [28, 29]. Ultimately, success may rely on the clinician's overall knowledge of psychopathology and response styles and the ability to integrate conflicting information regarding mental disorders and feigned presentation.

Another issue adding to the complexity of diagnosing malingering is the differentiation of malingering from factitious disorders. Similar to malingering, factitious disorders involve the intentional production of physical or psychological symptoms [1]. The key difference is the goal of factitious disorders is to assume the sick role in the absence of other incentives. Clinicians often struggle with assessing motivation and trying to determine the underlying rationale for the behavior. Differential diagnoses between malingering and factitious disorders should occur in two related steps: First, determine the occurrence of feigning using a validated instrument. If feigning is present, clinicians are then supposed to determine the underlying motivation [15, 30].

Neurocognitive Malingering

Malingering can extend into civil settings as well. Unlike forensic settings where individuals malinger to avoid trial or prison sentence, individuals often malinger in civil settings to receive monetary compensation. A prime example is personal injury litigation whereby an individual alleges that he or she received an injury of the mind or body. Given that compensation for personal injuries can be highly lucrative it is not surprising that rates of malingering in such cases have ranged from 20 to 35% [31].

Clearly the information presented earlier in this article regarding countertransference and assessment strategies remain salient; however, evaluating malingering in civil situations requires additional skill sets including assessing malingering on neuropsychological examinations (e.g., alleging brain damage). Malingering neurocognitive deficits is commonly seen when evaluating individuals in civil settings.

Cognitive Malingering

To understand cognitive malingering and know how to best diagnosis it, clinicians are advised to familiarize themselves with the criteria for malingering neurocognitive dysfunction (MND) functioning known as the *Slick criteria* [32]. The Slick criteria set forth in a seminal article [32] provided a definition of MND as "the volitional exaggeration or fabrication of cognitive dysfunction for the purpose of obtaining substantial material gain, or avoiding or escaping formal duty or responsibility..." (p. 552). The article allowed for gradients in MND ranging from definite to possible. These criteria are well reasonable and provide a fundamental foundation for diagnosing MND. To aid in the diagnostic process, measures specifically developed for MND are marketed and should be considered when cognitive malingering is expected.

Measures that Detect Cognitive Malingering

For the testing of MND, clinicians have many options; we focus only on few well-validated and frequently used measures due to space limitations. These measures often use chance responding for a forced-choice test and performing significantly lower than chance is indicative of poor effort and potential malingering. However, more sophisticated measures like the Validity Indicator Profile (VIP) [33] assesses for several issues relevant to MND and represent a major advancement in assessing for MND.

- Rey 15-Item Test consists of a 3×5 alphanumeric sequence that an individual is asked to reproduce. This is a simple measure that has continued to be very popular [34]; however, such popularity seems overstated and it may be best used to screen for cognitive malingering [35] as there have been reports of poor sensitivity, but good specificity. As such, this test does not appear appropriate for evaluating MND. An important consideration is not to use the test for individuals with mental retardation [35].
- Test of Memory Malingering [TOMM, [36]] is a forced-choice test, where the individual is presented with a series of pictures and later "forced" to pick which ones they previously viewed. The TOMM has shown some promise for use in forensic and civil evaluations [37, 38]; however, its cut score has been deemed to be high for some individuals with actual cognitive dysfunction and poor effort could be misinterpreted as malingering. Clinicians must differentiate reasons for poor performance, as low scores might be indicative of suboptimal effort.
- VIP [33] is a self-report test that has both verbal and nonverbal sections. The VIP has several advantages over its counterparts including three providing scores on three possibilities for poor performance: inconsistent, irrelevant, and suppressed. The latter is consistent with what would be considered MND. Over 1000 individuals were subjected to initial validation and 312 cases were cross validated [33]. The VIP has three scales, Inconsistent, Irrelevant, and Suppressed, to detect atypical performance. Notably, the Suppressed scale indicates formal malingering. The ability to differentiate among random responding,

irrelevant responding, and malingering is the real strength of the VIP. The VIP has demonstrated excellent properties in evaluating cognitive malingering [39, 40].

Conclusions

Mental health practitioners are encouraged to receive specialized training to understand the complexities of malingering as fully as possible. In the context of assessing malingering, clinicians should strive for diagnostic accuracy with the following:

1. Use only reliable and valid instruments with a proven track record of successfully differentiating bona fide patients from individuals engaging in deception.
2. Untangle psychopathology and true cognitive deficits from malingering through comprehensive assessments that include an evaluation of both response styles and actual deficits. Improve diagnostic accuracy through the use of collateral sources and extensive record reviews to buttress psychological assessment findings.
3. Use explanatory models, especially the adaptational and pathogenic models, to generate an understanding of situational aspects of feigning.
4. Understand that malingering is not "all or none" and should be viewed on a continuum. A prime example is partial malingering where an individual with a bona fide illness exaggerates his or her symptoms.

References

[1] American Psychiatric Association (2000). *Diagnostic and Statistical Manual of Mental Disorders*, 4th Edition, Text Revision (**DSM IV-R**), American Psychiatric Association Washington, DC.
[2] Cornell, D.G. & Hawk, G.L. (1989). Clinical presentation of malingerers diagnosed by experienced forensic psychologists, *Law and Human Behavior* **13**, 375–383.
[3] Vitacco, M.J., Rogers R., Gabel, J. & Munizza J. (2007). An evaluation of malingering screens with competency to stand trial patients: A known-groups comparison, *Law and Human Behavior*, **31**(3), 249–260.
[4] Boccaccini, M.T., Murrie, D.C. & Duncan, S.A. (2006). Screening for malingering in a criminal-forensic simple with the Personality Assessment Inventory, *Psychological Assessment* **18**, 415–423.
[5] Rogers, R. & Shuman, D.W. (2005). *Fundamentals of Forensic Practice: Mental Health and Criminal Law*, Springer, New York, NY.

[6] Rogers, R., Sewell, K.W., Grandjean, N.R. & Vitacco, M.J. (2002). The detection of feigned mental disorders on specific competency measures, *Psychological Assessment* **14**, 177–183.

[7] Vitacco, M.J. & Rogers, R. (2005). Assessment of malingering in correctional settings, in *Handbook of Correctional Mental Health*, C.L. Scott & J.B. Gerbasi, eds, American Psychiatric Press, Washington, DC, 133–154.

[8] Yates, B.D., Nordquist, C.R. & Schultz-Ross, A.R. (1996). Feigned psychiatric symptoms in the emergency room, *Psychiatric Services* **47**, 998–1000.

[9] Rogers, R. (1990). Models of feigned mental illness, *Professional Psychology* **21**, 182–188.

[10] Kucharski, T.L. & Duncan, S.A. (2006). Clinical and demographic characteristics of criminal defendants potentially misidentified by objective measures of malingering, *American Journal of Forensic Psychology* **24**, 5–20.

[11] Goldyne, A.J. (2007). Minimizing the influence of unconscious bias in evaluations: A practical guide, *Journal of the American Academy of Psychiatry and Law* **35**, 60–66.

[12] Ackerman, M. (2006). Forensic report writing, *Journal of Clinical Psychology* **62**, 59–72.

[13] Rogers, R., Sewell, K.W. & Goldstein, A. (1996). Explanatory models of malingering: A prototypical analysis, *Law and Human Behavior* **18**, 543–552.

[14] Rogers, R., Salekin, R.T., Sewell, K.W., Goldstein, A. & Leonard, K. (1998). A comparison of forensic and nonforensic malingerers: A prototypical analysis of explanatory models, *Law and Human Behavior* **22**, 353–367.

[15] Rogers, R., Bagby, R.M. & Dickens, S.E. (1993). *Structured Interview of Reported Symptoms, Professional Manual*, Psychological Assessment Resources, Odessa, FL.

[16] Butcher, J.N., Dahlstrom, W.G., Graham J.R., Tellegen A. & Kaemmer B. (1989). *Minnesota Multiphasic Personality Inventory-Second Edition Manual for administration and scoring*, University of Minnesota Press, Minneapolis, MN.

[17] Morey, L.C. (1991). *Personality Assessment Inventory*, Psychological Assessment Resources, Tampa, FL.

[18] Millon, T. (1994). *Millon Clinical Multiaxial Inventory-Third Edition (MCMI-III) Manual*, National Computer Systems, Minneapolis, MN.

[19] Hopwood, C.S., Morey, L.C., Rogers, R. & Sewell, K.W. (2007). Malingering on the personality assessment inventory: identification of specific feigned disorders, *Journal of Personality Assessment* **88**, 43–48.

[20] Rogers, R., Jackson, R.L., Sewell, K.W. & Salekin, K.L. (2005). Detection strategies for malingering: A confirmatory factor analysis of the SIRS, *Criminal Justice and Behavior* **32**, 511–525.

[21] Miller, H.A. (2001). *M-FAST: Miller-Forensic Assessment of Symptoms Test professional manual.* Psychological Assessment Resources, Odessa, FL.

[22] Vitacco, M.J., Jackson, R., Rogers, R., Neumann, C.S., Miller, H., Gabel, J. (2008). Detection strategies for malingering with the Miller Forensic Assessment of Symptoms Test: A confirmatory factor analysis of underlying dimensions, *Assessment*, **15**(1), 97–103.

[23] Widows, M.R. & Smith, G.P. (2004). *SIMS: Structured Inventory of Malingered Symptomatology Professional Manual*, Psychological Assessment Resources, Odessa, FL.

[24] Rogers, R., Sewell, K.W., Martin, M.A. & Vitacco, M.J. (2003). Detection of feigned mental disorders: A meta-analysis of the MMPI-2, *Assessment* **10**, 160–177.

[25] Strong, D.R., Greene, R.L. & Schinka, J.A. (2000). A taxometric analysis of MMPI-2 infrequency scales [F and F(p)] in clinical settings, *Psychological Assessment* **12**, 166–173.

[26] Strong, D.R., Glassmire, D.M., Frederick, R.I. & Greene, R.L. (2006). Evaluating the latent structure of the MMPI-2 F(p) scale in a forensic sample: A taxometric analysis, *Psychological Assessment* **18**, 250–261.

[27] Spitzer, R.L. & Endicott, J.. *Schedule of Affective Disorders and Schizophrenia-Change Version*, Biometrics Research, New York.

[28] Rogers, R., Jackson, R.L., Salekin, K.L. & Neumann, C.S. (2003). Assessing Axis I symptomatology on the SADS-C in two correctional samples: The validation of subscales and a screen for malingered presentations, *Journal of Personality Assessment* **81**, 281–290.

[29] Rogers, R. (2001). *Handbook of Diagnostic and Structured Interviewing*, Guilford Press, New York, NY.

[30] Vitacco, M.J. (2008). Syndromes associated with deception, in *Clinical Assessment of Malingering and Deception*, 3rd Edition, R. Rogers, The Guilford Press, New York, NY, 39–50.

[31] Mittenberg, W., Patton, C., Canyock, D. & Condit, D. (2002). Base rates of malingering and symptom exaggeration, *Journal of Clinical and Experimental Neuropsychology* **24**, 1094–1102.

[32] Slick, D.J., Sherman, E. & Iverson, G.I. (1999). Diagnostic criteria for malingered neurocognitive dysfunction: Proposed standards for clinical practice and research, *The Clinical Neuropsychologist* **13**, 545–561.

[33] Frederick, R.I. (1997). *Validity Indicator Profile, Test Manual*, Pearson Assessments, Minneapolis, MN.

[34] Slick, D.J., Jing, T.E., Strauss, E.H. & Hultsch, D.F. (2004). Detecting malingering: A survey of experts' practices, *Archives of Clinical Neuropsychology* **19**, 465–473.

[35] Reznek, L. (2005). The Rey 15-item memory test for malingering: A meta-analysis, *Brain Injury* **19**, 539–543.

[36] Tombaugh, T.N. (1996). *Test of Memory Malingering Professional Manual*, Multi-health Systems, New York.

[37] Greve, K.W., Bianchini, K.J. & Doane, B.M. (2006). Classification accuracy of the Test of Memory Malingering in traumatic brain injury: Results of a known-groups analysis, *Journal of Clinical and Experimental Neuropsychology* **28**, 1176–1190.

[38] Delain, S.L. & Ben-Porath, Y.S. (2003). Use of the TOMM in a criminal court assessment setting, *Assessment* **10**, 370–381.

[39] Frederick, R.I. (2002). Review of the Validity Indicator Profile, *Journal of Forensic Neuropsychology* **2**, 125–145.

[40] Frederick, R.I., Crosby, R.D. & Wynkoop, T.F. (2000). Performance of curve classification of invalid responding on the Validity Indicator Profile, *Archives of Clinical Neuropsychology* **15**, 281–300.

MICHAEL J. VITACCO

Malingering: Mental Retardation
see Mental Retardation: Death Penalty

Malpractice: Medical *see* Medical Malpractice

Malpractice Actions against Experts

Introduction

The term "malpractice," when describing expert behavior in professional dealings with third parties, has several connotations. In its popular understanding, it may be seen as a characterization of either negligent or intentional conduct that is considered harmful, inequitable, or fraudulent.

In professional practice, the term describes conduct that may expose the person guilty of such conduct to professional criticism by his peers in terms of sanctions within professional organizations to which the expert belongs. These sanctions may result in public or private reprimands, suspension or loss of membership privileges, expulsion from professional societies, and temporary or permanent loss of credentials or certifications. This form of malpractice is discussed in the separate article of **Ethics: Codes of Conduct for Expert Witnesses**.

The connotation in which the word "malpractice" is used in this article is as a legal term used in common law jurisdictions, particularly in the United States of America, to describe unlawful conduct that exposes an expert to possibly three different consequences: (i) a civil court action for damages caused to third parties while conducting professional duties; (ii) a criminal action brought by the government to punish defined criminal conduct such as fraud, theft, obstruction of justice, contempt of court, or similar crimes; or (iii) a quasi-criminal action brought by a governmental entity to restrict or remove a license to conduct a professional practice granted by public officials.

Since legal systems differ depending upon the country or jurisdiction, an in-depth exploration of malpractice becomes impossible within the confines of this work. For that reason, the possible legal consequences of professional misconduct are described only briefly here with reference to approaches taken by American courts and in the context of civil actions brought against experts.

Expert Malpractice – a Problem of National Scope

The development of a new cause of action designed to hold expert witnesses, like forensic scientists, doctors, and lawyers, responsible for their negligent professional behavior [1] has been driven by the growing recognition that expert negligence is not uncommon [2]. High-profile incidents have revealed failures in the application of some of the most well-established scientific techniques such as fingerprint identification [3, 4], DNA testing [5], and serologic analysis [6]. Other investigations have demonstrated that pathologists faked hundreds of autopsies [7] or committed grievous errors [8] in determining cause of death.

At present, the law does little to regulate the quality of expert testimony [9]. Nontort solutions offered by the scientific and legal communities to curb expert abuses include capping expert witness fees [10]; prescreening experts; using only court-appointed experts [11]; adhering to strict ethics codes [12]; instituting peer review [13]; and establishing a science court [14]. Additionally, it has been suggested that fraudulent experts be prosecuted [15].

The conventional wisdom long held that the principal safeguard against errant expert testimony is the opportunity for adversarial cross-examination [16]. In reality, however, most lawyers do a woefully inadequate job in cross-examining experts [17] due to a general reluctance to challenge experts in their own fields and improper trial preparation [18]. Finally, the vast majority of civil and criminal cases are settled or plea bargained prior to trial so that the expert may never be subjected to rigorous questioning during the adversary process.

To date, none of the nontort solutions offered to curb expert abuses have succeeded in accomplishing their goal. While attempts at self-regulation and court supervision may provide some deterrence, they do not compensate individuals harmed by negligent experts. This lack of effective solutions to expert negligence or intentional professional misconduct has led to the developing area of expert malpractice tort law.

The Tort of Expert Malpractice

The expert witness malpractice cause of action offers the most effective means of achieving the twin goals of compensating injured individuals and deterring future misconduct. As a result, the last two decades have seen a substantial increase in the number of tort actions against experts and their employers.

The four elements of an expert malpractice claim are (i) the existence of a duty owed to the plaintiff arising out of the relationship between the expert and the plaintiff; (ii) a negligent act or omission by the expert in breach of that duty; (iii) causation; and (iv) damages [19].

The premise of the cause of action is that, first, expert witnesses owe a duty to their clients. However, the duty does not end there. Expert witnesses also owe a duty to any foreseeable plaintiff who may be affected by the expert's conduct and who are likely to suffer damages due to a negligently rendered opinion. These duties are based upon their professional knowledge and skills and are similar to the duties owed by a doctor to a patient and a lawyer to a client. In this way, the specter of malpractice encourages experts to be careful, accurate, and compliant with "quality control" measures.

The standard of care for a forensic scientist is that of the reasonably prudent practitioner in the relevant scientific field [20]. Standards of professional practice and ethical codes help define the standard of care, and most disciplines within the forensic sciences have adopted such standards. In order to prevail, a plaintiff must prove that the expert did not adhere to the standard of a reasonably prudent expert in rendering an opinion, conducting an examination, or giving testimony. Ordinarily, an independent evaluation by a disinterested expert in the same field will be required to determine whether an expert deviated from the required standard of care.

A crucial element of the tort of malpractice is causation. Causation tests whether the defendant's actions were in fact connected to the plaintiff's injury, and whether the connection was close enough to allow compensation to the injured party. In some cases, it will be readily apparent that an expert's testimony alone "caused" the wrong. This is especially true when the expert evidence is the only determinative evidence presented in the litigation [21]. Studies have demonstrated that, despite jury instructions to the contrary, jurors give expert testimony greater weight than other evidence [22]. Thus, it is clear that financial injury to a potential plaintiff or conviction and incarceration of a potentially innocent individual who is prosecuted on the basis of an expert's opinion evidence,[a] are reasonably foreseeable consequences of expert negligence or intentional misconduct.

When a plaintiff proves that an expert has committed malpractice, the measure of damages that may be awarded include, though are not limited to (1) the difference between a full verdict of proven loss and the reduced verdict resulting from the expert's testimony; (2) the difference between a full settlement and the reduced settlement that resulted from the expert's misconduct; (3) the cost of the expert's investigation; and (4) the attorneys' fees for responding to the expert's testimony and in proving the misconduct [23].

Although traditionally experts were afforded absolute immunity in trial testimony and trial preparation, expert witness malpractice causes of action are gaining momentum [24]. Courts in New Jersey [25], Connecticut [26], Texas [27], California [28], Pennsylvania [29], Massachusetts [30], Louisiana [31], Vermont [32], and Missouri [33] are among the growing number of jurisdictions that have allowed plaintiffs to sue experts for malpractice. This trend has induced defendants to settle cases even when the jurisdiction has yet to recognize the cause of action [34].

Despite this trend, some jurisdictions continue to adhere to a policy of absolute immunity for expert witnesses [35]. Although witness immunity is an exception to the general rules of liability, and is traditionally extremely narrow in scope, a few courts have nevertheless shielded experts from civil liability for ordinary negligence by reasoning that (i) negligent mistakes or inaccuracies do not constitute perjury, or (ii) testimony and reports provided to courts are privileged [36]. Other courts have held that the expert witness who gives opinion evidence is the court's witness, and therefore enjoys immunity against all post-trial damage claims whether sued by a party or non-party to the action [37]. Such limitations are increasingly rare, however, and no court shields erring expert witnesses from perjury charges for willful deceptions, or from damage actions where the expert's conduct involved intentional or grossly negligent conduct.

There is a compelling argument to be made against expert immunity. First, the doctrine of immunity was not created to bar a suit against a professional who negligently performs services [38]. Moreover, when an expert is accused of malpractice, the real complaint is not with the testimony provided in court, but rather with the negligently produced out-of-court work product. By testifying, the expert merely publishes his negligence to the court. Absolute immunity should not be afforded to experts, who are neither judges nor their adjuncts, but merely third party participants in litigation. And the courts, the legal profession, and the forensic disciplines recognize that the trend is firmly toward permitting claims for damages resulting from negligent expert testimony.

Concerns that the proliferation of expert malpractice suits will have a chilling effect on the supply of willing forensic experts are misplaced. While the emergence of such a cause of action may chase the habitually negligent or incompetent expert from the field, this is, of course, a salutary by-product of the legal trend. Any additional impact on the supply of experts, or in the fees charged for their services, is not so compelling as to justify a public policy against recognizing the cause of action.

Conclusion

The interests of our system of justice in expert accountability and the full and accurate development of evidence in civil and criminal litigation are not served by protecting the incompetent or dishonest expert. The justice system as a whole benefits when expert malpractice actions are permitted, and the forensic sciences should enjoy greater respect and admiration when it is known that their members are accountable for their misdeeds.

While not universally recognized in American courts, malpractice actions against experts have been permitted in more and more jurisdictions and are occurring in greater numbers. This trend is likely to continue in the foreseeable future.

End Notes

a. Courts have awarded plaintiffs damages for illegal confinement due to legal malpractice, rejecting the argument that estimating the value of a person's loss of liberty is speculative. Geddie v. St. Paul Fire and Marine Ins. Co., 354 So. 2d 718 (La. App. 1978); Holliday v. Jones, 264 Cal. Rptr. 448 (Cal. App. 4 Dist. 1989) (awarding damages for emotional distress as a result of wrongful incarceration due to professional malpractice); In re Investig. of W. Va. St. Police Crime Lab, 438 S.E.2d, 509 (underlying civil suit settled for the state's $1 million insurance policy limit); see also, Restatement (Third) of the Law Governing Lawyers: Liability for Professional Negligence and Breach of Fiduciary Duty § 53 cmt. (g) (2000) ("emotional distress damages are . . . ordinarily recoverable when misconduct causes a client's imprisonment").

References

[1]   Hanson, R.K. (1996). Witness immunity under attack: disarming "Hired Guns", *Wake Forest Law Review* **31**, 497, 508–509; (Reviewing arguments in support of and in opposition to witness immunity for experts). See also Henderson Garcia, C. (1991). Expert witness malpractice: a solution to the problem of the negligent expert witness, *Mississippi College Law Review* **12**, 39.

[2]   Cooley, C.M. (2004). Reforming the forensic science community to avert the ultimate injustice, *Stanford Law and Policy Review* **15**, 381, 395–396 (Listing 21 recent exonerations where the underlying conviction was based on inaccurate or completely false testimony by forensic examiners). See also Giannelli, P.C. (2002). Fabricated reports, *Criminal Justice* **16**, 49 (discussing some of the recent "experts" who consistently fabricated reports and testimonies to achieve a particular bias).

[3] Stacey, R.B. (2004). A report on the erroneous fingerprint individualization in the Madrid train bombing case, *Journal of Forensic Identification* **54**, 706.

[4] Wax, S.T. & Schatz, C.J. (2004). A multitude of errors: The Brandon Mayfield case, *The Champion Magazine*, Sept./Oct.,6.

[5] Murray v. State, 692 So.2d 157, 159 (Fla. 1997); (Finding that State's expert "affirmatively misled" the trial court as to the general acceptance or reliability of PCR DNA methodology). See also Madigan, N. (2003). Houston's troubled DNA crime lab faces growing scrutiny, *The New York Times*, I20 (Detailing the results of an audit of the police DNA lab that found a number of problems with its methods; in response to the audit, the district attorney ordered a review of all convictions based on the lab's DNA analysis).

[6] State v. Woodall, 385 S.E.2d 253 (1989). Overturning rape conviction where serologist's evidence shown to be erroneous; In re Investig. of W. Va. St. Police Crime Lab., 438 S.E.2d 501, 509 (W. Va. 1993) (Report recommending that "[d]ue to the undisputed nature of the overwhelming evidence of misconduct on the part of [state serologist] Zain, . . ." 134 prisoners and parolees in whose cases the serologist had testified should be permitted to file petitions for post-conviction habeas corpus).

[7] Fricker, R.L. (1993). Pathologist's plea adds to turmoil, *ABA Journal* **79**, 24, 24. Fricker, R.L. (1993). Reasonable doubts, *ABA Journal* **79**, 39, 44 (the pathologist was reported to have a "reputation for providing the type of forensic evidence prosecutors needed," though his conclusions were later deemed "impossible" by qualified reviewing medical examiners).

[8] Nordheimer, J. (1993). In New Jersey slip-ups show autopsy system deficiencies, *The New York Times*, A1. This article describes a number of flawed autopsies by county medical examiners in two different New Jersey counties, including one case where a pathologist described bullet entrance and exit wounds, and its track through the brain, where it was later established that death was due to "blunt force injury" and that no evidence of a bullet wound existed, and a second case where a medical examiner concluded that a woman had died from alcohol poisoning and exposure, when a later autopsy established the woman had been strangled and raped.

[9] Peterson, J.L. & Murdock, J.E. (1989). Forensic science ethics: developing an integrated system of support and enforcement, *Journal of Forensic Sciences* **34**, 749. See also Austin v. American Assn. of Neurological Surgeons, 253 F.3d 967, 973 (7th Cir., 2001) ("[I]t is well known that expert witnesses are often paid very handsome fees, and common sense suggests that a financial stake can influence an expert's testimony, especially when the testimony is technical and esoteric and hence difficult to refute in terms intelligible to judges and jurors. More policing of expert witnesses is required, not less").

[10] Iowa Code Ann. § 622.72 (West 2006).

[11] Schroeder, O.C. & LeBlang, T.R. (2000). Court appointed experts, *Forensic Sciences* **1**, 18–1, 18–1–18–20, Cyril Wecht, Ed. Matthew Bender, N. Y. Explaining the role of the court-appointed expert; the statutory authorization for the court-appointed expert; the procedure for the appointment of the expert; the methods to discover the court-appointed expert's opinion; the weight accorded to the court-appointed expert's testimony; the use of court-appointed experts in civil and criminal trials; and finally, the constitutional issues related to appointing an expert; but see Struve, C.T. (2004). Doctors, the adversary system, and procedural reform in medical liability litigation, *Fordham Law Review* **72**, 943 (discussing a 1998 survey that indicated that in litigation involving complicated technical or scientific testimony only 16% of federal judges used court-appointed experts).

[12] http://www.cacnews.org/membership/handbook2006.pdf (Last accessed on Oct. 8. 2008).

[13] Carter, T. (2004). M.D. with a mission: a physician battles against colleagues he considers rogue expert witnesses, *ABA Journal* **90**, 40, 42. Advocating peer review in the courtroom for medical expert witnesses.

[14] Field, T.G., Jr., Kantrowitz, A., Cranor, C.F., Jacoby, I., Jasanoff, S., Mazur, A. & Cavicchi, J.R. (1993). Twenty-five year retrospective on the science court: a symposium, *Risk* **4**, 95–188. Containing a series of articles by advocates and detractors of the science court, including one by its "inventor"; see also Timmerbeil, S. (Spring 2003). The role of expert witnesses in German and U.S. civil litigation, *Annual Survey of International and Comparative Law* **9**, 163, 170 (discussing several proposals, including the science court, that addressed the concern that hired experts hindered the truth-seeking process of courts).

[15] In re Investig. of W. Va. St. Police Crime Lab, 438 S.E.2d, 501–509 (WV 1993). Harper, J. (1994). West Virginia court wants forensics expert prosecuted, *Houston Post* A22.

[16] Trower v. Jones, 520 N.E.2d 297 (Ill. 1988).

[17] Dowd, K.M. (1988). Expert Witnesses: Criminologist in the Courtroom, *The New England Journal on Criminal and Civil Confinement* **14**, 169, 171. Reviewing Anderson, P.A. & Winfree, L.T. (1987). *Expert Witnesses: Criminologist in the Courtroom*; Convicted by Juries, Exonerated by Science: Cases Studies in the Use of DNA Evidence to Establish Innocence After Trial, NIJ Research Report (June 1996) (Arguing that even improved science will not remedy the problem of inadequate legal counsel; of twenty-eight cases addressed in the study, had defense counsel sought the opinion of a competent expert or simply reviewed the case notes of the state's expert witnesses prior to trial, then the inconsistencies and inadequacies of these flawed testimonies could have been brought to light during the trial) (Available at http://www.ncjrs.org/txtfiles/dnaevid.txt (last visited on February 13, 2008)).

[18] Haddad, F.E. (1996). Admissibility of expert testimony, *Forensic Sciences* **1**(36), 1–21, 1–23, Cyril Wecht, Ed., Matthew Bender, N.Y. Stressing that the keys to an effective cross examination are (1) preparation and (2) becoming knowledgeable in the particular field.

[19] Keeton, W.P., Dobbs, D.B., Keeton, R.E. (1984). *Prosser and Keeton on Torts*, § 30, 5th Edition, Owen, D.G. (eds), West. 164–165. Dobbs, D.B. The Law of Torts § 114, 269 (West 2000); see also Daerr-Bannon, K.L. (2003). Cause of action for negligence or malpractice of expert witness, *Causes of Action 2d* **17,** 263 (adding that in a malpractice case against a friendly expert, the plaintiff must also prove that witness immunity is not applicable to the facts to avoid dismissal).

[20] LLMD of Michigan, Inc. v. Jackson-Cross Co., 740 A.2d 186, 191 (Pa. 1999). [t]he judicial process will be enhanced only by requiring that an expert witness render services to the degree of care, skill and proficiency commonly exercised by the ordinarily skillful, careful and prudent members of their profession; Masterson, L.R. (1998). Witness immunity or malpractice liability for professionals hired as experts? *The Review of Litigation* **17**, 393, 393.

[21] Frank, R.S. (1987). The essential commitment for a forensic scientist, *Journal of Forensic Sciences* **32**, 5. [t]he impact of the forensic scientist's conclusions affords no room for error, because such an error may be the direct cause of an injustice.

[22] Ludwig, K. & Fontaine, G. (1978). Effect of witnesses' expertness and manner of delivery of testimony on verdicts of simulated jurors, *Psychological Reports* **42**, 955. There are many cases that express concern that the special aura of reliability and credibility that surrounds an expert witness will cause the jury to neglect their fact-finding role. State v. Johnson, 681 N.W.2d 901, 906 (Wis. 2001); State v. Ward, 138 S.W.3d 245, 270 (Tenn. Crim. App. 2003); Franco v. State, 25 S.W.3d 26, 29 (Tex. App. 2000).

[23] Hansen, M. (2000). Experts are liable, too, *ABA Journal* **86**, 17, 17.

[24] Davis v. Wallace, 565 S.E.2d 386, 389–90 (W. Va. 2002).

[25] Levine v. Wiss & Co., 478 A.2d 397, 399 (N.J. 1984). Denying a court-appointed expert witness immunity; Weiss, L.S. (2004). Expert witness malpractice actions: emerging trend or aberration? *Practical Litigator* **15**(2), 27, 37 (discussing cases from other jurisdictions that recognize witness immunity if the expert was appointed by the court).

[26] Pollock v. Pahjabi, 781 A.2d 518 (Conn. Super. Ct. 2000).

[27] James v. Brown, 637 S.W.2d 914 (Tex. 1982).

[28] Mattco Forge, Inc. v. Arthur Young & Co., 60 Cal. Rptr. 2d 780 (Cal. App. 2 Dist. 1997).

[29] LLMD of Michigan, Inc., 740 A.2d 191 (Pa. 1999).

[30] Boyes-Bogie v. Horvitz, 14 Mass. L. Rptr. 208 (Mass. Super. 2001).

[31] Marrogi v. A.A. Mathews, 805 So. 2d 1118 (La. 2002).

[32] Politi v. Tyler, 751 A.2d 788 (Vt. 2000).

[33] Murphy v. A.A. Mathews, 841 S.W.2d 671 (Mo. 1992).

[34] DeBenedictis, D. (1994). Off-target opinions, *ABA Journal* **80**, 76, 76. Hospital and national drug laboratory settled on the eve of trial for undisclosed sums for misdiagnosing toxins in a baby's blood, which had resulted in the mother's murder conviction and imprisonment; In re Investigation of West Virginia State Police Crime Lab, *supra.*

[35] Bruce v. Byrne-Stevens & Associates Engineers, Inc., 776 P.2d 666 (Wash. 1989) Weiss, L.S. *Practical Litigator* N. **15**(2), 217, 30–31 (listing Washington as the only state where witness immunity still controls "friendly" experts and providing a detailed description of the *Bruce* decision); Diehl v. Danuloff, 618 N.W.2d 83 (Mich. App. 2000)(court-appointed expert enjoys quasi-judicial immunity as "an arm of the trial court"); Otero v. Warnick, 614 N.W.2d 177 (Mich. App. 2000)(holding that forensic odontologist for county medical examiner was not liable to a former criminal defendant because (1) as an employee of the medical examiner, the expert owed no duty to criminal defendants in performing his official duties, and (2) expert's testimony at trial was absolutely privileged provided it was relevant, material, and pertinent to the issue being tried).

[36] Saks, M.J. (1989). Prevalence and impact of ethical problems in forensic science, *Journal of Forensic Sciences* **34**, 772. Containing a summary of some cases involving litigation against expert witnesses.

[37] Bailey v. Rogers, 631 S.W.2d 784 (Tex. App. 3 Dist. 1982).. Compare Mattco Forge, Inc. v. Arthur Young & Co., 6 Cal. Rptr. 2d 781 (Cal. App. 2 Dist. 1992), on appeal after remand, 45 Cal. Rptr. 2d 581 (Cal. App. 2 Dist. 1995), on subsequent appeal, 60 Cal. Rptr. 2d 780 (Cal. App. 2 Dist. 1997) (holding that the California Civil Code's litigation privilege does not protect a negligent expert witness from liability to the party who hired the witness, though it would still shield experts that are court appointed, and would also shield expert witnesses from suit by opposing parties; Murphy, 841 S.W.2d at 679 (also holding that under Missouri law, privilege does not protect a negligent expert witness from liability to the party who hired the witness, though it would still shield experts that are court appointed, and would also shield expert witnesses from suit by opposing parties; Marrogi, 805 So. 2d, 1132 (broadening the scope of expert witness malpractice to include not only pretrial litigation services but also the expert's actual testimony during trial).

[38] Murphy, 841 S.W.2d 679 (Mo. 1992).. Holding that the policy behind witness immunity is not advanced by offering immunity for incompetent experts retained by a party to perform professional services including trial testimony; Marrogi, 805 So. 2d, 1132 (holding that the policy behind witness immunity is not advanced by offering immunity for incompetent experts retained by a party to perform professional services including trial testimony).

Related Articles

CAROL HENDERSON AND KURT W. LENZ

Management: Crime Scene *see* Crime Scene Management

Mandated Treatment: Mental Health *see* Treatment, Mandated: Mental Health

Mandatory Treatment *see* Therapeutic Jurisprudence

Marijuana as a Controlled Drug *see* Cannabis

Marks or Impressions of Manufactured Items

Introduction

Marks and impressions are regularly encountered at scenes of crime and may be produced by a vast number of objects such as tools, tires, footwear, and fabric. Marks produced by tools (*see* **Toolmarks**), tires (*see* **Tire Impressions**), and footwear are covered in separate articles. Marks left by fabrics can be encountered in a variety of situations. However, of particular interest is the fact that investigators frequently encounter glove marks when looking for fingermarks (*see* **Mass Grave Investigation**). When a gloved individual presses his or her hand on a surface, a residual mark may be left showing the pattern of the glove. This can result from dirty or greasy gloves, or even gloves that have been previously "contaminated" with body secretions or cosmetics. Negative marks can also occur from the removal of material from the surface, dust, for example. Glove marks can be two-dimensional or tri-dimensional, depending on the malleable nature, or not, of the recipient substrate.

Similar to shoe marks and tire marks, glove marks can be made of a combination of manufacturing and acquired features. The identifying power of glove marks will therefore depend on the quality of the mark (e.g., clarity) as well as the rarity of the fabric pattern and construction combined with the presence, or not, of random acquired features such as holes or wear and tear.

Glove marks may also help the investigator establish the "path" taken by an individual around the scene of crime. Furthermore, when clothing is pressed against a smooth surface, a latent mark is produced resulting in another type of fabric mark [1]. This is prevalent in motor vehicle hit and run accidents, where the examination of fabric impressions occurs when a segment of the vehicle comes into contact with the clothing of a pedestrian [2]. These marks may help determine the path taken by an individual, as well as the sequence of events that had taken place during the course of the crime.

Detection, Collection, and Examination of Fabric Impressions

Glove Marks

In the age of forensic science awareness, criminals are using gloves as a protective measure to prevent deposition of their fingerprints at a crime scene. Both leather gloves and fabric gloves are commonly utilized. Although leather gloves contain a natural fat, both types of gloves collect grease, sweat, and dirt through everyday wear. Further, at scenes of crime where blood is involved (such as homicide), the glove may be contaminated with blood. It is the presence of these materials that allow the pattern of the glove to be marked onto a surface [3]. Glove marks may be either latent or visible. Latent marks are "invisible" and can be found by performing a grazing angle search with a light source. It is important to remember that glove marks are much more fragile than fingermarks [1].

As glove marks are formed best on smooth surfaces, the powdering method can be used to increase the contrast between the latent deposit and the background surface. Either black or white powder may be used for the development process, which should be brushed on sparingly. If the powder is brushed on vaguely and in excess, the print detail will be destroyed [1]. Any glove mark found at the crime scene should be documented and evidence photography carried out. Photographing should be done with a camera set up on a tripod, taken perpendicular to the glove print to remove distortion and eliminate perspective (*see* **Crime Scene Photography: US Perspective**). The glove print must be photographed with and without a scale [3].

If possible, the entire object on which the glove print was found should be taken back to the laboratory for direct examination and comparison. However, if this is not possible, the glove print may be lifted with a gelatin lifter similar to that used for lifting fingermarks (*see* **Toolmarks**). If the glove mark is "negative" (such that the glove removes material off the surface, dust is an example [4]), it can be simply lifted using a black gelatin lifter.

A technique involving electrostatic attraction of the marks onto a plastic lifting film may also be used. This process is especially effective for faint glove marks on a colorful background [3]. Glove marks in blood can be enhanced and developed using reagents used for the detection and enhancement of fingermark in blood, such as amido black [5] for example, which is a stain sensitive to the presence of protein.

Comparison (or test) prints can be made from the suspect's glove, usually on glass or in some cases on the same material as the glove print deposit found at the crime scene. A number of comparison prints may be produced using varying degrees of pressure. Although producing a good-quality comparison print may be difficult, powders and polish should be avoided when making the print as minute details may be lost. Instead, breathing slightly on the finger of the glove may help improve results [3].

Fabric Marks

Fabric marks can be made with items such as clothing, socks, towels, and handkerchiefs. Although not as common as glove marks, fabric marks do arise during casework. Such marks are generally left on a surface if the fabric is thin and contains residual material such as moisture or is dirty. These marks are searched for and developed in the same way as for glove marks. Evidence photography is also carried out the same way as for glove marks; however, if the fabric print is adequately large, several photos must be taken.

The scale position and the angle of lighting should be altered for each photograph so that maximum detail of the fabric mark is documented [1]. Such marks should be compared with the suspect fabric exhibit, and the similarities and differences between the seams, structure of the fabric, and other oddities examined. For cases involving clothing impressions made on areas of a vehicle in a motor accident, one way of preserving the evidence is by photographing the fabric impression that was made on the segment of the vehicle. An exemplar is produced of the clothing article of interest, which is done using the previously described method. This exemplar is then used for direct 1 : 1 comparison with the photograph of the impression found on the motor vehicle [6].

Interpretation and Evidential Significance of Fabric Impressions

Glove Marks

When used as evidence, glove marks may demonstrate manufacturing (class) characteristics that show that the mark *could* have been made from a particular glove (i.e., nonexclusion). In some instances, glove marks show enough random acquired characteristics, such as distinctive holes, for example, that allow the examiner to conclude that a particular glove *did* leave the mark found at the scene (i.e., identification). Between these two conclusions, a qualified opinion may be given, where the value of the mark will depend on its quality as well as the rarity of the fabric pattern and construction combined with the presence, or not, of random acquired features. In any case, the presence of a meaningful (or unexplainable) difference between the mark and the test print allows the examiner to conclude that the mark *could not* have been made from a particular glove (i.e. exclusion).

In general, it is more common for an identification to be made with leather gloves than cloth gloves. Cloth gloves may exhibit tears and snags, or irregularities in the weave pattern due to the manufacturing process or material used. Leather gloves may show wrinkles and crease formations, which is more likely to leave a mark with a large number of comparative features. The presence of tears and cracks due to the random process of wear and tear may allow the mark to be identified, as exactly the same pattern of imperfections cannot be found on any two different gloves [3]. The difference between a cloth glove mark and a leather glove mark is the surface pattern. Leather gloves are made of the skin of an animal, which leaves unique marks on a surface not dissimilar to those left by fingerprints (Figure 1). Naturally, the patterns found on animal skin are not homogenous and vary from animal to animal. On the contrary, cloth marks are consistent for each type, and so the individual identification is more difficult to achieve. Furthermore, both leather and cloth gloves often mold to the finger tips of the individual, allowing another point of identification for the examiner. In rare cases, partial fingerprints can also be found within or superimposed with a glove print (occurring when there is a hole in the glove), obviously increasing the evidential value of the mark [1].

It should be noted that when a glove is seized in a case it should be collected and protected appropriately, as it may be possible to detect and examine finger marks or DNA recovered from inside the glove.

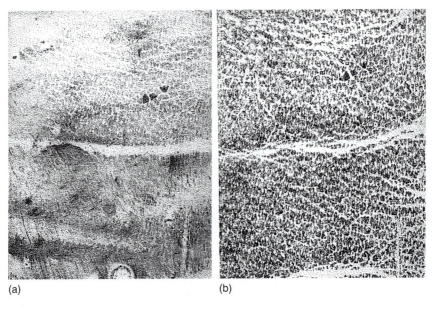

(a)   (b)

Figure 1 Comparison between a latent leather glove print (a) and the test print (b), showing the individual, minute characteristics of animal hide [1] [Reproduced with permission from Ref. 2. © IAI, 2000.]

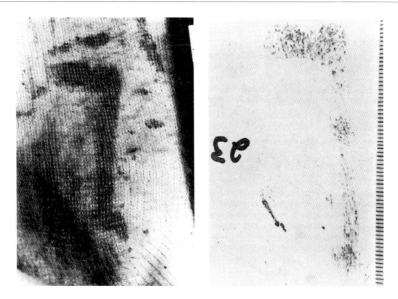

Figure 2 Comparison of bloodstain pattern on sock (reversed, 2:1 enlargement) and fabric impression enhanced with amido black stain (2:1 enlargement) [2] [Reproduced with permission from Ref. 6. © ASTM.]

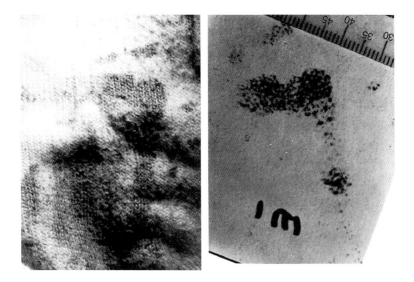

Figure 3 Comparison of the bloodstained sock and another fabric impression found at the crime scene, showing that the fabric tuft pattern on the sock was transferred onto the impression [Reproduced from Ref. 1. © Taylor and Francis Group, 2000.]

Fabric Prints

In most cases, fabric marks made by items such as towels and socks are hard to identify and individualize, reducing its evidential value. Unlike a glove mark, there is no definite boundary for the edges of the material. Comparing seam patterns or other surface patterns is difficult if the area on the item of interest that may have left the mark cannot be identified [1]. However, there has been a documented case involving the identification of fabric impressions made by a sock [2] (Figures 2, 3).

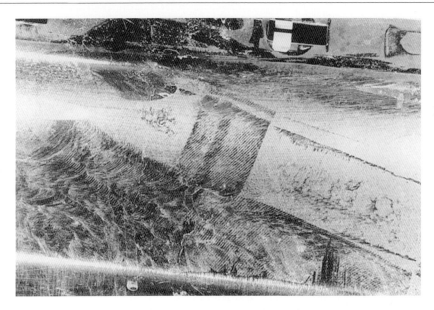

Figure 4   Impression found on the chrome bumper of a car after a motor vehicle accident involving a pedestrian [6] [Reproduced from Ref. 1. © Taylor and Francis Group, 2000.]

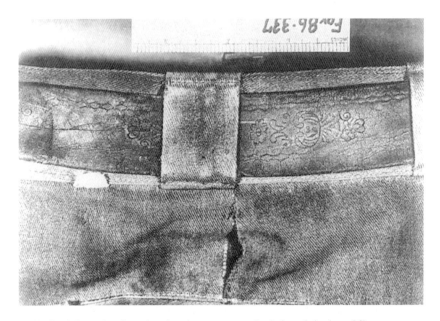

Figure 5   Pants and belt of the pedestrian, showing the pattern on the belt and the loop [6]

Fabric impressions were found at a homicide scene through the use of amido black stain (for marks in blood). After sequestering the suspect's bloodstained sock, it was discovered that the main bloodstain along with secondary bloodstains were in agreement with the impression found at the scene. Furthermore, the presence of four randomly placed raised tufts found on the sock corresponded with tuft markings found on the impression. The unique and random pattern as a result of the bloodstains and tufts was significant enough to trace the fabric impression to the suspect's socks [2].

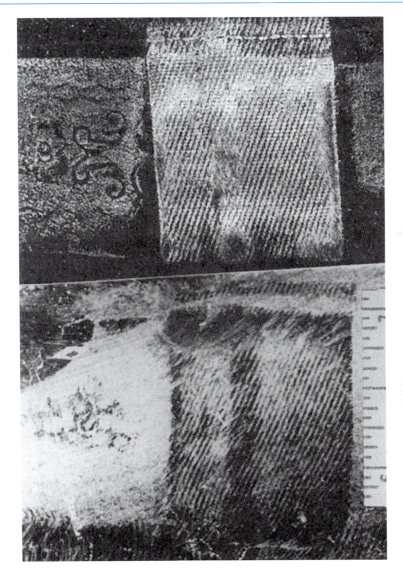

Figure 6 Juxtaposition of the belt and loop (top figure) with the corresponding region of fabric impression left on the chrome bumper (bottom figure) [6]

This example shows that the position and presence of unusual characteristics is enough to warrant an individual identification. The types of fabric impressions in such incidences as hit and run are also difficult to identify, as finding and preserving the fabric marks pressed into the vehicle is a tedious process. Although such impressions are not uncommon, it is rare to obtain evidence that permits identification of the clothing at the origin of the mark. However, an unusual case involving the individual identification

of a clothing impression on a motor vehicle has been reported [6]. A pedestrian was hit by a motor vehicle, thereby causing his death. Upon examination of the chrome bumper an impression was found. The sites on the impression corresponded with the weave pattern on the pedestrian's pants and the stitching and loop hole of his belt. The combination of the size and position of the clothing items and the inscription found on the belt, which was also transferred onto the impression, was very unusual and was the basis for the individual identification between the clothing and impression to be made [6] (Figures 4–6).

In most cases, fabric impressions provide class evidence, as it may be difficult to state that the marks had come from a given item excluding any other similar items. However, as for glove marks, the evidential value of fabric impressions will depend on the quality of the mark as well as the rarity of the fabric pattern and construction combined with the presence, or not, of random acquired features. As for glove marks, the presence of any meaningful (or unexplainable) difference between the fabric impression and the test print will allow the examiner to reach a conclusion of exclusion (i.e., the fabric impression *could not* have been made from the known fabric).

References

[1]   Fisher, B.A.J. (2000). *Techniques of Crime Scene Investigation*, 6th Edition, CRC Press.
[2]   Doller, W.D. (2000). An unusual case involving the individualization of fabric impressions made by a sock-clad foot, *Journal of Forensic Identification* **50**(5), 447–454.
[3]   Nickell, J. & Fischer, J.F. (1999). *Crime Science: Methods of Forensic Detection*, The University Press of Kentucky.
[4]   Cowger, J.F. (1992). *Friction Ridge Skin: Comparison and Identification of Fingerprints*, CRC Press.
[5]   Hussain, J. & Pounds, C.A. (1989). *The Enhancement of Marks in Blood: Part ii, A Modified Amido Black Staining Technique*, Report no. 685, Central Research Establishment, June, 1989.
[6]   Drummond, F.C. & Pizzola, P.A. (1990). An unusual case Involving the individualization of a clothing impression on a motor vehicle, *Journal of Forensic Sciences* **35**(3), 746–752.

SUSAN LUONG AND CLAUDE ROUX

Mass Grave Investigation

Mass Grave Definition

Mass graves are defined in various ways, most revolving around the number of people in a grave and what constitutes a "mass". This has ranged from two or more bodies that physically touch each other [1] to at least six individual bodies [2, 3]. Mant's [1] definition brings in the physical component that the bodies must be physically touching each other. Haglund [4] also feels that having remains in contact with each other is what makes mass graves different from other grave types, and uses that criterion in his definition.

Other definitions include the genesis of the grave. The United Nations Rapporteur interprets a mass grave as a location where three or more victims of extrajudicial, summary, or arbitrary executions were buried, not having died in combat or armed confrontations [5]. Schmitt [6, p. 279] defines a mass grave as "one that contains the remains of more than one victim who share some common trait connected with the cause and manner of death". He further goes on to state that "criminal mass graves contain the remains of a group of individuals who share some common trait that justified their assassinations in the eyes of the perpetrators" [6, p. 279]. A basic flaw in a definition of a mass grave that includes the genesis of the inhumation is that the investigator may never know whether they are dealing with a mass grave or not, if the genesis is not known. It is likely that this would lead to the need to find another term for such a grave where the reasons for the deaths are unknown.

A simple definition of a mass grave is that it contains four or more individuals buried at or about the same time. This is consistent with the definition of a mass murder in the *Crime Classification Manual* [7, p. 12] used by the Federal Bureau of Investigation. The Manual defines a mass murder as "a homicide involving four or more victims in one location and within one event" [7, p. 12]. A mass grave definition consistent with the standard definition of mass murder is simple and logical. The differentiation between a criminal mass grave and another type should rest on the result of the investigation, depending on whether the deaths were the result of a criminal act.

Mass Grave Taphonomy

Single and mass death sites have taphonomic differences. Graves with poor drainage and multiple layers of bodies tend to trap moisture, even if only the moisture from the decomposing remains themselves. This scenario accounts for the adipocere seen in mass graves created years or decades earlier. Undisturbed soils at the bottom of the grave trap water in the softer, unconsolidated soils of the grave fill and create conditions in which adipocere develops. This keeps the bodies in a moist environment, and they tend to saponify, as do remains under water. Thus, bodies in the center of a large body mass may be well preserved after years of burial. Where bodies are laid side by side in a single layer, the decomposition fluids leach into the soil and the bodies decompose in a manner more similar to a body in a single grave.

Thus, mass graves tend to create their own microenvironments toward preservation [4, 8]. Mant [8, p. 33] notes that in a mass grave the bodies in the center of the grave are much better preserved than in the periphery of the grave. Mant did his research after World War II, exhuming graves for the Nuremberg Tribunal. Also related to World War II were the 1943 German excavations in Poland investigating mass graves in the Katyn Forest. A professor of forensic medicine and criminology at Breslay University summarized the condition of the bodies at Katyn as follows:

> The stages of decay were found to vary in accordance with the position of the bodies in the pits. Whilst mummification had taken place on the top and at the sides of the mass of bodies, a humid process could be observed caused by the damp nearer the center Buhtz 1943 in [9, p. 142].

The German investigators attributed the preservation of the remains to the microenvironment created by the mass grave:

> In the mass graves at Katyn the murdered captives were packed so tightly together (either dead or dying) and sealed over with copious quantities of solid soil, that the putrification process was slowed considerably. For example, in the "L" shaped grave ... the initial interment was estimated to be almost 3000 bodies. These bodies were packed together so tightly that decaying and decomposing fluids of each body penetrated, imbibed, and infiltrated other dead bodies within the grave

(Official Statement Concerning the Mass Murder at Katyn 1943 as quoted in [10, p. 53]).

While it might seem contradictory to have mummified tissue, skeletonized remains, and adipocere tissue in the same grave, it happens in mass graves and is dependent on the moisture available to the remains. Moisture is essential for both decomposition and adipocere formation. In talking about mass graves excavated after World War II:

Adipocere formation depends on the hydrolysis of fat to fatty acids, and cannot take place without an adequate supply of water. This water is derived not only from the exterior of the body but also from the interior, dehydrating the underlying tissues and organs including the muscles themselves. Thus adipocere formation retards the action of putrefactive organisms.

It was found at exhumation, as would be anticipated from the above, that there was an outer layer of adipocere surrounding a layer of mummified muscle tissue. Some mummified muscle tissue was usually found incorporated in the deepest layers of adipocere [8, p. 45].

In the best of circumstances, relating the amount of adipocere formation to postmortem interval is difficult. Adipocere may appear as early as a few days following death [10, p. 101] and has been observed in burials as old as 122 years [11, p. 470]. Sledzik and Micozzi [12, p. 485] state that "presence of adipocere is an artifact of decomposition suggesting that a minimum length of time has passed since death, but it may not always be useful in determining the postmortem interval." In mass graves in particular, adipocere formation tells little about the length of the postmortem interval.

Mass Grave Investigation Strategy

The investigation of larger graves has a number of logistical challenges not seen in investigating smaller graves [2, 4, 13]. Maintaining access to the central remains for body removal, while cleaning the surrounding remains, can be a challenge. The large amounts of fill in the grave mean that the disposal of the soil removed from the grave must be carefully planned. As discussed above, a large mass of bodies creates differences in decomposition, which become more noticeable the larger the mass of the remains. Removing, as well as analyzing, remains in all stages of decomposition adds to the equipment and personnel needed, both in the field and the morgue. Other large graves may not have large body masses that create the differences in decomposition, but share the logistical challenges of a large excavation, adding to the logistical challenge. The larger the grave, the greater the range of preservation likely to be present.

Locating mass graves, like smaller graves, is often dependant on witness testimony [6]. Also, the same remote sensing technologies may apply (*see* **Length Measurement**), given the appropriate soil and topography conditions. In addition, the size of the graves makes them more likely to show up in aerial photography [2, pp. 120–121]. Given that large numbers of individuals were buried in the area and possibly executed there, and that it might have taken a number of people, as well as vehicles and equipment, to accomplish this, there is often surface evidence of a mass grave [6].

As with any archaeological feature, the outline and size should be defined before excavation. As the overburden is removed from a large grave, the excavator should look for the edges of the grave. This may be most easily done by placing two trenches, perpendicular to each other, over the grave (called *cross-trenching*). This should give the excavator an idea of the location of the sides of the grave. If the grave fill can be differentiated from the undisturbed soil, then the outline of the grave should be traced all around the edge. It sounds like common sense, but this will help keep the excavators from placing soil removed from one part of the grave on top of another part of the grave.

If the grave was dug using heavy machinery, it is probably going to take heavy machinery to remove the overburden to the depth of the remains. This will make it harder to look for tool marks or other indications of how the grave was dug. The excavators should look for teeth marks on the side of the grave showing the teeth of the original front-end loader or backhoe bucket. There may also be traces of a ramp that the machine used to access the bottom of the grave. On the ramp, or at the bottom, may be imprints of the tires, or treads, of the machine.

In some mass graves, the bodies are laid neatly side by side in rows in a long trench. In a case such as this, where the bodies were buried in an organized manner, the bodies can be numbered at one time, documented in sequence, and lifted in sequence.

Haglund and others [13] describe a method that worked satisfactorily on graves where the bodies were dumped in a disorganized manner. The excavators worked in two teams: a documentation team, and a body removal team. Working with groups of about 10 bodies at a time, the documentation team completed the mapping, notes, and photographs of the next 10 bodies to be removed on one side of the grave. If the bodies are not laid neatly in the grave, deciding on the next bodies to be removed takes some investigation to ensure which remains are

least encumbered by other remains. Bodies were not numbered until they were ready to be removed, in order to create fewer errors in numbering. It is possible to label two portions of the same body with different case numbers when the intervening portions of the remains are covered with soil or other bodies.

The body removal team then removed the remains from the grave. On fleshed remains, this sometimes entailed lifting limbs of some bodies in order to free the target remains. Skeletal remains presented more of a challenge, and portions of a single body sometimes needed to be documented and partially removed to get to the remains below. When this is done, then both the portion removed and the articulating portion left in the ground need to be carefully labeled. No more than two skeletons on each area should be partially removed, or confusion will inevitably result. At no point should personnel in the team change, if skeletons have been partially removed. The same people that partially removed one skeleton should remove the remainder of that same skeleton.

In graves where heavy machinery was used to bury the remains, it is not uncommon to find disassociated body parts. This also happens at sites where the remains were buried after they were partially decomposed. Should isolated body parts be found, they should be catalogued separately from the complete sets of remains. A "partial remains" log can be started that numbers the assemblage, gives the location, photograph numbers, and gives a brief description of the remains. Including the partial remains in the same numbering system as the complete remains is sure to lead to confusion during the examination when the partial remains are reunited with the remaining body parts.

Determining a Charge

Mass graves are (thankfully) relatively rare in domestic criminal cases. They tend to result from mass fatality incidents, either natural or cultural. Only the cultural incidents become forensic cases. The most common of these are war crimes, crimes against humanity, and genocide, and so a brief definition of each are discussed.

Genocide was defined as a crime after World War II in the 1948 Convention on the Prevention and Punishment of the Crime of Genocide. The definition of genocide set forth in the Convention is still definitive and used in the statutes of the Rwandan and Yugoslavian tribunals as well as the Rome Statute that established the International Criminal Court (ICC). The Convention defines genocide as a crime in either peace or war:

> any of the following acts committed with intent to destroy, in whole or in part, a national, ethnical, racial, or religious group, as such: killing members of the group; causing serious bodily or mental harm to members of the group; deliberately inflicting on the group conditions of life calculated to bring about its physical destruction in whole or in part; imposing measures intended to prevent births within the group; forcibly transferring children of the group to another group

(Convention on the Prevention and Punishment of the Crime of Genocide, United Nations. December 9, 1948).

The crime of genocide requires an intent to physically destroy a certain group of people. The court also requires that the group destroyed be a national, ethnical, racial, or religious group. Political dissidents and soldiers are not groups protected by the genocide convention. The forensic investigator considering genocide as a charge must attempt to determine whether there was intent to kill the deceased and that they belonged to a specific target group.

War crimes are violations of the international laws of war, a body of law known as the *International Humanitarian Law* (*IHL*). While limitations on armed conflict date at least as far back as the Chinese warrior Sun Tzu in the sixth century BC [14, p. 374], the Hague conventions of 1899 and 1907 codified much of the humanitarian law for the Western world. The Charter of the International Military Tribunal at Nuremberg defined war crimes as "violations of the laws or customs of war, including murder, ill-treatment, or deportation of civilians in occupied territory; murder or ill-treatment of prisoners of war (POWs); killing of hostages; plunder of public or private property; wanton destruction of municipalities; and devastation not militarily necessary" [14, p. 374].

Only intentional, grave breaches of the treaties are considered war crimes. If individuals violate the treaties, but do not commit a grave breach, then they have committed an illegal act, but not a war crime. Grave breaches of the conventions are defined as willful killing, torture or inhumane treatment (including medical experiments), willfully causing great suffering or serious injury to body or health, extensive destruction and appropriation of property not justified by military necessity and carried out unlawfully and wantonly, compelling a prisoner of war or civilian to serve in the forces of the hostile power, willfully depriving a prisoner of war or protected civilian of the rights of a fair and regular trial, unlawful deportation or transfer of a protected civilian, unlawful confinement of a protected civilian, and taking of hostages [14, p. 374]. In 1977, Protocol I of the Conventions expanded the definition of grave breaches to include certain medical experimentation, making civilians and undefended localities the object or inevitable victims of attack, the perfidious use of the Red Cross or Red Crescent emblem, transfer by an occupying power of parts of its population to occupied territory, unjustifiable delays in repatriation of POWs, apartheid, attack on historic monuments, and depriving protected persons of a fair trial [14, p. 374].

A crime against humanity has come to mean anything atrocious committed on a large scale [15, p. 107]. The term originated in the preamble of the 1907 Hague Convention, which was based on existing State practices that derived from the moral values that constituted the "laws of humanity". In 1945, the Nuremberg Charter, formally the Agreement for the Prosecution and Punishment of the Major War Criminals of the European Axis and Charter of the International Military Tribunal, first defined crimes against humanity in positive international law:

> Crimes against humanity: murder, extermination, enslavement, deportation, and other inhumane acts committed against civilian populations, before or during the war; or persecutions on political, racial or religious grounds in execution of or in connection with any crime within the jurisdiction of the Tribunal, whether or not in violation of the domestic law of the country where perpetrated [15, p. 107].

The statutes for the International Criminal Tribunal for the former Yugoslavia (ICTY) and the International Criminal Tribunal for Rwanda (ICTR) added rape and torture to the list of specific crimes included in crimes against humanity. The ICC added apartheid and enforced disappearances to the list [15, p. 108]. Crimes against humanity overlap with both genocide and war crimes. However, crimes against humanity can occur in either war or peace, unlike war crimes. Unlike genocide, they do not require the intent to "destroy in whole or in part" a specific group, but rather are part of a "widespread and systematic attack directed against any civilian population" (Rome Statute of the ICC, UN document A/Conf. 183/9, 17 July 1998, Art. 7).

The investigator, then, must show that the subjects of the attack are civilians and the incident is part of a systematic or widespread pattern, rather than an isolated incident. Widespread, according the to the ICTR court, is not defined geographically, but rather as an attack carried out against a "multiplicity of victims" [16, pp. 34, 35].

In framing a charge, the existence of the grave and the location of remains are the first indicator that a criminal act may have occurred. This proves that these people are not refugees, that they are not alive somewhere but unaccounted for, but that they are, indeed, dead. The demography of the grave also becomes of paramount importance. A grave full of adult males, dressed in military uniforms, may result from a postbattle cleanup. However, a grave full of woman and children in civilian clothing, suggests that something else occurred.

The artifacts in the grave and personnel effects are the best indicators of whether the individuals belonged to a specific target group. To decide on a charge, it may, in fact, be unnecessary to identify individuals, although international human rights groups consider the exhumation of the remains without an attempt to identify them and return the bodies to the families extremely unethical [17]. To determine a charge, what is needed is the knowledge that the bodies did or did not belong to a specific national, religious, ethnic, or military group. Clothing, identification papers, jewelry, and artifacts with the bodies are crucial in this regard.

Corroboration of Witness Testimony

In the forensic examination of a mass grave, as in any forensic investigation, witness information is of paramount importance and the forensic evidence often plays only a corroborative role. As Schmitt [6, p. 280] says, mass graves are seldom a secret. Often there are survivors to the massacre who come forward and tell their story. In the scene reconstruction of a mass grave scenario, everything, from the topography of the area to the location of materials in the grave, plays a part.

The ecological artifacts, or "ecofacts", in and near the site are important in reconstructing the events at the site. In the investigation of World War II graves in the Katyn Forest, the trees on the graves were used to help date the graves themselves [9]. So, it is helpful to be aware of the natural features of a site area and what they mean in relationship to the activities at the site.

The location of cartridge cases can be used to trace where individual shooters stood and how they moved throughout the area, through firearms identification analysis [18]. In an investigation in the village of Koreme, in the Kurdish portion of Iraq, investigators plotted each cartridge case found in an execution area, where 27 young Kurdish men had allegedly been killed by an Iraqi military execution squad. Of a total of 124 cases collected, the firing pin analysis identified a minimum of 7 individual weapons used in the execution. The weapon used was an AK-47, or similar weapon, which normally has a detachable magazine containing 30 rounds. The firearms analysis showed that one weapon fired a minimum of 37 rounds, requiring reloading during the executions [19]. Scott [19] was able to use the map of the cartridge cases to show that several weapons moved closer to the victims as they fired. At least two rounds were fired within 10 m of the victims by the same weapon that reloaded. This type of detail in scene processing and analysis is crucial in scene reconstruction and can be used as strong corroboration in witness testimony.

Summary

Definitions of mass graves include factors such as the number of bodies, whether they touch each other, and how the bodies came to be in the grave. This article suggests a definition of mass graves parallel to the definition of mass murder: mass graves are graves of four or more individuals buried at or about the same time.

Mass graves are different from single graves in the changes in how bodies decompose when in a mass and the logistical challenges in excavation. When bodies are piled up on top of each other, they decompose much differently than in a single grave, owing to accumulated water and body fluids. This variation in decomposition stage, as well as the sheer size of the graves, can make the exhumations logistically challenging.

Criminal mass graves rarely result from simple homicide, but often are a result of genocide, war crimes, or crimes against humanity. Determining a charge relies on attention to the cause and manner of death of decedents, grave demographics, artifacts, and personal effects. Attention to how the grave is dug and bodies are arranged can help to corroborate witness testimony on the sequence of events and mechanics of execution and body disposal.

References

[1] Mant, A.K. (1987). Knowledge acquired from post-war exhumations, in *Death, Decay, and Reconstruction: Approaches to Archaeology and Forensic Sciences*, A. Boddington, A.N. Garland & R.C. Janaway, eds, Manchester University Press, London.

[2] Connor, M.A. (2007). *Forensic Methods: Excavation for the Archaeologist and Investigator*, Altimira Press, New York.

[3] Skinner, M. (1987). Planning the archaeological recovery of evidence from recent mass graves, *Forensic Sciences International* **34**, 267–287.

[4] Haglund, W.D. (2002). Recent mass graves: an introduction, in W.D. Haglund & M.H. Sorg, eds, *Advances in Forensic Taphonomy: Method, Theory, and Archaeological Perspectives*, CRC Press, Baton Rouge, pp. 243–261.

[5] United Nations (1991). *Manual on the Effective Prevention and Investigation of Extra-Legal, Arbitrary and Summary Executions*, United Nations, New York.

[6] Schmitt, S. (2002). Mass graves and the collection of forensic evidence: genocide, war crimes, and crimes against humanity, in *Advances in Forensic Taphonomy: Method, Theory, and Archaeological Perspectives*, W.D. Haglund & M.H. Sorg, eds, CRC Press, Baton Rouge, pp. 277–292.

[7] Douglas, J.E., Burgess, A.W., Burgess, A.G. & Ressler, R.K. (1992). *Crime Classification Manual: A Standard System for Investigating and Classifying Violent Crimes*, Jossey-Bass Publishers, San Francisco.

[8] Mant, A.K. (1950). *A Study of Exhumation Data*, MD Thesis, University of London, London.

[9] FitzGibbon, L. (1977). *Katyn Massacre*, Corgi Books, London.

[10] Gill-King, H. (1997). Chemical and ultrastructural aspects of decomposition, in *Forensic Taphonomy: The Postmortem Fate of Human Remains*, W.D. Haglund & M.H. Sorg, eds, CRC Press, Baton Rouge, pp. 93–108.

[11] Manhien, M.H. (1997). Decomposition rates of deliberate burials: a case study of preservation, in *Forensic Taphonomy: The Postmortem Fate of Human Remains*, W.D. Haglund & M.H. Sorg, eds, CRC Press, Baton Rouge, pp. 469–481.

[12] Sledzik, P.S. & Micozzi, M.S. (1997). Autopsied, embalmed, and preserved human remains: distinguishing features in forensic and historic contexts, in *Forensic Taphonomy: The Postmortem Fate of Human Remains*, W.D. Haglund & M.H. Sorg, eds, CRC Press, Baton Rouge, pp. 483–495.

[13] Haglund, W.D., Connor, M.A. & Scott, D.D. (2001). The archaeology of contemporary mass graves, *Historical Archaeology* **35**(1), 57–69.

[14] Ratner, S.R. (1999). Categories of war crimes, in *Crimes of War: What the Public Should Know*, R. Gutman & D. Reiff, eds, W.W. Norton & Company, New York, pp. 374–376.

[15] Bassiouni, M.C. (1999). Crimes against humanity, in *Crimes of War: What the Public Should Know*, R. Gutman & D. Reiff, eds, W.W. Norton & Company, New York, pp. 107–108.

[16] Human Rights Watch (2004). Genocide, war crimes, and crimes against humanity, *Topical Digests of the Case Law of the International Criminal Tribunal for Rwanda and the International Criminal Tribunal for the Former Yugoslavia*, Human Rights Watch, New York.

[17] International Commission of the Red Cross (2002). *Special Issue: Missing Persons. International Review of the Red Cross*, p. 848.

[18] Scott, D.D. & Connor, M.A. (1997). Context delicti: archaeological work in forensic context, in *Forensic Taphonomy: the Postmortem Fate of Human Remains*, W.D. Haglund & M.H. Sorg, eds, CRC Press, Baton Rouge, pp. 27–38.

[19] Scott, D.D. (1993). Firearms identification of the Koreme execution site, in *The Anfal Campaign in Iraqi Kurdistan: The Destruction of Koreme*, Human Rights Watch, Washington, DC, pp. 103–107.

Further Reading

Lauck, J.H. (1988). *Katyn Killings: In The Record*, The Kingston Press, Clifton.

MELISSA CONNOR

Mass Murder *see* Homicide: Multiple (Behavior)

Massacre *see* Homicide: Multiple (Behavior)

Materials Science

Materials Engineering and Failure Analysis

The discipline of materials engineering and science spans the scope of the physical and chemical makeup of materials, the strength and other mechanical properties that are critical to appropriate decisions in product design, the relationships between and among materials, and finally, the analysis of actual or potential failures.

The primary forensic question in materials engineering and science is usually why a materials failure occurred. The exact reason will depend on the application, but four fundamental questions given in the following are frequently considered:

- When did the material fail in relation to a sequence of events? Did it fail and cause an event, or did it fail as a result of the event?
- Was design or manufacturing a factor?
- Was the choice of material a factor?
- Was inadequate maintenance a factor?

The materials engineer answers these questions using specific training in the relationships among material structure, properties, and processing, and their affect on material performance. The materials engineer also uses a variety of characterization techniques to determine these relationships.

The materials engineer's knowledge overlaps with other fields. The materials engineer must be familiar, for example, with civil engineering principles to establish stress states in materials under loading conditions, chemical engineering to determine the effect of environment on material properties, and mechanical engineering to understand how a particular part fits into an overall design.

In the forensic aspect, the materials engineer applies his understanding of materials to identify the root cause of material failures. The engineer is frequently called on to provide opinions in cases of product liability due to a materials failure. Typical cases include the failure of a variety of products, automobile or aircraft accidents, and industrial or residential construction defects.

When evaluating a materials failure, the materials engineer considers the relevant material properties.

Depending on the material in question and the type of failure, these properties can include mechanical properties such as strength, hardness, ductility, and toughness. Component design, stress state, and the effect of manufacturing defects, if present, must also be considered.

A variety of specialized references exist to assist the materials engineer in failure analysis. These include handbooks, testing protocols, and material specifications and standards.

Failure of Materials

The Stress–Strain Curve

Failure of materials in the extreme case is the fracture or permanent deformation of the material. Failure can also be any changes from the original or specified state of the material that prevent it from performing according to specification. Failure in this case includes mechanical changes such as temporary, elastic, or permanent, plastic, deformation, or the presence of defects that affect the expected mechanical properties.

To understand the processes of deformation and fracture, one must understand the mechanical properties of materials. The specific behavior of materials differs according to the type of material, but the defining properties are essentially the same. The important mechanical properties are given as follows:

- yield strength;
- tensile strength;
- percent elongation;
- Young's modulus;
- toughness;
- ductile or brittle behavior; and
- hardness.

These mechanical properties are tabulated for most engineering materials, including metals, plastics, and ceramics, and can be found in many print and on-line references, some of which are listed in the section "Information References" that deals with various information sources. For composites, bulk properties can be derived from the properties, volume fraction, and orientation of the constituents.

All of these properties, with the exception of hardness, can be directly determined from the stress–strain diagram of the material. A typical

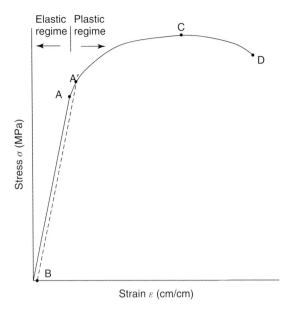

Figure 1 A typical stress–strain diagram for a metal

example of a stress–strain diagram for a metal is shown in Figure 1, and is discussed in the sections below.

The stress–strain diagram is obtained from a special type of materials characterization test called a *tensile test*. In a tensile test, an increasing load is applied to a specimen of the material being tested. As the load increases, the sample lengthens and deforms until fracture occurs. The changes in load and sample length with time are recorded, and converted into engineering stress and strain. From this data, the stress–strain diagram is created from which the mechanical properties of the material can be determined. Further details on the tensile test are provided in Section "Tensile Testing" (see Section "Materials Characterization").

Engineering Stress and Strain. Engineering stress, σ, is the amount of load, or force, per unit area applied to a material. Stress is commonly used instead of the force to remove the affect of material dimensions. For the same applied force, more deformation can be expected if the material being acted on has a smaller cross section, and less if the material has a larger cross section. The stress is defined as follows:

$$\sigma = \frac{F}{A_0} \qquad (1)$$

where F is the load at any given time and A_0 is the initial cross-sectional area of the specimen. Stress is expressed in units of megapascals (MPa), or as pounds per square inch (psi), in the English system of units, where 1 MPa = 145 psi.

Engineering strain, ε, is the change in length of a material under stress, in the direction of that applied stress. It is the change in length at any time compared to the initial length, and is calculated as follows:

$$\varepsilon = \frac{l_i - l_0}{l_0} = \frac{\Delta l}{l_0} \qquad (2)$$

where l_i is the length at any given time and l_0 is the initial specimen length. Strain is given in units of inches per inch (in./in.) or is stated as a percentage of the initial length ($\varepsilon \times 100\%$).

Deformation. When a load is applied to a material specimen, its dimensions will change in response. Depending on the amount of load, the deformation will be either temporary or permanent. For a small load, this deformation is temporary or elastic. Within the region of the material that is deforming elastically, inside the material itself, the bonds between atoms are being stretched. Atoms are displaced from their original positions and pulled away from each other, but no interatomic bonds are broken. In this case, when the load is removed, the bonds are no longer being stretched, and the atoms return to their equilibrium positions.

When a larger load is applied, the material will deform permanently or plastically. In this case, atoms are displaced far enough from their original positions that interatomic bonds are broken, and atoms move through the material. The movement of the atoms in response to the applied load results in permanent deformation.

These two regimes are shown on the stress–strain diagram of Figure 1. The linear region to the left of point A is the elastic region, and the nonlinear region to the right is the plastic region. As Figure 1 shows, plastic deformation only exists along with temporary elastic deformation.

The existence of the elastic and plastic deformation regimes has important implications for failure analysis. When an investigator examines a deformed component, the elastic portion of the deformation has recovered, and the actual deformation at the time of the event was greater than what is observed later.

The amount and significance of the elastic deformation can be determined from mechanical tests or from mechanical property data.

During a standard tensile test, changes in load or displacement are usually made slowly. When the load is applied rapidly, atoms have less time to move through the material. The effect is to make the material behave as if it were more brittle, in which case plastic deformation may be nonexistent.

Yield Strength. The yield strength of a material is the stress at which the material begins to deform plastically. Point A of Figure 1 is the demarcation point between elastic and plastic behavior. Below the yield stress, the material has only been elastically deformed. This elastic deformation can be compared to stretching a rubber band; if the stress is removed, the material returns to its original shape. If the yield stress at point A is exceeded, permanent deformation will occur. However, if a stress greater than the yield strength is applied and removed, recovery of the elastically deformed amount will take place; however, the plastic deformation will be permanent.

The exact point where the material behavior changes from elastic to plastic is not clear. Therefore, by convention, the yield strength is defined as the stress at a strain offset of 0.2% of the maximum measured strain before failure. As shown in Figure 1, the point on the x-axis where the strain is 0.2% of the maximum measured strain is located at point B. A line is drawn through that point, and parallel to the elastic portion of the stress–strain curve. The point, A', where that line crosses the stress–strain curve is defined as the yield strength.

Tensile Strength. The tensile strength is the maximum tensile stress that the specimen can bear. On the stress–strain curve, this occurs at point C, the point of greatest stress on the curve. As the load is constantly increased during the tensile test, after point C, nonuniform deformation will begin to occur, along with necking of the sample, leading rapidly to fracture, at point D. In other words, if the stress at point C is reached, the material will fail completely unless the force is immediately reduced.

Percent Elongation. Percent elongation is a measure of the amount of deformation in the specimen. Specifically, it is the ratio of the change in specimen length to the initial length, and is calculated using the equation for strain (Equation 2).

Young's Modulus. Young's modulus, also called the *modulus of elasticity*, indicates how much stress can be applied to the material before permanent deformation occurs. A mechanical analogy is the deformation of a spring under tension. When a load is placed on a spring, the spring deforms in direct proportion to the load. If a load is removed, the spring returns to its original length. If the load exceeding the stiffness of the spring is applied, the spring is stretched beyond its capability to rebound, and is permanently deformed. The Young's modulus is the slope of the linear region of the curve, from zero up to the yield stress, or

$$E = \frac{\sigma_y}{\varepsilon} \qquad (3)$$

where the strain is 0.02, by definition. The units of Young's modulus are megapascal.

Ductile or Brittle Behavior. The stress–strain curve can also reveal whether a material is ductile or brittle. As seen above, ductile materials, such as metals, undergo plastic deformation before failure; hence, failure occurs above the yield stress, and will result in permanent, plastic deformation of both the gross dimensions of the sample as well as the fracture surface. By contrast, with brittle materials little or no plastic deformation occurs. Typical stress–strain curves for ductile and brittle materials are shown in Figure 2.

Toughness. Toughness is a measure of the energy absorbed in the deformation until fracture of a material, and is measured as the area under the stress–strain curve. The units of toughness are joule per cubic meter.

Hardness. Hardness cannot be found directly from the stress–strain curve. It is determined by measuring the deformation resistance at the surface of the material. Several different methods are available for measuring hardness; however, all involve measuring the force required to press an indenter into a surface. Common methods are the Rockwell, Brinell, Knoop and Vickers hardness tests, and are specified by standards such as ASTM E18-05, E10-01, C730-98, and E92-82 [1].

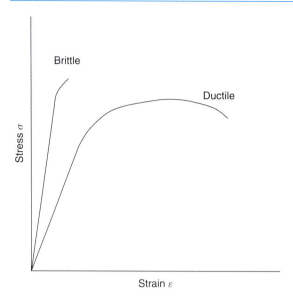

Figure 2 Typical stress–strain diagrams for a ductile and a brittle material

Hardness does correlate well with yield strength, since both yield strength and hardness measurements are taken when plastic deformation is just beginning. Tables and charts can be found in references such as the *ASM Metals Handbook* [2], which relate the yield strength of a metal to hardness.

Failure Modes

Fracture. The discussion until now has focused on ideal materials in a nominally defect-free state. Under those conditions, the material will fail when the tensile stress is exceeded. Materials in the real world can frequently contain defects or flaws, which may lower the strength of the material and lead to unexpected failure. The role of defects or flaws must be considered in failure analysis.

Defects can be material or geometric heterogeneities. Examples are inclusions, second phase particles, voids, machining marks, geometric variations, and miscellaneous surface flaws. These defects can act as stress concentrators, and by their geometry prevent the material from sustaining normal loading.

To demonstrate the effect of flaws on the strength of a material, a simple model of a flaw, a symmetrical crack, can be used. The crack is inside the material, and perpendicular to the direction of tensile loading. If the crack is small, it will be relatively stable. The

size of the crack may remain constant, or it may grow slowly, depending on the applied stress, any cyclic loading, and the morphology of the material.

This crack growth is occurring by ductile fracture mechanisms, where the term ductile indicates that the material at the crack tip is deforming. If the crack grows, once it reaches a critical length with respect to the direction of the applied stress, it becomes unstable. At the point of instability, the crack will rapidly propagate through the material, resulting in a fracture. The unstable crack growth occurs by brittle fracture, with little or no plastic deformation occurring at the fracture surface.

Since materials without any bulk defects can sustain stress up to their yield strength without deforming, the yield strength would seem to be an appropriate design criterion. When defects are present, however, the material can fail below the yield strength. To account for this, during design the yield strength is usually multiplied by a safety factor. The designed safety factor varies according to the application, but may be 1.5–2 times the yield strength. A material whose yield strength is above the resulting design strength can then be selected.

Choosing a material with a yield strength exceeding the expected stress is intended to protect against failure in three different ways:

- If the maximum stress is slightly or occasionally greater than expected, the stress will still remain within the design envelope as long as a safety factor is used.
- If the yield stress of the material is slightly below the anticipated strength, perhaps due to a processing problem, impurities or internal flaws, the applied stress will remain below the actual yield stress.
- In some materials, not prone to brittle fracture, if the tensile stress is exceeded, the material will fail, catastrophically and without warning. Since yield stress is used as the design criterion, rather than the tensile stress, if the yield stress is exceeded, the part will deform, and thus may provide warning of an incipient failure.

Fatigue. Variable loads, cycling between large and small, or from tension to compression, can lead to failure at stresses below the normal design strength of the component. This is called *fatigue failure*, and is caused by the simultaneous action of cyclic stress, tensile stress, and plastic strain. The cyclic stress starts the crack (nucleation); the tensile stress produces crack growth (propagation) until the remaining cross section of the part becomes too weak to sustain the load and quickly fails in overload.

The general features of a typical fracture surface can be seen in the photograph below (Figure 3).

The fluctuating tensile stress produces the striations shown in the figure, which are sometimes referred to as *beach marks* or *clamshell marks*. The presence of beach marks is a reliable evidence of

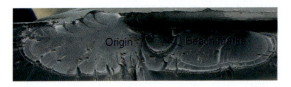

Figure 3 General features of a fatigue fracture, shown here in high-density polyethylene (HDPE). The fracture origin site can be located by tracing the center of curvature of the beach marks back to the root

fatigue crack propagation. However, depending on material and loading, the absence of fatigue striations does not mean that no fatigue occurred. The definitive call will depend upon the specifics of the material application and the events leading up to and following the failure, upon further examination under a high power optical microscope or scanning electron microscope (SEM) and upon fracture surface microstructure.

In cases where cyclic loading is present, the component must be designed to accommodate cyclic loads by setting the maximum load below an endurance load defined below. The $S-N$ curve is used for this purpose, where S stands for stress and N stands for the number of cycles.

The $S-N$ curve for steel, shown in Figure 4, illustrates that, as the stress decreases, the number of cycles before failure increases. In this figure, if the stress is kept below 50% of the fracture strength, then the metal is said to have an "infinite life", or is at least able to survive more than 10 million cycles. This stress level is called the *endurance level*. The

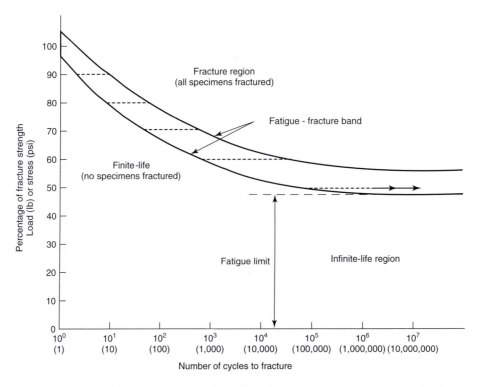

Figure 4 $S-N$ curves that typify fatigue test results for testing of medium-strength steels [Reproduced with permission from Ref. 3. © ASM International, 1986.]

American Society of Metals (ASM) Atlas of Fatigue Curves [3] may be referred to for the $S-N$ curves of particular metals.

Corrosion. Corrosion is an important mechanism of materials failure. Corrosion occurs when a metal interacts with the surrounding environment, and degrades as a result of electrochemical reaction. There are a number of specific types of corrosion; however, all follow the same basic process. Material is removed from the metal in the form of ions. This is called an *oxidizing*, or *anodic*, reaction. Ions are atoms that, in this case, have lost electrons. These lost electrons are taken up in a second reducing, or cathodic, reaction.

For corrosion to occur, three conditions described below must be present:

1. ionic pathway;
2. electrical pathway; and
3. a driving force.

The ionic pathway is generally moisture or an atmosphere with greater than 70% relative humidity. This allows the migration of the ions of corrosion.

The electrical pathway is any conducting pathway between the anode (oxidized area) and the cathode (reduced area).

The driving force may be two different metals in contact (galvanic driving force); a concentration difference such as an area of low oxygen potential on a pipe; or the difference stress in a metal part (so that the higher stress area tries to dissolve to lower its stress).

Generally, failure from corrosion is obvious in the initial inspection. To confirm corrosion and locate the root cause, it is useful to identify the required conditions listed above.

Materials Characterization

The forensic engineer or scientist specializing in materials has a variety of materials characterization techniques and protocols to use for explicitly testing or analyzing a failure. Standard testing protocols are defined by engineering and scientific organizations, such as the International Organization for Standardization (ISO) or the American Society of Testing and Materials (ASTM).

Mechanical Properties Characterization

Tensile Testing. Tensile testing methods, for example, ASTM E8, were originally developed to determine mechanical properties of metal specimens, although standard tests now exist for plastics (ASTM D638), ceramics (ISO 15490), and composites (ISO 527).

Two specimen configurations are preferred for the tensile test, one rectangular, and one cylindrical. For either configuration, the test specimen is tapered in the middle so that the cross-sectional dimensions are small compared to the length. The tapered section is called the *gauge length*. Owing to the smaller cross section in the gauge length, the stress is much higher there than anywhere else on the sample. Deformation is constrained to the gauge length, and failure will occur there, rather than where the testing fixture grips the specimen.

The sample is mounted in the tensile test instrument, held vertically by an upper and a lower grip. The lower grip is fixed, the upper on a movable crosshead. Load is applied by moving the upper crosshead upward. The specimen is elongated at a constant rate. Thus, the load and the cross-sectional area, and therefore the stress, change with time.

Internal load cells measure the applied force, from which the stress is calculated. Position sensors measure the crosshead location, from which the strain is determined. After the test is completed, the sample is removed from the fixture. In older test machines, load versus displacement is plotted continuously during the test with a pen plotter, and is then manually converted to a stress–strain curve. Modern instruments using computer control automatically generate the stress–strain curve.

Charpy Impact Test. The area under the stress–strain curve obtained in the tensile test corresponds to the toughness of the material. However, the area under the curve is dependent on the loading rate of the tensile test, which is typically very slow. The Charpy impact test, performed by ISO 179 or ASTM E23 methods, allows measurement of fracture toughness under dynamic conditions of rapid fracture.

A small rectangular sample with a cross section of $10\,mm \times 10\,mm$ is machined with a center notch on one of the rectangular faces. Just as the smaller cross-sectional area of the gauge length in the tensile test specimen ensures that the fracture will occur within that gauge length, the notch in the Charpy specimen ensures that impact fracture will occur at that notch.

The sample is placed in a test fixture consisting of a sample holder, a weighted pendulum, and a scale to measure the absorbed energy. The pendulum is raised and locked into place. On its release, the pendulum swings down and strikes the back, or unnotched, side of the specimen, breaking it.

The pendulum is almost frictionless, so without a specimen, the pendulum will swing back up to approximately the initial height. However, with a specimen in place, the pendulum swings to a lower height than it began at, as some of the kinetic energy of the pendulum is lost in breaking the specimen.

Therefore, the impact toughness measures the difference between the initial, potential, energy of the pendulum and its kinetic energy after breaking the sample. The Charpy impact energy is measured in foot-pounds.

Microstructural Characterization

Metallography. When alloying elements or impurities are present in a material, they may segregate into different regions, forming different structures or phases within the material. These structures can have a significant effect on the properties of the material. Many of these structures can be observed and identified with a microscope. If testing reveals that the mechanical properties of a material are different from the expected properties, it is frequently of interest to examine the structure of the material on a microscopic level. This examination often requires special sample preparation to reveal the microscopic features.

Originally developed to reveal the native microstructure of metals, cutting, mounting, polishing, and etching procedures exist to prepare specimens of any type of material for examination. The specimen preparation techniques are collectively grouped under the term *metallography*. The presence of flaws, such as inclusions or voids, and/or regions of differing elemental composition can frequently be identified by these methods. Preparation of a typical metal specimen is discussed below; preparation of other materials is substantially the same, although with different idiosyncratic challenges.

First, a specimen is cut to reveal a surface to examine. The typical specimen size is less than 1 inch by 1 inch. Cutting is best if done with a water- or oil-cooled cut-off wheel, to reduce any heat-induced changes. The mechanical cutting will necessarily create a zone of damage below the surface of the specimen, which will be removed later by polishing.

Once the specimen has been cut, it is encased in phenolic or an epoxy resin mixture. This hard mount will protect the sample and make polishing easier.

The mounted sample is then polished with various abrasives to remove the damaged surface zone. The polishing media starts out rough, with abrasive sandpaper of 120 or 240 grit size, and gets progressively finer, finishing with fine (0.3 µm) alumina or diamond polishing compound. In between polishing steps, the specimen surface is washed with soap and/or isopropyl alcohol and rinsed in an ultrasonic bath to remove any loose particles of the polishing media or sample fragments. It is also examined with a metallographic microscope to ensure the surface is smooth with no scratches.

Once a surface has reached the desired level of polish, chemical etching may be performed. Etching is the process of exposing a material to chemicals, such as acids, that preferentially remove materials of one phase or elemental composition with respect to other phases. This creates differences in surface height across the sample, which in turn, creates contrast during viewing with an optical microscope. Note that, owing to its different imaging technique, etching does not always produce contrast when the sample is viewed with an SEM.

Optical Microscopy. Information can frequently be gained about materials, especially fracture surfaces, from visual examination; however, it is frequently necessary to go to higher magnification to observe important features of a fracture surface or the distribution and morphology of different phases.

The typical magnification range of optical microscopy runs from 1 to 400 times the original size; 1000 times magnification is the upper limit of the magnification range for optical microscopes. When viewing fracture surfaces, which are typically rough, the depth of field, which is the ability of the microscope to keep the entire region being viewed in focus, can be a limiting factor. This is a function of the optics of the microscope, as well as of the behavior of light in general.

Electron Microscopy. When greater magnification than that provided by optical microscopy is required, an electron microscope can be used. The SEM is a common instrument, and one that provides images that are intuitive and easy to understand. Magnification ranges from 20 to above 20 000 times the original size.

In an optical microscope, an image is created by light reflected from, or transmitted through, a specimen, the focused through a lens, and into the eye. In the SEM, the image is created by bombarding the specimen surface with electrons. A beam of these primary electrons is scanned across the surface of the specimen. The primary electrons either reflect back from the specimen surface (as backscattered electrons), or eject electrons from the atoms in the specimen (secondary electrons). A specialized detector then detects the backscattered and secondary electrons. The signal collected by the detector is converted into an electrical signal that is proportional to the detected intensity; this electrical signal is then converted to a gray scale image that is displayed on a computer monitor. Magnification occurs when the primary electron beam is scanned across a small area of the samples, and the image of the scanned surface region is displayed on a larger computer screen. This image can be displayed, printed, or saved in digital format.

Common Failure Analysis Procedures

Many features of forensic materials failure investigation are the same, despite the type(s) of materials involved. Identification of the root cause of failure is key, as careful documentation of the details of the investigation and preservation of the materials are involved. However, owing to their different mechanical behavior and failure modes, different procedures are commonly used in failure analysis of metals, ceramics, plastics, and composites. Some examples of procedures required in a forensic investigation are presented below.

- **Metals**

The fracture surface must be preserved because the fracture surface contains the information on where the failure originated and how it occurred. The fracture origin is the point from which cracking begins which may occur because of damage or a defect in that area. The fracture surface may reveal information about the time to failure, as in fast failure by overload or gradual fatigue leading to overload of the remaining metal. The fracture surface can be examined by processes such as optical microscopy or SEM but normally should not undergo any testing which is destructive in nature. For items too large to allow study of the surface without cutting, the surface can be replicated using a rubber mold material that allows the replica to be examined without destruction of the original. Collections of fracture surface photographs can be found in the ASM references discussed in Section "Information References".

- **Ceramics and Glass**

In glass, the direction of the fracture movement from the origin can be determined by observing the rib marks, also called *Wallner lines*, which are found on the fracture surface. The rib marks, which appear as concentric ridges, are almost always concave toward the origin, in the direction from which the fracture initiated. Owing to the brittle nature of glassy materials, the failure mechanisms are complex; a reference such as Failure Analysis of Brittle Materials [4] may be consulted for more details.

- **Plastics**

The fracture surface of hard plastics has failure information like a metal. Plastics, unlike a metal, may be more strongly affected by the chemical environment and temperature it is exposed to. A plastic may fracture by simple overload, fatigue, creep or stress cracking. Creep fracture occurs some time after the application of a load to the plastic. Stress cracking occurs under a comparatively small load when the plastic is exposed to a chemically active environment. In all cases, a properly preserved surface can provide information as to the cause of the failure.

- **Composites**

Depending on the type, shape, and amount of fiber reinforcement and the type and properties of the matrix containing the fibers, the properties and characteristics of composites widely varies. Composite materials where fibers, such as glass or carbon, are bonded together are found in high strength, lightweight structures such as aircraft and sport car bodies. Composites also are found in fiberglass ladders and wood siding products used in construction where wood fibers are held in place by resins. Each composite is generally unique in its creation and individual in its characteristics. The most common composite failures are due to delamination (separation) of the fiber mats because of failure of the adhesive, or misorientation of the fiber mats due to design or manufacture.

Information References

A number of reference sources, including handbooks and textbook references, provide background and details on the materials science and engineering concepts introduced in this article. Callister's text [5] is popular for undergraduate courses in materials engineering, and provides an accessible overview of the relevant principles. Deiter [6] or Courtney [7] provide in depth information on metallurgy and failure modes of materials. For corrosion, Uhlig's text [8] is covers both corrosion mechanisms and prevention methods.

The expert will frequently consult the publications of the ASM [9]. ASM publishes a 21-volume series of handbooks, on various aspects of materials engineering and science, including but not limited to metals. Handbooks of particular interest are Volume 10 (Materials Characterization) [10], Volume 11 (Failure Analysis and Prevention) [11], Volume 13B (Corrosion: Materials) [12] and Volume 19 (Fatigue And Fracture) [13]. A selection of articles from these handbooks, specific to metals, is contained in the previously discussed Metals Handbook [2].

As previously discussed, accepted materials property testing methods are standardized by both the ASTM [1] and the ISO [14]. Descriptions of specific methods or standards are available for purchase through both organizations. For validation of methods and consistency of results, it is preferable to follow a standard method when an appropriate one is available.

References

[1]   American Society of Testing and Materials (ASTM). Handbooks and standards are updated on a regular basis. The issuing organisations can provide information on the most current version. See www.astm.org for latest version information.

[2]   Davis, J. (ed) (1999). *Metals Handbook*, 2nd Edition, ASM International.

[3]   Boyer, H. (ed) (1986). *ASM Atlas of Fatigue Curves*, ASM International.

[4]   Frechette, V. (1990). *Failure Analysis of Brittle Materials: Advances in Ceramics*, Wiley, Vol. 28.

[5]   Callister, W. (2006). *Materials Science and Engineering: An Introduction*, 7th Edition, Wiley.

[6]   Deiter, G. & Bacon, D. (1989). *Mechanical Metallurgy*, 3rd Edition, McGraw-Hill.

[7]   Courtney, T. (2005). *Mechanical Behavior of Materials*, 2nd Edition, Waveland Pr.

[8]   Uhlig, H. (1985). *Corrosion and Corrosion Control*, 3rd Edition, Wiley-Interscience.

[9]   American Society of Metals (ASM). See www.asminternational.org for latest version information.

[10]   Whan, R. (ed) (1986). *ASM Handbook Volume 10: Materials Characterization*, 9th Edition, ASM International.

[11]   Powell, G. & Mahmoud, S. (1986). *ASM Handbook Volume 11: Failure Analysis and Prevention*, 9th Edition, ASM International.

[12]   Cramer, S. (ed) (2005). *ASM Handbook Volume 13B: Corrosion: Materials*, ASM International.

[13]   Dimatteo, N. (1996). *ASM Handbook Volume 19: Fatigue And Fracture*, ASM International.

[14]   International Organization for Standardization (ISO). See www.iso.org for latest version information.

Related Articles

Microscopy: Light Microscopes
Reconstruction: Accident

Anastasia D. Micheals and Robert N. Anderson

Matrix: DNA

Contemporary forensic DNA identification systems utilize a panel of fluorescent dyes to identify specific fragments, alleles, or nucleotides. Commonly, four or five dyes are used simultaneously. As the excitation of a particular fluorescent dye indicates a specific forensic outcome, it is essential that the detections systems have high specificity in their ability to isolate a particular dye or color. As there is some overlap in the emission spectra of the dyes that are simultaneously utilized, there is a need to filter out the "background" color that is drawn up with each individual dye. The technique applied is referred to as *multicomponent analysis* or *color deconvolution* [1].

A set of standards is run, each of which is labeled with one of the individual dyes that are to be utilized in the test system. Computer software is then able to analyze the fluorescence data from each dye and assess the amount of overlap contributed by the other dyes of the system. As each dye analyzed generates data for each of the other dyes, collectively, the dataset is referred to as a *matrix* or *matrix file*. Matrix files differ for different sets of dyes and different electrophoresis systems and instruments. They are also subject to slight variation if there is a change in environmental conditions (such as temperature) and they should be regenerated for different batches of polymer or polyacrylamide (if using slab-gel systems).

The application of the matrix file occurs after the raw fluorescence data has been collected; it is usually applied automatically as one of the first steps of analysis. Applying the matrix has the effect of optimizing the signal from each dye, which sharpens the image and simplifies interpretation. A common artifact associated with this aspect of profile interpretation is known as *pull-up* and it occurs when there is incomplete separation of the spectra of two or more dyes. This creates spurious peaks of different colors that are effectively drawn up under the true peak. Pull-up is most likely to occur when the sample is overloaded, or off scale.

Reference

[1] Butler, J.M. (2005). *Forensic DNA Typing: Biology, Technology and Genetics of STR Markers*, Elsevier Academic Press, Burlington, MA.

SIMON J. WALSH

Medical Effects of Alcohol *see* Alcohol: Behavioral and Medical Effects

Medical Malpractice

Introduction

Medical malpractice charges are nearly as old as medicine. Already in the Codex Hammurapi (1700 B.C.), punishment in cases of medical malpractice was described [1, 2].

The *Constitutio Criminalis Carolina* (1532 A.D.) contains a separate chapter on medical malpractice (Chapter XXIX), and in this chapter, notions such as negligence, causality, and expert evidence can be found.

From the seventeenth to the nineteenth century it was mainly experts in forensic medicine who dealt with medical malpractice in their textbooks [1–3], e.g., Paolo Zacchia (1584–1659). In his book *Quaestionum–Medico legalium cura* (1621–1635) the sentence, "Medicus errat ommitendo et commitendo" can be found, which means that damage to the patient can not only be caused by doing something wrong but also by omitting to do the right. For a long time medical malpractice was a subject that was not frankly discussed within the medical community and public. A change was caused by the U.S. report "to err is human" (1999) [4], although

Table 1   Adverse events in hospitalized patients – an international comparison[a]

Study and place of study	Number of investigated cases	Adverse events (%)	Potentially preventable adverse events (%)
New York	31 000	3.7	–
Colorado and Utah	14 321	2.9	58
Australia	14 179	16.6	51
London	1014	10.8	46
New Zealand	6579	12.9	63

[a] According to [7]

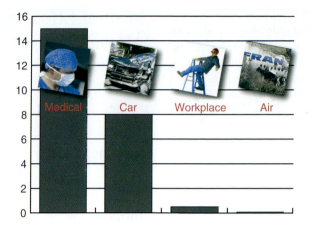

Figure 1   Incidence of annual accidental deaths in the United Kingdom (in thousands)

the message "Errare humanum est" is not new [5, 6]. But it was mainly the estimated cost caused by adverse events and medical malpractice that was surprising (Table 1). On the basis of Anglo-American studies, an estimation of adverse events in hospitalized patients in Germany was carried out. Taking into account the 16.5 million hospitalizations a year (in 2001), 31 600–83 000 deaths were estimated to be due to adverse events [7]. This would mean that more people would die as a consequence of wrong medical diagnosis or therapy than as a result of colon cancer (20 200), breast cancer (18 000), pneumonia (17 800), and traffic accidents (7700). For the United Kingdom, similar figures have been arrived at (Figure 1).

However, speaking about mishaps during medical care, adverse events, and medical malpractice requires a strict consideration of the terminology since epidemiologic research and law have different understandings of similar terms [8–12]. In the following, some aspects of medical malpractice will be addressed, which are based on international studies and also on experiences in Germany since some nationwide statistical data are available.

Definitions

Meanwhile, different institutions have proposed different definitions, e.g., the European Council, WHO, etc. [8, 9, 11–13].

Examples of definitions are given below:

An adverse event (AE) is a noxious and unintended response.

A preventable adverse event (PAE) is a noxious and unintended response that might have been prevented.

A negligent adverse event (NAE) is a noxious and unintended response due to a break of duty of care. An NAE is an equivalent of medical malpractice.

In penal law, medical malpractice is mainly defined as an AE (injury, harm) due to medical negligence. Medical negligence is defined as a preventable mistake caused by a breach of duty of care. Furthermore, there must be a causal connection between the mistake and injury, and in most jurisdictions this causal connection has to be proved without reasonable doubt.

In civil law, medical malpractice is defined as follows: "The defendant (doctor) owed duty of care to the plaintiff (patient). The doctor breaches the duty of care by failing to adhere to the standard of care expected. The standard is the quality that would be expected of a reasonable practitioner in similar circumstances. This breach of duty caused an injury to the patient." Furthermore, for epidemiologic research a definition of medical error is of importance.

Error may be error in planning or execution. An error of execution is the failure of a planned action to be completed as intended, whereas an error of planning is the use of a wrong plan to achieve an aim.

Epidemiology

Clear data on the epidemiology of medical malpractice are lacking. However, in the United States,

United Kingdom, and Australia, several studies were conducted concerning AE, PAE, and NAE but mostly only in hospitalized patients [14–36]. For ambulant medical care, hardly any data are available.

It is well known that only a small proportion of misadventures are on record, while the majority of misadventures or injuries do not become known [7, 11, 12, 37]. This fact is often illustrated by an iceberg model of accidents and errors (Figures 2 and 3).

The German Alliance of Patient Safety has carried out a systematic review of papers on the incidence of AEs, errors, etc. [33, 35]. Studies fulfilling the following criteria were included:

- original papers with data from January 1995 to December 2005;
- data collected on a well-defined reference group of patients;
- papers in which at least one of the following relevant criteria had been checked:

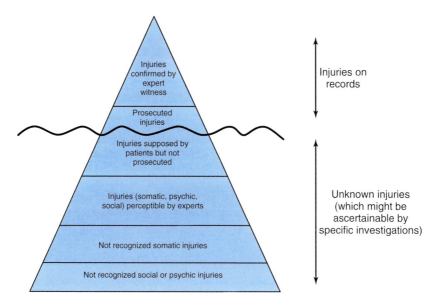

Figure 2   Types of injuries and probability of detection

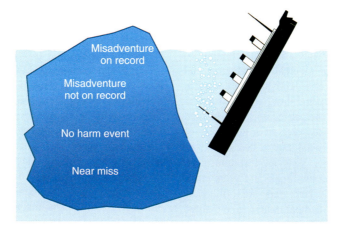

Figure 3   Iceberg model if accidents and errors

- AE
- PAE
- NAE
- errors
- near misses.

Each paper must contain a clear description of how the data were evaluated. Furthermore, clear data on factors like proportion, ratio, incidence rates must be evident. From more than 25 000 studies in PubMed and Embase, 151 studies from 25 countries with 7 686 166 patients fulfilled these criteria. The review revealed a dependency of the frequency of reported AEs, PAVs, and NAEs on the sample size: the higher the sample size, the lower the frequency. Furthermore, there was no influence of the geographic origin of the study; so the results may be more or less representative for countries with a "western" standard in health care. Among hospitalized patients, AEs can be expected in 5–10%, PAEs in 2–4%, NAEs in about 1%, and lethal outcome in about 0.1%. This would mean that on the basis of epidemiologic studies for hospitalized patients in Germany, 880 000–1 750 000 AEs, 350 000–700 000 PAEs, 175 000 NAEs, and 17 500 lethal cases would be expected. These data on the mortality due to AE and PAE were confirmed in a recent review of the German Alliance of Patient Safety [34]. According to this review, mortality due to PAE is 0.1% of all hospitalized patients. This would mean that in Germany with 17 million hospitalized patients per year, 17 000 lethal cases have to be expected. However, only a small proportion of these cases raise legal discussions. For most countries, data on the frequency of medical malpractice claims are not available. For Germany, it is estimated that only 1500–2000 cases a year are investigated by the public prosecutor [38]; these are mainly cases where death is thought to have occurred because of medical malpractice, and by a legal autopsy the cause and manner of death have to be cleared. In penal law, it is estimated that one investigation by the prosecutor is performed per 60 000 inhabitants, one piece of information of a prosecutor on 90 000 inhabitants [38]. On average, only eight cases per year are brought to a penal court, with four convictions and four stays of proceedings. For civil law, data are not available on the frequency of medical malpractice claims, but estimations speak of about 15 000 claims per year [39–41].

Every doctor is obliged to have a liability insurance. Data from the liability insurance companies are, however, not available [41, 42]. One insurance company with 108 000 insured doctors reported about 4500 incidents a year, with a settlement of cases in 30%, going to a civil court 10%, and medical malpractice confirmed at court in 4% [7].

In Germany, most claims of medical malpractice are dealt with at the arbitration committees of the medical councils. More than 30 years ago the medical councils formed these arbitration committees to make medical malpractice claims possible without applying to the courts [39, 43–50]. More than 10 000 cases per year are dealt with at the arbitration committees, and in 30% cases patient claims are confirmed.

Data of the Arbitration Committees

Since the data by the arbitration committees of the medical councils are well documented and evaluated either locally by the responsible medical chamber or nationwide by the German medical chamber, some details shall be addressed.

At the present moment, nine arbitration committees exist in Germany (Baden-Wuerttemberg, Bavaria, Hesse, Northrhine, Northern Germany, Saarland, Saxony, Westphalia, Rhineland-Palatinate). These arbitration committees have annual meetings and have recently evaluated their material nationwide (Medical Error Reporting System, MERS) [39, 43, 50]. The data of the nine arbitration committees are shown in Table 2. The largest arbitration board is that of the Northern German chambers in Hanover, and the smallest is that of Saarland. Table 2 gives details and numbers of applications per year, mode of settlement, and decisions [43].

Doctors in hospital are more often concerned with medical malpractice claims than those in private practice (Table 3). The most frequent complaints were on surgical therapy, followed by postoperative care, diagnostic imaging, informed consent, etc. (Table 4). The most frequent diagnoses resulting in malpractice claims are coxarthrosis, gonarthrosis, and fractures of lower leg and ankle (Table 5).

The bodily damages caused by medical malpractice can be classified as follows (Figure 4): no damage, minor damage, passing damage, permanent damage, and death [49]. Results concerning the severity of damages shown in Figure 4 are

Table 2 Official statistics on the work of the German committees of experts and arbitration boards (year 2004)[a]

	Baden-Wuerttemberg	Bavaria	Hesse	Northrhine	Northern Germany	Saarland	Saxony	Westphalia–Lippe	Rhineland-Palatinate	Total
1. Total no. of applications of the past year	976	828	860	1793	4040	128	380	1777	362	11 144
2. No. of old applications not yet settled	677	729	747	2042	3887	79	143	1106	319	9729
3. No. of settled applications of last year	1057	770	793	1885	4211	119	395	1617	364	11 211
4. No. of applications still open at the end of the reporting year	596	787	813	1950	3716	88	128	1267	317	9662

(continued overleaf)

Table 2 (*continued*)

II Mode of settlement of claims of last year	Baden-Wuerttemberg	Bavaria	Hesse	Northrhine	Northern Germany	Saarland	Saxony	Westphalia–Lippe	Rhineland-Palatinate	Total
1. Withdrawn by applicant or not followed up because of lack of interest	72	87	91	158	345	13	3	103	39	911
2. Refused because of incompetence	137	30	14	110	68	6	2	94	17	478
3. Rejected because of unenforceability of error in treatment or doctor's duty to inform	24	9	8	0	1	0	0	8	2	52
4. Rejected because of the lapse of the application term	0	20	9	50	0	2	0	36	17	134
5. Rejected because hospital operator not governed by public law	1	0	0	0	7	0	0	3	5	16

or other case of public liability										
6. Rejected because of expert opinion	0	2	1	0	0	0	0	5	0	
7. Rejected because of preliminary proceedings, lawsuit, or legally binding court decision	17	12	13	30	42	3	8	25	2	152
8. Not decided because of appeal of one party	46	108	64	48	812	5	10	90	11	1194
9. Settled because of advising information	60	5	6	0	116	0	100	0	5	292
10. Rejected or not accepted for decision because of other reasons	0	4	8	111	0	5	8	43	20	199

(continued overleaf)

Table 2 (*continued*)

III	Baden-Wuerttemberg	Bavaria	Hesse	Northrhine	Northern Germany	Saarland	Saxony	Westphalia–Lippe	Rhineland-Palatinate	Total
Remaining cases accepted for decision on the merits										
1. Total	700	493	548	1378	2820	85	264	1210	246	7744
2. Error in doctor's duty to inform approved	6	12	14	25	25	0	2	4	1	89
3. Error in doctor's duty to inform questionable because of controversial facts	0	23	0	15	0	0	0	22	3	63
4. Medical malpractice and causality for injury approved	117	105	131	353	725	16	62	167	60	1736

										Total
5. Medical malpractice approved, causality negated	171	15	25	76	266	2	28	35	4	622
6. Medical malpractice approved, causality not clarified	0	7	6	28	0	0	0	16	6	63
7. Medical malpractice and error in doctor's duty to inform negated	406	359	370	830	1804	64	172	961	170	5136
8. Alternative verdict (as far as not included in 2 or 5)	0	6	2	51	0	0	0	5	2	66
9. Arbitration proposal (as far as not included in 1 and 7)	0	0	0	0	0	3	0	0	0	3

[a] Taken from [43]

Table 3   Medical malpractice and site of treatment[a]

Medical malpractice and site of treatment	Doctor's practice	Hospital
Site of treatment	2432	5303
Medical malpractice/inadequate informed consent confirmed	657	1336
Inadequate informed consent confirmed	27	45

Medical specialty 2006			
Doctor's practice		Hospital	
General practitioner	389	Traumatic surgery orthopedics	1063
Orthopedic surgery	336	General surgery	943
General surgery	249	Orthopedic surgery	629
Gynecology	239	Gynecology	418
Internal medicine	218	Internal medicine	395
Traumatic surgery orthopedics	190	Anesthesiology and intensive care	179
Ophthalmology	149	Urology	166
Radiology	98	Neurosurgery	164
Dermatology and venereal diseases	79	ENT	134
Urology	71	Obstetrics	134

[a] Taken from [43]

Table 4   Claims by patients[a]

Claims by patients	2006	2005
Total no. of decisions on the merits	6751	7320
Total no. of claims (based on total no. of decision on the merits, maximum 4 claims/decision)	11 949	10 496
Most frequent claims		
Surgical therapy, performance	2998	
Postoperative therapy	861	
Diagnostic imaging	858	
Informed consent, risk	654	
Diagnostics, anamnesis, examination	636	
Therapy, conservative	599	
Diagnostics, general	539	
Therapy, pharmaceutics	477	
Indication	474	
Type of surgical therapy	397	

[a] Taken from [43]

Table 5   Most frequent diagnoses resulting in malpractice claims[a]

Most frequent diagnoses resulting in malpractice claims	2006
Decisions all together (total no.)	6751
Most frequent diagnoses	
Coxarthrosis (degenerative arthritis of hip joint)	225
Gonarthrosis	170
Fracture of lower leg and ankle	155
Fracture of forearm	130
Breast cancer	130
Intervertebral disk degeneration, lumbar	115
Traumatic injury of the knee	103
Deformity of toes/fingers	100
Degenerative injury of the knee	96
Femoral fracture	94

[a] Taken from [43] The table specifies the 10 most frequent diagnoses according to frequency. For all proceedings, a (correct) diagnosis (*ex post*) is referred to; for cases with more than one diagnosis, only the most important one is taken into consideration

based on the material of the arbitration committee in Northrhine [49].

The frequency of confirmed medical malpractice differs between doctors in private practice and hospital doctors as well as from discipline to discipline (Table 6). Medical malpractice is more often confirmed in doctors in private practice than in hospital doctors. Disciplines that are at special risks are general surgery, gynecology, and trauma surgery [43].

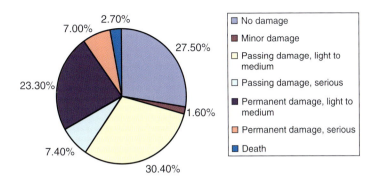

Figure 4 Bodily damage caused by medical malpractice (taken from [49]) [Reproduced with permission from Ref. 35. © Ärzteblatt, 2007.]

Medical malpractice claims have increased over the last few years (Figure 5). The error rate differs widely between the different arbitration boards (Figure 6). The arbitration board in North Rhine has the highest error rate (39%), and the board in Saarland the lowest (22%) [47].

While in Bavaria just 51 claims per 1 million residents are registered per year, other areas of Germany have many more claims per 1 million residents, e.g., North Rhine or Northern Germany [47] (Figure 7). While in Bavaria just 2 errors per 1000 physicians per year are confirmed, this rate is much higher in other German areas (Figure 8).

The probability to be charged for medical malpractice differs by the factor 3 for different regions of Germany. The probability that a medical malpractice is confirmed differs even by a factor of 6.

Data from the Files of Institutes of Forensic Medicine

The arbitration committees deal predominantly with living patients [48, 49]. Lethal cases are a special subgroup and the best available data source are the files of the Institutes of Forensic Medicine [51–58]. Therefore, this special subgroup shall be addressed separately, especially since death is the severest outcome of medical malpractice.

From a separate retrospective analysis of medical malpractice claims in lethal cases, it is known that the number of cases has increased in the past years [57, 58]. Concerning medical malpractice claims in lethal cases, a doubling of cases could be observed (from 300 to 600 cases a year) in the cooperating German Institutes of Forensic Medicine (Figure 9). The

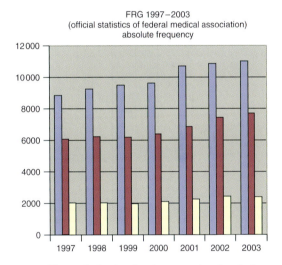

Figure 5 Medical malpractice claims, cases accepted for decision, and the number of confirmed medical malpractice over the years (from [47]) [Reproduced from Ref. 21. © Springer, 2005.]

autopsy rate due to medical malpractice claims varied between the institutes from 2.4 to 20%. That means that in some institutes every fifth autopsy was due to medical malpractice claims. Obviously, the prosecutor has a wide range of discretionary powers.

Hospital doctors are more often confronted with medical malpractice claims than doctors in private practice.

The medical disciplines concerned are surgery followed by internal medicine, general practice

Table 6 Medical malpractice charges: Arbitration committee North Rhine[a]

Medical disciplines and locations of medical care

1.1.2005–31.12.2005	n	In %	Medical malpractice confirmed (n)	In %		n	In %	Medical malpractice confirmed (n)	In %
Doctors in private practice[b]	593	100.00	189	31.8	Doctors in hospitals[b]	1236	100.00	335	27.1
Orthopedic surgery[c]	86	14.50	17	19.7	General surgery[d]	264	21.36	85	32.2
General surgery[d]	76	12.82	29	38.1	Trauma surgery	175	14.16	57	32.5
Gynecology and obstetrics	70	11.80	27	38.6	Orthopedic surgery[c]	146	11.81	26	17.8
General practitioner	66	11.13	20	30.3	Gynecology and obstetrics	141	11.41	36	25.5
Internal medicine[d]	52	8.77	13	25	Internal medicine[d]	95	7.69	24	25.2
Urology	43	7.25	16	37.2	Urology	45	3.64	11	24.4
Radiology	30	5.06	22	73	Anesthesiology	37	2.99	7	18.9
ENT	30	5.06	6	20	Vascular surgery	37	2.99	8	21.6
Ophthalmology	26	4.38	2	7.7	Cardiology	32	2.59	7	21.8
Dermatology	18	3.04	5	27.7	ENT	30	2.43	6	20

[a] Taken from [49]
[b] One doctor per private practice
[c] Formerly orthopedics and reconstructive surgery
[d] Without subspecialization

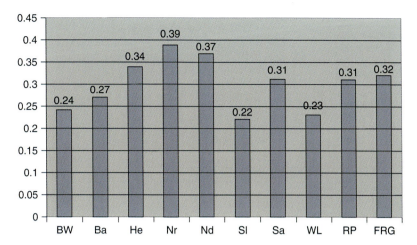

BW, Baden-Wuerttemberg; Ba Bavaria; He, Hesse; Nr, North Rhine-Westphalia;
WL, Westphalia Lippe; Nd, arbitration board of Northern Germany; Sl, Saarland;
Sa, Saxony; RP, Rhineland-Palatinate; FRG, Federal Republic of Germany

Figure 6 Error rates according to different arbitration boards and committies of experts in Germany (according 1998–2003) [Reproduced from Ref. 21. © Springer, 2005.]

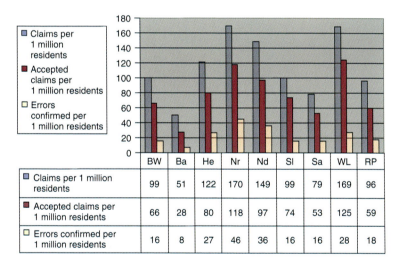

Figure 7 Claims, accepted claims, and confirmed errors per federal state per 1 million residents and year (averaged 1998–2003) (according to [47]) [Reproduced from Ref. 21. © Springer, 2005.]

and anesthesiology (Table 7). The cause of accusation was mostly conservative therapy, followed by surgical therapy, endoscopy, and intensive care (Table 8). There are different classifications of the types of mistakes, e.g. (see also Figure 10),

- medical malpractice, mistakes in information, documentation, and medication errors; and

- machine/medical product and organization.

In a separate evaluation of medical malpractice claims in lethal cases, medical malpractice charges were subdivided as follows:

1. negligence (omitting the necessary treatment)
   - insufficient diagnostics

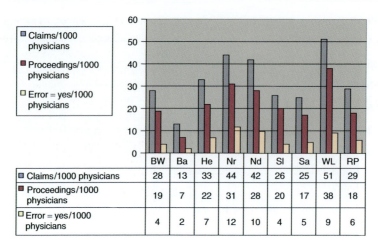

	BW	Ba	He	Nr	Nd	Sl	Sa	WL	RP
Claims/1000 physicians	28	13	33	44	42	26	25	51	29
Proceedings/1000 physicians	19	7	22	31	28	20	17	38	18
Error = yes/1000 physicians	4	2	7	12	10	4	5	9	6

Figure 8   Claims, accepted claims, and errors per 1000 working physicians per year (averaged 1998–2003) (according to [47]) [Reproduced from Ref. 21. © Springer, 2005.]

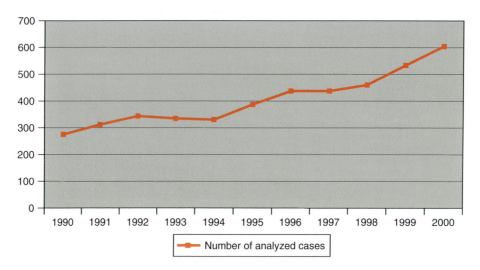

Figure 9   Number of autopsies in cases of suspected medical malpractice over the years

- delayed reaction to postoperative complications
- delayed admission to hospital and to intensive care unit

2. Complications in/or after surgery
   - intraoperative complications
   - exitus in tabula
   - complications concerning endoscopic operations
   - postoperative complications (bleeding, suture insufficiency, peritonitis)

3. Wrong treatment
   - transfusion reaction (transfusion of ABO-incompatible blood)
   - telephone diagnostics (therapeutical recommendations by telephone without visiting the patient)
   - further wrong treatment (retained instruments)

4. Mistake in care
   - insufficient prophylaxis of decubital ulcers
   - insufficient thrombosis prophylaxis

– wrong positioning during operation
5. Adverse drug event, medication errors
   – wrong drug
   – wrong dose
   – wrong application/administration
   – wrong frequency
   – disregarding drug allergy
   – misinterpretation of order given
   – illegible order.

Table 7   Medical disciplines concerned

Medical disciplines	Cases
Surgical disciplines	1272
Internal medicine	699
Practitioners	434
Anesthesiologists	156
Gynecologists and obstetricians	151
Orthopedic surgeons	126
Psychiatrists/neurologists	117
Pediatricians	86
ENT (ear, nose, and throat) specialists	72
Urologists	66
General practitioners	20

From patients and relatives, mostly the accusation is for negligence of a doctor, followed by complications within surgical therapy, wrong therapy, and medication errors (Table 9).

In nearly 40% of cases, the cause of the preliminary proceedings was the classification of the manner of death as "unclear" or "unnatural" in the death certificate (Table 10). Only in 20%, a complaint by relatives is the cause of the preliminary proceedings. Of special interest is the fact that medical malpractice is more often confirmed in doctors in private practice than in clinicians (Table 11). This is of importance since most epidemiological investigations on AE, PAE, and NAE are confined to hospitalized patients. For doctors in private practice

Table 8   Cause of accusation

Cause of accusation	
Conservative therapy	2604
Surgical therapy	1737
Endoscopy	232
Intensive care	88
Naturopathic treatment/alternative medicine	18

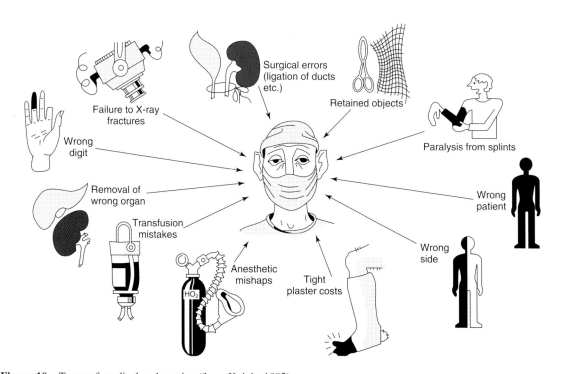

Figure 10   Types of medical malpractice (from Knight 1992)

Table 9   Classification of accusation

Type of accusation	Cases	Percentage (%)
Negligence	2158	48.5
Medication error, adverse event due to drug therapy	557	12.5
Complications within surgical therapy	1472	33.1
Wrong therapy	766	17.2
Mistake in care	320	7.2
Accusation not specified	153	3.4

Table 10   Causes of preliminary proceedings according to the analyzed documents

Cause of preliminary proceedings	Number of cases (%)
Manner of death "unclear" or "unnatural" in death certificate	1715 (38.5)
Cause of proceedings is unknown	1303 (29.3)
Complaint of offense by relatives (including friends and carers)	831 (18.7)
Complaint of a cotreating or post-treating physician	271 (6.1)
Complaint of offense by relatives as well as "manner of death unclear" or "unnatural" in the death certificate	190 (4.3)
No formal preliminary proceeding by the prosecutor, but proceeding to clear cause and manner of death	73 (1.6)
Self-complaint of the physician(s)	21 (0.5)
Complaint by the patient himself before death	18 (0.4)
Complaint by staff (especially nursing staff)	10 (0.2)
Anonymous complaint of offense	9 (0.2)
Other	9 (0.2)

Table 11   Occupational group and number of approved medical malpractice and approved medical malpractice with approved causality for death

Occupational group	Number of approved medical malpractice	Approved medical malpractice with confirmed causality
Clinicians	7.8	3.5
Doctor in private practice	14.7	5.2
Nursing staff	20.3	9.3
Emergency service doctor	11.9	4.7
A group of doctors	12.6	4.0

Table 12   Distribution of malpractice charges by duration and site of treatment

Site of treatment	Treatment day 1	Treatment days 2–5	Treatment >days 5
Hospital	10	45	138
Home visit	58	8	26

Although surgery is the discipline with most accusations of medical malpractice, the rate of confirmed medical malpractice with approved causality is rather low, with 3.1%. Another difference between doctors in private practice and hospital doctors is that the interval between beginning of treatment and claim of medical malpractice is comparatively short in the case of doctors in private practice but longer in hospital doctors (Table 12). Apparently, death after short outpatient consultations place physicians at higher risk for malpractice charges.

In prospective clinical studies, medication errors make up a great part of AEs; medication errors are, however, underrepresented in other files of medical malpractice.

Adverse Drug Events

In epidemiological studies on adverse events, the most frequently seen iatrogenic injuries are nosocomial infections and adverse drug events [32, 59, 60]. However, these complications are not found in a comparable frequency in the files of the Institutes of Forensic Medicine, arbitration committees, liability

and nursing staff, the rate of approved medical malpractice is 14.7 and 20.3%, respectively, much higher than for clinicians.

Table 13 Results of medical malpractice proceedings

	Ulsenheimer	Althoff/ Solbach 1984 (Aachen)	Mallach *et al.* 1993 (Tübingen)	Peters 2000 (Düsseldorf)[a]	Orben 2004	Bonn 2005[a]
Total	245	90	410	194 (297 accused)	601 (751 accused)	210 accused
Closing or acquittal	162 (66.1%)	80 (88.9%)	358 (87.3%)	89%	709 (94.4%)	183 (87.1%)
Sentence or settlement based on Section 153a StPO	66 (26.9%)	10 (11.1%)	52 (12.7%)	6%	42% (5.6%)	16 (7.6%)

[a] Partially the proceedings have been settled otherwise or have not yet been closed at the moment of data collection
Most preliminary proceedings are closed according to Section 170 Abs. 2 Strafprozessordnung (StPO; code of criminal procedure); that means that either no medical malpractice is evident, or the causal connection could not be proved with certainty. Only in 5–12% the doctor is either sentenced or the preliminary criminal proceeding is closed according to Section 153 a StPO (payment of an administrative fine). The higher frequency of sentences or settlement after paying an administrative fine in the material of Ulsenheimer (Table 13) is due to the fact that he, as a specialized solicitor, sees only cases that are quite severe

insurance companies, and health insurance companies [61–67].

Adverse drug reaction is a noxious and unintended response to a drug occurring at a conventional dose and used for disease in prophylaxis, diagnosis, therapy, or modification of physiological functions.

Adverse drug event is an adverse drug reaction and/or event caused by medication errors.

For instance, on the basis of a Scandinavian study [59], 50 000 lethal cases of adverse drug reactions would be expected in Germany just for hospitalizations in internal medicine; 28 000 fatal outcomes would be classified as preventable [60]. Obviously, there is a large gap between the frequency of fatalities based on epidemiological studies and those coming to the public attention. The types of medical malpractice in drug therapy are [65, 66] as follows:

- disregarding drug allergy
- mix-up of electrolyte solutions (KCl instead of NaCl)
- inadequate substitution of drug addicts
- wrong dose, especially in renal insufficiency, when antineoplastic drugs are given
- wrong administration of drugs (e.g., intrathecal administration of Vincristin when simultaneously different chemotherapeutics are given).

The typical patients in fatal adverse drug events are old, multidiseased patients using multiple drugs

already on arrival at the hospital, very often receiving an additional four or more drugs during hospitalization. These patients have very frequently combined severe cardiac and pulmonary diseases.

Outcome of Medical Malpractice Claims

Not only are clear epidemiological data on the international frequency of medical malpractice claims missing from the literature but data on the outcome of such claims are also absent. For Germany, cases dealt with at the arbitration committees are well documented, and the success rate for medical malpractice claims is about 30% (see also Table 2 and Figures 5–8). In penal law, most preliminary criminal proceedings are closed according to Section 170 code of criminal procedure (i.e., that fault was either ruled out or could not be proved). Thus, there is either no medical malpractice, or the causal connection between medical malpractice and fatal outcome could not be proved with the necessary certainty [38, 68–71] (Table 12).

Conclusions

AEs in medical malpractice have gained importance because of their frequency as well as the socioeconomic costs and public and political attention. Organizations such as the Council of Europe or World

Health Organization have published recommendations on management of patient safety and prevention of AEs in health care [8, 13].

According to recent surveys of the German Alliance of Patient Safety among hospitalized patients, AEs can be expected in 5–10% of patients, PAEs in 2–4%, NAEs in 1%, and lethal outcome in about 0.1% [33–35].

Medical malpractice claims dealt with at the German arbitration committees are successful for the patient in one-third of the cases. The files of the Institutes of Forensic Medicine are indispensable for the epidemiology of AEs and improvement of patient safety for several reasons [58]:

First, the most dramatic cases are perhaps seen in forensic medicine – death due to medical malpractice[5, 6];
Second, since most studies on adverse events focus on hospitalized patients, the files of the forensic institutes cover the ambulant sector of health care as well.

Forensic pathologists can also contribute to an increase in patient safety since malpractice claims can provide a rich source of data concerning a small number of serious events [72]. A thorough evaluation of serious incidents, although less sophisticated than a root cause analysis, produces far more information than a usual hospital reporting system. Identification and evaluation of errors as well as reporting of errors may also contribute to the prevention of errors. This, among other medical disciplines, is also a task of forensic medicine [13].

References

[1]   Dettmeyer, R., Preuß, J. & Madea, B. (2004). Malpractice – role of the forensic pathologist in Germany, *Forensic Science International* **144**, 265–267.

[2]   Wagner, H.J. (1981). Zur historischen Entwicklung des Berichts "Ärztlicher Kunstfehler", *Zeitschrift Für Rechtsmedizin* **56**, 303–306.

[3]   Virchow, R. (1870). *Kunstfehler der Ärzte*. Aktenstücke des Reichstags des Norddeutschen Bundes 5, 12–15, Berlin.

[4]   Kohn, L.T., Corrigan, J.M. & Donaldson, M.S. (eds) (2001). *To Err is Human. Building a Safer Health System*, National Academy Press, Washington, DC.

[5]   Madea, B. & Dettmeyer, R. (2006). Behandlungsfehler und Medizinschadensfälle – nicht nur ein Thema der Rechtsmedizin, *Editorial Rechtsmedizin* **16**, 353–354.

[6]   Madea, B. & Dettmeyer, R. (2007). *Medizinschadensfälle und Patientensicherheit. Häufigkeit, Begutachtung, Prophylaxe*, Deutscher Ärzteverlag, Köln.

[7]   Gutachten (2003). des Sachverständigenrates für die Konzertierte Aktion im Gesundheitswesen. Bundesrat-Drucksacke 143/03 vom 26.02.2003. Band I, Kapitel 4, S 131 ff.

[8]   Council of Europe, Committee of Ministers (2006). *Recommendations REC7 of the Committee of Ministers to Member States on Medical Management of Patient Safety and Prevention of Adverse Events in Health Care*. http://www.coe.int/T/E/Social_Cohesion/Health. Cited 23 Oct 2006.

[9]   Holzer, E., Thomeczek, C., Hauke, E., Conen, D. & Hochreithener, M.A. (2005). *Patientensicherheit. Leitfaden für den Umgang mit Risiken im Gesundheitswesen*. Facultas, Wien.

[10]   Merry, A. & McCall Smith, A. (2001). *Errors, Medicine and the Law*, Cambridge University Press.

[11]   Thomeczek, C., Bock, W., Conen, D., Ekkernkamp, A., Everz, D., Fischer, G., Gerlach, F., Gibis, B., Gramsch, E., Jonitz, G., Klakow-Franck, R., Oesingmann, U., Schirmer, H.-D., Smentkowski, U., Ziegler, M. & Ollenschläger, G. (2004). Das Glossar Patientensicherheit – Ein Beitrag zur Definitionsbestimmung und zum Verständnis der Thematik "Patientensicherheit" und "Fehler in der Medizin", *Gesundheitswesen* **66**, 833–840.

[12]   Thomeczek, C., Rohe, J. & Ollenschläger, G. (2007). Das unerwünschte Ereignis in der Medizin, in *Medizinschadensfälle und Patientensicherheit. Häufigkeit – Begutachtung – Prophylaxe*, B. Madea & R. Dettmeyer (Hrsg) Deutscher Ärzte-Verlag, Köln, 13–20.

[13]   World Alliance of Patient Safety (WHO) (2005). *Draft Guidelines for Adverse Event Reporting and Learning Systems*. http://www.who.int/patientsafety/events/05/Reporting_Guidelines.pdf.

[14]   Bennett, R.G., O'Sullivan, J., DeVito, E.M. & Remsburg, R. (2000). The increasing medical malpractice risk related to pressure ulcers in the United States, *Journal of the American Geriatrics Society* **48**, 73–81.

[15]   Brennan, T.A., Leape, L.L., Laird, N.M., Localio, R.A. & Hiatt, H.H. (1990). Incidence of adverse events and negligent care in hospitalized patients, *Transactions of the Association of American Physicians* 137–144.

[16]   Brennan, T.A., Leape, L.L., Laird, N.M., Hebert, L., Localio, A.R., Lawthers, A.G., Newhouse, J.P., Weiler, P.C. & Hiatt, H.H. (1991). Incidence of adverse events and negligence in hospitalized patients. Results of the Harvard Medical Practice Study I, *New England Journal of Medicine* **324**(6), 370–376.

[17]   Brennan, T.A., Sox, C.M. & Burstin, H.R. (1996). Relation between negligent adverse events and the outcomes of medical-malpractice litigation, *New England Journal of Medicine* **335**(26), 1963–1967.

[18]   Brennan, T.A. (2000). The Institute of Medicine report on medical errors – could it do harm? *New England Journal of Medicine* **342**(15), 1123–1125.

[19] Brenner, J.R., Lucey, L.L., Smith, J.J. & Saunders, R. (1998). Radiology and medical malpractice claims: a report on the practice standards claims survey of the physician insurers association of America and the American college of radiology, *American Journal of Radiology* **171**, 19–22.

[20] Chopra, V., Bovill, J.G. & Spierdijk, J. (1990). Accidents, near accidents and complications during anaesthesia, *Anaesthesia* **45**, 3–6.

[21] Dean, B., Schachter, M., Vincent, C. & Barber, N. (2002). Causes of prescribing errors in hospital inpatients: a prospective study, *The Lancet* **359**, 1373–1378.

[22] Dean, B., Schachter, M., Vincent, C. & Barber, N. (2002). Prescribing errors in hospital inpatients: their incidence and clinical significance, *Quality and Safety in Health Care* **11**, 340–344.

[23] Ebbesen, J., Buajordet, I., Erikssen, J., Brors, O., Hilberg, T., Svaar, H. & Sandvik, L. (2001). Drug-related deaths in a department of internal medicine, *Archives of Internal Medicine* **161**, 2317–2323.

[24] Karcz, A., Holbrook, J., Auerbach, B., Blau, M.I., Bulat, P.I., Davidson, A., Docimo, A.B., Doyle, M.J., Erdos, M.S., Friedmann, M., Green, E.D., Hobbs, E.T., Iseke, R.J., Josephson, G.W., Kline, J., Moyer, P., Shea, D.J., Soslow, A.R., Testarmata, A.M. & Woodward, A.C. (1990). Preventability of malpractice claims in emergency medicine: a closed claims study, *Annals of Emergency Medicine* **19**(8), 865–873.

[25] Karcz, A., Korn, R., Burke, M.C., Caggiano, R., Doyle, M.J., Erdos, M.J., Green, E.D. & Williams, K. (1996). Malpractice claims against emergency physicians in Massachusetts: 1975–1993, *American Journal of Emergency Medicine* **14**(4), 341–345.

[26] Leape, L.L. (2000). Institute of medicine medical errors figures are not exaggerated, *Journal of the American Medical Association* **284**, 95–98.

[27] Leape, L.L. (2002). Reporting of adverse events, *New England Journal of Medicine* **347**(20), 1633–1638.

[28] Leape, L.L., Brennan, T.A., Laird, N.M., Lawthers, A.G., Localio, A.R., Barnes, B.A., Hebert, L., Newhouse, J.P., Weiler, P.C. & Hiatt, H. (1991). The nature of adverse events in hospitalized patients: results of the Harvard Medical Practice Study II, *New England Journal of Medicine* **324**(6), 377–384.

[29] Leape, L.L., Lawthers, A.G., Brennan, T.A. & Johnson, W.G. (1993). Preventing medical injury, *Quality Review Bulletin* 144–149.

[30] Leape, L.L., Bates, D.W., Cullen, D.J., Cooper, J., Demonaco, H.J., Gallivan, P.T., Hallisey, R., Ives, J., Laird, N., Laffel, G., Nemeskal, R., Petersen, L., Porter, K., Servi, D., Shea, B.F., Small, S.D., Sweitzer, B.J., Thomson, B.T. & Vander Vliet, M. (1995). System analysis of adverse drug events, *Journal of the American Medical Association* **274**, 35–43.

[31] Leape, L.L., Epstein, A.M. & Hamel, M.B. (2002). A series on patient safety, *New England Journal of Medicine* **347**(16), 1272–1274.

[32] Pirmohamed, M., James, S., Meakin, S., Grenn, C., Scott, A.K., Walley, T.J., Farrar, K., Park, B.K. & Breckenridge, A.M. (2004). Adverse drug reactions as cause of admission to hospital: prospective analysis of 18 820 patients, *British Medical Journal* **329**, 15–19.

[33] Schrappe, M. (2006). *Aktionsbündnis Patientensicherheit*. Agenda Patientensicherheit 2006.

[34] Schrappe, M. (2007). *Aktionsbündnis Patientensicherheit*. Agenda Patientensicherheit 2007.

[35] Schrappe, M. & Lessing, C. (2007). Zur Häufigkeit von Medizinschadensfällen, in *Medizinschadensfälle und Patientensicherheit. Häufigkeit – Begutachtung – Prophylaxe*, B. Madea & R. Dettmeyer (Hrsg), eds, Deutscher Ärzte-Verlag, Köln, pp. 21–32.

[36] Studdert, D.M., Thomas, E.J., Burstin, H.R., Zbar, B.I.W., Orav, E.J. & Brennan, T.A. (2000). Negligent care and malpractice claiming behaviour in Utah and Colorado, *Medical Care* **38**(3), 250–260.

[37] Thomeczek, C. & Ollenschläger, G. (2006). Fehlermeldesysteme – aus jedem Fehler auch ein Nutzen? Bedeutung von Fehler-und "Incident-Reporting-Systems "in Industrie und Medizin, *Rechtsmedizin* **16**, 355–360.

[38] Orben, S.T. (2004). *Rechtliche Verantwortung für Behandlungsfehler. Hallesche Schriften zum Recht*, Carl Heymanns Verlag KG, Köln, Band 19.

[39] Berner, B. (2007). Tätigkeit der Gutachterkommissionen und Schlichtungsstellen in Deutschland, in *Medizinschadensfälle und Patientensicherheit. Häufigkeit – Begutachtung – Prophylaxe*, B. Madea & R. Dettmeyer (Hrsg), eds, Deutscher Ärzte-Verlag, Köln, pp. 33–38.

[40] Hansis, M.L. & Hansis, D.E. (2001). *Der ärztliche Behandlungsfehler*. 2 Aufl. ecomed Landsberg.

[41] Hansis, M.L. & Hart, D. (2001). Medizinische Behandlungsfehler in Deutschland, *Gesundheitsberichterstattung des Bundes* **4**, 1–15.

[42] Weidinger, P. (2007). Behandlungsfehlervorwürfe und Regulierungspraxis der Haftpflichtversicherer, in *Medizinschadensfälle und Patientensicherheit. Häufigkeit – Begutachtung – Prophylaxe*, B. Madea & R. Dettmeyer (Hrsg), eds, Deutscher Ärzte-Verlag, Köln, pp. 39–52.

[43] Bundesärztekammer (2005). Tätigkeitsbericht 2005. Kapitel 7, Ärztliche Berufsausübung, 368–370. For further information see also: Statistische Daten der BÄK. http://www.baek.de/downloads/ gutachterkommissionenstatistik2006.pdf.

[44] Carstensen, G. (1990). Erfahrungen einer ärztlichen Gutachterkommission bei Behandlungsfehlern, *Zeitschrift für die Gesamte Versicherungswirtschaft* **79**, 42–53.

[45] Dettmeyer, R. & Madea, B. (2001). Iatrogene Schäden, Behandlungsfehler und Behandlungsfehlerbegutachtung, in *Handbuch Gerichtliche Medizin*, B. Madea & B. Brinkmann, eds, Springer-Verlag, Berlin-Heidelberg, New York, Tokio, Bd. 2, pp. 1457–1492.

[46] Eissler, M. (2004). Auswertung der Ergebnisse der Gutachterkommission für Fragen ärztlicher Haftpflicht bei der Landesärztekammer Baden-Württemberg für das Jahr 2002, *MedR Medizinrecht* 429–433.

[47] Eissler, M. (2005). Die Ergebnisse der Gutachterkommissionen und Schlichtungsstellen in Deutschland – ein bundesweiter Vergleich, *MedR Medizinrecht* **23**(5), 280–282.

[48] Laum, H.D. & Beck, L. (2003). Großes Interesse im Ausland an außergerichtlicher Schlichtung – Gutachterkommission für ärztliche Behandlungsfehler bei der Ärztekammer Nordrhein zieht positive Bilanz des Berichtszeitraums 2001/2002 – Kürzere Dauer der Verfahren, *Rheinisches Ärzteblatt* **57**, 19–20.

[49] Laum, H.D. & Beck, L. (2007). Vertrauensbeweis von Patienten und Ärzten. Die Ergebnisstatistik der Gutachterkommission spricht für die weiterhin hohe Akzeptanz ihrer Arbeit bei den Verfahrensbeteiligten, *Rheinisches Ärzteblatt* **1**, 15–18.

[50] Merten, M. (2007). Risikomanagement. Den Ursachen auf der Spur, *Deutsches Ärzteblatt* **104**, A1140–A1142.

[51] Bove, K.E. & Iery, C. (2004). The role of the autopsy in medical malpractice cases. I. A review of 99 appeals court decisions, *Archives of Pathology and Laboratory Medicine* **126**, 1023–1031.

[52] Dettmeyer, R., Egl, M. & Madea, B. (2005). Medical malpractice charges in Germany – role of the forensic pathologist in the preliminary criminal proceeding, *Journal of Forensic Sciences* **50**, 423–427.

[53] Kirch, W. & Schafii, C. (1996). Misdiagnosis at a university hospital in four medical eras, *Medicine (Baltimore)* **75**(1), 29–40.

[54] Kirch, W., Shapiro, F. & Fölsch, U.R. (2004). Health care quality: misdiagnosis at a university hospital in five medical eras. Autopsy-confirmed evaluation of 500 cases between 1959 and 1999/2000: a follow-up study, *Journal of Public Health* **12**, 154–161.

[55] Kricher, T., Nelson, J. & Burdo, H. (1985). The autopsy as a measure of accuracy of the death certificate, *New England Journal of Medicine* **313**, 1263 ff.

[56] Madea, B. & Dettmeyer, R. (2003). Ärztliche Leichenschau und Todesbescheinigung, *Deutsches Ärztebl* **100**, A3161–A3179.

[57] Preuß, J., Dettmeyer, R. & Madea, B. (2006). Begutachtung behaupteter letaler Behandlungsfehler im Fach Rechtsmedizin. Bundesweite Multicenterstudie, *Rechtsmedizin* **16**, 367–382.

[58] Preuß, J., Dettmeyer, R. & Madea, B. (2005). *Begutachtung Behaupteter Letaler und Nicht Letaler Behandlungsfehler im Fach Rechtsmedizin. Bundesweite Multicenterstudie im Auftrag des Bundesministeriums für Gesundheit und Soziales (BMGS)*. http://www.bmg.bund .de/cln_041/nn_599776/sid_22070317BA8CF91EC8A7 A1BA5BEAD9D7/SharedDocs/Publikationen/ Forschungsberichte/f-338,param=.html_nnn=true.

[59] Erster Deutscher Kongress für Patientensicherheit bei medikamentöser Therapie. Focus: Arzneimitteltherapie im Krankenhaus. 19.-20. April 2005,. Saarbrücken, unter anderem mit folgenden Vorträgen: Erikksen J: Tod durch Arzneimitteltherapie im Krankenhaus – Ergebnis und Konsequenzen der norwegischen Studie. Bates D: Medikamentionsfehler nicht negieren sondern vermeiden: Praxiserprobte Konzepte am Brigham and Womans Hospital in Boston – einem der 10 besten Krankenhäuser der USA.

[60] Schurrer, J.U. & Frölich, J.C. (2003). Zur Häufigkeit und Vermeidbarkeit von tödlichen unerwünschten Arzneimittelwirkungen, *Internist* **44**, 889–895.

[61] Lauterberg, J. & Mertens, A. (2007). Behandlungsfehler-Management in der Gesetzlichen Krankenversicherung am Beispiel der AOK, in *Medizinschadensfälle und Patientensicherheit. Häufigkeit – Begutachtung – Prophylaxe*, B. Madea & R. Dettmeyer (Hrsg), eds, Deutscher Ärzte-Verlag, Köln, pp. 57–64.

[62] Lignitz, E. & Mattig, W. (1989). *Der Iatrogene Schaden*, Akademie-Verlag, Berlin.

[63] Madea, B. (1994). Adverse drug reaction and medical malpractice, *Proceedings of the 16th Congress International Academy of Legal Medicine and Social Medicine*, Springer, Berlin.

[64] Madea, B. (1996). Rechtliche Aspekte der Arzneimitteltherapie – Aufklärung über Arzneimittel – Neben- und Wechselwirkungen, in *Innere Medizin und Recht*, B. Madea, U.J. Winter, M. Schwonzen & D. Radermacher (Hrsg), eds, Blackwell Wissenschaftsverlag, Berlin-Wien, pp. 28–49.

[65] Madea, B., Hennsge, C. & Lignitz, E. (1994). Fahrlässige Tötung durch medikamentöse therapie, *Rechtsmedizin* **4**, 123–131.

[66] Madea, B., Preuß, J., Musshoff, F. & Dettmeyer, R. (2006). Behandlungsfehlervorwürfe bei Arzneimitteltherapie – Gutachterliche Aspekte, in *Kausalität. Forensische Medizin, Toxikologie, Biologie, Biomechanik und Recht*, G. Kauert, D. Mebs & P. Schmidt (Hrsg), eds, Berliner Wissenschaftsverlag, pp. 77–99.

[67] Thomsen, H. (2006). Behandlungsfehler und Risikomanagement im AOK Institut Medizinschaden, *Rechtsmedizin* **16**, 361–366.

[68] Madea, B., Vennedey, Ch., Dettmeyer, R. & Preuß, J. (2006). Ausgang strafrechtlicher Ermittlungsverfahren gegen Ärzte wegen Verdachts eines Behandlungsfehlers, *The Deutsche Medizinische Wochenschrift* **131**(38), 2073–2078.

[69] Madea, B., Preuß, J., Vennedey, Ch. & Dettmeyer, R. (2007). Begutachtung von Behandlungsfehlervorwürfen im Strafverfahren, in *Medizinschadensfälle und Patientensicherheit. Häufigkeit – Begutachtung – Prophylaxe*, B. Madea & R. Dettmeyer (Hrsg), eds, Deutscher Ärzte-Verlag, Köln, pp. 105–120.

[70] Ulsenheimer, K. (1987). Ein gefährlicher Beruf: Strafverfahren gegen Ärzte, *Medizinrecht* **5**, 207–216.

[71] Ulsenheimer, K. (2007). Risikomanagement als Schadensprophylaxe aus der Sicht des Juristen, in *Medizinschadensfälle und Patientensicherheit. Häufigkeit – Begutachtung – Prophylaxe*, B. Madea & R. Dettmeyer (Hrsg), eds, Deutscher Ärzte-Verlag, Köln, pp. 185–196.

[72] Dettmeyer, R., Driever, F., Becker, A., Wiestler, O.D. & Madea, B. (2001). Fatal myeloencephalopathy due to

accidental intrathecal vincristin administration – a report of two cases, *Forensic Science International* **122**, 60–64.

[73]   Knight, B. (1992). Legal Aspects of Medical Practice. *Churchhill Livingstone, Edinburgh.*

Further Reading

Faure, M. & Koziol, H. (Hrsg.) (eds) (2003). *Cases on Medical Malpractice in a Comparative Perspective*, Springer-Verlag, Heidelberg-Berlin.

Madea, B. & Waider, H. (1995). Ärztliche Offenbarungspflicht iatrogener Schädigungen, *Fortschritte der Medizin* **113**, 247–149.

Related Articles

Expert Opinion in Court: Civil Law Jurisdictions (France, Germany, Italy, and Spain)
Malpractice Actions against Experts

BURKHARD MADEA

Medical Records *see* Mental Status: Examination

Medical Treatment: Capacity to Consent to *see* Capacity to Consent to Medical Treatment

Memory *see* Deception: Truth Serum, Eyewitness Testimony

Memory: Adult *see* Eyewitness: Suggestibility of

Memory: Reconstructive

Memories Are Not Fixed

When we try to remember the past, we do not replay an event like a video camera might do. Memories are also not like books stored on a shelf, only to be opened and read the same each time. Rather we "reconstruct" what happened, sometimes by drawing inferences about what happened, or piecing together information that seems plausible. This is why memory is referred to as *reconstructive* in nature. Reconstruction is the process by which people build a memory of a past event at the time they are trying to remember it.

Sir Frederic C. Bartlett was one of the first researchers to champion the reconstructive nature of memory, as is described in his classic 1932 book *Remembering* [1]. To demonstrate how memory was a reconstructive process he had subjects read an unusual story and then asked them to recall it from memory at varying intervals that ranged from minutes to hours or even years. Sometimes he asked people to tell the story to another person, who told it to another and so on. Bartlett found that the story was often not well remembered, and that people made systematic errors when they tried to recall it or tell it to someone else. For example, they tried to make the story more coherent than it really was, and they often added details that were not part of the original story. He also found that as subjects reconstructed the story from memory, accurate recall was the exception rather than the rule.

Bartlett's experiments challenged the belief that memories were stored as static unchanging traces in the brain and that recall meant merely reexciting, or stimulating, these traces. The act of remembering is the end result of a complex process that begins when information is first presented and is stored in the mind. That complex process involves a number of stages that are fundamental to how memory works.

How Memory Works

There are three essential stages in the memory process: acquisition, retention, and retrieval [2]. Acquisition is the first stage: when an individual first experiences an event, devotes attention to it, and encodes it into memory. Retention is the second stage and it refers to the passage of time that occurs between the original event and recollection of the event. The final stage of the process is retrieval, when the individual tries to remember the event (or reconstruct it). Errors can enter memory at any or all of these three stages.

During the acquisition stage, errors can be introduced when details of the event are not properly encoded and stored in long-term memory. In order to recall an event, an individual must first devote attention to it. When a person distorts information at the acquisition stage, the errors are sometimes called *constructive* errors. With poor lighting or long distances or a minimal chance to view the material, errors are more likely to occur.

Errors can also occur during the retention stage of memory. The length of time that passes between the initial encoding of an event and the recall of that event affects how much detail will be recalled. In 1885, Ebbinghaus conducted classic experiments documenting how recall deteriorates over time [3]. Using only himself as a subject, Ebbinghaus memorized lists of non-sense syllables and tested his recall over time. He found that forgetting occurs rapidly at first and then becomes more gradual as time goes on; these results were then plotted onto his now famous "forgetting curve".

The passage of time weakens our memory for an event and makes us more susceptible to errors. One way that errors can be introduced is through the acquisition of misleading information, a phenomenon known as the *misinformation effect* [4]. In studies of the misinformation effect, subjects witness a complex event such as a car accident and half are subsequently provided with misleading information about the event. In one study that used a car accident as the target event, participants in the misinformation group were given the suggestion that the traffic sign seen in the event was a yield sign instead of the stop sign that was actually seen. When later asked to provide a description of the initial event, participants who received the misleading information were less accurate than those who had not been exposed to any misinformation. These participants incorrectly claimed that they had seen a yield sign. The longer the time interval between witnessing the event and the introduction of the misinformation, the more memory for the initial event was impaired.

At the retrieval stage, memory for the target event can be altered by the way that questions are worded [2]. Even the change of a single word can affect memory for an event. In one study, participants were shown a short film of a car crash and then were given a questionnaire about the events that they had just seen. When participants were asked, "Did you see the broken headlight"?, significantly more of the participants reported that they had seen the broken headlight, a detail that was not in the film, than when participants were asked, "Did you see a broken headlight"? The change from "a" to "the" makes a significant difference because the use of the word "the" suggests that the item exists.

In another study on the influence of question wording, participants watched an automobile accident and then were asked about the speed of the cars involved in the accident. A question like "How fast were the cars going when they smashed into each other"? led to higher estimates of speed than the question "How fast were the cars going when they hit each other"? Moreover, the "smashed" question led people to be more likely to claim that they saw broken glass in the accident, a detail that did not occur. It is also important to note that once an individual recalls an event in a particular way, this is the new construction of the event.

These errors reveal something about the reconstructive nature of memory. When people hear the word "smashed", it is commensurate with a severe accident, one that occurred at higher speeds, and thus they infer that the speed was higher. Moreover, since broken glass is often associated with severe accidents they may infer that it occurred and think, in this case wrongly, that they saw it.

Another line of work that shows the reconstructive nature of memory is work on "pragmatic inference" [5]. A pragmatic inference is an assertion that leads people to believe that they experienced something that was not actually experienced. When people were presented with a statement like "The karate champion hit the cement block", they will often remember hearing "The karate champion broke the cement block". This is not a logical inference; the champ could have hit the block but not broken it. However, many people will draw the inference and misremember what they heard.

People also can come to remember autobiographical events that never happened. These wholly fabricated incidents are known as *rich false memories* [4].

In one study, the relatives of subjects created scenarios and implanted false memories of being lost for an extended time in a shopping mall and being rescued by an elderly person, at the age of six. This procedure for planting false memories has come to be known as the *lost-in-the-mall* technique. Using strong suggestion, people have been led to remember falsely that they were lost as a child, that they were attacked by an animal, or that they nearly drowned and had to be rescued by a lifeguard.

Rich false memories can also be planted through the use of other techniques such as guided imagination, suggestive dream interpretation, hypnosis, and the use of doctored photographs. These techniques have produced false memories in approximately 30% of the people who receive the suggestion. One criticism of the memory implantation studies is that the participants may be recalling actual memories, not false ones. In order to counter this criticism, researchers have successfully demonstrated that people can also be given impossible memories like meeting Bugs Bunny at Disneyland.

Source monitoring errors also highlight the reconstructive nature of memory. Source monitoring errors refer to the phenomenon of recalling someone or something but forgetting the source of the original object of recall [6]. For example, you may recognize a face but be unable to remember where you first encountered the person. In most cases, this failure to recall the source of the original memory does not have major implications, but for those accused of criminal acts, the consequences can be quite serious. In one known case, a psychologist was accused of rape based on the victim's detailed recollection of her attacker [3]. He was later cleared when it was discovered that he was on live television at the time, which the victim was watching during her attack. She recalled his face clearly but had misattributed the source.

Errors of source attribution can also occur when we are attempting to create something wholly our own. *Cryptomnesia* refers to the act of unknowingly attributing the work of someone else to oneself [3]. Without meaning to, people occasionally plagiarize other works or adopt the memories of other people as their own. Carl Jung reported on this phenomenon in the early 1900s noting that Friedrich Nietzsche had taken part of a story written by the German physician and poet Kerner. In a more recent case, Kaavya Viswanathan, a Harvard sophomore and author, claimed that her plagiarism from two novels by Megan McCafferty was entirely unconscious and unintentional.

On occasion, we sometimes unintentionally adopt the memories of siblings or close others. Common memories that have been adopted from someone else are for achievements or suffered misfortunes. We recall these events as happening to us, and are genuinely surprised when we discover that these memories are not ours. The memories that we are least likely to appropriate are those pertaining to wrongdoing, perhaps because of our self-serving biases. The adoption of another person's memory is not an intentional act but rather, it reflects the reconstructive nature of memory and how errors can insert themselves in our recollections. Knowing that these errors can occur unintentionally should make us less irritated and more forgiving when we observe them.

To reiterate, memories may sometimes become less clear over time, but they also change for other reasons. They are continually constructed and reconstructed, and for these reasons will often differ from genuine reality. Unfortunately, without independent objective corroboration, there is no way to assess whether a memory is accurate or not.

Applications

The courtroom is one arena where the reconstructive nature of memory is apparent. Eyewitnesses are frequently the cornerstone of the prosecution's case against a defendant, and provide compelling evidence to jurors (*see* **Eyewitness Testimony**; **Interrogative Suggestibility**; **Memory: Repressed**; **Eyewitness: Suggestibility of**). Yet eyewitness testimony is often mistaken, and such mistakes can be disastrous. Analyses of wrongful convictions, where individuals have been exonerated on the basis of DNA, have shown that the major cause is faulty eyewitness memory [7]. When a witness takes the stand and professes certainty about the defendant's guilt, it is powerful evidence. Unfortunately, confidence is not equal to accuracy and confidence can be inflated by many factors. One such factor is confirmatory feedback. When an individual is given positive feedback about the identification that they have made, they become more confident about their choice. The feedback need not even be verbal, as in a remark "Good job, you picked the suspect". Even a nod can serve as positive feedback, and artificially inflate a witness's confidence, making them more compelling when they testify in court.

Rich false memories can also appear in the courtroom. In one case, a sheriff's deputy named Paul Ingram confessed to sexually abusing his daughters and being involved in a satanic cult that involved animal sacrifice and infanticide [8]. Ingram was highly suggestible and was imprisoned despite a lack of evidence indicating that the cult even existed. Sadly, Ingram is not the only individual who has been imprisoned or had a life destroyed by false memories. In the early 1980s, dozens of individuals were swept up in accusations of child abuse involving satanic cults. Most, but not all, of these people have been released from prison but the emotional scars of the accusations remain.

Memory is inherently a reconstructive process, one that works well in most cases but can occasionally result in errors with dire consequences. Since memory errors can have such serious consequences, it is important that we keep in mind that memory is malleable. When we seek to recall, we seek to reconstruct and errors can occur at any stage.

References

[1]   Bartlett, F.C. (1932). *Remembering*, Cambridge University Press, London.

[2]   Loftus, E.F. (1996). *Eyewitness Testimony*, Harvard University Press, Cambridge.

[3]   Schacter, D.L. (2001). *The Seven Sins of Memory: How the Mind Forgets and Remembers*, Houghton Mifflin, Boston.

[4]   Loftus, E.F. (2005). Planting misinformation in the human mind: a 30-year investigation into the malleability of memory, *Learning & Memory* **12**, 361–366.

[5]   Chan, J.C.K. & McDermott, K.B. (2006). Remembering pragmatic inferences, *Applied Cognitive Psychology* **20**(5), 633–639.

[6]   McNally, R.J. (2005). *Remembering Trauma*, The Belknap Press of Harvard University Press, Cambridge.

[7]   Doyle, J.M. (2005). *True Witness: Cops, Courts, Science, and the Battle Against Misidentification*, Palgrave Macmillan, New York.

[8]   Ofshe, R. & Watters, E. (1994). *Making monsters: False memories, Psychotherapy, and Sexual Hysteria*, University of California Press, Berkeley.

TIAMOYO PETERSON AND ELIZABETH F. LOFTUS

Memory: Repressed

Memory, Repressed

The term "repression" was popularized by Sigmund Freud in the late nineteenth century. By Freud's account, repression consisted of individuals making certain events that elicited painful or disruptive effects on the psyche inaccessible as a defense mechanism for the self. Although the term and various definitions of repression have existed for more than a century, there has been essentially no substantial proof that massive repression exists. There are, however, alternative explanations for what looks like "repression". Some individuals do not think about unpleasant experiences and are later reminded of them. This is not repression, but ordinary forgetting and remembering. Moreover, some individuals can have false memories planted in their minds as a result of suggestion, giving the appearance that an event was not being remembered (*see also* **Eyewitness: Suggestibility of**; **Hypnosis and Memory**; **Recollective Accuracy of Traumatic Memories**).

Despite the lack of verifiable proof of massive repression [1, 2], allegations of repression can have dramatic consequences. The existence of repressed and recovered memories became a fierce topic of debate due to alleged cases of childhood sexual abuse (CSA), many of which involved memories recovered by suggestive therapy techniques. A number of these cases resulted in legal battles and families being torn apart. This entry offers a brief overview and history of the repressed memory debate, legal claims and cases that resulted from the debate, and research that has attempted to examine the existence of repression.

Surge in Recovered Memories and their Effects

Media Contribution

Claims of recovered memories of CSA blossomed in the late 1980s and early 1990s. Accusations of CSA, including claims of satanic ritual abuse, peaked in the two-year period of 1991–1992. Since the early 1990s, the number of CSA accusations as a result of recovered memories has steadily declined. The media undoubtedly contributed to the surge in repressed memories that were recovered in therapists' offices throughout North America. A notable case that was brought into the public eye as a result of the media coverage was a murder case involving George Franklin.

In 1990, George Franklin stood trial for a murder that had occurred more than 20 years earlier. Franklin was accused of murdering Susan Nason, a friend of his daughter, Eileen. Although Eileen was 8 years old at the time of her friend's murder, her testimony was key. Eileen testified that she had witnessed her father murder her friend and repressed the memory for 20 years. When her "memory" returned in the late 1980s, she contacted the police. George Franklin was found guilty of murder based solely on Eileen's testimony of her recovered memory. It was the first time that an American citizen had been tried and convicted of a murder on the basis of a recovered memory.[a]

In addition to the media coverage of trials involving recovered memories, a number of people began to write self-help books to assist victims of CSA. One of these books, *The Courage to Heal* by Ellen Bass and Laura Davis, encouraged victims to recover memories of abuse and to confront alleged molesters. There were a number of supporters of *The Courage to Heal*; however, there were also those who criticized its message. The critics contended that it caused widespread harm to many innocent people – both the alleged perpetrators, and the accusers whose lives may have been negatively affected by false accusations. Bass and Davis have no formal training in psychiatry or psychology, and some critics have argued that their book encourages the recovery of memories that may not be true. Because *The Courage to Heal* has sold over 800,000 copies, many people feel that it has contributed greatly to the surge in the number of recovered memory cases by engendering people to embrace their recovered memories, regardless of the existence of corroborative evidence of abuse.

Statute of Limitations

Another development that fueled the controversy over repressed memory concerned changes in how claims of repression were handled by the judicial system. Washington State was the first state to toll the statute of limitations for repressed memory cases. This meant that people with newly recovered memories of CSA had three years from the time of remembering to sue their parents, other relatives, or any alleged molesters. A number of other states followed Washington's example, and as a result, thousands of lawsuits were filed.

Most provisions applicable to victims of CSA fall into the categories of "minority tolling" and "delayed discovery doctrine". A tolling doctrine postpones the date from which a statutory period begins. In the case of minority tolling, a statute might run three years after the child turns 18, the legal age of majority. This delay is thought to be beneficial because some children may not feel comfortable coming forward to report abuse while still under the care of their abuser.

The delayed discovery doctrine has typically been used in cases involving medical malpractice. For example, the statute of discovery would be extended for a patient who had surgery and later realized that her abdominal pain resulted from her doctor failing to remove a sponge during a prior surgery. Thus, at the time it was determined that the sponge was causing the abdominal pain, the statute of limitations for a malpractice suit would begin to accrue. Those in support of applying the delayed discovery doctrine in recovered memory cases purport that such a medical malpractice claim is analogous to an individual who alleges recovery of CSA memories in that the source of their pain would be realized when the memories are recovered. Such an individual would have some number of years from the date they assert the memory was recovered in which to pursue legal action.

Because the statutes of limitations were tolled, a number of victims were able to sue their alleged abusers more easily. As a result, thousands of cases were brought to the courtroom. Soon there became another way in which repressed memories made their appearance in the court. People who were accused of CSA sued their accusers' therapists for planting false memories of childhood abuse that led to the original accusations. In addition, some patients who had "recovered" memories of abuse began to realize that those memories were not true. These patients retracted their claims and many of them sued their therapists. They are categorized into the group known as "Retractors".

Retractors

There have been a number of CSA accusers who have reestablished family relationships and acknowledged that their prior accusations were false. These retractors typically blame their therapists for suggesting to them that they were victims of CSA and for encouraging memory recovery through questionable therapeutic techniques such as guided imagery, "truth serums" (sometimes termed *Amytal interviews*), and hypnosis.

In 1997, a landmark case ensued in which a retractor sued her therapist who helped her "recover" memories of CSA. Ms. Burgus, a patient of Dr. Braun's, originally sought treatment for postpartum depression, but was diagnosed as having multiple personalities. Dr. Braun believed that her symptoms resulted from sexual and ritual abuse including cannibalism and torture. He purported that this abuse was the cause of her forming multiple personalities. Even though Ms. Burgus had no recollection of the sexual and ritual abuse, Dr. Braun encouraged her to try and remember these instances of abuse through hypnosis. Ms. Burgus eventually realized that these allegations were not true. She retracted her previous abuse accusations and sued her former therapists, including Dr. Braun and the hospital. The lawsuit was settled for 10.6 million dollars.

False Memory Syndrome

Although therapy helps a number of people, it can have detrimental effects in cases involving recovered memories. This is particularly true in situations where there is no history of sexual abuse. For example, when a daughter accuses her father of child abuse, the family can be devastated. Often it forces other family members to choose sides; this has caused some families to become torn apart as a result of "recovered" memories (for the landmark legal case in this area see *Ramona v. Ramona*, No. 61898, California Superior Court, Napa County, 1994; reported in Johnston, Moira (1997) *Spectral Evidence*. Boston: Houghton Mifflin).

In addition to causing strain on family life, patients may develop new symptoms unrelated to the primary concern for which the patient sought therapy in the first place. These symptoms include false beliefs and memories of having been abused, a syndrome now referred to as *False Memory Syndrome*. This syndrome is characterized by flashbacks, which include detailed memories, and even hallucinations and delusions of the abuse. Thus, the patient believes that she has specific recollections of abuse that may not have occurred.

Families and professionals who saw the need to prevent the spread of False Memory Syndrome formed an organization in 1992 called the False Memory Syndrome Foundation (FMSF). The FMSF also supports the reconciliation of families who were torn apart by claims of repressed and recovered CSA.

Research in the Field

Like the topic itself, research in the field of repressed and recovered memories has been controversial. There are several different methodologies that have been used to study such alleged memories. The most common types of studies are retrospective, prospective, and case histories. Retrospective studies rely on the self-report of alleged abuse years after the actual event was said to have happened. Prospective studies use later self-reports of alleged abuse, but attempt to corroborate the abuse through various channels such as police reports or social worker reports. Lastly, case histories rely on data collected from an individual's personal experience. In general, most of the data has been collected from women who were alleged victims of CSA.

In one example of a retrospective study, researchers Briere and Conte [3] asked participants, who were recruited by their therapists, if there was ever a time in which they failed to remember their first instance of abuse. Those who reported forgetting the abuse at some point reported that the abuse occurred at a very young age compared to the reported age of the participants who claimed continuous memories of abuse. Overall, more than half of the participants reported that there was some point in time that they did not remember the abuse. However, from this study, it is problematic to conclude that repression exists. Not specifically remembering an event does not necessarily constitute massive repression. In fact, this lack of remembering can easily be accounted for by ordinary forgetting. Because of this, the results of this particular study cannot be satisfactorily interpreted, nor can they be considered adequate proof that memories can be repressed.

Another researcher, Melchert [4], conducted a retrospective study to clarify the confusing findings of earlier studies. In a nonclinical sample of individuals, of those reporting physical, emotional and/or sexual abuse, around half reported that they did not have continuous memories of the abuse. Many participants in this study who claimed to not remember being abused later reported that they either consciously avoided thinking about the abuse, could have remembered the abuse if they had been reminded, or did not realize that the abusive acts against them were in fact abuse until a later time.

Another strategy for examining "repression" involves the use of a prospective design. Here, there is documentation made by an agency or individual (e.g., social worker) at the time of or shortly after the alleged CSA occurred. Some time after the abuse has been reported, individuals are contacted to determine what they remember about their prior claims of abuse.

In a prospective study conducted by Williams [5], women were contacted 17 years after CSA had been reported to authorities. Of these participants, 38% failed to recall the previously reported abuse to the interviewer. Thus, some consider this study to be a prime example of evidence that memories of CSA may be repressed. However, critics assert that participants may have remembered the abuse, but may have not wanted to discuss such an uncomfortable event with the interviewer. Additionally, in this study the younger the participant was at the time of the reported abuse, the less likely they were to remember the incident. This difference in remembering due to age could be explained by childhood amnesia, which is discussed later in this entry. More recently, in another prospective study conducted by Goodman and colleagues [6], only 8% of participants who had previously reported abuse failed to report remembering the abuse at the later interview. Even the rather low percentage could be the result of unwillingness to tell rather than inability to remember.

Another method for examining repression is with individual case histories. Some mental health professionals report on a patient who they claim had a repressed and recovered memory. The case of "Jane Doe" is a famous case history within the field of repressed and recovered memories [7, 8]. In the mid-1980s Jane Doe's parents filed for divorce and engaged in a vicious battle over custodial rights of Jane. As a result of this custody dispute, Jane, who was 6 years old at the time, was psychologically evaluated. A psychiatrist supported the abuse accusation, and Jane's father obtained custody while Jane's mother lost the rights of visitation.

In 1995, when Jane Doe was 17 years old, the same psychiatrist videotaped Jane again. At first Jane failed to remember being abused by her mother and then, during the same videotaped session, she appeared to spontaneously recover memories of the abuse. The psychiatrist asserted that this particular case was solid evidence of traumatic amnesia and recovery of memory. Following this claim, some critics who questioned the validity of this case history investigated other facts surrounding the reported abuse of Jane to determine whether this case offered conclusive evidence for repression. These investigators discovered that Jane had discussed the alleged abuse on many occasions between the first and second video tapings, thus undermining any claim of repression. Additionally, documented facts were brought to light that suggested that Jane may have not been abused by her mother at all.

Alternative Explanations for Repression

There are a number of possible sources from where richly detailed memory reports may come. The reports of victims who have claimed to recover memories could reflect true memories that have simply been forgotten by normal memory processes. The "recovery" of these memories may have been triggered by a retrieval cue. Another explanation is that the memories could reflect lies. Finally, it is possible that these memories are the result of therapists' suggestions and other activities in group therapy sessions that planted false beliefs.

True Memories

Instances where individuals claim to have recovered memories may actually entail ordinary forgetting and remembering. For example, an individual may remember an event that occurred at a much later date that they had not thought of in a long time. This true memory may be brought to mind by a trigger in the environment, such as a particular setting. However, this would be a case of ordinary forgetting and not repression and recovery of a memory. Additionally, failing to think about an event such as sexual abuse for any given amount of time does not necessarily mean that the memory for the event was repressed. In any given case in which a person reports recovering a memory, the statement could be an accurate reflection of the individual's experience; however, it may be an instance of ordinary forgetting.

False Memories

It can be difficult to discriminate true memories from false ones; however, there are a few situations where we can say with near certainty that the reported recovered memory is false. For example, some people have claimed that they remembered abuse inflicted upon them before they were two years old. There have even been people who claim to have recovered memories of abuse that occurred when they were six months old. As adults we do not have concrete and reliable episodic memories for events that occurred in the first couple years of our lives. This phenomenon is known as "childhood amnesia". Therefore, it can be concluded that these very early "memories" are almost certainly false.

For those individuals whose recovered memories cannot be explained by childhood amnesia, research on suggestibility and the malleability of memory may explain their situations. Researchers have shown that humans are rather susceptible to forming false memories. In addition, a number of individuals believe those memories to be true and even embellish upon the details of those false memories. In research where rich false memories have been planted, a significant minority of subjects have been led through suggestion to believe that they had experiences like being lost in a shopping mall [9] or being attacked by a vicious animal [10]. These studies have shown that people are even susceptible to embracing false memories as their own. Once planted, the individual can report the false event with a great deal of detail, confidence, and emotion.

Conclusion

After decades of research in the field, there is little, if any, substantial evidence that massive repression exists. Moreover, there are other possible explanations for what might look like the recovery of a repressed memory. These include ordinary forgetting or being subjected to suggestible circumstances. Given the massive evidence that has been gathered on the malleability of memory, it should not be surprising that at least some individuals who purport they have recovered memories of past abuse may have actually formed false memories.

End Notes

a. George Franklin served six and half years in prison before his conviction was eventually overturned.

References

[1]   Holmes, D.S. (1994). Is there evidence for repression? Doubtful, *The Harvard Mental Health Letter* **10**, 4–6.
[2]   Pope Jr, H.G. & Hudson, J.I. (1995). Can individuals "repress" memories of childhood sexual abuse? An examination of the evidence, *Psychiatric Annals* **25**, 715–719.
[3]   Briere, J. & Conte, J.R. (1993). Self-reported amnesia for abuse in adults molested as children, *Journal of Traumatic Stress* **6**, 21–31.
[4]   Melchert, T.P. (1996). Childhood memory and a history of different forms of abuse, *Professional Psychology: Research and Practice* **27**, 438–446.
[5]   Williams, L.M. (1994). Recall of childhood trauma: a prospective study of women's memories of child sexual abuse, *Journal of Consulting and Clinical Psychology* **62**, 1167–1176.
[6]   Goodman, G.S., Ghetti, S., Quas, J.A., Edelstein, R.S., Alexander, K.W., Redlich, A.D., Cordon, I.M. & Jones, D.P.H. (2003). A prospective study of memory for child sexual abuse: new findings relevant to the repressed-memory controversy, *Psychological Science* **14**, 113–118.
[7]   Loftus, E.F. & Guyer, M.J. (2002). Who abused Jane Doe? The hazards of the single case history, *Skeptical Inquirer* **26**(3), 24–32.
[8]   Loftus, E.F. & Guyer, M.J. (2002). Who abused Jane Doe? The hazards of the single case history, *Skeptical Inquirer* **26**(4), 37–40, 44.
[9]   Loftus, E.F. & Pickrell, J.E. (1995). The formation of false memories, *Psychiatric Annals* **25**, 720–725.
[10]   Porter, S., Yuille, J.C. & Lehman, D.R. (1999). The nature of real, implanted, and fabricated memories for emotional childhood events: Implications for the recovered memory debate, *Law and Human Behavior* **23**(5), 517–537.

Nicci B. Fowler, Kally J. Nelson
and Elizabeth F. Loftus

Memory Accuracy *see*
Recollective Accuracy of Traumatic Memories

Mental Health Courts

Introduction

In a perfect world we should not need mental health courts, let alone a literature about them. But we do. Realistically, in a less than perfect world we should perhaps aspire to see mental health courts as part of our future but not as the full "answer to the problem" as they are currently seen. "The problem" is that over the past 15–20 years the criminal courts have had to contend with ever-increasing numbers of mentally disordered individuals coming through the courthouse doors. This article describes the basics of mental health courts, how they operate, and examines how and why these courts have become an integral part of both the criminal justice and mental healthcare systems.

Background

The provision of mental healthcare services in most Western European and North American communities has witnessed a steady decline over the past number of decades. Beginning with the deinstitutionalization movement occurring in the later half of the twentieth century, adequate mental healthcare services became increasingly scarce. The reality today is no different; mental healthcare systems are generally underfunded and overexpended. There has been a movement toward community-based treatment of major mental illness, which in many instances appears to be insufficient. Despite what was promised, the money saved with the closure of hospitals has typically not been reinvested in community treatment. At the same time, while it is acknowledged that community-based mental healthcare is an important component of the mental healthcare system, it cannot address the needs of many of the more seriously afflicted individuals.

It goes without saying that decreasing mental healthcare services does not lessen the needs of those members of our society who rely on such services. For these individuals closed doors and long-wait lists have offered little. Regrettably, those unable to receive adequate services often find themselves attracting the attention of the criminal justice system, leaving that system to "sort out the mess".

The effects of our emancipated mental healthcare system are varied; however, a site where it has had a particularly acute impact has been the criminal justice system. Being the social safety net of last resort, the criminal justice system has swelled with mentally disordered accused and has struggled to meet the rising demands placed upon it. In some jurisdictions, mentally disordered accused entering the criminal justice system has increased at a rate in excess of 10% per year over the past dozen years [1].

Unfortunately, the criminal justice system has become the surrogate mental healthcare provider in most societies. A *criminalization* of mental illness has occurred: a shifting of responsibility onto the criminal justice system for the provision of basic mental healthcare services.

Understandably, the criminal justice system has not delivered. The criminal justice system was neither designed nor intended to address society's responsibility to the mentally disordered individual. Even a basic familiarity with the traditional criminal justice system will reveal that it is no substitute. Undoubtedly, it is worse. Accused with mental disorders languish in detention centers and correctional facilities. They often fail to receive much needed treatment, typically feel alienated and marginalized, and generally have a difficult time regaining normal functioning once entwined in the system. The regression in treatment and rehabilitation, along with an overreliance on warehousing the mentally ill in penal settings, is a deplorable anachronism that harkens back to before the development of asylum care. Ironically, we presently find ourselves where we were situated 200 years ago trying to get the mentally ill out of the prisons and criminal justice system. We have come full circle.

Mental Health Courts: A Response

Mental health courts are a response to this reality. Recognizing the criminalization process that has occurred, these courts have sought to reverse the misplaced responsibility for the provision of mental

healthcare services. These courts have various objectives, which include the targeting of accused with mental disorders, and have as their mandate one or more of the following objectives:

1. "diversion" of accused who have been charged with minor to moderately serious criminal offenses and offering them an alternative;
2. expediting the pretrial processes of assessing fitness to stand trial;
3. treatment of operative mental disorders; and
4. a slowing of the so-called revolving door.

Through successful participation in a treatment program overseen by a mental health court team, some accused can avoid conviction and sentence, as they are "diverted" back into the civil mental healthcare system. This model is based upon the earlier established drug courts. The court "intervenes" at a discrete point in time along the criminal justice continuum. Some jurisdictions have included diversion as a component of their mental health court but have attempted to also intervene at multiple postarrest junctures and to a much larger population of mentally disordered accused.

Mental Health Courts – A Broadly Defined Category

Despite sharing similar objectives, there are many models that claim the label of a "mental health court". Accordingly, when considering these courts it is important to gain an appreciation for the scope of what is being referred to. Different courts have different (or multiple) entry points in the criminal prosecution process, different entrance requirements, objectives, and outcomes. Nevertheless, very generally speaking, mental health courts are all attempting a rehabilitative response to what would otherwise have been criminally sanctioned behavior. The general philosophy driving this approach is quite simple – the traditional response to aberrant behavior where it is substantially the product of mental disorder is both ineffective and inappropriate.

Therapeutic Jurisprudence

In beginning to appreciate mental health courts, it is necessary to understand the principles of therapeutic jurisprudence (*see* **Therapeutic Jurisprudence**). It is a theory which holds that the law should be administered and applied in a way that incorporates therapeutic goals. It advocates use the justice system in a manner which addresses the underlying factors that may lead an individual to come into contact with the law. It is a vehicle to obtaining a better societal response to proscribed behaviors.

This novel approach to criminal justice has particular relevance to mentally disordered accused in today's society.

We know that many mentally disordered accused often "end up" in the criminal justice system. Often they are charged with minor and nonviolent offenses. Many times the factors that place these accused in the justice system could more effectively be addressed in ways other than imposing traditional criminal justice sanctions. It is this normative foundation that explains why mental health courts often focus on treatment of mental health systems, housing, substance addictions, job training, and other matters in preference to such traditional options as jail, fines, and probation.

Restorative Justice

The creation of mental health courts also resonates with the principles and ideological foundation of the restorative justice movement. Restorative justice is a view of justice that centers on repairing the harm and relational disruption caused by criminal behavior. One of restorative justice's key tenets is to foster the involvement of all stakeholders, including the community, to restore victims and offenders to intact, contributing members of society. Mental health courts play a key role in this restorative process by rerouting accused to both treatment and a place in the community, and by enlisting the community to provide care and supervision for an afflicted individual deserving of both compassion and intervention. Given the frequency with which family and others close to a mentally disordered accused become his or her victims, a therapeutic outcome is more likely to reflect victims' wishes that offenders be dealt with in a compassionate, humane, and ultimately more socially protective way, notwithstanding their having been victimized by the accused.

The First Mental Health Courts

The first mental health courts began as grass root initiatives in the mid-1990s. Early versions, as mentioned above, found inspiration from the success of

drug courts – an emerging brand of court dedicated to accused with substance addictions. On a very basic level, drug courts operate by offering accused an option: avoid serving a sentence for a drug-related offense by completing a drug-treatment program.

As judicial initiatives, drug courts were quickly lauded as helping to break addiction cycles. By adopting principles of therapeutic jurisprudence and focusing upon addiction as opposed to crime, these courts were assisting the participants avoid subsequent drug offenses. The success of the treatment model espoused by drug courts spawned a parallel idea for accused with mental disorders.

Like drug courts, the first mental health courts in the United States found promise in offering treatment instead of punishment. Their ability to effectively remove individuals from the criminal justice system through the provision of services demonstrated an important reality: for many accused, minor offenses may more accurately represent an inability to control or manage their mental health symptoms as opposed to deliberate criminality.

The increasing appeal of specialty courts and a growing awareness that the traditional criminal justice system was failing individuals with mental disorders have combined to legitimize the emergence of mental health courts. And come they have. The onset has been remarkable; despite only appearing within the past decade or so, they now number in excess of 200 within North America alone. Beyond the courts that currently exist, numerous jurisdictions are actively pursuing implementation.

The first known program in Canada that addressed the issue of mentally disordered accused in the criminal justice system appears to have been in Toronto, Ontario, Canada. The "Diversion of Mentally Disordered Accused" became a program that was officially part of the Crown Policy Manual in 1994. This program is most like the programs referred to as "mental health courts" in the United States. In addition to this program, a mental health court has been created to deal with a broader range of issues. Diversion is just one option in the court's range of options and therapeutic armamentarium. The mental health court operating in Toronto houses a diversion program but intervenes at various other postarrest junctures to assist all mentally disordered accused, regardless of the offense charged, whether or not "diversion" will ultimately become an option.

The Operation of a Mental Health Court

Understanding the operation of a mental health court requires an appreciation of both the mental health court team and the eligibility of accused for program participation.

While the "nuts and bolts" of mental health courts will vary, integral to the functioning of a mental health court is a multidisciplinary team approach. Judges and lawyers are supplemented by any number of psychiatrists, psychologists, case workers, and social workers who collaborate on how the particular needs of the accused can effectively be met. The various disciplines represented in these teams form a concentrated resource which facilitates the court's operation.

Each court maintains a formal or informal policy outlining the type of accused eligible for the court. Typically, participation in the "diversion" component of a mental health court is reserved for individuals with mental disorders charged with minor to moderately serious offenses. Nevertheless, certain courts also provide services that do not involve eligibility requirements. As an example, the Toronto mental health court addresses the pretrial issues of fitness to stand trial and treatment of underlying mental disorder for all accused, regardless of the seriousness of the offense. As well, the court may order assessments to determine the issue of criminal responsibility. On a voluntary basis it will also entertain resolutions and bail hearings.

In most mental health courts in the United States, eligible and consenting accused are given a choice: participate in a treatment program and have your criminal charges stayed, dropped, or reduced, or proceed in the regular stream. The treatment program is strictly voluntary, and accused are most often able to opt out at any time. The approach in Canada has been somewhat different. The primary focus is with respect to assessing fitness to stand trial and providing treatment. The accused's participation in this aspect of the court's operation is not voluntary. Thereafter, once fit to stand trial, whether the accused elects to remain with the court for a bail hearing, participate in "diversion", or resolve the matter with a guilty plea is the accused's option.

Accused who elect to participate in the mental health court will typically be required to comply with an individually tailored treatment program designed by the mental health court team.[a] The benefit of a multidisciplinary team is that treatment can take a variety of forms and is not limited to medication, but can include psychological therapies, educational training, occupational training, housing and access to social services, budgetary counseling, etc.

As previously noted, a primary goal of mental health courts is to reconnect and reintegrate individuals in need of treatment to the appropriate services. In this way, mental health courts form bridges to various services within the community. Assisting individuals manage their mental disorders through the provision of mental health and social services reduces the likelihood of subsequent offenses, and in this way mental health courts also seek to curb the disproportionately high rate of recidivism in this segment of the population. With a reduction in recidivism, the courts also make communities safer places to live. There are now studies that support the previously intuitive projection that mental health courts do, indeed, reduce recidivism rates [2].

That the behaviors that resulted in the accused's appearance before the court were not contrived by him or her to be criminal in nature in the usual sense, and more likely reflect one or more mental disorders, is a foundational premise of a mental health court. All of the court's personnel are inevitably guided by the premise that, but for the accused's mental disorder or condition (and attendant socioeconomic decline), he or she would not likely have become involved in the conduct before the court. The corollary to this premise is that no professional or worker from either the legal or mental health arenas should become involved in a mental health court unless he or she is philosophically oriented to a therapeutic outcome, and this is so notwithstanding public protection considerations.

Mental health courts consequently do not share the hard-hitting adversarial atmosphere associated with most criminal courts; actually, mental health courts hardly feel like courts at all. An informal atmosphere aimed at putting the participants at ease and fostering an environment conducive to discussion is a feature common to all mental health courts.

General Observations and Caveats

The recent emergence of mental health courts has transformed the criminal justice landscape for mentally disordered accused. While traditionally one general criminal court served any type of offender, today mental health courts represent one of many specialized "problem-solving" courts in existence to serve specific types of offenders with special needs, including drug courts, domestic violence courts, aboriginal courts, and prostitution courts. The speed with which mental health courts have emerged cannot be understated. A mere 10 years ago none was reported to be in existence, while today well over 200 mental health courts exist in North America alone.

It can be stated that mental health courts have emerged out of frustration and an abhorrence of the realities faced by mentally disordered accused. Lengthy delays for fitness assessments, a cast of courtroom players untrained and/or unfamiliar with the realities of mental illness, and a prison system more prone to exacerbate than to manage, only begin to enumerate the list. These courts are often held to be direct commentaries on the failure of the traditional justice system to meet the needs of mentally disordered accused.

The mental health court movement in North America appears to be proceeding on the assumption that these courts represent the answer. In the United States, a congressional commitment to the funding of an additional 100 mental health courts in 2001 evidences this belief. Currently in Canada there exists a strong impetus in many provinces to create these courts.

Yet, it is ironic that if one were to design the optimal mental healthcare delivery system it is unlikely that too many professionals would conclude that judges, courts, and the criminal justice system at large are the best vehicle. Judges and lawyers as mental health service brokers? Unfortunately, our systems, both the mental health and criminal justice system, are the product of evolution rather than design. They have evolved like any other complex organism. Unable to turn back the clock, the question remains: what of mental health courts? The unfortunate reality is that mentally disordered accused are in ever-increasing numbers dropped at the courthouse door.

It is accepted that there will continue to be a need for mental health courts in the criminal justice system – but hopefully the need will be reduced in the context of our ultimate solution. Even if overhauls of the mental healthcare system reduce the numbers of mentally disordered accused coming in to the criminal justice system as they are presently recognized, it is clear that the courts should endeavor to respond more appropriately to this population.

Mental health courts may be the mechanism for that better response within the criminal justice system.

The question to ask then is how to proceed; how, and what, should we learn from the short existence of mental health courts? A distillation of the accumulating literature [3] permits a listing of the features of mental health courts which should be avoided, those which we should strive to include, and general observations regarding mental health court's role in the justice system.

Mental health courts did not emerge in a vacuum. They represent an evolutionary response to an escalating need to deal more effectively with the growing numbers of mentally ill entering the criminal justice system. Their existence is a reflection of decades of erosion of the civil mental healthcare system's ability to completely fulfill its role and a testament to the expression "necessity is the mother of invention."

Mental health courts are an example of the justice system's ability to respond to a societal problem in a nontraditional, yet more effective, manner. The traditional punishment-based response of the criminal justice system to individuals who are in need of correction has failed both society and the mentally disordered accused and is, in fact, counterproductive. As an example of therapeutic jurisprudence, mental health courts attempt to get at the underlying root causes of undesirable behavior. They are an example of therapeutic jurisprudence in action.

Mental health courts should have no "entrance ticket" other than a willingness on the part of the accused to attempt change. It is inappropriate to require an accused entering a diversion program to enter a guilty plea or to accept criminal responsibility. It is antithetical to both the goal of "decriminalization" and the notion that the accused we are diverting are being diverted because their otherwise criminal activity is more reasonably seen as the product of their mental disorder. To dangle the prospect of leniency in front of the mentally disordered accused and promise that lenient outcome only if he pleads guilty completely undermines the voluntariness of the plea.

Participation in a diversion program should be voluntary. Setting aside the philosophical debate as to what is truly voluntary, an accused should be permitted to enter or leave a diversion program at will. It is well established that motivation is the lynchpin for change. It is equally well established that it is rather pointless to waste rehabilitative time, resources, and effort on an individual who is not a willing participant.

Noncompliance with a diversion program should not attract criminal sanctions. For the reasons noted above, there is little point in *forcing* an accused to comply with a treatment regime. Noncompliance should, first of all, be visited with further reassurance and support. Perhaps alternative therapeutic courses should be considered. Relapse is a normal, expected feature of rehabilitation. It should not attract penalties. If after all supportive options have been exhausted the accused is showing no interest in participating, they should be permitted to withdraw and return to the regular prosecutory stream. A mentally disordered accused should not be punished for attempting a therapeutic avenue, but failing.

A second reason for not including criminal sanctions as a response to noncompliance is that it is inconsistent with the principal objective of decriminalizing the mentally disordered accused.

Upon completion of the diversion program the accused should avoid a criminal conviction. The objective is to "divert" the accused out of the criminal justice system. Therefore, once society's intervention has been successfully complied with, the accused should be rewarded with the avoidance of a criminal conviction. Again, this is consistent with the primary objective of decriminalizing the mentally disordered individual.

Diversion programs should, as much as possible, divert the accused back in to the civil mental health-care system. In order to avoid a two-tier mental healthcare system with one perceived to be superior, it is seen as preferable to rely upon one universal system. Diversion programs constitute another entry portal, but the resources should not be dependent upon outstanding criminal charges. It should not be one system for the "bad" and one system for the "good". Such a system may actually serve to increase the arrest rates of mentally disordered individuals if the police believe that the only or best way to secure treatment for the individual is to introduce him to the criminal justice system.

The duration of a diversion program should be a function of clinical improvement rather than participation for a fixed period of time. If the objective of the diversion program is to reintegrate the accused back in to society once sufficiently stable, it does not seem logical to connect completion or "success" to a time line. The duration of time spent in the

diversion program should naturally vary from individual to individual.

Counsel should be mandatory for all accused entering a diversion program. Given the problematic considerations of "capacity" to consent to assessment and treatment and the general issues of voluntariness, to some extent the court can take comfort when the accused is represented by counsel. For vulnerable accused, such as mentally disordered accused, the assignment of counsel is a layer of protection and comfort that should be included as a matter of routine.

The expectations of the diversion program should be explicitly stated. Of course, if an accused is to be a voluntary participant, it is imperative that the accused understand precisely what it is that he is agreeing to participate in. A very good practice adopted by some courts is the creation of a "contract" wherein the particulars of the diversion plan are clearly articulated and agreed to. This may serve a useful purpose in refreshing all party's memories as to what was agreed. Again, the agreement can be modified, as necessary, in that most rehabilitative programs are to a large extent a matter of trial and error. In addition to assisting the mentally disordered accused, clearly defined goals and objectives can provide focus for the service providers within the court.

Any jurisdiction contemplating a diversion program or mental health court should not see that as a singular or unidimensional response to the problem of mentally disordered individuals coming in to the criminal justice system. The need for a mental health court should often be seen as symptomatic of a "sick" civil mental healthcare system. A full review and overhaul of the civil mental healthcare system will also reduce the extent to which the mental health court will be relied upon as a principal delivery vehicle. It makes little sense to divert an accused back to a civil system that was not adequate in the first place. As well, it is apparent that precharge diversion and the identification of high-risk individuals may be preferable to postarrest diversion. Accordingly, mental health courts comprise only one response within a range of solutions. Optimally, these courts should simply form one part of a larger strategy; it is inappropriate to view mental health courts as a panacea to the range of problems that have given rise to the existence of these courts.

Every diversion program or mental health court should strive to include a plan for evaluation. A confluence of factors and barriers has served to frustrate research into the functioning and efficacy of mental health courts. To counter this reality, it is important for mental health courts to be diligent in data collection and to collect data ranging from the volume of accused coming through the system to recidivism rates. Monitoring a program in a systematic way will provide useful information as to which components are efficacious and which ones are not.

A court-based diversion plan should incorporate as many community "partners" as possible. The success of a diversion program will inevitably be, in part, determined by how robustly the community is supporting the plan. In many ways the effectiveness of a mental health court can be predicted by the strength of the essential services found in the community. By having both forensic and nonforensic programs and community agencies in the diversion scheme, mental health courts will provide for a better transfer of the accused out of the criminal justice system and back in to the community.

All professionals participating in the diversion program or mental health court should receive specialized training. Training is an important aspect of a mental health court to ensure that participants are approaching the task of diversion from the same perspective, and having the same objectives ensures that the team will function more consistently. As an example, it is not uncommon for different factions within a mental health court to view "success" differently, such that the accused will be confronted with a confusing and frustrating set of expectations. Again, consistency and effectiveness require all mental health court staff to be fully apprised and "on the same page".

Trained judges, lawyers and prosecutors, clinicians, and other court personnel, are on the forefront of a new and challenging area of service provision and study. They are often in the best position to understand the complex relationship between mental disorder and criminality, and the plight of the mentally ill in the criminal justice system. Their knowledge and experience provides them with an opportunity to play a unique educative role within their own community, or other communities looking to put a mental health court in place.

Families and friends of the accused should be included in the diversion process to the greatest extent possible. Where possible, and where appropriate, mental health courts should strive to enlist the support of friends and family so that the accused will experience a consistently supportive environment within which he may progress. Individuals close to the accused can also be recruited as "therapists" and sources of information with respect to progress as well as relapse.

Upon completion of a diversion program a continuation of treatment and support in the community must be guaranteed. It is pointless to invest in a court-based diversion program only to have all the supports put in place withdrawn upon completion. Involvement with a mental health court should not lead to a dead end but hopefully should represent a bridge to the recipient of essential services on a going-forward basis. Again, this points to the desirability of having one universal mental healthcare system that supports all mentally disordered individuals regardless of whether they are presently before the courts.

Mental health courts should intervene at multiple junctures. It is submitted that a comprehensive mental health court should assist the accused at multiple junctures, not just "diversion". This view strikes as both obvious and inevitable in light of the various mental health concerns that often arise at any point from the inception to conclusion of a criminal prosecution. Commencing at the point of arrest, a specialty court can assist the mentally disordered accused with bail hearings, the assessment of fitness, treatment orders, keep-fit orders, uncomplicated criminal responsibility matters, disposition hearings, guilty pleas, and sentencing as well as the business of diversion. While diversions are typically focused on "outcomes", the mentally disordered accused has unique concerns at many junctures in the prosecution process which can be addressed by a mental health court.

End Notes

a. At the same time, some jurisdictions have a fixed 'program' of a fixed duration in which all candidates enroll. It is the author's view that individually fashioned regimens adjusted to the individual's particular needs are more likely to be successful.

References

[1]   Schneider, R.D. (2000). 7*A Statistical Survey of Provincial and Territorial Review Boards*, Federal Department of Justice, Ottawa.

[2]   Kaplan, A. (2007). Mental health courts reduce incarceration, save money, *Psychiatric Times* **24**(8), 1–3.
[3]   Schneider, R.D., Bloom, H. & Heerema, M. (2006). *Mental Health Courts: Decriminalizing the Mentally Ill*, Irwin Law, Toronto.

Related Articles

Therapeutic Jurisprudence

RICHARD D. SCHNEIDER

Mental Health Evaluations: Malingering in *see* Malingering: Forensic Evaluations

Mental Health Practitioners: Threat to *see* Violence Risk Assessment for Mental Health Professionals

Mental Health Treatment: Mandated *see* Treatment, Mandated: Mental Health

Mental Health Treatment: Right to *see* Treatment, Right to: Mental Health

Mental Health Treatment: Right to Refuse *see* Treatment, Right to Refuse: Mental Health

Mental Illness *see* Psychopathology: Terms and Trends

Mental Illness: Criminalization of *see* Criminalization of the Mentally Ill

Mental Retardation

Over the years, there have existed many definitions of mental retardation, each of which has been revised based on the new knowledge and/or the changing perceptions of scholars in the field (see Reference [1] for an overview). At present, there exist three primary definitions that have been put forth by the following organizations: (i) American Association on Intellectual and Developmental Disabilities (AAIDD, formerly the American Association on Mental Retardation (AAMR)), (ii) the American Psychiatric Association (APA), and (iii) the World Health Organization (WHO). There are similarities among the three definitions, but there are also differences that can result in different ways of portraying the disorder. In the following paragraphs, the reader is provided a glimpse into the construct of mental retardation as put forth by each organization; for a more comprehensive description, the reader is encouraged to consult the primary sources (see below for details) and current authoritative texts, such as Jacobson *et al.* [2] and Switzky and Greenspan [3].

American Association on Intellectual and Developmental Disabilities (AAIDD)

According to the AAIDD [4], mental retardation is defined as "disability characterized by significant limitations both in the intellectual functioning and in adaptive behavior as expressed in conceptual, social, and practical adaptive skills. This disability originates before the age of 18" (p. 8). The AAIDD does not identify any one measure of intelligence as necessary for diagnostic purposes, nor does it require the use of a particular measure of adaptive behavior. Instead, the organization states that the measures must be standardized using the general population and be appropriate for their intended use [1].

As noted in the manual, the following five assumptions are essential to the application of this definition.

1. Limitations in present functioning must be considered within the context of community environments typical of the individual's age peers and culture.
2. Valid assessment considers cultural and linguistic diversity as well as differences in communication, sensory, motor, and behavioral factors.
3. Within an individual, limitations often coexist with strengths.
4. An important purpose of describing limitations is to develop a profile of needed supports.
5. With appropriate personalized supports over a sustained period, the life functioning of the person with mental retardation generally will improve (p. 8).

American Psychiatric Association (APA)

Similar to the definition put forth by the AAIDD, in the Diagnostic and Statistical Manual, fourth edition, text revision (DSM-IV-TR) the APA conceptualizes mental retardation as a disability that is characterized by deficits in both the intellectual functioning and adaptive behavior that are manifest before the age of 18. Specifically, the diagnosis of mental retardation is made if all of the following criteria are met [5].

1. Significantly subaverage intellectual functioning; an intelligence quotient (IQ) of approximately 70 or below on an individually administered IQ test (for infants, a clinical judgment of significantly subaverage intellectual functioning).

2. Concurrent deficits or impairments in present adaptive functioning (i.e., the person's effectiveness in meeting the standards expected for his or her age by his or her cultural group) in at least two of the following areas: communication, self-care, home living, social/interpersonal skills, use of community resources, self-direction, functional academic skills, work, leisure, and health and safety.
3. The onset is before the age 18 ([5]; p. 49).

A feature of the diagnosis that was dropped by the AAIDD but maintained by the APA is severity of impairment. Specifically, according to the APA, mental retardation falls along a continuum of severity. The four levels of severity identified by the APA are based on the measured IQ: (i) mild, (ii) moderate, (iii) severe, and (iv) profound. The diagnosis of mental retardation, severity unspecified may be applied when there is strong evidence to support the diagnosis, but the individual cannot be tested using a standardized measure of intelligence.

International Classification of Diseases (ICD; 10th Edition)

Unlike the definitions put forth by the AAIDD and the APA, the WHO provides only a description of the disorder and not the means by which to diagnose it [6]. As noted in the International Classification of Diseases (ICD)-10, mental retardation is

... a condition of arrested or incomplete development of the mind, which is especially characterized by impairment of skills manifested during the developmental period, skills which contribute to the overall level of intelligence, i.e., cognitive, language, motor, and social abilities. Retardation can occur with or without any other mental or physical condition.

Degrees of mental retardation are conventionally estimated by standardized intelligence tests. These can be supplemented by scales assessing social adaptation in a given environment. These measures provide an approximate indication of the degree of mental retardation. The diagnosis will also depend on the overall assessment of intellectual functioning by a skilled diagnostician.

Intellectual abilities and social adaptation may change over time, and, however, poor, may improve as a result of training and rehabilitation. Diagnosis should be based on the current levels of functioning (p. 369–370).

Similar to APA, ICD-10 describes mental retardation as a condition that falls along a continuum from mild to profound mental retardation based on the IQ score. Again, the ICD-10 does not provide specific information regarding how to diagnose the condition but instead provides a method by which mental retardation can be classified and traced via medical databases.

It is important to note that some experts in the field of mental retardation disagree with the way it is currently defined. For example, according to Greenspan and Switzky [7], "Mental retardation (MR) is an invented bureaucratic category, currently undergoing radical rethinking and likely renaming, that includes many biological-based brain disorders, but is itself determined through functional criteria (e.g., IQ below a certain level) that are purely arbitrary" (p. 19). Given the ever-changing models and definitions of intellectual disabilities, it is critical that individuals interested in mental retardation stay abreast of advancements in the field.

Etiology

Like many disorders, mental retardation does not have a single identifiable etiological factor. As described in the 2002 AAMR manual, the etiology of mental retardation is conceptualized as multifactorial and is composed of four broad categories of risk factors: (i) biomedical, (ii) social, (iii) behavioral, and (iv) educational. These four factors do not function in isolation, but instead are thought to interact across the life of the individual and across generations [4]. In fact, in each category there exist many distinct factors that can cause deficits in intellectual functioning. For instance, chromosomal disorders (e.g., Down syndrome), maternal illness, birth injury, and traumatic brain injury are all factors found in the biomedical domain. In the social domain are risk factors such as poverty, domestic violence, lack of adequate stimulation, and institutionalization. Maternal drug and alcohol use, parental smoking, parental rejection of the caretaking role, and social deprivation are examples of behavioral risk factors. Finally, parental intellectual ability, lack of preparation for parenthood, inadequate education services, and inadequate family support have been identified as educational risk factors.

In their review of epidemiological studies on the etiology of mental retardation, McLaren and Bryson [8] found that as many as 50% of the population of individuals diagnosed with mental retardation had more than one causal risk factor. It is important to note that the presence of any one risk factor, or perhaps even a combination of many risk factors, does not mean that an individual has mental retardation. The diagnosis of mental retardation requires observable impairments in functional abilities, regardless of etiology, and in about half of the cases of mental retardation, the etiology is not known [9]. It is important to be aware that the absence of an identifiable risk factor or etiology does not mean that an individual does not have mental retardation.

Assessment of Mental Retardation

The Intelligence Quotient. As is clear from the definitions of mental retardation, an individual's level of intellectual functioning must be established before a diagnosis can be made. To do this, an individual must be administered a standardized measure of intellectual functioning that provides an IQ. Although there are many tests of intelligence, the most commonly used, individually administered, and well-standardized tests are the *Wechsler Adult Intelligence Scale – Fourth Edition* [10] the *Wechsler Intelligence Scale for Children – Fourth Edition* [11], and the *Stanford-Binet Intelligence Scales – Fifth Edition* (SB5) [1]. For diagnostic purposes, the most important index of functional ability is the overall, or Full Scale, IQ.

The AAIDD and APA both require an IQ of approximately 70 or below for a diagnosis of mental retardation. A score of 70 places an individual approximately two standard deviations below the mean of the general population at the time the test was developed.[a] When accounting for standard error of measurement, this cutoff score may be as high as 75.

Adaptive Functioning. As previously noted, in addition to the IQ criterion, a diagnosis of mental retardation requires concomitant deficits in adaptive behavior. In brief, adaptive behaviors are everyday skills, such as walking, talking, grooming, cooking, cleaning, and participating in school or work. These abilities are learned over time in the context of one's home and community, and they represent skills that are necessary to function within that context. It is important to emphasize that adaptive behaviors develop over the course of time and with experience, and thus individuals are evaluated against their same age peers. To measure adaptive skills, adaptive behavior scales have been developed and normed on individuals with and without intellectual disabilities. These scales require that an informant, typically a parent, teacher, or other individual who is very familiar with the individual's daily level of functioning, rate the person of interest on a variety of skills. For instance, the informant may rate the extent to which the individual follows directions or balances a checkbook along a continuum ranging from "Never Does or Can't Do" to "Always Does or Can Do Without Assistance".

For the diagnosis of mental retardation, the AAIDD definition requires that "significant limitations in adaptive behavior should be established through the use of standardized test measures normed on the general population, including people with disabilities and people without disabilities. On these standardized measures, significant limitations in adaptive behavior are operationally defined as performance that is at least two standard deviations below the mean on either (a) one of the following three types of adaptive behavior: conceptual, social, or practical, or (b) an overall score on a standardized measure of conceptual, social, and practical skills" ([4], p. 14). Like the AAIDD, the APA [5] recommends the use of standardized measures in the assessment of adaptive behavior. That said, it is well recognized that in some instances quantitative analysis of functional abilities is either inappropriate or does not provide enough information to make a determination. In addition to standardized, quantitative measures, both the AAIDD and the APA state that the final determination of mental retardation requires the use of multiple sources of information and clinical judgment.

There exist numerous scales of adaptive behavior that can be used for the purposes of diagnosis, classification, and planning for supports; no single measure is best for all the three. Examples of adaptive functioning scales commonly used in the assessment of mental retardation include the Scales of Independent Behavior – Revised Full Scale (SIB-R) [12], the *Adaptive Behavior Assessment System – Second Edition (ABAS-II)* [13], and the *Vineland*

Adaptive Behavior Scales – Second Edition (VABS-II) [14]. It is important to note that, regardless of the measure chosen, the utility of the information obtained is limited by the quality of the information provided by the rater [4, 15].

Mental Retardation and Everyday Life

As previously mentioned, mental retardation is characterized by problems in everyday life or adaptive functioning and the extent of these difficulties varies with the severity of retardation. Difficulties in adaptive functioning may be evident in social, conceptual, and/or practical areas [4]. There exist many misconceptions about how to conceptualize adaptive behavior for diagnostic purposes. First, some believe that adaptive behavior is measured by estimates of abilities or potential, but it is the individual's actual performance that is important. Second, adaptive behavior is typical behavior that reflects an individual's ability to function on a day-to-day basis. It is not measured by isolated successes or failures. Third, adaptive behavior is performance in one's community, not in restricted settings, such as prison or therapeutic treatment programs. Fourth, the definition of mental retardation does not require that a cause of impairment be identified; diagnosis is determined by the presence of significant deficits in intellectual functioning and concomitant deficits in adaptive behavior that are evident before the age of 18.

As previously noted, there are hundreds of identified causes of mental retardation, but the cause for any individual is often not known. This is particularly true for individuals with IQs in the 60s who usually do not have a medical syndrome that is known and do not have an obviously different appearance or manner. For instance, people with mild mental retardation have significant limitations in achieving independence, but they have fewer difficulties and require less support or assistance than people with more severe levels of retardation.

With regard to support, it is typical for individuals with mild mental retardation to receive informal help from family members or neighbors, rather than from provider agencies, and it is quite likely that they have, or have had, gainful employment in jobs that require limited decision making or judgment. In most instances, individuals with mild mental retardation require support from others to manage money and make major life decisions. Few people in this category require a legal guardian, and many marry and have meaningful social relationships. In fact, it is common for these individuals to be active participants in their communities, and as a result, they are vulnerable to exploitation by others. Further, it is more common for people with mild or perhaps moderate mental retardation to be engaged in criminal activity, than it is for those with more severe levels of impairment.

As the degree of mental retardation becomes more severe, the need for formal supports from an agency, such as a local mental health center or other provider, becomes greater. People with moderate or severe mental retardation are more likely to require supervision for most, if not all, of their day. As a result of this greater supervision and less personal freedom, they are less likely to be exploited in the community or to become involved in criminal activity. Nevertheless, these individuals are subject to exploitation, often by care providers. For instance, men may be exploited for their labor, or women may be exploited for sexual favors.

In contrast to individuals with mild mental retardation, individuals with more severe degrees of impairment are likely to have an identifiable medical or environmental cause for their retardation (e.g., Down syndrome and/or fetal alcohol syndrome) and to need specialized medical care. These individuals are also more likely to have serious behavior problems that require professional services. Problems of aggression, self-injury, self-stimulation, property destruction, and other disruptive behavior can limit individuals' opportunities for integrated community living. These problem behaviors are sometimes associated with mental illnesses that coexist with mental retardation [16].

Services and Supports

The services and supports available today are more varied and individualized than in the past; the following are just a few examples. The federal Individuals with Disabilities Education Improvement Act (IDEIA) of 2004, Public Law 108–446, mandates individualized services from birth to the age of 22. The Early Intervention Program for Infants and Toddlers with Disabilities (Part C) under IDEIA serves children from birth to the age of two. The IDEIA also mandates services and describes procedures for services during the school years through age 22.

Students are provided an Individualized Education Program (IEP) and a transition plan to smooth the path from school to community living and work. Children and adults in the United States identified with mental retardation are eligible for Medicaid [17], which provides medical and a wide variety of other lifetime services.

In adulthood, many people with mild mental retardation are not identified by any service agency and, thus, receive only informal supports from family, neighbors, and employers. This is not surprising as these individuals show fewer deficits and demonstrate a higher level of skill in some of the more obvious areas of functioning (e.g., work, leisure, and social relationships). It is important to note that the majority of individuals with mental retardation, at all levels of functioning, reside with their parents or other family members throughout their lives. Residential care is typically reserved for more impaired individuals.

The most significant trend in services in recent years has been away from uniform programs that are designed to serve large numbers of people with disabilities and toward individualized services that reflect the desires and abilities of each person. People who receive formal services from a public or private provider agency typically participate in a person-centered planning process. The result is a written, person-centered plan (PCP) that describes the services and supports best suited to that individual. The plan typically includes residential, work, and personal living considerations for the individual, and it is reviewed and revised regularly. PCPs are characterized by emphasis on living in the most integrated setting that is appropriate to the person and honoring the choices of the person with regard to residence, work, social supports, health care, community participation, recreation, and other personal preferences.

Personal planning commonly occurs in the area of residential care. Over the past few decades, the emphasis has moved from "housing" individuals with mental retardation in large institutions, toward providing them with opportunities for more independent living with individualized services in smaller settings [18]. In keeping with one's PCP, the most appropriate residential option is chosen from a range that includes small group homes, supported apartments, semi-independent living, and home ownership. All of these models of residential services require trained staff members who provide individualized supports.

A significant challenge to fulfilling the ideal of individualized residential living is the need for direct support personnel who can provide varied individualized services, often around the clock.

With regard to employment, state vocational rehabilitation agencies assist people in obtaining competitive or supported employment. These services begin in adolescence with planning for transition from school to work. People with mild mental retardation typically have basic functional academic skills and do not have physical disabilities that would limit their work opportunities. These individuals often thrive in jobs that do not require abstract thinking or decision making. They may, however, require more supervision than the average worker, and they may require support in managing their money.

Individuals with moderate or severe mental retardation are often good candidates for supported employment. In this model, the worker has assistance in learning and in performing the job for as long as needed. In some instances, the assistant or job coach can be faded out as the worker becomes more independent. In other instances, the job coach may be needed permanently. As the severity of mental retardation increases, the individual is more likely to have significant motor limitations (e.g., cerebral palsy), significant health problems (e.g., seizure disorder), or significant communication problems that interfere with work and require more assistance and/or shorter work hours. Regardless of severity of disability, the trend in employment services in recent years has been toward competitive or supported employment in real community jobs and away from sheltered workshops and other work in isolated and separate settings.

The use of community services provides a final example of how individual planning or person-centered planning can be implemented for the betterment of the individual. Services and supports in a PCP may come from "natural supports", such as family members or neighbors, or from formal provider agencies. Medicaid largely dictates the rules for services for such agencies in the United States, and the sources of funding are typically a mix of Medicaid, state, and local government, private payers, and charity. The PCP is intended to support the greatest degree of personal independence that the person wishes and can achieve. This goal may be difficult to achieve, because many adults with mental retardation are socially isolated. Their natural support network is limited to their families and paid service providers. To expand the individual's social network, the PCP describes strategies to increase the individual's participation in meaningful activities each day. Adults with mental retardation have typically led very sedentary lifestyles, and the result has been prevalent obesity and associated health problems. The PCP is designed to prevent such problems through a healthy and active lifestyle that includes access to health care and emphasis on personal choice.

In summary, the construct of mental retardation is ever evolving. At the time of writing, the 11th edition of the AAIDD manual is underway and is likely to recommend changes in methods of assessment, methods of prevention, and the identification and implementation of needed supports. Though there is a new DSM under construction, it is unlikely that the two agencies will come together to create one conceptualization of mental retardation. Historically, the DSM has followed in the footsteps of AAIDD, and based on the timeline,[b] it is likely that the fifth version of the DSM will closely mirror AAIDD's 2002 conceptualization.

End Notes

[a.] In recent years it has been shown that IQ scores for the general population, as measured by the Wechsler scales, have been increasing by 0.3 points per year. This phenomenon has been termed the *Flynn effect* and has resulted in much debate regarding the accuracy of IQ scores over time and how best to interpret scores obtained on tests with outdated norms. The interested reader may want to refer to the following publications for a more detailed description of the phenomenon and the controversy surrounding it [19].

[b.] DSM-V is expected to be commercially available in 2011.

References

[1]   Roid, G.H. (2003). *Stanford-Binet Intelligence Scales*, 5th Edition, Riverside, Itaska, IL.

[2]   Jacobson, J.W., Mulick, J.A. & Rojahn, J. (eds) (2007). *Handbook of Intellectual and Developmental Disabilities*, Springer, New York.

[3]   Switzky, H. & Greenspan, S. (eds) (2006). *What is Mental Retardation? Ideas for an Evolving Disability in the 21st Century*, American Association on Mental Retardation, Washington, DC.

[4]   American Association on Mental Retardation (2002). *Mental Retardation: Definition, Classification, and Systems of Supports*, 10th Edition, American Association on Mental Retardation, Washington, DC.

[5]   American Psychiatric Association (2000). *Diagnostic and Statistical Manual of Mental Disorders*, 4th Edition, text revision, American Psychiatric Association, Washington, DC.

[6]   World Health Organization (1993). *International Statistical Classification of Diseases and Related Health Problems*, 10th Edition, World Health Organization, Geneva.

[7]   Greenspan, S. & Switzky, H. (2003). Execution exemption should be based on actual vulnerability not disability label, *Ethics and Behavior* **13**, 19–26.

[8]   McLaren, J. & Bryson, S.E. (1987). Review of recent epidemiological studies of mental retardation: prevalence, associated disorders, and etiology, *American Journal on Mental Retardation* **92**, 243–254.

[9]   McDermott, S., Durkin, M.S., Schupf, N. & Stein, Z.A. (2007). Epidemiology and etiology of mental retardation, in *Handbook of Intellectual and Developmental Disabilities*, J.W. Jacobson, J.A. Mulick & J. Rojahn, eds, Springer, New York, pp. 3–40.

[10]   Wechsler, D. (2008). *Wechsler Adult Intelligence Scale*, 4th Edition, Psychological Corporation, Harcourt Brace, San Antonio, TX.

[11]   Wechsler, D. (2003). *Wechsler Intelligence Scale for Children*, 4th Edition, Psychological Corporation, Harcourt Brace, San Antonio, TX.

[12]   Bruininks, R., Woodcock, R.W., Weatherman, R.F. & Hill, B.K. (1996). *SIB-R: Scales of Independent Behavior – Revised*, Riverside, Itaska, IL.

[13]   Harrison, P.L. & Oakland, T. (2003). *ABAS-II: Adaptive Behavior Assessment System*, 2nd Edition, Psychological Corporation, San Antonio, TX.

[14]   Sparrow, S.S., Balla, D.A. & Cicchetti, D.A. (2005). *Vineland Adaptive Behavior Scales*, 2nd Edition, Pearson Assessments, Minneapolis.

[15]   Beail, N. (2003). Utility of the Vineland Adaptive Behavior Scales in diagnosis and research with adults who have mental retardation, *Mental Retardation* **41**, 286–289.

[16]   Fletcher, R., Loschen, E., Stavrakaki, C. & First, M. (eds) (2007). *Diagnostic Manual – Intellectual Disability (DM-ID): A Textbook of Diagnosis of Mental Disorders in Persons with Intellectual Disability*, NADD Press, Kingston, NY.

[17]   National Research Council (2002). Mental retardation: determining eligibility for social security benefits. Committee on Disability Determination for Mental Retardation, in *Division of Behavioral and Social Sciences and Education*, D.J. Reschly, T.G. Myers & C.R. Hartel, eds, National Academy Press, Washington, DC.

[18]   Prouty, R., Lakin, C. & Coucouvanis, K. (2007). In 2006, fewer than 30% of persons receiving out-of-home residential supports lived in homes of more than six residents, *Intellectual and Developmental Disabilities* **45**, 289–292.

[19]   Kanaya, T., Scullin, M.H. & Ceci, S.J. (2003). The Flynn Effect and U.S. policies: the impact of rising IQ scores on American society, *The American Psychologist* **58**, 778–790.

KAREN L. SALEKIN AND J. GREGORY OLLEY

Mental Retardation: Death Penalty

In 2002, the US Supreme Court held in a 6–3 decision in the landmark case of *Atkins v. Virginia* [1] that the execution of offenders with mental retardation violates the Eighth Amendment's prohibition against cruel and unusual punishments. The Court reversed its 5–4 decision 13 years earlier in *Penry v. Lynaugh* [2], which held that the Eighth Amendment's ban on cruel and unusual punishments did not categorically prohibit the execution of offenders with mental retardation.

The Court's holding in *Atkins* was based on several stems of reasoning, including public policy justifications in support of capital punishment and the extent to which they apply to individuals who have mental retardation [3]. The Court found that a "national consensus" had developed against the execution of individuals with mental retardation based on the fact that (i) many state legislatures had previously voted "overwhelmingly" in favor of the prohibition, (ii) there was a "complete absence" of states that had reinstated the death penalty for offenders with mental retardation, and (iii) the practice of executing offenders with mental retardation was uncommon, even in those states that allowed such executions.

In the 13 years between the *Penry* and *Atkins* decisions, only five states (i.e., Alabama, Louisiana, South Carolina, Texas, and Virginia) had carried out executions of offenders who were suspected to have mental retardation [1, 4], which was documented to be as many as 44 individuals [5]. The Court remarked that it was not the number of states that prohibited the practice that was significant, but it was the "consistency of the direction of change" that the Court found to be "powerful evidence that today our society views mentally retarded offenders as categorically less culpable than the average criminal". The Court also considered opposition to such executions expressed by religious and professional organizations, disapproval by the world community, and polling data that showed a "widespread consensus" among Americans who were against such executions.

Citing the scientific literature extant at the time [6, 7], the Court noted that although those with mental retardation may be competent to stand trial and know the wrongfulness of their criminal acts, because of their impairments, "they have diminished capacities to understand and process information, to communicate, to abstract from mistakes and learn from experience, to engage in logical reasoning, to control impulses, and to understand reactions of others". Drawing on other research findings in the field [8, 9], the Court also noted that individuals with mental retardation "often act on impulse rather than pursuant to a premeditated plan, and that in group settings they are followers rather than leaders". The Court concluded that the deficiencies of those with mental retardation "do not warrant an exemption from criminal sanctions, but do diminish their personal culpability".

The Court also considered how the underlying justifications of the death penalty – retribution and deterrence – apply to offenders with mental retardation [3]. The Court reasoned that "the lesser culpability of the mentally retarded offender surely does not merit that form of retribution". Similarly, the Court recognized that because of their cognitive and behavioral impairments that render them less morally culpable, those with mental retardation are also less likely able to "process the information of the possibility of execution as a penalty and, as a result, control their conduct based upon that information." As such, the Court further noted, "Nor will exempting the mentally retarded from execution lessen the death penalty's deterrent effect with respect to offenders who are not mentally retarded."

Finally, the Court expressed concern that as a group, defendants with mental retardation "face a special risk of wrongful execution," not only because they may confess to crimes they did not commit [9] but also because of their lesser ability to provide defense counsel with meaningful assistance, their tendency to serve as poor witnesses, and their demeanor, which may create an erroneous impression that they lack remorse for their crimes.

Following the *Atkins* decision, courts in death penalty jurisdictions have begun to call upon mental

health professionals to evaluate offenders in capital murder cases to assist the trier of fact in making a determination of mental retardation. Mental health professionals may be requested to render an expert opinion about mental retardation in so-called "*Atkins* hearings" at different stages of legal proceedings, which may occur pretrial, at the sentencing phase, or during postconviction appeals. However, the assessment of mental retardation in death penalty cases presents many challenges for forensic experts. In addition, the results of informal surveys of psychologists' professional practices in *Atkins* cases suggest great variability in the assessment methods used to diagnose mental retardation [10, 11].

A comprehensive review of the assessment of mental retardation in death penalty cases is beyond the scope of this chapter. The focus here is to (i) provide an overview of death penalty statutes on mental retardation in the United States, (ii) describe the contemporary definitions of mental retardation, (iii) discuss the diagnosis of mental retardation in death penalty cases, and (iv) review the available research on malingered mental retardation.

Death Penalty Statutes on Mental Retardation

Currently, there are 37 states, in addition to the federal government and the US military, which have the death penalty [12] (*see also* **Death Penalty and Age**). The 13 states that do not have the death penalty are Alaska, Hawaii, Iowa, Maine, Massachusetts, Michigan, Minnesota, New York, North Dakota, Rhode Island, Vermont, West Virginia, and Wisconsin. The District of Columbia also does not have the death penalty. At the time of *Penry*, only two states, Georgia and Maryland, had enacted laws that prohibited the execution of individuals with mental retardation. In the 13 years between *Penry* and *Atkins*, 16 other states enacted statutes barring such executions [1, 12]. The 18 states that had statutes that barred execution of those with mental retardation at the time of *Atkins* were Arizona, Arkansas, Colorado, Connecticut, Florida, Georgia, Indiana, Kansas, Kentucky, Maryland, Missouri, Nebraska, New Mexico, New York (except for murder by a prisoner), North Carolina, South Dakota, Tennessee, and Washington [12]. In 1988, when the Congress enacted legislation reinstating the federal death penalty, it excluded the execution of those with mental retardation [3].

After the *Atkins* ruling, eight more death penalty states revised their statutes to provide definitions of mental retardation. The states are California, Delaware, Idaho, Illinois, Louisiana, Nevada, Utah, and Virginia [12]. Because the *Atkins* Court provided little guidance to the states on how to develop rules to determine which offenders have mental retardation, there is significant variability across these pre- and post-*Atkins* state statutes. Twelve death penalty states apparently have yet to develop statutes for determining mental retardation in *Atkins* cases: Alabama, Mississippi, Montana, New Hampshire, New Jersey, Ohio, Oregon, Oklahoma, Pennsylvania, South Carolina, Texas, and Wyoming. Although some of these states have statutes that define mental retardation for the purpose of civil commitment and/or guardianship, it is unclear how these statutes may apply in *Atkins* cases. Other states, such as Mississippi, have adopted the *Atkins* decision in case law [13].

Definitions of Mental Retardation

Mental retardation has been defined by professional organizations in the field (*see also* **Mental Retardation**). The American Association on Intellectual and Developmental Disabilities (AAIDD) (formerly the American Association on Mental Retardation (AAMR)) has published four major versions of its definition since 1961. The 2002 version is the most recent. The American Psychiatric Association (APA) has also published four major versions of its *Diagnostic and Statistical Manual of Mental Disorders*. The 2000 version (*DSM-IV-TR*) [14] is the most recent.

Many state legislatures enacted statutes based on the 1983 American Association on Mental Deficiency (former name for AAMR) definition of mental retardation [3]: "Mental retardation refers to significantly subaverage general intellectual functioning existing concurrently with deficits in adaptive behavior and manifested during the developmental period" [15]. In 1992, the AAMR revised its definition with an emphasis on refining the adaptive functioning component of the previous version:

> Mental retardation refers to substantial limitations in present functioning. It is characterized by significantly subaverage intellectual functioning, existing concurrently with related limitations in two or more of the following applicable adaptive skill areas: communication, self-care, home living, social skills,

community use, self-direction, health and safety, functional academics, leisure, and work. Mental retardation manifests before age 18 [16].

The 1992 AAMR definition was one of the definitions cited in *Atkins* and was adopted by several state legislatures in the 1990s [3]. However, it has been criticized for lacking empirical research support and theoretical grounding [17]. The APA's current definition in the *DSM-IV-TR* [14] contains language similar to the 1992 AAMR definition and also was one of the definitions cited in *Atkins*. The AAMR revised its definition in 2002 [18] and this version also focuses on describing adaptive functioning: "Mental retardation is a disability characterized by significant limitations both in intellectual functioning and in adaptive behavior as expressed in conceptual, social, and practical adaptive skills. This disability originates before age 18." Ellis [3] has suggested that the 2002 AAMR definition is most appropriate, because it contains the three essential components of all definitions cited in the *Atkins* decision. The 2002 AAMR definition also has been described as being more consistent with contemporary thinking and research on the assessment of adaptive behavior [19].

Diagnosis of Mental Retardation in Death Penalty Cases

Regardless of which definition is used to diagnose mental retardation, it is essential that the assessment methods used are consistent with the standards of professional practice [3, 20], particularly in capital murder cases, because there is no other assessment in which the stakes are higher. Because the population of individuals with mental retardation consists mostly of those who function in the mild range of impairment [14] and their impairments are often not immediately observable, accurate diagnosis for this subpopulation is difficult [19]. Some commentators [21, 22] have suggested that misdiagnosis may stem from a lack of understanding of the definition of mental retardation and failure to properly assess each diagnostic criterion.

Despite differences across the definitions of mental retardation, all have three common clinical components: (i) significant deficits in intellectual functioning; (ii) related deficits in adaptive functioning; and (iii) manifestation of deficits during the developmental period.

Intellectual Functioning

Current definitions of mental retardation require that an individual demonstrate significant limitations in intellectual functioning as measured by standardized psychometric instruments [14, 18]. This is operationally defined in the *DSM-IV-TR* [14] definition as an intelligence quotient (IQ) score of ~70 or below, or two standard deviations below the statistical mean. Because of the measurement error associated with intelligence test scores (±5 points), it is possible to diagnose mental retardation based on an IQ score of 75 or below [14].

There are three individually administered intelligence tests that are generally accepted measures of mental retardation for adults. They are the *Wechsler Adult Intelligence Scale – Fourth Edition* (*WAIS-IV*) [23]; the *Stanford-Binet Intelligence Scale – Fifth Edition* (*SB-5*) [24]; and the *Kaufman Adolescent and Adult Intelligence Test* (*KAAIT*) [25]. Group-administered intelligence tests, such as the *Revised Beta* [26], have been widely used as screening tests in correctional facilities [21, 27]. However, only global measures of intelligence are appropriate for diagnosing mental retardation [19] and are considered by many practitioners as the "gold standard" in assessments of mental retardation in death penalty cases [10].

The interpretation of IQ scores depends heavily upon the examiner's clinical judgment. Factors related to the examinee's behavior during the testing process, such as fatigue, effort, motivation, and attempts to malinger intellectual deficits can threaten the validity of scores. In addition, practice effects can be caused by repeated administrations of the same intelligence test in a short period. This problem may occur frequently in *Atkins* proceedings in which multiple experts administer the same intelligence test to offenders within a relatively brief timeframe. It is not uncommon to find differences in an individual's IQ scores over time. Such differences in IQ scores may occur on multiple administrations of the same test, scores on different editions of the same test, and scores on different tests [27].

Comparisons of IQ scores also can be misleading because of the "Flynn effect", which means there is a tendency for IQ scores to increase in the general population over time [28–30]. Thus, an individual's IQ may be artificially increased as a function of when the intelligence test was administered. The Flynn effect has become a topic of much debate, particularly with regard to the practice of adjusting individual IQ scores in capital cases. Some authors [31–34] have advocated modifying individual test scores to correct for the Flynn effect. Others [35] have argued that such modification of individual IQ scores is not an accepted professional practice. Harcourt Assessment, the publisher of the Wechsler tests, does not endorse the recommendation to modify *WAIS-III* scores to account for the Flynn effect [36].

Adaptive Functioning

The *adaptive behavior prong of the diagnosis of mental retardation* suggests that intellectual deficits are accompanied by real-world disabling effects on an individual's functioning [3]. Adaptive behavior has been described as the most problematic part of the definition of mental retardation [19] and may also be the least understood [37]. Some psychologists and legal professionals tend to view adaptive behavior only in terms of practical daily living skills. However, for those who function in the mild range of mental retardation, deficits are more likely to exist in the areas of social and conceptual skills [19].

Several standardized instruments have been developed to assess adaptive behavior, such as the *Vineland Adaptive Behavior Scales II* (*VABS II*) [38], *Adaptive Behavior Assessment System – Second Edition* (*ABAS-II*) [39], and the *Scales of Independent Behavior – Revised* (*SIB-R*) [40], each of which has been normed on the general population including those with intellectual disabilities. Although these instruments are commonly used in the field, they have been criticized for inadequately assessing the constructs of gullibility and naiveté, which are common characteristics of individuals with mental retardation [41]. Some experts occasionally use the *Street Survival Skills Questionnaire* (*SSSQ*) [42] in death penalty cases to assess defendants' adaptive functioning [10]. The *SSSQ* has been criticized [19] as an inappropriate measure of adaptive deficits because it is a test of knowledge, rather than performance, and it emphasizes practical skills and not conceptual or social skills.

Most adaptive behavior scales are intended to measure an individual's current functioning in the community. This creates methodological problems for assessments of adaptive functioning with incarcerated populations, particularly those who have been on death row for many years. In such cases, the examiner must perform a retrospective assessment of adaptive functioning. However, concerns exist regarding the validity of retrospective assessments of adaptive behavior [43]. Some authors [44] have called for the development of a "penologically normed" instrument to assess adaptive functioning for incarcerated populations. To date, there is no such instrument available, and information about an inmate's prison behavior normed on other inmates would not contribute to a valid diagnosis of mental retardation. Because there is no perfect method to retrospectively assess adaptive behavior, experts must rely on a mixture of imperfect information and clinical judgment [19].

Age of Onset

The "third" component of all definitions of mental retardation requires that the disability be manifested during the developmental period [14, 18]. Many states have defined this as prior to age 18, although some states have extended the age to 22 [3, 12]. This prong of the definition distinguishes mental retardation from other disabilities that may occur later in life, such as traumatic brain injury and dementia, and it also helps to identify defendants in death penalty cases who may attempt to feign mental retardation [3, 45].

Malingered Mental Retardation

In his dissenting opinion in *Atkins* [1], Justice Scalia expressed concern about the possibility that individuals can "readily feign" mental retardation. This issue also has been raised in Mississippi case law, which has explicitly addressed the need for assessments of malingering in *Atkins* claims. In *Foster v. State* [46], the Mississippi Supreme Court required the use of the *Minnesota Multiphasic Personality Inventory-2* (*MMPI-2*) [47] to assess malingering in *Atkins* cases. However, the *MMPI-2* was designed to identify malingered mental illness, not mental retardation. It also has been criticized as an invalid measure of malingering for those with mental retardation because of its required eighth grade reading level [48]. Nevertheless, great pressure has been placed upon psychologists to assess malingering in *Atkins* cases (*see also* **Malingering: Forensic Evaluations**).

Malingered Cognitive Deficits

Few studies have investigated the validity of malingering measures for those with mental retardation. The studies that are available have produced mixed results. In a study by Hurley and Deal [49] using a sample of individuals with IQ scores between 50 and 78, subjects were administered four measures of malingering, which included one that assesses feigned psychiatric disorders, the *Structured Interview of Reported Symptoms* (*SIRS*) [50], and three measures of malingered memory: the *Test of Memory Malingering* (*TOMM*) [51], the *Rey 15-Item Memory Test* [52], and the *Rey Dot Counting Test* (*RDCT*) [53]. The findings did not support the use of three of the four measures with a population with mental retardation. The authors recommended that one (*RDCT*) undergo further evaluation for its effectiveness as a screening measure. On the other hand, a study by Simon [54] with a sample of 21 adjudicated forensic inpatients with comorbid Axis I disorders and mental retardation supported the use of the *TOMM* [51] for assessing malingering with individuals with mental retardation.

Goldberg and Miller [55] administered the *Rey-15 Item Memory Test* [52] to individuals with severe psychiatric disorders and those with mental retardation. Although the cut scores worked well for the psychiatric patients, they were ineffective for those with mental retardation. Similarly, Hayes *et al.* [56] administered three measures of malingering, including the *Rey 15 Item Memory Test* [52], the *M-Test* [57], and the *Rey Dot Counting Test* [53] to 38 subjects in a maximum-security forensic hospital who had been diagnosed with mental retardation. On the basis of the results, the researchers concluded that the battery of tests contributed nothing to the identification of malingering in defendants with mental retardation. Conversely, Schretlen and Arkowitz [58] used a combination of measures, including validity scales of the *MMPI-2* [47], two scores on the *Bender Gestalt* [59], and an experimental measure to identify individuals feigning insanity or mental retardation. The researchers found that the combination of measures accurately identified most of the subjects who feigned mental retardation.

Although several more recent studies investigating the use of effort measures with populations of persons with mental retardation have been published in the last year, these studied also have produced rather mixed results [60–62].

Malingered Adaptive Deficits

To date, only one study has investigated the susceptibility of measures of adaptive behavior to malingered responding. Doane and Salekin [63] investigated whether collateral informants could feign adaptive deficits on the *ABAS-II* [39] and the *SIB-R* [40] within the context of a death penalty case. The results indicated that both measures were susceptible to feigning by collateral informants. The *ABAS-II* was extremely vulnerable to exaggeration of deficits, and this response style was not easily detected. Subjects were not as adept at feigning mental retardation on the *SIB-R*, and the response style was easily detected.

In summary, few studies have investigated the validity of assessments of malingered mental retardation, especially malingered adaptive deficits. Similarly, most instruments designed to detect malingered cognitive deficits lack normative data for populations who have mental retardation and have not been validated for the purpose of detecting malingered mental retardation. Therefore, concerns regarding false positives exist with such instruments, because individuals with mental retardation may produce scores suggestive of malingering when they are not. Further research is needed to determine how to appropriately assess both malingered adaptive skills and feigned intellectual deficits in populations with mental retardation.

Conclusion

In light of the US Supreme Court's decision in *Atkins v. Virginia* [1], courts in death penalty jurisdictions are faced with the challenge of determining whether offenders in capital murder cases have mental retardation. Bonnie [64] observed that one of the "striking aspects" of the Court's decision in *Atkins* is that the constitutional prohibition against the execution of offenders with mental retardation is framed in the language of a "clinical diagnosis". Thus, expert opinions by mental health professionals play a critical role in the legal determination of mental retardation in *Atkins* cases, because the court's decision may depend heavily on an expert's diagnosis.

Standards that govern the admissibility of scientific evidence [65] not only require that forensic experts' methodology be generally accepted in the field, but expert opinions also must be based on knowledge, skill, experience, training, and education. However, few mental health professionals have

extensive training in both forensic evaluation and mental retardation [66]. In addition, the mandates of some *Atkins* statutes defy principles of psychological assessment and can create ethical dilemmas for psychologists who serve in the role of experts in such cases [67].

In 2005, Division 33 of the American Psychological Association (Mental Retardation and Developmental Disabilities) formed an *Ad Hoc* Committee [68] to identify issues related to mental retardation and the death penalty and to clarify psychologists' role in *Atkins* proceedings. Several seminal articles have since been published that describe the controversies surrounding assessments in *Atkins* cases and provide recommendations for best practice [66, 69, 70]. Experts in the fields of forensic evaluation and mental retardation must continue working together to ensure that assessments of mental retardation in death penalty cases meet the highest standard of professional practice, as the outcome of these evaluations is literally a matter of life or death.

References

[1] Atkins v. Virginia, 536 U.S. 304 (2002).

[2] Penry v. Lynaugh, 492 U.S. 302 (1989).

[3] Ellis, J.W. (2003). Mental retardation and the death penalty: A guide to legislative issues, *Mental and Physical Disability Law Reporter* **27**, 11–24.

[4] Keyes, D.W., Edwards, W.J. & Perske, R. (1997). People with mental retardation are dying legally, *Mental Retardation* **35**, 59–63.

[5] Keyes, D.W., Edwards, W.J. & Perske, R. (2002). People with mental retardation are dying, legally: At least 44 have been executed, *Mental Retardation* **40**, 243–244.

[6] McGee, J. & Menolascino, F. (1992). The evaluation of defendants with mental retardation in the criminal justice system, in *The Criminal Justice System and Mental Retardation*, R.W. Conley, R. Luckasson & G.N. Bouthilet, eds, Paul Brookes Publications, Baltimore.

[7] Appelbaum, K.L. & Appelbaum, P.S. (1994). Criminal justice related competencies in defendants with mental retardation, *Journal of Psychiatry and Law* **14**, 483–503.

[8] Ellis, J. & Luckasson, R.A. (1985). Mentally retarded criminal defendants, *George Washington Law Review* **53**, 414–493.

[9] Everington, C. & Fulero, S.M. (1999). Competence to confess: Measuring understanding and suggestibility of defendants with mental retardation, *Mental Retardation* **37**, 212–220.

[10] Macvaugh, G.S. & Grisso, T. (2006). Assessment of mental retardation in death row inmates: A survey of

professional practices, *Paper Presented at the Conference of the American Psychology-Law Society, March 2006*, St. Petersburg.

[11] Everington, C. & Olley, J.G. (2004). An analysis of forensic psychological evaluations in capital cases involving defendants with mental retardation: Has Atkins made a difference? *Paper Presented at the Conference of the American Psychology-Law Society, March 2004*, Scottsdale.

[12] Death Penalty Information Center. Retrieved from website: www.deathpenaltyinfo.org (accessed on, 2007).

[13] Chase v. State, 873 So.2d 1029 (Miss. 2004).

[14] American Psychiatric Association (2000). *Diagnostic and Statistical Manual of Mental Disorders*, 4th Edition, Text Revision. American Psychiatric Association, Washington, DC.

[15] American Association on Mental Deficiency (1983). *Classification in Mental Retardation*, 8th Edition, American Association on Mental Deficiency, Washington, DC.

[16] American Association on Mental Retardation (1992). *Mental Retardation: Definition, Classification, and Systems of Supports*, 9th Edition, American Association on Mental Retardation, Washington, DC.

[17] Greenspan, S. (1997). Dead manual walking? Why the 1992 definition needs redoing, *Education and Training in Mental Retardation and Developmental Disabilities* **32**, 179–190.

[18] American Association on Mental Retardation (2002). *Mental Retardation: Definition, Classification, and Systems of Supports*, 10th Edition, American Association on Mental Retardation, Washington, DC.

[19] Everington, C. & Olley, J.G. (2008). Implications of *Atkins v. Virginia*: Issues in defining and diagnosing mental retardation, *Journal of Forensic Psychology Practice* **8**(1), 1–23.

[20] Olvera, D.R., Dever, R.B. & Earnest, M.A. (2000). Mental retardation and sentences for murder: Comparison of two recent court cases, *Mental Retardation* **38**, 228–233.

[21] Baroff, G.S. (1991). Establishing mental retardation in capital cases: A potential matter of life and death, *Mental Retardation* **29**, 343–349.

[22] Keyes, D.W., Edwards, W.J. & Derning, T.J. (1998). Mitigating mental retardation in capital cases: Finding the "invisible" defendant, *Mental and Physical Disability Law Reporter* **22**, 529–539.

[23] Wechsler, D. (2008). *Wechsler Adult Intelligence Scale*, 4th Edition, Psychological Corporation, San Antonio.

[24] Roid, G.H. (2003). *Stanford-Binet Intelligence Scales*, 5th Edition, Riverside, Itaska.

[25] Kaufman, A.S. & Kaufman, N.L. (1993). *Kaufman Adolescent and Adult Intelligence Test*, American Guidance Service, Circle Pines.

[26] Kellogg, C.E. & Morton, N.W. (1978). *The Revised Beta Examination (Beta II)*, The Psychological Corporation, San Antonio.

[27] Baroff, G.S. (2003). Establishing mental retardation in capital cases: An update, *Mental Retardation* **41**, 198–202.

[28] Flynn, J.R. (1984). The mean IQ of Americans: Massive gains 1932 to 1978, *Psychological Bulletin* **95**, 29–51.

[29] Flynn, J.R. (1998). WAIS-III and WISC-III IQ gains in the United States from 1972 to 1995: How to compensate for obsolete norms, *Perceptual and Motor Skills* **86**, 1231–1239.

[30] Kanaya, T., Scullin, M. & Ceci, S. (2003). The Flynn effect and U.S. policies, *American Psychologist* **58**, 778–790.

[31] Flynn, J.R. (2006). Tethering the elephant: capital cases, IQ, and the Flynn Effect, *Psychology Public Policy and Law* **12**, 170–189.

[32] Greenspan, S. (2006). Issues in the use of the "Flynn Effect" to adjust IQ scores when diagnosing MR, *Psychology in Mental Retardation and Developmental Disabilities* **31**, 3–7.

[33] Greenspan, S. (2007). Flynn-adjustment is a matter of basic fairness: Response to Roger B. Moore, Jr, *Psychology in Mental Retardation and Developmental Disabilities* **32**, 7–8.

[34] Flynn, J.R. (2007). Capital offenders and the death sentence: A scandal that must be addressed, *Psychology in Mental Retardation and Developmental Disabilities* **32**, 3–7.

[35] Moore, R.B. (2006). Modification of individual's IQ scores is not accepted professional practice, *Psychology in Mental Retardation and Developmental Disabilities* **32**, 11–12.

[36] Weiss, L. (2007). *Technical Report: Response to Flynn*, Harcourt Assessment, Retrieved from website: http://harcourtassessment.com/NR/rdonlyres/98BBF5D2-F0E8-4DF6-87E2-51D0CD6EE98C/0/WAISIII_TR_lr.pdf.

[37] Everington, C. & Keyes, D. (1999). Diagnosing mental retardation in criminal proceedings: The importance of documenting adaptive behavior, *Forensic Examiner* **8**, 31–34.

[38] Sparrow, S.S., Balla, D.A. & Cicchetti, D. (2005). *Vineland Adaptive Behavior Scales II*, Pearson Assessments, Minneapolis.

[39] Harrison, P.L. & Oakland, T. (2003). *ABAS II: Adaptive Behavior Assessment System*, 2nd Edition, The Psychological Corporation, San Antonio.

[40] Bruininks, R.H., Woodcock, R.W., Weatherman, R.F. & Hill, B.K. (1996). *SIB-R: Scales of Independent Behavior – Revised*, Riverside, Itaska.

[41] Greenspan, S. & Switzky, H.N. (2003). Execution exemption should be based on actual vulnerability, not disability label, *Ethics and Behavior* **13**, 19–26.

[42] Lindenhoker, D. & McCarron, L. (1983). *The Street Survival Skills Questionnaire*, McCarron-Dial Systems, Dallas.

[43] Brodsky, S.L. & Galloway, V.A. (2003). Ethical and professional demands for forensic mental health professionals in the post-*Atkins* era, *Ethics and Behavior* **13**, 3–9.

[44] Weiss, K.J., Haskins, B.H. & Hauser, M.J. (2004). Commentary: *Atkins* and clinical practice, *Journal of*

The American Academy of Psychiatry and the Law **32**, 309–313.

[45]   Bonnie, R.J. & Gustafson, K. (2007). The challenge of implementing *Atkins v. Virginia*: How legislatures and courts can promote accurate assessments and adjudications of mental retardation in death penalty cases, *Richmond Law Review* **41**, 811–860.

[46]   Foster v. State, 848 So.2d 175 (Miss. 2003).

[47]   Hathaway, S. & McKinley, J.C. (1989). *The Minnesota Multiphasic Personality Inventory (MMPI-2)*, Merrill/Prentice Hall, Columbus, Ohio.

[48]   Keyes, D.W. (2004). Use of the Minnesota multiphasic personality inventory (MMPI) to identify malingering mental retardation, *Mental Retardation* **42**, 151–153.

[49]   Hurley, K.E. & Deal, W.P. (2006). Assessment instruments measuring malingering used with individuals who have mental retardation: Potential problems and issues, *Mental Retardation* **44**, 112–119.

[50]   Rogers, R., Bagby, R.M. & Dickens, S.E. (1992). *Structured Interview of Reported Symptoms: Professional Manual*, Psychological Assessment Resources, Odessa, FL.

[51]   Tombaugh, T.N. (1996). *Test of Memory Malingering (TOMM) Manual*, Multi-Health Systems, New York.

[52]   Lezak, M. (1995). *Neuropsychological Assessment*, 3rd Edition, Oxford University Press, New York.

[53]   Boone, K., Lu, P. & Herzberg, D. (2002). *The Dot Counting Test*, Western Psychological Services, Los Angeles.

[54]   Simon, M.J. (2007). Performance of mentally retarded forensic patients on the Test of Memory Malingering, *Journal of Clinical Psychology* **63**, 339–344.

[55]   Goldberg, J.O. & Miller, H.R. (1986). Performance of psychiatric inpatients and intellectually deficient individuals on a task that assesses the validity of memory complaints, *Journal of Clinical Psychology* **42**, 43–46.

[56]   Hayes, J.S., Hale, D.B. & Gouvier, W.M. (1997). Do tests predict malingering in defendants with mental retardation? *Journal of Psychology* **131**, 575–576.

[57]   Beaber, R.J., Marston, A., Michelli, J. & Mills, M.J. (1985). A brief test for measuring malingering in schizophrenic individuals, *American Journal of Psychiatry* **142**, 1478–1481.

[58]   Schretlen, D. & Arkowitz, H. (1990). A psychological test battery to detect prison inmates who fake insanity or mental retardation, *Behavioral Sciences and The Law* **8**, 75–84.

[59]   Bender, L. (1938). *A Visual Motor Gestalt Test and Its Clinical Use*, The Orthopsychiatric Association, New York.

[60]   Graue, L.O., Berry, D.T.R., Clark, J.A., Sollman, M.J. Cardi, M., Hopkins, J. & Werline, D. (2007). Identification of feigned mental retardation using the new generation of malingering detection instruments: Preliminary findings, *The Clinical Neuropsychologist* **21**, 929–942.

[61]   Marshall, P. & Happe, M. (2007). The performance of individuals with mental retardation on cognitive tests assessing effort and motivation, *The Clinical Neuropsychologist* **21**, 826–840.

[62]   Dean, A.C., Victor, T.L., Boone, K.B. & Arnold, G. (2008). The relationship of IQ to effort test performance, *The Clinical Neuropsychologist* **22**, 705–722.

[63]   Doane, B.M. & Salekin, K.L. (in press). Susceptibility of current adaptive behavior measures to feigned deficits, *Law and Human Behavior*.

[64]   Bonnie, R.J. (2004). The American Psychiatric Association's resource document on mental retardation and capital sentencing: Implementing *Atkins v. Virginia*, *Journal of The American Academy of Psychiatry and the Law* **32**, 304–308.

[65]   Daubert v. Merrell Dow Pharmaceuticals, Inc., 509 U.S. 579 (1993).

[66]   Olley, J.G. (2006). The assessment of adaptive behavior in adult forensic cases: Part 2: The importance of adaptive behavior, *Psychology in Mental Retardation and Developmental Disabilities* **32**, 7–8.

[67]   Duvall, J.C. & Morris, R.J. (2006). Assessing mental retardation in death penalty cases: Critical issues for psychology and psychological practice, *Professional Psychology, Research and Practice* **37**, 658–665.

[68]   Olley, J.G., Greenspan, S. & Switzky, H. (2006). Division 33 *ad hoc* committee on mental retardation and the death penalty, *Psychology in Mental Retardation and Developmental Disabilities* **31**, 11–13.

[69]   Olley, J.G. (2006). The assessment of adaptive behavior in adult forensic cases: Part 1, *Psychology in Mental Retardation and Developmental Disabilities* **32**, 2–4.

[70]   Olley, J.G. (2007). The assessment of adaptive behavior in adult forensic cases: Part 3: Sources of adaptive behavior information, *Psychology in Mental Retardation and Developmental Disabilities* **33**, 3–6.

GILBERT S. MACVAUGH, III, KAREN L. SALEKIN AND J. GREGORY OLLEY

Mental Status: Examination

Introduction

No complex activity can be studied without good bookkeeping. Yet even the best system demands adequate judgment and individual initiative.
      –Adolf Meyer "Motto" [1]

The Mental Status Examination (MSE) refers to the structured reporting of information systematically obtained by the clinician regarding an individual's mental state at the time of the interview. The MSE is usually presented as a separate section of the evaluation, distinct from the individual's biographical history or anamnesis (childhood, education, employment, relationships, and other history) and distinct from information regarding past psychiatric history, substance abuse, and history of medical illness. The MSE summarizes findings that are obtained through systematic assessment at the time of the interview. The examiner may rely upon direct observation as well as the individual's spontaneous statements, responses to inquiry regarding present symptoms and responses to specific test questions (of cognitive function, for example).

Historical Background of the Mental Status Examination

Although the format of the MSE was codified by the Swiss-American psychiatrist Adolf Meyer in 1902 [1, 2] in a privately printed pamphlet, some treatises from the nineteenth century present case reports or vignettes by describing the patient's symptomatology and findings on examination in a structured manner, using the categories that comprise the MSE as we know it today. As recently as the 1960 s, psychiatrists debated the value of the MSE, leading up to studies of the reliability of findings on different elements of the MSE. Today, in the English-speaking world, the usefulness of the MSE is accepted by consensus and it is taught as a standard part of the training of psychologists and psychiatrists.

Purposes of the Mental Status Examination

The primary purpose of performing a MSE is to aid in establishing a diagnosis of the individual's current state. This may include the determination of acute symptomatology in the context of longstanding illness as well as the assessment of the individual's risk of imminent harm to himself or others. Although the MSE is generally performed the most thoroughly by mental health professionals, the MSE is relevant in medical specialties other than psychiatry, because a patient's mental state may have bearing on the reliability of information given in the subjective account of his or her history, medical or otherwise ([3], pp. 5–6).

The aim of the MSE as recorded in a clinical treatment note or a forensic report is to communicate information to a reader. The MSE can be viewed as analogous to the physical examination, in that it provides a structured assessment of the person's present condition and a coherent, organized presentation of the data. A psychiatrist may make use of the MSE to remind herself on a future office visit of how the patient appeared the time before. A doctor on call may refer to the MSE to determine whether a patient was stable earlier in the day; he will then record his own examination along with the details of his management of the situation, so that the patient's psychiatrist will know the details of the patient's condition overnight.

In the forensic setting, a MSE conveys the evaluee's mental state at the time of the examination and thereby provides a context and support for the expert's findings in the evaluation. In an assessment of Competence to Stand Trial, for example, the recording of the defendant's present mental condition allows the expert to refer back to these elements in the writing of her opinion. In adversarial proceedings, the MSE allows the trier of fact to assess whether differences in expert opinion may be in part explained by differences in mental state at separate points in time.

Conducting the Mental Status Examination

Similarities Between the MSE in Clinical Treatment and Forensic Settings

Both types of interview require clinical skill in order to obtain the necessary information to complete an assessment. Information pertaining to the MSE is obtained in the context of a larger interview process that includes the history of past psychological symptoms, treatment, and personal history. Although clinicians view the MSE as a specific examination that takes place during a particular portion of the interview (usually after the individual's account of her history and pertinent background information) the clinician obtains data that contribute to the MSE throughout the entire face-to-face contact time with the person being evaluated. Development of rapport is important as is tact and a nonjudgmental attitude, as the interviewee may be reluctant to speak about symptoms such as hallucinations, delusions, fears, or suicidal ideas (SI). The clinician should also be attentive to his own potential bias or his personal reactions to the individual, which may lead to avoidance of necessary exploration of the interviewee's responses to questions.

Differences Between the MSE in Clinical Treatment and Forensic Settings

Clinical treatment interviews and forensic evaluations serve different purposes, and the MSE is partly shaped by elements specific to each context. A succinct summary of the major differences between treatment interviews and forensic interviews may be found in Melton *et al.* [4] The differences most pertinent to the MSE *per se* concern the examiner's attitude and the degree of validity of the interviewee's self-report in forensic settings. These are addressed briefly below:

Confidentiality. Unlike the treatment interview, a forensic interview is likely to result in a written report to a legal entity (attorney, court, or administrative agency) responsible for deciding an issue that has required clarification by an expert. Despite the nonconfidentiality warning given at the beginning of the interview, the examiner's necessary use of clinical interviewing skills may put the evaluee at ease, leading the evaluee to have the impression that the examiner is in a helping role. This may encourage the individual to reveal information about current symptoms that he may later realize is not in his best interest. On the contrary, some evaluees are acutely aware of the nonconfidential nature of the content of the MSE and may purposefully or unintentionally misrepresent, distort or falsify their responses to the examiner's questions, or withhold information (*see* **Malingering: Forensic Evaluations**). One of the ethical challenges of forensic practice involves the task of maintaining an appropriate balance between scepticism and neutrality, on the one hand, and empathy and tact on the other.

Therapeutic Versus Medicolegal Aims. Related to the issue of malingering is the awareness on the part of both examiner and evaluee of the legal questions that form the backdrop and purpose of the interview. Unlike the treatment interview, with its emphasis on therapeutic aims and problem solving in the patient's current circumstances, the MSE in a forensic

interview contributes to forming an opinion on a legal issue. Additionally, the forensic question posed to the evaluator sometimes entails an assessment of cause and effect, further changing the role of the MSE. An evaluee may believe that it is in his best interest to exaggerate symptoms reported in the MSE, because he is asserting emotional damages in a tort claim. Or an evaluee may seek to give the impression of having few if any pathological symptoms at present in order to support a claim in favor of fitness for return to work.

Categories of the Mental Status Examination

An essential feature of the MSE is its systematic nature. The clinician may observe a number of elements important in the MSE during the subjective, narrative portion of the interview, while the interviewee is giving an account of his past history and the issues leading up to the request for evaluation, either with the aim of treatment or for legal purposes. Nevertheless, the systematic organization of the MSE allows the examiner to review the major components of the individual's current mental state in a more thorough fashion, and helps to avoid the omission of questions regarding significant areas of mental functioning that would otherwise not be formally assessed.

Table 1 represents the major categories of the MSE, which are usually assessed by most clinicians in the English-speaking community. We define in broad outline the meanings of the technical terms that describe these categories, referring the reader to more comprehensive, detailed treatises which are available [3, 5].

The panoply of tests and possible questions that a clinician may use to assess elements of each of the categories described in Table 1 is wide, and each examiner has his preferences. There is no standardized set of tests and questions for performing the MSE, though, as stated above, consensus exists regarding the areas of mental functioning that should be included.

A Note on the Mini Mental State Examination

Although a number of the tests used to assess items on the cognitive portion of the MSE overlap with or

Table 1   Main categories of the mental status examination

Appearance, attitude, and behavior	This section of the report includes description of the individual's physical appearance (clothing, tattoos, or piercing), hygiene and physical movement (such as tics, visible side effects of medications, agitation, or slowness). The individual's degree of cooperation with the interview and his interaction style may also be noted.
Mood and affect	Mood refers to the person's description of her general emotional state (e.g., sad, happy, or nervous) and may be reported as a direct quote. Affect refers to the clinician's observation of the outward emotional expression, including the appearance of sadness or elation, range and variability of expression, and the appropriateness of emotions in relation to the content of the individual's speech.
Speech and language	A person's speech may be described on the basis of ease of flow, spontaneity, rate, and volume. The examiner may also comment on whether the individual is difficult to interrupt or speaks as though under pressure. Included here are comments on speech and language abnormalities, such as stuttering, slurring, or use of invented words.
Thought process and content	Thought process refers to the flow of ideas and whether the thinking is disjointed or coherent. The examiner may note whether the individual has a tendency to give answers in a circuitous manner or tends to express vaguely associated thoughts without coming back to the topic at hand.
	Thought content refers to the person's preoccupations, obsessions or delusions, as well as nondelusional paranoid or grandiose ideas.
	This section also includes the presence or absence of suicidal and homicidal ideas.
Perception	The presence or absence of perceptual abnormalities is noted here and may include hallucinations (when the individual reports a perception involving one of the five senses, in the absence of real stimuli) or illusions (when a true stimulus is misinterpreted or distorted).
Cognition	This section includes the person's level of consciousness (awake, alert, or sleepy), assessment of immediate and short-term memory, concentration and ability for abstract thinking. The individual's awareness of current events and general knowledge is also reported here.
Insight and judgment	Insight refers to the individual's understanding of his condition. The term is primarily used to describe his awareness and acceptance of having a psychiatric disorder, though it may also be used to indicate awareness of his legal situation.
	Judgement refers to the person's ability to use logical reasoning to respond to situations, and is often formally tested through hypothetical scenarios as well as assessed through observation of recent behavior and responses in the interview.

are identical to items on the rating scale known as the *Mini Mental State Examination* (*MMSE*), these two evaluations should not be confused. The MMSE was devised by Folstein *et al.* in 1975 [6] as a means of providing rapid and clinically feasible assessment of whether an individual may be suffering from an organic brain disorder. The MMSE is scored on a scale of a maximum of 30 points, and provides an impression as to whether further formal testing is required. It does not assess the noncognitive

areas covered in the MSE. The full MMSE is not considered to be an inherent part of the MSE, though some clinicians may choose to perform it routinely in each evaluation by personal preference.

The Mental Status Examination in Medical Records

In the recording of a MSE in the medical record, the examiner usually assumes that any reader has the same level of technical knowledge as the examiner himself. The writer often uses commonly accepted abbreviations (AH for auditory hallucinations, SI for suicidal ideas) and frequently does not write in complete sentences (Affect – constricted, inappropriate).

The level of detail included in the MSE varies according to the clinician's familiarity with the patient and according to the findings that may bear emphasis when a record is being created to communicate with other practitioners. Upon first contact in the outpatient setting, or at the time of admission, the MSE is recorded in detail. At subsequent outpatient follow-up visits or on subsequent evaluations in the hospital, an MSE may cover very briefly those portions of the examination that are unremarkable or unchanged. A change in clinical condition, or emergency coverage, on call for example, may stimulate the examiner to record greater detail. In general, the majority of clinicians comment on each of the main categories of the MSE in the record following any assessment of the patient. It is common practice to remark on the presence or absence of suicidal or homicidal ideas during the interview in making a record of each contact with the patient.

It is important to keep in mind that although mental health professionals tend to be aware that what they write in the medical record may someday appear in court, legal proceedings are not the main purpose of the medical record. An attorney should not attempt to interpret abbreviations, scrawls, and shorthand that are rife in the medical record without the assistance of a medical expert. Although this may seem obvious, the point also extends to the gathering of data, in that attorneys should not attempt to sort and select medical records, which are often obtained from multiple sources and can be voluminous, prior to forwarding the material to an expert for technical assessment. A set of documents that is as complete as possible – and as legible as possible (i.e., sufficiently dark photocopies) – is indispensable to the expert in formulating an opinion.

The Mental Status Examination in Forensic Reports

The recording of the MSE in the context of legal proceedings follows guidelines for all forensic reports: technical terms must be "translated" into language comprehensible to a lay reader remaining all the

while coherent for assessment by another forensic examiner who may be called upon to comment on the findings. Because the MSE represents one of the most highly technical parts of the forensic report, the task of translation into lay language poses particular challenges. Descriptions should be sufficiently detailed so as to evoke for the reader a mental impression of the state of the individual at the time of evaluation. In the case of positive (abnormal) findings or findings that differ from prior descriptions of the person, examples are useful.

An MSE should be performed at each meeting with the evaluee, though repetition of the cognitive examination is usually unnecessary unless there are intervening factors between interviews (e.g., changes in medication, or an observed difference in performance in the interview). This MSE should be recorded for each interview date, in order to convey the consistency or lack thereof in the individual's mental state overtime. If the evaluee is seen on three occasions, the examiner should comment on the MSE on each of the three dates, briefly if there is no significant change, and at greater length if there are major differences.

The narrative description of the MSE in a forensic report should follow the same outline, including the same categories as that of the clinical MSE. This ensures that another clinical examiner, hired by the opposing side or brought into the case at a later point by the same attorney, is able to follow a predictable sequence familiar to all clinicians.

The writing of the MSE is also an occasion for the examiner to identify the evidence that will be included to support the determination of a diagnosis and opinion. The MSE is a chance for the examiner to systematically assess the evidence that is present at the time of the interview, in reference to the legal questions on which he has been asked to opine.

Is the Mental Status Examination "Objective"?

The river where you set your foot just now is gone – those waters giving way to this, now this.

– Heraclitus, "Fragments" [7]

We stated earlier that the MSE is analogous to the physical examination in other branches of medicine. However, psychiatric symptoms are in general more apt to vary between evaluations than physical findings such as a tumor or a broken bone. More so than in general medicine, findings on the psychiatric examination may vary between examiners and at different points in time. This is relevant in legal proceedings, where discrepant expert opinions are subject to comparison and cross-examination.

In a 1961 article, Rosenzweig *et al.* presented findings from a study of the agreement between evaluators and consistency over time in findings on the MSE. They found that "while reliability (agreement) was not significantly influenced by individual bias in interpretation of concepts or by individual capacity to make observations it was significantly influenced by individual differences in interviewing technique" ([8], p. 1107). This suggests that if examiners are observing the same phenomenon, they are likely to record it in a similar manner, but that those elements of the MSE that require the examiner to elicit specific responses are susceptible to greater variation, depending upon the interviewer's focus and approach in asking questions.

Numerous factors may influence the result of the MSE, including the interviewee's degree of fatigue or willingness to be forthcoming, the examiner's interview style and technique, the setting where the interview occurs, etc. The evaluee's mental condition is subject to change over time, due to worsening or improvement of his mental illness, the effects of medication and the presence or absence of life stressors. The MSE is an assessment of present mental state and to some extent, differing expert opinions may reflect differing data at the time of evaluation. Nevertheless, as Ross and Leichner point out, "[t]he MSE is one of the tightest areas of clinical psychiatry, and its assessment is reliable both when the assesor's responses are restricted to highly discrete, operationalized items and in global, qualitative assessment" ([9], p. 111) even where the examiners' vocabulary in the description of details vary.

Conclusion

The MSE is a useful means of organizing clinical data concerning an individual's mental condition at the time of examination. The MSE refers to a particular time in the clinical interview when present state information is reviewed in a systematic manner, as well as to the written recording of this information, along with other observations obtained during face-to-face contact with the patient or forensic evaluee.

References

[1]   Meyer, A.. (1951). Outlines of examinations; privately printed, 1918, in *The Collected Papers of Adolf Meyer, Volume III: Medical Teaching*, E.E. Winters, ed, The Johns Hopkins Press, Baltimore, pp. 224–258.

[2]   Keller, M.B. & Manschreck, T.C. (1981). The bedside mental status examination – reliability and validity, *Comprehensive Psychiatry* **22**(5), 500–511.

[3]   Trzepacz, P.T. & Baker, R.W. (1993). *The Psychiatric Mental Status Examination*, Oxford University Press, New York.

[4]   Melton, G.B., Petrila, J., Poythress, N.G. & Slobogin, C. (1997). *Psychological Evaluations for the Courts: A Handbook for Mental Health Professionals and Lawyers*, 2nd Edition, The Guilford Press, New York, p. 42.

[5]   Othmer, E., Othmer, S.C., Othmer, J.P. (2005). *Psychiatric Interview, History, and Mental Status Examination. Kaplan & Sadock's Comprehensive Textbook of Psychiatry*, 8th Edition, B.J. Sadock & V.A. Sadock, eds, Lippincott Williams & Wilkins, Philadelphia, pp. 794–826.

[6]   Folstein, M.F., Folstein, S.E. & McHugh, P.R. (1975). 'Mini-mental state': a practical method for grading the cognitive state of patients for the clinician, *Journal of Psychiatric Research* **12**(3), 189–198.

[7]   Haxton, B. (translator) (2001/2003). *Heraclitus. 41 Fragments*, Penguin Books, New York.

[8]   Rosenzweig, N., Vandenberg, S.G., Moore, K. & Dukay, A. (1961). A study of the reliability of the mental status examination, *American Journal of Psychiatry* **117**, 1102–1108.

[9]   Ross, C.A. & Leichner, P. (1988). Residents performance on the mental status examination, *Canadian Journal of Psychiatry* **33**, 108–111.

Further Reading

Taylor, M.A., Abrams, R., Faber, R. & Almy, G. (1980). Cognitive tasks in the mental status examination, *Journal of Nervous and Mental Disease* **168**(3), 167–170.

Suzanne Yang and Delaney M. Smith

Methanol *see* Alcohol: Use, Abuse, Tolerance, and Dependency

Method: Error *see* Error Rates in Forensic Methods

Microchemistry

Microchemistry, also known as *chemical microscopy*, was defined by Emile Chamot in elementary chemical microscopy as, "the application of the microscope to the solution of chemical problems". He also explained that microchemistry is chemistry on a small scale. The American microchemist, Benedetti-Pichler, defined microchemistry as the development, correlation, and systematization of the methods for handling small quantities of material, and for the observation of their properties. The scientific discipline of microchemistry has a rich and storied history going back to Pliny (23–79 AD), who describes an iron sulfate test. Microchemistry has been practiced for over 180 years, long before the development of instrumental methods. Microchemical tests provide a rapid and inexpensive way to obtain chemical data from microscopic size particles. Many rather simple tests have been developed to qualitatively analyze cations, anions, and functional groups. Francois-Vincent Raspail (1794–1878) is often recognized as the founder of chemical microscopy and the first true microchemist. In 1827, Raspail published results of his work on silica in Spongilla and calcium oxalate in the starch of monocotyledons. It is within this publication that he introduces the term *chemical microscopy*. Friedrich Emich (1860–1940) and Fritz Pregl (1860–1930) from the Technical University of Graz, Austria were the preeminent microchemists in Europe. The earliest complete book dealing with microchemistry was from an American, Theodore G. Wormley, The Microchemistry of Poisons, in 1867. There are many other exceptional scientists that have advanced chemical microscopy, an incomplete list of these individuals include E. Boricky, A. Streng, K. Haushofer, C. Klement, A. Renard, H. Behrens, A.C. Hutsse, C. Hinrichs, N. Schoorl, J. Donau, P.D.C. Kley, O. Tunmann, H. Molisch, C.W. Mason, L. Rosenthaler, L. Kofler, A. Kofler, F. Schneider, W. McCrone, H. Schaeffer, H. Keune, C. Fulton, E. Jungreis, Palenik, S., and J. Delly [1].

Practicing scientists working in chemistry, microanalysis, and serology can rely on many sources of literature in microchemistry. The classic texts by E.M. Chamot and C. W. Mason, Volumes 1 and 2, the Handbook of Chemical Microscopy [2] are essential. They were originally published in 1930–1931, and have gone through several editions and reprints. C. Fulton's Modern Microcrystal Test for Drugs [3] is a usefully text employed in drug identification. E. Jungreis' book, Spot Test Analysis, defines tests for clinical, environmental, forensic, and geochemical applications [4]. A large volume of periodical literature is available. There are three journals devoted to microchemistry: Mikrochemie (1923–1952), Mikrochimica Acta (1953-), and the Microchemical Journal (1957-). The Microscope (1937-) is an excellent source of literature on microchemistry, such as J. Hollifield's 2003 article, "Characterization of Squaric Acid Precipitates" [5] and T. Hopen and J. Kilbourn's article "Characterization and Identification of Water-Soluble Explosives" [6]. Many useful microchemical tests and spot tests have been developed over the years and incorporated into books, articles, and manuals in areas as diverse as paper and textile fiber analysis, explosives, drug chemistry, and food microscopy (*see* **Explosion Debris: Laboratory Analysis of**). Spot tests are color or precipitate reactions resulting from mixing an unknown and a test reagent on a ceramic or glass plate having a series of depressions (a spot plate). The fifth edition of the *Merck Index* describes over 4510 named reactions [7].

Long before the advent of instrumental chemical analysis "chemical microscopes" were employed to critically examine and identify materials in the physical world. These microscopes were based upon the petrographic microscope (used in the examination of mineralogical specimens) design first developed by Henry Fox Talbot in the 1840s. The microscope was equipped with Nicol prisms that polarized light. A circular rotating stage with a Vernier scale was employed to measure crystallographic angles. These microscopes are essentially the same type used today, referred to as *polarized light microscopes* (*PLM*), and are used in all modern forensic laboratories around the world (*see* **Microscopy: Low Power**; **Microscopy: High Power**). For most observations, a $10\times$ objective and a $10\times$ ocular, giving a total magnification of $100\times$ is adequate. Occasionally, a $40\times$ objective may be used giving a total magnification of 400×. Scientists must have a good foundation in the basic principles of polarized light microscopy to understand what they are looking at and the terminology used to describe the crystals. Even no reactions or the formation of a precipitate but no crystals tell something about the material being tested.

Other equipment useful in microchemical testing include known chemically pure reagents, a small glass rod with a 3–4-mm smooth tip, glass or porcelain spot plates, disposable capillary pipettes, microscope slides, and spatulas [8].

Microchemical tests, also known as *microcrystal tests*, are used in both organic and inorganic characterization and identification of unknowns. E. G. C. Clarke states, in Isolation and Identification of Drugs [9], the value of crystal tests: "The microcrystal test is unsuitable as a primary method of identification of an unknown compound, as it does not lend itself to form the basis of an identification scheme. Its real value is as a means of final identification to confirm a provisional diagnosis made from chromatographic or spectrometric evidence, its extreme simplicity, the rapidity of which may be performed, and its high degree of specificity, rendering it ideal for this purpose". When properly performed, microcrystal testing is a useful tool for the analytical chemist. As with any other analytical tool it has its advantages and limitations. It is fast, requires very little sample, is often nondestructive (in that the tested material can be recovered), can distinguish among the isomers of some compounds, and, for many compounds, is highly specific. Some disadvantages are that when first starting, the analyst must test many compounds to learn what the products are and which reagents work best. Analysts must learn how to be consistent in reporting what they see, i.e., the written description of the crystals or drawings of the crystals must be reported in the same manner, there is no printout of the results (although with the advent of digital microphotography this problem can be eliminated), and some closely related compounds may give the same type of crystals.

The basic techniques of microcrystal testing and the examination of many substances encountered in forensic analysis are well documented in Volume II of Chamot and Mason. Microcrystal testing of materials requires getting the material in question to react with specific reagent(s) to obtain insight as to the composition of the material or to identify the substance. The nature of the material being examined, and, often,

experience determine the method used. In inorganic microchemical analysis, ions of the material being tested need to be brought into solution. For most reactions water is used as the solvent. The solubility of the test material gives clues in identification. For example, sodium chloride rapidly dissolves in water whereas sulfur does not. Other times the solvent may need to be slightly basic or acidic. To perform a solubility test, a single particle (or a few particles) is placed on a microscope slide next to a very small drop of solvent. The solvent can be first placed on a glass rod and gently tapped to the microscope slide releasing the solvent. While using the stereobinocular microscope one of the test particles is pushed into the solvent and the solubility, if any, is recorded. If solubility is not observed, gentle heating over a small flame and quick microscopical observation reveal the status of solubility. Another direct method to observe solubility is "huffing" on a single crystal with warm breath. The heat and moisture from the mouth may be all that is needed to dissolve a particle. Chamot and Mason give three microscopical methods for the addition of reagents to test drops. Method I is the method most commonly used. The reagent and test particle are dissolved in separate drops of water on a microscope slide. They are joined together using a glass rod forming a narrow channel between the two drops. Diffusion occurs as the two drops contact each other forming precipitates and, or, characteristic crystals. Method II introduces a large crystal of the reagent to the test drop to form crystals. In method III, the reagent solution is drawn in a narrow channel across a dry film, obtained by evaporating to dryness a solution of the substance to be tested. A drop of the test solution is placed on a clean slide and a drop of the reagent is then placed near the dried material. Using a glass rod or a platinum needle, a small line of the reagent solution is pulled across the dried film being careful not to inundate the entire dried area and examine the crystals. The hanging drop method is another elegant test using sublimation to form crystals. A drop of the test solution, a portion of the dried material, or material containing the unknown substance is placed on a microscope slide, and a cut glass ring from a test tube is placed over it. A drop of another material that causes the sample to volatilize is added. A drop of the test reagent is placed on a coverslip, which is then inverted and placed over the opening (Figure 1). The volatilized material rises and reacts with the reagent. This is a good method when one has a mixture and cannot develop identifiable crystals with any of the other methods and the compound of interest is known to volatilize.

Coupled with microcrystalline tests are spot tests (color tests), the basis of many tests by law enforcement agencies to test street drugs to determine what they may be. However, in the hands of the trained microscopist, many of these tests are very specific and provide detailed information. F. Feigl's books on inorganic and organic spot tests are some of the principle reference books useful when conducting these tests [10, 11]. The Merck Manual, fifth edition, is another good reference for finding tests for specific materials. These tests can be used to determine the

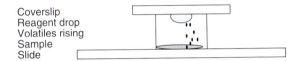

Coverslip
Reagent drop
Volatiles rising
Sample
Slide

Figure 1   Schematic diagram of a sublimation cell used in the hanging drop method

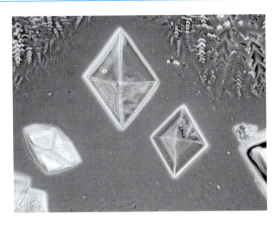

Figure 2   Recrystallization of sodium nitrate from a drop of water. Original magnification 200×

presence of metals, chemical compounds (inorganic and organic), certain elements, anions, cations, materials in food products, building materials, poisons, plant material, etc. Feigl based his tests on reactions that produced a macroscopic color; however,

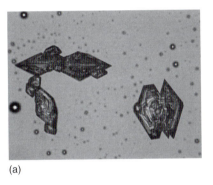

(a)

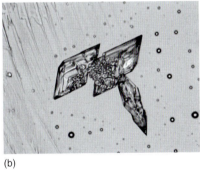

(b)

Figure 3   Sulfur recrystallized from chloroform. Original magnification 200×

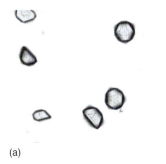

(a)

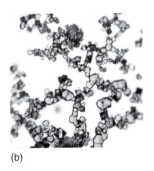

(b)

Figure 4   Isotropic octahedral crystals indicate the presence of ammonium. (a) magnification 200×; (b) 100×

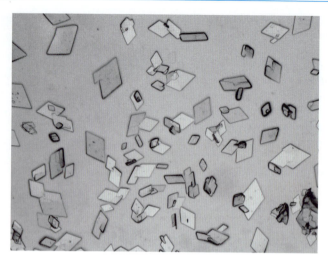

Figure 5   Yellow organic paint pigment using the sublimation cell. Original magnification 200×

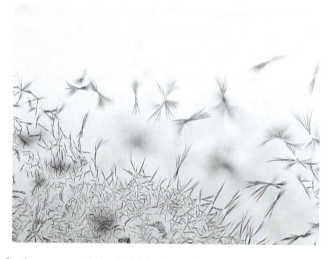

Figure 6   Takayama test for the presence of blood. Original magnification 200×

when these tests are conducted on a microscale, the reactions need to be viewed using the PLM. Often the colored product forms a precipitate that may crystallize forming distinctive crystals that can be characterized.

Microchemical tests and spot tests are used by forensic scientists in a number of disciplines. Examples of some of these tests are included with photomicrographs to convey the science and art of microscopy.

In the analysis of explosive residue, microchemical tests are often used (*see* **Explosion Debris:** **Laboratory Analysis of**). Inorganic water-soluble explosive oxidizers can be identified by the direct addition of a particle into a small drop of water on a microscope slide. By allowing a known particle to dissolve and recrystallize, characteristic well-formed crystals of the oxidizer can be quickly identified (Figure 2). Sulfur, an ingredient in black powder, can be recrystallized from methylene chloride or chloroform and its characteristic bipyramidal crystals observed (Figure 3). Ammonium can be identified by the hanging drop method. A few grains of the test chemical such as ammonium perchlorate, are placed

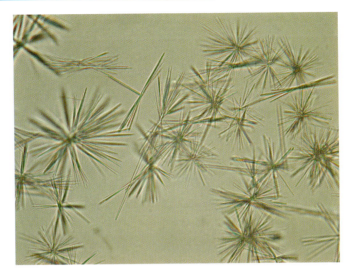

Figure 7 Colorless needles of gypsum, which formed in the presence of calcium. Original magnification 200×

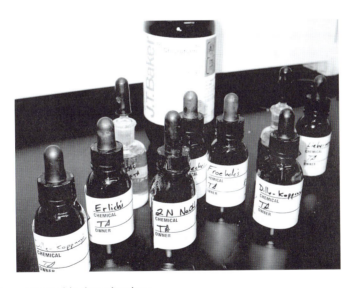

Figure 8 A group of reagents used in drug chemistry

onto a microscope slide and covered with one drop of 2N sodium hydroxide. One drop of platinic chloride solution is placed on the underside of a coverslip and then placed over the glass ring. Soon isotropic octahedra indicative for the presence of ammonium, forms (Figure 4). Many organic paint pigments can be identified by placing a test particle on a microscope slide that is covered with a small cut test tube ring of glass in which a coverglass is placed on top (*see* **Paint**). The slide is placed on a hot plate and

as the sample heats crystalline sublimation products form on the underside of the coverglass (Figure 5).

In the examination of microscopic flakes of material suspected to be blood, the Takayama test can be used. A portion of a suspected blood flake is placed on a microscope slide and covered with a coverslip. One or two drops of the Takayama reagent (prepared using sodium hydroxide, pyridine, glucose, and distilled water) are instilled under the coverslip. The slide is warmed for approximately 30 s on a hot

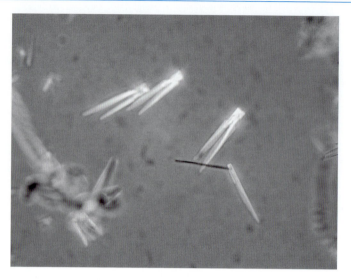

Figure 9   Gold chloride solution in phosphoric acid showing distinctive "clothe-pin" crystals indicative of methamphetamine. Original magnification 400×

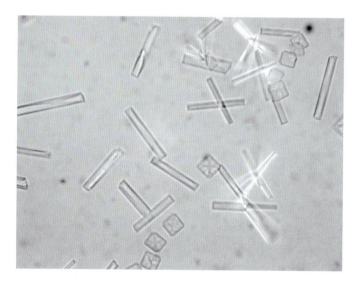

Figure 10   Gold chloride solution in phosphoric acid showing distinctive crystals indicative of dl-amphetamine. Original magnification 400×

plate. The presence of needle-shaped or rhomboid hemochromogen crystals (Figure 6) indicates a positive test for the presence of blood. This test is reported to react positive with as little as 0.001 ml of blood or 0.1 mg of hemoglobin. To test for the presence of calcium, a particle of suspected calcite ($CaCO_3$) is dissolved in a small drop of dilute hydrochloric acid. The evolution of carbon dioxide bubbles indicates CO_2 is being liberated. Using method I, a drop of dilute sulfuric acid is added. Observation along the edges yields birefringent colorless needles of gypsum ($CaSO_4 2H_2O$), which form in the presence of calcium (Figure 7). Many microchemical tests and reagents have been developed for the identification of drugs (Figure 8). Commonly used microchemical tests in drug chemistry include the use of gold chloride in phosphoric acid to confirm the presence of methamphetamine (Figure 9) and dl-amphetamine (Figure 10).

In spite of the continuing value of microcrystalline tests, lack of training and modern tendency to rely on instrumentation results in them being used less in forensic laboratories than some years ago.

References

[1]   Delly, J.G. (2006). *The Literature of Classical Micro-chemistry, Spot Tests, and Chemical Microscopy*, The Eyepoint, http://www.Modern Microscopy.com.

[2]   Chamot, E.M. (1938/1940). *Handbook of Chemical Microscopy*, John Wiley & Sons, New York, Vol. 1 and 2.

[3]   Fulton, C. (1969). Modern microcrystal test for drugs, in *The Identification of Organic Compounds by Microcrystalloscopic Chemistry*, Wiley Interscience, New York.

[4]   Jungreis, E. (1997). *Spot Test Analysis: Clinical, Environmental, Forensic, and Geochemical Applications*, 2nd Edition, John Wiley & Sons.

[5]   Hollifield, J. (2003). Characterization of squaric acid precipitates, *The Microscope* **51**(2), 81–103.

[6]   Hopen, J.T. & Kilbourn, J.H. (1985). Characterization and identification of water soluble explosives, *The Microscope* **33**, 1–22.

[7]   Merck (1940). Chemical, clinico-chemical reactions, tests and reagents, in *The Merck Index*, A 367 page table (623–990), 5th Edition, Merck Publishing.

[8]   Delly, J.G. (2006). *Essentials of Polarized Light Microscopy*, 3rd Edition, McCrone Associates, College of Microscopy.

[9]   Clarke, E.G.C. (1969). *Isolation and Identification of Drugs*, The Pharmaceutical Press, London, Reprinted 1971.

[10] Feigl, F. (1958). *Spot Tests in Inorganic Analysis*, 5th Edition, E.O. Ralph, ed, Elsevier, Amsterdam.

[11] Feigl, F. (1966). Spot tests in organic analysis, in *Collaboration with Vinzenz Anger*, E.O. Ralph, ed, 7th Edition, Elsevier, Amsterdam.

WILLIAM M. SCHNECK

Microsatellites

Prior to the 1980s, forensic genetic testing targeted polymorphic protein and blood group marker systems, for example ABO blood grouping and human leukocyte antigens (HLAs). These methods were limited by their low level of polymorphism and the relatively large amount of high-quality biological material required [1]. Also, there was limited analysis of biological material other than blood.

In 1980, Wyman and White used the restriction nuclease *Eco*RI to demonstrate variation in length between individuals at one particular noncoding locus on chromosome 14 [2]. The digested DNA was separated on a gel and detected by Southern blot analysis using a radioactive probe. This type of analysis was called *restriction fragment length polymorphism* (RFLP). This was the first example of a DNA marker that could be used to distinguish between individuals.

In 1985, Jeffreys *et al.* described a new type of polymorphic DNA marker termed *minisatellites* or *variable number tandem repeats* (VNTRs). Minisatellites are composed of sequences varying from 15 to 50 bp in length, repeated tandemly up to a total length of 20 kb [3]. It was this DNA technology that was first used in a criminal investigation (see Case study 1).

Case Study 1 This is a study of two murder investigations involving teenage girls in Leicester, England, in the mid-1980s. Owing to the case circumstances, investigators thought they were perpetrated by the same individual. Subsequently, a 17-year-old male confessed to the latter murder but denied involvement in the first. Using minisatellite technology, Professor Jeffreys was able to show that the biological materiel was left behind by the same person and that the man who had previously confessed could not be this person. A mass screen was undertaken with DNA sampled from 600 men from surrounding villages. A local baker, Colin Pitchfork, was eventually charged and convicted of the murders [4].

However, minisatellite analysis using RFLP was time consuming, difficult to interpret, and required over 50 ng of DNA.

In the 1990s, forensic DNA analysis advanced again to utilize PCR technology. PCR was originally applied forensically to HLA DQα and subsequently to minisatellites (known as *amplified fragment length polymorphisms, AMP FLPs*). PCR analysis of

VNTRs was quicker and required only approximately 5 ng of DNA; however, the resulting fragments of DNA were still relatively large [5].

By reducing the targeted repeat sequence, the amplified product is smaller and therefore less prone to be affected by sample degradation as many forensic samples may be. For this reason, microsatellites or short tandem repeats (STRs) amplified via the PCR became the preferred method for many forensic laboratories in the mid-1990s (*see* **Short Tandem Repeats**). STRs are lengths of DNA 2–5 nucleotides in length repeated tandemly. Their short length, variability between different individuals, and their ability to be amplified via PCR make them extremely useful as forensic DNA markers. Refer to **Short Tandem Repeats** for a more thorough discussion.

References

[1] Gill, P., Jeffreys, A.J. & Werrett, D.J. (1985). Forensic application of DNA 'Fingerprints', *Nature* **318**, 577–579.

[2] Wyman, A.R. & White, R. (1980). A highly polymorphic locus in human DNA, *Proceedings of the National Academy of Sciences* **77**(11), 6754–6758.

[3] Jeffreys, A.J., Wilson, V. & Thein, S.L. (1985). Hypervariable 'minisatellite' regions in human DNA, *Nature* **314**, 67–73.

[4] Napper, R. (2000). A national DNA database. The United Kingdom experience, *Australian Journal of Forensic Sciences* **32**, 65–70.

[5] Helmuth, R., Fildes, N., Blake, E., Luce, M.C., Chimera, J. & Madej, R. (1990). HLA-DQα allele and genotype frequencies in various human populations, determined by using enzymatic amplification and oligonucleotide probes, *American Journal of Human Genetics* **47**, 515–523.

JO-ANNE BRIGHT

Microscopy: FTIR

Introduction

Infrared spectroscopy is a technique widely practiced by forensic scientists and analytical chemists in general. The principle behind the technique is to shine infrared radiation onto a specimen and record the way in which it absorbs the radiation. The way in which this is done is by using a device called an *infrared spectrometer*, which, in it simplest implementation, irradiates the specimen at any one time with only a single wavelength of light in the infrared range. After absorption at that wavelength has been measured and recorded the spectrometer moves on to another wavelength, absorbance is recorded, and so on, until the entire infrared range has been covered. In classical instruments, this requires the spectrometer to make use of a device that works like a prism, and slits that reject radiation around the wavelength being measured. A graph of the magnitude of absorbance at each wavelength is referred to as that *specimen's infrared spectrum*. In general, other types of light (or electromagnetic radiation) can be absorbed by specimens as well, for example visible light is absorbed by a number of objects, resulting in a physical manifestation we know as color. The reason why infrared radiation, in particular, is useful in an analytical chemistry sense is because its absorbance arises from the interaction between the radiation and the many different connections (or bonds) between the atoms that make up the molecules that make up the specimen. What distinguishes one type of molecule from another is the types of atoms they contain and the arrangement in which the atoms are bonded to each other. As infrared spectroscopy is very sensitive to the bonds and the atoms present in molecules, it is a very powerful technique for analyzing materials to identify the molecules that make it up. By comparison, visible light absorption is much less sensitive to the atoms and bonds present in molecules, therefore it has much less analytical power. This can be appreciated by considering, for example, three objects with exactly the same shade of red, such as an apple, paint on a car, and a piece of dyed fabric. All three objects exhibit identical visible light spectra, but as the molecules of the chemicals responsible for the color are all different, their patterns of absorption of infrared light (i.e., their infrared spectra) are all different.

The infrared absorbance experiment described earlier is conducted in the laboratory by shining a beam of infrared radiation of about 10–15 mm in diameter onto the specimen. This is not a limitation if the objective of the exercise is to analyze a drug seizure or a large sample of paint or liquid. However, a substantial amount of evidentiary material is small or microscopic. A variant of infrared spectroscopy, which arises because there is a lower limit to the size of specimen that can be handled by standard laboratory equipment, is called *infrared microscopy* (or more correctly *infrared microspectrometry*). In infrared microspectroscopy, the infrared beam of large diameter is reduced in size to about 0.2 mm, and then caused to interact with the microscopic specimen. The infrared radiation emerging from the specimen and its vicinity is magnified and passed on to a detector. Three general types of equipment can be used for microspectroscopy: a beam condenser, which is an accessory that is attached to a standard spectrometer and makes use of its infrared beam and detector; an infrared microscope accessory, which also attaches to a standard spectrometer, but carries its own detector; and an infrared microspectrometer, which is an instrument that only operates on the microscopic domain. Beam condensers, although inexpensive, are difficult to use for trace evidence and do not produce good results for very small specimens, for this reason they are not commonly used in modern forensic laboratories. The other two accessories produce a much smaller beam at the specimen. The beam is circular, but it can be trimmed into square or rectangular shapes by curtains that can be drawn across the beam (these are referred to as a *diaphragm* or an *aperture*) before it is focused onto the specimen. This is important because fibers and many microscopic particles are not circular. Perhaps the most important feature as far as the analyst is concerned is that infrared microscope accessories and microspectrometers allow the specimen to be viewed and moved around at the focal point of the condensed infrared beam, and allow the size and orientation of diaphragms to be adjusted so that a region of interest within the specimen is analyzed, rather than the entire specimen.

In forensic science infrared microspectroscopy is used for the examination of microscopic particles of paint, rubber, explosives, and plastic, individual textile fibers, individual crystals of drugs and diluents, and individual textile fibers. Although it can be used for the examination of minerals (such as extenders in paint), it is not used for the examination of glass or metallic particles. Although there were early attempts at infrared microspectroscopy, its widespread popularity has only emerged in the last two decades owing to the widespread release of Fourier transform spectrometers. In conventional spectrometers, as described earlier, only single wavelengths of radiation are presented to the specimen at any one time. The wavelength selection process is not very efficient, with the result that only a very dim beam interacts with the specimen. If this beam is passed through a microscope to interact with a very tiny specimen, it is very difficult to measure the small levels of absorbance involved. In Fourier transform instruments, the entire range of infrared radiation is presented at high brightness to the specimen. The signal received from the specimen is a sum of all absorbances over all wavelengths over the entire infrared region, and a special mathematical procedure, called *Fourier transformation*, is used to "unscramble" the summed data into the infrared spectrum (*see* **Paint**; **Examination of Fibers and Textiles**; **Drug Analysis**).

Forensic scientists use infrared spectroscopy in two, nonexclusive general ways. Firstly, for the purposes of identification, the infrared spectrum of an unknown specimen is searched against entries on a spectral database until a "match" is found. In the case of a mixture of compounds, infrared spectroscopy is relatively straightforward in that the spectrum of the mixture is simply a direct combination or sum of the spectra of the individual components. Secondly, infrared spectroscopy is also used in a comparative sense, that is, to examine whether two pieces of material might share a common origin (for example comparison of a foreign fiber retrieved from a victim and fibers from a garment worn by a suspect). Some limitations of infrared spectroscopy are that some materials do not absorb infrared light at all (for example, common salt, metals, etc.), it is not a good technique for the detection of traces within a material (for example, explosives residues within water or soil), and sometimes it can be difficult to distinguish between members of a particular class of materials (for example, within the nylon textile fiber class, it is difficult to distinguish between nylon 6 and nylon 6, 6).

Infrared Transmission Microspectroscopy

Figure 1 depicts the important features found in an infrared microspectrometer or a microscope accessory functioning in transmission mode. The "lenses" in these devices are manufactured from paired convex and concave mirrors, because infrared radiation is absorbed by glass, and it is impractical to make

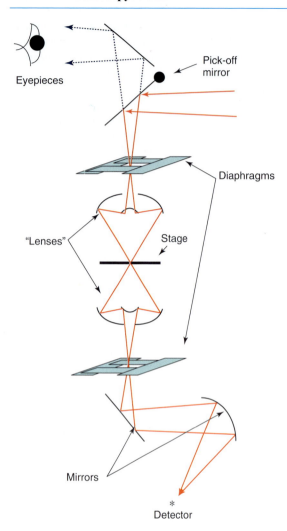

Figure 1 Schematic diagram of a typical infrared microspectrometer or infrared microscope accessory. The solid arrows and lines indicate the path for infrared radiation, while the dashed lines and arrows indicate the path for visible light to the observer once the pickoff mirror has been swung to the vertical position. Each "lens" comprises a concave mirror and a convex mirror depicted by the black lines. Not all microscopes have the diaphragm situated between the stage and the detector (termed a redundant diaphragm) [Reproduced from Ref. 3. © Taylor and Francis Group, 1999.]

lenses from material that is transparent to infrared radiation. Each diaphragm is made from four thin sheets of material opaque to infrared radiation that can be moved independently across the beam. At the center of the device is a stage upon which the

specimen is mounted. X, Y, and Z controls allow the stage to be moved in three orthogonal directions in space so that the specimen can be placed into the center of the beam and brought into the focal point of the beam. The pickoff mirror can be swung into the position shown in Figure 1, which allows the infrared beam to pass through the specimen for analysis, or it can be swung vertically so that the specimen can be viewed through the eyepieces at high magnification, positioned appropriately, and a diaphragm set up. Further discussion of infrared microscopes and their application to forensic science can be found in [1–3].

Figures 2(a and b) illustrate the function of the diaphragm. Figure 2(a) depicts the situation where the diaphragm curtains are fully retracted, which results in a circular beam of maximum diameter illuminating the specimen. Obviously a substantial portion of the beam reaches the detector having not passed through the specimen. Radiation that has not passed through the specimen but reaches the detector is referred to as "stray' radiation and its intrusion into spectroscopy is not desirable. To reduce the amount of stray radiation the diaphragm can be configured as shown in Figure 2(b), where the specimen is illuminated with a small, appropriately shaped spot of radiation. Figure 3 depicts two spectra recorded from the same single polyethylene terephthalate (also know as PET or "polyests") textile fiber. The spectrum in (a) was recorded with a diaphragm established as depicted in Figure 2(a) (i.e., high stray light), while that in (b) was recorded using a diaphragm as shown in Figure 2(b) (lower stray light). The effect of stray light is that peaks do not attain their true relative heights, and this is called *photometric inaccuracy*.

Although the spectrum in Figure 3(b) is good, it is still not perfect photometrically; this arises because of the effects of a phenomenon known as *diffraction*. When any radiation is caused to pass through an opening or passes close by an opaque edge, bending of the radiation (diffraction) takes place. The amount of bending is inversely proportional to the frequency of the illuminating radiation; infrared being of a frequency lower than visible light bends more, and low frequency infrared (i.e., that recorded at the "right hand side" of spectra) bends more than high frequency infrared. As a consequence, even though the diaphragm in Figure 2(b) casts a sharp shadow on the specimen to the human eye (which operates

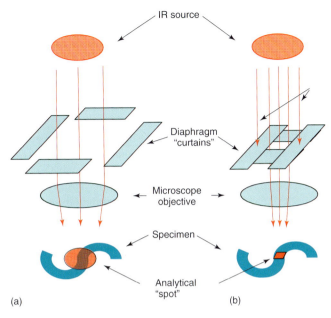

Figure 2 (a) Shows an infrared microscope with a textile fiber on the specimen stage. The curtains of the diaphragm are moved back away from the infrared beam path and as a consequence a spot of maximum size falls on to the fiber. Much of the beam does not interact with the specimen and goes on to reach the detector as stray radiation. (b) Depicts the situation where the curtains of the diaphragm are adjusted to trim off stray radiation [Reproduced from Ref.3. © Taylor and Francis Group, 1999.]

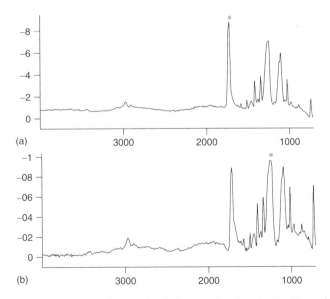

Figure 3 Spectrum (b) was collected from a single polyethyleneterephthalate textile fiber using an infrared microscope configured as shown in Figure 2(a) (i.e., with no diaphragm). Spectrum (a) was acquired from the same fiber with the microscope configured as shown in Figure 2(b). Note the differences between the two spectra with regard to the absolute absorbance values for the peaks (e.g., the two largest peaks, marked with asterisks, have values of about 0.1 and 0.8), of the two largest peaks in each spectrum (marked with an asterisk), the fact that the two maxima are at different frequencies, and the apparent "magnification" of small peaks in spectrum (b) [Reproduced with permission from reference [3], p. 189.]

using comparatively high frequency visible radiation), when infrared radiation is used to illuminate the specimen the shadow is not distinct. Figure 4 is a refinement of Figure 2(b) showing diffracted radiation and an approximation of the "shadow" of two opposite edges of the diaphragm imaged through the optics of an infrared microscope as "seen" by the specimen. Diffraction causes more stray light to reach the specimen than the size of the diaphragm would suggest. Any attempt to completely eliminate stray light is accompanied by compromises and diminishing returns. It is of course possible to reduce the size of the diaphragm to compensate for diffraction, but as indicated in Figure 4, diffraction does not stop at a certain point beyond the edge of the diaphragm, it continues indefinitely, albeit at a rapidly diminishing magnitude. For relatively large specimens (greater than about 30–40 μm in size), it is an effective tactic to configure a diaphragm to be about 5–10 μm smaller than the specimen and eliminate a large proportion of the stray light; reducing the size further reduces stray light further, but by ever diminishing returns. This is not recommended for specimens much smaller than about 30 μm as the reduction in the size of the diaphragm starts to severely attenuate the intensity of the radiation presented to the specimen, which is translated into a reduction in the signal to noise ratio of the spectral data, with the result that small peaks can disappear into the baseline. Depending upon the microscope used, a different diaphragm configuration (called *dual remote diaphragms*, as depicted in Figure 1) can be employed to improve the situation, but in any event, for very small specimens a compromise must be drawn between signal to noise ratio and rejection of stray light; it must be assumed that some residual stray light is present and its potential spectral contribution appreciated. In forensic comparisons it is a wise precaution to ensure that spectra of questioned and reference specimens are collected under conditions of equivalent stray light (i.e., specimens of approximately the same dimensions, and diaphragms of approximately the

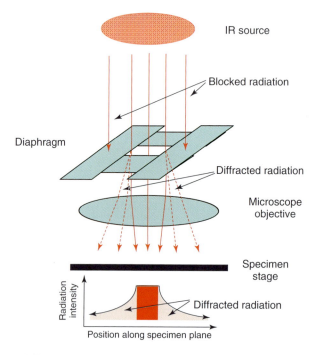

Figure 4 This diagram shows diffracted infrared radiation (dotted red arrows) that "bends" past the diaphragm established for a specimen as shown in Figure 2(b). An exaggerated approximation of the intensity of radiation across the specimen stage is depicted in the graph below. Instead of a sharp shadow (i.e., a rapid drop to zero intensity) beyond the edge of the fiber a more gradual drop to zero takes place. All the radiation that contributes to the pink zone in the graph reaches the detector as stray radiation

same dimensions). If these precautions are taken, the analyst can be certain that spectral differences between different specimens reflect a genuine compositional difference between the specimens and not spectral artifacts (i.e., these precautions guard against Type 1 errors, or false elimination of association, stray light effects are very unlikely to lead to Type 2 errors, or false association). Efforts should also be taken to minimize stray light during the recording of spectra for spectral libraries and chemometric datasets, otherwise poor matching/clustering might result.

In the case of a homogeneous specimen, such as a chip of single layer paint, the main consequence of diffraction in infrared microspectroscopy is photometric inaccuracy arising from stray light. In the case of a heterogeneous specimen, such as a cross-section of multilayer paint, the consequences of diffraction are a little more serious. Figure 5 refines the situation in Figure 4 with the diaphragm established to isolate the light gray central paint layer from adjacent dark gray and clear layers. As in Figure 4, diffracted infrared radiation strikes beyond where the diaphragm suggests it should. In this situation, however, instead of the diffracted radiation traveling through air and reaching the detector as stray radiation, it travels through adjacent paint layers and on to the detector, with the result that the acquired spectrum mostly relates to the blue layer but contains contributions from the adjacent layers. Again, with large specimens it is desirable to arrange the diaphragm well away from any interface with adjacent layers, but again it is also not an effective option with smaller specimens. For additional material relating to the effects of diffraction and stray radiation upon infrared microspectroscopy see [3–5].

For infrared transmission analysis of polymeric materials, and others that strongly absorb infrared radiation, it is desirable that the thickness of the specimen does not exceed $10-20\,\mu$m. If the specimen is much thicker than, then the possibility arises that the infrared beam at some frequencies will be completely absorbed, and this leads to photometric inaccuracies much greater than those arising from stray light and diffraction. It is usually the case that forensic specimens, even single textile fibers, exceed the desirable thickness, so it is usual in infrared transmission microspectroscopy to treat the sample in some way to make it thinner. The use of a microtome, crushing the specimen between diamond

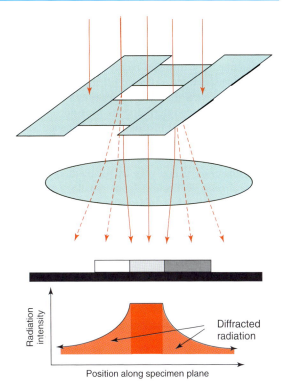

Figure 5 This diagram shows a cross section of three-layer paint placed under an infrared microscope with the diaphragm established on the interfaces between the light gray central layer and the adjacent clear and dark gray layers. As in Figure 4, the diffracted radiation and its intensity across the sample stage are depicted as dotted lines and light shading, respectively. Diffracted radiation passes through the clear and dark gray layers, carrying their spectral characteristics to the detector

anvils, pressing or rolling it, or carefully slicing sections away using a scalpel or microknife are all effective. A collateral benefit of crushing or rolling the specimen is that it makes it wider; this allows for the usage of bigger diaphragms and therefore allows for better rejection of stray light.

Infrared Reflectance Microspectroscopy

Infrared microspectroscopy is not restricted to transmission techniques. By the use of mirrors it is possible to collect the infrared radiation reflected from the surface of the specimen and transfer it to the detector to acquire reflectance spectral data. For thin or transparent specimens, it is also possible to mount them on a highly reflective substrate, such as aluminum foil or a gold coated glass microscope slide, and collect not only the radiation reflected from the surface of the specimen but also the radiation that has passed through the specimen, reflected off the substrate, and then traveled back through the specimen. This technique is sometimes referred to as *transflection*, as it is a mixture of transmission and reflectance spectroscopy. In this technique, the specimen thickness is effectively doubled as far as transmission is concerned, therefore it is a very useful method for very thin specimens. Reflection (and transflection) spectroscopy produces baseline artifacts (dips) that can be corrected using a mathematical function called a *Kramers–Kronig transformation*. Most spectrometer manufacturers offer software applications that perform this transformation.

Another technique of use to the forensic scientist is attenuated total reflectance (ATR) spectroscopy. In this technique, the beam from the microspectrometer is directed into a special crystal and caused to reflect internally off a face of the crystal. At the point of reflection a small proportion of the beam exists beyond the face of the crystal. This so-called evanescent wave can interact with material in contact with the surface of the crystal, and if the material absorbs in the infrared region then the reflected beam is slightly attenuated as a result. Figure 6 illustrates the essential features of ATR spectroscopy. The reflected beam is measured with and without the material in contact with the crystal and the difference between the two states yields the ATR spectrum. The distance that the evanescent wave emerges from the crystal depends upon the frequency of the incident radiation; low frequency radiation emerges further than high frequency radiation. As a result, low frequency infrared radiation interacts with a specimen placed in contact with the crystal more strongly compared to high frequency infrared radiation. Compared to a transmission spectrum of the same substance, an ATR spectrum shows an ever increasing intensification of peaks toward the right hand side of the spectrum (i.e., to the low frequency end). This means that if ATR spectra are to be compared against transmission spectra, there has to be some correction of the ATR data; this also can be done using software. The actual distance that the evanescent wave emerges from the surface of the crystal is very small (the order of microns), and therefore it only penetrates a very short distance into the specimen. Obviously ATR spectroscopy is very surface sensitive; this must be borne in mind if specimens are contaminated on their surface, weathered, or laminated. In practice, ATR microspectroscopy is very simple. Microscopes can be configured with an accessory crystal fitted to the objective, or special objectives can be purchased. The specimen is placed on a strong substrate onto the stage of the microscope, the region of the specimen to be analyzed is selected and then, using the Z control of the stage, the specimen is brought into contact with the ATR crystal. It is preferable that the microscope has some means by which the pressure brought to bear on the specimen is controlled, otherwise it is possible to damage components by using too much force, or collect poor data as a result of insufficient pressure.

Infrared Microspectral Imaging

Infrared microspectral imaging involves collection of many infrared spectra at many positions (called *pixels*) across the specimen The image is produced by selecting a frequency of interest (or a frequency range of interest), software then represents each pixel as a coloured spot the brightness of which is proportional to the infrared absorption at the frequency of interest at each pixel. As the image originates from the abundance and distribution of functional groups (measured by means of their characteristic infrared group frequencies) within the specimen, it illustrates the spatial distribution of chemically equivalent and chemically distinct regions in the specimen. Infrared microspectral imaging, therefore, can be very informative. As the image relates directly to

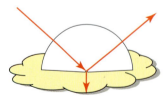

Figure 6 This diagram depicts a hemispherical attenuated total reflectance crystal of an infrared microscope pressed against a piece of paint. The infrared beam traveling from the source to the detector via the crystal is depicted by the solid arrows. At the point of reflection off the face of the crystal a small portion of the beam emerges from the face of the crystal (the evanescent wave, depicted as the small arrow) and interacts with the paint

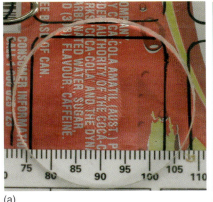 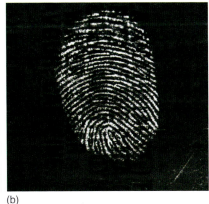

(a)   (b)

Figure 7 (a) The image was collected using visible light. It shows a fingerprint (circled) deposited on a Coke™ beverage can that has been treated with Superglue™ resin. (b) The image is a mosaic of over 1000 individual 700 μm² infrared images of the fingerprint displaying absorbance intensity at 1789 cm⁻¹ (the C=O stretch frequency of Superglue™), Image supplied by B Reedy and M Tahtouh, Centre of Forensic Science, University of Technology Sydney, Sydney, Australia [Reproduced with permission from B Reedy and M Tahtouh, University of Technology Sydney.]

chemical information within the specimen, infrared microspectral imaging is most frequently referred to as *infrared chemical imaging*, or sometimes as *hyperspectral imaging*.

Prior to about 1995, the only way to construct chemical images was to place the specimen under an infrared microscope, establish a diaphragm delineating a certain portion of the specimen (say a 20 μm × 20 μm area), collect a spectrum of that pixel, move the specimen 20 μm in some direction and record another pixel spectrum, and keep repeating the process until the desired area on the specimen has been analyzed. Even though this was usually accomplished with the aid of an automated microscope stage, it was a time-consuming process and low fidelity images were usually produced. In modern instruments, instead of a single detector an array of many detectors (such as 256, 1024, or 4096) arranged in a square pattern (called a *focal plane array*) is used to collect a set of spectra simultaneously from a square array of pixels (such as 256, 1024, or 4096) in the specimen. As all spectra are acquired simultaneously, focal plane array mapping is very rapid. Furthermore, images can be acquired at high spatial resolution without a requirement for apertures. If it is important to image an area larger than the field of view of the microscope then a motorized stage can be employed to move the specimen to an adjacent location and collect another data image set. Data image sets can then be displayed together to form a mosaic image of the specimen. The potential that microspectral infrared imaging offers to forensic science has been demonstrated through its successful application to fingerprint visualization [6, 7] and paint examination [8]. Figure 7 shows the greatly enhanced contrast possible with infrared microspectral imaging. The image on the left shows a fingerprint enhanced by Superglue™ fuming and photographed using visible light. The fingerprint (circled) is barely visible. The infrared image, on the right, displays the relative intensity of infrared absorbance at 1789 cm⁻¹ at each pixel in a mosaic of over 1000 smaller infrared images. The infrared image has such high contrast between the background (a Coke™ beverage can) and the fingerprint because the background paint has very little absorbance at 1789 cm⁻¹ while the superglue has a very strong absorbance.

References

[1] Humecki, H.J. (ed) (1995). Practical spectroscopy, *Practical Guide to Infrared Microspectroscopy*, Marcel Dekker, New York, Vol. 19.

[2] Roush, P.B. (ed) (1987). *The Design, Sample Handling, and Applications of Infrared Microscopes*, ASTM STP 949, American Society for Testing and Materials, Philadelphia.

[3] Kirkbride, K.P. & Tungol, M.W. (1999). Infrared microspectroscopy, in *Forensic Examination of Fibers, 2nd Edition*, J. Robertson & M. Grieve, eds, Taylor & Francis, London, pp. 179–222.

[4] Sommer, A.J. & Katon, J.E. (1991). Diffraction-induced stray light in infrared microspectroscopy and its effects on spatial resolution, *Applied Spectroscopy* **45**, 1633–1640.

[5] Messerschmidt, R.G. (1995). Minimizing optical nonlinearities in infrared microspectroscopy, In *Practical Guide to Infrared Microspectroscopy*, *Practical Spectroscopy*, H.J. Humecki, ed, Marcel Dekker, New York, Vol. 19, pp. 1–39.

[6] Tahtouh, M., Despland, P., Shimmon, R., Kalman, J.R. & Reedy, B.J. (2007). The application of infrared chemical imaging to the detection and enhancement of latent fingerprints: method optimization and further findings, *Journal of Forensic Science* **52**, 1089–1096.

[7] Crane, N.J., Bartick, E.G., Schwartz Perlman, R. & Huffman, S. (2007). Infrared spectroscopic imaging for noninvasive detection of latent fingerprints, *Journal of Forensic Science* **52**, 48–53.

[8] Flynn, K., O'Leary, R., Lennard, C., Roux, C. & Reedy, B.J. (2005). Forensic applications of infrared chemical imaging: multi-layered paint chips, *Journal of Forensic Science* **50**, 832–841.

K. PAUL KIRKBRIDE

Microscopy: Hair *see* Hair: Microscopic Analysis

Microscopy: High Power

A microscope is an instrument designed to extend man's visual capability, i.e., to make visible even the minute details that cannot be seen with the naked eye [1].

A *compound* microscope is one that provides magnification in two stages by means of an *objective* and an *eyepiece*. The term is not restricted to high magnification or high power microscopes, as low power microscopes are also compound microscopes. However, when the term *compound microscope* is used, many people think of the classical transmitted light microscope such as that shown in Figure 1. Today such an instrument can be used in a wide variety of forms, including inverted microscopes and with numerous forms of transmitted and epi-illumination

allowing the observation of surface features and the ability to "see through" the specimen. In order to obtain successful outcomes, sample preparation is usually required. This can be complex and involve making thin sections (or cell preparations) and using a variety of chemical staining techniques.

It is beyond the scope of this article to explain the optical theory underlying image formation in a compound microscope. The reader is referred to [2] for the more detailed treatment of this topic. The end result is that the observer normally sees a magnified, virtual, and inverted image.

The term *high power* refers to the ability to visualize the specimen at overall magnifications of up to $1,000\times$. This is achieved with objective lens magnification of up to $100\times$ and an eyepiece magnification of generally $10\times$. The normal total magnification is not necessarily the *effective* magnification as the latter depends on the microscope being properly set up to achieve the full *resolving power* of the objective.

The RMS Dictionary defines resolving power as "the ability to make points or lines which are closely adjacent in an object distinguishable in an image. High resolving power implies that the resolved distance is small".

In order to achieve maximum resolution, the full numerical aperture (NA) of lens systems has to be achieved. Figure 2 shows the concept of NA. Briefly, if the maximum possible resolving power of an objective is to be achieved, then the maximum cone of light entering the objective must be achieved. This requires that the sub stage *condenser* is properly focused.

The highest possible NA can be achieved only with an oil immersion objective for the reasons shown in Figure 2. Maximum NA depends on the microscope being properly set up which includes correct illumination of the object. Two forms of illumination to be commonly used are called, *critical illumination* and *Köhler illumination*, where the latter is the preferred method of illumination. Assuming the microscope is correctly set up, then NA critically depends on the type and quality of objective lens. Typically, objective lenses are complex multilens systems with correction for spherical and chromatic aberrations. A typical nonresearch instrument has *achromat* lenses. These are corrected for red and blue color aberration. *Apochromatic* lenses also are corrected for blue–violet color aberration. It is also possible to correct for field curvature to provide a flat

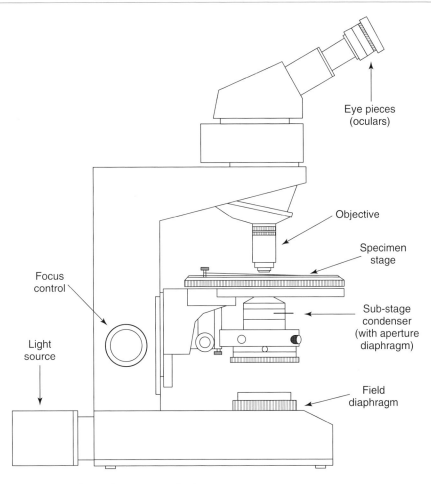

Figure 1 Main components of a modern compound microscope

field. Such lenses are called *plan*. Hence, in a high grade research compound microscope, the objectives are plan apochromat lenses with an NA in the order of 1.00 for 40× and 1.30 for 100× oil immersion. A typical achromat, dry objective at 40× would have an NA of 0.60–0.65.

The substage condenser also has a multilens system. Low cost microscopes have a two lens Abbe type condenser and higher cost microscopes have a more complex aplanatic condenser which is corrected for spherical aberration. To achieve objective NA of 1.4, a fully corrected oil immersion achromatic type condenser is required.

Finally, several types of *eyepiece* are also available. Typically today, a *compensating* eyepiece is found in which the eyepiece is designed to correct for lateral chromatic error.

Modern microscopes are designed and manufactured for ease of use and have features such as *parcentration* (ensuring that as objectives are changed the center of the visual field remains the same) and *parfocality* (ensuring focusing can be achieved as objectives are changed with a minimum of fine adjustment).

In most modern microscopes, the illuminating system is built into the base of the microscope. In low cost microscopes this is usually a precentred halogen bulb. In more expensive microscopes, a tungsten light source is common with the capability to center the light sources.

The standard set up for routine high power microscopic examination is *brightfield* microscopy in which direct light passes through the specimen, enters the objective, and illuminates the background

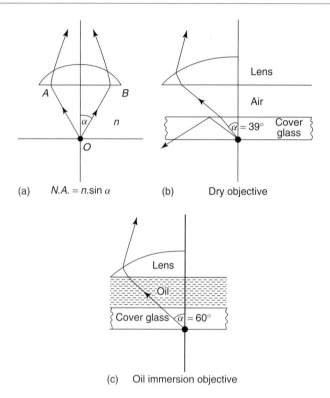

(a)   N.A. = n.sin α

(b)   Dry objective

(c)   Oil immersion objective

Figure 2   (a) A diagram to represent the concept of numerical aperture (NA), *n* is the refractive index of the medium (usually air) between the object O and the lens, *α* is half the angle of acceptance *AOB*. (b) Path of light rays in a dry objective of NA 0.95. The maximum value of *α* is 39° due to refraction at the air/cover glass interface. Rays with a greater obliquity are totally reflected at the surface of the cover glass. (c) Path of light rays in an oil immersion objective of NA 1.3. The value of *α* is now increased to 60° since there is now no air/glass interface refraction [Reproduced with permission from Edward Arnold Ltd. © 1976 [3].]

against which the image is seen. In order to visualize the image, there has to be a difference in the refractive index (RI) of the specimen and the mountant in which the specimen is placed; usually covered by a glass cover slip. For example, the measurement of the RI of glass is based on using a mountant whose RI changes as it is heated; for hair microscopy, the choice of mountant is critical if the internal structure of the hair is to be seen. For some samples, it can help to increase contrast by closing the iris diaphragm in the sub stage condenser. However, for very transparent specimens, there are a number of specialist techniques such as *dark field* microscopy and *phase contrast* microscopy, which provide images with a high degree of contrast. These techniques, especially phase contrast, are widely applied in biology but are not frequently used in routine forensic work.

Other specialist forms of microscopy include *fluorescence* microscopy and *polarizing* microscopy. Epi or incident fluorescence is commonly used in the forensic examination of fibers. Transmission fluorescence has been applied in aspects of forensic biology. It is beyond the scope of this article to describe the theory of polarizing microscopy. In brief, it makes use of the *optical* properties of some samples, (anisotropic) to "twist" polarized light. Casartelli [4] has described in simple terms how a polarized light microscope works. Although there are differing views within the forensic community as to the role of polarizing microscopy, there is no doubt that polarizing microscopy is still a valuable technique adding an analytical dimension to the microscope. The McCrone Particle Atlas [5] gives an insight into the extremely wide range of possible applications of this technique for forensic work.

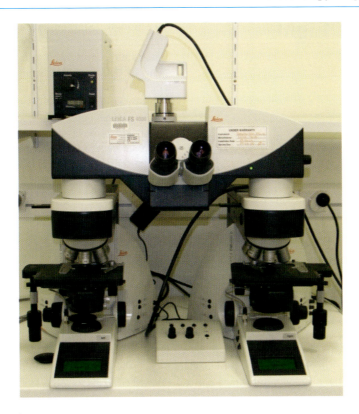

Figure 3   Comparison microscope

Finally, the forensic world makes use of comparison microscopy (see Figure 3) in which two microscope systems are linked by a system of prisms to present their images into a single binocular comparison eyepiece such that two images can be directly compared side by side. This technique is used in the forensic examination of fiber and hairs. Most of the current modern microscopes have the capability of being linked to image capture systems.

In conclusion, the compound light microscope is a versatile and indispensable piece of equipment. As a general recommendation, "simple is best". A less expensive microscope with limited options is often fit for purpose and is more preferred for routine use. This is especially the case where very little formal training is offered in basic microscopy. To achieve even close to the theoretical performance of any microscope, it must be kept clean and regularly serviced and maintained. Add to this an understanding of the basic theory of image formation, and how to use a microscope, and there is no reason why anyone cannot make effective use of microscopy.

References

[1]   Anon (1989). *RMS Dictionary of Light Microscopy*, Oxford University Press – Royal Microscopical Society.
[2]   De Forest, P.R. (2002). Foundation of forensic microscopy, in *Forensic Science Handbook*, 2nd Edition, R. Saferstein, ed, Prentice Hall, New Jersey, Vol. 1, Chapter 5, pp. 215–319.
[3]   Bradbury, S.L. (1976). *The Optical Microscope in Biology*, Arnold, London.
[4]   Casartelli, J.D. (1969). *Microscopy for Students*, 2nd Edition, McGraw Hill, London.
[5]   McCrone, W.C., Draftz, R.G. & Delly, J.G. (1967). *The Particle Atlas*, Ann Arbor Science Publishers.

Further Reading

Houck, M.M., Bowen, R. An argument for light microscopy – a review of forensic microscopy for trace evidence analysis. *Forensic Science Review* **17**, 1–15. 2005.

JAMES ROBERTSON

Microscopy: Light Microscopes

Introduction

This article is intended to cover the fundamentals of light microscopy. A microscopical examination may be the only instrumental technique needed to identify a piece of evidence, provide direction for further analysis, or compliment other instrumental techniques.

The microscope is used in many forensic disciplines including firearms identification, serological examinations, drug chemistry, and trace evidence. It is in the discipline of trace evidence where the light microscope has found its greatest use in the characterization, identification, and comparison of particulate material. The trace evidence analyst may encounter limitless types of particulate matter including fibers, hairs, paint, explosives, pollen, soil, glass, and tape. The use of the light microscope provides valuable information in the examination of trace particulate and its exclusion in any examination would be inconceivable.

Stereomicroscopy

Stereomicroscopes, sometimes referred to as *dissecting microscopes*, are microscopes that produce a magnified image of a specimen that is upright, laterally correct and with a perception of depth – exactly the way the eye sees in normal vision. The stereomicroscope is of particular importance in forensic examinations because the 3-D image, the extended depth of field, and long working distance facilitate inspection, sorting, preparation, and dissection of evidence. In many cases, these instruments can also provide enough information to identify the sample.

Design

In normal vision or when using a stereomicroscope, the brain combines two off-axis images to generate one image that is not only two dimensional but also has the perception of depth. There are two types of stereomicroscopes produced today – the *Greenough* design and the *Common Main Objective* design.

Greenough Stereomicroscope. The Greenough stereomicroscope dates from the later part of the nineteenth century and uses two completely independent optical axes that are set approximately 14° apart (Figure 1). Because the left and right optical paths must maintain critical alignment throughout the entire optical path, it is impossible for the user to insert and remove accessory items such as coaxial illuminators, epi-fluorescence or add a port for documentation. However, it is possible to produce highly corrected optics, including apochromatic lenses, at relatively low cost. Many laboratory-grade stereomicroscopes are Greenough instruments and are quite adequate for examinations and sorting of evidence.

Common Main Objective Stereomicroscope. The common main objective (CMO) stereomicroscope features two parallel optical axes (one for each eye) from the eyepieces down through the main body. At the common main objective, each optical path turns inward to view the specimen at slightly different angles (Figure 2). This type of microscope also produces a stereoscopic 3-D image, but with an important advantage over the Greenough design.

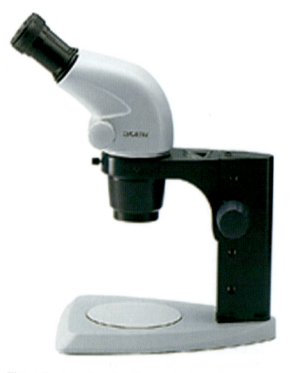

Figure 1   A modern day Greenough stereomicroscope

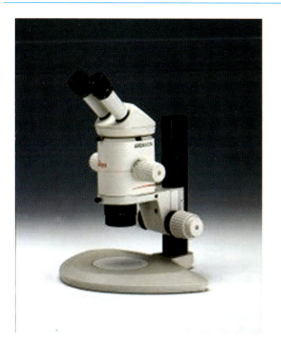

Figure 2 A modern day common main objective stereomicroscope

Since the optical paths are parallel, the image in a CMO instrument that is above the main body and below the observation tube is projected at infinity. Thus, the CMO stereomicroscope can accommodate a wide range of accessories, which can be easily inserted and removed by the user. These accessories include multiple photo/video ports, coaxial illuminators, and epi-fluorescence illuminators, often in combinations. Additionally, the observation tube that contains the eyepieces can be easily interchanged to accept other special purpose observation tubes that have eyepieces set at unique angles, eyepiece tubes that tilt for ergonomic advantages, or eyepiece tubes with long extensions to increase the distance of the observer from the specimen.

Magnification and Resolution

The total magnification of a stereomicroscope is a function of the eyepiece magnification, the main objective (if a CMO instrument) or the supplementary objective (if a Greenough instrument), the magnification factor of any intermediate accessory, and the magnification setting of the main body of the microscope. It is possible with some CMO stereomicroscopes to extend the total visual magnification to nearly 1000X, although the resolving power of any stereomicroscope is limited primarily to the numerical aperture of the main objective, which is at most approximately 0.2 and yields a maximum useful visual magnification of about 200X. Refer to the section "Brightfield" for a more detailed discussion on magnification, numerical aperture, and resolution.

Accessories

The accessories for CMO stereomicroscopes are extensive and allow these instruments to examine the internal structures of evidence in transmitted light and their surface details in incident light. Illumination sources include fiber optic bundles and ringlights as well as fixed and adjustable LED sources. Components for polarization, darkfield, epi-fluorescence, and digital documentation may be added to expand the functionality. Stereomicroscopes may be used with compact incident light stands for the examination of small pieces of evidence or they may be attached to elaborate heavy-duty stands for the detailed inspection of clothing or other large objects such as an automobile.

Limitations of the Stereomicroscope

Because the image projected through either side of a stereomicroscope is not perpendicular to the specimen plane, the left and right edges of a flat sample are out of focus when the center is in sharp focus. This is generally not a noticeable problem at lower magnifications and when the instrument is used for observation of samples that have a significant amount of surface relief. However, when the stereomicroscope is used for video discussion or documentation, only one side of the stereo image is diverted to the camera. Since either side is off-axis, accommodations must be made for this nonperpendicular view. With CMO instruments, the major manufacturers offer carriers that shift the position of one side of the microscope over the center of the main objective. The view obtained with this uniaxial instrument is perpendicular to the specimen plane and uses the center portion of the main objective which offers more optical correction than the lens periphery. This uniaxial position also provides the most accuracy when an eyepiece micrometer or computer software is used for measuring.

Brightfield Microscopy

A brightfield (biological) microscope with ordinary (unpolarized) illumination can be utilized to characterize, identify, and compare many types of particles encountered by the trace evidence microscopist. Although we see later that a polarized light microscope will give additional properties one can use to characterize and identify particles, unpolarized light may be employed to characterize physical features and to determine average optical properties of particles. Hairs, diatoms, and pollen grains are a few examples of particles that can be identified solely based on their physical characteristics when utilizing brightfield microscopy. Also, unpolarized light can be used to determine the refractive index (RI) and the color of particles that have a single RI (isotropic) as well as determine the average RI and the average color of particles that have more than one RI (anisotropic).

Concepts in the Design of the Light Microscope

To effectively use a microscope, a microscopist must know how to configure and adjust a microscope plus have a basic understanding of light and how it interacts with matter. The following discussion of microscopy is intended to be a simple primer that provides an introduction to light and the components of a contemporary compound microscope.

Light. The portion of the electromagnetic spectrum that the human eye detects as light is the range of wavelengths of energy from approximately 380 to 750 nm. The eye recognizes the shorter wavelengths of light as the colors violet to blue, the intermediate wavelengths as the colors green to yellow, and the longer wavelengths as the colors orange to red. Furthermore, the human eye interprets an increase in the amplitude of this wave as an increase in intensity or brightness of the light (Figure 3).

The interaction of light with matter provides specific information that can be used to characterize and identify particles during a microscopical examination. Also, the interaction of light with the components of a microscope directly affects the quality of the information revealed in the resulting magnified image. The principal interactions of light with matter which are discussed here are reflection, refraction, and dispersion.

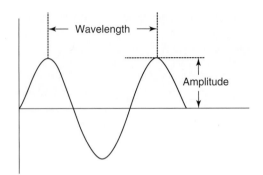

Figure 3 Diagram Figure showing wavelength and amplitude for a ray of light

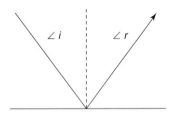

Figure 4 Specular reflection

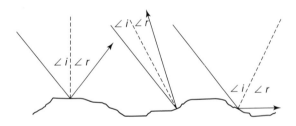

Figure 5 Diffuse reflection

Reflection. Specular reflection occurs when light strikes a smooth surface (Figure 4). The angle at which the light leaves the surface is equal to the angle at which it arrives and, therefore, the angle of reflection (r) is equal to the angle of incidence (i).

Diffuse reflection occurs when light strikes an irregular surface and the rays are reflected in different directions. Diffuse reflection still obeys the laws of reflection as the angle of reflection is still equal to the angle of incidence (Figure 5). How light is reflected off a material using incident light can provide valuable information when characterizing and comparing samples.

Refraction. Refractive index (*n*) is the ratio of the speed of light in a vacuum to the speed of light in a transparent medium. When light enters a medium having a different RI at any angle other than perpendicular to the surface, the light will not only change velocity but also direction. This change in direction, or bending of light, is known as *refraction*. Refraction is governed by Snell's law that states

$$n_r/n_i = \sin i / \sin r \qquad (1)$$

where n_r is the RI of the refractive medium, n_i is the RI of the incident medium, $\sin i$ is the sine of the angle of incidence, and $\sin r$ is the sine of the refraction.

Therefore, as light passes from a medium of lower to one of a higher RI, the incident ray of light will be refracted toward the normal to the interface then away from the normal to the interface as it passes from a higher to lower RI medium (Figure 6). Furthermore, as the difference between the two refractive indices increases, the amount the light ray is refracted also increases. The refraction of light as it passes through the optical components of a microscope is an essential function of the microscope lenses in the formation of a magnified image.

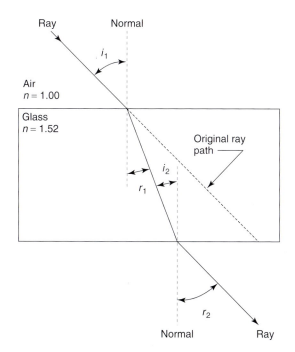

Figure 6   Refraction of light

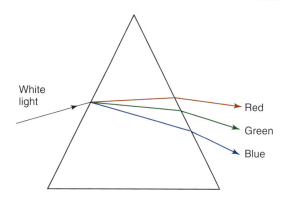

Figure 7   Dispersion of white light through a glass prism

Dispersion. Dispersion is the change in RI of a transparent substance as a function of the wavelength of light resulting in the separation of white light into its component wavelengths or colors (Figure 7). The RI is usually lower for longer wavelengths (red) and higher for shorter wavelengths (blue). The dispersion of white light as it passes through the optical elements of a microscope results in a degraded image quality and requires correction or compensation for this aberration.

Magnification.   A simple magnifier helps the eye focus an object that is closer than 10 in (25 cm), which is the normal reading distance for the eye. When the object is moved closer to the eye, its visual angle is increased and the object can be focused by the eye when a positive lens is placed between the eye and the object (Figure 8). Magnification can be expressed in several ways but one simple relationship is:

$$\text{Magnification} = \text{image size}/\text{object size} \qquad (2)$$

A compound microscope uses an objective lens positioned close to the specimen to produce a magnified real image of the object. The eyepiece functions as a simple magnifier and further magnifies the real image produced by the objective. Therefore, the final magnification to the observer is the product of the objective magnification, the eyepiece magnification, and any intermediate tube factor that may be present in the microscope.

Objectives.   The objective is the lens system nearest the specimen and can have a series of complex lens

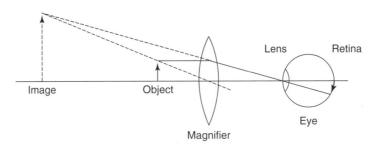

Figure 8 Diagram of simple magnification

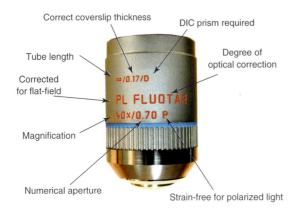

Figure 9 Objective nomenclature

elements. The objective provides the primary magnification and in part defines the resolution of the final image. Objectives are designed as having different magnifications and numerical apertures. The resolution of the microscope, which is the ability to discern fine structure or minute particles spaced closely together, is a function of the objective and the condenser. The nomenclature engraved on the body of the objective provides useful information regarding magnification, numerical aperture, and intended usage (Figure 9). For example, a 0.17 value means that the objective must be used with a coverglass of 0.17 mm thickness or the image will not be as sharp due to spherical aberration.

Eyepieces.   The eyepiece provides a magnified secondary image of the primary image produced by the objective. Eyepieces having different magnifications and field-of-view indexes are available. The field-of-view index of the microscope eyepiece is the diameter in millimeters of an internal diaphragm which is used to match the level of correction of the objectives being used. Eyepieces with wide field-of-view indexes require objectives with more extensive correction for flatness of field or the periphery of the image will be out of focus. The 10X magnification eyepiece is the most widely used eyepiece and is available with a field-of-view index from 18 to 25.

Condenser.   The primary function of the substage condenser in a transmitted light microscope is to concentrate and focus the light evenly across the field of view. Laboratory and research grade microscopes must be able to achieve Köhler illumination which requires an adjustable condenser. Condensers for brightfield observation techniques may span the entire magnification range from a 1.25X objective to a 100X objective and have a mechanism that permits a top condensing lens to be swung in the light path for objective magnifications of 10X and above. This dual function allows the condenser to evenly illuminate large fields at low magnification and smaller fields at higher magnification.

Special use condensers for phase contrast, polarization, darkfield, and differential interference contrast (DIC) provide the necessary components to achieve these special contrasting techniques. Since the highest numerical aperture possible with a dry condensing system is 0.90, condensers are available that allow immersion oil to be placed on the underside of the specimen slide to couple the condenser optically to the specimen allowing condenser numerical apertures up to 1.4.

Illuminators.   Most microscopes today use built-in or directly coupled illumination sources, often with a power supply providing variable intensity control that is integrated into the microscope stand. The primary illumination source for transmitted light is a low-voltage tungsten halogen bulb with high intensity wattages from 20 to 100. Light emitting diodes (LEDs) are being used in some microscopes because they produce a bright white light with an exceptionally long life.

Although a routine bench microscope may not have provisions for adjustment of the filament, the light produced is sufficient to properly illuminate the specimen and render high quality images. Research level instruments have the lamp located in an attached housing that provides for critically positioning the filament in the center of the optical axis, independently controlling a secondary image of the filament produced by a reflecting mirror behind the bulb, and precisely focusing the filament for Köhler illumination.

Numerical Aperture.   As the focal length of the front element of an objective becomes shorter (closer to the object) as is required to increase the magnification of the objective, the angle of acceptance of the image forming rays (angular aperture) is increased (Figure 10). The numerical aperture is a measure of the light gathering ability of a lens system and determines the resolving power and depth of field. Generally, objectives with the shortest working distance have the highest magnification and the greatest angular apertures (AA). The numerical aperture can be calculated using the formula:

$$NA = n \sin \frac{AA}{2} \qquad (3)$$

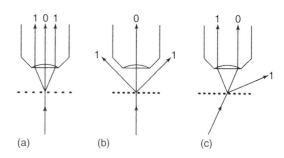

Figure 11   Diffraction of light through fine structure

where n is the RI of the space between the front element of the objective (or top element of the condenser) and the microscope slide.

Diffraction.   In the late nineteenth century, Ernst Abbe demonstrated that there is a correlation among diffraction, numerical aperture, resolution, and the RI of the medium between the specimen and the front lens of the objective. A series of diffracted rays are produced when light interacts with a specimen and as the detail in the specimen becomes finer, the angle of the diffracted rays increase (Figure 11). To resolve detail in a specimen, one needs to capture the direct ray and at least one of the first-order diffracted rays. However, the image quality improves as more of the diffracted rays are captured. Also, the shorter wavelengths of light (blue) produce a smaller diffraction angle than the longer wavelengths of light (red) resulting in greater resolution for shorter wavelengths.

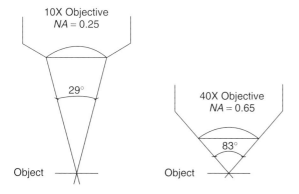

Figure 10   Diagram showing acceptance angle for two objectives having a different magnification and numerical aperture

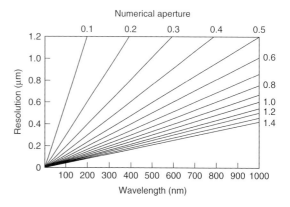

Figure 12   Diagram showing the relationship among wavelength, numerical aperture, and resolution

Resolving Power. The numerical aperture of an objective and the condenser along with the wavelength of light used to illuminate the sample determines the resolving power of the microscope. Resolving power is the ability of an optical system to make two closely spaced points (fine detail) visible as separate entities. Therefore, a resolving power of 1 μm means that two point-shaped particles at a 1 μm distance from each other will just be distinguishable as separate objects. A graph depicting the relationship among wavelength, numerical aperture, and resolving power is provided in Figure 12.

Contrast. If a magnified image is to be of value, the details of the structure of the specimen must be observable. While a microscope may be resolving the fine details of a specimen, these details are of no value unless there is sufficient contrast for the eye to detect the structure. Contrast may be enhanced by mounting the sample in a medium with a different RI, by the use of colored stains, or by simply closing down the aperture diaphragm. However, as the aperture diaphragm is closed down, the resolution significantly decreases. It is a good practice to observe specimens with the aperture diaphragm in different positions. Also, optical or illumination contrasting techniques such as darkfield, Rheinberg, phase contrast, differential interference contrast (DIC), or modulation contrast can be employed. It is the appropriate combination of resolution, contrast, and magnification that provides the microscopist with an image with sufficient detail to provide useful information.

Finite and Infinity Microscopes. The two designs for compound microscopes are finite tube length and infinity corrected tube length (Figure 13). While both systems can produce high-quality images, the infinity corrected system is now the most commonly available optical design for laboratory and research grade instruments. A microscope with infinity corrected optics allows for accessory components to be added such as incident light illuminators for opaque specimens or epi-fluorescence illumination, polarizers, and compensators without degrading the image. Many contemporary bench microscopes and all older instruments are of the finite tube length design.

Objective Aberrations. A perfect converging lens causes all of the light rays emitting from a point on one side of a lens to be converged (focused) on the

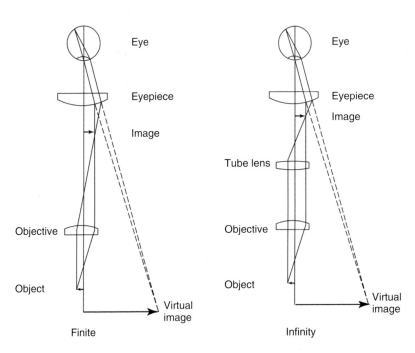

Figure 13 Ray path through a finite corrected microscope (left) and an infinity corrected microscope (right)

other side of the lens and produces an exact image of the original point. In practice, all lenses suffer from aberrations and, in fact, these imperfections impair the ability of the lens to produce that exact copy of an object. Of the six primary aberrations, spherical and chromatic affect the entire field while coma, astigmatism, curvature of field, and distortion affect the quality of the off-axis or peripheral image. To a degree, all of these aberrations can be reduced to a level at which they no longer adversely interfere with visual observation. The extent to which a microscope is corrected for these aberrations determines its performance and subsequent cost.

Particle Characterization – Unpolarized Light

Before any microscopical examination can begin, one must ensure that the microscope is properly aligned and adjusted for Köhler illumination. Depending on the microscope being utilized, the centering and focusing of the lamp filament may not be possible to obtain true Köhler illumination. This is because many manufacturers have eliminated the ability to center and focus the lamp filament and have introduced a diffuser into the light path. Once Köhler illumination is achieved, particles are characterized and identified based on the properties that are observed and measured. This is first accomplished using unpolarized light or with plane polarized light utilizing a single polar and finally with crossed (two) polars.

Sample Preparation. Samples are prepared for microscopical examination by placing them between a microscope slide and coverglass (coverslip) and using a liquid (mounting medium) of choice. The mounting medium may be a temporary medium that will evaporate away such as water or a suitable organic liquid. Xylene was commonly used in past years as a temporary medium, but its use today has been restricted in some laboratories. A stain may also be used as mounting medium. Some common stains that may be used include: Graff C stain or Selliger's stain to characterize and identify cellulose fibers; iodine solution or Betadine solution to detect starch grains and gelatinized starch particles; and malachite green in nitrobenzene to detect and identify clay particles.

A standard oil having a known RI is another mounting medium that can be used, such as Cargille refractive index liquids (Cargille Laboratories, Cedar Grove, NJ, USA). A standard oil having a RI of 1.66 is usually employed for general particle characterization and for the examination of the heavy mineral fraction (density $> 2.89\,\mathrm{g\,cc^{-1}}$) in a soil sample. A liquid having a $RI = 1.550$ is usually favored to characterize and identify minerals in the light fraction (density $< 2.89\,\mathrm{g\,cc^{-1}}$). Many fiber microscopists prefer a liquid having a $RI = 1.525$.

There are many permanent mounting media to choose from including Permount™, Meltmount™, Entellan™, and Norland Optical Adhesive™. Aroclor™ has been used in the past years as a mounting medium but is not readily available today. As can be seen, there are numerous mounting media to choose from and which mounting medium one will use greatly depends on the sample and the information one wishes to obtain from the examination.

Particle Morphology. Under examination, the first characteristic one will notice is the physical features of the particles. General terms should be used to describe particles unless one understands precise descriptions that are used in specialized fields (crystallography, wood taxonomy, mineralogy, paleontology, etc.) and can be applied correctly. Also, the microscopist will project a more visual image of the particle observed under the microscope using descriptive terms such as irregular, spherical, acicular, granular, platy, fibrous, or tabular. Also, interfacial angles between crystal faces can be measured if present.

Particle Size. The next characteristic one may determine is particle size. The size of a particle may help to distinguish between two particles that have similar morphologies such as corn starch and rice starch, the former having an average diameter twice that of latter. Also, particle size is an important consideration when comparing particles contained in two different samples.

Particle size can be either estimated or measured precisely. The particle size is estimated by comparing the particle to the diameter of the field of view. A 10X objective has a field of view of approximately 2.2 mm or 2200 μm, whereas a 40X objective has a field of view around 0.54 mm or 540 μm. Precise particle measurements can be made using a calibrated eyepiece scale, which is located in the front focal plane of the eyepiece and is therefore superimposed on the field of view. One can calibrate the eyepiece

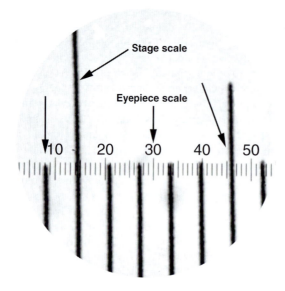

Figure 14   Image of the eyepiece scale superimposed over the stage micrometer scale

scale using a stage micrometer. For the stage micrometer shown in Figure 14, each division is equal to 10 μm. Note that 42 eyepiece divisions equals 6 stage micrometer divisions or 60 μm. Therefore, each eyepiece scale division for this objective equals 1.4 μm. Since the diameter of the field of view varies with each objective, the eyepiece scale must be calibrated for each objective so the particle size can be measured accurately using any objective.

Refractive Index.   Refractive index as previously defined is the ratio of the velocity of light in a vacuum to the velocity of light passing through a transparent medium. The RI will always be greater than 1.00 and determination of the RI (or RIs) is an important aspect in the identification of transparent particles. Also, it is important to remember that the RI varies with the wavelength of light (dispersion) and it is understood that the RI value usually reported is at 589 nm (n_D) unless otherwise noted.

The degree of observed contrast (dark edges) of a particle is a measure of the RI of the particles relative to the RI of the medium. The particle contrast will increase as the difference in RI increases between the particle and the medium. If the particle has colored borders it means that the particle and medium have the same RI at some wavelength near or in the visible

region of light. If the particle is "invisible" then the liquid and the particle have the same RI.

With a little practice, one can judge the difference between the RI of the particle and the RI of the liquid by the amount of contrast observed. If the contrast is low, one can estimate that the particle and the liquid have a RI difference that ranges from ±0 to 0.04. If the contrast is moderate, then the difference of the two RIs is estimated to be somewhere between ±0.04 and 0.12. If the contrast is high, the difference between the particle and liquid RIs is greater than 0.12. To "calibrate" your eye, one should estimate the amount of contrast in a consistent manner with the aperture diaphragm closed down (smallest opening).

The degree of contrast observed for a particle in a liquid does not demonstrate if the particle has a higher or lower RI than the mounting medium. Even though there are several ways to determine which has a higher RI, the Becke line technique is commonly conducted to quickly determine whether the particle or the liquid has the higher RI. The Becke line is a bright halo that is observed near the boundary of a particle which moves in and out of the particle as the particle is brought through good focus. This halo is the result of the concentration of light due to the refraction (light changing direction) at the interface of the particle and mounting medium having different refractive indices. The light will be bent toward the normal (an imaginary line perpendicular to the surface) as it enters a transparent medium of higher RI and away from the normal as it enters a medium of lower RI. As you focus above the plane of best focus (increase the distance between the objective and particle) the Becke line will move into the particle if it has a higher RI or will move into the liquid if it has a higher RI (Figure 15). The aperture diaphragm should be closed down when conducting the Becke line test and the movement of the fine focus must be slight.

Isotropic particles (noncrystalline particles and cubic crystals) have a single RI and this index will be observed whether unpolarized or plane polarized light is employed. However, anisotropic particles (crystals with more than one RI) have either two principal RIs (uniaxial) or three principal RIs (biaxial). The two principal RIs for uniaxial crystals are noted as ω and ε. For biaxial crystals, the three principal RIs are noted as α, β, and γ. Also, anisotropic fibers have two different refractive indices: RI parallel to the length ($n_{\parallel}$) and perpendicular to the length ($n_{\perp}$).

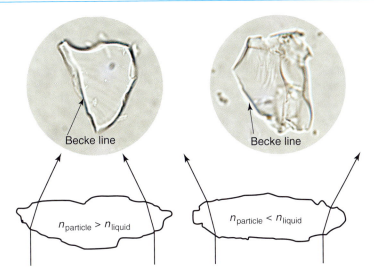

Figure 15 Ray diagram and images showing the Becke line slightly above best focus for a particle having a higher refractive index than the mounting medium (left) and for a particle having a refractive index lower than the mounting medium (right)

With unpolarized light we will observe an average RI (n_{iso}) for anisotropic particles. For most anisotropic crystals, the average RI can be calculated using the formula:

$$n_{iso} = \frac{1}{3}(2\omega + \varepsilon) \quad \text{or} \quad n_{iso} = \frac{1}{3}(\alpha + \beta + \gamma) \quad (4)$$

And for anisotropic fibers:

$$n_{iso} = \frac{1}{3}(n_{\parallel} + 2n_{\perp}) \quad (5)$$

One advantage of looking at the average RI (n_{iso}) of anisotropic particles is that the average RI will be observed regardless of the orientation of the particle. Determining and comparing the average RI of anisotropic particles is a useful technique when characterizing a sample containing different types of textile fibers as well as for the detection of trace components in a sample. A list of n_{iso} values for fibers is provided by Gaudette in "The Forensic Aspects of Textile Fiber Examination". If a particle/fiber of interest is found by using unpolarized light, polarized light (plane or crossed) can be quickly inserted into the light path so additional optical properties can be determined.

Dispersion Staining. Dispersion staining is a powerful technique that one can employ to find the RI relationship between transparent particles and the mounting medium. Dispersion staining colors are observed when a particle and a liquid have different dispersion curves (plot of RI with wavelength) but have a common RI. This technique is useful for the identification of particles where the RI data is known and is especially useful for the detection of a component in a "needle-in-a-haystack" type of examination.

The dispersion staining technique employs an opaque annular stop or central stop located in the back focal plane of the objective (Figure 16). This stop enhances the color that is observed at the border of the particle and liquid. The color of the particle at the border will depend on where the liquid and the particle have the same RI. Wavelengths of light at the intersection of the dispersion curves for the particle and liquid will not be deviated and will pass through the opening of the annular stop but will be blocked if employing the central stop. The other wavelengths of light will be deviated and be blocked by the annular stop but will pass through the opening of the central stop if employed. The degree of deviation of the wavelengths of light will depend on the differences in the dispersion curves of the particle and liquid. As one would expect, the dispersion staining colors become more vivid if the particle and liquid have very different dispersion curves (Figure 17).

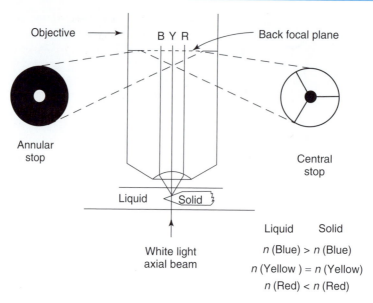

Figure 16 Diagram of the dispersion staining objective with the annular and central stop [Reproduced with permission from McCrone Research Institute.]

Table 1 Dispersion staining colors. λ_0 notes where the particle and the liquid have the same RI[a]

Matching λ_0 (nm)	Annular stop colors	Central stop colors	
		In focus	Becke line
<420	Blue–black	Light yellow	Faint gold + violet
430	Blue–violet	Yellow	Faint gold + violet
455	Blue	Golden yellow	Faint gold + violet
485	Blue–green	Golden–magenta	Yellow + violet
520	Green	Red–magenta	Violet + orange
560	Yellow–green	Magenta	Blue violet + red orange
595	Yellow	Blue–magenta	Blue + red
625	Orange	Blue	Blue
660	Orange–red	Blue–green	Green
>680	Brown–red	Pale blue	Pale green

[a]Reproduced with permission from McCrone Research Institute

The central stop method is generally preferred since the complementary dispersion staining colors are observed on a darkfield. Table 1 shows the colors observed at various matching wavelengths using the annular stop and central stop.

One can plot the dispersion curve for a particle by plotting the matching RI observed in several different liquids (Figure 18). To accomplish this, one must know the dispersion data for the liquids. This plot will provide the RI not only at n_D but also at n_F (486 nm) and n_C (656 nm), the other two refractive indices commonly listed in literature.

Alternately, one can plot a dispersion staining curve in a series of liquids and obtain the n_D value for a particle without knowing the dispersion data for the liquids. This is accomplished by plotting a horizontal line at the n_D value for the different liquids (Figure 19). However, only the RI at 589 nm (n_D) has any direct RI value to literature values. The RIs at the other wavelengths along the dispersion staining

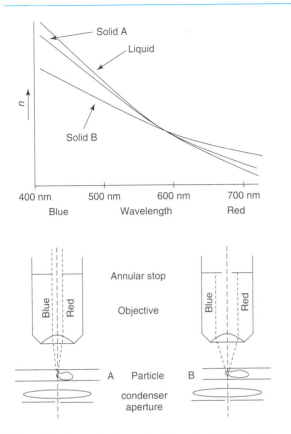

Figure 17 Ray paths through a dispersion staining objective using an annular stop corresponding to the dispersion curves for solid A and for solid B mounted in the same liquid

curve do not provide the actual RI of the particle. Therefore, to determine the actual RI for the particle at any wavelength other than n_D (589 nm), one needs to replot the dispersion staining curve using the actual known dispersion data for the liquids. In addition, dispersion curves are generally plotted with a linear wavelength scale whereas for dispersion staining curves the wavelength scale is plotted as $1/\lambda^2$. Plotting the wavelength as $1/\lambda^2$ generally provides a straighter line for the dispersion staining curve. For more information on dispersion staining, one should consult the *Polarized Light Microscopy* manual by McCrone, McCrone, and Delly.

Other Characteristics. If present, other characteristics may be noted including (but not limited to) color, transparency, and surface features. The color of the particle may be the first feature noted and can be observed with transmitted and/or reflected light. The color of a particle is the result of selective absorption of certain wavelengths of light. Only the average transmission color will be observed with unpolarized light for transparent particles with more than one RI. It can be seen later that the use of plane polarized light (single polar) will provide additional information for colored particles which have more than one RI.

Some particles may not transmit all the illuminating light and are translucent rather than transparent. This translucent characteristic may be due to optical discontinuities within the particle which scatter light through refraction and/or reflection as light travels through the particle. These optical discontinuities may be the result of different orientation of internal grain structure, impurities, or inclusions such as air bubbles. It may also be the result of surface features which are more apparent when the RI of the particle and liquid differ greatly.

The surface of the particle is another important feature used to characterize and compare particles. Transmitted light is used to observe the surface of a transparent or translucent particle by focusing on the top and bottom surfaces. However, with opaque particles, a reflected light illuminator is employed. General descriptive terms may include smooth, dimpled, fractured, rough, pitted, and nodular.

Polarized Light Microscopy

The polarized light microscope (PLM) is a powerful analytical instrument for the forensic trace analyst. The polarizing microscope can be applied to almost any type of trace evidence and will increase the number of identification characteristics one can determine for a particle under investigation. The PLM differs from a biological microscope in that it has a polarizer (polar) located in the substage condenser, an analyzer (second polar) located above the stage, a circular stage, strain free objectives, a crossline eyepiece, and a slot for inserting compensators in the body tube. The most common compensator is the full-wave (530 nm) compensator, but it is desirable to have a quarter-wave (137 nm) compensator and a variable compensator. Also, the stage and/or objectives should be centerable.

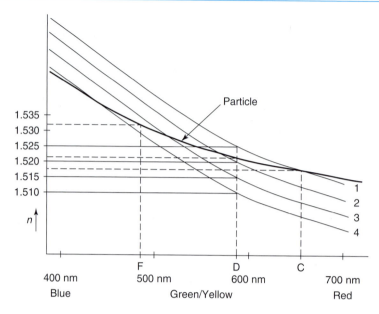

Figure 18 Dispersion curve plot for a particle mounted in four different liquids. The refractive index values are $n_F = 1.532$, $n_D = 1.522$, and $n_C = 1.517$

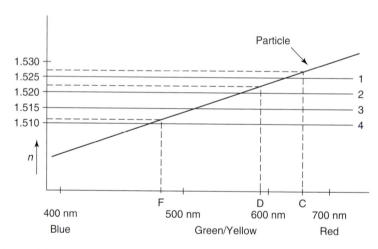

Figure 19 Dispersion staining curve for the particle in Figure 16. The dispersion staining values are $n_F = 1.511$, $n_D = 1.522$, and $n_C = 1.527$

Particle Characterization – Single Polar

As noted in the section "Brightfield", without any polarizer (polar) in the system one can observe only the average color and RI of anisotropic particles. This is because ordinary light is unpolarized and vibrates in a multitude of different directions perpendicular to the propagation direction of travel. Since optical properties will vary with the vibration of the light in an anisotropic particle, one must employ plane polarized light to observe and measure these variations.

Plane polarized light is obtained by using a polarizing filter. When unpolarized light passes through a polarizing filter, the light will exit vibrating in a single (privileged) direction perpendicular to the direction of travel (Figure 20). Now with the employment of

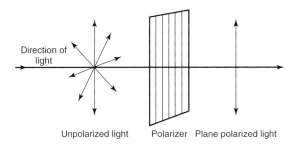

Figure 20 Unpolarized light passing through a polarizing filter resulting in plane polarized light

a single polar, one will be able to measure different optical properties of an anisotropic material as a function of the vibration direction of the light passing through the particle. Therefore, utilizing PLM will increase the number of optical properties that one can determine when characterizing and identifying particles. Before one measures the different properties of a particle, it is necessary to have a well centered stage and check the alignment of the polarizer and analyzer which are normally aligned perpendicular to each other.

Refractive Indices. With plane polarized light, more than one RI can be observed for anisotropic particles. The RIs one will observe will depend on the orientation of the particle and the alignment of the RIs with the polarizer. Fibers are discussed first since they lay flat on the microscope slide and show their two principle indices: the RI parallel ($n_{\parallel}$) to the fiber length and the RI perpendicular ($n_{\perp}$) to the fiber. When the length of the fiber is aligned parallel to the polarizer, the $n_{\parallel}$ RI will be observed

(Figure 21a). If one rotates the stage and aligns the fiber perpendicular to the polarizer, than the $n_{\perp}$ will be observed (Figure 21b). If one rotates the stage so neither of the RIs coincides with the polarizer, than the light will be vectorially split between the two RIs and will be split equally when the fiber is aligned at a 45° angle to the polarizer (Figure 21c). When the fiber is aligned parallel or perpendicular to the polarizer, the respective RIs can be estimated or precisely determined using immersion methods or by employing the dispersion staining technique. Note that the polyester fiber shows higher contrast when the fiber is aligned east–west (parallel RI) and is a quick way to check that your polarizer is also aligned east–west.

Unlike fibers, which show their longitudinal view, most crystals show a randomly oriented view when mounted on a microscope slide. The optical indicatrix helps us to understand how the RI varies depending on the vibration direction of light through a crystal. The indicatrix is a 3-D model whose radii are proportional to the RI values perpendicular, or nearly so, to the direction of light and, therefore, assumes a different solid geometrical form depending on the RIs of a crystal. Thus, for an isotropic (cubic or noncrystalline) particle which has a single refractive index, all the radii would be of equal length and will result in the simplest indicatrix having the form of a sphere (Figure 22). If one would cut a section at any angle through the center of the indicatrix, a circular section would be obtained having a circumference equidistant at all points from the center of the sphere. Therefore, one would observe a single RI for light traveling perpendicular to any circular section no matter the vibration direction of the light.

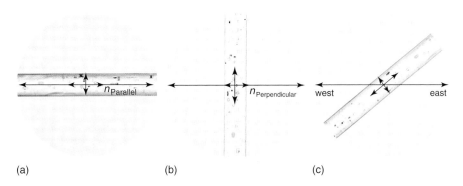

(a)   (b)   (c)

Figure 21 Three different orientations of a polyester fiber viewed with an east-west polarizer. Note the chance of contrast in the different views. The RI of mounting medium is 1.525

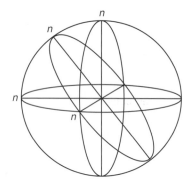

Figure 22 Isotropic indicatrix

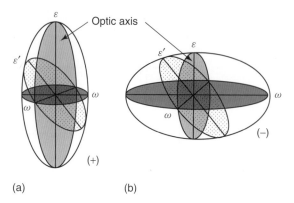

Figure 23 Uniaxial indicatrix: (a) prolate ellipse where $\varepsilon > \omega$ (positive optic sign) and (b) oblate ellipse where $\varepsilon < \omega$ (negative optic sign)

For uniaxial (tetragonal and hexagonal) crystals, the indicatrix takes on an elliptical form with the maximum and minimum magnitude of the radii equal to the two principal indices, ε and ω. If the $\varepsilon > \omega$ (+) optic sign the shape of the ellipsoid will be prolate (Figure 23a) and if $\varepsilon < \omega$ (−) optic sign the shape of the ellipsoid will be oblate (Figure 23b).

For all uniaxial crystals, the ε RI coincides with the optic axis. The optic axis is a unique axis and if one cuts a section though the center of the indicatrix perpendicular to the optic axis, a circular section

(shaded dark gray) will be obtained as shown in Figure 23. Plane polarized light traveling along the optic axis will vibrate in this circular section containing only the ω RI. Therefore, a uniaxial crystal in this orientation would behave as an isotropic crystal since only the ω RI will be observed (Figure 24a) and the contrast for the crystal will remain constant with plane polarized light as you rotate the stage.

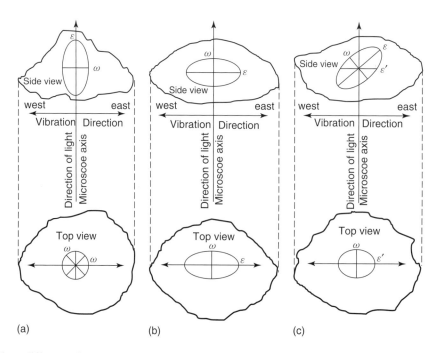

Figure 24 Three different orientations with the uniaxial indicatrix superimposed in the different views

For a section cut through the center of a uniaxial indicatrix parallel to the two principal indices, ε and ω, a principal ellipse (shaded light gray) will be obtained as seen in Figure 23. Therefore, if the propagation direction of the plane polarized light is perpendicular to this section, one will observe either the ε RI or the ω RI when one or the other is aligned parallel to the vibration direction of the polarized light (Figure 24b). If the stage is rotated so neither principal RI is parallel with the polarizer, as previously discussed, the plane polarized light will be split vectorially between the two principal RIs and equally when they are positioned at a 45° angle from the polarizer. Also, with a crystal in this orientation the contrast will change as the stage is rotated and the degree of contrast change will be dependent on the differences in the RIs between ε, ω and the mounting medium.

An ellipse will be obtained if a section (textured plane) is cut at a diagonal angle through the center of an indicatrix as shown in Figure 23. This elliptical cross section will contain the ω and ε' RIs. An ε' RI can be any multitude of RIs between ε and ω and which ε' RI will be observed is dependent on the orientation of the crystal. If the propagation direction of plane polarized light is perpendicular to an elliptical section, one will observe either the ω RI or the ε' RI when one or the other is aligned parallel to the vibration direction of the polarized light (Figure 24c). If the stage is rotated so neither RI is parallel with the polarizer, the plane polarized light will be split vectorially between the two RIs and equally when they are positioned at a 45° angle from the polarizer. Also, as mentioned above, when one rotates the stage with a crystal in this orientation the contrast will change and to what degree will depend on the differences in the RIs of ω, ε' and the mounting medium. How to easily locate the RIs for a randomly oriented crystal is discussed in the crossed polarized light section.

For biaxial (orthorhombic, monoclinic, and triclinic) crystals, the indicatrix is a triaxial ellipsoid defined by the three principal indices α, β, and γ. By definition, α is the lowest RI, γ is the highest RI, and β is the intermediate RI that lies somewhere between α and γ. As one can see in Figure 25a, light traveling parallel to γ will vibrate in the plane (shaded dark gray) containing α and β, light traveling parallel to α will vibrate in the plane (shaded gray) containing β and γ, and light traveling parallel to β will vibrate in

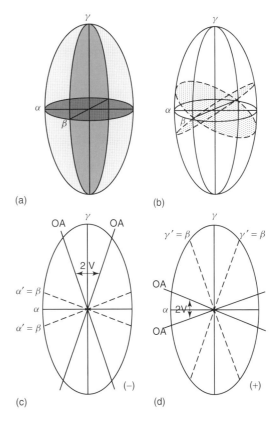

Figure 25   Biaxial Indicatrix

the plane (shaded light gray) containing α and γ. In the plane (shaded light gray) containing α, the lowest RI, and γ, the highest RI, there are radii equal to β RI. Therefore, there are two sets of radii that would describe two circular planes containing only the β RI in the biaxial indicatrix (Figure 25b). Light traveling perpendicular to the two circular planes would travel along the optic axes which lie in the ellipsoid plane containing α and γ. If the β RI is closer to α RI, the crystal has a positive (+) optic sign (Figure 25c). However, if the β RI is closer to the γ RI, the crystal has a negative (−) optic sign (Figure 25d). The RIs between α and β are noted as α' and RIs between β and γ are noted as γ'.

As with uniaxial crystals, one can superimpose the RIs within a crystal to understand and/or predict optical characteristics that one might observe during the examination of a particle (Figure 26). Again, how to easily locate the RIs for a randomly oriented crystal will be discussed in the crossed polarized section.

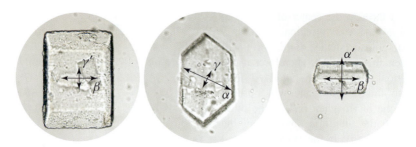

Figure 26   Three views of a sucrose crystal with the RIs superimposed in the different views

The RIs of anisotropic particles can be estimated or precisely determined using immersion methods or by employing the dispersion staining technique.

Color – Pleochroism and Dichroism.   Pleochroism observed with plane polarized light provides an additional diagnostic characteristic. Pleochroism is the general term for the phenomenon of colored anisotropic particles that absorb different wavelengths of light depending on the vibration direction through the particle. Dichroism is the proper term that refers to uniaxial crystals and many dyed fibers that show two colors with plane polarized light. All colored anisotropic particles show pleochroism but at times the change in color may be too faint to detect. Colored isotropic particles and colorless particles do not show pleochroism.

Employing plane polarized light, all one needs to do to observe pleochroism/dichorism is to rotate the stage while viewing a colored anisotropic crystal or a dyed fiber which displays this effect (Figure 27). When observing pleochroism, one should note the change of color corresponding to any physical features such as a crystal face, cleavage plane, or fiber length. The strongest absorption color usually corresponds to the highest RI direction but the asbestos mineral crocidolite is an exception to this rule.

Particle Characterization – Crossed Polars

With crossed polars, one will greatly increase the number of identification characteristics that can be determined for a particle under investigation. Crossing the polars will allow one to determine the degree of birefringence, observe different types of extinction, determine the sign of elongation, and observe interference figures. As previously discussed, it is very important to insure that the polars are properly aligned with the eyepiece crosslines and the stage is well centered.

Wave Interference.   Two waves having the same wavelength and traveling along the same propagation direction will interfere to produce a resultant wave having the same wavelength whose amplitude is the vector sum of the original two waves. However, it is important to understand the difference in how the resultant wave and interference colors are produced by two rays vibrating in the same plane or by two waves after vibrating in perpendicular planes.

Retardation of Waves Polarized in the Same Plane. If two waves, having the same wavelength and traveling in the same direction, are vibrating in the same plane and one wave is retarded from the other

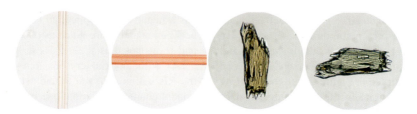

Figure 27   Dyed fiber showing dichorism (left two images) and a hyperstene crystal showing pleochroism (right two images)

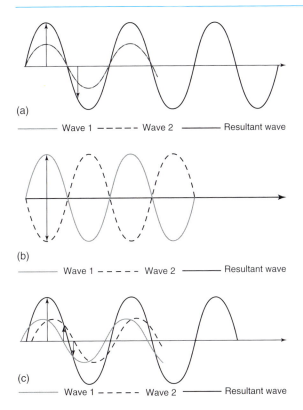

(a)

——— Wave 1 – – – – – Wave 2 ——— Resultant wave

(b)

——— Wave 1 – – – – – Wave 2 ——— Resultant wave

(c)

——— Wave 1 – – – – – Wave 2 ——— Resultant wave

Figure 28 Interference between two waves traveling in the same plane and along the same path produce the resultant wave shown when one wave is retarded by (a) $n\lambda$, (b) $n\lambda + \lambda/2$, and (c) $n\lambda = \lambda/8$. [Illustration by David Diener]

wave resulting in a path difference 1λ, 2λ, or any $n\lambda$ (where n is an integer) the two waves will be in phase. This will result in constructive interference and the resultant wave will appear brighter since the amplitude of the resultant wave is twice the amplitude of the original rays (Figure 28a). However, if two waves, having the same wavelength and traveling in the same direction, are vibrating in the same plane and one wave is retarded from the other wave so the path difference is $\lambda/2$, $1\lambda + \lambda/2$, $2\lambda + \lambda/2$, or any $n\lambda + \lambda/2$, the two waves will destructively interfere. The resultant wave will have zero amplitude and this wavelength will be eliminated (Figure 28b). Furthermore, if two waves, having the same wavelength and traveling in the same direction, are vibrating in the same plane and one ray is retarded some distance other than $n\lambda$ or $n\lambda + \lambda/2$, the resultant wave produced will be

a combination of both constructive and destructive interference (Figure 28c).

Interference Colors Produced by Two Waves Vibrating in the Same Plane. If two beams of white light interfere in the same plane as described above, some wavelengths will be eliminated while other wavelengths will be intensified. As a result, a series of colors known as *interference colors* will be produced and the resultant color will be dependent on the phase difference for the different wavelengths of light. This phenomenon produces what is commonly referred to as *thin film interference colors*, also known as *Newton's colors*. These colors are frequently seen when white light incident on a thin transparent film is reflected from the top and bottom surfaces, resulting in the reflected rays interfering with each other. Soap bubbles, a layer of oil on water, and thin deposits on a reflective substrate are a few examples that commonly show thin film interference colors.

Retardation of Waves Polarized in the Perpendicular Planes. When plane polarized light enters an anisotropic crystal which is oriented so the two indices (major or prime) are at a 45° angle from the polarizer, the wave will be resolved and vectorially split equally into two waves traveling in two mutually perpendicular planes. As a result, the slow wave (higher RI) will be retarded from the fast wave (lower RI). When both rays exit the crystal, they will continue to vibrate in perpendicular planes and will interfere with each other at the analyzer to produce a resultant wave vibrating in a single plane that is the vector sum of the two parent waves. If the two waves for a particular wavelength have a path difference of 1λ, 2λ, 3λ, or any $n\lambda$, the resultant wave will vibrate in the same plane as the original wave. The analyzer, which is a second polarizer located above the crystal whose privileged vibration direction is perpendicular to the polarizer, will block this wavelength of light (Figure 29a). However, if for a particular wavelength the two waves vibrating in two mutually perpendicular planes have a path difference of $\lambda/2$, $1\lambda + \lambda/2$, $2\lambda + \lambda/2$, or any $n\lambda + \lambda/2$, the resultant wave will vibrate in a plane particular to the polarizer vibration direction. Therefore, the analyzer will allow this wavelength of light to be transmitted through the analyzer (Figure 29b).

Furthermore, when a path difference for a particular wavelength has been separated $\lambda/4$, $1\lambda + \lambda/4$,

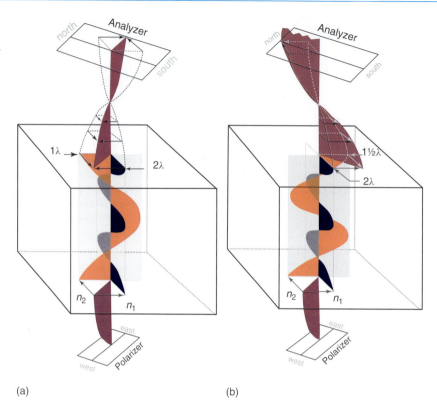

(a)   (b)

Figure 29 Interference (a) between two waves after emergence from a crystal when one wave is retarded by 1λ. Note the resultant wave is polarized in the same plane as the polarizer and would be completely be extinguished by the analyzer. Interference (b) between two waves after emergence from a crystal when one wave is retarded by 1/2λ. Note the resultant wave is polarized in the same plane as the analyzer and would be completely be transmitted by the analyzer. For illustration purposes, the waves are shown interfering before they reach the analyzer which allows for an easier understanding of the interaction of light when it reaches the analyzer. [Illustration by David Diener]

$2\lambda + \lambda/4$, or any $n\lambda + \lambda/4$, the resultant wave will vibrate in a circular, cork screw fashion and only 50% of this wavelength will be passed (transmitted) by the analyzer. And, if the path difference is any other value than $n\lambda$, $n\lambda + \lambda/2$, $n\lambda + \lambda/4$, which is normally the case, the resultant wave will vibrate in an elliptical fashion and some percentage of the resultant wave will be passed by the analyzer. The percent transmission of light by the analyzer for different phase differences is illustrated in Figure 30.

Interference Colors Produced by Two Waves Vibrating in Perpendicular Planes. If illuminated with white light, an anisotropic crystal viewed between crossed polars where the light vibrates along the two indices, a series of polarization (interference) colors will be observed as a result of unequal

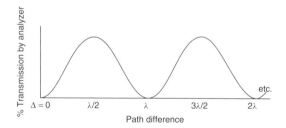

Figure 30 Percent transmission of light by the analyzer depending on the phase difference (retardation) after passage through a birefringent crystal with crossed polars

transmission by the analyzer of the different wavelengths of light as previously described. The interference colors of the particle will be brightest when the two indices are positioned at a 45° angle from the vibration direction of the polarizer. These interference colors are commonly referred to as *polarization colors* or *retardation colors*.

Birefringence. Birefringence is the numerical difference of the two refractive indices $(n_2 - n_1)$ for an anisotropic particle in a particular view. These indices for a crystal may be principal or prime indices and for a fiber $(n_\parallel - n_\perp)$. When the birefringence value is stated in literature, it is the maximum difference between the indices of a fiber or crystal unless otherwise stated. The interference color one sees between crossed polars is due to retardation (r) of the different wavelengths of light and is the result of the relationship between birefringence (B) and thickness (T) of the material under investigation. It is very important to remember that the thickness of the material is not the linear distance measured in the plane of the preparation but the thickness along the microscope axis.

This relationship is expressed as $r = 1000BT$ and is plotted graphically in the Michel–Levy chart that was first published in 1889, and a microscopist can determine any one of the values if the other two are known (Figure 31). Referring to the Michel–Levy chart, one can see that thickness increases as you move up the left ordinate. The retardation (path difference) increases as you go to the right and the colors become paler. The birefringence for a particle can be determined by moving up the diagonal line where an observed retardation color and known thickness intersect. Glass fibers of any thickness would be black on a black field with crossed polars since glass has one RI and light travels through the particle at a single velocity. However, a 10 μm fiber showing a first-order red color would have a birefringence of 0.055

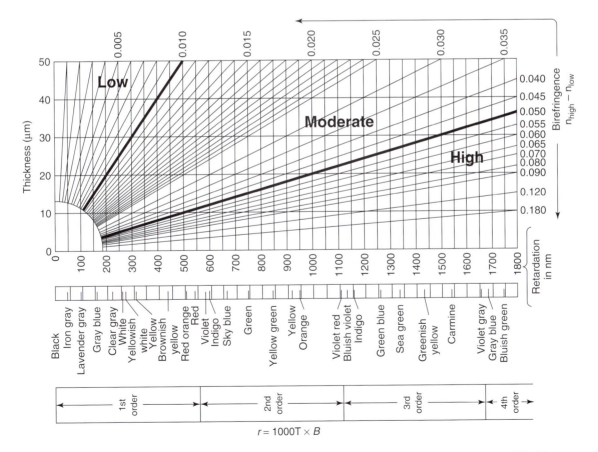

Figure 31 A black and white Michel–Levy chart showing the relationship among retardation, thickness, and birefringence. One can obtain a color Michel–Levy chart from most of the references listed in the bibliography

and a $10\,\mu m$ fiber showing a third-order red color would have a birefringence of 0.170. Some particles will not follow the Michel–Levy series of retardation colors but will show anomalous polarization colors and when recognized it is a unique identifying characteristic.

Extinction. Particles will be brightest between crossed polars when the two indices are in a particular view. As one rotates the stage, the particle will usually go dark every 90°, a circumstance known as *extinction*. There are different types of extinction one can observe for a particle (Figure 32). Most particles will show complete or uniform extinction and may show parallel, symmetrical, or oblique extinction.

Some particles will not uniformly go to complete extinction but will show nonuniform extinction. Undulose extinction shows areas of extinction that move progressively across the particle in a fanlike motion as the stage is rotated. Polycrystalline crystals will show areas of extinction due to the random orientation of the crystals to each other.

Other particles may not show any extinction. Cotton fibers may not show good extinction due to the different orientations of the overlaying top and bottom layer of the collapsed fiber. Some particles in a particular view may show dispersion of extinction and the different "extinction" colors are dependent on the wavelength of light (Figure 33). When recognized, it is a unique identifying characteristic.

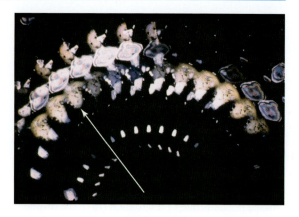

Figure 33 Photomicrograph of RDX by Dr. Walter C. McCrone with a crystal (arrow) showing dispersed extinction when viewed with crossed polars. The photomicrograph is a series of 12 exposures with the stage being rotated several degrees between each exposure. Note the crystal does not go to complete extinction but displays a series of colors from blue to purple to yellow. The RDX crystal above the crystal showing dispersed extinction has a different orientation and shows complete extinction [Reproduced with permission from McCrone Research Institute.]

Sign of Elongation. By convention, a fiber has a positive (+) sign of elongation if $n_{\parallel} > n_{\perp}$ and a negative (−) sign of elongation if $n_{\parallel} < n_{\perp}$. One can quickly determine if the fiber has a (+) or (−) sign of elongation by using a compensator. Compensators are usually marked with an arrow with a γ or Z symbol

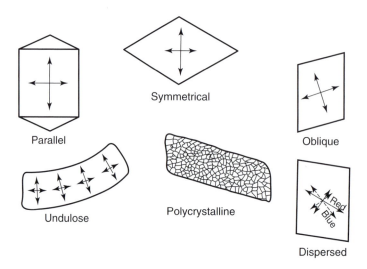

Figure 32   Different types of extinction [Reproduced with permission from McCrone Research Institute.]

to indicate the slow component (higher RI) direction. Commonly used compensators to determine the sign of elongation include the first-order red plate having a retardation of 530 nm and the quarter-wave plate having a retardation of 137 nm.

Utilizing crossed polars, the retardation colors are noted for a fiber that is aligned parallel to the slow component direction of the compensator. When a first-order red plate is inserted, the retardation will change by 530 nm and the two retardations (fiber and compensator) will be added or subtracted (lower RI from the higher RI). Addition means the two slow components are parallel and the fiber has a (+) sign of elongation (i.e., $n_\parallel > n_\perp$). Subtraction means the slow component of the fiber is perpendicular to the slow component of the compensator and the fiber has a (−) sign of elongation (i.e., $n_\parallel < n_\perp$).

For example, if a gray blue (150 nm) retardation color is observed with crossed polars for a fiber aligned parallel to the slow component of the compensator and turns blue (680 nm) when the 530 nm compensator is inserted, then the two retardations have added and the fiber has a (+) sign of elongation. However, the fiber has a negative sign of elongation if it turns yellow (380 nm). Higher-order retardation colors observed with crossed polars will appear more pale when the compensator is inserted for a fiber that has a (+) sign of elongation and brighter for a (−) sign of elongation. Wollastonite, a fibrous mineral, may show (+) or (−) sign of elongation because the β RI is parallel to the length of the fiber. When α (or α') RI is perpendicular to the length, the fiber will have a (+) sign of elongation and a (−) sign of elongation when γ (or γ') RI is perpendicular to the fiber length.

Interference Figures. An interference figure is an important diagnostic feature that is formed by rays that travel along different directions within the crystal. Interference figures are observed by examining the back focal plane of the objective using a Bertrand lens, a phase telescope, or by removing an eyepiece and inserting a pinhole eye cap. Unfortunately, most crystals have orientations that provide interference figures that are of little diagnostic value. However, if one can recognize a crystal in the orientation that will provide a useful figure, one can determine a number of optical properties such as if the crystal is uniaxial or biaxial, the location of the principal refractive indices, and the optic sign. Low retardation colors observed on highly birefringent crystals provide the best interference figures.

An objective having a numerical aperture of at least 0.65 is required to obtain an interference figure and the aperture diaphragm needs to be opened to provide a full cone of light to the objective. An example of a centered uniaxial interference figure is provided and a centered biaxial figure is provided in Figure 34. One should be aware of the value of interference figures even though a more in depth discussion is not possible here but one can investigate a number of references listed in the bibliography such as *Optical Crystallography* by F. Donald Bloss for more information.

Fusion Methods

Fusion methods many times can be included when characterizing a sample. Most of the time, a sample can be heated over an alcohol lamp and characteristic crystals that develop from the melt state can be observed. Also, a hot stage can be attached to the microscope and used to accurately determine the melting point of a particle under investigation. Many microscopists use the hot stage to distinguish between polymers like low density and high density polyethylene as well as nylon 6 and nylon 6,6.

Fusion methods can be used to characterize not only organic compounds but also some inorganic compounds. For example, ammonium nitrate has four crystal phases above room temperature: an orthorhombic crystal phase from room temperature to 32 °C, a second biaxial crystal phase from 32 to 84 °C, a tetragonal crystal phase from 84 to 125 °C, and finally a cubic crystal phase which melts at 170 °C. Using a polarized light microscope, it is truly a spectacular sight to view a sample going from room temperature to a melted state and from a melted

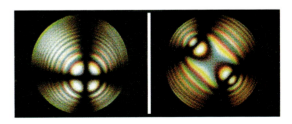

Figure 34 Interference figures: uniaxial (left) and biaxial (right) [Reproduced with permission from McCrone Research Institute.]

state back to room temperature. For more information on fusion methods one should consult the *Polarized Light Microscopy* manual by McCrone, McCrone and Delly as well as *Fusion Methods* by McCrone.

Microchemical Tests

Microchemical tests aid in the identification of particles under investigation and should not be overlooked by the forensic microscopist. These tests can be applied to both inorganic compounds (e.g., explosives) and organic compounds (e.g., drugs) and many times a microchemical test will provide more information about a particle under investigation (e.g., valence state) than other modern instrumental methods. Microchemical tests are particularly useful because they are quickly and easily conducted, their sensitivity requires only a minute amount of sample, and they are easy to perform.

Most microchemical tests are based on the formation of characteristics crystals that develop using a selected reagent and are normally carried out on a microscope slide without a coverslip using a 10X objective. An in-depth discussion on microchemical methods is not possible in this article and one should consult references such as the *Handbook of Chemical Microscopy, Volume 1 and 2*, by Chamot and Mason as well as "Microchemical Reactions in Particle Identification" by S. Palenik in the *Particle Atlas, Volume 5*, for a detailed presentation on microchemical methods.

Fluorescence Microscopy

Since the early 1980s, fluorescence microscopy has become a common analytical tool employed in the trace evidence section of many forensic laboratories. This technique is a sensitive and simple analytical tool that can be employed to characterize and compare many different types of trace evidence such as paints, cosmetics, fibers, adhesives, plastics, and mineral grains in soil samples. Fluorescence microscopy is a nondestructive method that can quickly provide information which cannot be obtained by other types of instrumentation. This article addresses only reflected or incident light (also referred to as *Epi*) fluorescence since it is the type of fluorescence microscopy used today. A simple diagram of a reflected light fluorescence microscope showing the ray paths for illuminating and imaging the specimen is provided in Figure 35.

Fluorescence

Luminescence is the term used to describe nonthermal radiation of longer wavelength (lower energy) that is emitted when energy of shorter wavelength (higher energy) is absorbed by some materials. The fluorescent material may be inorganic or organic and the emitted radiation (luminescence) is usually in the visible region of light. The energy stimulation can be ion, X-ray, electron, or photon radiation. Luminescence can also be produced by chemical reactions

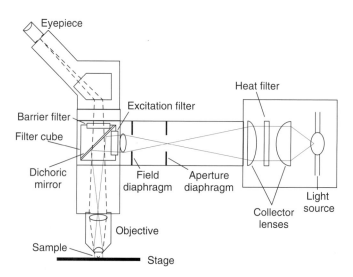

Figure 35   Schematic diagram showing the illuminating and imagining ray path through a fluorescent microscope

or by mechanical action. Depending on the type of primary excitation, different descriptive terms may be used to describe the luminescence: e.g., ionoluminescence (ion), Roentgenoluminescence (X-ray), cathodoluminescence (electron), and photoluminescence (photon).

Luminescence can be further subdivided into phosphorescence and fluorescence. Phosphorescence is generally characterized by continued luminescence after the excitation stops and fluorescence ceases instantaneously when the excitation stops. Fluorescence can also be subdivided into primary fluorescence (auto) and secondary fluorescence. Primary fluorescence is the ability to emit luminescence without any treatment or staining. Secondary fluorescence requires staining the specimen with a dye (e.g., fluorchrome). Normally, only primary fluorescence will be of interest in the examination of trace evidence.

Illuminators

There are two types of light sources used for fluorescence microscopy which are the pressure mercury lamp and the xenon lamp. The high-pressure mercury lamp produces a rather noncontinuous energy distribution with most of its energy output concentrated in several narrow bands (Figure 36). The xenon lamp produces a more continuous spectrum from the ultraviolet to the near infrared and closely resembles characteristics of visible light (Figure 37). In addition to being able to produce a more continuous energy spectrum, xenon lamps can be switched on and off without waiting for the lamp to warm-up or cool down. Various output powers are available for these

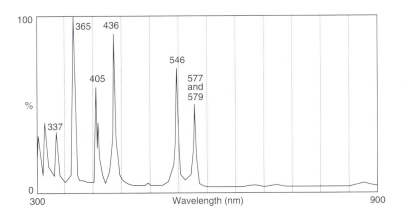

Figure 36 Spectral output for mercury lamp

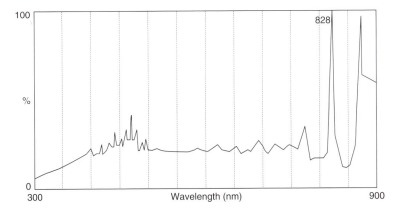

Figure 37 Spectral output for xenon lamp

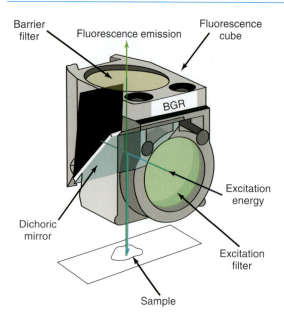

Figure 38 Cutaway view showing the components of a fluorescent filter cube

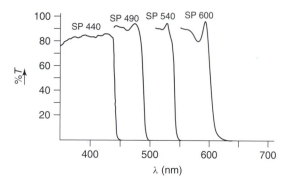

Figure 39 Typical transmission curves for several short-pass excitation filters. The nomenclature denotes the cut-off wavelength at 50% maximum transmission

lamps, but generally 100 W mercury lamps and 75 W xenon lamps are used for the examination of trace evidence samples. Before starting any examination, one needs to ensure that the microscope has been properly aligned and adjusted so that the illumination field provides the best image quality.

Optical Cube

Besides the alignment of the microscope, the proper selection of the filters contained in the cube is an important factor in determining the intensity of the fluorescence image observed though the microscope. The optical cube or filter cube contains the excitation filter, the dichroic mirror (DM), and the barrier filter (Figure 38). Manufacturers today offer a variety of fluorescence cubes containing different filter and mirror combinations, and it is important to understand the purpose of each component of the cube. The filters and mirror in a cube allow certain wavelengths of light to be transmitted, reflected, or absorbed and the correct configuration will maximize the fluorescence intensity of the sample being examined.

Excitation Filter. The excitation or exciter filter (EX) allows shorter wavelengths of light from the

illuminator to pass through while longer wavelengths are suppressed. As one would expect, the purpose of this filter is to transmit only the wavelengths of illumination that will effectively excite the specimen and eliminate longer wavelengths of light that would obscure any fluorescence from the specimen. The filter may have simple nomenclature designating the wavelength range that is passed (transmitted) such as UV or U for ultraviolet, B for blue, G for green or may have a more detailed nomenclature specifying the wavelength range that is passed by the filter. Shortpass (SP) filters that transmit shorter wavelengths yet block longer wavelengths were used in the past for the excitation filter. The nomenclature typically used for these filters denotes the cut-off wavelength that is located at 50% maximum transmission (Figure 39). Today, however, bandpass (BP) filters, or bandpass interference filters (BPIF) are utilized almost exclusively for the excitation filter. BP filters typically have a nomenclature which denotes the center wavelength of the transmission and may note the bandwidth at half of the maximum transmission (Figure 40). BP filters can further be designated as wideband or narrowband filters. As suggested by S. Palenik in "Microscopical Examination of Fibers", wideband filters would be a better choice for the forensic microscopist since they are considering a wide range of materials that may fluoresce over a broad range of wavelengths.

Dichroic Mirror. The shorter wavelengths of excitation illumination will be reflected toward the specimen by the DM, also referred to as the *chromatic beam splitter* (BS). The DM is positioned at a 45°

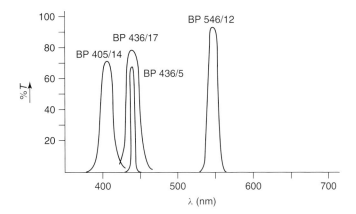

Figure 40 Typical transmission curves for several bandpass excitation filters. The nomenclature denotes the center wavelength of transmission and the bandwidth at 50% maximum transmission

in the optical light path. At the same time, the unwanted longer wavelengths of light will be transmitted through the DM and absorbed on the interior black coated surface of the cube. Once the excitation wavelength reaches the specimen, the emitted fluorescent wavelengths from the sample and some of the unabsorbed excitation wavelength(s) of light will be reflected back toward the DM. The longer fluorescent wavelengths will be transmitted through the DM toward the eyepiece and the unabsorbed and unwanted excitation wavelengths will be reflected back to the lamp. This unique ability of the DM to reflect the shorter wavelengths and pass longer wavelengths is accomplished with the use of a thin-film interference coated piece of glass. Current DMs can pass and reflect light with 90% efficiency. The typical nomenclature for a DM will denote the wavelength (located at 50% maximum transmission) at which shorter wavelengths will be reflected by the mirror and longer wavelengths will be passed (Figure 41).

Barrier Filter. The last filter in the cube is the barrier (BA) or emitter (EM) filter. Since the wavelength ranges transmitted for the excitation filter and the DM may slightly overlap, the barrier filter is needed to block any harmful ultraviolet excitation light and effectively transmit only the fluorescence emitted by the sample. A barrier filter can be either a longpass (LP) filter or BP filter. Longpass filters allow wavelengths longer than their cut-on point to be transmitted and the nomenclature for these filters denotes the cut-on wavelength that is located at 50% maximum transmission (Figure 42).

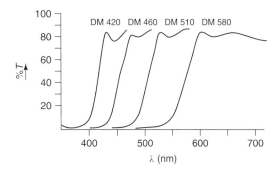

Figure 41 Typical transmission curves for several dichroic mirrors. The nomenclature denotes the cut-on wavelength at 50% maximum transmission

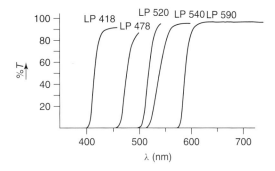

Figure 42 Typical transmission curves for several barrier filters. The nomenclature denotes the cut-on wavelength at 50% maximum transmission

A simple ray diagram showing the function of each component in a filter is provided in Figure 43

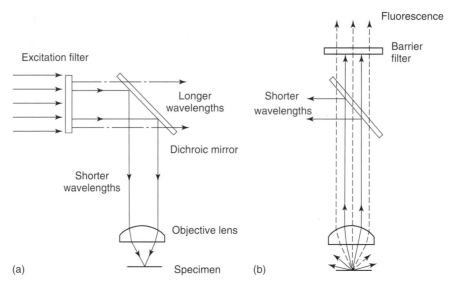

Figure 43 Schematic diagram showing the function for the different components of a fluorescence filter cube. Excitation rays (a) and fluorescence emission (b)

and an example of a typical transmission curve for a filter cube is provided in Figure 44.

Cathodoluminescence

Furthermore, it is worth noting that the use of cathodoluminescence (CL) microscopy is gaining

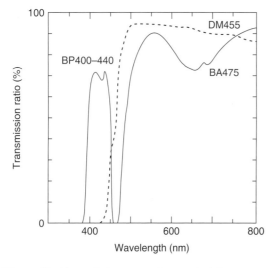

Figure 44 Transmission curves for a typical fluorescence filter cube

popularity in forensic laboratories. As mentioned at the beginning of this section, cathodoluminescence is the fluorescence (luminescence) obtained by excitation of the sample using electrons instead of photons. Accessories for the scanning election microscope (SEM) can be obtained to observe cathodoluminescence or one can outfit a light microscope with a small vacuum specimen chamber containing a cold-cathode electron gun. An example of a paint sample observed utilizing reflected visible light, fluorescence, and cathodoluminescence is provided in Figure 45. For more information on cathodoluminescence, one may consult "Applications of Cathodoluminescence in Forensic Science" by S. Palenik and J. Buscaglia in *Forensic Analysis on the Cutting Edge: New Methods for Trace Evidence Analysis.*

Comparison Microscopy

Comparison microscopes are used extensively in a forensic laboratory to compare pieces of evidence to a known specimen. Although comparison microscopes are employed in the examination of bullets, cartridge cases, or toolmarks, this type of examination is also used to compare trace evidence such as hairs, fibers, paint chips, and other types of particles that may

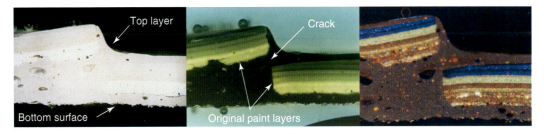

Figure 45 Embedded cross section of a multilayered white paint sample from an old building. The last application of white paint flowed through the crack in the paint and migrated under the older layers of paint. Images (from left to right) are reflected (ordinary) light, fluorescence, and cathodoluminescence

become separated from a source and accidentally left at the scene of a crime.

Design

The most critical part of a comparison microscope is the optical bridge that connects the optical paths of two side-by-side microscope systems. This bridge consists of multiple prisms arranged in such a manner to allow the magnified images from the left and right sides to be viewed simultaneously with a fine "hairline" split between the two fields of view. Depending on the complexity of the instrument, the prisms can be adjusted either mechanically or by motors so that the hair-line is moved horizontally in the field of view to expose more or less of one side of the image or to superimpose the left and right images over each other.

The comparison microscope used for firearms, toolmarks and documents is configured for low visual magnifications from 2X to 120X and uses incident (reflected) illumination. A system used for trace evidence comparisons uses two compound microscopes usually equipped for intermediate visual magnifications from 40X to 600X and with brightfield and polarized transmitted illumination (Figure 46). Microscopes for fiber comparisons are now often supplied with epi-fluorescence components for comparison of known and questioned materials at selected excitation and emission wavelengths.

Acknowledgment

The authors would like to thank Ms Natasha Neel with the Bureau of Alcohol, Tobacco, Firearms, and Explosives and Mr Christopher Taylor with the US Army Criminal Investigation Laboratory who reviewed many versions of this article and provided a number of valuable suggestions. A special thanks to Mr Stephen Garten with the Bureau of Alcohol, Tobacco, Firearms, and Explosives who helped prepare figures, compile references, and review various versions of this document. Also, the authors dedicate this article to the late Dr Walter C. McCrone, our mentor and good friend, who encouraged and helped many forensic microscopists worldwide.

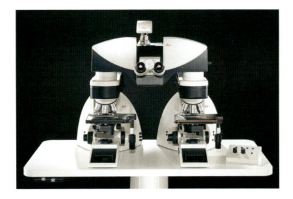

Figure 46 Modern trace evidence comparison microscope

Further Reading

Stereomicroscopy

DeForest, P.R. (2005). Foundations of forensic microscopy, in *Forensic Science Handbook*, R. Saferstein, ed, Prentice Hall, Englewood Cliffs, pp. 416–528.

McCrone, W.C. (1991). Light microscopy, in *Physical Methods of Chemistry*, B.W. Rossiter & J.F. Hamilton, eds, John Wiley & Sons, New York.

McCrone, W., McCrone, L. & Delly, J. (1978). *Polarized Light Microscopy*, McCrone Research Institute, Chicago.

Needham, G. (1958). *The Practical Use of the Microscope*, Springfield, Thomas.

Nikon (2007). Nikon microscopyu: stereomicroscopy [Online], http://www.microscopyu.com/articles/stereomicroscopy/index.html.

Petraco, N. & Kubic, T. (2004). *Microscopy for Criminalists, Chemists, and Conservators*, CRC Press, Boca Raton.

Brightfield Microscopy

Abramowitz, M. (2003). *Microscope Basics and Beyond*, Olympus America, New York, Vol. 1.

Bradbury, S. & Bracegirdle, B. (1998). *Introduction to Light Microscopy*, BIOS Scientific Publishers, Oxford.

Davidson, M. & Abramowitz, M. Optical microscopy [Online], http://www.olympusmicro.com/primer/microscopy.pdf.

DeForest, P.R. (2005). Foundations of forensic microscopy, in *Forensic Science Handbook*, R. Saferstein, ed, Prentice Hall, Englewood Cliffs, pp. 416–528.

Houck, M. & Siegel, J. (2006). Microscopy, *Fundamentals of Forensic Science*, Academic Press, Amsterdam, pp. 79–98.

McCrone, W.C. (1991). Light microscopy, in *Physical Methods of Chemistry*, B.W. Rossiter & J.F. Hamilton, eds, John Wiley & Sons, New York, pp. 343–443.

McCrone, W., McCrone, L. & Delly, J. (1978). *Polarized Light Microscopy*, McCrone Research Institute, Chicago.

Needham, G. (1958). *The Practical Use of the Microscope*, Springfield, Thomas.

New York Microscopical Society (1989). *Glossary of Microscopical Terms and Definitions*, 2nd Edition, New York Microscopical Society, New York (this is currently available from the McCrone Research Institute in Chicago).

Nikon (2007). Nikon microscopyu: introduction to polarized microscopy [Online], http://www.microscopyu.com/articles/polarized/polarizedintro.html.

Nikon (2007). Nikon microscopyu: concepts and formulas in microscopy [Online], http://www.microscopyu.com/articles/formulas/formulasindex.html.

Petraco, N. & Kubic, T. (2004). *Microscopy for Criminalists, Chemists, and Conservators*, CRC Press, Boca Raton.

Zeiler, H. (1973). *The Optical Performance of the Light Microscope*, 2 parts, McCrone Research Institute, Chicago.

Polarized Light Microscopy

Benedetti-Pichler, A. (1942). *Introduction of the Microtechnique of Inorganic Analysis*, John Wiley & Sons, New York.

Bloss, F. (1999). *An Introduction to the Methods of Optical Crystallography*, Mineralogical Society of America, Washington, DC.

Chamot, E. & Mason, C. (1931). *Handbook of Chemical Microscopy*, Wiley, New York (Vol. 2 is currently available from The McCrone Research Institute in Chicago) 2 vols.

DeForest, P.R. (2005). Foundations of forensic microscopy, in *Forensic Science Handbook*, R. Saferstein, ed, Prentice Hall, Englewood Cliffs, pp. 416–528.

Dyar, M.D., Gunter, M.E. & Tasa, D. (2006). Optical mineralogy, in *Mineral and Optical Mineralogy*, Mineralogical Society of America, pp. 81–102.

Hartshorne, N. & Stuart, A. (1970). *Crystals and the Polarizing Microscope*, American Elsevier Science, New York.

Houck, M. & Bowen, R. (2005). An argument for light microscopy – a review of forensic microscopy for trace evidence analysis, *Forensic Science Review* **17**(1), 1.

Houck, M. & Siegel, J. (2006). Microscopy, in *Fundamentals of Forensic Science*, Academic Press, Amsterdam, pp. 79–98.

Kile, D. (2003). *The Petrographic Microscope: Evolution of a Mineralogical Research Instrument*, The Mineralogical Record, Arizona.

McCrone, W. (1957). *Fusion Methods in Chemical Microscopy*, Interscience Publishers, New York (this is currently available from the McCrone Research Institute in Chicago).

McCrone, W.C. (1979). Particle analysis in the crime laboratory, in *The Particle Atlas*, W.C. Mc.Crone, J.G. Delly & S.J., Palenik, eds, Ann Arbor Science Publishers, Ann Arbor, p. 1379 (this is currently available on CD from the McCrone Research Institute in Chicago) Vol. 5.

McCrone, W.C. (1987). *Asbestos Identification*, Ann Arbor Science Publishers, Ann Arbor.

McCrone, W.C. (1991). Light microscopy, in *Physical Methods of Chemistry*, B.W. Rossiter & J.F. Hamilton, eds, John Wiley & Sons, New York, pp. 343–443.

McCrone, W., McCrone, L. & Delly, J. (1978). *Polarized Light Microscopy*, McCrone Research Institute, Chicago.

Nikon (2007). Nikon microscopyu: introduction to polarized microscopy [Online], http://www.microscopyu.com/articles/polarized/polarizedintro.html.

Olympus (2007). Olympus microscopy resource center: specialized microscopy techniques – polarized light microscopy [Online], http://www.olympusmicro.com/primer/techniques/polarized/polarizedhome.html.

Palenik, S.J. (1979). Microchemical reactions in particle identification, in *The Particle Atlas*, W.C. Mc.Crone, J.G. Delly & S.J. Palinik, eds, Ann Arbor Science Publishers, Ann Arbor, pp. 1175–1184 (this is currently available on CD from the McCrone Research Institute in Chicago) Vol. **5**.

Palenik, S. (1988). Microscopy and microchemistry of physical evidence, in *Forensic Science Handbook*, R. Saferstien, ed, Prentice Hall, Englewood Cliffs, pp. 161–208.

Petraco, N. & Kubic, T. (2004). *Microscopy for Criminalists, Chemists, and Conservators*, CRC Press, Boca Raton.

Stoiber, R. & Morse, S. (1994). *Crystal Identification with the Polarizing Microscope*, Chapman and Hall, New York.

Viney, C. (1990). *Transmitted Polarized Light Microscopy*, McCrone Research Institute, Chicago.

Wahlstrom, E. (1979). *Optical Crystallography*, John Wiley and Sons, New York.

Fluorescence Microscopy

Abramowitz, M. (1993). *Fluorescence Microscopy: The Essentials*, Olympus American, New York.

Birk, G. (1984). *Instrumentation and Techniques for Fluorescence Microscopy*, Wild Leitz (Australia) Pty, Sydney.

Herman, B. (1998). *Fluorescence Microscopy*, BIOS Scientific Publishers, Oxford, 2 Vols.

Holz, H. *Worthwhile Facts About Fluorescence Microscopy*, Zeiss Publication.

Marshall, D. (1988). *Cathodoluminescence of Geological Materials*, Unwin Hyman, London.

Nikon (2007). Nikon microscopyu: fluorescence microscopy [Online], http://www.microscopyu.com/articles/fluorescence/index.html.

Olympus (2007). Olympus microscopy resource center: specialized microscopy techniques – fluorescence microscopy [Online], http://www.olympusmicro.com/primer/techniques/fluorescence/fluorhome.html.

Palenik, S. (1999). Microscopical examination of fibers, in *Forensic Examination of Fibres*, J. Robertson & M. Grieve, eds, CRC Press, Boca Raton, p. 153.

Palenik, C. & Buscaglia, J. (2007). Applications of cathodoluminescence in forensic science, in *Forensic Analysis on the Cutting Edge*, R. Blackledge, ed, John Wiley & Sons, New Jersey, pp. 141–174.

Reichman, J. (2000). *Handbook of Optical Filters for Fluorescence Microscopy*, Chroma Technology Corp, Rockingham.

Semrock 2000. 2007 Catalog.

Spring, K. & Davidson, M. Introduction to fluorescence microscopy [Online], http://www.microscopyu.com/articles/fluorescence/fluorescenceintro.html.

Comparison Microscopy

Ernst Leitz Wetzlar (1986). *Bulletin for the Forensic Laboratory – Comparison Microscope*, R. Beck, ed, Ernst Leitz Wetzlar.

Needham, G. (1958). *The Practical Use of the Microscope*, Springfield, Thomas.

Petraco, N. & Kubic, T. (2004). *Microscopy for Criminalists, Chemists, and Conservators*, CRC Press, Boca Raton.

THOMAS J. HOPEN AND MALCOLM DAVIS

Microscopy: Low Power

Microscope is an instrument designed to extend man's visual capability, i.e., to make visible even the minute details that can not be seen with the naked eye [1].

On the basis of the early pioneering study on microscopy in the sixteenth century, the first real microscope was made in the seventeenth century by Antony van Leeuwenhoek. Nonetheless, Leeuwenhoek, using this simple microscope, which was little more than a magnifying glass, discovered bacteria and spermatozoa and he built 400 microscopes in his lifetime! From this "single lens" microscope evolved the *compound microscope*, which simply means more than one lens so that the image magnified by one lens can be magnified by another. Today the term *microscope* is generally used to refer to a compound microscope, where the lens closer to the object being viewed is the *objective* lens while that closer to the eye of the observer is the *eyepiece*. Despite the apparent complexity of research level microscopes, they are in essence simple. They are also probably the most poorly understood and badly used of all laboratory instruments. The stereo microscope is a compound microscope. A typical high-quality stereo microscope is shown in Figure 1. In fact it comprises two compound microscopes, which are aligned side-by-side at the correct visual angle to provide a true stereoscopic image. Most stereo microscopes in laboratories today have a common main objective, and as the "workings" of the microscope are housed in a single body, it is not obvious that there are two optical systems present. Older Greenough type systems had two completely separate optical systems. Not all low-magnification binocular (two eyepieces) microscopes are stereo microscopes. Low-cost, low-magnification microscopes for students often have a single objective and image forming system, with a beam splitter delivering an image to both eyepieces. These microscopes do not produce a stereo image.

Current stereo microscopes have many attractive properties:

- they have a long working distance (the distance between the specimen and the objective lens);
- an upright nonreversed image (i.e., the image is seen in the same direction as it sits on the stage, facilitating sample movement and magnification);
- the image has a genuine three dimensional feel;
- little sample preparation usually required;
- various types of illumination can be used including transmitted light and overhead or incident light of several types (ring light, angled reflected light);
- large field of view; and
- can be attached to an arm enabling the examination of larger objects.

Modern instruments can also be set up for polarizing and fluorescence applications.

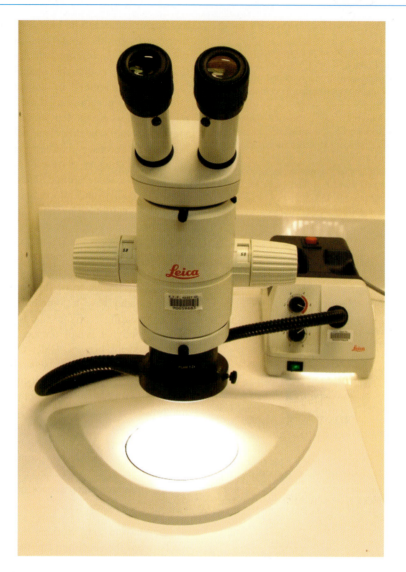

Figure 1   Stereo microscope

The useful magnification range is typically between 2.5× and a maximum of 100×. More expensive instruments often have a zoom capability.

The stereo microscope can be considered to be an extension of the human eye allowing the observer to see more details. In forensic work, stereo microscopes are mainly used to investigate the microscopic details of large objects, such as clothing, down to small fibers, soil, plant material, glass, paint, and other possible physical evidence contained in recovered debris.

There are probably no areas of forensic endeavor where low-power microscopy does not have a role to play.

With most new instruments, video or still digital cameras can be attached enabling the examiner to record images for inclusion in case notes or in case reports.

Training in the use of low-power microscopes is strongly recommended if they are to be used to their full potential. However, even a relatively inexperienced individual can make reasonably effective use of simple low-power microscopes. This is not the case with high-power microscopes.

Reference

[1] Anon (1989). *RMS Dictionary of Light Microscopy*, Oxford University Press – Royal Microscopical Society.

Further Reading

De Forest, P.R. (2002). Foundation of forensic microscopy, in *Forensic Science Handbook*, 2nd Edition, R. Saferstein, ed, Prentice Hall, New Jersey, Vol. 1, Chapter 5, pp. 215–319.

Houck, M.M. & Bowen, R. (2005). An argument for light microscopy – a review of forensic microscopy for trace evidence analysis. *Forensic Science Review* **17**, 1–15.

JAMES ROBERTSON

Microscopy: Scanning Electron Microscopy

Introduction

The invention of the electron microscope gave rise to the discovery of infinite entities, so far invisible, by optical microscopes. The use of electrons made it possible to overcome the optical limits of light. Nowadays, electron microscopy is a well-established technique and is widely used for forensic science purposes. With resolution in the nanometer and Angstrom range, electron microscopy and scanning probe microscopy are two of the most powerful microscopy techniques available today.

According to the imaging mechanism, the family of electron microscopes consists of the transmission electron microscope (TEM), the scanning transmission microscope (STEM), the scanning electron microscope (SEM), and the environmental SEM (ESEM). The Nobel prize-winning TEM was first developed, followed by the SEMs [1, 2]. The TEMs, TEM as well as STEM, are less in use for forensic observations because of the limitation of specimen thickness ($<1\,\mu m$ thick).

The first SEMs were constructed in the 1930s and 1940s and have since then been constantly developed into very high-resolution instruments and this development lead to the invention of the ESEM, which allowed the observation of specimens that were, until then, impossible to submit to a classical SEM because of its high-vacuum environment.

The SEM is a very versatile instrument for the visualization of very small objects, the study of surface morphology, thanks to its resolution and excellent depth of field as well as its spectroscopic possibilities (Figure 1a, b). Like optical microscopes, the SEM measures only the X and Y dimensions of a sample, contrary to scanning probe microscopes (SPMs) that measure the Z dimension as well.

The SEM operates with an electron beam that interacts with the sample and generates several signals that are detected and processed to form the image [3]. Given that the electrons interact with the molecules of air, the electron beam has to be produced and travel in a vacuum, avoid trajectory deviations.

SEM: Functioning and Image Mechanisms

SEMs consist of five main parts: the electron source, the electron column with a series of electromagnetic lenses, the sample chamber, the signal processing part constituted of several detectors, the signal processing devices, and the image visualization devices such as a monitor (Figure 2). An elaborated pumping system is attached to the microscope, keeping the microscope and its parts under vacuum (ranging from 10^{-4} to about 10^{-10} Torr).

Electron Source

The electron beam can be generated by either a thermoionic source or a field emission (FE) source. The first kind produces electrons when heated and the second type generates electrons when an intense electric field is applied to it. These sources are part of an assembly – the electron gun. The two different systems cannot be interchanged. However, the choice of the source influences the performance of the SEM, i.e., the quality of its electron beam as well as its probe size. The FE source produces a monochromatic beam (small electron energy spread), where thermoionic sources have a greater electron

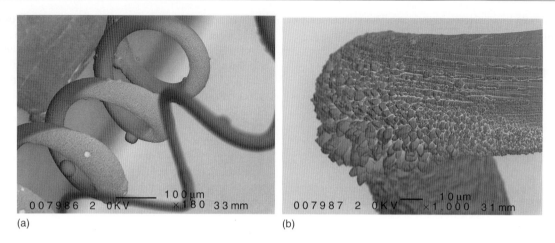

Figure 1   The high depth of field and high resolution allow having a sharp general view (a) or detail view (b) of a filament of a broken car light bulb

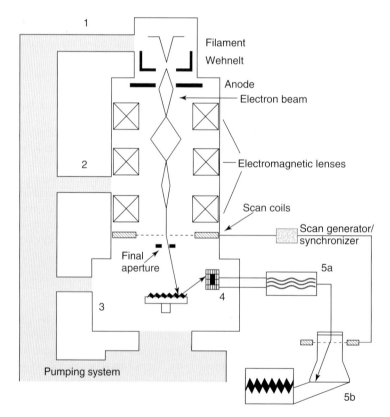

Figure 2   Schema of a conventional SEM: 1. Electron source (thermoionic gun); 2. electron column; 3. sample chamber; 4. detectors; 5a. Signal processing devices (e.g., photomultiplier, amplifier, etc.); and 5b. visualization system (monitor and computer)

energy range. The gun operates under vacuum is common to both the systems (10^{-4}–10^{-9} Torr).

The function of the electron gun, independent of the type, is to focus the electrons coming off the source and to direct this beam into the electron column and finally to the sample. To achieve this, the electron source is incorporated into a gun assembly, which acts as a lens to focus the emitted electrons. The assembly basically consists of a cathode and an anode. However, the design of the gun is different for thermoionic sources and field emission sources.

Thermoionic Gun. This gun consists of three elements: the electron emitting material (commonly called *filament*), the Wehnelt, and the anode (Figure 3).

These three parts form the so-called triode where the filament is the cathode. The Wehnelt has a potential that is more negative – the bias voltage – than the cathode itself. The bias voltage is variable and is used for controlling the emission of electrons from the filament. A high bias voltage restricts the emission to a small area, thereby reducing the total emitted current. A low bias voltage increases the size of the emitting area on the filament and thus the total emission current. The Wehnelt creates a negative field that makes the emitted electron converge to a point called a crossover situated between the Wehnelt and the anode (Figure 3). This crossover determines the size of the final probe diameter and thereby the resolution of the microscope. The Wehnelt acts as a simple electrostatic lens – the first lens in the

microscope. The crossover is determined by the type of filament, the electric field between the cathode and the anode, and the exit angles of the electrons from the filament. The heating current and the Wehnelt bias voltage have to be set in order to operate at saturation condition (i.e., the smallest beam diameter with an even bright spot).

The filament in a thermoionic gun has to be either of a high-melting point material or with a low work function (i.e., necessary energy for the electrons to escape). In practice, tungsten with its high melting temperature (3660 K) and rare-earth boride crystal such as lanthanum hexaboride (LaB_6) or cerium hexaboride (CeB_6) are used. The tungsten filament has either a hairpin shape or is pointed, to minimize the emitting area. Tungsten filaments are heated directly, where rare-earth boride crystals are indirectly heated by a bonding material surrounding the crystal, such as carbon or rhenium. This type of filament can be used in standard tungsten SEM if the vacuum system is upgraded. Tungsten filaments need a vacuum of around 10^{-4} Torr where boride crystals require a higher vacuum (around 10^{-6}–10^{-7} Torr).

Field Emission Gun. FE guns are much simpler than thermoionic ones. They consist of a cathode and two anodes (Figure 4).

A very fine tungsten tip with a radius of <100 nm constitutes the cathode. This sharp tip is submitted to a strong electric field (>10^{-7} V/cm) that lowers the work function barrier sufficiently for electrons to tunnel out of the tungsten. This electric field is

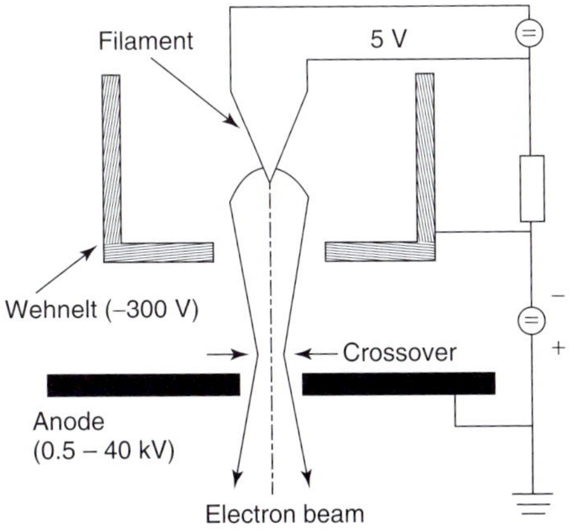

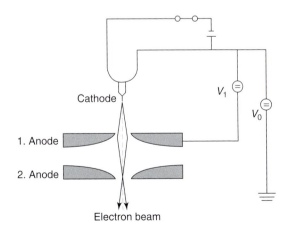

Figure 3 Schema of a thermoionic gun with a hairpin-shaped filament

Figure 4 Schema of a cold field emission gun (V_0, acceleration bias; V_1, extraction bias)

Table 1 Comparison of the resolution in function of the electron gun system:

kV	Tungsten (nm)	LaB$_6$ (nm)	Field emission	
			CFE (nm)	TFE (nm)
0.5	80	50	15	
1.0	40	25	5	15
30.0	4	3	1.5	2

(CFE: cold field emission; TFE: thermal field emission). The spatial resolution depends on the type of electron gun, the electron-optical system and the extent to which the material interacts with the electron beam. The values are indicative and depend on the instrument

achieved by the first anode. The work of the second anode is to accelerate the electrons to 100 kV or more. The combined fields of the anodes act like a more refined electrostatic lens to produce a crossover. The second anode controls the effective probe size and position. In this system, the tungsten is operated at ambient temperature and that is why the process is called a *cold field emission*. This requires a high vacuum of about 10^{-9} Torr, preventing the tungsten tip from rapid surface contamination. The vacuum can be lowered when heating the tip. The thermal energy assists in the electron emission and the surface contaminations are not the same. For such *thermal field emission*, the tungsten tip is coated of zirconia (ZrO_2), which lowers the work function of the tungsten and therefore enhances the electron emission. This makes it possible to use a broader tip than for the cold FE. This type is called *Schottky* emitters.

Electron Column

Once the electron beam has left the electron gun, it is guided to the sample by a series of electromagnetic lenses. The lenses direct and condense the electron beam to its final size of about 2–80 nm (depending on the acceleration voltage). The electron beam is divergent after passing through the anode plate and must be collimated by condenser lenses and apertures into a relatively parallel stream. This is achieved by electromagnetic lenses. In fact, the lenses beyond the electron gun demagnify the image of the crossover in the electron gun. Electrons can be directed and focused by electrostatic fields (e.g., electron gun) or magnetic fields. Most electron microscopes are equipped with electromagnetic lenses because of their lower inherent aberrations. The resolution of a SEM

is a function of the final electron beam diameter and the acceleration voltage and, as a consequence, of the type of electron gun. The resolution of a FE-SEM is better than that of a thermoionic gun SEM (Table 1). The limit of resolution is reached when the current within the electron probe is insufficient to produce a usable signal. Given the small size of the probe beam, the depth of field is high compared to a conventional light microscope (hundreds of times more).

Lenses. The lenses in electron microscopes are electromagnetic lenses (except the gun lens in the FE gun that is an electrostatic lens). A magnetic lens consists of a coil of copper wires inside the iron pole pieces. A current through the coils creates a magnetic field (force lines are symbolized by the circles in Figure 5) in the bore of the pole pieces. Where the circuit is interrupted (the gap), the magnetic field goes out into the vacuum and creates the lens field that is used for focusing the electron beam.

The rotationally symmetric magnetic field is inhomogeneous, i.e., it is weak in the center of the gap and becomes stronger close to the bore. Therefore, electrons close to the center are less strongly deflected than those passing the lens far from the axis. The overall effect is that a beam of parallel electrons is focused into a spot (so-called *crossover*). An electron passing through this field perpendicular to these field lines moves in a curved trajectory because there is a force on the electron created by the electron's movement in the magnetic field. It results in a helical trajectory and a rotation of the image. The focal length of the lens is controlled by the current in the lens coil. The focal length decreases as the current increases (the electrons are more deviated) or the acceleration voltage decreases.

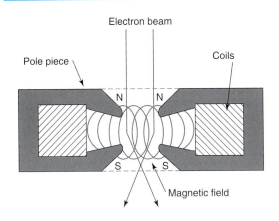

Figure 5 Schema of an electromagnetic lens (cross section)

The SEMs employ one or several condenser lenses to demagnify the diameter of the electron beam. The final lens in the column is the objective lens. Its role is to focus the image by controlling the movement of the probe crossover along the optical axis (Z-axis) of the column. The design of this lens generally incorporates space for the scanning coils, the stigmator (for correction of astigmatic lens defaults), and the beam-limiting aperture. This lens either includes the specimen (i.e., the specimen is placed inside the lens) or not (i.e., the specimen is placed outside the lens, in the case of large specimens).

Scanning Devices. In a SEM, the electron beam is not stationary on the specimen but moves in a raster on the specimen surface. The electron probe scans across the specimen in two perpendicular (X and Y) directions.

The deflection system is integrated in the last lens, the objective lens, or is situated just above it (Figure 2). The scanning coils, mounted in sets of two above another, create magnetic fields (positive and negative). The electrons in the beam will be attracted by the positive field and repelled by the other, leading to a deflection toward the positive coil. The beam moves over the specimen surface line by line in an X, Y raster covering a rectangular area. The raster is generated by the line and frame generators that feed the scan coils with the appropriate current leading to magnetic fields of different strength according to the scan size. The scan process is continuous and once

one sequence is finished, a new frame is immediately started.

The output of the two scan generators is also applied to the deflection coils of a display device, typically a TV-type cathode-ray tube (CRT) on which the SEM image will appear. Since the electron beams in the SEM column and in the CRT are scanning in synchronism, for every point on the specimen (within the raster-scanned area) there is a corresponding point on the display screen. In a modern SEM, the scan signals are generated digitally by computer. The image is acquired pixel by pixel.

The signal which modulates the image brightness can be derived from any property of the specimen which is caused by (or changes in response to) electron bombardment (cf. below "image mechanism").

Magnification Process. It is convenient here to consider the magnification process. Unlike light microscopes or TEMs, the magnification is not achieved by means of lenses but is the ratio of the linear size of the viewing screen to the linear size of the raster on the specimen. The image on the screen has a fixed size given by the display screen and is bigger than the raster area on the specimen; the magnification (M) is

$$M = \frac{\text{Scan distance* in the image}}{\text{Scan distance* on the specimen}}$$

(* length of the scanned line)

Magnification is therefore controlled by the current supplied to the X, Y scanning coils, and not by objective lens power. The magnification of a SEM ranges from $10\times$ or less to $1\,200\,000\times$ or more (depending on the SEM type and the operation mode, i.e., high, low, or environmental vacuum) (Figure 6).

Sample Chamber

Unlike the sample stage of a conventional optical microscope, the sample chamber in a SEM is a confined space and cannot be directly operated by hands. The chamber is constructed in order to be directed by the means of devices allowing moving, tilting (range of -5 to $\pm70^\circ$), and rotating the specimen. This requires a very fine tuned mechanical system that provides small and continuous motions (mm to $<0.01\,\mu m$) in the X, Y, and Z directions as well as

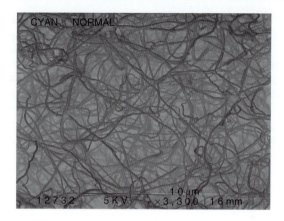

Figure 6 Cyanoacrylate deposit on a fingerprint ridge

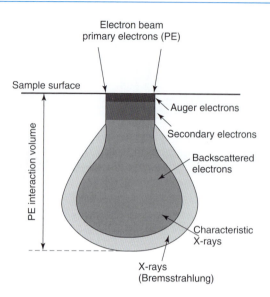

Figure 7 The interaction volume depends on several parameters (acceleration voltage, atomic number of the sample elements, and the sample density)

an almost absolute stability of the object. The eucentric goniometer stage is nowadays fully motorized. The size of the chamber determines the size of the specimen. In general, forensic SEMs have a rather big chamber (up to around 400 mm left to right) in which a big object can fit and be moved (moving area up to about 150 mm × 150 mm for X/Y movements and up to 65 mm for Z movements). Standard SEMs have a rather small chamber, allowing movements of 10 mm × 10 mm. If the sample to submit has bigger dimensions, the area of interest has to be cut out (modification of the evidence). Small objects are normally mounted on specimen holders of different shapes and sizes (often with diameters of around 12 mm) according the type of stage. The chamber is constructed in order to withstand the necessary vacuum for the electron beam (high vacuum around 10^{-4} Torr or more). It also hosts all devices necessary for the caption and processing of the output signals.

Electron Interaction and Image Mechanisms

The incident electron beam will generate several reactions once it penetrates the specimen surface. The beam strikes the specimen point by point. Several interactions occur, providing the signals that form the image or give material information about the specimen. The incident electrons interact both elastically and inelastically with the specimen, forming the limiting interaction volume from which the various types of radiation emerge, including backscattered, secondary and absorbed electrons, characteristic and Bremsstrahlung X-rays,

and in some materials, cathodoluminescence radiation (emission of photons), and Auger electrons (Figure 7).

By measuring the magnitudes of these signals with suitable detectors, a determination of certain properties of the specimen (topography, composition, crystallography, electrical conductivity, etc.) can be made at the single location where the electron beam strikes. All interactions occur together but can be selected individually by using the appropriate detector. Not all detectors are usually present on a single instrument. The size, depth, and shape of the interaction volume depend on the density of the material being investigated and the beam velocity (acceleration voltage) (Figure 8). The interaction volume takes a shape between a pear or teardrop and a hemisphere. The resulting signals are either electrons or photons. The first category is primarily used for the image and the second category of signals is mainly taken for spectroscopic information.

Imaging Signals. Secondary electrons (SEs) are the most common signal used for investigations of surface morphology. They are produced as a result of interactions, i.e., inelastic scatter between primary electrons (incident beam electrons) and the weakly bound electrons in the conduction band of the sample.

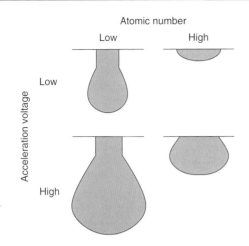

Figure 8 Influence of the acceleration voltage of the primary electrons in function of the atomic number of the sample elements

These electrons are knocked out of their orbitals and, if sufficient near the sample surface, escape as SEs. The SEs are low-energy electrons ($<50\,\mathrm{eV}$) and only those formed near the sample surface (within a few nanometers) have enough energy to escape and to be detected (Figure 7). The energy is obtained when they collide with a primary electron.

The other phenomenon that occurs is the elastic scatter between the primary electrons and the atoms of the sample. The electrons are diffracted by the atomic fields within the specimen and backscatter out of the sample surface. Because their trajectory changes they might travel out of the specimen. The

backscattered electrons (BSEs) have energy of up to that of the primary electrons and are emitted from approximately the top 40% of the area of the teardrop or hemisphere (Figure 7). The BSE come from deeper regions in the specimen and because of the diffraction (spread of the electron beam) within the specimen material the image resolution is inferior.

An SE reproduces the morphology of the surface, whereas the BSE creates shadows (topography information) because of the straight trajectory and atomic number contrast (composition information) (Figure 9a, b).

BSE are often used in analytical SEM along with the spectra made from the characteristic X-rays. Because the intensity of the BSE signal is strongly related to the atomic number (Z) of the specimen, BSE images can provide information about the distribution of different elements in the sample as well as the crystallographic structure of the specimen.

The caption of both the signals (SE and BSE) can be achieved by one or two separate detectors. The most commonly used detector is the *Everhart–Thornley electron detector*, which is sensitive to both the signals [4]. It consists of a scintillator, a light pipe, and a photomultiplier tube. This type of detector is not very efficient for BSE signals. That is why often a second dedicated detector is installed for the caption of only the high-energy BSE. Scintillator backscatter detectors, solid-state diode detectors (semiconductors), or channel plate detectors can be fitted.

The amplified electrical signal output is displayed as a two-dimensional intensity distribution on an analogue cathode ray tube (monitor), or subjected

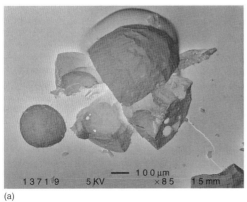

(a)

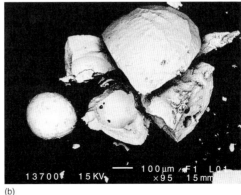

(b)

Figure 9 Comparison between a SE and a BSE image: the surface details of soldering particles in SE mode (a) disappear in BSE mode (b)

to analogue-to-digital conversion and displayed and saved as a digital image. The brightness of the signal depends on the number of SE and/or BSE electrons reaching the detector.

Spectroscopic Signals: X-Rays, Auger Electrons, and Light.   The other signals (characteristic X-rays, cathodoluminescence radiation, and Auger electrons) that occur when bombarding a material with an electron beam are used less for imaging purposes than they are for analytical needs.

The most frequently used analytical method in association with the SEM is an X-ray spectrometer. X-rays are emitted when the electron beam removes an inner shell electron from the sample, causing a higher energy electron to fill the shell and release energy in form of photons (X-ray) or Auger electrons. These X-rays are characteristic of the difference in energy between the two shells and of the atomic structure of the element from which they are emitted. Therefore, these X-rays are characteristic for each element and are used to identify the composition and measure the abundance of elements in the sample (Figure 7). The emitted X-rays are detected and processed by two methods by using two characteristics associated with light (wave and energy quantum). The same applies to X-rays. They can be detected either by their wavelength or by their energy. The latter technique, energy dispersive X-ray spectroscopy (EDX), is most commonly associated to the SEM. In the case of the detection of the X-ray energy, the photons are detected by a semiconductor (silicon doped with lithium) that converts the energy of the X-ray into a proportional electrical charge. This analogue impulsion is amplified, digitalized, and then treated in a multiple channel analyzer. Each impulsion is attributed according to its charge to a predefined channel. The information is accumulated in a histogram and displayed on a monitor. The simultaneous counting of all the photons in the range of $0-20 \, \text{keV}$ allows to acquire in one step a spectrum of all elements, within limits, of a sample (Figure 11b). This gives a quick overview of a sample composition. However, the accuracy of EDX spectrum is affected by several limitations. The qualitative analysis does not include all the elements from the periodic table. It is restricted from boron ($Z = 5$) to uranium ($Z = 92$). Another limitation is given by its lack of specificity, with respect to the oxidation state of complex anions. Quantitative analysis

is compromised by secondary fluorescence (higher energy X-rays excite the emission of X-rays of lower energy in a sample) causing the emission of more X-rays of an element than really present and overlapping peaks. A semi-quantitative analysis is more appropriate for this type of X-ray analysis, contrary to the wavelength dispersive X-ray spectroscopy (WDX).

This method allows the measuring of the wavelength of the emitted X-ray from the sample. X-ray diffraction is a powerful tool to study both the X-ray spectra and the arrangement of atoms in crystals. The X-ray wavelength is determined by irradiating a known single crystal at a precise angle. The single crystal diffracts the photons in accordance to the Bragg's law and is collected by a detector (proportional counter or scintillation counter). The crystal is positioned in equal distance to the specimen and to the detector. The crystal with known spacing is chosen. These planes reflect different wavelengths at different angles. The detector can discriminate one angle from another and attribute the corresponding wavelength. Only one element at the time can be determined. WDX counts only the X-rays of a single wavelength, not producing a broad spectrum of wavelengths or energies. Several crystals are necessary to cover the whole range of X-rays. This generally means that the element must be known to find a crystal capable of diffracting it properly. Although this technique is more sensitive than the EDX, it is less applicable in forensic science, because the sample composition has to be known and its surface has to be plane and polished, parameters that are encountered only rarely among forensic samples.

Although SEM-EDX has few restrictions, it is a very versatile and efficient technique for elemental analysis. The combination of high magnification and the possibility to analyze the target is very useful, especially in forensic science.

The next two spectroscopic techniques are encountered less in forensic applications, but they can be associated with the SEM. Instead of X-ray emission, the excess energy is transferred to a third electron from a further outer shell, prompting its ejection. This ejected species is called an *Auger electron* (Figure 7), and the method for its analysis is known as *Auger electron spectroscopy* (*AES*). The Auger electron has a specific characteristic energy that depends on the type of atom and the chemical environment in which the atom was located. Auger spectrometry is a widely used surface analysis technique.

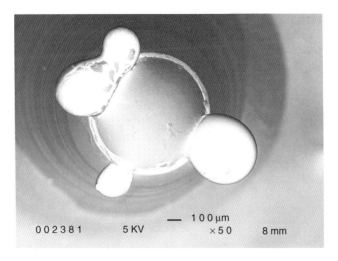

Figure 10   The influence of a high vacuum on a wet sample: the ink contained in the ink reservoir is pressed out of the ball housing and forms the drops around the tip of a ballpoint pen

Inelastic scatter can generate the emission of light (UV–visible–IR), the so-called *cathodoluminescence*. This phenomenon occurs when an electron is promoted from the valence band into the conduction band, leaving behind a hole. When an electron and a hole recombine, it is possible for a photon to be emitted. It happens for materials with a band gap structure and is useful for the characterization of semiconductors, insulators, certain minerals, glasses, and biological specimens. The radiation is detected with an appropriate photomultiplier for the photon-energy range of interest.

Sample Preparation

As mentioned above, classical SEMs operate in a vacuum environment and with an electron beam. This has a dramatic influence on a sample that cannot withstand the pressure of about 10^{-4} Torr or more (e.g., hydrated, oily, and out gassing samples) and/or is not conductive (Figure 10).

The chamber size might also have its influence and need a resizing of the sample, which might be a handicap for forensic investigations (disruption of the sample integrity). The problem of non-conductivity can be overcome by applying a conductive coat to the sample. Non-oxidation metals such as gold, platinum, palladium, and carbon are used. They are conductive and chemically stable (no oxidation) and inert. The metals are deposited on the sample by low-vacuum

sputter coating or by high vacuum evaporation (carbon). The coat is some nanometers thick. Carbon coating is appropriate if the sample has not only to be visualized but also to be analyzed (carbon is not detected by EDX). The coating prevents the accumulation of static electric charge on the specimen during electron irradiation. Another reason for coating, even when there is more than enough conductivity, is to increase signal and improve contrast and resolution. For hydrated samples, they have to be dried or frozen before being submitted to the chamber vacuum, which may modify its morphology. If coating, drying, or freezing is required, then the SEM observation has to be done at the end of an observation sequence. Optical characteristics are altered by the coat. To overcome both the problems (vacuum incompatibility and insulating surface) without modifying the sample, one has to use a low-voltage beam of the FE-SEM and/or an ESEM. The latter even allows visualizing the samples in a nearly atmospheric pressure.

Environmental SEM

The ESEM has been invented with the aim to develop a SEM that accepts virtually any specimen regardless of composition and provides a high-resolution SE image (Figure 11a). The ESEM unites all this requirements. Commercial ESEMs have been introduced in the late 1980s and early 1990s. Ten years of research

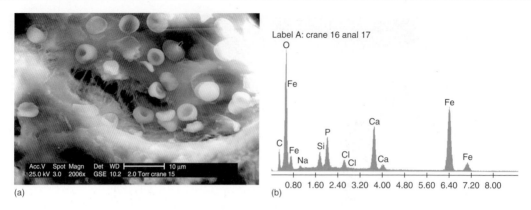

Figure 11   ESEM image (a) of hemoglobin cells around a crane fracture and their EDX analysis (b)

and development were necessary for the creation of such an instrument as well as for the discovery of a new signal detection method [5]. Although the ESEM has partially the same setup as the conventional SEM, the main problem was to find a solution allowing the use of an electron beam in a high-pressure ambience without contaminating the electron gun chamber and the electron column and ultimately to still detect the emitted signals (SE, BSE, X-rays, etc.). The problem of keeping the upper parts (gun and electron column) of the SEM in high vacuum is overcome through the use of a differential pumping technique. A series of chambers at increasing pressure along the beam path are linked by small apertures. Dedicated pumps at each stage maintain the required pressure gradient and stop contaminants from reaching the clean upper column. The sample chamber can then be maintained at a relatively high pressure (10–20 Torr) while the electron optical column is differentially pumped to keep the vacuum adequately high at the electron gun. Several stages of differential pumping system are built in the final aperture lens. The pressure is regulated by the flow of gas (inert gas and/or water vapor). The high-pressure region around the sample in the ESEM neutralizes charge and provides an amplification of the SE signal. Positively charged ions generated by the beam interactions with the gas help to neutralize the negative charge on the specimen surface. The pressure of gas in the chamber can be controlled, and the type of gas used can be varied according to the need. The detectors of the emitted signals are different from those described for the conventional SEM. The conventional SE detector (Everhart–Thornley detector)

cannot be used in the presence of gas because of an electrical discharge (arcing) caused by the kilovolt bias associated with this detector. In lieu of this, an environmental secondary detector (ESD) is used [6]. It takes advantage of the ionization behavior of the low-pressure gases found in the specimen environment. Gas ionization is induced by a moderate electric field, forcing collision between highly mobile SEs and neutral gas molecules. It results in a multiplication of the secondary signal and at the same time the positive ions neutralize the electrical charges at the specimen surface.

For the backscattered electron, the conventional BSE detection means have been adapted to operate in the gaseous conditions of the ESEM. The characteristic elemental X-rays also produced in the ESEM can be detected by the same detectors used in the conventional SEM (Figure 11a, b).

Modern ESEMs have a "three-in-one" concept. Three different vacuum modes (high, low, and environmental vacuum) can be chosen with one instrument according to the specimen vacuum sensitivity. They are equipped with the conventional detectors (when working in high vacuum; 10^{-4} Torr and more an Everhart–Thornley for SE, solid state for BSE) as well as the dedicated environmental detectors as described for low vacuum. These instruments still have an excellent resolution range (3.5 nm at 30 kV in all vacuum modes, <15 nm in low-vacuum mode at 3 kV).

The possibility to work in a vacuum of about 20 Torr makes it possible to add some optional devices such as a Peltier cooled stage (-20 to $+50\,^{\circ}$C), a heating stage (for temperatures up to $1500\,^{\circ}$C) and

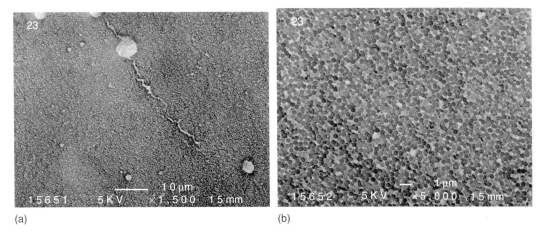

(a)   (b)

Figure 12   Aspect of a gel pen ink stroke (a) and (b) under different magnifications

a cryo transfer system (for *in situ* investigations) for the observation of sample behavior under temperature changes.

Forensic Utility of SEMs

With the commercialization of ESEM, there is no limit to its use in forensic science. The ESEM has demonstrated its near universal applicability, combining the high resolution and depth of field of the SEM with the flexibility and ease of the light microscope. Whenever something small has to be studied, the SEM is certainly the microscope to choose [7]. The only limit is that optical properties and characteristics cannot be studied, as well as the aspect of the sample in transparency. In case of a non-pigmented water-based ink stroke leaving no deposit on the paper (when the ink is completely absorbed by the fibers), it cannot be seen by SEM. This limits the application for line crossing problems [8]. See also the relevant article about intersecting lines in this encyclopedia.

The magnification range from macro to micro allows zooming in and out of details of the sample, with an extreme ease and with a resolution and depth of field never obtained by the conventional light microscopes (Figure 12a, b).

The additional spectroscopic tools make the SEM a powerful analytical instrument, allowing a target compositional analysis. The area of interest can be selected and analyzed. This makes the technique essential for gunshot residues (GSRs), because of its

capability to analyze discrete particles in the sample. The analysis is nowadays fully automated and the position of each analyzed particle is recorded. This makes the localization and verification of each analyzed particle very convenient. An advantage is that the particles are directly taken from the support (e.g., suspect) by the SEM holder equipped with a carbon-coated adhesive. No further sample preparation is required prior to the SEM/EDX analysis. This minimizes the risk to lose particles while handling.

The elements constituting the GSR can originate from the primer, the bullet, a coating or jacket on the bullet, cartridge components, and previous residues in the barrel. The characteristic particles for Sinoxid primers contain the metal elements lead, barium, antimony, and calcium [9, 10]. The heavy metal particles in a lead-free primer (e.g., Sintox^{TM} ammunition commercialized by Dynamit Nobel AG) are replaced by the elements titanium and zinc [10, 11]. Particles from the bullet are composed of copper, zinc, nickel, mild steel, and lead (in metallic form).

The samples usually contain many other particles that are of no particular interest (contaminations from the support); the particles of interest have to be "selected" before being analyzed. This is done by the backscattered detector, which is calibrated in relation to the Z (atomic number) and not to the video intensity. The particles are detected based on their average atomic number falling within a predefined Z range in relation to primer compositions, which tend to have particles with intrinsically high average Z. Therefore, searching for "bright particles only" is eliminated. The older systems are based on this method, which of course lacks selectivity. The GSR particles are $0.5–10\,\mu m$ in size (usually $0.5–2\,\mu m$). Therefore, the automated search and analysis of a sample, i.e., a defined area on the sample holder surface, take quite some time but is much faster and reliable than a manual search of primer residue particles.

In case of a positive result (i.e., particles containing the above-mentioned elements in combination), its interpretation is not evident. The combinations Pb/Sb/Ba and Sb/Ba are considered to be characteristic for Sinoxid primer residues [12]. However, other sources might produce particles with same combinations [13–15]. In view of these findings, the morphological aspect of the found particles becomes important and might allow to support stronger the hypothesis of GSR particles than particles generated from another source than a firearm. GSR particles have a spherical morphology. Not to forget also the memory effect when firing different ammunitions from the same firearm that might produce mixed compositions of GSR particles [10, 11, 16]. More details about GSR can be found as a separate specific contribution in this encyclopedia.

The combined abilities of the SEM to resolve fine structures and determine their elemental composition are an indispensable aid in the examination of small items of trace evidence. There is no doubt that the SEM is extremely useful and the list of its forensic applications is endless. However, the only inconvenience of the technique is still its price.

References

[1]   Ruska, E. (1934). Ueber Fortschritte im Bau und in der Leistung des magnetischen Elektronenmikroskopes, *Zeitschrift für Physik* **87**, 580–602.

[2]   Ruska, E. (1980). *The Early Development of Electron Lenses and Electron Microscopy*, S. Hirzel Verlag, Stuttgart.

[3]   Goldstein, J., Newbury, D., Echlin, P., Joy, D., Lyman, C., Echlin, P., Lifshin, E., Sawyer, L. & Michael, J. (2003). *Scanning Electron Microscopy and X-ray Microanalysis*, Springer, New York.

[4]   Everhart, T.E. & Thornley, R.F.M. (1960). Wide-band detector for micro-microampere low-energy electron currents, *Journal of Scientific Instruments* **37**, 246–248.

[5]   Danilatos, G.D. (1988). Foundations of environmental scanning electron microscopy, *Advances in Electronics and Electron Physics* **71**, 109–250.

[6]   Danilatos, G.D. (1990). Theory of the gaseous detector device in the ESEM, *Advances in Electronics and Electron Physics* **78**, 1–102.

[7]   Mazzella, W.D. & Khanmy-Vital, A. (2003). A study to investigate the evidential value of bluer gel pen inks, *Journal of Forensic Sciences* **48**, 419–424.

[8]   Khanmy-Vital, A., Kasas, S. & Dietler, G. (2001). The use of atomic force microscopy to determine the sequence of crossed lines, *Problems of Forensic Sciences* **66**, 401–412.

[9]   Zeichner, A. & Levin, N. (1997). More on the uniqueness of gunshot residue (GSR) particles, *Journal of Forensic Sciences* **42**, 1027–1028.

[10]   Khanmy, A. & Gallusser, A. (1995). Influence of weapon cleaning on the gunshot residues from heavy metal free ammunition, *Advances in Forensic Sciences* **3**, 60–65.

[11]   Gunaratnam, L. & Himberg, K. (1994). The identification of gunshot residues particles from lead-free Sintox ammunition, *Journal of Forensic Sciences* **39**, 532–536.

[12]   Wallace, J.S. & McQuillan, J. (1984). Discharge residues from cartridge-operated industrial tools, *Journal of Forensic Science Society* **24**, 495–508.

[13]   Mosher, P.V., McVicar, M.J., Randall, E.D. & Sild, E.H. (1998). Gunshot similar particles produced by fireworks, *Canadian Society of Forensic Science Journal* **31**, 157–168.

[14]   Garofano, L., Capra, M., Ferrari, F., Bizzaro, G.P., DiTullio, D., Dell'Olio, M. & Ghitti, A. (1999). Gunshot residue – further studies on particles of environmental and occupational origin, *Forensic Science International* **103**, 1–21.

[15]   Torre, C., Mattutino, G., Vasino, V. & Robino, C. (2002). Brake linings: a source of non-GSR particles containing lead, barium and antimony, *Journal of Forensic Sciences* **47**, 494–504.

[16]   Zeichner, A., Levin, N. & Springer, E. (1991). GSR particles formed by using different types of ammunition in the same firearm, *Journal of Forensic Sciences* **36**, 1020–1026.

AITA KHANMY-VITAL

Mini-STRs

Disclaimer: The opinions and assertions contained herein are solely those of the authors and are not to be construed as official or as views of the US Department of Defense, the US Department of the Army, or the Armed Forces Institute of Pathology.

For well over a decade, short tandem repeat (STR) markers have played an important role in advancing the field of forensic DNA typing (*see* **Short Tandem Repeats**). In the United States, there are two commercial companies that produce multiplex STR kits used by forensic laboratories: Applied Biosystems (Foster City, CA) and Promega Corporation (Madison, WI). Each company has produced a "megaplex" autosomal STR kit containing 16 markers: the 13 Combined DNA Index System (CODIS) loci [1, 2]. 2 markers specific to each company's kit, and the amelogenin marker for sex determination. Both 16-plex kits have amplicon sizes ranging from 100 to 450 base pairs (bp). The availability of commercial kits has helped to standardize the STR markers used by the forensic community.

The conventional STR kits perform well when an optimal quantity (approximately 1 ng) of high-quality DNA is used, exhibiting peak height balance both within loci (heterozygous alleles) and between each marker. However, biological evidence at crime scenes is often exposed to the elements and/or microbial agents that may cause DNA to degrade. Inhibitor molecules, such as heme in blood or humic acid in soil, can also copurify with DNA and prohibit the generation of a full STR profile. Degradation and inhibition may result in amplification failure especially of high-molecular weight loci, resulting in a "partial profile" in which only a subset of the core 13 CODIS loci are obtained (*see* **DNA: Degraded Samples**). The loss of multiple forensic markers as a result of degradation and inhibition reduces the overall statistical significance of any observed match. If a biological sample is too highly degraded for STR analysis, the forensic scientist

may have to turn to mitochondrial DNA (mtDNA), which can be expensive and time consuming to test, and may result in limited information, especially for common mtDNA haplotypes (*see* **Mitochondrial DNA: Profiling**).

One strategy to recover the genetic information lost due to DNA degradation would be to reduce the size of the PCR (Polymerase Chain Reaction) amplicons for the "larger" loci. By designing PCR primers to bind closer to the core tandem repeat (Figure 1), it is possible to create a smaller PCR product, a "mini-STR", while still retaining the core repeat information. The reduced-size PCR amplicon then has a greater chance (relative to conventional STR primers) of generating a profile when genetic material is degraded.

Emergence of Mini-STRs as a Forensic Tool

During the mid-1990s, Dr John Butler (presently at the National Institute of Standards and Technology, NIST) and his colleagues at GeneTrace Systems developed a system to rapidly genotype STR profiles using matrix-assisted laser desorption/ionization time-of-flight (MALDI/TOF) mass spectrometry. The rapid detection of multiple unlabeled PCR products using MALDI/TOF represented a significant reduction in sample processing and analysis time as compared to standard STR profiling. One limitation of the MALDI/TOF technology, however, was related to the size of PCR fragment analyzed; amplicons larger than 140 bp were difficult to resolve with the method. To make the commonly used forensic STR

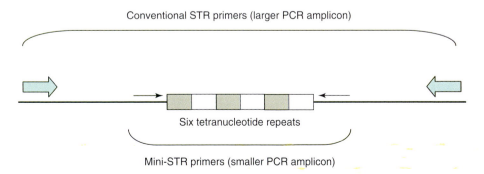

Conventional STR primers (larger PCR amplicon)

Six tetranucleotide repeats

Mini-STR primers (smaller PCR amplicon)

Figure 1   An example of a mini-STR compared to conventional STR primers. The mini-STR primers are adjacent to the six nucleotide repeats producing a smaller PCR product compared to the conventional STR primers

markers more amenable to MALDI/TOF detection, Butler and colleagues redesigned the primers to create smaller amplicons. Significantly, Butler and colleagues noted in their 1998 publication that these reduced-size amplicons could be utilized to increase the recovery of STR profiles from degraded samples [3, 4].

A few years later, laboratories began publishing information on reduced-size PCR amplicons for (mostly CODIS) loci [5–8]. These early studies demonstrated the forensic potential of mini-STRs, sometimes with very significant results. For example, Hellmann *et al.* [5] reduced the amplicon size of the TPOX locus by 160 bp to test telogen hairs. This group was able to recover the correct genotype over 77% of the time compared to only about 18% of the time with conventional primers – a fourfold improvement.

Additional advances in mini-STR research and application also came as a result of the terrorist attack on the World Trade Center (WTC) towers on September 11, 2001. Shortly after the attacks, the New York Office of the Chief Medical Examiner (NY-OCME) was charged with the task of identifying the nearly 3000 victims of the disaster. Knowing that many of the samples recovered from the crime scene would be highly degraded and of poor quality, the NY-OCME investigated new technologies, such as single nucleotide polymorphism (SNP) typing and reduced-size STR amplicons, to increase the success rate on the compromised samples. Through work at NIST and a private laboratory (the Bode Technology Group) all of the core CODIS markers were redesigned as mini-STRs [9]. Protocols were developed and validated at NIST [9], and samples from the disaster were tested at the Bode Technology Group [10]. Mini-STRs proved to be valuable for the identification efforts: nearly 20% of the 850 DNA-only identifications from the WTC disaster were made using mini-STRs [11].

Following the success of mini-STRs in recovering genetic information from CODIS loci, additional research into other markers of forensic interest has included autosomal loci unlinked to the CODIS markers [12]. Additional markers not linked to the CODIS loci can be useful for resolving complex paternity cases such as incest. A set of X-chromosome mini-STRs [13] have been developed for select forensic scenarios where linked X-STR markers can provide

additional discrimination relative to autosomal loci. Finally, Y-chromosome mini-STRs [14] have been developed to amplify male-specific loci (*see* **Y-Chromosome Short Tandem Repeats**).

In 2007, the first commercial mini-STR kit, AmpF*ℓ*STR® MiniFiler™ (Applied Biosystems), became available to the forensic community. A 9-plex, MiniFiler™ includes amelogenin and eight of the largest loci from the AmpF*ℓ*STR® Identifiler® and SGM Plus® (Applied Biosystems) STR typing kits. The MiniFiler™ amplicon sizes generally range up to 250 bp (290 bp for the extended FGA locus alleles), and represent an approximate 30–200 bp size reduction as compared to the Identifiler® and SGM Plus® amplicons for the included loci. In addition to the reduced-size amplicons, the MiniFiler™ amplification protocol, which increases (relative to other AmpF*ℓ*STR® kits) the number of thermal cycles to 30, and proprietary amplification buffer, which already contains the DNA polymerase, are kit optimizations designed to overcome inhibition and recover loci from compromised samples. MiniFiler™ is thus intended for use as a supplement to other megaplex STR kits when an insufficient number of loci are recovered, or as a stand-alone kit when extremely limited sample quantities would prevent multiple attempts to develop a genetic profile [15].

A second commercial mini-STR kit, PowerPlex® S5 (Promega Corporation), is also now available to forensic practitioners. Like MiniFiler™, the S5 kit utilizes small amplicons (under 260 bp) and a proprietary amplification buffer optimized to overcome inhibition. In contrast to MiniFiler™, however, PowerPlex® S5 includes only four loci in addition to amelogenin. Rather than as a means to recover additional loci when large-amplicon loci fail, the S5 kit is marketed as a reliable, lower-cost exclusionary tool for criminal casework and population screening.

Challenges to Mini-STR Development

With the availability of commercially available mini-STR kits, many forensic laboratories can now take advantage of using these markers on casework samples without the need to produce "in-house" multiplexes that must pass high quality control standards for use in forensic casework. However, challenges remain to the development and use of both in-house and commercial mini-STR kits. These include repeat size limitations, limited multiplex real estate, and the potential for profile discordance as a result of primer design.

Some of the current CODIS loci are difficult to develop as true mini-STRs because of the size of the repeat region. For example, the FGA locus has a rather large allele spread – ranging from 17 to 33 repeats (and up to 51 repeats among the extended alleles). A large allele spread is advantageous for a high-diversity marker, but successful amplification of a 50 tetranucleotide repeat (200 bp) along with an additional 40–50 bp for the flanking primer sequence (240–250 bp total amplicon) in a highly degraded sample is unlikely. Ideally, mini-STR multiplexes would be composed of markers with amplicons sizes no larger than 150 bp.

However optimal from a profile recovery standpoint, the restriction of mini-STRs to amplicons sizes less than 150 bp greatly limits the number of markers that can be tested in a four or five fluorescent dye system. To overcome the limited multiplex real estate, a few multiplexes, with each dye channel containing 1–2 mini-STR markers, could be constructed for use in tandem. However, a disadvantage to typing with multiple assays is the consumption of additional, often limited, DNA template. This could be especially problematic when typing samples under "low copy number" conditions where multiple replicates are required for data analysis and interpretation [16, 17] (*see* **Low Copy Number DNA**). Although a greater number of fluorescent dyes could be used to increase the number of loci amplified in a single reaction, this is not at present a viable option because of capillary electrophoresis (CE) detection limitations.

Alternately, nonnucleotide linker molecules that shift the electrophoretic mobility of the amplified product could be used to construct a mini-STR multiplex with more than 1–2 markers per dye channel. For example, suppose that two mini-STR loci, A and B, have the amplicon size ranges 72–112 and 96–136 bp, respectively. In constructing a multiplex, it would be necessary to position these two loci in separate dye channels since there is potential for overlap between the higher molecular weight alleles of locus A and the lower molecular weight alleles of locus B. Using non-nucleotide linkers equivalent to approximately 2.5 bp [18], the addition of 10 such linkers between the primer and the fluorescent dye for locus B would shift the apparent size of the

amplicon by +25 bp. As a result, locus B would migrate at 121–161 bp and provide enough separation to be included in the same dye channel as locus A. Although non-nucleotide linker molecules can increase the electrophoretic separation between overlapping loci as described, there is a limit to the number of linkers that can be added to a primer and still result in consistently high-quality data.

Primer design presents an additional challenge to the development of mini-STRs from standard STR loci. A necessity for the creation of reduced-size STR amplicons is a clean sequence region flanking the repeat motif. Not all of the industry-standard STR markers have clean flanking regions, which can make the design of mini-STRs a challenge, and may result in nonconcordant alleles when typing the same loci with different STR multiplexes. For example, the CODIS marker D7S820 has a polyT stretch found 13 nucleotide bases downstream of the core tetranucleotide repeat. Designing a primer adjacent to the repeat and avoiding the polyT repeat would potentially miss a number of microvariants created by the addition (X.1) or subtraction (X.3) of thymidine nucleotides in this region. In other words, if a sample tested with a conventional kit typed as a 15.1 allele, a mini-STR designed to avoid this polyT region (through placement of an amplification primer between the core repeat and the T-stretch) would result in a 15 allele.

There are several additional ways in which newly designed STR primers may result in allele discordance with standard STR typing kits. For example, suppose that at some STR locus an individual is genotyped as 4, 5 using a commercial kit. We shall focus only on the chromosome possessing the "5" allele (Figure 2, bottom allele). Interestingly, this particular allele has six core repeats. but between the core repeat and the forward primer of the commercial kit is a 4 bp deletion on the chromosome. The net effect of this deletion (equivalent to a single tetranucleotide repeat) is that the commercial kit scores this allele as having five repeats (Figure 2A; the sample types as a 4, 5). If the newly designed mini-STR primer is designed to hybridize between the commercial kit primer and the 4 bp deletion, then both genotypes will be concordant (Figure 2B; the sample types as a 4, 5). If, however, the mini-STR primer binding site includes the 4 bp deletion region, it is possible that little or no hybridization will occur. This would be especially true if the 3′ end of the

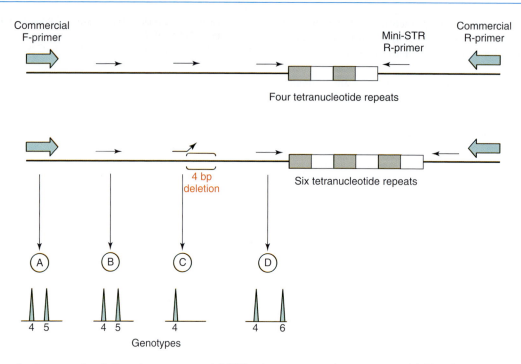

Figure 2 An example of discordance among mini-STR primers compared to a commercial kit. The top chromosome has four tetranucleotide repeats and the bottom chromosome has six tetranucleotide repeats. In the flanking region of the forward primer, there is a 4 bp deletion. Amplification using the commercial STR primers (A) results in a genotype of 4, 5 the deletion effectively "subtracts" one of the core repeats. (B) The mini-STR primer binding site is also outside of the 4 bp deletion region, and produce a 4, 5 genotype. (C) The 3' end of the mini-STR primer produces no PCR product from the bottom chromosome resulting in a "null allele" genotype of 4, 4 and be discordant with the conventional kit. (D) The mini-STR primer is adjacent to the core repeat and is well within the 4 bp deletion, the genotype will be 4, 6 and be discordant with the conventional kit

mini-STR primer did not match the target sequence on the chromosome. If a "null allele" were to result due to the primer binding site mutation (Figure 2C; the sample types as 4, 4), the mini-STR genotype will be discordant with the kit genotype. Finally, if the mini-STR primer is adjacent to the core repeat and thus well within the 4 bp deletion, the genotype resulting from the mini-STR amplification will be 4, 6 (Figure 2D) and again discordant with the conventional kit.

Because of the mutations that result in insertions, deletions, and SNPs in the flanking regions of forensic STRs, laboratories should always test any new mini-STR primer set against the conventional kit on a set of population samples to assure concordance between the two systems. In most cases discordance is not a major issue since typically only one allele of the total 26 CODIS alleles would be affected. That is, a moderate stringency database search would

still identify a profile typed with the conventional kit when compared to the mini-STR-generated profile with a single allele difference.

Conclusions

Mini-STRs have already proven effective for the recovery of genetic information from highly compromised samples, such as those encountered in mass disasters (*see* **Disaster Victim Identification**). Beyond the increased power of discrimination offered by the recovery of more genetic loci, mini-STRs have also proven valuable for the sorting and reassociation of highly commingled remains [17] from mass graves according to the International Commission on Missing Persons [19]. The European forensic community has recently recommended that current forensic loci should be reduced in size as much as possible and that new mini-STRs be incorporated into the next generation STR multiplexes to increase the number of shared Interpol loci [20, 21]. In the future, mini-STRs may play an important role in the analysis of forensic evidence normally reserved for mtDNA analysis, such as skeletal remains [22] and shed telogen hairs [23]. The potential utility of mini-STRs is high and their frequency of use in forensic casework is likely to increase as both new and familiar autosomal, X-chromosome, and Y-chromosome loci are designed with reduced-size amplicons.

References

[1] FBI's Combined DNA Index System (CODIS) Homepage; http://www.fbi.gov/hq/lab/codis/index1.htm.

[2] Budowle, B, Moretti, T.T., Niezgoda, S.J. & Brown, B.L. (1998). CODIS and PCR-based short tandem repeat loci: law enforcement tools. *Proceedings of the Second European Symposium on Human Identification*, June 1998. Innsbruck, Austria, Madison, WI. Promega Corporation. pp. 73–88. http://www.promega.com/geneticidproc/eusymp2proc/17.pdf.

[3] Butler, J.M., Li, J., Shaler, T.A., Monforte, J.A. & Becker, C.H. (1998). Reliable genotyping of short tandem repeat loci without an allelic ladder using time-of-flight mass spectrometry, *International Journal of Legal Medicine* **112**(1), 45–49.

[4] Butler, J.M. & Becker, C.H. (2001). *Improved Analysis of DNA Short Tandem Repeats with Time-of-Flight Mass Spectrometry*, Science and Technology Research Report, National Institute of Justice, available at: http://www.ncjrs.gov/pdffiles1/nij/188292.pdf.

[5] Hellmann, A., Rohleder, U., Schmitter, H. & Wittig, M. (2001). STR typing of human telogen hairs—a new approach, *International Journal of Legal Medicine* **114**(4–5), 269–273.

[6] Wiegand, P. & Kleiber, M. (2001). Less is more—length reduction of STR amplicons using redesigned primers, *International Journal of Legal Medicine* **114**(4–5), 285–287.

[7] Ohtaki, H., Yamamoto, T., Yoshimoto, T., Uchihi, R., Ooshima, C., Katsumata, Y. & Tokunaga, K. (2002). A powerful, novel, multiplex typing system for six short tandem repeat loci and the allele frequency distributions in two Japanese regional populations, *Electrophoresis* **23**(19), 3332–3340.

[8] Tsukada, K., Takayanagi, K., Asamura, H., Ota, M. & Fukushima, H. (2002). Multiplex short tandem repeat typing in degraded samples using newly designed primers for the TH01,CSF1PO,and vWA loci, *Legal Medicine (Tokyo)* **4**, 239–245.

[9] Butler, J.M., Shen, Y. & McCord, B.R. (2003). The development of reduced size STR amplicons as tools for

analysis of degraded DNA, *Journal of Forensic Science* **48**(5), 1054–1064.

[10] Holland, M.M., Cave, C.A., Holland, C.A. & Bille, T.W. (2003). Development of a quality, high throughput DNA analysis procedure for skeletal samples to assist with the identification of victims from the World Trade Center attacks, *Croatian Medical Journal* **44**, 264–272.

[11] Biesecker, L.G., Bailey-Wilson, J.E., Ballantyne, J., Baum, H., Bieber, F.R., Brenner, C., Budowle, B., Butler, J.M., Carmody, G., Conneally, P.M., Duceman, B., Eisenberg, A., Forman, L., Kidd, K.K., Leclair, B., Niezgoda, S., Parsons, T.J., Pugh, E., Shaler, R., Sherry, S.T., Sozer, A. & Walsh, A. (2005). DNA Identifications after the 9/11 World Trade Center attack, *Science* **310**(5751), 1122–1123.

[12] Coble, M.D. & Butler, J.M. (2005). Characterization of new miniSTR loci to aid analysis of degraded DNA, *Journal of Forensic Sciences* **50**(1), 43–53.

[13] Asamura, H., Sakai, H., Kobayashi, K., Ota, M. & Fukushima, H. (2006). MiniX-STR multiplex system population study in Japan and application to degraded DNA analysis, *International Journal of Legal Medicine* **120**(3), 174–181.

[14] Park, M.J., Lee, H.Y., Chung, U., Kang, S.C. & Shin, K.J. (2007). Y-STR analysis of degraded DNA using reduced-size amplicons, *International Journal of Legal Medicine* **121**(2), 152–157.

[15] Mulero, J.J., Chang, C.W., Lagacé, R.E., Wang, D.Y., Bas, J.L., McMahon, T.P. & Hennessy, L.K. (2008). Development and validation of the AmpFlSTR MiniFiler PCR Amplification Kit: a MiniSTR multiplex for the analysis of degraded and/or PCR inhibited DNA, *Journal of Forensic Science* **53**(4), 838–852.

[16] Gill, P., Whitaker, J., Flaxman, C., Brown, N. & Buckleton, J. (2000). An investigation of the rigor of interpretation rules for STRs derived from less than 100 pg of DNA, *Forensic Science International* **112**(1), 17–40.

[17] Irwin, J.A., Leney, M.D., Loreille, O., Barritt, S.M., Christensen, A.F., Holland, T.D., Smith, B.C. & Parsons, T.J. (2007). Application of low copy number STR typing to the identification of aged, degraded skeletal remains, *Journal of Forensic Science* **52**(6), 1322–1327.

[18] Butler, J.M. (2005). *Forensic DNA Typing: Biology and Technology behind STR Markers*, 2nd Edition, Academic Press, London.

[19] Parsons, T.J., Huel, R., Davoren, J., Katzmarzyk, C., Milos, A., Selmanovic, A., Smajlovic, L., Coble, M.D. & Rizvic, A. (2007). Application of novel "mini-amplicon" STR multiplexes to high volume casework on degraded skeletal remains, *Forensic Science International: Genetics* **1**, 175–179.

[20] Gill, P., Fereday, L., Morling, N. & Schneider, P.M. (2006a). The evolution of DNA databases – recommendations for new European loci, *Forensic Science International* **156**, 242–244.

[21] Gill, P., Fereday, L., Morling, N. & Schneider, P.M. (2006b). Letter to editor – new multiplexes for Europe: amendments and clarification of strategic development, *Forensic Science International* **163**, 155–157.

[22] Opel, K.L., Chung, D.T., Drabek, J., Tatarek, N.E., Jantz, L.M. & McCord, B.R. (2006). The application of miniplex primer sets in the analysis of degraded DNA from human skeletal remains, *Journal of Forensic Sciences* **51**(2), 351–356.

[23] Müller, K., Klein, R., Miltner, E. & Wiegand, P. (2007). Improved STR typing of telogen hair root and hair shaft DNA, *Electrophoresis* **28**(16), 2835–2842.

MICHAEL D. COBLE AND REBECCA S. JUST

Miranda Rights: Capacity to Waive *see* Capacity to Waive Miranda Rights

Miranda Warnings *see* Deception: Truth Serum

Missing Persons and Paternity: DNA

Introduction

Matching DNA profiles have proved to be of great value in forensic science when they link a person to evidence associated with a crime. The chance of a coincidental match between the profiles of two different people is so small that matches are rightly regarded as strong evidence. This has led to the increasing use of searches for a particular profile in databases of profiles previously obtained by law enforcement agencies. These forensic applications make little appeal to an essential nature of DNA profiles – genetic markers are heritable, meaning that a parent passes on one copy of his or her marker genes to a child. This leads to the similarity of profiles between related individuals and the application of DNA profiling to parentage disputes and missing person searches. The strength of the evidence from matching or partially matching profiles depends in large degree on the degree of relatedness of the people whose DNA is examined and calculations can be complex. There is simplification, however, in the situation where the people are not inbred and where their population can be regarded as being in a state of evolutionary equilibrium. These simplifications are described in this article.

The calculations described here are all within the framework of likelihood ratios of the probabilities of an observed set of DNA profiles under alternative hypotheses about the relatedness of the people whose DNA has been examined.

Measures of Inbreeding and Relatedness

The use of DNA profiles in parentage and missing persons situations rests on the comparisons of profiles from people who may be related. The greater the degree of relatedness, the more likely it is that profiles will be similar but it is necessary to be able to quantify such statements. Are father and son more related than are two brothers? How can profiles from two men be used to favor the explanation that they are brothers over the claim they are unrelated? Such questions require a means for attaching numbers to the degree of relatedness, and these numbers refer to the chance that alleles, the components of DNA profiles, are identical by descent.

People are related when they have ancestors in common and this means that relatives may share genes – the genes that descended from those ancestors. Two copies, or alleles, of the same genetic marker that have descended from the same ancestral allele are said to be identical by descent (ibd). Two individuals that have ibd alleles are said to be related, and individuals that receive ibd alleles from their parents are said to be inbred. In the classical theory of population genetics, there is an implied reference population: ibd alleles are copies of the same allele in the reference population and their histories further back in time are not considered. The probability that an allele taken at random from one individual is ibd to an allele taken at random from another individual is the coancestry coefficient θ of those two individuals. The inbreeding coefficient F of a child has the same value as the coancestry θ of its parents.

There is a simple "path-counting" method for determining coancestry coefficients. For individuals X and Y, the number of individuals in the path linking them through their common ancestor(s) A is written as α. This number includes the individuals themselves. If F_A is the inbreeding coefficient of the ancestor, generally zero, the coancestry coefficient is given by $\theta_X = \sum_A (0.5)^\alpha (1 + F_A)$. For people related on only the maternal or paternal side of their family, there is likely to be only one ancestor A and the simplest example is that of parent Y and child X. Their common ancestor is Y and their coancestry is $(0.5)^2 = 0.25$. If Z is one of the parents of Y, then the grandparent (Z)–grandchild (X) coancestry is $(0.5)^3 = 0.125$, and so on. The two paths linking full-sibs X and Y through their parents G and H are XGY and XHY so $\theta_{XY} = (0.5)^3 + (0.5)^3 = 0.25$.

The equality of the coancestries for parent–child and full-sib pairs suggest that a more detailed quantification of relatedness is needed, and the first step is to use the number of pairs of alleles two relatives have that are ibd. There can be zero, one, or two such pairs depending on whether the individuals are unrelated, unilineal relatives (e.g., parent–child) or bilinear relatives (e.g., full-sibs). This description requires that an individual's two alleles are not themselves ibd. Calculating the probabilities k_0, k_1, k_2 that two individuals have 0, 1, 2 ibd pairs is fairly straightforward. If X has alleles a, b and Y has alleles c, d then it is necessary to ask how many of the four pairs ac, ad, bc, bd are ibd. If c is the allele that is copied by parent Y to transmit to child X, then it must be that either a or b is ibd to c. There are no other ibd relationships and $k_0 = 0, k_1 = 1, k_2 = 0$. If a, c are the alleles that full-sibs have received from parent G and b, d are the alleles they receive from parent H, then each of these pairs has equal chances of being copies of the same or different parental alleles and so being ibd or not. This leads to $k_0 = 0.25, k_1 = 0.50, k_2 = 0.25$. The coancestry coefficient θ is a summary of the three k coefficients: $\theta = k_1/4 + k_2/2$. Values of these measures are shown in Table 1 for some common relatives. Note that they all refer to the unobservable property of identity by descent. It is the expected values for those degrees of relatedness that are shown in the table.

Table 1 Identity by descent measures for noninbred relatives

Relationship	k_2	k_1	k_0	θ
Identical twins	1	0	0	$\frac{1}{2}$
Full sibs	$\frac{1}{4}$	$\frac{1}{2}$	$\frac{1}{4}$	$\frac{1}{4}$
Parent/child	0	1	0	$\frac{1}{4}$
Half-sibs	0	$\frac{1}{2}$	$\frac{1}{2}$	$\frac{1}{8}$
First cousins	0	$\frac{1}{4}$	$\frac{3}{4}$	$\frac{1}{16}$
Unrelated	0	0	1	0

The k-coefficients are sufficient for describing the relatedness for noninbred individuals. There is a more elaborate set of 15 coefficients for the situation with inbreeding when any two or three of four of the alleles carried by two people may be ibd. These coefficients were discussed in a review by Weir *et al.* [1]. For a random-mating population and genetic markers that have reached a state of equilibrium between the opposing evolutionary force of genetic drift that reduces genetic variation and the force of mutation that increases variation, all 15 of these more complicated ibd measures can be expressed in terms of the quantity θ. This θ is the probability that any two alleles in a population are ibd and it refers to the effect of past evolutionary events rather than immediate family membership. The probability that any three alleles are ibd is $2\theta^2/(1 + \theta)$ and the chance that any four alleles are ibd is $6\theta^2/[(1 + \theta)(1 + 2\theta)]$. The probability that two pairs of alleles are ibd (whether or not all four are ibd) is $\theta^2(1 + 5\theta)/[(1 + \theta)(1 + 2\theta)]$. These results were all derived by Evett and Weir [2].

Frequencies of sets of alleles

Setting up a set of identity measures was the first step in allowing observed DNA profiles to be used to make inferences about relatedness of the people represented by those profiles. Identity measures describe the relationship and they can also be used to express how likely it is that two people with a specified degree of relatedness have particular profiles. In other words, if the relationship is known, then the profile types can be predicted. Some results from statistical theory can then be used to reverse the argument: if the profiles are known, what can be inferred about the relatedness?

Identity by descent cannot be observed, but the ibd probabilities allow the probabilities of sets of alleles to be expressed as functions of allele frequencies. Without any inbreeding or relatedness, the probability P_{ii} that an individual is homozygous for allele A_i is given by the Hardy–Weinberg result $P_{ii} = p_i^2$ where p_i is the frequency of the allele. The genotype frequency P_{ij} for heterozygote $A_i A_j$ is $P_{ij} = 2p_i p_j, j \neq i$.

For individuals with inbreeding level F, these Hardy–Weinberg frequencies are modified to $P_{ii} = p_i^2 + F p_i (1 - p_i)$ and $P_{ij} = 2(1 - F) p_i p_j$. Of more importance in the present context are the probabilities that two related individuals have specified genotype frequencies. The probability that two noninbred members of the same family are both homozygous $A_i A_i$ has to take into account that they may share zero, one, or two pairs of alleles ibd. This means that their four copies of allele A_i may represent four, three, or two independent (non-ibd) alleles. The required probability is

$$\Pr(A_i A_i, A_i A_i) = k_0 p_i^4 + k_1 p_i^3 + k_2 p_i^2 \quad (1)$$

and the complete set of probabilities is shown in Table 2.

To take into account the evolutionary relatedness quantified by the parameter θ, there is a very convenient result first described in the forensic context by Balding and Nichols [3]. The probability that an allele is of type A when n_A of the previous n alleles examined were of that type is $[n_A \theta + (1 - \theta) p_A]/[1 + (n - 1)\theta]$ and this can be called the *Dirichlet sampling formula*. For the first allele

Table 2 Genotype-pair probabilities for noninbred relatives (different subscripts denote different alleles)

Genotype pair	Probability
$A_i A_i, A_i A_i$	$k_2 p_i^2 + k_1 p_i^3 + k_0 p_i^4$
$A_i A_i, A_j A_j$	$k_0 p_i^2 p_j^2$
$A_i A_i, A_i A_j$	$k_1 p_i^2 p_j + 2k_0 p_i^3 p_j$
$A_i A_i, A_j A_k$	$2k_0 p_i^2 p_j p_k$
$A_i A_j, A_i A_j$	$2k_2 p_i p_j + k_1 p_i p_j (p_i + p_j) + 4k_0 p_i^2 p_j^2$
$A_i A_j, A_i A_k$	$k_1 p_i p_j p_k + 4k_0 p_i^2 p_j p_k$
$A_i A_j, A_k A_l$	$4k_0 p_i p_j p_k p_l$

examined, the probability is just p_A. The probability an allele is A, given that an A has already been seen, is $[\theta + (1 - \theta) p_A]$ so the chance they are both A is $p_A[\theta + (1 - \theta) p_A] = p_A^2 + \theta p_A (1 - p_A)$. The "background" or "evolutionary" relatedness produces the same effect as an inbreeding coefficient of $F = \theta$.

The probability that an allele is A, given that the previous two alleles were A, is $[2\theta + (1 - \theta) p_A]/(1 + \theta)$ and this is of immediate use in paternity testing: it is the probability that a random man provides paternal allele A, given that the alleged father is homozygous for the allele (but see Table 4).

As one further example, the probability that an allele is A, given that the previous three alleles examined were also A, is $[3\theta + (1 - \theta) p_A]/(1 + 2\theta)$. In the forensic context where a crime stain, left by the perpetrator, is of type AA this leads to the probability that a suspect is also of type AA:

$$\Pr(AA|AA) = \Pr(A|AAA) \Pr(A|AA)$$
$$= \frac{[3\theta + (1 - \theta) p_A][2\theta + (1 - \theta) p_A]}{(1 + \theta)(1 + 2\theta)} \quad (2)$$

Note the use of the conditional probability symbol $|$.

The results just described for relatives, meaning familial relationships among people in the same family or evolutionary relatedness among people in the same population, are employed in the likelihood ratios for comparing alternative hypotheses about sets of observed DNA profiles. Whether the context is in the forensic situation involving a suspect and a crime stain, or the parentage situation of a child and an alleged father, or the missing person situation involving a stain or some remains and the relatives of the missing person, there is the evidence E of two or more DNA profiles and there are alternative hypotheses H that specify the relationship(s) among the sources of those profiles. One hypothesis, H_p, may be identity in the forensic case, father–child in the parentage case, and sibships in the missing person case. An alternative, H_d, may be unrelatedness in each case. The strength of the evidence is expressed as a likelihood ratio LR = $\Pr(E|H_p)/\Pr(E|H_d)$.

The identity measures and expressions for joint genotypic probabilities also allow another type of calculation that has recently arisen in studies of databases [4]. When all profiles in a database are compared to all other profiles, there are often quite striking degrees of similarity observed. It is helpful to be able to predict the degree of such similarity, taking into account familial and evolutionary relatedness, in order to determine whether or not the observed similarities indicate any unusual features of the database. To date, the observations have been consistent with expectations [4], and these expectations are now described.

The probability P_2 that two profiles match is [4]

$$P_2 = \sum_i \Pr(A_i A_i, A_i A_i) + \sum_i \sum_{j \neq i} \Pr(A_i A_j, A_i A_j)$$

$$= \sum_i \Pr(A_i A_i A_i A_i) + 2 \sum_i \sum_{j \neq i} \Pr(A_i A_i A_j A_j)$$

$$= \frac{1}{D} [6\theta^3 + \theta^2 (1 - \theta)(2 + 9 S_2) +$$

$$2\theta (1 - \theta)^2 (2 S_2 + S_3) + (1 - \theta)^3 (2 S_2^2 - S_4)] \quad (3)$$

The first line specifies the genotypes, the second shows the corresponding sets of alleles, and the third shows the value from the Dirichlet assumption. Random mating is assumed for the second line. The third line employs the notation $S_k = \sum_i p_i^k, k = 2, 3, 4$ and $D = (1 + \theta)(1 + 2\theta)$. Partial matches occur when two individuals share one allele at a locus, rather than the two required for a match. The probability that two individuals partially match is

$$P_1 = 2 \sum_i \sum_{j \neq i} \Pr(A_i A_i, A_i A_j)$$

$$+ \sum_i \sum_{j \neq i} \sum_{k \neq i, j} \Pr(A_i A_j, A_i A_k)$$

$$= 4 \sum_i \sum_{j \neq i} \Pr(A_i A_i A_i A_j)$$

$$+ 4 \sum_i \sum_{j \neq i} \sum_{k \neq i, j} \Pr(A_i A_i A_j A_k)$$

$$= \frac{1}{D} [8\theta^2 (1 - \theta)(1 - S_2) + 4\theta (1 - \theta)^2 (1 - S_3)$$

$$+ 4(1 - \theta)^3 (S_2 - S_3 - S_2^2 + S_4)] \quad (4)$$

with the same meaning for the three rows as for P_2. Finally, for two individuals to mismatch, i.e., have no alleles in common,

$$P_0 = \sum_i \sum_{j \neq i} \Pr(A_i A_i, A_j A_j)$$

$$+ 2 \sum_i \sum_{j \neq i} \sum_{k \neq i, j} \Pr(A_i A_i, A_j A_k)$$

$$+ \sum_i \sum_{j \neq i} \sum_{k \neq i, j} \sum_{l \neq i, j, k} \Pr(A_i A_j, A_k A_l)$$

$$= \sum_i \sum_{j \neq i} \Pr(A_i A_i A_j A_j)$$

$$+ 2 \sum_i \sum_{j \neq i} \sum_{k \neq i, j} \Pr(A_i A_i A_j A_k)$$

$$+ \sum_i \sum_{j \neq i} \sum_{k \neq i, j} \sum_{l \neq i, j, k} \Pr(A_i A_j A_k A_l)$$

$$= \frac{1}{D} [\theta^2 (1 - \theta)(1 - S_2)$$

$$+ 2\theta (1 - \theta)^2 (1 - 2 S_2 + S_3)$$

$$+ (1 - \theta)^3 (1 - 4 S_2 + 4 S_3 + 2 S_2^2 - 3 S_4)] $$

$$(5)$$

If, in addition to membership in the same population, two individuals have family relatedness described by k_0, k_1, k_2:

$$\Pr(\text{Match}) = k_2 + k_1 [\theta + (1 - \theta) S_2] + k_0 P_2$$

$$\Pr(\text{Partial Match}) = k_1 (1 - \theta)(1 - S_2) + k_0 P_1$$

$$\Pr(\text{Mismatch}) = k_0 P_0 \quad (6)$$

It is important to stress that these matching probabilities P_0, P_1, P_2 do not refer to specific profiles. They represent similarities over all profile types and so they apply to studies of databases rather than to specific parentage or missing person situations.

Parentage Testing

The usual situation in paternity disputes is that mother, child, and alleged father are genotyped. The alleged father is declared "not excluded" if he carries an allele that is inferred to be the child's paternal allele and the strength of the evidence against him is quantified as the paternity index PI. The two simplest explanations for the genetic evidence E are

H_p: the alleged father is the father.
H_d: the alleged father is not the father.

and the paternity index is

$$PI = \frac{\Pr(E|H_p)}{\Pr(E|H_d)} \qquad (7)$$

If there is a prior probability π_0 of paternity, the posterior probability π should be changed to Bayes' theorem:

$$\frac{\pi}{1-\pi} = PI \times \frac{\pi_0}{1-\pi_0} \qquad (8)$$

The PI can be expressed in terms of probability of genotype G_C of child, conditional on genotypes G_M, G_{AF} of mother, and alleged father:

$$
\begin{aligned}
PI &= \frac{\Pr(G_C|G_M, G_{AF}, H_p)\Pr(G_M, G_{AF}|H_p)}{\Pr(G_C|G_M, G_{AF}, H_d)\Pr(G_M, G_{AF}|H_d)} \\
&= \frac{\Pr(G_C|G_M, G_{AF}, H_p)}{\Pr(G_C|G_M, G_{AF}, H_d)} \qquad (9)
\end{aligned}
$$

since the adult probabilities do not depend on the hypotheses. Provided the mother and alleged father are not related, so that the child's maternal and paternal alleles A_M and A_P are independent, it is more convenient to work with the alleles than the child's genotype. Noting that A_M depends only on the mother's genotype:

$$
\begin{aligned}
PI &= \frac{\Pr(A_M A_P|G_M, G_{AF}, H_p)}{\Pr(A_M A_P|G_M, G_{AF}, H_d)} \\
&= \frac{\Pr(A_M|G_M, H_p)\Pr(A_P|A_M, G_M, G_{AF}, H_p)}{\Pr(A_M|G_M, H_d)\Pr(A_P|G_M, G_{AF}, H_d)} \\
&= \frac{\Pr(A_P|A_M, G_M, G_{AF}, H_p)}{\Pr(A_P|G_M, G_{AF}, H_d)} \qquad (10)
\end{aligned}
$$

because $\Pr(A_M|G_M)$ does not depend on H.

Suppose first that familial or evolutionary relatedness is not considered. Under explanation H_p, the alleged father has provided the paternal allele, of type A_i say, and the probability of the allele is 1.0 or 0.5, depending on whether he is homozygous or heterozygous for that allele. Under explanation H_d some other man, the true father TF, has provided the paternal allele and the probability of this unknown man providing the paternal allele is just the population allele frequency p_i. The PI is $1/p_i$ or $1/(2p_i)$ for homozygous $A_i A_i$ or heterozygous $A_i A_j$ alleged fathers.

Alleged father related to true father

There are situations, including those of incest, where the alternative hypotheses involve relatives. There may be reason to suspect that either the alleged father or his brother is the true father of a child. The two hypotheses become

H_p: the alleged father is the father.
H_d: the alleged father is related to the father.

and then it is necessary to determine the probability of the paternal allele, given that it came from a relative of the alleged father. Provided there is no inbreeding, the calculations follow from the joint probabilities for relatives given in Table 2 and are shown in Table 3. These lead to the probabilities of paternal allele A_i under H_d that it came from a relative, and the PI values are $1/[2\theta_{AT} + (1 - 2\theta_{AT})p_i]$ for homozygous alleged fathers and $1/\{2[\theta_{AT} + (1 - 2\theta_{AT})p_i]\}$ for heterozygous alleged fathers. The quantity θ_{AT} is the coancestry of alleged and (under H_d) true fathers.

It is also possible to construct a likelihood ratio for a different pair of alternative explanations for situations when the alleged father is either deceased or

Table 3 Paternity index calculations when H_d is that alleged father is related to the father. (The paternal allele is A_i and A_j, A_k are any other distinct alleles.)

Alleged father	$\Pr(A_i|H_p)$	Relative	$\Pr(\text{Relative}|\text{Alleged father})$	$\Pr(A_i|H_d)$
$A_i A_i$	1.0	$A_i A_i$	$(k_0 p_i^4 + k_1 p_i^3 + k_2 p_i^2)/p_i^2$	1.0
		$A_i A_j$	$(2k_0 p_i^3 p_j + k_1 p_i^2 p_j)/p_i^2$	0.5
$A_i A_j$	0.5	$A_i A_i$	$(2k_0 p_i^3 p_j + k_1 p_i^2 p_j)/(2p_i p_j)$	1.0
		$A_i A_j$	$[4k_0 p_i^2 p_j^2 + k_1 p_i p_j(p_i + p_j) + 2k_2 p_i p_j]/(2p_i p_j)$	0.5
		$A_i A_k$	$(4k_0 p_i^2 p_j p_k + k_1 p_i p_j p_k)/(2p_i p_j)$	0.5

otherwise not available for testing but his relative can be tested. If X is the tested man, the hypotheses are

H_p: X is a relative of the father Y.
H_d: X is unrelated to the father Y.

If the degree of relatedness in H_p is specified by θ_{XY}, then the PI, often called the *Avuncular Index*, when the paternal allele is A_i is $[1 - 2\theta_{XY} + 2\theta_{XY}/p_i]$ when the tested man is homozygous $A_i A_i$, $[1 - 2\theta_{XY} + \theta_{XY}/p_i]$ when the tested man is heterozygous $A_i A_j$, and it is $(1 - 2\theta_{XY})$ when the tested man does not carry A_i.

Evolutionary relatedness

For populations in which there is a (low) level of relatedness of individuals because of the evolutionary history of the population, there is a need to consider the relatedness of mother, alleged father, and father. This does not affect $\Pr(A_P|G_M, G_{AF}, H_p)$ because that is determined by the genotype of the alleged father. Under H_d, however, the Dirichlet sampling

Table 4 Paternity Index values for a population with evolutionary relatedness. (Different subscripts denote different alleles)

G_M	G_C	A_M	A_P	G_{AF}	PI
$A_i A_i$	$A_i A_i$	A_i	A_i	$A_i A_i$	$\dfrac{1+3\theta}{4\theta+(1-\theta)p_i}$
				$A_i A_j$	$\dfrac{1+3\theta}{2[3\theta+(1-\theta)p_i]}$
	$A_i A_j$	A_i	A_j	$A_j A_j$	$\dfrac{1+3\theta}{2\theta+(1-\theta)p_j}$
				$A_i A_j$	$\dfrac{1+3\theta}{2[\theta+(1-\theta)p_j]}$
				$A_j A_k$	$\dfrac{1+3\theta}{2[\theta+(1-\theta)p_j]}$
$A_i A_k$	$A_i A_i$	A_i	A_i	$A_i A_i$	$\dfrac{1+3\theta}{3\theta+(1-\theta)p_i}$
				$A_i A_k$	$\dfrac{1+3\theta}{2[2\theta+(1-\theta)p_i]}$
	$A_i A_j$	A_i	A_j	$A_j A_j$	$\dfrac{1+3\theta}{2\theta+(1-\theta)p_j}$
				$A_i A_j$	$\dfrac{1+3\theta}{2[\theta+(1-\theta)p_j]}$
				$A_j A_l$	$\dfrac{1+3\theta}{2[\theta+(1-\theta)p_j]}$

formula can be used. The probability of the paternal allele depends on the four alleles already seen: those of the mother and the alleged father. The resulting PI values are shown in Table 4.

Missing Person Calculations

Many of the issues involved in missing person calculations are the same as those for paternity disputes. Instead of a paternal allele being known, a biological sample from the missing person is available. Suppose a person is missing; the genetic evidence E consists of the genotype from a sample that has come from some person X who may be the missing person Y, together with the genotypes from the spouse M and child C of the missing person. Two explanations of the evidence are

H_p: the sample is from the missing person.
H_d: the sample is not from the missing person.

A general approach for calculating the likelihood ratio is to work with probabilities of genotypes conditional on those in the previous generation(s):

$$
\begin{aligned}
LR &= \frac{\Pr(E|H_p)}{\Pr(E|H_d)} \\
&= \frac{\Pr(G_C, G_M, G_X|H_p)}{\Pr(G_C, G_M, X|H_d)} \\
&= \frac{\Pr(G_C|G_M, G_X, H_p)\Pr(G_M, G_X|H_p)}{\Pr(G_C|G_M, G_X, H_d)\Pr(G_M, G_X|H_d)} \\
&= \frac{\Pr(G_C|G_M, G_X, H_p)}{\Pr(G_C|G_M, H_d)}
\end{aligned}
\tag{11}
$$

since the genotype of the child does not depend on that of X when H_d is true (ignoring evolutionary relatedness within the population). This likelihood ratio is the same as in the paternity case where X is alleged to be the father of child C who has mother M. Similar extensions can be made to allow for X to be a relative of the missing person, or to allow for evolutionary relatedness among all members of a population.

It may be the case that people apart from the spouse and child of the missing person are typed. The general procedure is the same: the probabilities of the set of observed genotypes under two explanations are compared. Suppose the parents P, Q as well as the child C and spouse M of the missing person Y are typed, and that a sample is available that has come from some person X thought under H_p to be Y. Under explanation H_d, the sample from X did not come from Y, and therefore the genotype of X does not depend on the genotypes of P and Q and the genotype of C does not depend on the genotype of X.

$$
\begin{aligned}
LR &= \frac{\Pr(E|H_p)}{\Pr(E|H_d)} \\
&= \frac{\Pr(C, M, X, P, Q|H_p)}{\Pr(C, M, X, P, Q|H_d)} \\
&= \frac{\Pr(C|M, X, P, Q, H_p)\,\Pr(M, X, P, Q|H_p)}{\Pr(C|M, X, P, Q, H_d)\,\Pr(M, X, P, Q|H_d)} \\
&= \frac{\Pr(C|M, X, H_p)\,\Pr(M, X|P, Q, H_p)}{\Pr(C|M, P, Q, H_d)\,\Pr(M, X|P, Q, H_d)} \\
& \qquad \frac{\Pr(P, Q|H_p)}{\Pr(P, Q|H_d)} \\
&= \frac{\Pr(C|M, X, H_p)\,\Pr(M|H_p)\,\Pr(X|P, Q, H_p)}{\Pr(C|M, P, Q, H_d)\,\Pr(M|H_d)\,\Pr(X|H_d)} \\
&= \frac{\Pr(C|M, X, H_p)\,\Pr(X|P, Q, H_p)}{\Pr(C|M, P, Q, H_d)\,\Pr(X|H_d)}
\end{aligned}
\tag{12}
$$

An example is shown in Table 5.

Evolutionary relatedness can be accounted for by modifying the terms involving allele frequencies. In this case, the term $\Pr(X|H_d)$ needs to take into account the alleles already seen in P, Q, M, and C. For the example in Table 5, where $X = A_1 A_3$, this probability is that of obtaining A_1 after having seen two copies of A_1 and A_2 and one copy of A_3, A_4, A_5 and A_6, and then of obtaining A_3 after having seen

three copies of A_1, two copies of A_2, and one copy of A_3, A_4, A_5 and A_6. From the Dirichlet sampling formula, this probability is

$$
\begin{aligned}
&\Pr(A_1 A_3 | A_1 A_1 A_2 A_2 A_3 A_4 A_5 A_6) \\
&\quad = \frac{2\theta + (1-\theta)p_1}{1 + 8\theta}\,\frac{\theta + (1-\theta)p_3}{1 + 7\theta}
\end{aligned}
\tag{13}
$$

As a final example, consider the case where profiles are available from one parent P, four siblings S, the spouse M, and a child C of a missing person, as well as from a sample X that may be from that missing person. Sample profiles are shown in Table 6. Write the evidence as $E = (C, M, X, S, P)$ and the hypotheses H_p, H_d that X is or is not from the missing person. It is necessary to introduce the untyped parent Q and add over all possible genotypes for this parent that are consistent with P and S under H_d, and consistent with P, S, X under H_p. The probability of any specific genotype of Q does not depend on the hypotheses. The general procedure is still to write the probabilities for people conditional on those in the previous generations:

$$
\begin{aligned}
LR &= \frac{\Pr(C, M, X, S, P|H_p)}{\Pr(C, M, X, S, P|H_d)} \\
&= \frac{\sum_Q \Pr(C, M, X, S, P|Q, H_p)\,\Pr(Q|H_p)}{\sum_Q \Pr(C, M, X, S, P|Q, H_d)\,\Pr(Q|H_d)} \\
&= \frac{\sum_Q \Pr(C|M, X, S, P, Q, H_p)}{\sum_Q \Pr(C|M, X, S, P, Q, H_d)} \\
&\qquad \frac{\Pr(M, X, S, P|Q, H_p)\,\Pr(Q)}{\Pr(M, X, S, P|Q, H_d)\,\Pr(Q)} \\
&= \frac{\sum_Q \Pr(C|MXH_p)\,\Pr(M|H_p)}{\sum_Q \Pr(C|MSPQH_d)\,\Pr(M|H_d)} \\
&\qquad \frac{\Pr(XSP|QH_p)\,\Pr(Q)}{\Pr(X|H_d)\,\Pr(SP|QH_d)\,\Pr(Q)} \\
&= \frac{\sum_Q \Pr(C|MXH_p)\,\Pr(XS|PQH_p)}{\sum_Q \Pr(C|MPQH_d)\,\Pr(X|H_d)} \\
&\qquad \frac{\Pr(P|QH_p)\,\Pr(Q)}{\Pr(S|PQH_d)\,\Pr(P|QH_d)\,\Pr(Q)} \\
&\qquad + \\
&= \frac{\Pr(C|M, X, H_p)\sum_Q \Pr(X, S|P, Q, H_p)}{\Pr(X|H_d)\sum_Q \Pr(C|M, P, Q, H_d)} \\
&\qquad \frac{\Pr(Q)}{\Pr(S|P, Q, H_d)\,\Pr(Q)}
\end{aligned}
\tag{14}
$$

Table 5 An example of a missing person calculation.

Child	G_C	$A_1 A_2$
Sample	G_X	$A_1 A_3$
Spouse	G_M	$A_2 A_4$
Mother	G_P	$A_1 A_5$
Father	G_Q	$A_3 A_6$
$\Pr(C|M, X, H_p)$	$=$	$\frac{1}{4}$
$\Pr(X|P, Q, H_p)$	$=$	$\frac{1}{4}$
$\Pr(C|M, P, Q, H_d)$	$=$	$\frac{1}{8}$
$\Pr(X|H_d)$	$=$	$2p_1 p_3$
LR	$=$	$\frac{1}{4p_1 p_3}$

Table 6 An example of a missing person calculation

P	mother, with genotype A_3A_4
S	sibs, with genotypes $A_2A_4, A_2A_4, A_2A_4, A_3A_4$
Q	untyped father who must have genotype A_2A_3 or A_2A_4
M	spouse, with genotype A_5A_6
C	child, with genotype A_3A_5
X	sample, with genotype A_3A_3

$$\Pr(C|M, X, H_p) = 1/4$$

$$\Pr(X, S|P, Q, H_p) = \begin{cases} \dfrac{1}{1024}, & Q = A_2A_3 \\ 0, & Q = A_2A_4 \end{cases}$$

$$\Pr(X|H_d) = p_3^2$$

$$\Pr(C|M, P, Q, H_d) = \begin{cases} \dfrac{1}{2}, & Q = A_2A_3 \\ \dfrac{1}{4}, & Q = A_2A_4 \end{cases}$$

$$\Pr(S|P, Q) = \begin{cases} \dfrac{1}{256}, & Q = A_2A_3 \\ \dfrac{1}{256}, & Q = A_2A_4 \end{cases}$$

$$\Pr(Q) = \begin{cases} 2p_2p_3, & Q = A_2A_3, \\ 2p_2p_4, & Q = A_2A_4 \end{cases}$$

$$LR = \frac{(1/4) \times (1/1024) \times 2p_2p_3}{(p_3^2)[(1/2) \times (1/256)2p_2p_3 + (1/4) \times (1/256)2p_2p_4]}$$

$$= \frac{1}{4p_3(2p_3 + p_4)}$$

Details for the specific profiles are shown in Table 6.

Discussion

Interpreting DNA evidence for situations involving parentage or missing person identification rests on the profile probabilities for sets of related individuals. When relatedness is a consequence of membership in the same family, there is a set of three parameters that are the probabilities two people share zero, one, or two pairs of ibd alleles. For the relatedness resulting from the shared evolutionary history of all members of a population, there is a convenient formulation in terms of a general coancestry coefficient θ. This formulation has become widely used in single-contributor forensic calculations and it should also be used in paternity calculations. The identification of remains in missing person situations can be quite complicated when many family members are typed, but the use of likelihood ratios to compare evidence probabilities under alternative hypotheses provides a general approach. The probabilities need to be written for individuals in one generation conditional on individuals in previous generations.

Relatedness coefficients allow the probabilities of DNA profiles for sets of individuals to be written out explicitly. Although increasing relatedness is expected to result in increasing profile similarity, the probability expressions in Tables 1 and 2 make it clear that even unrelated people may have very similar profiles, whereas related people may have quite dissimilar profiles. For example, unrelated people may both be homozygous A_1A_1 at a locus and full-sibs may have completely different genotypes A_1A_1, A_2A_2. It is more appropriate to compare evidence probabilities under alternative hypotheses than it is to have arbitrary rules that deny the possibility of relatedness, once some threshold level of allelic dissimilarity is reached.

Acknowledgment

This work was supported in part by NIH grant GM 75091.

References

[1] Weir, B.S., Anderson, A.D. & Hepler, A.B. (2006). Genetic relatedness analysis: modern data and new challenges, *Nature Reviews Genetics* **7**, 771–780.

[2] Evett, I.W. & Weir, B.S. (1998). *Interpreting DNA evidence–statistical genetics for forensic scientists*, Sinuaer Associates, Sunderland.

[3] Balding, D.J. & Nichols, R.A. (1994). DNA profile match probability calculations: how to allow for population stratification, relatedness, database selection and single bands, *Forensic Science International* **64**, 125–140.

[4] Weir, B.S. (2007). The rarity of DNA profiles, *Annals of Applied Statistics* **1**, 358–370.

Related Articles

Mitochondrial DNA: Interpretation

Short Tandem Repeats: Interpretation

BRUCE S. WEIR

Mistaken Identification *see* Eyewitness Lineups: Identification from

Mitigation Testimony

Despite a growing consensus against the death penalty in the United States, there still exist a large number of people that believe in the use of capital punishment. Problematic to some is the holding in *Witherspoon v. Illinois* [1], which guaranteed that only those individuals that are willing to impose the death penalty be allowed to serve as jurors in capital litigation. As such, imposition of the death penalty may not be readily influenced by issues that have led to the decrease in support for the death penalty (e.g., wrongful executions, lack of deterrent value), and these individuals may be more inclined to give the death sentence than would many people in the general population.

In 1979, the United States Supreme Court (USSC) upheld the use of guided discretion in the application of the death sentence for specific crimes in a bifurcated trial; the first stage requires the jury to determine guilt or innocence, and the second to determine sentence after consideration of aggravating and mitigating circumstances (see, for example, [2–4]). In brief, aggravating circumstances are factors that define and narrow the class of defendants

eligible for the death penalty (*Zant v. Stephens* [5]), and mitigating circumstances are factors that decrease a capital defendant's culpability to the level at which the death penalty is considered undeserved. In order to proceed with the option of death, the state must prove that one or more statutory aggravating factors exists.

In most states, aggravating circumstances are delineated by statute and include factors that can be separated into four categories: (i) defendant characteristics (e.g., whether the defendant was previously convicted of another capital offense or a felony involving the use or threat of violence to the person not limited to the following factors of the crime and/or the defendant); (ii) elements of the crime (e.g., the defendant knowingly created a great risk of death to many persons; the capital offense was especially heinous, atrocious, or cruel compared to other capital offenses); (iii) motive for the crime (e.g., the capital offense was committed for pecuniary gain; the capital offense was committed to disrupt or hinder the lawful exercise of any governmental function or the enforcement of laws; and (iv) victim characteristics (e.g., the murdered individual was an on-duty peace officer who was killed in the course of performing his official duties and the defendant knew, or should have known, that the victim was a peace officer; the defendant was an adult and the murdered person was an unborn child in the womb at any stage of its development) [6]. While the number of statutory aggravating circumstances varies by state, all states, however, place the burden of proof at the level of beyond a reasonable doubt.

In contrast to aggravating factors, mitigating factors are not limited to those defined by statute, but instead include "any aspect of character or record, and any circumstance of the offense that might serve as a basis for a sentence less than death" [7]. In its decision in *Wiggins v. Smith* [8] the USSC unequivocally stated that failure to investigate and present mitigating evidence during the sentencing phase of a capital trial violates the defendant's Sixth Amendment right to effective assistance of counsel. In *Wiggins*, the defense had found, but failed to present, mitigating circumstances including, but not limited to, severe neglect and physical abuse, sexual abuse, and borderline mental retardation. In the majority opinion, Justice Sandra Day O'Connor opined that "Had the jury been able to place [Wiggins's] excruciating life history on the mitigating side of the scale, there is a reasonable probability that at least one juror would have struck a different balance" (p. 536).

Jury Decision Making in Capital Litigation

At the most basic level, the concepts of mitigating and aggravating circumstances are easily understood: a mitigating circumstance lessens a defendant's moral culpability and goes against a sentence of death, and an aggravating circumstance increases a defendant's moral culpability and may be used to support the imposition of the death sentence. Despite the apparent simplicity of the constructs, research has consistently shown that jurors' ability to apply these concepts during capital litigation is impaired (e.g., [9–13]). In their evaluation of comprehension of capital sentencing instructions in California, Haney and Lynch [14] identified significant problems in this arena. In their sample of college educated individuals, only 15% were able to provide a legally correct definition of aggravation, 12% could provide a correct definition of mitigation, and a mere 8% provided correct definitions of both terms. Perhaps the most concerning findings were that 30% of the sample provided completely incorrect definitions of mitigation and, after being read jury instructions three times, 11% of the sample was unable to provide a definition of mitigation. In 1997, Haney and Lynch [15] again evaluated the comprehension of jury instructions with respect to the value of providing jurors with explicit definitions of the constructs. The results of this study demonstrated that the inclusion of explicit definitions did nothing to improve overall comprehension.

Garvey [16] addressed an important question in capital litigation, specifically, what impact, if any, do certain factors have on jury decision making in capital cases. Using data from the Capital Jury Project (CJP)[a], Garvey found that the following factors made it more likely that a juror would impose the death penalty: (i) the murder was particularly heinous; (ii) the victim of murder was a child; (iii) the defendant lacked remorse; and (iv) the defendant was identified to be a risk for future dangerousness. Conversely, doubt regarding guilt, a defendant's youthfulness, the presence of mental retardation, and other factors that are outside of the defendant's control (e.g., mental illness) were found to be strong mitigators. Of import was that jurors assigned almost no weight to developmental factors such as child abuse or a background of extreme poverty.

Though studies on lay persons' knowledge regarding developmental risk factors have not yet been conducted, it is possible that the limited significance that jurors placed on these factors is related to lack of understanding regarding the long-term impact of negative life events. In a study that evaluated juror's perceptions of expert testimony, Sundby [17] found that most jurors held negative views about experts, and in particular defense experts. The data demonstrated the presence of three major concerns regarding defense experts, who provide mitigation testimony: (i) jurors believed that such experts lack objectivity; (ii) jurors do not believe that experts have the ability to explain human behavior; and (iii) jurors believe that experts fail to make the critical connection between the psychological principles and the defendant's behavior. Jurors clearly need more than just a recitation of traumatic life experiences and the delivery of a sad story. What jurors need is an explanation of how adverse life events impacted the development of the defendant and how such adversity can be linked to their status as a capital defendant.

Risk, Protective Factors, and Resilience: A Developmental Approach to Mitigation

The sheer magnitude of the outcome of the sentencing decision in capital litigation warrants exploration into the best method to communicate jurors. It is the opinion of this writer that presentation of a defendant's life history within the context of theories of developmental psychopathology is critical, as it provides jurors with a context to understand the defendant's life history. The rationale behind this belief lies in the fact that the capital defendant is similar to any other person in that they have a developmental history. Their developmental trajectory was influenced and shaped by numerous intervening events that either served to hinder or enhance positive growth and development.

In the field of developmental psychology, these life events have been identified under the terms *risk factors* and *protective factors*, respectively. From the developmental perspective, "maladaption is viewed as evolving through the successive adaptations of persons in their environments. It is not something a person 'has' or an ineluctable expression of an endogenous pathogen. It is the complex result of a myriad of risk and protective factors operating overtime" [18, p. 251].

Risk factors

At the most basic level, a risk factor is a predictor that has been scientifically demonstrated to have a strong link to adverse outcomes such as delinquency, adult antisocial behavior, substance abuse, unemployment, and violence. A recent study [19] investigated the precursors to serious and chronic delinquency, as well as youth violence, and from these data were able to identify a number of risk and protective factors. Included among the many risk factors were such things as perinatal difficulties, family history of criminal behavior and substance abuse, early exposure to violence, economic deprivation, media portrayals of violence, academic failure and lack of commitment to school, and low intelligence.

It is well accepted that there is no single risk factor, or a set of risk factors, that is necessary or sufficient to produce an adverse outcome. In fact, years of research has unequivocally shown that outcomes worsen as the number of risk factors increases (*see*, for example, [20–24]). For example, longitudinal studies have shown that children and adolescents diagnosed with conduct disorder demonstrate broad-based dysfunction over multiple domains. In his review of the literature, Kazdin [25] linked seven categories of dysfunction in adulthood to a prior diagnosis of conduct disorder. Specifically, data from multiple studies have shown that these individuals are more likely to (i) experience psychiatric disturbances; (ii) engage in criminal behavior; (iii) have limited occupational success; (iv) function poorly in school; (v) have impaired marital relationships; (vi) isolate from others; and (vii) experience poor physical health. Not surprisingly, these areas of dysfunction are common among death-row inmates [26].

Protective Factors

While the lives of capital murder defendants tend to be laden with risk factors such as poverty, early exposure to illicit drugs and violence, physical abuse, and ineffective parenting [26], in even the most disadvantaged of systems, an individual is typically exposed to one or more protective factors (e.g., a teacher or coach who takes an interest in the child;

an opportunity to engage in community recreation; a family member who notices danger in the home and takes the child in). For the past three decades, the importance of prevention has been recognized, and researchers and policy makers have been dedicated to finding ways to increase access to protective factors; the goal of such intervention is to foster resilience in at-risk children and adolescents (see below for a presentation of the concept of resilience).

The push toward prevention is exemplified in a study funded by the National Institute on Drug Abuse that identified protective factors that can help prevent high-risk youths from engaging in delinquent behavior and illicit substance use [27]. The authors of this study found that resistance to both illicit substance use and delinquency was directly related to the accumulation of protective factors across multiple domains of an adolescent's life. Some of the protective factors identified in the study include appropriate parental supervision, mutual connectedness between parent and child, a commitment to education by both child and parent, association with a peer group that has conventional values, parental approval of one's peer group, positive self-esteem, and child involvement in pro-social activities.

Resiliency

Perhaps the main obstacle to presenting mitigation testimony is the fact that jurors, though similar in that they have matured in response to internal and external forces, are different from capital litigants in that they have somehow succeeded (even if only marginally so) in the presence of some adversity. In the developmental psychology literature, this construct has been referred to as *resiliency* and has been used to explain how individuals that were raised in the same environment can demonstrate highly disparate life trajectories.

Resilience has been defined as a "dynamic developmental process reflecting evidence of adaptation despite significant life adversity" [28]. As previously mentioned, studies have demonstrated that the presence of any single risk factor does not cause adverse outcomes. Instead, it is the convergence of risk factors that leads to widespread dysfunction, and it is the presence of protective factors that fosters resilience (see, for example, [29, 30]).

It has become apparent that resilience in adulthood is related to a number of factors such as having had more resources and fewer adversities early in life. Exposure to effective parenting, having had a greater number of positive relationships with adult role models, and there being a longer time between the birth of siblings have been found to buffer the negative impact of adverse life events (e.g., [31, 32]). These findings, among others, underscore the critical role of protective factors in the developmental process.

Expert Testimony on Mitigation

Searching for and understanding the role of protective factors has dual purposes in mitigation. First, like most people, the capital defendant will have had exposure to one or more protective factors over the course of their life. This may be the influence of a teacher, involvement in a coping skills program, or perhaps the presence of supportive parents. The usefulness of the identification of protective factors lies not in their presence, but in their impact on the life course of the defendant. It may be that there were opportunities for change via counseling or involvement in extracurricular activities, but that these protective factors were not powerful enough to overcome the impact of the risk factors. Second, there are cases in which protective factors are absent from the life of the defendant and this fact must be made apparent to the jury.

Furthermore, the court must be made aware that the defendant's life trajectory may have been different had someone come forward and intervened on behalf of the individual, or had their life experience included positive influences such as access to prosocial peer groups, financial stability, or a safe living environment. During the presentation of mitigation, it is important to clearly delineate what could have been done to change the defendant's life course, what was done to assist in the process of change, and what tools were readily available yet not implemented.

With respect to expert testimony on mitigation, it is imperative that the mental health practitioner is knowledgeable of the risk factors experienced by the defendant and be able to discuss the impact of these risk factors in relation to interventions that were or were not implemented. Of course, individual risk factors would need to be evaluated over the life course, and be discussed with respect to cumulative stress and the interaction among factors.

While perhaps not obvious, the issue of resiliency is of great import in capital mitigation. Clearly, millions of people experience adverse life events, but it is only the rare few who engage in capital crime. In order for mitigation to be successful, the trier of fact must be convinced that the defendant's experience of similar life events was unique, and that it was the uniqueness of the defendant's response that provides an explanation for the violent behavior.

In addition to having a comprehensive understanding of developmental psychopathology, it is critical that the mental health professional is aware that juror decision making does not occur in a vacuum; instead, information is acquired, manipulated, and maintained in the context of each juror's life experience. Similar to decision making in other realms, individuals that are asked to make decisions in the legal arena are doing so, at least in part, on the basis of schemas. In other words, the knowledge that they have accumulated from previous interactions over many years has a direct influence on how jurors think and respond (e.g., [33]). As such, the strength of mitigation evidence is at least in part related to the relationship between the defendant, the crime, and the pre-existing schemata of each juror.

In situations in which jurors' schemata are based on biased or inaccurate information that are detrimental to the defendant, the power of mitigation testimony is likely to be greatly reduced. As such, mental health professionals must enter the courtroom ready to discuss stereotypes and to present information that challenges the myths that may surround the character and life history of the defendant.

Putting it all in Context: *Moore v. Parker*

The lack of understanding of the complexity of presenting mitigating circumstances was highlighted in a recent decision by the US Court of Appeals for the Sixth Circuit. In the case of *Moore v. Parker* [34], the Court affirmed the district court's denial of Moore's writ of *habeas corpus* that was based on ineffective assistance of counsel. With regard to the penalty phase, Moore brought forth the following claims: "his attorneys erred by (1) allegedly spending only about three percent of their preparation time on the penalty phase; (2) remaining unaware of ninety-five letters sent to the first court supporting him, which could have led them to more mitigating evidence and (3) not having another psychologist examine him after the first on they selected proved to be a fraud."

In response, Judges Boggs and Cook found that the testimony of four witnesses that testified to Moore's troubled upbringing (i.e., the defendant, Moore's aunt, Moore's prison "boss", and a Reverend that had only a brief conversation with Moore) and one psychologist (not hired to conduct a mitigation evaluation) was sufficient for the purposes of mitigation.[b] Judge Boggs affirmed the lower court's ruling, at least in part, on the basis of the finding that strong mitigators were presented to the jury. Included among them were "severe abuse and neglect", "his mother stabbing his father and to his having grown up in numerous foster homes and institutions", "his mother's alcoholism and his father's abusiveness", "his abuse and neglect in foster homes and institutions," and "watching his father hitting his mother so hard that his father broke his hand in three places." Judges Boggs and Cook agreed with the district court in their view that the testimony of the psychologist "cast Moore as an easily angered, impulsive, out of control emotional leech with poor judgment" and such testimony would have been detrimental to his case.

What is pointed out in the dissent is that Moore's dangerousness was not placed in the context of his chaotic and abusive upbringing. Furthermore, Judge Martin unequivocally stated that had the jury been presented with a "graphic description of Moore's atrocious childhood" there exists a reasonable probability that the jury may have come to a different decision at sentencing.

As aptly discussed in Douglas Rau's review of *Moore v. Parker* [35], it is clear that Judges Boggs and Cook were focused on whether or not mitigation testimony would engender sympathy from the jury. In their narrow conceptualization of the goal of mitigation, the judges lost sight of the fact that sympathy does not arise solely from presentation of positive defendant attributes in the face of adversity. To the contrary, in a capital case sympathy is more likely to be engendered by the presentation of the horrible and unfathomable aspects of an individual's upbringing that help to explain how the defendant came to be the potentially dangerous, frightening, and unpredictable person that committed murder. As stated by Judge Martin, expressed mitigation specialists are "qualitatively different from lay witnesses and can translate complex information into testimony that will assist the jury in reaching its determination."

End Notes

[a.] The Capital Jury Project is an ongoing program of research on the decision making of capital jurors. The project began in 1991 by a consortium of university-based researchers and is supported with funds from the National Science Foundation.

[b.] In his dissent, Judge Martin noted that only Moore and his aunt spoke of the issue of childhood, not four witnesses as noted by Judges Boggs and Cook.

References

[1] Witherspoon v. Illinois, 391 U.S. 510 (1968).
[2] Gregg v. Georgia, 428 U.S. 153 (1976).
[3] Jurek v. Texas, 428 U.S. 262 (1976).
[4] Proffitt v. Florida, 428 U.S. 242 (1976).
[5] Zant v. Stephens, 462 U.S. 862, 878 (1983).
[6] Acker, J.R. & Lanier, C.S. (1994). "Parsing this lexicon of death": aggravating factors in capital sentencing statutes, *Criminal Law Bulletin* **30**, 107–153.
[7] Lockett v. Ohio, 438 U.S. 586 (1978).
[8] Wiggins v. Smith, 539 U.S. 510 (2003).
[9] Bentele, U. & Bowers, W.J. (2002). How Jurors decide on death: guilt is overwhelming; aggravation requires death; and mitigation is no excuse, *Brooklyn Law Review* **66**, 1013–1080.
[10] Costanzo, M. & Costanzo, S. (1992). Jury decision making in the capital penalty phase: legal assumptions, empirical findings, and a research agenda, *Law and Human Behavior* **16**, 185–201.
[11] Diamond, S.S. (1993). Instructing on death: psychologists, juries, and judges, *American Psychologist* **48**, 423–434.
[12] Haney, C., Sontag, L. & Costanzo, S. (1994). Deciding to take a life: capital juries, sentencing instructions, and the jurisprudence of death, *Journal of Social Issues* **50**, 149–176.
[13] Lynch, M. & Haney, C. (2000). Discrimination and instructional comprehension: guided discretion, racial bias, and the death penalty, *Law and Human Behavior* **24**, 337–358.
[14] Haney, C. & Lynch, M. (1994). Comprehending life and death matters: a preliminary study of California's capital penalty instructions, *Law and Human Behavior* **18**, 411–436.
[15] Haney, C. & Lynch, M. (1997). Clarifying life and death matters: an analysis of instructional comprehension and penalty phase arguments, *Law and Human Behavior* **21**, 575–595.

[16] Garvey, Stephen P. (1998). Aggravation and mitigation in capital cases: what do jurors think? *Columbia Law Review* **98**, 1538.

[17] Sundby, S.E. (1994). The jury as critic: an empirical look at how capital juries perceive expert and lay testimony, *Virginia Law Review* **83**, 1109–1188.

[18] Sroufe, L.A. (1997). Psychopathology as an outcome of development, *Development and Psychopathology* **9**, 251–268.

[19] Herrenkohl, T.I., Maguin, E. & Hill, K.G. (2000). Developmental risk factors for youth violence, *Journal of Adolescent Health* **26**, 176–186.

[20] Coie, J.D., Watt, N.F., West, S.G., Hawkins, J.D., Asarnow, J.R. & Markman, H.J., Ramey, S.L., Shure, M.B. Long, B. (1993). The science of prevention, *American Psychologist* **48**, 1013–1022.

[21] Deater-Deckard, K., Dodge, K. & Bates, J.E. (1998). Multiple risk factors in the development of externalizing behavior problems: group and individual differences, *Development and Psychopathology* **10**, 469–493.

[22] Egeland, B., Carlson, E. & Sroufe, L.A. (1993). Resilience as process, *Development and Psychopathology* **5**, 517–528.

[23] Garmezy, N. & Masten, A.S. (1991). The protective role of competence indicators in children at risk, in *Life-Span Developmental Psychology: Perspectives on Stress and Coping*, E.M. Cummings, A.L. Greene & K.H. Karraker, eds, Lawrence Erlbaum Associates, Hillsdale, England, pp. 151–174.

[24] Masten, A.S. & Wright, M.O. (1997). Cumulative risk and protection models of child maltreatment, in *Multiple Victimization of Children: Conceptual, Developmental, Research and Treatment Issues*, B.B.R. Rossman & M.S. Rosenberg, eds, Haworth Press, Binghampton, pp. 7–30.

[25] Kazdin, A.E. (1997). Conduct disorder across the lifespan, in *Developmental Psychopathology: Perspectives on Adjustment, Risk, and Disorder*, S.S. Luthar, J.A. Burack, D. Cicchetti & J.R. Weisz, eds, Cambridge University Press, pp. 248–272.

[26] Cunningham, M.D. & Vigen, M.P. (2002). Death row inmate characteristics, adjustment, and confinement: a critical review of the literature, *Behavioral Sciences and the Law* **20**, 191–210.

[27] Smith, C., Lizotte, A.J., Thornberry, T.P. & Krohn, M.D. (1995). Resilient youth: identifying factors that prevent high-risk youth from engaging in delinquency and drug use, in *Delinquency and Disrepute in the Life Course*, J. Hagan, ed, Greenwich, CT, pp. 217–247.

[28] Rau, D. (2007). The scope of mitigation in the death penalty. *Journal of the American Academy of Psychiatry and the Law* **35**, 135–136.

[29] Cicchetti, D. (2003). Forward, in *Resilience and Vulnerability: Adaptation in the Context of Childhood Adversities*, S.S. Luthar, ed, Cambridge University Press, New York, p. XX.

[30] Garmezy, N. (1985). Stress-resistant children: the search for protective factors, in *Recent Research in Developmental Psychopathology*, J.E. Stevenson, ed, (*Journal of Child Psychology and Psychiatry* Book Supplement No. 4), Pergamon Press, Oxford, pp. 213–233.

[31] Rutter, M. (1985). Resilience in the face of adversity: protective factors and resistance to psychiatric disorder, *British Journal of Psychiatry* **147**, 598–611.

[32] Masten, A.S. & Powell, J.L. (2003). A resilience framework for research, policy, and practice, in *Resilience and Vulnerability: Adaptation in the Context of Childhood Adversities*, S.S. Luthar, ed, Cambridge University Press, New York, pp. 1–25.

[33] Werner, E. & Smith, R. (2001). *Journey From Childhood to Midlife: Risk, Resiliency, & Recovery*, Cornell University Press, New York.

[34] Fiske, S.T. & Taylor, S.E. (1984). *Social Cognition*, Addison-Wesley, Reading.

[35] Moore v. Parker, 425 F.3d 250 (6th Cir., 2005).

Further Reading

People v. Taylor, No. 123 (N.Y. Ct. App. filed Oct. 23, 2007).

People v. LaValle (3 N.Y.3d 88).

Baze v. Rees, 217 S.W. 3d 207, 209 (Ky. 2006), cert. granted, 76 U.S.L.W. 3154 (U.S. Sept. 25, 2007). (No. 07–5439).

http://www.gallup.com

National Omnibus Poll (2007). as cited in http://www.death penaltyinfo.org/article.php?did = 2163#DPIC07).

KAREN L. SALEKIN

Mitochondrial DNA: Interpretation

Introduction

The general principles of interpretation of mtDNA evidence have been detailed previously [1]; we follow the same principles and nomenclature here. Any mtDNA investigation seeks to address whether or not the donor of a reference sample (K) could be the donor, or a maternal relative of the donor, of a questioned sample (Q). The sequences obtained from the samples K and Q are referred to as SK and SQ, respectively.

Despite intense interest and many attempts to detect it, paternal inheritance of human mtDNA has only been demonstrated reliably in a single instance ([2]; for a critique of studies claiming to demonstrate paternal inheritance of mtDNA, see [3]). Therefore, for the purposes of forensic interpretation of mtDNA evidence, we assume strict maternal inheritance.

What Constitutes a Match between *K* and *Q*?

If the result of the mtDNA analysis is that *K* and *Q* have the same sequence, this observation supports the contention that these samples have a common maternal origin. If *K* and *Q* have different sequences, then the contention of a common maternal origin is not supported by the observation. However, if the difference between *K* and *Q* is slight, the interpretation is not straightforward as the mutation rate of mtDNA is an order of magnitude greater than that of nuclear DNA. Differences in mtDNA sequence can be observed both between maternal relatives (e.g., [4]) and within a single individual (e.g., [5–9]). Two main approaches to evaluating whether an "inclusion", an "exclusion", or an "inconclusive" result is reported have been adopted. The first is a simple rule-set based on the number of differences between the samples: if no differences between the samples are observed, an inclusion is reported, if one difference is observed, the result is declared inconclusive and if two or more differences are observed, an exclusion is reported [10].

In the second approach, the general framework of the likelihood ratio (LR) is applied [1, 11, 12]:

Probability of the evidence | *K* and *Q* have the same maternal origin
──────────────────────────────────────
Probability of the evidence | *K* and *Q* have different maternal origins

$$= \frac{\Pr(E|H_p)}{\Pr(E|H_d)} \qquad (1)$$

In this approach, any uncertainty about whether or not the mtDNA samples originated from the same maternal lineage is reflected in the numerator of the LR. Thus, if the sequences match exactly, the numerator would approach 1; if the sequences differ at many positions, the numerator tends toward 0, resulting in exclusion. For sequences, which differ at a single base or a small number of bases, the numerator is intermediate, depending on the mutation rate at the particular base(s) in question, the body tissue from which *K* and *Q* originate, and the number of generations separating the donors of these samples. Data

regarding the mutability of individual mtDNA bases is accumulating, with some of the most useful information coming from phylogenetic analyses, which enable distinction to be made between bases that are highly polymorphic due to recurring mutations at highly mutable sites and those that are polymorphic because an ancient mutation has reached appreciable frequency in one or more populations (e.g., [13–16]). Several large studies of heteroplasmic segregation within (e.g., [5–9]) and between (e.g., [4]) individuals provide data to inform the assessment of impact of the body tissue and that of the generational divide, respectively.

Commonly Used Methods for Assessing Evidential Strength When an Inclusion is Reported

All methods for assessing evidential strength rely on population databases to gauge how common or rare is the sequence in question. Databases are considered in detail in the section "Databases".

The Counting Method

Many practitioners rely on the "counting method" to illustrate to the court the relative strength of a mtDNA match. In this method, the number of sequences matching that of the crime scene and suspect observed in the available databases is reported, together with the size of the databases. This method has the advantage of simplicity, and relies on no population genetics assumptions. For common haplotypes, it gives a relatively good estimate of the match probability, providing the database is relevant. However, for haplotypes that have not previously been observed in the database, the practitioner must ensure that the court is not left with the impression that failure to observe a haplotype in a database of, for example, several thousand sequences, indicates that the strength of the observed match is on a par with an autosomal DNA match such as a short tandem repeat (STR) match.

Upper Bound Frequency Estimation

Some have therefore extended the approach to calculate an upper 95% confidence interval for the frequency estimate. Following Holland and Parsons [12], this is calculated as

$$p = 1 - \alpha^{1/n} \qquad (2)$$

where $\alpha = 0.05$ for a 95% confidence interval.

Confidence intervals can also be calculated for frequency estimates for haplotypes that have previously been observed. Again following [12], this is calculated as

$$p \pm \sqrt{\frac{p(1-p)}{n}} \qquad (3)$$

where n is the database size.

However, this method is unlikely to give a robust estimate of the confidence interval in most instances, as the normal approximation is poor when p is small [12].

An alternative approach is to add the observations of the sequence in the case to the database, in an approach similar to that advocated by Balding and Nichols [17] for addressing sampling error. Under the assumption of innocence, the profile from the crime sample and that from the reference sample do not originate from the same individual; the calculation is therefore

$$p = \frac{(x+2)}{(n+2)} \qquad (4)$$

where x is the number of observations of the sequence and n is the database size [1].

Buckleton *et al.* [11] have suggested that the correct estimator for haploid genomes should be:

$$p = \frac{(x+1)}{(n+2)} \qquad (5)$$

However, we contend that the estimator is intended to provide a common sense method to ensure that the strength of evidence is not overstated, given that the sequence has been observed (twice) in the case, even if not in the reference database, so prefer to adopt the more conservative and intuitive formula as originally stated [1]. Nevertheless, when either is fed into an LR, the result converges (Tables 1 and 2).

Table 1 $SQ = SK = $ [146C, 16129A, 16189C] (quoted as differences to the revised Cambridge Reference Sequence [18]); database searches carried out using www.empop.org

Method	Sampling correction	Count in Austrian Caucasian database	Result from Austrian Caucasian data	Count in Western European Caucasian database	Result from Western European Caucasian database
Counting method	None	0/273	No matching sequences found in 273 Austrians	0/3830	No matching sequences found in 3830 Western Europeans
Upper bound frequency estimation	$p = 1 - \alpha^{1/n}$ [12]	0/273	0.011	0/3830	0.0008
	$p = (x+2)/(n+2)$ [1]	0/273	0.007	0/3830	0.0005
	$p = (x+1)/(n+2)$ [11]	0/273	0.004	0/3830	0.0003
Likelihood ratio	$p = 1 - \alpha^{1/n}$ [12] $LR = 1/P$	0/273	91.6	0/3830	1279
	$p = (x+2)/(n+2)$ [1] $LR = 1/P$	0/273	137	0/3830	1916
	$LR = (n+3)/(x+2)$ $p = (x+1)/(n+2)$ [11]	0/273	138	0/3830	1916
Database structure method [17]	None	0/101	392	0/3830	Not calculated as κ unknown

Table 2 $SQ = SK = $ [263G, 340T, 523del, 524del] (quoted as differences to the revised Cambridge Reference Sequence [18])

Method	Sampling correction	Count in Austrian Caucasian database	Result from Austrian Caucasian data	Count in Western European Caucasian database	Result from Western European Caucasian database
Counting method	None	1/273	One matching sequence found in 273 Austrians	1/3830	One matching sequence found in 3830 Western Europeans
Upper bound frequency estimation	$p + \sqrt{(p(1-p)/n)}$ [12]	1/273	0.007	1/3830	0.0005
	$p = (x+2)/(n+2)$ [1]	1/273	0.011	1/3830	0.0008
	$p = (x+1)/(n+2)$ [11]	1/273	0.007	1/3830	0.0005
Likelihood Ratio	$p + \sqrt{(p(1-p)/n)}$ [12] $LR = 1/P$	1/273	137	1/3830	1915
	$p = (x+2)/(n+2)$ [1] $LR = 1/P$	1/273	92	1/3830	1277
	$LR = (n+3)/(x+2)$ $p = (x+1)/(n+2)$ [11]	1/273	92	1/3830	1278
Database structure method [19]	n/a			Not calculated as this method is for previously unobserved haplotypes only	

The Likelihood Ratio Approach

The general formulation of the LR is given in the section "What Constitutes a Match between K and Q". In adopting the LR approach, an estimate of the likelihood of the evidence conditional on K and Q having different maternal origins must come from some estimate of the frequency of the observed sequence in a relevant population. This estimate may be achieved *via* the counting method, or an extension of this method to correct for sampling error as described in the previous section.

The LR approach has the significant advantage of enabling the evidence to be considered as a whole: evaluation of whether or not K and Q match (section "What Constitutes a Match between K and Q") and evaluation of how frequently the sequences occur are weighed against each other, not considered in

isolation. The usefulness of such an approach is best illustrated by examples as follows (updated from [1]):

1. SK and SQ match exactly, and there are no sequences the same or very similar to these in the database. The findings therefore support the proposition that K and Q have the same maternal origin. The counting method, a frequency estimate or a likelihood ratio (corrected for sampling error and distribution of mtDNA types in the population if necessary) could be used to assist the court in assessing the strength of support for this hypothesis.

2. SQ and SK differ by a single, frequently mutating base; neither sequence has previously been observed in the database, but there are other sequences in the database differing by a single base. The findings support the proposition that SQ and SK have a common maternal origin, but

the strength of this support is lower than that in example 1; this reduction is by a factor approximating the substitution rate, plus an additional small reduction to allow for the possibility that one of the similar sequences in the database may have the same maternal origin, albeit invoking an additional mutation.

3. *SQ* and *SK* are identical, both showing a heteroplasmic base at a site not known to be a mutation "hotspot";[a] the sequence (with either base at the heteroplasmic position) has not previously been observed in the database. The findings support the proposition that *Q* and *K* have the same maternal origin; this support is enhanced relative to that in example 1, by a factor approximating the substitution rate at the heteroplasmic base.

4. *SQ* and *SK* differ by a single base at which substitution has previously been observed, but which does not appear to be a mutation "hotspot"; *SQ* has been observed once in a database of 100 sequences, *SK* has not been observed before and there is an additional sequence in the database that differs from *SK* at a mutation "hotspot". There is significant uncertainty surrounding estimates for both the numerator and the denominator, but on balance, the *LR* is not likely to be significantly different to 1 and the result would be reported as inconclusive.

5. *SQ* and *SK* differ at a position that appears from phylogenetic and familial mutation rate estimates to be stable; *SQ* and *SK* have both been observed several times in the database. The findings support the proposition that *Q* and *K* have different maternal origins, and an exclusion is effectively reported.

Methods Not Yet Commonly Adopted

Strength of Evidence Calculation Based on Database Structure (Proportion of Singleton Haplotypes)

Brenner [19] proposed a method for calculating the evidential strength of rare Y chromosome haplotypes; this method is equally applicable to mtDNA evidential strength calculations where the crime sample has a previously unobserved haplotype

$$\Pr(T = SQ) \leq \frac{(1 - \kappa)}{n} \qquad (6)$$

where *T* is the haplotype of an innocent suspect for whom the probability of a chance match is being calculated; *SQ* is the crime scene profile; and *K* is the proportion of samples in the database that are singletons.

Hence, for example in a database where $\kappa = 80\%$,

$$\Pr(T = S) \leq \frac{1}{5n} \qquad (7)$$

which in the simplest case of an exact match between crime scene profile and suspect profile results in a likelihood ratio

$$LR = \frac{1}{\Pr(T = S)} \geq 5n \qquad (8)$$

Thus, as long as the crime sample is added to the database, the *LR* can be significantly greater than the size of the database. Incorporating sampling corrections and development of the method to allow for heteroplasmy and mutation have not yet been reported.

Phylogenetic Method for Calculating Match Probability

A method for evaluating match probabilities, taking into account the genealogical tree, which reflects the ancestral relationships between the sequences in a database has been reported by Wilson *et al.* [20]. This type of model can potentially take account of demographic issues such as population structure, thus avoiding the criticisms of Salas *et al.* [13], who also advocate phylogenetic approaches.

In essence, the coalescent model [21] and models for population growth and subdivision, together with mutation rate information specify the Bayesian prior distributions for the genealogical tree underlying a sample of DNA sequences. Inference about aspects of this tree is on the basis of its posterior distribution, given the observed data.

The authors used Monte Carlo Markov Chain (MCMC) algorithms for the analysis, in which the tree consisted of *n* (database size) +1 (crime scene profile) observed sequences. A new branch connecting an unobserved sequence, *x*, of an alternative possible culprit with an unknown mtDNA sequence with the tree *via* a new node, *z*, was introduced (see Figure 1; from [20]). At each iteration of the algorithm, the probability that the sequence *x* matches *s* was calculated, conditional on the location and state

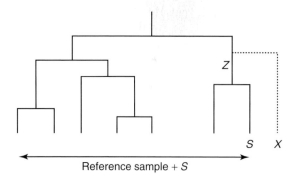

Figure 1 From [20]: Representation of the maternal genealogy of $n = 6$ individuals in an anonymous reference database, together with the suspect, s, and a further individual, x, regarded as an alternative suspect of unknown mtDNA type: the node labeled z corresponds to the most recent woman ancestral to both x and at least one of the other $n = 1$ individuals [Reproduced from Ref.16. © Elsevier, 2005.]

of the node z. The average of these conditional probabilities over 10^5 MCMC outputs approximates the match probability (P_m).

Using this algorithm under the standard coalescent (no population growth or subdivision), this match probability was calculated for the following:

1. the most common haplotype;
2. a haplotype not previously observed, but very similar to the most common haplotype; and
3. a haplotype not previously observed and very different to any observed haplotype.

from a dataset of mtDNA minisequence haplotypes in British Caucasians, Afro-Caribbeans, and Asians [22]. These match probabilities were compared with frequency estimates generated using the counting method amongst $n + 1$ observed sequences, and very similar results were obtained. Counter intuitively the match probability of the dissimilar haplotype in the Afro-Caribbean and Asian datasets was higher than that for the haplotype most similar to the most common haplotype.

The authors concluded that the counting method was usually, although not always, a conservative method. The coalescent model with growth gave similar results, but the model with population splitting was not applied. It would be a profitable area of research for mtDNA interpretation to use similar phylogenetic methods to study the effects of population

substructure and establish the circumstances under which the counting method is not conservative.

Databases

Database Relevance and Availability

The availability of relevant databases is critical to the forensic interpretation of mitochondrial data. Whereas the shuffling of preexisting variants by recombination is the principal source of the discriminating power of autosomal STR multiplexes, mtDNA variation only arises through *de novo* mutation events, which are destined to remain associated with the genetic background of the progenitor molecule. Consequently the frequency of a mitochondrial haplotype cannot be predicted by simple multiplication of the relevant allele frequencies at each polymorphic site as for autosomal STRs, but must be determined by direct observation of the entire haplotype within a database.

The strength of mitochondrial evidence is heavily dependant upon the size of the database, particularly when a novel haplotype is involved; unfortunately the haploid nature of the mitochondrial genome also increases its susceptibility to genetic drift leading to higher F_{st} values and greater variation between geographically and ethnically distinct populations. This in turn necessitates the construction of databases for each subpopulation that may give rise to an evidential sample in order that the appropriate strength of evidence can be derived. Furthermore, the greater cost and complexity of sequencing combined with the difficulty of acquiring samples from the appropriate populations generally means that the available databases are often small or derive from populations that do not faithfully reflect the composition of the potential source gene pool. Many laboratories have little option but to make use of databases from areas outside of their jurisdiction. In cosmopolitan populations, where significant migration over a number of generations is the rule, it is likely that the typically general population databases available are sufficiently representative of the population from which the offender originated. Studies of mtDNA variability within and between European populations have confirmed this trend for most European cosmopolitan populations [23], although the resolution of this analysis would not detect localized differences in, for example, small village populations.

Mitochondrial sequence databases covering differing portions of the genome have been compiled for both forensic and academic purposes typically covering both HVI and HVII regions (e.g., Federal Bureau of Investigation (FBI)/Scientific Working Group on DNA Analysis Methods (SWGDAM): http://www.fbi.gov/hq/lab/fsc/backissu/april2002/miller1.htm [24] & European DNA Profiling Group (EDNAP) mtDNA Population Database (EMPOP): http://www.empop.org [25]); Mitomap: http://www.mitomap.org/ [26]) with a rapidly increasing but still limited number of whole genome sequences becoming available (http://www.genpat.uu.se/mtDB/ [27]). Although it is becoming clear that many highly informative Single Nucleotide Polymorphisms (SNPs) are located within the coding regions and much effort is being applied to detecting these in an efficient way (e.g., [28]), database size and the limited quantities of crime stain material generally confines casework sequencing to the hypervariable regions, which are most likely to discriminate between potential sources. Variant sites are typically recorded as changes from the revised Cambridge Reference Sequence [18] allowing comparisons between databases, but one should note that the span of the regions examined may not correspond precisely between data sets. Phylogenetic studies on the basis of this accumulated data have highlighted great variability in mutation rate, subsequent persistence, and distribution of variation at different bases (e.g., [13–16]). The two hypervariable regions being noncoding have fewer functional constraints and therefore can tolerate the greatest polymorphism; some sites are particularly unstable and are frequently heteroplasmic, including two poly C regions, which are inclined to slippage. Such regions are variable upon many branches of the phylogenetic tree due to recurrent mutation, while many slower mutating sites are polymorphic only in a single lineage.

Knowledge of the phylogenetic relationships between populations on the basis of their patterns of haplogroup sharing has greatly increased our understanding of the complex genetic origins of ethnic subpopulations. Many mitochondrial clades are strongly associated with geographic regions and have been used to trace the migration of humans from Africa to colonize the world. Demographic studies have highlighted several instances in which different patterns of genetic contribution are apparent for females (mtDNA) and males (Y chromosome), this being apparent in many Hispanic populations where the indigenous female contribution is very strong, but much reduced with respect to Y chromosomes, where European origins predominate but the extent to which this is apparent depends on the population being examined [29, 30].

Recent periods of mass migration, either forced or by choice, have greatly altered the mtDNA gene pool of many regions but care must be taken to ensure that databases, which appear to share similar ethnic origins, either from the continent of origin or resulting from dispersals to other parts of the globe, are indeed reliable substitutes. Similarly tribal or caste differences may exist even among indigenous people, which should be accounted for by ensuring that sampling accurately reflects the current composition of the area in question.

Database formats range from simple tables in published papers through to sophisticated online databases. The level of checking prior to publication may also vary from a single automated sequence read per sample through to duplication of sequencing using primers on both strands upon templates derived from separate duplicate extractions or polymerase chain reactions (PCRs) with witnessing of all manual stages. Online databases such as FBI/SWGDAM (http://www.fbi.gov/hq/lab/fsc/backissu/april2002/miller1.htm) and EMPOP (http://www.empop.org) are openly accessible and have been updated with additional samples or corrections as appropriate, indeed the EMPOP database includes the sequence electropherograms to aid confirmation of profile quality and accuracy [31]. Full details of the sample's geographic and ethnic origin are submitted so that its relevance to an enquiry can be fully determined. Furthermore, all potential contributors have to correctly genotype a number of quality control samples before their samples are uploaded and every haplotype is checked using the Network phylogenetic software package (http://www.fluxus-technology.com/) to screen for potential sequencing or transcription errors.

Concerns Regarding Database Quality

A series of publications have used the phylogenetic approach to highlight the likely occurrence of errors in the majority of databases (e.g., [32–34]). While genuine recurrence of mutations at hypervariable positions results in small reticulations within phylogenetic networks in which the temporal order of mutations cannot be determined, when groups of closely spaced variants reoccur on widely separated branches of the network, this has usually provided evidence of artificial recombination resulting from errors during the transcription of data or mix-ups with tubes, which have "recombined" HVI and HVII regions from different individuals [35]. When individual slow-mutating sites show variants on widely separated branches this highlights sequences, which should be checked for accuracy but may in fact be authentic. The majority of errors are thought to occur during transcription of data to the published tables and their frequency is therefore reduced by software packages that reduce the amount of human intervention. Other potential causes include degraded samples in which contaminant DNA overwhelms an unduplicated PCR reaction, or a primer binding site polymorphism, which knocks out amplification of the authentic sequence.

Further sources of error include base shifts in tabulated data, where the positions relative to the revised cambridge reference sequence (rCRS) are incorrect; these can involve shifts of a single base, by several positions (often 10 or 100), or into an adjacent column. Phantom mutations, where unlikely transversions appear in sequences may be owing to transcription errors or problems with the sequencing chemistry, which result in hard to interpret positions [33]. Reference bias, where a change from the rCRS is overlooked and therefore goes unreported, and base mis-scoring when transversions are mis-recorded as the more common transitions also occur frequently (all discussed in detail in [32]). Virtually all of these errors could be avoided by duplication of the sequence using primers on both strands, the independent comparison of these sequences with the reference and their recording in two different formats e.g., motif and dot table, which can subsequently be compared electronically to highlight any discrepancies [31, 34].

As errors have been highlighted by these publications in widely used databases such as the SWG-DAM Mitochondrial DNA Database, much effort has been made to purge these and test what effect they may have had on reports produced with the imperfect data. Budowle *et al.* [36] argue that sequencing errors have largely been eliminated owing to improved chemistries, equipment and software and

the widespread adoption of duplication by forensic laboratories as outlined in International Society for Forensic Genetics (ISFG) guidelines [37]. Using up-to-date casework techniques discrepancies are exceedingly rare demonstrating that these safeguards successfully eliminate the vast majority of potential errors. They also conclude that the impact on reporting is marginal. The likely effect of any error is to create a new haplotype that does not already exist in nature, therefore assuming the error rate is low it merely reduces the true size of the database by the proportion of profiles, which contain errors. Although there is no justification for complacency and every effort should be made to rigorously control and improve the accuracy of databases used in forensics, it is unlikely that the error levels that had existed would have counteracted the conservative allowances that are made for database size.

Database Size

How large should a database be? Clearly this depends on many factors, primarily the diversity within the population. This has been modeled by Pereira *et al.* [38] using samples from a database of 549 individuals from across Portugal in comparison with 1 200 Germans from a single village [39]. While haplotype diversity peaked with samples of 300 in Portugal and 400 in the German sample, the number of haplotypes continued to rise almost linearly. The proportion of Portuguese haplotypes that were unique for HVI declined from around two-thirds when the sample size was 50 to about a third in the full database of 549, while for HVII the decline was much faster from 39.0% to 14.9% as the smaller number of polymorphic sites in this region are subject to a higher rate of recurrent mutation. When both HV regions are considered together the proportion of unique sequences remained above 50% even in the full database and modeling suggests that a sample size in excess of 1 300 would be required to reduce the proportion of novel haplotype observations below 5% among each subsequent addition of 100 samples. Given that the Portuguese population is less diverse than Central Europeans, it is clear that in most instances databases ideally need to number in the thousands before they cease to reveal a substantial number of previously unobserved haplotypes.

Worked Examples

To illustrate the practical impact of using the different interpretation methods and databases described earlier, the methods detailed have been applied to two example sequences, using two databases, both drawn from the EMPOP database: 273 Austrian Caucasians and 3830 Western Europeans. The phylogenetic method was not included, as the algorithms were developed for minisequence data, not full sequence data; computationally, full sequence data are more challenging. Additionally, for the database structure method, only 101 Austrian Caucasians were considered, as the structure of this dataset had previously been published [40].

End Notes

a. Hotspots are regions of the genome (usually single bases or short homopolymeric runs) that have greatly increased mutation rates to the extent that the same mutation is found in several different haplotypic backgrounds due to recurrent mutation.

References

[1] Tully, G., Bär, W., Brinkmann, B., Carracedo, A., Gill, P., Morling, N., Parson, W. & Schneider, P. (2001). Considerations by the European DNA profiling (EDNAP) group on the working practices nomenclature and interpretation of mitochondrial DNA profiles, *Forensic Science International* **124**, 83–91.

[2] Schwartz, M. & Vissing, J. (2002). Paternal inheritance of mitochondrial DNA, *New England Journal of Medicine* **347**, 576–580.

[3] Bandelt, H.-J., Kong, Q.-P., Parson, W. & Salas, A. (2005). More evidence for non-maternal inheritance of mitochondrial DNA? *Journal of Medical Genetics* **42**, 957–960.

[4] Parsons, T.J., Muniec, D.S., Sullivan, K., Woodyatt, N., Alliston-Greiner, R. Wilson, M.R., Berry, D.L., Holland, K.A., Weedn, V.W., Gill, P. & Holland, M.M. (1997). A high observed substitution rate in the human mitochondrial DNA control region, *Nature Genetics* **15**, 363–368.

[5] Sullivan, K.M., Alliston-Greiner, R., Archampong, F.I.A., Piercy, R., Tully, G., Gill, P. & Lloyd-Davies, C. (1996). A single difference In mtDNA control region sequence observed between hair shaft and reference samples from a single donor, *Proceedings of the Seventh International Symposium on Human Identification, Scottsdale (AZ), Promega Corporation*, pp. 126–129.

[6] Wilson, M.R., Polansky, D., Replogle, J., DiZinno, J.A. & Budowle, B. (1997). A family exhibiting heteroplasmy in the human mitochondrial DNA control region

reveals both somatic mosaicism and pronounced segregation of mitotypes, *Human Genetics* **100**, 167–171.

[7] Calloway, C.D., Reynolds, R.L., Herrin, G.L. & Anderson Jr, W.W. (2000). The frequency of heteroplasmy in the HVII region of mtDNA differs across tissue types and increases with age, *American Journal of Human Genetics* **66**, 1384–1397.

[8] Tully, L.A., Parsons, T.J., Steighner, R.J., Holland, M.M., Marino, M.A. & Prenger, V.L. (2000). A sensitive DGGE assay reveals a high frequency of heteroplasmy in hypervariable region one of the human mitochondrial DNA control region, *American Journal of Human Genetics* **67**, 432–443.

[9] Paneto, G.G., Martins, J.A., Longo, L.V., Pereira, G.A., Freschi, A. & Alvarenga, V.L. (2007). Heteroplasmy in hair: differences among hair and blood from the same individuals are still a matter of debate, *Forensic Science International* **173**, 117–121.

[10] Scientific Working Group on DNA Analysis Methods (2003). Guidelines for mitochondrial DNA (mtDNA) nucleotide sequence interpretation, *Forensic Science Communications* **5**, at http://www.fbi.gov/hq/lab/fsc/backissu/april2003/swgdammitodna.htm.

[11] Buckleton, J., Walsh, S. & Harbison, S. (2005). Nonautosomal forensic markers, in *Forensic DNA Evidence Interpretation*, J. Buckleton, C.M. Trigg & S. Walsh, eds, CRC Press, Florida, pp. 299–339.

[12] Holland, M. & Parsons, T. (1999). Mitochondrial DNA sequence analysis – validation and use for forensic casework, *Forensic Science Review* **11**, 21–50.

[13] Salas, A., Bandelt, H.-J., Macaulay, V. & Richards, M.B. (2007). Phylogenetic investigations: the role of trees in forensic genetics, *Forensic Science International* **168**, 1–13.

[14] Galtier, N., Enard, D., Radondy, Y., Bazin, E. & Belkhir, K. (2006). Mutation hotspots in mammalian mitochondrial DNA, *Genome Research* **16**, 215–222.

[15] Gurven, M. (2000). How can we distinguish between mutational "hotspots" and "old sites" in human mtDNA samples? *Human Biology* **72**, 455–471.

[16] Allard, M.W., Polanskey, D., Miller, K., Wilson, M.R., Monson, K.L. & Budowle, B. (2005). Characterization of human control region sequences of the African American SWGDAM forensic mtDNA data set, *Forensic Science International* **148**, 169–179.

[17] Balding, D.J. & Nichols, R.A. (1994). DNA profile match probability calculation: how to allow for population stratification relatedness database selection and single bands, *Forensic Science International* **64**, 125–120.

[18] Andrews, R., Kubacka, I., Chinnery, P., Lightowlers, R., Turnbull, D. & Howell, N. (1999). Reanalysis and revision of the Cambridge reference sequence for human mitochondrial DNA, *Nature Genetics* **23**(2), 147.

[19] Brenner, C. (2006). Evidential strength of a rare haplotype, *Oral presentation at: DNA in Forensics*, 28-30 September, Innsbruck.

[20] Wilson, I.J., Weale, M.E. & Balding, D.J. (2003). Inferences from DNA data: population histories evolutionary processes and forensic match probabilities, *Journal of the Royal Statistical Society A* **166**, 155–201.

[21] Kingman, J.F.C. (1982). The coalescent, *Stochastic Processes and their Applications* **13**, 235–248.

[22] Tully, G., Sullivan, K.M., Nixon, P., Stones, R.E. & Gill, P. (1996). Rapid detection of mitochondrial DNA sequence polymorphisms using multiplex solid-phase fluorescent minisequencing, *Genomics* **16**, 97–159.

[23] Melton, T., Wilson, M., Batzer, M. & Stoneking, M. (1997). Extent of heterogeneity in mitochondrial DNA of European populations, *Journal of Forensic Science* **42**, 437–446.

[24] Monson, K.L., Miller, K.W.P., Wilson, M.R., DiZinno, J.A. & Budowle, B. (2002). The mtDNA Population Database: an integrated software and database resource for forensic comparison, *Forensic Science Communications* http://www.fbi.gov/hq/lab/fsc/backissu/april2002/miller1.htm **4**.

[25] Parson, W., Brandstätter, A., Alonso, A., Brandt, N., Brinkmann, B., Carracedo, A., Corach, D., Froment, O., Furac, I., Grzybowski, T., Hedberg, K., Keyser-Tracqui, C., Kupiec, T., Lutz-Bonengel, S., Mevag, B., Ploski, R., Schmitter, H., Schneider, P., Syndercombe-Court, D., Sørensen, E., Thew, H., Tully, G. & Scheithauer, R. (2004). The EDNAP mitochondrial DNA population database (EMPOP) collaborative exercises: organization results and perspectives, *Forensic Science International* **139**(2–3), 215–226.

[26] Ruiz-Pesini, E., Lott, M.T., Procaccio, V., Poole, J.C., Brandon, M.C. & Mishmar, D. (2007). An enhanced MITOMAP with a global mtDNA mutational phylogeny, *Nucleic Acids Research* **35**(Database issue), D823–D828.

[27] Ingman, M. & Gyllensten, U. (2006). mtDB: Human Mitochondrial Genome Database a resource for population genetics and medical sciences, *Nucleic Acids Research* **34**(Database issue), D749–D751.

[28] Coble, M.D., Vallone, P.M., Just, R.S., Diegoli, T.M., Smith, B.C. & Parsons, T.J. (2006). Effective strategies for forensic analysis in the mitochondrial DNA coding region, *International Journal of Legal Medicine* **120**, 27–32.

[29] Allard, M.W., Polanskey, D., Wilson, M.R., Monson, K.L. & Budowle, B. (2006). Evaluation of variation in control region sequences for Hispanic Individuals in the SWGDAM mtDNA data set, *Journal of Forensic Science* **51**(3), 566–573.

[30] Hammer, M.F., Chamberlain, V.F., Kearney, V.F., Stover, D., Zhang, G. & Karafet, T. (2006). Population structure of Y chromosome SNP haplogroups in the United States and forensic implications for constructing Y chromosome STR databases, *Forensic Science International* **164**(1), 45–55.

[31] Brandstatter, A., Niederstatter, H., Pavlic, M., Grubwieser, P. & Parson, W. (2007). Generating population data for the EMPOP Database – An overview of the mtDNA sequencing and data evaluation processes considering 273 Austrian control region sequences as example, *Forensic Science International* **166**, 164–175.

[32] Bandelt, H.J., Lahermo, P., Richards, M. & Macaulay, V. (2001). Detecting errors in mtDNA data by phylogenetic analysis, *International Journal of Legal Medicine* **115**, 64–69.

[33] Brandstatter, A., Sanger, T., Lutz-Bonengel, S., Parson, W., Beraud-Colomb, E. & Wen, B.J. (2005). Phantom mutation hotspots in human mitochondrial DNA, *Electrophoresis* **26**(18), 3414–3429.

[34] Salas, A., Carracedo, C., Macaulay, V., Richards, M. & Bandelt, H.-J. (2005). A practical guide to mitochondrial DNA error prevention in clinical forensic and population genetics, *Biochemical and Biophysical Research Communications* **335**, 891–899.

[35] Bandelt, H.J., Salas, A. & Lutz-Bonengel, S. (2004). Artificial recombination in forensic mtDNA population databases, *International Journal of Legal Medicine* **118**(5), 267–273.

[36] Budowle, B., Polanskey, D., Allard, M.W. & Chakraborty, C. (2004). Addressing the use of phylogenetics for the identification of sequences in error in the SWGDAM Mitochondrial DNA Database, *Journal of Forensic Science* **49**(6), 1256–1261.

[37] Bär, W., Brinkmann, B., Budowle, B., Carracedo, A., Gill, P. & Holland, M. (2000). DNA Commission of the International Society for Forensic Genetics: guidelines for mitochondrial DNA typing, *International Journal of Legal Medicine* **113**(4), 193–196.

[38] Pereira, L., Cunha, C. & Amorim, A. (2004). Predicting sampling saturation of mtDNA haplotypes: an application to an enlarged Portuguese database, *International Journal of Legal Medicine.* **118**, 132–136.

[39] Pfeiffer, H., Forster, P., Ortmann, C. & Brinkmann, B. (2001). The results of an mtDNA study of 1200 inhabitants of a German village in comparison to other Caucasian databases and its relevance for forensic casework, *International Journal of Legal Medicine* **114**, 169–172.

[40] Parson, W., Parsons, T.J., Scheithauer, R. & Holland, M.M. (1998). Population data for 101 Austrian Caucasian mitochondrial DNA d-loop sequences: application of mtDNA sequence analysis to a forensic case, *International Journal of Legal Medicine* **111**, 124–132.

Related Articles

Databases

Mitochondrial DNA: Profiling

Short Tandem Repeats

GILLIAN TULLY AND JON WETTON

Mitochondrial DNA: Profiling

Introduction

Mitochondrial deoxyribonucleic acid (mtDNA) analysis is a routine adjunct to crime scene investigation. Introduced in the early 1990s to aid with the identification of military remains, and implemented since then by the Armed Forces DNA Identification Laboratory in Rockville, Maryland, in all military conflicts [1], it was first used in criminal justice proceedings by the FBI in 1996 in *Tennessee v. Paul William Ware* [2]. In that case, a single hair located in the throat of a victim linked Ware to a homicide. MtDNA provides a valuable locus for forensic DNA typing in certain circumstances, especially for skeletal remains, shed hairs, or hair fragments, and degraded samples of all types. In general, it is used when short tandem repeat (STR) testing is not possible owing to limited or degraded nuclear DNA because mtDNA is naturally abundant and resistant to degradation [3]. MtDNA cannot be a unique identifier, as can nuclear DNA, due to its pattern of maternal inheritance, nor does it have the statistical power of a nuclear DNA match; as such, it is used as supplementary circumstantial evidence in criminal cases. MtDNA analysis has played a large role in the identification of missing persons when applied to skeletal remains.

Mitochondrial DNA Biology

Deoxyribonucleic acid (DNA) is found in two locations in all human cells except red blood cells (*see* **DNA**). Nuclear deoxyribonucleic acid (nuDNA), inherited from both parents, makes up 26 pairs of chromosomes in the nucleus. Mitochondrial deoxyribonucleic acid (mtDNA), inherited only from the mother, is located in the mitochondria, small, peanut-shaped cytoplasmic organelles that generate cellular energy. The full complement of nuDNA has about 3 billion of the four chemical bases of DNA (adenine, guanine, thymine, and cytosine, abbreviated as A, G, T, and C; also known as *nucleotides*) in a linear array within the chromosomes. Human mtDNA contains approximately 16 569 nucleotides in a small circular molecule. Whereas each cell contains two copies of nuDNA, there are hundreds to thousands of mtDNA molecules within dozens to hundreds of mitochondria per cell, depending on the particular tissue. With some exceptions, all tissues in an individual are homogeneous for the single mtDNA type, or sequence, of DNA nucleotides in that individual's mtDNA molecules.

The mtDNA types, sequences, or "profiles" present among humans have been generated by mutational changes occurring in this DNA over many generations. All living humans can be linked by their profiles into a single large tree and share a common maternal ancestor; those individuals with similar types are most closely clustered in the tree. MtDNA reflects the biogeographical ancestry of a particular maternal lineage. For example, certain types may be readily recognizable as having originated in Asia, Africa, or Europe. MtDNA is passed intact from a mother to all her children; males inherit their mother's mtDNA but do not pass it on to their children. For this reason, all maternally related individuals share the same mtDNA profile.

The natural abundance of mtDNA is the key to its forensic utility. MtDNA recovery from small or degraded biological samples is greater than nuDNA recovery owing to the high copy number (there are many mitochondria in a cell, but one nucleus) and because the molecule's small circular structure may protect it from damage by heat, humidity, acidity, and ultraviolet (UV) light. In addition, nuDNA in naturally shed hairs and hair shafts is extremely limited even when these samples are freshly collected [4].

The mtDNA molecule codes for 13 proteins, two ribosomal RNAs, and 22 transfer RNAs, and also contains a 1122 bp "non-coding" region, sometimes called *the control region* or *D-loop*, which is forensically informative [5]. The DNA sequence differs so much among individuals in two "hypervariable" sections of the control region that the likelihood of choosing two people at random with the same mtDNA sequence is very low [6]. About 8–12 nucleotide differences would be observed between two maternally unrelated individuals for the regions that are analyzed, comprised of DNA sequence about 700 bp long [7].

Candidates for forensic mtDNA typing analyses are as follows: (i) shed hairs with no follicle, tissue, or root bulb attached, (ii) hair shaft fragments, (iii) bones or teeth that have been subjected to long periods of high acidity, high temperature, or high humidity, (iv) stain or swab material that has been unsuccessfully typed for nuDNA markers, and (v) tissue (skin, muscle, organ) that has been unsuccessfully typed for nuDNA markers. While mtDNA typing of blood, semen, and saliva crime scene stains from clothing and floors is possible, it is likely that mixtures will be obtained due to the extreme sensitivity of this form of typing in samples that, unlike hairs and bones, are difficult to clean before DNA extraction. On the other hand, degraded samples collected from near-sterile or UV radiation–exposed surfaces, such as the exterior of a vehicle, may easily provide single-source mtDNA profiles.

The Analytical Process

An mtDNA analysis begins when total genomic DNA is extracted from biological material such as a tooth, blood sample, or hair. Extraction methods, such as grinding of hair or bone or complete dissolution of proteinaceous material are designed and validated in order to optimize the yield of DNA for specific sample types. In addition, the external surfaces of samples are thoroughly cleaned via sanding with a rotary drill bit (for bones) or ultrasonic water baths (for hairs). Approximately 2 cm of a single hair is used in the average case, though success has been achieved with much less; for skeletal remains, approximately 0.1–0.5 g of bone is used [8, 9].

Following extraction, the polymerase chain reaction (PCR) is used to amplify the two hypervariable portions of the noncoding region using flanking primers. Primers are small bits of DNA that identify and hybridize to or adhere to the ends of the region one wishes to PCR amplify, therefore targeting a region for amplification. Primer pairs have been designed and manufactured to encompass virtually any region of mtDNA in humans, and may include "mini-primer pairs" that can recover the smallest fragments of DNA from a degraded sample, usually under 150 bp in length [10] (see also **DNA: Degraded Samples**).

Because the natural abundance of mtDNA as well as the creation of PCR product introduces many copies of mtDNA into the laboratory, care is taken to eliminate the introduction of exogenous (contaminating) DNA during both the extraction and amplification steps by methods such as the use of prepackaged sterile equipment and reagents, aerosol-resistant barrier pipette tips, gloves, masks, and lab coats, separation of pre- and post-amplification areas in the lab using dedicated reagents for each, ultraviolet irradiation of equipment, and autoclaving of tubes and reagent stocks. In forensic casework, questioned samples are processed at different times than known samples and in different laboratory rooms. Most importantly, several negative controls that would indicate the presence of contamination introduced during testing are run in parallel with all samples. Overall, contamination is more of a concern for the mtDNA laboratory than the nuclear DNA laboratory, but each laboratory determines through internal validation studies how contamination and its control, detection, and interpretation can impact casework and still result in a defensible outcome [11].

When adequate amounts of PCR product are amplified from the two hypervariable regions, as determined from either a yield gel or other detection method, sequencing reactions are performed. These chemical reactions use each PCR product as a template to create a new complementary strand of DNA in which some nucleotides are labeled with dye. The strands created at this stage are then separated according to size by an automated sequencer that uses a laser to "read" the sequence. Where possible, the sequences of both hypervariable regions (called *HV1* and *HV2*) are determined on both strands of the double-stranded DNA molecule and in overlapping PCR products, with sufficient redundancy to confirm the nucleotide sequence that characterizes that particular sample.

Two forensic analysts independently assemble the mtDNA sequence and then compare it to a standard published reference sequence called *the revised Cambridge Reference Sequence* (rCRS, [12, 13]), denoting all the nucleotide differences. The entire process is then repeated with a known sample, usually blood, saliva, or a buccal swab, collected from a known individual. The sequences from both samples, about 780 nucleotides each, are compared to determine if they match. Depending on data quality or ambiguities, portions of the analysis may be repeated.

Heteroplasmy

Heteroplasmy is defined as the presence of two or more types of mtDNA within an individual

[14]. There are two forms of heteroplasmy: length heteroplasmy and site (or sequence) heteroplasmy. The baseline state of mtDNA composition in humans, with the exception of individuals with tissue-specific mitochondrial diseases, is homoplasmy. That is, the overwhelming majority of mtDNA-containing cells within an individual contain the same 16 569 bp mtDNA molecule throughout. The exception to this dominant state of uniformity is the frequent occurrence of length heteroplasmy in certain control region strings of cytosine residues ("C-stretches"), which creates populations of mtDNA molecules in each cell that differ slightly in length. Length heteroplasmy occurs in about 50% of all individuals. Site or sequence heteroplasmy, where at a single nucleotide address there are two different DNA bases such as T and C, has been observed in approximately 1% of blood samples and 10–15% of hair samples, with other tissues such as bone believed to be intermediate with respect to frequency. Some degree of heteroplasmy exists in all individuals; precisely how detectable and abundant it is becomes the focus of the forensic DNA practitioner. Guidelines are derived from each laboratory's validation studies to allow for conservative interpretations of heteroplasmy such that false failures to exclude cannot occur when it is present.

Interpretation

The FBI's Scientific Working Group on DNA Analysis Methods (SWGDAM) Guidelines for mtDNA Nucleotide Sequence Interpretation ((http://www.fbi.gov/hq/lab/fsc/backissu/april2003/swgdammitodna.htm) state:

> The following guidelines may be used in most cases:
>
> - Exclusion
>   If there are two or more nucleotide differences between the questioned and known samples, the samples can be excluded as originating from the same person or maternal lineage.
>
> - Inconclusive
>   If there is one nucleotide difference between the questioned and known samples, the result will be inconclusive.
>
> - Cannot Exclude
>   If the sequences from questioned and known samples under comparison have a common base

at each position or a common length variant in the HV2 C-stretch, the samples cannot be excluded as originating from the same person or maternal lineage.

In the event of a "cannot exclude" result, the SWGDAM mtDNA database (http://www.fbi.gov/hq/lab/fsc/backissu/april2002/miller1.htm) is searched for the mitochondrial sequence that has been observed for the samples. At present, the SWGDAM database of human mtDNA sequences has around 5000 sequences available for a search of a casework sequence, but an increase to over 10 000 samples is expected within one to two years. The current convention in the event of a failure to exclude is for the analyst to report the number of times the observed sequence is present in the database in order to estimate its relative frequency in the population. A frequency statistic is calculated, and a 95 or 99% confidence interval is placed around the estimated frequency to account for the inherent uncertainty in the frequency calculation since one would never be able to type all living humans [1]. This convention of using the upper-bound frequency provides a very conservative approach to estimating how many individuals at most would be expected to have a particular type. For example, a novel type (one that has not been observed previously in the database) would be estimated to occur at most in 6 in 10 000 individuals based on the size of the database currently being used.

While around 60% of all mtDNA types appear to be rare (occurring a single time) in each of the FBI's ethnic sub-databases (individuals claiming to be African or of African origin, Asian or of Asian origin, Caucasian or of European origin, or Hispanic), there is one mtDNA sequence that is seen in around 7% of Caucasians. Interestingly, the frequency of this type has remained fairly stable as the database has grown over the last 10 years. However, almost two-thirds of the newly typed samples have novel sequences; therefore, all the mtDNA variation present in the general human population has not yet been identified. One exception to the high diversity that is present within ethnic databases has been observed: due to founder effects, mtDNA diversity in native Americans is limited, and certain types in this group are observed at high frequencies [15].

In addition to the SWGDAM database, over 20 000 human mtDNA control region sequences have been characterized by anthropologists and forensic scientists (see the many references to human mtDNA populations that have been studied at http://www.mitomap.org/, as well as [16]). In general, the pattern observed in most populations around the world, with the exception of some populations of anthropological interest, is that most of the sequences are uncommon, and few types are present at frequencies greater than 1%. Because of this fact, it is possible to exclude greater than 99% of a population as potential contributors of a sample in most cases, except where one is dealing with a more common type. In contrast, a multilocus nuclear DNA typing profile provides vastly superior discriminatory power and statistics that permit source attribution. For this reason, mtDNA can never provide the resolution of individuality that nuDNA typing can.

As mentioned above, mtDNA is maternally inherited, so that any maternally related individuals would be expected to share the same mtDNA sequence. This fact is useful in cases where a long deceased or missing individual is not available to provide a reference sample but any living maternal relative might do so. Because of meiotic recombination and the diploid (biparental) inheritance of nuDNA, the reconstruction of a nuDNA profile from even first-degree relatives of a missing individual is rarely this straightforward. This feature has allowed some important historical mysteries to be solved, such as the identification of the remains of the assassinated Romanov family [17], the Vietnam Unknown Soldier [18], and American outlaw gunfighter Wild Bill Longley [19]. However, the maternal inheritance pattern of mtDNA might also be considered problematic. Because all individuals in a maternal lineage share the same mtDNA sequence, mtDNA cannot be considered a unique identifier. In fact, apparently unrelated individuals might share an unknown maternal relative at some distant point in the past. For this reason, it is important that judges, attorneys, and juries in criminal proceedings are educated about the maternal inheritance pattern of mtDNA.

Nonforensic Uses

While mtDNA is useful for forensic examinations, it has also been used extensively in two other major scientific realms. First, there are a number of serious inherited diseases caused by deleterious mutations in gene-coding regions of the mtDNA molecule [20]. In addition, molecular anthropologists have been using mtDNA for three decades to examine both the extent of genetic variation in humans and the relatedness of populations all over the world [21]. An mtDNA maternal inheritance pattern can reveal ancient population histories, which might include migration patterns, expansion dates, and geographic homelands. MtDNA has been recovered from several Neanderthal skeletons, and the resulting population genetics studies have allowed anthropologists to conclude that modern humans do not share a close relationship with Neanderthals in the human evolutionary tree [22]. The general methods for performing all mtDNA analyses, including forensic methods, are identical to those used in molecular biology laboratories all over the world for studying DNA from any living organism. There are several thousand published articles on mtDNA available at http://www.mitomap.org/.

Laboratory Practices

MtDNA analysis is offered by the FBI in their Quantico facility as well as in four regional laboratories. Several private commercial labs also offer testing, as do the Armed Forces DNA Identification Lab, University of North Texas Health Science Center, Office of the Chief Medical Examiner in New York, and California Department of Justice. Most, if not all, of these laboratories are guided in application of mtDNA analysis by federal Quality Assurance Standards for DNA testing and various accrediting bodies.

MtDNA matching has become an extremely valuable resource for the FBI's National Missing Person DNA Database program. Under this program, maternal relatives submit samples for typing and inclusion to the database for eventual comparison to profiles obtained from recovered skeletal remains.

Although mtDNA is still undergoing admissibility hearings in some jurisdictions, several hundred cases have been litigated in over one-half of the United States since 1996. All convictions in which mtDNA has played a role have been upheld at the appellate level (*see also Frye v. United States*). For more information on court cases and appellate decisions, see http://www.denverda.org/DNA/Mitochondrial_DNA_Legal_Decisions.htm.

A complete tutorial on mtDNA is available online at http://dna.gov/training/otc/ through the President's DNA Initiative. This course was specifically developed for officers of the court.

References

[1] Holland, M.M. & Parsons, T.J. (1999). Mitochondrial DNA sequence analysis – validation and use for forensic casework, *Forensic Science Reviews* **11**, 21–50.

[2] Davis, C.L. (1998). Mitochondrial DNA: State of Tennessee v. Paul Ware, *Profiles in DNA* **1**, 6–7.

[3] Budowle, B., Adams, D.E., Comey, C.C. & Merrill, C.R. (1990). Mitochondrial DNA: a possible genetic material suitable for forensic analysis, in *Advances in Forensic Sciences*, H.C. Lee & R.E. Gaensslen, eds, Year Book Medical Publishers, Chicago, IL, pp. 76–97.

[4] Wilson, M.R., Polanskey, D., Butler, J., DiZinno, J.A., Replogle, J. & Budowle, B. (1995). Extraction, PCR amplification and sequencing of mitochondrial DNA from human hair shafts, *Biotechniques* **18**, 662–669.

[5] Taanman, J.-W. (1999). The mitochondrial genome: structure, transcription, translation, and replication, *Biochimica et Biophysica Acta* **1410**, 103–123.

[6] Vigilant, L., Stoneking, M., Harpending, H., Hawkes, K. & Wilson, A.C. (1991). African populations and the evolution of human mitochondrial DNA, *Science*, **253**, 1503–1507.

[7] Budowle, B., Wilson, M.R., DiZinno, J.A., Stauffer, C., Fasano, M.A., Holland, M.M. & Monson, K.L. (1999). Mitochondrial DNA regions HVI and HVII population data, *Forensic Science International* **103**, 23–35.

[8] Melton, T. & Nelson, K. (2005). Forensic mitochondrial DNA analysis of 691 casework hairs, *Journal of Forensic Sciences* **50**, 73–80.

[9] Nelson, K. & Melton, T. (2007). Forensic mitochondrial DNA analysis of 116 casework skeletal samples, *Journal of Forensic Sciences* **52**, 557–561.

[10] Gabriel, M.N., Huffine, E.F., Ryan, J.H., Holland, M.M. & Parsons, T.J. (2001). Improved mtDNA sequence analysis of forensic remains using a "mini-primer set" amplification strategy, *Journal of Forensic Sciences* **46**, 247–253.

[11] Carracedo, A., Bär, W., Lincoln, P., Mayr, W., Morling, N., Olaisen, B., Schneider, P., Budowle, B., Brinkmann, B., Gill, P., Holland, M., Tully, G. & Wilson, M. (2000). DNA Commission of the International Society for Forensic Genetics: guidelines for mitochondrial DNA typing, *Forensic Science International* **110**, 79–85.

[12] Andrews, R.M., Kubacka, I., Chinnery, P.F., Lightowlers, R.N., Turnbull, D.M. & Howell, N. (1999). Reanalysis and revision of the Cambridge Reference Sequence for human mitochondrial DNA. *Nature Genetics* **23**, 147.

[13] Anderson, S., Bankier, A.T., Barrell, B.G., de Bruijn, M.H.L., Coulson, A.R., Drouin, J., Eperon, I.C. Nierlich, D.P., Roe, B.A., Sanger, F., Schreier, P.H., Smith, A.J.H., Staden, R. & Young, I.G. (1981). Sequence and organization of the human mitochondrial genome, *Nature* **290**, 457–465.

[14] Melton, T. (2004). Mitochondrial DNA heteroplasmy, *Forensic Science Reviews* **16**, 1–20.

[15] Budowle, B., Allard, M.W., Fisher, C.L., Isenberg, A.R., Monson, K.L., Stewart, J.E.B., Wilson, M.R. & Miller, K.W.P. (2000). HVI and HVII mitochondrial DNA data in Apaches and Navajos, *International Journal of Legal Medicine* **116**, 212–215.

[16] Parson, W., Brandstätter, A., Alonso, A., Brandt, N., Brinkmann, B., Carracedo, A., Corach, D., Froment, O., Furac, I., Grzybowski, T., Hedberg, K., Keyser-Tracqui, C., Kupiec, T., Lutz-Bonengel, S., Mevag, B., Ploski, R., Schmitter, H., Schneider, P., Syndercombe-Comb, D., Sorensen, E., Thew, H., Tully, G. & Scheithauer, R. (2004). The EDNAP mitochondrial DNA population database (EMPOP) collaborative exercises: organisation, results, and perspectives, *Forensic Science International* **139**, 215–226.

[17] Gill, P., Ivanov, P.L., Kimpton, C., Piercy, R., Benson, N., Tully, G. Evett, I., Hagelberg, E. & Sullivan, K. (1994). Identification of the remains of the Romanov family by DNA analysis, *Nature Genetics* **6**, 130–135.

[18] Daoudi, Y., Morgan, M., Diefenbach, C., Ryan, J., Johnson, T., Conklin, G., Duncan, K., Smigielski, K., Huffine, E., Rankin, D., Mann, R., Holland, C., McElfresh, K., Canik, J., Armbrustmacher, V. & Holland, M. (1998). Identification of the Vietnam Tomb of the Unknown Soldier: the many roles of mitochondrial DNA, in *Proceedings of the Ninth International Symposium on Human Identification*. Promega Corporation, Scottsdale, AZ.

[19] Owsley, D.W., Ellwood, B.B. & Melton, T. (2006). Search for the grave of William Preston Longley, hanged Texas gunfighter, *Historical Archaeology* **40**, 50–63.

[20] Wallace, D.C., Brown, M.D. & Lott, M.T. (1999). Mitochondrial DNA variation in human evolution and disease, *Gene* **238**, 211–230.

[21] Stoneking, M. (1990). Mitochondrial DNA variation and human evolution, in *Human Genome Evolution*, M. Jackson, T. Strachan & G. Dover, eds, BIOS Scientific Publishers, Oxford, pp. 263–281.

[22] Krings, M., Stone, A., Schmitz, R.W., Krainitzki, H., Stoneking, M. & Pääbo, S. (1997). Neandertal DNA sequences and the origin of modern humans, *Cell* **90**, 1–12.

TERRY MELTON

Mixture Interpretation: DNA

Introduction

A mixed DNA profile is obtained when two or more contributors provided biological material to an evidentiary sample that has been analyzed. Here, only routine STR analysis techniques will be considered. With a STR profile, the presence of a mixture becomes obvious when more than two alleles are detected at a given locus.

DNA mixture interpretation is a complex and contentious field. There are a number of unsettled issues in the interpretation of mixtures and current methods, while adequate, leave clear room for improvement. In this section, we will outline current methods for interpretation and also highlight those areas where further research would benefit our science.

The primary division in modern interpretation methods lies between those who seek to

1. extract from the mixed DNA profile, when feasible, a single (unmixed) profile of interest and report it using the statistical techniques used for single stain calculation (*see* **Short Tandem Repeats: Interpretation**);
2. report an exclusion probability (often termed *random man not excluded* (RMNE) or *combined power of exclusion* (CPE)); and
3. report a likelihood ratio.

Much discussion has occurred debating these points, with views often very strongly held. This is unusual as the pros and cons of each method are well known and little new information has been added to the debate in recent years.

The peak heights present in mixtures are assumed to be approximately proportional to the amount of DNA from each contributor, and there is considerable empirical evidence for this. However, the correlation is only approximate and may be affected by degradation, stutter, and stochastic effects. The larger of two contributors is termed the *major contributor* and is assumed to be the source of the largest peaks. The smaller contributor is termed the *minor*. In a three-person mixture, the contributors may be present in quantities described by the terms *major, minor,* and *trace*.

It is also possible that two contributors are present in approximately equal proportion. In such cases, the mixture may be termed a $1:1$ mixture.

Treating the Mixture as a Single Stain

If the profile in question is a clear major minor and the major is the profile of evidential interest, then it is acceptable to interpret the mixture as if it was an unmixed stain as long as care is taken regarding a potential factor of 2. Consider the situation where the stain may be explained as mixture of the suspect as the major and an unknown minor then under the defense hypothesis two unknowns are required to explain the mixture. In such cases, the unmixed stain calculation will err in favor of the prosecution by a factor of 2. This is known as the *Whitaker effect* [1–4].

Random Man Not Excluded

A frequentist method in common use is often termed *Random Man not Excluded*. In its simplest implementation it gives the probability that a random man has both his alleles contained within the mixture. Hence, for a mixture that shows the alleles abc and d the genotypes aa, ab, ac, ad, bb, bc, bd, cc, cd, and dd are not excluded.

Formally, if the mixture has alleles $A_1 \ldots A_n$ then the exclusion probability at locus l, (PE_l) is $PE_l = 1 - \left(\sum_{i=1}^{n} p(A_i) \right)^2$ if Hardy–Weinberg equilibrium is assumed. By writing $\sum_{i=1}^{n} p(A_i) = p$, we can obtain $PE_l = 1 - p^2$. If Hardy–Weinberg equilibrium is not assumed, Budowle gives $PE_l = 1 - \left(\sum_{i=1}^{n} p(A_i) \right)^2 - \theta \sum_{i=1}^{n} p(A_i) \left(1 - \sum_{i=1}^{n} p(A_i) \right)$. We can write this as $PE_l = 1 - p^2 - \theta p(1 - p)$. The use of the equivalent of NRC II recommendation 4.1 [5] leads to $PE_l = 1 - p^2 - \theta \sum_{i=1}^{n} p_i (1 - p_i)$, which differs slightly. The PE across multiple loci (PE) is calculated as $PE = 1 - \prod_l (1 - PE_l)$.

The advantages of such an approach are that

1. it does not assume a number of contributors;
2. it can report a statistic for mixtures that are lower quality than reportable under an LR approach; and
3. it is easier to explain.

Extensions to this approach essentially use judgment or a set of rules to generate a list of possible unknown genotypes. The assumptions used to generate this list may include assuming a number of contributors and a conditioning profile. Once the list of possible genotypes is generated, the combined probability of inclusion (CPI, the complement of CPE) is generated by summing the estimated probabilities of the included genotypes. RMNE is assigned as 1-CPI. Typically, the genotype probabilities are estimated using the product rule but this is not a requirement.

There is a debate at the adequacy of using RMNE as a meaningful statistics (see EFS entry by Balding). If we agree that a balanced and fair assessment of the evidence is only achieved through the use of a likelihood ratio, hence by addressing the evidence both under H_p and H_d, then RMNE statistics does not represent an appropriate expression of the weight of evidence. This is because (i) the numerator is not assessed and (ii) the proposition for the denominator implies a loose concept of a random man and the evidence is assessed without taking into account of the profile of the suspect at hand.

Likelihood Ratio-Based Approaches

The first stage in the development of a likelihood ratio for mixtures is the establishment of the two hypotheses. Even using sublevel 1 hypotheses (see EFS entry by this can be problematic and requires the use of judgment and an awareness of the case circumstances [6–11]). Issues include, but are not restricted to

- assigning a number of contributors and
- determining whether any contributors can be safely assumed to be present under both the prosecution and defense hypotheses. Contributors that are assumed to be present are termed *conditioning* contributors.

One of the more common two person mixtures is one that can be explained as containing the DNA of the suspect and the complainant. In such a case, the hypotheses may be

H_p: the DNA in the crime stain is from the suspect and the complainant and

H_d: the DNA in the crime stain is from an unknown person and the complainant.

In this case, the conditioning contributor is the complainant. The unknown person is termed *the unknown*.

If E is used to represent the DNA results obtained in the case, then the LR is $p(E|H_p)$ divided by $p(E|H_d)$.

Assigning the Number of Contributors

Assignment of the number of contributors is undertaken from the number of alleles observed with some attention paid to peak balances. The number of alleles per locus is an important parameter but it should not be the only criterion used [12, 13]. It is important to have an understanding of stuttering and of genetic phenomena such as trisomy, gene duplication, and somatic mutation [4]. Mixtures where an evidential profile is sufficiently low in peak height that dropout may have occurred should be treated as low-template profiles. Hence most of the discussion here will assume that dropout is not an issue (for more information on such artifacts, see EFS entry on low template DNA).

Typically, the number of contributors is assigned as the minimum number required to explain the mixed profile. Hence a profile containing at most two alleles per locus is assigned as containing one contributor unless peak balances suggest that a second contributor is present. A profile containing at most four alleles per locus is assigned as a two-person mixture. Profiles containing five or more alleles are termed *higher order mixtures*.

Interpretation of higher order mixtures can be problematic but is simplified if conditioning contributors may be assumed and if one profile is clearly a major contributor. If it cannot be simplified, it is advised to refrain from undertaking any calculation.

Once the number of contributors is assigned, the hypotheses generated and the presence of any conditioning contributors determined that the next step is to list the possible genotypes for any unknown contributors. This may be achieved either considering peak height or not.

Considering Only Qualitative Data

If no consideration is to be made of peak height, then the methods of Weir *et al.*, Fung and Hu, and Curran *et al.* return the likelihood ratio either utilizing the product rule (Weir *et al.*), NRC II recommendation

4.1 (Fung and Hu) or recommendation 4.2 (Curran *et al.*) [14–20].

Although LR computation varies in function of the propositions involved, this discussion can be pursued on the basis of a case with a two-person mixture that can be explained as containing a complainant and a suspect (H_p) or as the complainant and an unknown person (H_d). The arguments can be extended without loss of generality to other pairs of propositions. In this case, the LR is always in the form of one divided by the sum of the random match probabilities for the collection of all the possible genotypes for the unknown person. The summation under the denominator assessment implies an equally weighted contribution for each potential genotype. This is justified by the fact that the model explicitly does not take into account peak areas.

The Curran *et al.* method is embodied in the software DNAMIX II and is suitable for casework use. It does not take account of peak heights and cannot handle dropout. Since it does not utilize all the available information it has the expected performance of understating the evidence if H_p is true and overstating it if H_d is true. Recall that this is the expected performance of any method that does not utilize all the available evidence. Certain rules based on peak height may be applied to identify those situations where the approach may be nonconservative and appropriate action may then be taken. This is especially true when the peak areas would suggest that a combination of the designated contributors is not supported if the H_p is true. By default, the above methods assign a probability of 1 to the numerator of the likelihood ratio and concentrate on the estimation of the denominator. That default value may not always be supported by the data.

Beecham and Weir (in draft) have developed a method to add a sampling uncertainty consideration to the method of Curran *et al.* [14] This approach is embodied the software DNAMIX III (available at http://statgen.ncsu.edu/~gwbeecha/).

The work by Fung and Hu [19] led also to the development of dedicated software, also in case involving relatives [21] (available at http://www.hku.hk/statistics/EasyDNA/).

Considering Peak Heights

If peak heights are to be considered then the list of possible unknown genotypes is modified by eliminating those combinations that are expected to give a poor fit to the peak heights. Consider the situation where we have a conditioning profile, say the complainant, who has genotype ab. The peak heights $a = 1000, b = 2000, c = 1000$ are very unlikely if the unknown contributor is genotype ac. Hence the genotype ac is eliminated as a possibility for the unknown. This elimination process may proceed by the judgment of an experience caseworker or according to a set of rules. One set of such rules has been published [22] and is embodied in the software suite Fss-I[3]. Three types of rules are typically used on the basis of (i) expected peak imbalance, (ii) expected mixing proportion between the two contributors, and (iii) expected allelic dropout. Currently, appropriate treatments have been given to two-person mixtures only. In this case, the LR is on the form of one divided by the sum of the random match probabilities for the collection of all the genotypes for the unknown person that have passed the rules.

The situation where a minor evidential profile is present in an assumed two-person mixture and dropout is possible can be handled by careful application of judgment or the rules. Typically, possibilities for the unknown are expanded to include one or two unobserved alleles. The possibility of two unobserved alleles returns a likelihood ratio of 1 for this locus and is not always conservative (see the recent case against Garside and Bates [23]). The possibility of one unobserved allele is typically handled using the $2p$ rule [24] or its subpopulation corrected variants. However, any profile where dropout is possible is really low-template DNA (LTDNA) and the LTDNA style of interpretation should be applied [25].

Once the set of possible unknown genotypes has been determined the likelihood ratio may be developed using either the product rule or one of the subpopulation correction options (see EFS entry by Balding). The approaches outlined above are commonly referred to as *binary*, because the decision on accepting or rejecting a given combination amount to assign a weight of 1 or 0 in the likelihood ratio calculation. It is not a full probabilistic approach as early advocated by Evett, Gill and Lambert [26] and continued by Perlin and Szabady [27], but it constitutes a promising step toward it. However, the use of a binary model should be undertaken having in mind a clear understanding of its limits. As mentioned for the techniques not involving peak areas, the analyst needs to make sure that the genotype of the suspect is the best supported option (taking into account peak areas) under the numerator proposition and that all reasonable genotypes are included in the denominator [28, 29].

Standard

There has been a substantial move amongst the European Network of Forensic Science Institutes toward setting standards for interpretation of mixtures, see [28, 30].

Issues in Mixture Interpretation

Currently, there are a number of areas in DNA mixture interpretation, which are under active research. This includes methods to handle the uncertainty in the number of contributors, dealing with dropout, automation of the process, and a more effective use of the peak height information. Of particular interest is the research involving Bayesian networks that may bring intuitive ways to handle the complexity of mixture interpretation [31].

References

[1] Evett, I.W. (1987). On meaningful questions: a two-trace transfer problem, *Journal of the Forensic Science Society* **27**, 375–381.

[2] Triggs, C.M. & Buckleton, J. (2003). The two trace transfer problem revisited, *Science and Justice* **43**(3), 127–134.

[3] Meester, R. & Sjerps, M. (2003). The evidential value in the DNA database search controversy and the two-stain problem, *Biometrics* **59**(3), 727–732.

[4] Buckleton, J.S., Triggs, C.M. & Walsh, S.J. (2004). *DNA Evidence*, CRC Press, Boca Raton.

[5] NRC_II (1996). *National Research Council Committee on DNA Forensic Science, The Evaluation of Forensic DNA Evidence*, National Academy Press, Washington, DC.

[6] Cook, R., Evett, I.W., Jackson, G., Jones, P.J. & Lambert, J.A. (1998). A hierarchy of propositions: deciding which level to address in casework, *Science and Justice* **38**(4), 231–240.

[7] Cook, R., Evett, I.W., Jackson, G., Jones, P.J. & Lambert, J.A. (1999). Case pre-assessment and review in a two-way transfer case, *Science and Justice* **39**(2), 103–111.

[8] Cook, R., Evett, I.W., Jackson, G., Jones, P.P. & Lambert, J.A. (1998). A model for case assessment and interpretation, *Science and Justice* **38**(3), 151–156.

[9] Cook, R., Evett, I.W., Jackson, G. & Rogers, M. (1993). A workshop approach to improving the understanding of the significance of fibres evidence, *Journal of the Forensic Science Society* **33**(3), 149–152.

[10] Evett, I.W., Gill, P.D., Jackson, G., Whitaker, J. & Champod, C. (2002). Interpreting small quantities of DNA: the hierarchy of propositions and the use of Bayesian networks, *Journal of Forensic Sciences* **47**(3), 520–530.

[11] Evett, I.W., Jackson, G. & Lambert, J.A. (2000). More on the hierarchy of propositions: exploring the distinction between explanations and propositions, *Science & Justice* **40**(1), 3–10.

[12] Buckleton, J.S., Curran, J.M. & Gill, P. (2007). Towards understanding the effect of uncertainty in the number of contributors to DNA stains, *Forensic Science International Genetics* **1**(1), 20–28.

[13] Paoletti, D.R., Doom, T.E., Krane, C.M., Raymer, M.L. & Krane, D.E. (2005). Empirical analysis of the STR profiles resulting from conceptual mixtures, *Journal of Forensic Sciences* **50**, 1361–1366.

[14] Curran, J.M., Triggs, C.M., Buckleton, J.S. & Weir, B.S. (1999). Interpreting DNA mixtures in structured populations, *Journal of Forensic Sciences* **44**(5), 987–995.

[15] Weir, B.S., Triggs, C.M., Starling, L., Stowell, L.I., Walsh, K.A.J. & Buckleton, J.S. (1997). Interpreting DNA mixtures, *Journal of Forensic Sciences* **42**(2), 213–222.

[16] Evett, I.W. & Weir, B.S. (1998). *Interpreting DNA Evidence – Statistical Genetics for Forensic Scientists*, Sinauer Associates, Sunderland.

[17] Evett, I.W., Buffery, C., Willott, G. & Stoney, D.A. (1991). A guide to interpreting single locus profiles of DNA mixtures in forensic cases, *Journal of the Forensic Science Society* **31**(1), 41–47.

[18] Fung, W.K. & Hu, Y.Q. (2000). Interpreting DNA mixtures based on the NRC-II recommendation 4.1, *Forensic Science Communications* **2**(4), http://www.fbi.gov/programs/lab/fsc/backissu/oct2000/fung.html.

[19] Fung, W.K. & Hu, Y.Q. (2001). The evaluation of mixed stains from different ethnic origins: general result and common cases, *International Journal of Legal Medicine* **115**, 48–53.

[20] Fung, W.K. & Hu, Y.Q. (2002). The statistical evaluation of DNA mixtures with contributors from different ethnic groups, *International Journal of Legal Medicine* **116**, 79–86.

[21] Hu, Y.Q. & Fung, W.K. (2003). Evaluating forensic DNA mixtures with contributors of different structured ethnic origin: a computer software, *International Journal of Legal Medicine* **117**(4), 248–249.

[22] Bill, M., Gill, P., Curran, J., Clayton, T., Pinchin, R., Healy, M. & Buckleton, J. (2005). PENDULUM – a guideline based approach to the interpretation of STR mixtures, *Forensic Science International* **148**, 181–189.

[23] R. v Garside and Bates, (2006). *EWCA Crim 1395*, Royal Courts of Justice, London.

[24] Buckleton, J. & Triggs, C.M. (2006). Is the 2p rule always conservative? *Forensic Science International* **159**, 206–209.

[25] Gill, P., Whitaker, J.P., Flaxman, C., Brown, N. & Buckleton, J.S. (2000). An investigation of the rigor of interpretation rules for STR's derived from less that 100 pg of DNA, *Forensic Science International* **112**(1), 17–40.

[26] Evett, I.W., Gill, P.D. & Lambert, J.A. (1998). Taking account of peak areas when interpreting mixed DNA profiles, *Journal of Forensic Sciences* **43**(1), 62–69.

[27] Perlin, M.W. & Szabady, B. (2001). Linear mixture analysis: a mathematical approach to resolving mixed DNA samples, *Journal of Forensic Sciences* **46**(6), 1372–1377.

[28] Gill, P., Brown, R.M., Fairley, M., Lee, L., Smyth, M., Simpson, N., Irwin, B., Dunlop, J., Greenhalgh, M., Way, K., Westacott, E.J., Ferguson, S.J., Ford, L.V., Clayton, T. & Guiness, J. (2008). National recommendations of the technical UK DNA working group on mixture interpretation for the NDNAD and for court going purposes, *Forensic Science International: Genetics* **2**(1), 76–82.

[29] Clayton, T.M. & Buckleton, J.S. (2004). Mixtures, in *Forensic DNA Evidence Interpretation*, CRC Press, Boca Raton, pp. 217–274.

[30] Gill, P., Brenner, C.H., Buckleton, J.S., Carracedo, A., Krawczak, M., Mayr, W.R., Morling, N., Prinz, M., Schneider, P.M. & Weir, B.S. (2006). DNA commission of the international society of forensic genetics: recommendations on the interpretation of mixtures, *Forensic Science International* **160**, 90–101.

[31] Cowell, R.G., Lauritzen, S.L. & Mortera, J. (2008). Probabilistic modelling for DNA mixture analysis, *Forensic Science International: Genetics Supplement Series* **1**(1), 640–642.

JOHN S. BUCKLETON

M'Naghten Standard of Insanity *see* Insanity: Defense

M'Naghten's Rule *see* Behavioral Science Evidence

Modeling: Fire *see* Fire Modeling and Its Application in Fire Investigation

Modeling: Trauma Causation in Vehicle Accidents *see* Trauma Causation: Analysis of Automotive

Molestation *see* Child Sexual Abuse Accommodation

Morphogenesis of Fingerprints *see* Friction Ridge Skin: Morphogenesis and Overview

MtDNA *see* Mitochondrial DNA: Profiling

Multiple Personalities *see* Dissociative Disorders

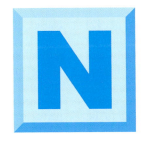

Narcoanalysis *see* Deception: Truth Serum

Narcotics: Amphetamine *see* Amphetamine

Narcotics: Benzodiazepines *see* Benzodiazepines

Narcotics: Cannabis *see* Cannabis

Narcotics: Cocaine *see* Cocaine

Narcotics: Opiods *see* Opioids

Natural Causes of Sudden Death: Noncardiac

Respiratory

Pneumonia

Prior to the discovery of antibiotics, one-third of all people who developed pneumonia subsequently died from the infection. Until the introduction of antibiotics, pneumonia was the most common cause of death in the United States and, perhaps, worldwide. Since the advent of antibiotics, the situation has changed radically.

More often than not, pneumonia-related deaths do not occur quickly. Respiratory and/or systemic symptoms and signs are often present before death occurs. Occasionally, the forensic pathologist may be confronted with cases of sudden unexpected death (SUD), which are the sequel of a fulminant course of a previously undiagnosed pneumonia.

Children represent a special population; in a series of 265 autopsies of children with SUD, the main cause was disease of the respiratory system (total 113 cases, 42.6%, included lobular pneumonia (28.3%), aspiration pneumonia (24.8%), and viral pneumonia (16.8%). The high predominance of respiratory deaths is probably explained by the relative immaturity of children's lungs, and the fact that the body's resistance is reduced [1].

Many cases of SUD in infancy can be adequately explained after performing a careful postmortem examination (*see* **Autopsy**). Vennemann *et al.* [2] reported that, in Germany, 2910 infants died in 2004, and of these 394 babies died suddenly and unexpectedly. The authors of that report investigated a three-year population-based, case–control study, in Germany (1998–2001). A total of 455 deaths were reviewed and 51 (11.2%) were found to be unexplained. Most of these deaths were due to respiratory or generalized sepsis, and, of course, a number of different viruses and bacteria have been suggested as causative agents of sudden infant death syndrome (SIDS), though this connection has never been conclusively established.

Bacterial Pneumonia

Acute bacterial infection of the lungs is still one of the commonest causes of death, especially in the very young and very old, but often its presence is due to the existence of some other secondary to some other debilitating process. For example, bacterial pneumonia is a major cause of morbidity and mortality among transplant recipients.

The onset of bacterial pneumonia varies from sudden to gradual. The patient experiences shaking chills, high fever, sweating, shortness of breath, chest pain, and a cough that produces thick, greenish or yellow phlegm. Acute respiratory insufficiency and/or severe sepsis may cause death in these subjects [3]. And, while there are case reports describing rapid symptom progression, SUD from pneumonia is rare [4, 5].

Some evidence for respiratory tract infection is common among infants dying suddenly. For example, Lin reported that in his autopsy series of sudden infant death, 28.3% of the decedents had lobular pneumonia [1]. Epidemiologic evidence indicates that SIDS is associated with *Bordetella pertussis* infection. Nicoll and Gardner [6] examined postperinatal infant deaths resulting from respiratory causes and SIDS. All these cases occurred in England and Wales between 1968 and 1984; they estimated an excess mortality rate for undiagnosed pertussis of 460–700 deaths. Similarly, Cherry calculated 362 excess infant deaths caused by pertussis [7]. Data from Sweden and Norway indicate a direct correlation between the incidence of pertussis and the occurrence of SIDS [8]. In another study, Heininger *et al.* [9] enrolled 254 infants with SUDs; an autopsy diagnosis of SIDS was made in 76% of the infants. In the remaining subjects,

causes of death were respiratory or other infections (14%), congenital anomalies or organ failures (4%), aspiration (2%), or accidents or traumatic events (4%). During a standardized autopsy, nasopharyngeal specimens and tracheal specimens were obtained for polymerase chain reaction (PCR) assays to detect B pertussis. PCR results were positive for B pertussis for 12 case subjects (5.1%) (all with SIDS or respiratory infections).

Generally, bronchopneumonia and pneumonia are characterized by widespread patchy areas of inflammation that begin as a widely dispersed bronchitis and bronchiolitis; focal areas of pneumonia then develop in the centers of the acini. The consolidated areas are generally larger and more numerous in the lower lobes where they may be several millimeters across. Small beads of yellow mucous can often be expressed from the bronchioles on the cut surface of the lung. In severe cases, patches of consolidation may become confluent. Once the bacteria reach the alveoli they elicit an acute inflammation, with copious exudation of fluid and migration of neutrophils into the alveoli [10]. In lobar pneumonia (as in the case of pneumococcal infection), the changes are uniform throughout the affected lobe.

Viral Pneumonia

Half of all cases of pneumonia are believed to be caused by viruses. More viruses are being identified as the cause of respiratory infection, and though most attack the upper respiratory tract, some produce pneumonia, especially in children. Most cases of viral pneumonia are mild and get better without treatment, but some cases are more serious and require hospitalization. People at risk for more serious viral pneumonia typically have impaired immune systems such as people with HIV, transplant patients, young children (especially those with heart defects), the elderly, and those that immunocompromised for whatever reason.

Viral pneumonia is caused by several different viruses, including influenza, parainfluenza, adenovirus, rhinovirus, herpes simplex virus, respiratory syncytial virus, hantavirus, and cytomegalovirus. The initial symptoms of viral pneumonia are the same as influenza symptoms: fever, dry cough, headache, muscle pain, and weakness. Increasing breathlessness may also occur; fever may be present. Viral pneumonia may be complicated by an invasion of bacteria, with all the typical symptoms of bacterial pneumonia. Sometimes the clinical course is quite uneventful and viral infection only recognized with the occurrence of SUD.

Cases of fatal varicella pneumonia have been described in adult patients [11–13]. Fatal influenza infection can be caused by influenza pneumonia alone, by respiratory complications caused by bacterial superinfection [14], or by extrapulmonary influenza-associated manifestations such as myocarditis or encephalopathy. Complication rates of influenza infection, as well as for all the other virus infections, are highest in immunosuppressed patients, diabetics or individuals with other severe metabolic illnesses, and people older than 65 years. Case reports of fatal, sudden death due to influenza pneumonia have been described in the literature [14, 15].

Many viral infections may result in life-threatening complications in healthy children and many cases of a SUD of children due to viral pneumonia have been reported [16–20].

It can become difficult to unequivocally diagnose the underlying disease, especially if incipient stages and/or general infections are involved. Interstitial pneumonia, as caused by viruses, is defined histologically, but in its early stages the changes can be nonspecific; detection of the virus would therefore be required to verify the diagnosis [21, 22]. In viral pneumonia, the lungs appear bulky, and may be hyperemic (overfilled with blood). Bloodstained, frothy fluid oozes freely from the cut surface. Areas of hemorrhage are present and may be extensive. The mucosa of the bronchial tree is very hyperemic. The histological pattern is characterized by interstitial pneumonitis, with extensive alveolar collapse, and filling of remaining alveoli with fluid and desquamated epithelial cells. Alveolar epithelial damage is common in viral pneumonia; it causes the formation of hyaline membranes [10].

Mycoplasma Pneumonia

The vast spectrum of diseases caused by *Mycoplasma pneumoniae* includes pharyngitis, sinusitis, tracheobronchitis, pneumonia, myocarditis, pancreatitis, hepatitis, arthritis, and meningoencephalitis. Such infections are generally benign and often run a sub-clinical course; it is estimated that less than 5% of the cases of mycoplasma pneumonia are severe enough to require admission to a hospital. A very small number of fatal sudden mycoplasma pneumonia cases have been reported [23, 24].

Mycoplasma pneumonia generally produces widespread bronchiolitis and interstitial pneumonia similar to that caused by many respiratory viruses. The bronchiolitis sometimes progresses to epithelial ulceration. Lymphocytic infiltration of the walls of alveolar ducts and alveoli characterizes the interstitial pneumonia while edema fluid, red blood cells, and macrophages are found in many groups of alveoli and some alveoli may contain hyaline membranes [10].

Acute Interstitial Pneumonitis

A particular form of interstitial pneumonia is acute interstitial pneumonitis (AIP), a fulminant disease culminating in acute respiratory failure and often death. First described by Hamman and Rich [25], AIP is a life-threatening respiratory disease of unknown cause that occurs in patients of both genders equally; generally, it occurs in previously healthy people with no significant medical history. Patients report a prodromal (before main symptoms) illness lasting several days with fever, nonproductive cough, malaise, followed by the acute onset of progressive shortness of breath, which rapidly evolves to respiratory failure. Other signs and symptoms that may be present include cyanosis, crackles, wheezing, hemoptysis, diaphoresis, and hypotension [26, 27]. The radiological and histological patterns are those of acute respiratory distress syndrome (ARDS); however, AIP differs from ARDS because, in the former, there is an absence of known inciting events and multiorgan failure does not occur. While mortality in all patients with ARDS has decreased over the years, there have been no analogous reports of an improvement in survival rates for patients with AIP; in every reported series, the hospital mortality has been >50% [28].

We have previously reported a fatal case of AIP in a 15-year-old boy with sudden death [29]. The postmortem diagnosis was made on the basis of the convergence of clinical onset and course, anatomical, pathological, and radiological findings, as well as the exclusion of each known cause of ARDS, in particular infections, confirmed by negative results of microbiological analysis, and of immunohistochemical and laboratory tests for the detection of more common respiratory virus.

The exact pathogenesis of AIP remains a mystery; thus, the diagnosis of AIP remains a diagnosis of exclusion. The differential diagnosis includes infectious pneumonia, ARDS, drug-induced lung disease, acute pancreatitis, congestive heart failure (CHF), connective-tissue disease, and other acute forms of interstitial lung disease.

The histological features of AIP, as seen in open lung biopsies or autopsies, are those of diffuse alveolar damage (DAD), a nonspecific pattern of acute lung injury deriving from numerous causes, which shows both epithelial and endothelial injury. Histological lung examination generally shows the typical findings of DAD: alveolar septa mildly thickened by edema and capillary congestion, alveolar edema, hyaline membranes lining the denuded alveolar walls, hyperplastic Type 2 pneumocytes, alveolar infiltrates of polymorphonuclear neutrophilic leukocytes, pigmented macrophages, monocytes and plasma cells, and fibrin thrombi in small arteries.

Thromboembolism

Thromboembolism encompasses two interrelated conditions that are part of the same spectrum, deep venous/vein thrombosis (DVT) and pulmonary embolism (PE). Obstruction of blood flow to one or more arteries of the lung occurs when a thrombus lodged in a pulmonary vessel breaks free and travels to the lung. Almost all clinically important PEs are the result of a DVT occurring in the deep veins of the lower extremities, proximal to and including the popliteal veins. However, emboli also can originate from the pelvic veins, the inferior vena cava, and even the upper extremities. PE and thromboembolic disease represent major health problems worldwide. The diagnosis is often difficult to establish and is frequently missed. De Bakey [30] published a review after critical evaluation of more than 375 000 postmortem cases and more than 3 000 000 clinical cases of PE that had been reported around the world over the preceding half a century. He concluded that there was great confusion over true incidence of PE. Fifty years later, the true incidence of thromboembolic disease is still not known [31].

Risk factors for venous thromboembolism include patients age, surgery, trauma, hospital or nursing home confinement, active malignant neoplasm with, or without, concurrent chemotherapy, central vein catheterization or transvenous pacemaker,

prior superficial vein thrombosis, varicose veins, and neurological disease with extremity paresis. Compared to residents in the community, hospitalized residents have over a 150-fold increased incidence of acute venous thromboembolism. Those hospitalized for medical illness and those hospitalized for surgery account for cases of thromboembolism in almost equal proportions. The incidence in nursing home residences independently accounts for over one-tenth of all venous thromboembolism diseases in the community. The risk among surgery patients can be further stratified on the basis of patients age, type of surgery, and the presence of active cancer. The incidence of postoperative venous thromboembolism is increased for surgery patients who are 65 years of age or older. High-risk surgical procedures include neurosurgery, major orthopedic surgery of the leg, thoracic, abdominal or pelvic surgery for malignancy, renal transplantation, and cardiovascular surgery. Active cancer accounts for almost 20% of all cases of venous thromboembolism occurring in the community. The risk appears to be higher for patients with pancreatic cancer, lymphoma, malignant brain tumors, cancer of the liver, leukemia, and colorectal and other digestive cancers. Prior superficial vein thrombosis is an independent risk factor for subsequent DVT or PE, remote from the episode of superficial thrombophlebitis. Long-haul (>6 h) air travel is associated with a slightly increased risk for venous thromboembolism. Among women, additional risk factors for venous thromboembolism include oral contraceptive use and hormone therapy, pregnancy, and the postpartum period. Other conditions associated with venous thromboembolism include heparin-induced thrombocytopenia, myeloproliferative disorders (especially polycythemia rubra vera and essential thrombocythemia), intravascular coagulation and fibrinolysis/disseminated intravascular coagulation (ICF/DIC), nephrotic syndrome, paroxysmal nocturnal hemoglobinuria, thromboangitis obliterans (Buerger's disease), thrombotic thrombocytopenic purpura, Bechet's syndrome, systemic lupus erythematosis, inflammatory bowel disease, homocystinuria, and possibly hyperhomocysteinemia [32]. Heart failure is another well-known risk factor for thromboembolism.

The spectrum of disease produced by thromboembolism ranges from clinically unsuspected or clinically unimportant to massive embolism causing death. Untreated acute proximal DVT accounts for clinical PE in 33–50% of patients. Mortality in untreated PE is approximately 30%: about one-third of PE cases are fatal. Data indicate that more than one half of all cases of thromboembolism remain undiagnosed. The clinical diagnosis of pulmonary thromboembolism is notoriously inaccurate, with many cases either wrongly diagnosed (overdiagnosed) or missed (underdiagnosed). Autopsy is still regarded as the diagnostic gold standard (*see* **Autopsy**). The accuracy of antemortem diagnosis of PE is within the range of just 10–30% [31]. DVT and PE are very often undiagnosed in life, especially in children dying SUDs.

The prevalence of PE at autopsy varies widely in different published autopsy series, from not less than 10% in unselected material [33]; in 20% of all hospitalized patients [34]; in 20–60% of adult autopsies [35]; in more than half of all autopsies [36]; in about 10% of adults who die suddenly in hospital [37]; approximately 3.5% of all hospital deaths [38]; 1% in the general population of hospital patients; and 30% in patients dying after severe burns, trauma, or fractures [39]. The incidence of PE at autopsy is strongly influenced by the nature of the population surveyed (age and nature of patients, i.e., surgical, oncological, gerontological), by the mode of selection for postmortem examination and, in particular, by the care with which the autopsy is performed [31].

At autopsy, gross examination will reveal embolus in the main pulmonary vascular tree; segmental or subsegmental pulmonary arteries are affected in most of the cases and are more prevalent in nonfatal pulmonary thromboembolism (PTE). On the other hand, emboli in the main arteries, as well as in arteries of the trunk and above, are more prevalent in fatal PTE. Pulmonary infarctions that appear as dark areas where the air space has become filled with blood are frequently seen. They are commonly multiple.

Thrombosis of the deep leg veins is often detected at gross examination as the source of embolism. However, the absence of thrombus from these veins does not exclude them as the site of thrombosis since dislodgement and embolization may leave no residual disease.

Amniotic Fluid Embolism

Amniotic fluid embolism (AFE) is a rare but potentially fatal complication of pregnancy with an incidence approximately between 1 in 8000 and 1 in 80 000 pregnancies. The first reported case of AFE was documented in 1926 [40]. It was first recognized as a syndrome in 1941, when two investigators described the presence of fetal mucin and squamous cells during postmortem examination of the pulmonary vasculature in women who had unexplained obstetric deaths [41]. Since then, many studies, case reports, and series have been published in an attempt to elucidate the etiology, risk factors, and pathogenesis of this obstetric complication [42].

The true incidence of AFE is not known. There are many reasons for this. Firstly, there are a number of inaccuracies in reporting the cause of maternal death. Secondly, the presentation can be variable and the number of nonfatal or subclinical episodes is unclear. Finally, in those patients who do survive or in whom no autopsy was performed, it is often quite difficult to confirm the diagnosis [43]. AFE is one of the leading causes of death during labor and the first few postpartum hours, and it remains a deadly, unpreventable, and unpredictable obstetric emergency. Recent data suggest mortality rates approach 61%. Most patients do not survive the initial course and die within five days. Of those patients who survive, neurologic impairment is common [44]. Other authors refer an associated mortality rate up to 90% [45]. The fetal mortality rate, although better than the maternal rate, is a dismal 21%. Fifty percent of the surviving neonates experience permanent neurological injury. Predisposing factors traditionally associated with AFE include placental abruption, uterine overdistention, fetal death, trauma, tumultuous or oxytocin-stimulated labor, multiparity, advanced maternal age, and rupture of membranes. However, in numerous demonstrated cases of AFE, none of these conditions or demographic characteristics were present [46].

The syndrome appears to be initiated after maternal intravascular exposure to fetal material that is contained in the amniotic fluid. Many hypotheses have been proposed to explain the pathophysiology of this condition. Clark *et al.* [47] contend that AFE more closely resembles an anaphylactic reaction to fetal debris than an embolic event, and they propose the term *anaphylactoid syndrome of pregnancy*. Recently, bradykinin, released in association with DIC, has been considered as an important contributor to the severe hypotension that is manifested with AFE [48, 49]. The literature also contains evidence that AFE may not be a true embolic event resulting from the physical obstruction of the pulmonary vasculature. The high degree of variability in symptoms, the lack of characteristic findings on radiological exam, the absence of a dose–response effect on symptoms, and the occasional occurrence of coagulopathies are not entirely consistent with a physical block to the circulation, at least not as the main mechanism of disease. An alternative hypothesis is that fetal antigen leaking into the maternal circulation might activate the complement cascade. This rare immune response may be initiated by an obscure pathological antigen, or by common antigens presented uncommonly – in amount, timing, or frequency of entry into the maternal circulation [50, 51].

Presenting symptoms may vary; common clinical features include shortness of breath, altered mental status followed by sudden cardiovascular collapse, DIC, and maternal death.

The entry criteria in the National Registry for AFE [47] include

1. acute hypotension or cardiac arrest;
2. acute hypoxia, defined as dyspnea, cyanosis, or respiratory arrest;
3. coagulopathy, defined as laboratory evidence of intravascular consumption or fibrinolysis or severe clinical hemorrhage in the absence of other explanations;
4. onset during dilatation and evacuation, labor, cesarean delivery, or within 30 min postpartum;
5. absence of any other significant confounding condition or potential explanation for the signs and symptoms observed.

Although labor and delivery appear to be the greatest risk period [52], AFE has been reported in the second trimester and as having a delayed presentation [53], up to 36 h postpartum [54].

The diagnosis of AFE is very difficult even at autopsy (see **Autopsy**; **Histology**). It is a commonly held misconception that the presence of fetal debris in the pulmonary circulation is diagnostic of an amniotic fluid embolus. In fact, fetal debris can be found in the pulmonary circulation in a predominance of patients who underwent a normal labor, and AFE is only identified in 78% of those patients who meet the criteria for the diagnosis of AFE [43, 47, 55].

Some authors have suggested that AFE may be the result of anaphylactic reactions to fetal antigens, and that the major part of this clinical syndrome

is the result of mast cell degranulation followed by the release of histamine, tryptase, and other mediators. It has been suggested that the identification and distribution of mast cell tryptase within the pulmonary tree is a useful criteria for the diagnosis of fatal AFE. In a previous report, Fineschi *et al.* [56] demonstrated a numerical increase of pulmonary mast cells in the subjects who died of AFE compared with that of the control groups. Many other reports add further supporting evidence to the concept of AFE as an anaphylactoid syndrome of pregnancy [57–59].

Macroscopic autopsy findings in AFE are usually insignificant; neither are macroscopic findings generally found either. Postmortem diagnosis is based on histological demonstration of amniotic fluid components (fetal squames, lanugo, and mucin) in pulmonary blood vessels that can be demonstrated by various staining methods (Alcian blue, Attwood). Evaluation of pulmonary mast cell tryptase using immunohistochemistry as well as measurement of serum tryptase level as markers of mast cell degranulation are recommended in all cases of suspected AFE-related death.

Morbid Obesity

Obesity and overweight are defined as an accumulation of excess body fat, to an extent that may impair health. A crude population measure of excess fat is the body mass index (BMI), a person's weight (in kilograms) divided by the square of his or her height (in meters). WHO defines overweight as a BMI of 25 or more, and obesity as a BMI of 30 or greater. Obesity is a complex pathological condition that affects virtually all age and socioeconomic groups and threatens to overwhelm both developed and developing countries. WHO's latest projections indicate that globally, in 2005, approximately 1.6 billion adults (age 15+) were overweight, and that at least 400 million adults were obese. WHO further projects that by 2015, approximately 2.3 billion adults will be overweight and more than 700 million will be obese. At least 20 million children under the age of 5 years were overweight globally in 2005. Contrary to conventional wisdom, the obesity epidemic is not restricted to industrialized societies; in developing countries, it is estimated that over 115 million people suffer from obesity-related problems.

Overweight and obesity lead to serious health consequences. Risk increases progressively as BMI increases. In fact, there is evidence that, on a population level, the risk of chronic disease increases progressively as average BMI increases above 21. Obesity is associated with numerous comorbidities such as cardiovascular disease (CVD), Type 2 diabetes, hypertension, certain cancers, and sleep apnea [60]. A relationship exists between BMI and all-cause mortality also in adolescence [61]. In conclusion, the mortality associated with untreated morbid obesity is significant, manyfold that of the normal population and exceeds the risk of surgical intervention [62].

Even in the absence of comorbidity, when adipose tissue accumulates in excess, a variety of adaptations/alterations in cardiac structure and function occur, as do changes in metabolism [63], Obesity may affect the heart through its influence on known risk factors such as dyslipidemia, hypertension, glucose intolerance, inflammatory markers, obstructive sleep apnea/hypoventilation, and the prothrombotic state, as well as through yet-unrecognized mechanisms. As a whole, overweight/obesity predisposes, or is at least associated with, numerous cardiac complications such as coronary heart disease (CHD), heart failure, and sudden death through its impact on the cardiovascular system (*see* **Cardiac and Natural Causes of Sudden Death**).

Obese subjects have an increased risk of arrhythmias and sudden death, even in the absence of cardiac dysfunction, and the risk of sudden cardiac death with increasing weight is seen in both genders. In the Framingham study, the annual sudden cardiac mortality rate in obese men and women was estimated to be ≈ 40 times higher than the rate of unexplained cardiac arrest in a matched nonobese population.

Moreover, a prolonged QT_c interval was observed in $\approx 30\%$ of subjects with impaired glucose tolerance, and there is a positive association between BMI and QT_c. When visceral obesity or insulin levels increase, sympathovagal balance may be the best explanation for changes in QT_c. The clinical significance of obesity-associated QT prolongation and the mechanisms involved remain speculative. Moreover, because extremely obese patients often have a dilated cardiomyopathy, fatal arrhythmias may be the most frequent cause of death [61]. In conclusion, subjects with morbid obesity have high rates of sudden, unexpected cardiac deaths and the literature is rich in reports of cases of SUD in morbidly obese subjects [64–66].

Hematological Disorders

Hemoglobinopathies

Hemoglobinopathy is a type of genetic defect that results in abnormal structure of one of the globin chains of the hemoglobin molecule. The most common hemoglobinopathy is sickle-cell disease (SCD). In the United States today, 1 of every 650 African-Americans (0.15%), greater than 50 000 individuals, suffers from sickle-cell disease. In addition, almost 2 million patients, representing 8% of the African-American population, are affected by sickle-cell trait being heterozygous for the sickle-cell gene [67].

The most common causes of death in the sickle-cell population include infection/sepsis, acute chest syndrome (ACS) (clinical term defined by new pulmonary infiltrate on chest radiography, accompanied by fever, chest pain, and variety of respiratory symptoms, including wheezing, coughing, and tachypnea), sudden cardiac death, cerebrovascular accident, and renal failure. Among all reported causes of death in sickle-cell disease, age-specific patterns are well documented. In sickle-cell infants and children, sepsis, predominantly pneumococcal, represents a leading cause of death, followed by acute splenic sequestration. In the adult sickle-cell population, mortality is much more commonly associated with ACS, sickle-cell pain crises, and/or cardiac failure [68–70].

More than 20% of sickle-cell patients develop fatal acute or chronic pulmonary complications. The acute pulmonary sequelae, including ACS, thromboembolism, lung edema, fat/bone marrow embolism, and vaso-occlusive crisis, account for a large proportion of sudden deaths among sickle-cell patients [71, 72]. In a recent report on 306 autopsies of patients with sickle-cell disease, the most common cause of death for all sickle variants and for all age groups was infection (33–48%). The terminal infection was heralded by upper respiratory tract syndromes in 72.6% and by gastroenteritis in 13.7%. The most frequent portal of entry in children was the respiratory tract but, in adults, it was a site of severe or chronic organ injury. Other causes of death included stroke 9.8%, therapy complications 7.0%, splenic sequestration 6.6%, pulmonary emboli/thrombi 4.9%, renal failure 4.1%, pulmonary hypertension (PHT) 2.9%, hepatic failure 0.8%, massive hemolysis/red cell aplasia 0.4%, and left ventricular failure 0.4% [73].

Sudden and unexpected death in this population is not rare [74]; Manci *et al.* reported that death was frequently sudden and unexpected (40.8%) or occurred within 24 h after presentation (28.4%), and was usually associated with acute events (63.3%) [73]. Darbari *et al.* [75] reported that leading circumstances of death in 141 autopsies of adult SCD included PHT (26.2%), renal failure (22.6%), infection (18.4%), thromboembolism (14.9%), cardiac diagnoses (12.0%), cirrhosis (11.3%), pneumonia or ACS (9.9%), bleeding (7.8%), and iron overload (7.0%); in 23.4% of cases, death was sudden.

In sickle-cell disease, sudden death frequently occurs during exertion and is characterized by rhabdomyolysis, heat stroke, and cardiac arrhythmia; this entity has been widely reported in literature where many cases of sudden death associated with sickle-cell disease or sickle-cell trait have been described in affected soldiers during military basic training, in athletes during training, and in previous healthy subjects during exertion [76–83].

Military recruits, pilots, and subjects exposed to hypoxic stress such as high altitude, and experiencing sudden cardiorespiratory collapse as a result of sickle-cell trait have been described [84].

Many hypotheses have been offered to explain the high rate of sudden death in SCD. Involvement of autonomic nervous dysfunction in sudden death has been reported in various diseases and it has been suggested that this may be the case in sickle-cell anemia as well [85]. Heat stress, dehydration, viral illness, and poor physical conditioning have all been identified as factors, which may contribute to exertional rhabdomyolysis and sudden death in SCD, suggesting a multifactorial etiology [80]. Dehydration, hypoxia, acidosis, and physical exertion are known aggravating factors for sudden death in sickle-cell trait, because that can initiate a vaso-occlusive sickle-cell crisis. Others have proposed a role for some coexisting disease such as diabetes [86].

Of particular interest to the forensic pathologist, illicit drug use, especially cocaine and morphine, both of which are recognized triggers of global hypoxic events, may lead to the sickling of red blood cells, with consequent vaso-occlusion and lung edema has been and, in fact, such a sequence has been reported as explaining a case of sudden death [87].

Only few autopsy studies of sickle-cell patients have addressed patterns of pathologic pulmonary involvement that are very often recognizable in SCD [70, 88, 89]. When pulmonary involvement is present, it is usually in the form of PHT, first detected at autopsy with various grade of changes (from reversible to irreversible), consisting in mild-to-severe medial hypertrophy and muscularization of pulmonary arterioles. The lungs from many of these individuals manifest intimal fibroelastosis of small- and medium-sized pulmonary arteries. Small muscular arteries can show dilatation and may form plexiform lesions. Cardiomegaly may be also present. In Graham's study [67], almost two-third of the cases had significant pulmonary findings at autopsy (71.4%). The most frequent postmortem pulmonary findings were pulmonary edema (47.6%), followed by thromboembolism (38.1%), fat emboli (33.3%), PHT, grades I–IV (33.3%), and microvascular vaso-occlusive thrombi (28.5%). Oppenheimer and Esterly found autopsy evidence of pulmonary thromboemboli in 66%.

In conclusion, data from literature indicate a high rate of occurrence of pulmonary findings (fat embolism, PHT, and cardiac right ventricular hypertrophy) in a large percentage of SDC patients presenting with sudden death. Histological examination may reveal widespread vaso-occlusive sickling of red blood cells in the brain, heart, liver, kidneys, adrenal glands, thyroid gland, intramyocardial coronary arteries, skeletal muscles, pancreas, testis, and spleen.

Leukemia

Leukemia is a neoplastic disease that arises in blood-forming tissue such as the bone marrow and causes large numbers of blood cells to be produced and enter the bloodstream. The leukemias form a very heterogeneous group of neoplasms, which differ both in clinical course (acute or chronic), and blood cell line that affected. Depending on these factors, patients with leukemia may have a number of symptoms, such as fevers or night sweats, frequent infections, weakness or tiredness, headache, bleeding and bruising easily, pain in the bones or joints, swelling or discomfort in the abdomen (from an enlarged spleen), swollen lymph nodes, especially in the neck or armpit, and weight loss.

SUD secondary to undiagnosed neoplasia is extremely uncommon in adults, with a reported incidence between 0.17% [90] and 0.58% [91]. Acute leukemia, as well as bronchogenic carcinoma, gastric adenocarcinoma, and adenocarcinoma of the urinary bladder, are the most common tumors causing SUD in adults [92]. Death has been attributed to a variety of mechanisms, including hemorrhage, thromboembolism, and widespread tumor dissemination.

Cases of SUDs due to splenic rupture in subjects with undiagnosed chronic leukemia have been described [93]: acute cardiovascular failure [94], intracardiac thrombosis [95], and pulmonary complications [96].

In acute leukemia, symptoms appear rapidly and progress quickly. As in chronic leukemia, sudden death is reported both in adults and children [97], sometimes occurring after a period of complete remission of the disease [98, 99]. Sudden unexpected death due to neoplastic disease in infancy and childhood (SUDNIC) is extremely uncommon. The most common causes of SUDNIC are tumors affecting vital structures, such as the heart and brainstem, and include primary cardiac tumors, primary CNS neoplasms, and fatal CNS hemorrhage secondary to hematopoietic neoplasms [100, 101]. Other less common causes of sudden death in children with leukemia may involve intracerebral infiltration or hyperviscosity and leukostasis [101]. Whybourne et al. [102] reported a case in which sudden death was the first manifestation of lymphoblastic leukemia in a 16-week-old boy; at autopsy, no evidence of intracranial hemorrhage was found. Infiltration of multiple organs (myocardium, lungs, etc.) was detected. The mechanism of mortem was retraced to the diffuse infiltration of myocardium probably predisposing to arrythmias, favored also by the diffuse infiltration of the lungs leading to a condition of hypoxia. Recently, Somers et al. [103] reviewed a 20-year autopsy cases ($n = 4926$); 8 cases of SUDNIC were identified in which postmortem diagnoses included 2 cases of acute leukemia (1 myelogenous, 1 lymphoblastic). Finally, it has recently been recognized that some form of treatment for leukemia may, themselves, cause SUD.

In conclusion, data from literature demonstrate that infants, children, and adults may have minimal or no symptoms in the presence of leukemic disease and highlight the need for a thorough autopsy examination in all cases of SUD. Arsenic tetroxide is now often used in the treatment of acute promyelocytic leukemia, and it appears to be an effective agent. However, its use is sometimes accompanied by sudden death because arsenic disrupts the normal function of potassium channels, leading to QT prolongation and torsades des pointes [104].

Metabolic Disorders

Diabetes

Diabetes mellitus (DM) is an etiologically and clinically heterogeneous group of metabolic disorders that share the common feature of hyperglycemia. Long-term hyperglycemia produces tissue damage, which ultimately manifests itself as microvascular disease, macrovascular disease, and neuropathy. Since 1991, when the British Diabetic Association initated a study of unexplained deaths in young patients with Type 1 DM [105], evidence has correlated the so-called dead-in-bed syndrome with diabetes. What characterized this kind of death is that it occurs at night and the patients are found dead in an undisturbed bed the next morning. Patients had gone to bed in apparent good health, and subsequent autopsy consistently revealed no cause of death (of course, the study was undertaken before it was possible to screen ion channel disease postmortem, and no doubt that some of the children included in the original study did suffer from some form of inherited long QT syndrome (LQTS) syndrome. See below). Nocturnal hypoglycemia is common among Type 1 diabetic patients; however, the precise mechanism by which hypoglycemia may cause sudden death remains uncertain. The suddenness of death in these patients implicated a possible cardiac cause. Many hypotheses have been proposed to explain the "dead-in-bed syndrome": undetected autonomic neuropathy, hypoglycemia-induced disturbances in cardiac electrophysiology, and other factors are probably involved in the sudden death of young diabetic patients.

However, the definite cause of the "dead-in-bed" syndrome continues to be a subject of further speculation and investigation (Figure 1) [106].

Cardiovascular autonomic neuropathy (CAN) encompasses damage to the autonomic nerve fibers that innervate the heart and blood vessels, resulting in abnormalities in heart rate control and vascular dynamics; it has been widely studied as a risk factor for sudden death in patients with DM [107, 108].

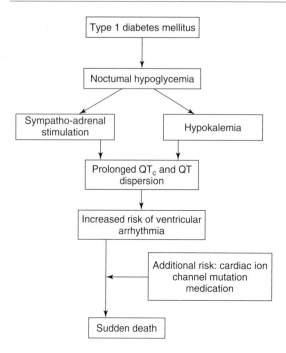

Figure 1 Hypothesis for "dead-in-bed syndrome" in Type 1 diabetes mellitus

One potential cause may be severe but asymptomatic ischemia, which can induce lethal arrhythmias. QT prolongation may also predispose individuals to life-threatening cardiac arrhythmias and sudden death. It has been shown that predisposition to arrhythmias and an association with mortality may also be related to intracardiac sympathetic imbalance [109, 110]. However, the significance of CAN as an independent cause of sudden death has been questioned recently. In the Rochester Diabetic Neuropathy Study, the investigators found that all cases of sudden death in individuals with and without diabetes had severe coronary artery disease (CAD) or left ventricular dysfunction. They suggested that although CAN could be a contributing factor, it was not a significant independent cause of sudden death. Heart failure is, however, common in individuals with diabetes; it is identified in these patients by the presence of neuropathy, even in those without evidence of CAD or left ventricular dysfunction [108]. The association of CAN in the absence of coronary disease and cardiomyopathy requires further study [111].

It is well known that DM is an independent risk for CVD: the association between diabetes and

incidence of CAD is widely reported in the literature. In the United States, diabetes is referred to as the most prevalent factor placing patients at risk for coronary events [112]. Furthermore, patients with DM have increased risk for ventricular arrhythmia that is thought to be secondary to CAD or CHF. Susceptibility to dysrhythmias in diabetic hearts is a very debatable issue. Diabetes is an independent risk for cardiac arrythmias in addition to other CVDs [113, 114]. QT prolongation is associated with SUD in the diabetic populations [115]. In a large study, Mohaved *et al.* [116] founded that patients with DM have significantly higher prevalence of ventricular fibrillation independent of CAD or CHF, which, in part, may explain the higher risk of sudden death in these patients.

Furthermore, patients with DM have a hyperco-agulable state that is of multifactorial origin. Many coagulation factors, such as fibrinogen, d-dimer, and von Willebrand factor may become elevated in diabetics. At the same time, there is decreased fibrinolysis along with platelet hyperaggrebility and endothelial dysfunction. Tsai *et al.* [117] founded DM as an independent risk for venous thromboembolism in a large population including both genders. Mohaved *et al.* [118] founded that DM is strongly associated with PE and PHT independent of CAD, CHF, or smoking.

In cases where diabetes is related to the occurrence of sudden death, gross necropsy examination may reveal signs of coronary plaques and coronary stenoses. The kidneys may show smaller size and granular surface. Histologically, the earliest detectable change in glomerular structure is the thickening of the basement membrane. Postmortem biochemistry of vitreous humor is a worthwhile adjunct to routine postmortem screening. Apart from the determination of glucose level in vitreous fluid, the determination of hemoglobin A1c considered as a definitive indicator of prolonged hyperglycemia has been proposed as a useful tool in postmortem diagnosis of diabetes [119].

Alcoholic Ketoacidosis

The entity of alcoholic ketoacidosis (AKA) was first described by Dillon *et al.* [120]. AKA affects chronic alcoholics and is characterized by metabolic acidosis with increased anionic gap. A typical patient with AKA has a history of chronic alcohol abuse (*see* **Alcohol: Use, Abuse, Tolerance, and Dependency**; **Alcohol: Interaction with Other Drugs**; **Alcohol: Behavioral and Medical Effects**) and recent binge drinking, followed by the abrupt cessation of alcohol consumption. Clinical findings of AKA are very similar to those of diabetic ketoacidosis, but hyperglycemia and glycosuria are generally absent. AKA is due to the accumulation of D-β-hydroxybutyrate and acetoacetic acid. The accumulation is probably the result of various factors such as volume depletion (vomiting, decreased fluid intake) and starvation having a lipolytic effect. As the previous alcoholic intake has an inhibitory effect on fatty acid oxidation, a higher level of fatty acids will be available. When fatty acids are presented to the liver faster than they can be oxidized, it results in a surplus of acetyl–CoA. The excess of acetyl–CoA is converted into β-hydroxy-β-methyl-glutaryl-CoA, which is cleaved to form acetyl–CoA and free acetoacetic acid. Some of the acetoacetic acid is reduced to D-β-hydroxybutyrate and a small amount is decarboxylated to acetone [121].

In uncomplicated AKA, the prognosis may be good, but several complications could be present (lactic acidosis, acute pancreatitis, Wernike's encephalopathy, etc.). AKA may be a life-threatening condition and it is a significant factor in at most a small minority of alcoholic deaths [122]. Fatalities of chronic alcoholics where the cause of death could not be determined by thorough autopsy, histology and toxicology including determination of alcohol concentration are described [123]; in those cases, ketoacidosis and lactic acidosis were assumed to be the cause of death. In such cases of unexpected and unexplained deaths in chronic alcoholics, measurement of ketone bodies in vitreous humor or pericardial fluid using clinical laboratory methodologies is recommended. In particular, β-hydroxybutyric acid (β-HBA) should be considered as the diagnostic marker of choice for the postmortem determination of AKA and as the cause of death [124].

Hypoglycemia

Since the introduction of insulin into diabetes care in 1921, hypoglycemia (HoG) emerged as a very complex concern. Some medications (all insulins, all insulin secretagogs) can cause HoG. There is particular concern about the drug metformin: most

experts suggest that metformin monotherapy does not cause clinically relevant HoG under usual circumstances, but it might under unusual circumstances. Such circumstances include combined therapy with metformin and insulin or insulin secretagogs (I/IS).

Many conditions make patients more sensitive to I/IS and predispose to HoG: leanness and youth, physical activity, first trimester of pregnancy and the immediate postpartum period, impaired liver function and alcoholism (depleted glycogen stores), impaired renal function (prolonged half-life insulin), counter-regulatory hormone failure (adrenals, glucagon, and growth hormone), autonomic neuropathy, previous hypoglycemia, being unaware of hypoglycemia, total parental nutrition, and poor metabolic control [125].

The scientific literature quotes very different values for the incidence of mortality due to HoG, which ranges in insulin-treated diabetic patients (high-risk populations) from 2 to 4% [125].

The exact mechanism by which hypoglycemia causes sudden death remains uncertain. One explanation of HoG-related sudden death is that hypoglycemia directly causes disturbances in cardiac electrophysiology, which may provoke malignant tachydysrhythmias. There have been reports of premature ventricular contractions, atrial arrhythmias, and ischemic ECG changes during hypoglycemia [126–128]. Moreover, there is evidence that insulin-induced hypoglycemia causes an acquired form of long QT syndrome. In addition to QT_c prolongation during hypoglycemia, QT dispersion (the difference between the longest and shortest QT interval on a 12-lead ECG) increases [129, 130].

In conclusion, the sudden death of a diabetic patient treated with I/IS creates a unique diagnostic problem. A high level of suspicion based on circumstantial evidence must alert the forensic pathologists on hypoglycemia as a probable cause of death (Figure 2) [125].

Postmortem diagnosis of HoG as a cause of sudden death can be proved by testing glucose levels in blood or spinal or vitreous fluid. The measurement of the ketone body β-hydroxybutyrate (β-HBA) may also help in the investigation of cases where hypoglycemia is suspected [131].

Thyroiditis

In forensic medicine, the study of thyroid function and disease is important in cases of sudden death [132–135].

Consideration	Lower risk, less probability	Higher risk, greater probability
Age	Older	Young
Duration of diabetes	Short	Long
Control as judged by the levels of CBG, hemoglobin AIc, and fructosamine	Suboptimal	Optimal
Adjusts to late meals and activity	Yes	No
History of frequent episodes of hypoglycemia	No	Yes
History of being unaware of hypoglycemia	No	Yes
Keeps a CBG diary	Yes	No
Keeps follow-up appointments	Yes	No
Frequency of CBG testing	Frequent	Rare or never

Figure 2   Considerations for assessing risk of hypoglycemia or, if applicable, estimating the probability that hypoglycemia caused idiopathic or accidental sudden death

Cases of sudden death associated with undiagnosed chronic thyroiditis are described [136–138]. An unusual case of fatal heatstroke in a young woman discovered unconscious in a sauna has been reported in which a preexisting Hashimotos thyroiditis was revealed at autopsy [139]. Moreover, an association between lymphocytic myocarditis and lymphocytic thyroiditis in a case of sudden death involving a 40-year-old man with no known medical history has also been reported [140].

Reports in the literature also raise the possibility of thyroid disease, in particular silent (painless) thyroiditis, may be an underlying cause of SUDs. Routine microscopy of the thyroid gland is therefore advocated in cases of SUD. It has also been suggested that postmortem measures of thyroid hormones

(thyroxine [T4] and triiodothyronine [T3]) and the pituitary hormone known as *thyroid-stimulating hormone* (*TSH*) may be useful diagnostic tools in cases of SUDs [141].

Anaphylaxis

Anaphylaxis was first described in the scientific literature about 100 years ago by Portier and Richet, who reported that their attempts to immunize dogs against the sting of jellyfish with actinia extract instead brought about an acute anaphylactic episode. In the extreme or classic form, anaphylaxis typically involves the cutaneous, respiratory, cardiovascular, and gastrointestinal systems, target organs all heavily populated with mast cells. Its presentation is often more enigmatic, with variable target organ involvement and expression of symptoms.

In 1998, a Joint Task Force on Practice Parameters defined anaphylaxis as an "immediate systemic reaction caused by rapid, IgE-mediated immune release of potent mediators from tissue mast cells and peripheral basophils". Aggregation of FceRI by allergen-driven cross-linking of receptor-bound IgE activates mast cells and basophils to release mediators that induce the pathophysiologic features of the anaphylactic response. Initial sensitization occurs through a highly coordinated series of steps involving a variety of cell types and mediators, which is affected by environmental exposure and complex genetic factors. Anaphylactic reactions are distinguished from anaphylactoid reactions, which "mimic signs and symptoms of anaphylaxis, but are caused by non-IgE-mediated release of potent mediators from mast cells and basophils" [142].

The most common etiologies of anaphylactic reactions include allergic responses to food, drug (medications, biologics, and vaccines), insect sting, and latex. Also exercise (jogging, walking, tennis, dancing, etc.) can lead to typical anaphylaxis. The pathogenesis and true incidence of exercise-induced anaphylaxis remain unknown. Finally, another form of anaphylaxis consists of the so-called idiopathic anaphylaxis, whose diagnosis is one of exclusion. The exact incidence of idiopathic anaphylaxis is unknown, but several studies estimate that nearly 20% of cases of anaphylaxis are idiopathic. There are no clinically distinguishing features (although 33% of cases are nocturnal), and it may be fatal.

Anaphylaxis is an uncommon cause of sudden death. In many cases, no specific macroscopic or microscopic findings are detected at autopsy. The most common finding is nonspecific pulmonary congestion and edema, but features suggesting an allergic reaction (cutaneous erythema, urticaria, laryngeal and/or pharyngeal edema) may be present. The presence of petechial hemorrhages is another nonspecific postmortem finding as is brain swelling. Generally, histological examinations will disclose mucosal edema, inflammation with eosinophilia, epithelial sloughing in the bronchial tree, cerebral edema, and polyvisceral stasis [143, 144].

In the presence of a clinical history suggestive for anaphylaxis-related death, postmortem measurement of serum tryptase levels can be a useful diagnostic aid. Tryptase, a neutral protease, is the major protein component of mast cell secretory granules. An elevated serum tryptase level is considered to be a specific marker for systemic mast cell activation, which is a central feature of anaphylaxis. In addition to this, because this enzyme has a longer serum half-life than other chemical mediators like histamine, the measurement of serum tryptase level is reported to be useful for postmortem as well as antemortem diagnosis of anaphylaxis [145–147]. Finally, in SIDS, one possible explanation hypothesized some 40 years ago is an anaphylactic reaction to protein components such as cow's milk [148, 149]. It was suggested that sensitized infants might suffer a fatal anaphylactic reaction if recently ingested cow's milk was regurgitated and inhaled during sleep. The question is still under debate [150]. New evidence is provided for an increased degree of mast cell activation in infants whose death was classified as SIDS. The stimuli for mast cell degranulation in these infants remains unclear, but the potential for anaphylaxis to have occurred in a proportion of cases of SIDS must be considered [151–154].

Infection

Massive adrenal hemorrhage (Waterhouse–Friderichsen syndrome) is an uncommon, but usually fatal, consequence of overwhelming sepsis [155]. Despite the predominant association with meningococcal infection, there are numerous other well-recognized etiologies, including sepsis resulting from other organisms, and noninfectious causes, such as anticoagulant treatment, antiphospholipid syndrome, trauma, and spontaneously occurring or postoperative adrenal hemorrhage. Gram-negative organisms, including klebsiella, pasturella, and *Hemophilus influenzae*, have all been reported to precipitate the syndrome. There are fewer reports of Waterhouse–Friderichsen syndrome following infection with Gram-positive bacteria. The clinical picture is generally characterized by sudden onset shock, pyrexia, cyanosis, dyspnea, and purpura, with adrenal hemorrhage. Unexpected death can occur as sequel of a rapidly progressive course of a previously undiagnosed infection [156–159].

At necropsy skin rashes will be evident, as will signs of upper airway infection, bronchopneumonia, and evidence of meningitis. Hemorrhage, elsewhere, may coexist with a massive adrenal hemorrhage, which is a more characteristic finding. Microscopic examinations generally reveal hemorrhages involving all layers of the adrenal glands with secondary cell necrosis. Measurement of serum procalcitonin concentration (PCT) may be a useful aid [160]. In fact, it is well known that in bacteremia and sepsis, PCT levels are highly elevated (>10 ng ml^{-1} in sepsis), and therefore PCT is a well-established clinical parameter in the diagnosis of systemic infection of bacterial origin [161].

References

[1]   Lin, S. (2006). Analysis of 265 autopsies of sudden death in children, *Journal of Clinical Forensic Medicine* **13**(6–8), 293–295.

[2]   Vennemann, M., Bajanowski, T., Butterfass-Bahloul, T., Sauerland C., Jorch, G., Brinkmann, B. & Mitchell, E.A. (2007). Do risk factors differ between explained sudden unexpected death in infancy and sudden infant death syndrome?, *Archives of Disease in Childhood* **92**(2), 133–136.

[3]   Kellum, J.A., Kong, L., Fink, M.P., Weissfeld, L.A., Yealy, D.M., Pinsky, M.R., Fine, J., Krichevsky, A., Delude, R.L. & Angus, D.C. (2007). Understanding the inflammatory cytokine response in pneumonia and sepsis, results of the Genetic and Inflammatory Markers of Sepsis (GenIMS) Study, *Archives of internal medicine* **167**(15), 1655–1663.

[4]   Escoffery, C.T. & Shirley, S.E. (2002). Causes of sudden natural death in Jamaica, a medicolegal (coroner's) autopsy study from the University Hospital of the West Indies, *Forensic Science International* **129**(2), 116–121.

[5]   Batalis, N.I., Caplan, M.J. & Schandl, C.A. (2007). Acute deaths in nonpregnant adults due to invasive streptococcal infections, *The American Journal of Forensic Medicine and Pathology* **28**(1), 63–68.

[6]   Nicoll, A. & Gardner, A. (1988). Whooping cough and unrecognised postperinatal mortality, *Archives of Disease in Childhood* **63**, 41–47.

[7]   Cherry, J.D. (1984). The epidemiology of pertussis and pertussis immunization in the United Kingdom and the United States: a comparative study, *Current Problems in Pediatrics* **14**, 1–78.

[8]   Lindgren, C., Milerad, J. & Lagercrantz, H. (1997). Sudden infant death and prevalence of whooping cough in the Swedish and Norwegian communities, *European Journal of Pediatrics* **156**, 405–409.

[9]   Heininger, U., Kleemann, W.J. & Cherry, J.D. (2004). A controlled study of the relationship between *Bordetella pertussis* infections and sudden unexpected eaths among German infants, *Pediatrics* **114**(1), e9–e15.

[10]   Corrin, B. (2000). *Pathology of the Lungs*, Churchill Livingstone Edition.

[11]   Burton, G.G., Sayer, W.J. & Lillington, G.A. (1966). Varicella pneumonitis in adults: frequency of sudden death, *Diseases of the Chest* **50**(2), 179–185.

[12]   Gregorakos, L., Myrianthefs, P., Markou, N., Chroni, D. & Sakagianni, E. (2002). Severity of illness and outcome in adult patients with primary varicella pneumonia, *Respiration; International Review of Thoracic Diseases* **69**(4), 330–334.

[13]   Popara, M., Pendle, S., Sacks, L., Smego Jr, R.A., Mer, M. (2002). Varicella pneumonia in patients with HIV/AIDS, *International Journal of Infectious Diseases* **6**(1), 6–8.

[14]   Tsokos, M., Zöllner, B. & Feucht, H.H. (2005). Fatal influenza A infection with *Staphylococcus aureus* superinfection in a 49-year-old woman presenting as sudden death, *International Journal of Legal Medicine* **119**, 40–43.

[15]   Drescher, J., Zink, P., Verhagen, W., Flik, J. & Milbradt, H. (1987). Recent influenza virus A infections in forensic cases of sudden unexplained death, *Archives of Virology* **92**(1–2), 63–76.

[16]   An, S.F., Gould, S., Keeling, J.W. & Fleming, K.A. (1993). Role of respiratory viral infection in SIDS: detection of viral nucleic acid by *in situ* hybridization, *Journal of Pathology* **171**(4), 271–278.

[17]   Bajanowski, T., Wiegand, P., Cecchi, R., Pring-Akerblom, P., Adrian, T., Jorch, G. & Brinkmann, B. (1996). Detection and significance of adenoviruses in cases of sudden infant death, *Virchows Archieve* **428**(2), 113–118.

[18]   Hoang, M.P., Ross, K.F., Dawson, D.B., Scheuermann, R.H. & Rogers, B.B. (1999). Human herpesvirus-6 and sudden death in infancy: report of a case and review of the literature, *Journal of Forensic Sciences* **44**(2), 432–437.

[19]   Pfeiffer, H., Varchmin-Schultheiss, K. & Brinkmann, B. (2006). Sudden death in childhood due to varicella pneumonia: a forensic case report with clinical implications, *International Journal of Legal Medicine* **120**, 33–35.

[20]   Dettmeyer, R., Sperhake, J.P., Müller, J. & Madea, B. (2008). Cytomegalovirus-induced pneumonia and myocarditis in three cases of suspected sudden infant death syndrome (SIDS): diagnosis by immunohistochemical techniques and molecularpathologic methods, *Forensic Science International* **174**(2–3), 229–233.

[21]   Bajanowski, B., Rolf, G., Jorch, B. & Brinkmann, B. (2003). Detection of RNA viruses in sudden infant death (SID), *International Journal of Legal Medicine* **117**, 237–240.

[22]   Fernandez-Rodriguez, A., Ballesteros, S., de Ory, F., Echevarria, J.E., Alvarez-Lafuente, R., Vallejo, G. & Gomez, J. (2006). Virological analysis in the

diagnosis of sudden 156 children death:, a medico-legal approach, *Forensic Science International* **161**, 8–14.

[23] Chan, E.D. & Welsh, C.H. (1995). Fulminant mycoplasma pneumoniae pneumonia, *The Western Journal of Medicine* **162**, 133–142.

[24] Daxboeck, F., Eisl, B., Burghuber, C., Memarsadeghi, M., Assadian, O. & Stanek, G. (2007). Fatal mycoplasma pneumoniae pneumonia in a previously healthy 18-year-old girl, *Wiener Klinische Wochen-schrift* **119**(11–12), 379–384.

[25] Hamman, L. & Rich, A. (1935). Fulminating diffuse interstitial fibrosis of the lungs, *Transactions of the American Clinical and Climatological Association* **51**, 154–163.

[26] Vourlekis, J.S., Brown, K.K. & Schwarz, M.I. (2001). Acute interstitial pneumonitis: current understanding regarding diagnosis, pathogenesis, and natural history, *Seminars in Respiratory and Critical Care Medicine* **22**(4), 399–408.

[27] Vourlekis, J.S. (2004). Acute interstitial pneumonia, *Clinics in Chest Medicine* **25**(4), 739–747.

[28] Quefatieh, A., Stone, C.H., Di Giovine, B., Toews, G.B. & Hyzy, R.C. (2003). Low hospital mortality in patients with acute interstitial pneumonia, *Chest* **124**, 554–559.

[29] Turillazzi, E., Di Donato, S., Neri, M., Riezzo, I. & Fineschi, V. (2007). An immunohistochemical study in a fatal case of acute interstitial pneumonitis (Hamman–Rich syndrome) in a 15-year-old boy presenting as sudden death, *Forensic Science International* **173**, 73–77.

[30] De Bakey, M.E. (1954). A critical evaluation of the problem of thromboembolism: collective review, *Surgery, Gynecology and Obstetrics* **98**, 1–27.

[31] Steiner, I. (2007). Pulmonary embolism – temporal changes, *Cardiovascular Pathology* **16**, 248–251.

[32] Heit, J.A. (2006). The epidemiology of venous thromboembolism in the community: implications for prevention and management, *Journal of Thrombosis and Thrombolysis* **21**(1), 23–29.

[33] Woolf, N. (1998). *Pathology Basic and Systemic*. London, WB Saunders.

[34] Riede, U.N., Schaefer, H.E. & Wehner, H. (1998). *Allgemeine und Spezielle Pathologie*, 2nd Edition, Stuttgart, Georg Thieme Verlag.

[35] Kissane, J.M. (1985). *Anderson's Pathology*, 8th Edition, St. Louis, Mosby.

[36] Rubin, E. & Farber, J.L. (1994). *Pathology*, 2nd Edition, Philadelphia, Lippincott.

[37] Damjanov, I. (2002). *Pathology Secrets*. Philadelphia, Hanley & Belfus.

[38] Braunstein, H. (1987). *Pathology*, 2nd Edition, St. Louis, CV Mosby.

[39] Kumar, V., Abbas, A.K. & Fausto, N. (2005). *Robbins and Cotran Pathologic Basis of Disease*, 7th Edition, Elsevier Saunders.

[40] Meyer, J.R. (1926). Embolus pulmonar-caseosa, *Brazilian Journal of Medical and Biological Research* **2**, 301–303.

[41] Steiner, P.E. & Luschbaugh, C.C. (1941). Maternal pulmonary embolism by amniotic fluid, *Journal of the American Medical Association* **117**, 1245–1254.

[42] Stafford, I. & Sheffield, J. (2007). Amniotic fluid embolism, *Obstetrics and Gynecology Clinics of North America* **34**(3), 545–553.

[43] Davies, S. (2001). Amniotic fluid embolus: a review of the literature, *Canadian Journal of Anaesthesia* **48**, 88–98.

[44] Martin, R.W., Amniotic fluid embolism, *Clinical Obsetrics and Gynecology* (1996). **39**(1) 101–106.

[45] Cunningham, G.F., Gant, N.F., Leveno K.J., Gelstrap L.C., Hawth J.C. & Wenstrom K.D. (eds). (2001). Obstetrical hemorrhage. in *Williams's Obstetrics*, New York, McGraw-Hill.

[46] Perozzi, K.J. & Englert, N.C. (2004). Amniotic fluid embolism. An obstetric emergency, *Critical Care Nurse* **24**, 56–61.

[47] Clark, S.L., Hankins, G.D.V., Dudley, D.A., Dildy, G.A. & Porter, T.F. (1995). Amniotic fluid embolism: analysis of the national registry, *American Journal of Obstetrics and Gynecology* **172**, 1158–1169.

[48] Lurie, S., Feinstein, M. & Mamet, Y. (2000). Disseminated intravascular coagulopathy in pregnancy: thorough comprehension of etiology and management reduces obstetricians' stress, *Archives of Gynecology and Obstetrics* **263**, 126–130.

[49] Robillard, J., Gauvin, F., Molinaro, G., Leduc, L., Adam, A. & Rivard, E. (2005). The syndrome of amniotic fluid embolism: a potential contribution of bradykinin, *American Journal of Obstetrics and Gynecology* **193**, 1508–1512.

[50] Benson, M.D., Kobayashi, H., Silver, R.K., Oi, H., Greenberger, P.A. & Terao, T. (2001). Immunologic studies in presumed amniotic fluid embolism *Obstetrics and Gynecology* **97**(4), 510–514.

[51] Benson, M.D. (2007). A hypothesis regarding complement activation and amniotic fluid embolism, *Medical Hypotheses* **68**(5), 1019–1025.

[52] Fletcher, S.J. & Parr, M.J.A. (2000). Amniotic fluid embolism: a case report and review, *Resuscitation* **43**, 141–146.

[53] Malhotra, P., Agarwal, R., Awasthi, A., Das, A. & Behera, D. (2007). Delayed presentation of amniotic fluid embolism: lessons from a case diagnosed at autopsy, *Respirology (Carlton, Vic)* **12**(1), 148–150.

[54] Devriendt, J., Machayekhi, S. & Staroukine, M. (1995). Amniotic fluid embolism: another case with non-cardiogenic pulmonary oedema, *Intensive Care Medicine* **21**, 698–699.

[55] Martin, S.R. & Foley, M.R. (2006). Intensive care in obstetrics: an evidence-based review, *American Journal of Obstetrics and Gynecology* **195**, 673–689.

[56] Fineschi, V., Gambassi, R., Gherardi, M. & Turillazzi, E. (1998). The diagnosis of amniotic fluid embolism: an immunohistochemical study for the quantification of pulmonary mast cell tryptase, *International Journal of Legal Medicine* **111**(5), 238–243.

[57] Farrar, S.C. & Gherman, R.B. (2001). Serum tryptase analysis in a woman with amniotic fluid embolism. A case report, *The Journal of Reproductive Medicine* **46**(10), 926–928.

[58] Nishio, H., Matsui, K., Miyazaki, T., Tamura, A., Iwata, M. & Suzuki K. (2002). A fatal case of amniotic fluid embolism with elevation of serum mast cell tryptase, *Forensic Science International* **126**, 53–56.

[59] Rainio, J. & Penttila, A. (2003). Amniotic fluid embolism as cause of death, in a car accident – a case report, *Forensic Science International* **137**, 231–234.

[60] Bouldin, M.J., Ross, L.A., Sumrall, C.D., Loustalot, F.V., Low, A.K. & Land, K.K. (2006). The effect of obesity surgery on obesity comorbidity, *The American Journal of the Medical Sciences* **331**, 183–193.

[61] Poirier, P., Giles, T.D., Bray, G.A., Hong, Y., Stern, J.S., Pi-Sunyer, F.X. & Eckel, R.H. (2006). Obesity and cardiovascular disease: pathophysiology, valuation, and effect of weight loss, *Circulation* **113**, 898–918.

[62] Oluseun, A., Sowemimo, S.M., Yood, J.C., Moore, J., Huang, M., Ross, R., McMillian, U., Ojo, P. & Randolph, B.R. (2007). Natural history of morbid obesity without surgical intervention, *Surgery for Obesity and Related Diseases* **3**, 73–77.

[63] Poirier, P., Martin, J., Marceau, P., Biron, S. & Marceau, S. (2004). Impact of bariatric surgery on cardiac structure, function and clinical manifestations in morbid obesity, *Expert Review of Cardiovascular Therapy* **2**, 193–201.

[64] Drenick, E.J. & Fisler, J.S. (1988). Sudden cardiac arrest in morbidly obese surgical patients unexplained after autopsy, *American Journal of Surgery* **155**(6), 720–726.

[65] Rössner, S., Lagerstrand, L., Persson, H.E. & Sachs, C. (1991). The sleep apnoea syndrome in obesity: risk of sudden death, *Journal of Internal Medicine* **230**(2), 135–141.

[66] Duflou, J., Virmani, R., Rabin, I., Burke, A., Farb, A. & Smialek, J. (1995). Sudden death as a result of heart disease in morbid obesity, *American Heart Journal* **130**(2), 306–313.

[67] Graham, J., Mosunjac, M., Hanzlick, R.L. & Mosunjac, M. (2007). Sickle cell lung disease and sudden death: a retrospective/prospective study of 21 autopsy cases and literature review, *The American Journal of Forensic Medicine and Pathology* **28**(2), 168–172.

[68] Thomas, A.N., Pattison, C. & Serjeant, G.R. (1982). Causes of death in sickle cell disease in Jamaica, *British Medical Journal* **285**, 633–635.

[69] Gray, A., Anionwu, E.N., Davis, S.C. & Brozovic M. (1991). Patterns of mortality in sickle cell disease in the United Kingdom, *Journal of Clinical Pathology* **44**, 459–463.

[70] Adedeji, M.O., Cespedes, J., Allen, K., Subramony C & Hughson, M.D. (2001). Pulmonary thrombotic arteriopathy in patients with sickle cell disease, *Archives of Pathology and Laboratory Medicine* **125**, 1436–1441.

[71] Dail, D.H. & Hammar, S.P. (1993). *Pulmonary Pathology*, 2nd Edition, New York, Springer-Verlag, 685–691.

[72] Knight, J., Murphy, T. & Browning, I. (1999). The lung in sickle cell disease, *Pediatric Pulmonology* **28**, 205–216.

[73] Manci, E.A., Culberson, D.E., Yang, Y.M., Gardner, T.M., Powell, R., Haynes Jr, J., Shah, A.K. & Mankad, V.N. (2003). Causes of death in sickle cell disease: an autopsy study, *British Journal of Haematology* **123**(2), 359–365.

[74] Platt, O.S., Brambilla, D.J., Rosse, W.F., Milner, P.F., Castro, O, Steinberg, M.H. & Klug, P.P.. The correct title is Martality in sickle cell disease. Life expectancy and risk factors for early death. (1994a). Mortality in sickle cell disease, *The New England journal of Medicine* **330**, 1639–1644.

[75] Darbari, D.S., Kple-Faget, P., Kwagyan, J., Rana, S., Gordeuk, V.R. & Castro, O. (2006). Circumstances of death in adult sickle cell disease patients, *American Journal of Hematology* **81**(11), 858–863.

[76] Diggs L.W. (1984). The sickle cell trait in relation to the training and assignment of duties in the armed forces: III. Hyposthenuria, hematuria, sudden death, rhabdomyolysis, and acute tubular necrosis, *Aviation, Space, and Environmental Medicine* **55**(5), 358–364.

[77] Sateriale, M. & Hartm P. (1985). Unexpected death in a black military recruit with sickle cell trait: case report, *Military Medicine* **150**(11), 602–605.

[78] Kerle, K.K. & Nishimura, K.D. (1996). Exertional collapse and sudden death associated with sickle cell trait, *Military Medicine* **161**(12), 766–767.

[79] Evans, P. & Murray, M.J. (1997). Sudden exertional death and sickle cell trait, *American Family Physician* **55**(3), 784.

[80] Wirthwein, D.P., Spotswood, S.D., Barnard, J.J. & Prahlow, J.A. (2001). Death due to microvascular occlusion in sickle-cell trait following physical exertion, *Journal of Forensic Sciences* **46**(2), 399–401.

[81] Bock, H., Seidl, S., Hausmann, R. & Betz, P. (2004). Sudden death due to a haemoglobin variant, *International Journal of Legal Medicine* **118**(2), 95–97.

[82] Channa Perera, S.D. & Pollanen, M.S. (2007). Sudden death due to sickle cell crisis during law enforcement restraint, *Journal of Forensic and Legal Medicine* **14**, 297–300.

[83] Mitchell, B.L. (2007). Sickle cell trait and sudden death – bringing it home, *Journal of the National Medical Association* **99**(3), 300–305.

[84] Thogmartin, J.R. (1998). Sudden death in police pursuit, *Journal of Forensic Sciences* **43**(6), 1228–1231.

[85] Romero Mestre, J.C., Hernández, A., Agramonte, O. & Hernández, P. (1997). Cardiovascular autonomic dysfunction in sickle cell anemia: a possible risk factor for sudden death?, *Clinical Autonomic Research* **7**(3), 121–125.

[86] Schütt, M. & Meier M. (2005). Sudden death in sickle cell trait: could coexistent diabetes play a role? *Medical Hypotheses* **64**(1), 217.

[87] Gerber, N. & Apseloff, G. (1993). Death from a morphine infusion during sickle cell crisis, *The Journal of Pediatrics* **123**, 322–325.

[88] Oppenheimer, E.H. & Esterly, J.R. (1971). Pulmonary changes in sickle cell disease, *The American Review of Respiratory Disease* **103**, 858.

[89] Haque, A.K., Gokhale, S., Rampy, B.A., Adegboyega, P., Duarte, A. & Saldana, M.J. (2002). Pulmonary hypertension in sickle cell hemoglobinopathy: a clinicopathological study of 20 cases, *Human Pathology* **33**, 1037–1042.

[90] DiMaio, S.M., DiMaio, V.J. & Kirkpatrick, J.B. (1980). Sudden, unexpected deaths due to primary intracranial neoplasms, *The American Journal of Forensic Medicine and Pathology* **1**, 29–45.

[91] Gezelius, C. & Eriksson, A. (1988). Neoplastic disease in a medicolegal autopsy material: a retrospective study in northern Sweden, *Zeitschrift fur Rechtsmedizin* **101**, 115–130.

[92] Luke, J.L. & Helpern, M. (1968). Sudden unexpected death from natural causes in young adults: a review of 275 consecutive autopsied cases, *Archives of Pathology* **85**, 10–17.

[93] Nestok, B.R., Goldstein, J.D. & Lipkovic, P. (1988). Splenic rupture as a cause of sudden death in undiagnosed chronic myelogenous leukaemia, *The American Journal of Forensic Medicine and Pathology* **9**(3), 241–245.

[94] de Fijter, C.W., Schuur, J., Potter van Loon, B.J., Kingma, W.P. & Schweitzer, M.J. (1996). Acute cardiorespiratory failure as presenting symptom of chronic lymphocytic leukaemia, *The Netherlands Journal of Medicine* **49**(1), 33–37.

[95] Beaubien, E.R., Wilson, T.W. & Satkunam, N. (1998). Sudden death in a patient with chronic lymphocytic leukaemia, *Canadian Medical Association Journal* **159**(9), 1123–1125.

[96] Ahmed, S., Siddiqui, A.K., Rossoff, L., Sison, C.P. & Rai, K.R. (2003). Pulmonary complications in chronic lymphocytic leukaemia, *Cancer* **98**(9), 1912–1917.

[97] Aragona, M. & Aragona F. (2000). Unexpected death by leukostasis and lung leukostatic tumors in acute myeloid leukemia. Study of four cases, *Minerva Medica* **91**(10), 229–237.

[98] Lascari, A.D., Pearce, J.M. & Swanson, H. (1997). Sudden death due to disseminated cryptococcosis in a child with leukemia in remission, *Southern Medical Journal* **90**(12), 1253–1254.

[99] Hitosugi, M., Fukui, K., Takatsu, A., Harada, T., Homori, M. & Kawano, K. (1998). An autopsy case of sudden death caused by untreated sepsis after complete remission of acute promyelocytic leukaemia, *Nihon Hoigaku Zasshi* **52**(6), 355–359.

[100] Tsuda, N., Oka, R., Kajino, H., Kajino, M. & Okuno, A. (2000). Sudden death of a patient in complete remission after anthracycline therapy for acute lymphoblastic leukaemia, *Pediatrics International* **42**(3), 319–321.

[101] Byard, R.W. (2004). *Sudden Death in Infancy and Childhood*, 2nd Edition, Cambridge, Cambridge University Press, 643.

[102] Whybourne, A., Zillman, M.A., Miliauskas, J. & Byard, R.W. (2001). Sudden and unexpected infant death due to occult lymphoblastic leukaemia, *Journal of Clinical Forensic Medicine* **8**(3), 160–162.

[103] Somers, G., Smith, C.R., Perrin, D.G., Wilson, G.J. & Taylor, G.P. (2006). Sudden unexpected death in infancy and childhood ue to undiagnosed neoplasia: an autopsy study, *The American Journal of Forensic Medicine and Pathology* **27**(1), 64–69.

[104] Drolet, B., Simard, C. & Roden, D.M. (2004). Unusual effects of a QT-prolonging drug, arsenic trioxide, on cardiac potassium currents, *Circulation* **109**(1), 26–29.

[105] Tattersall, R.B. & Gill, G.V. (1991). Unexplained sudden death of type 1 diabetic patients, *Diabetic Medicine* **8**, 49–58.

[106] Start, R.D., Barber, C., Kaschula, R.O. & Robinson, R.T. (2007). The 'dead in bed syndrome' – a cause of sudden death in Type 1 diabetes mellitus, *Histopathology*. **51**(6), 843–845.

[107] Weston, P.J. & Gill, G.V. (1999). Is undetected autonomic dysfunction responsible for sudden death in Type 1 diabetes mellitus? The dead in bed syndrome revisited, *Diabetic Medicine* **16**, 626–631.

[108] Suarez, G.A., Clark, V.M., Norell, J.E., Kottke, T.E., Callahanm M.J., O'Brien, P.C., Low. P.A. & Dyck, P.J. (2005). Sudden cardiac death in diabetes mellitus: risk factors in the Rochester diabetic neuropathy study, *Journal of Neurology, Neurosurgery, and Psychiatry* **76**(2), 240–245.

[109] Kahn, J.K., Sisson, C. & Vinik, A.I. (1988). Prediction of sudden cardiac death in diabetic autonomic neuropathy, *Journal of Nuclear Medicine* **29**, 1605–1606.

[110] Stevens, M., Dayanikli, F., Raffelm D., Allman, K., Standford, T., Feldman, E., Wieland, D., Corbett, J. & Schwaiger, M. (1988). Scintigraphic assessment of regionalized defects in myocardial sympathetic intervation and blood flow regulation in diabetic patients with autonomic neuropathy, *Journal of the American College of Cardiology* **31**, 1575–1584.

[111] Vinik, A.I. & Ziegler, D. (2007). Diabetic cardio-vascular autonomic neuropathy, *Circulation* **115**(3), 387–397.

[112] Mazzone, T. (2007). Prevention of macrovascular disease in patients with diabetes mellitus: opportunities for intervention, *The American Journal of Medicine* **120**(9 Suppl 2), S26–S32.

[113] Movahed, M.R., Hashemzadeh, M. & Jamal, M. (2005a). Diabetes mellitus is a strong, independent risk for atrial fibrillation and flutter in addition to other cardiovascular disease, *International Journal of Cardiology* **105**(3), 315–318.

[114] Movahed, M.R., Hashemzadeh, M. & Jamal, M. (2005b). Increased prevalence of third-degree atrioventricular block in patients with type II diabetes mellitus, *Chest* **128**(4), 2611–2614.

[115] Giunti, S., Bruno, G., Lillaz, E., Gruden, G., Lolli, V., Chaturvedi, N., Fuller, J.H., Veglio, M. & Cavallo-Perin, P. (2007). Incidence and risk factors of prolonged QTc interval in type 1 diabetes: the EURODIAB Prospective Complications Study, *Diabetes Care* **30**(8), 2057–2063.

[116] Movahed, M.R., Hashemzadehm M., Jamal, M. (2007). Increased prevalence of ventricular fibrillation in patients with type 2 diabetes mellitus, *Heart and Vessels* **22**(4), 251–253.

[117] Tsai, A.W., Cushman, M., Rosamond, W.D., Heckbert, S.R., Polak, J.F. & Folsom, A.R. (2002). Cardiovascular risk factors and venous thromboembolism incidence: the longitudinal investigation of thromboembolism etiology, *Archives of Internal Medicine* **162**, 1182–1189.

[118] Movahed, M.R., Hashemzadeh, M. & Jamal, M. (2005c). The prevalence of pulmonary embolism and pulmonary hypertension in patients with Type II diabetes mellitus, *Chest* **128**, 3568–3571.

[119] Khuu, H.M., Robinson, C.A., Brissie, R.M. & Konrad, R.J. (1999). Postmortem diagnosis of unsuspected diabetes mellitus established by determination of decedent's hemoglobin A1c level, *Journal of Forensic Sciences* **44**(3), 643–646.

[120] Dillon, E.S., Dyer, W.W. & Smelo, L.S. (1940). Ketone acidosis in nondiabetic adults, *The Medical Clinics of North America* **24**, 1813–1822.

[121] Thomsen, J.L., Felby, S., Theilade, P., Nielsen, E. (1999). Alcoholic ketoacidosis as a cause of death in forensic cases, *Forensic Science International* **75**, 163–171.

[122] Pounder, D.J., Stevenson, R.J. & Taylor, K.K. (1998). Alcoholic ketoacidosis at autopsy, *Journal of Forensic Sciences* **43**(4), 812–816.

[123] Brinkmann, B., Fechner, G., Karger, B. & DuChesne, A. (1998). Ketoacidosis and lactic acidosis – frequent causes of death in chronic alcoholics?, *International Journal of Legal Medicine* **111**(3), 115–119.

[124] Iten, P.X. & Meier M. (2000). Beta-hydroxybutyric acid – an indicator for an alcoholic ketoacidosis as cause of death in deceased alcohol abusers, *Journal of Forensic Sciences* **45**(3), 624–632.

[125] Koch, B. (2006). Selected topics of hypoglycemia care, *Canadian Family Physician* **52**(4), 466–471.

[126] Collier, A., Mathews, D.M., Young, R.J. & Clarke, B.F. (1987). Transient atrial fibrillation precipitated by hypoglycaemia: two case reports, *Postgraduate Medical Journal* **63**, 895–897.

[127] Lindstrom, T., Jorfeldt, L., Tegler, L. & Arnquist, H.J. (1992). Hypoglycaemia and cardiac arrhythmias in patients with Type 2 diabetes, *Diabetic Medicine* **9**, 536–541.

[128] Baxter, M.A., Garewal, C., Jordan, R., Wright, A.D. & Nattrass, M. (1995). Hypoglycaemia and atrial fibrillation, *Postgraduate Medical Journal* **66**, 981.

[129] Heller, S.R. (2002). Abnormalities of the electrocardiogram during hypoglycaemia: the cause of the dead in bed syndrome?, *International Journal of Clinical Practice. Supplement* **129**, 27–32.

[130] Robinson, R.T.C.E., Harris, N.D., Ireland, R.H., Lee, S., Newman, C. & Heller, S.R. (2003). Mechanisms of abnormal cardiac repolarization during insulin-induced hypoglycemia, *Diabetes* **52**, 1469–1474.

[131] Denmark, L.N. (1993). The investigation of beta-hydroxybutyrate as a marker for sudden death due to hypoglycemia in alcoholics, *Forensic Science International* **62**(3), 225–232.

[132] Simson Jr, L.R. (1976). Thyrotoxicosis: postmortem diagnosis in an unexpected death, *Journal of Forensic Sciences* **21**, 831–832.

[133] Terndrup, T.E., Heisig, D.G. & Garceaum, J.P. (1990). Sudden death associated with undiagnosed Graves disease, *The Journal of Emergency Medicine* **8**, 553–555.

[134] Randall, B.B. (1992). Fatal hypokalemic thyrotoxic periodic paralysis presenting as the sudden, unexplained death of a Cambodian refugee, *The American Journal of Forensic Medicine and Pathology* **13**, 204–206.

[135] Guthrie, G.P., Hunsaker III, J.C., O'Connor, W.N. (1987). Sudden death in hypothyroidism, *The New England journal of Medicine* **317**(1291), 1–5.

[136] Edston, E. (1996). Three sudden deaths in men associated with undiagnosed chronic thyroiditis, *International Journal of Legal Medicine* **109**(2), 94–97.

[137] De Letter, E.A., Piette, M.H., Lambert, W.E. & De Leenheer, A.P. (2000). Medico-legal implications of hidden thyroid dysfunction: a study of two cases, *Medicine, Science, and the Law* **40**(3), 251–257.

[138] Vestergaard, V., Drostrup, D.H. & Thomsen, J.L. (2007). Sudden unexpected death associated with lymphocytic thyroiditis, *Medicine, Science, and the Law* **47**(2), 125–133.

[139] Siegler, R.W. (1998). Fatal heatstroke in a young woman with previously undiagnosed Hashimoto's thyroiditis, *Journal of Forensic Sciences* **43**(6), 1237–1240.

[140] Lorin De La Grandmaison, G., Izembart, M., Fornes, P., Paraire, F. (2003). Myocarditis associated with Hashimoto's disease, a case report, *International Journal of Legal Medicine* **117**(6), 361–364.

[141] Edston, E., Druid, H., Holmgren, P. & Öström, M. (2001). Postmortem measurements of thyroid hormones in blood and vitreous humor combined with histology, *The American Journal of Forensic Medicine and Pathology* **22**(1), 78–83.

[142] Sampson, H.A., Munoz-Furlong, A., Bock, S.A., Schmitt, C., Bass, R., Chowdhury, B.A., Decker, W.W., Furlong, T.J., Galli, S.J., Golden, D.B., Gruchalla, R.S., Harlor, Jr, A.D., Hepner, D.L., Howarth, M., Kaplan, A.P., Levy, J.H., Lewis, L.M., Lieberman, P.L., Metcalfe, D.D., Murphy, R., Pollart, S.M., Pumphrey, R.S., Rosenwasser, L.J., Simons, F.E., Wood, J.P. & Camargo, C.A., Symposium on the definition and management of anaphylaxis: summary report, *The Journal of Allergy and Clinical Immunology* (2005). **115**, 584–591.

[143] Pumphrey, R.S.H. & Roberts, I.S.D. (2000). Postmortem findings after fatal anaphylactic reactions, *Journal of Clinical Pathology* **53**, 273–276.

[144] Greenberger, P.A., Rotskoff, B.D. & Lifschultz, B. (2007). Fatal anaphylaxis: postmortem findings and associated comorbid diseases, *Annals of Allergy, Asthma and Immunology* **98**(3), 252–257.

[145] Yunginger, J.W., Nelson, D.R., Squillace, D.L., Jones, R.T., Holley, K.E., Hyma, B.A., Biedrzycki, L., Sweeney, K.G., Sturner, W.Q. & Schwartz, L.B. (1991). Laboratory investigation of deaths due to anaphylaxis, *Journal of Forensic Sciences* **36**, 857–865.

[146] Ansari, M.Q., Zamora, J.L. & Lipscomb, M.F. (1993). Postmortem diagnosis of acute anaphylaxis by serum tryptase analysis, *American Journal of Clinical Pathology* **99**, 101–103.

[147] Schwartz, L.B. (2006). Diagnostic value of tryptase in anaphylaxis and mastocytosis, *Immunology and Allergy Clinics of North America* **26**, 451–463.

[148] Parish W.E., Barrett, A.M., Coombs, R.R.A., Gunther, M. & Camps, F.E. (1960). Hypersensitivity to milk and sudden death in infancy, *Lancet* **II**, 1106–1110.

[149] Parish, W.E., Richards, C.B., France, N.E. & Coombs, R.R.A. (1964). Further investigations on the hypothesis that some cases of cot death are due to a modified anaphylactic reaction to cows' milk, *International Archives of Allergy and Applied Immunology* **24**, 215–243.

[150] Nishio, H. & Suzuki, K. (2004). Serum tryptase levels in sudden infant death syndrome in forensic autopsy cases, *Forensic Science International* **139**(1), 57–60.

[151] Platt, M.S., Yunginger, J.W., Sekula-Perlman, A., Irani, A.M.A., Smialek, J., Mirchandani, H.G. & Schiwartz, L.B. (1994b). Involvement of mast cells in sudden death syndrome, *The Journal of Allergy and Clinical Immunology* **94**, 250–256.

[152] Hagan, L.L., Goetz, D.W., Revercomb, C.H. & Garriott, J.G. (1998). Sudden infant death syndrome: a search for allergen hypersensitivity, *Annals of Allergy, Asthma and Immunology* **80**, 227–231.

[153] Edson, E., Gidlund, M., Wickman, H., Ribbing & van Hage-Hamsten, M. (1999). Increased mast cell tryptase in sudden infant death – anaphylaxis, hypoxia or artefact?, *Clinical and Experimental Allergy* **29**, 1648–1654.

[154] Buckley, M.G., Variend, S., Walls, A.F. (2001). Elevated serum concentrations of b-tryptase, but not a-tryptase, in sudden infant death syndrome (SIDS). An investigation of anaphylactic mechanisms, *Clinical and Experimental Allergy* **31**, 1696–1704.

[155] Varon, J., Chen, K., Sternbach, G.I. (1998). Rupert Waterhouse and Carl Friderichsen, adrenal apoplexy, *The Journal of Emergency Medicine* **16**, 643–647.

[156] Doherty, S. (2001). Fatal pneumococcal Waterhouse-Friderichsen syndrome, *Emergency Medicine (Fremantle, W.A.)* **13**(2), 237–239.

[157] Tsokos, M. (2003). Fatal Waterhouse-Friderichsen syndrome due to *Ewingella Americana* infection, *The American Journal of Forensic Medicine and Pathology* **24**(1), 41–44.

[158] Hamilton, D., Foweraker, H.J. & Gresham, G.A. (2004). Waterhouse-Friderichsen syndrome as a result of non-meningococcal infection, *Journal of Clinical Pathology* **57**(2), 208–209.

[159] Adem, P.V., Montgomery, C.P., Husain, A.N., Koogler, T.K., Arangelovich, V., Humilier, M., Boyle-Vavra, S. & Daum, R.S. (2005). *Staphylococcus aureus* sepsis and the Waterhouse-Friderichsen syndrome in children, *The New England journal of Medicine* **353**(12), 1245–1251.

[160] Tsokos, M. (2002). Postmortem measurement of serum procalcitonin concentration in Waterhouse-Friderichsen syndrome, *Virchows Archieve* **441**(6), 629–631.

[161] Tsokos, M., Reichelt, U., Nierhaus, A. & Puschel, K. (2001). Serum procalcitonin (PCT): a valuable biochemical parameter for the post-mortem diagnosis of sepsis, *International Journal of Legal Medicine* **114**, 237–243.

Further Reading

McGee, J.O.D., Isaacson, P.G. & Wright, N.A. (1992). *Oxford Textbook of Pathology*, Oxford University Press, Oxford.

Sampson, U.A., Muñoz-Furlong, A., Bock, A., *et al.* (2005). Symposium on the definition and of anaphylaxis, summary report, *The Journal of Allergy and Clinical Immunology* **115**, 584–591.

VITTORIO FINESCHI AND EMANUELA
TURILLAZZI

Neuropsychological Assessment

Neuropsychological assessment refers to the application of standardized psychological measurement techniques to determine the relationship between brain impairment and its cognitive and behavioral concomitants (*see also* **Head Injury: Neuropsychological Assessment**). Forensic neuropsychological assessment is the use of such techniques in responding to official or legal questions. Forensic neuropsychologists are increasingly being called upon to provide opinions in a wide range of types of legal referrals. A recent count of citations of the word "neuropsychologist" in a database of court decisions yielded a large and growing count of cases involving neuropsychological consultation. Forensic issues were recently identified as the most-researched areas in the field of neuropsychology, with recent exponential growth in the number of studies and articles referencing forensic matters, such as malingering assessment (*see* **Malingering: Forensic Evaluations**).

Choice and Credentialing of the Neuropsychological Expert

The clinical neuropsychologist is typically a clinical psychologist who is also trained in the neurosciences and clinical neurology, and who has completed appropriate postdoctoral training and experience in the field of neuropsychology. Definitions of clinical neuropsychologists have been published by Division 40 (neuropsychology) of the American Psychological Association (APA) [1] and by the National Academy of Neuropsychology [2]. These definitions define clinical neuropsychologists as being licensed psychologists with appropriate graduate training in psychology, neuropsychology, and/or the neurosciences and at least two years of supervised postdoctoral experience. The Division 40 definition includes review by one's peers as a test of these competencies, and specifically references diplomate status as the "clearest evidence" that competence as a clinical neuropsychologist is met.

The choice of a forensic neuropsychological expert should take these issues of training and credentialing into account. One should also consider the neuropsychologist's experience with the disorder in question. For example, in cases involving closed head injuries, a neuropsychologist with experience in working with head injury patients in a rehabilitation setting may be preferred. The neuropsychologist's history as a forensic expert should also be taken into account. Some attorneys may prefer to choose neuropsychologists with a substantial history of testifying in court, while others may prefer experts who have little or no track record as an expert witness. In any event, a neuropsychologist who has consistently testified in prior cases for both the plaintiff and the defense, or the prosecution and the defense in criminal matters, is a plus. Consider also the neuropsychologist's capacity for teaching or educating the court and/or jury regarding the clinical issues that are apparent in the case. Reports should be written in an accessible, straightforward style with normal language and avoidance of highly technical terms as much as possible.

Admissibility of Neuropsychological Evidence

Properly credentialed neuropsychologists are able to serve as expert witnesses in most jurisdictions (*see also* **Expert Opinion: United States**). In some states, such as North Carolina and Georgia, there has been case law limiting neuropsychologists from expressing opinions regarding the medical causation of brain injuries. In Georgia, this issue was remedied with legislation. In most states, however, courts have consistently found that neuropsychologists are qualified to render opinions regarding the causation and pathology of brain insults. The Iowa Supreme Court case decision in *Hutchison v. American Family Mutual Insurance Company* provides an outline for the use of neuropsychological testimony in court, including that neuropsychologists are qualified to diagnose the general state of the brain and the causation of brain pathology. The *Daubert v. Merrell Dow Pharmaceuticals, Inc.* (*see also* **Daubert v. Merrell Dow Pharmaceuticals**) case sets out key principles for the admission of scientific evidence and expert testimony in courts: whether the technique can be tested (falsifiability), has the technique been published (peer review), is there an acceptable error rate, whether the techniques have gained general acceptance in the scientific field, and whether there is a published guide or manual to govern the use of the instrument. In general, most of the widely used neuropsychological tests meet these standards; indeed, neuropsychology as a profession, because of its emphasis on empirical methods of assessment and long tradition of careful research, seems ideally suited to meet *Daubert* challenges in court.

The American Academy of Neurology [3] has produced official guidelines affirming the value of neuropsychological assessment in the practice of neurology. Professional psychological practice organizations, such as the National Academy of Neuropsychology and the American Academy of Clinical Neuropsychology, have published guidelines for performing forensic neuropsychological assessments. These guidelines are intended to describe the "most desirable and highest level of professional conduct", as opposed to other documents such as APA's *Ethical Principles of Psychologists and Code of Conduct*, which simply describe standards for competent and adequate conduct. These guidelines indicate that neuropsychologists working for a third party, such as an insurance company, attorney, or the court, must inform the examinee of the nature of the evaluation, the neuropsychologist's duty to remain objective, and the destination of the report that will be produced. The presence of a clinician–patient relationship must not be implied, but disavowed. The examination must be conducted in a manner adequate to answer the questions posed by the referral source. The measurement procedures must meet standards for psychometric accuracy, including the presence of acceptable reliability, validity, and appropriate normative standards. The potential for motivational bias must be addressed in the testing, and the report should reflect a reasoned, knowledgeable assessment of potential biasing issues in the assessment. Interpretations of test results that appear to deviate from normal levels must take into account other information as well, such as information about the patient's history, information from the direct observation of the patient, the functional abilities of the patient, and the nature of the potential neuropsychological syndromes that could account for the test findings.

The Uses and Utility of Neuropsychological Assessment

Neuropsychological assessment is often indicated when questions about cognition or brain–behavior relationships are raised during the course of a medical evaluation that are not explicable by history, mental status observations, radiological techniques, or laboratory techniques alone. The neuropsychologist is typically called upon when a complex set of symptoms and behaviors dictates in-depth measurement and observation of an individual's neurocognitive function and/or neurobehavioral characteristics. In the forensic realm, neuropsychological assessment is often sought when an allegation of brain injury or brain dysfunction is relevant to a given legal question.

The potential types of forensic referrals are many and varied. In the criminal forensic area, these include questions of trial competence in individuals with suspected neurocognitive impairment; criminal responsibility evaluations in defendants with suspected brain dysfunction or severe mental illness; evaluations to determine other criminal competencies, such as competence to waive one's Miranda rights or waive one's rights to appeal; evaluations to determine factors relevant to sentence mitigation; and evaluations to determine the appropriateness for transfer of a juvenile's case to an adult court. In the civil realm, a nonexhaustive list would include evaluations in personal injury cases in situations of alleged brain injuries, evaluations of injured employees in workers' compensation cases, alleged dementia or memory problems in disability applicants, and evaluation of civil competencies, such as evaluation of testamentary capacity or ability to manage one's affairs in the case of an allegedly demented older individual.

Neuropsychologists are often called upon to estimate whether a brain-injured individual has returned to a prior level of function, such as when confronted with the question of whether the patient can return to work. This is an issue of great interest in many medicolegal situations, relevant to the estimation of compensable impairment in workers' compensation injuries, or damage liability in personal injury cases. For example, after receiving a left frontal contusion, a professional editor may expect to encounter difficulty in tasks that tap verbal reasoning, whereas a skilled machinist might be just as debilitated from a comparable right-hemisphere lesion.

Examination of these referrals often hinges upon comparison of current test results with premorbid abilities. Premorbid function can be assessed informally by taking a careful history including prior educational achievement, occupations, daily activities, hobbies, and personal achievements. Both actuarial and assessment techniques also exist that allow estimation of prior function. Prior intelligence can be predicted within a degree of error by mathematical regression techniques, utilizing demographic information such as educational level, occupational history, age, and region of the country. Reading ability is highly resistant to most acquired cognitive disorders, with the exception, of course, of alexia. Thus reading skill is a good marker of prior function. Other cognitive skills that can be assessed with the neuropsychological evaluation tend to remain constant, even with significant cortical insults. The most powerful techniques are those that mathematically combine both psychometric data with demographic estimation techniques (e.g., Wechsler Test of Adult Reading, Oklahoma Premorbid Intelligence Assessment).

Another important set of referral questions addresses the patient's level of residual functional capacity after recovery. Normal resumption of activities of daily living, socialization, and performance in work-like settings may not be possible depending on age, course of illness, severity of injury, and the presence of concomitant psychiatric illness. These are functional questions that may be best answered by a combination of assessment techniques, including administering formalized tests (see next section), observing the patient in demanding environments, interviewing the family, and taking a complete history of the illness.

Neuropsychological Assessment Instruments

The most recent version of a popular handbook for neuropsychologists reviews more than 160 tests which have found their way into common use among neuropsychologists Straus *et al.* [4], and these are only a small subset of the tests available commercially or in the research literature. Instead of attempting to present specific tests to the reader, categories and representative examples of neuropsychological tests will be described here, in order to convey a sense of the range and utility of neuropsychological testing.

Intelligence Tests in Neuropsychological Assessment

A comprehensive intelligence test, usually the Wechsler test appropriate to the age of the patient, often

serves as the backbone of most neuropsychological evaluations. Comprehensive intelligence tests have the advantage of carefully developed norms and the fact that they tap many key neurocognitive abilities (e.g., verbal expression, processing speed, visual analytic skills). Because of the development of the standardization samples on these tests, it is also possible to account for the expected effects of such variables as educational level and ethnicity, if desired. A disadvantage is the fact that comprehensive intelligence quotient (IQ) scores and summary index scores tend to be resistant to changes caused by neurocognitive disorders. Partially, this is due to the fact that neurocognitive disorders rarely cause generalized dysfunction except in the more severe cases. Also, intelligence tests are not weighted heavily with executive function and memory tests; the tests are shown to be most sensitive to cortical dysfunction. Indeed, it is not unusual for an early to mid-stage Alzheimer's patient to be relatively debilitated due to memory loss, but score near-normal limits on most sections of the Wechsler Adult Intelligence Scale, or for a Pick's Disease (an illness involving deterioration of executive functioning and personality change due to brain degeneration) patient to exhibit grossly inappropriate behavior but to have an average or better IQ.

Folstein Mini-Mental State Examination (MMSE)

The Mini-Mental State Examination (MMSE) is a universally recognized neuropsychological test that is widely used by psychiatrists, psychologists, neurologists, and geriatric practitioners. This test taps several cognitive functions including orientation, word memory, naming, verbal comprehension, writing, and drawing. Benefits of the MMSE are the instant recognizability of the test and the fact that so many clinicians across differing disciplines can readily interpret its scores. Unfortunately, it is also short on items tapping executive function, and its memory section, as generally administered, is crude. This test is often supplanted with tests that have additional memory and executive items to allow greater sensitivity to senile dementia and a broader range of assessed functions (e.g., Modified MMSE; Dementia Rating Scale).

Halstead–Reitan Neuropsychological Test Battery

The Halstead–Reitan Neuropsychological Test Battery (HRNTB) contains many of the most commonly used neuropsychological tests. It originated from the work of Ward Halstead, who in 1947 at the University of Chicago published his observations of several hundred case studies of patients who had frontal lobe damage. By using 10 scores, Halstead blindly distinguished patients with confirmed brain lesions from control subjects. Reitan [5], a student of Halstead, modified the battery in 1955 to identify lateralizing features of patient performances such as motor deficits expected in subtle stroke, the effect of temporal lobe epilepsy on memory, and the loss of abstraction ability associated with frontal damage. Reitan also modified the original battery to include tests that would accurately measure aphasia and variations of normal aging. An extensive norming project [6] has provided an excellent source of demographically corrected norms for the tests.

The Halstead Impairment Index is a global measure of brain dysfunction in neuropsychology backed by research and a wide degree of acceptance. Most normal subjects are able to pass 60–100% of the tests included in the Index. Patients who have moderate impairments may be within the normal range on only 30–60% of the tests, and those with severe dysfunction on less than 30%. From continued use of the battery over the decades, 3 of the original 10 scores were dropped because of questionable validity. The Index includes seven scores within the following five subtests:

1. Category Test

The Category Test is an abstract reasoning task consisting of 180 items. The patient is required to use mental flexibility and problem solving to form concepts, utilizing feedback from the examiner about the accuracy of their attempts.

2. Tactual Performance Test

The Tactual Performance Test is a test requiring the integration of multiple cognitive skills: spatial skills, spatial memory, dexterity, processing speed, and planning ability. The patient is blindfolded and placed before a board with cutouts into which blocks can be inserted. The patient is then asked to place the blocks in the cutouts, first using the dominant hand, then the nondominant hand, then both. Then the patient is asked to draw a representation of the board from memory. Since more than 40% of the brain's processing power is devoted to visual processing, removal of vision presumably cripples the efficiency with which the patient can approach the task. For the brain-injured patient, excessive time is often required to complete this task. The lateralized nature of the test allows some comparison of relative hemispheric efficiency.

3. Finger Tapping Test

Finger Tapping is a test of fine motor speed. Five consecutive 10 s trials are obtained with the dominant and nondominant index fingers, and then compared to norms. Injury to either region of motor cortex, as well as injuries affecting overall cortical efficiency, can result in degraded scores on this task.

4. Rhythm Test

The Rhythm Test originated from the Seashore Measures of Musical Talent test, in which the patient is asked to differentiate between 30 pairs of rhythmic patterns. These pairs are presented in rapid succession on a tape recorder, and the patient must distinguish whether they are the same or different.

5. Speech Sounds Perception Test

The Speech Sounds Perception Test involves 60 spoken nonsense words that are administered by audiotape. The patient is required to underline the corresponding printed response on an answer sheet, measuring verbal discrimination and sustained attention.

General Neuropsychological Deficit Scale

In addition to the seven scores provided by five index subtests, other subtests from the HRNTB are used to represent patients' performances on the General Neuropsychological Deficit Scale (GNDS). Subtests used to contribute to this scale, in addition to those in the Index, include the Lateral Dominance Examination, Grip Strength, the Sensory-Perceptual Examination, Tactile Form Recognition, the Trail Making Test Parts A and B, and the Aphasia Screening Test. The GNDS, much like the Impairment Index, provides a global impairment rating but takes into account 42 variables, thereby increasing reliability. Clinical judgment also allows the clinician to take into account variables in the interpretation of data related to the level and pattern of performance, pathognomonic signs, and laterality. In practice, though, the entire HRNTB is rarely given, with the neuropsychologist instead relying upon subtests of the battery scored with the help of the demographically corrected norms, described above.

Functions Measured in Neuropsychological Assessments

Sensorimotor Ability

Many neuropsychologists administer a partial neurological examination as part of their overall assessment. Depending on the referral questions, the sensorimotor assessment may include informal testing of olfactory function, visual fields, auditory perception, stereognosis (tactile appreciation of objects), and cerebellar function (e.g., heel-to-shin testing, alternating hand movements). As mentioned above, standardized testing of strength, motor speed (hand and foot tapping), and fine motor control are generally a component of the examination.

Attention and Concentration

After ensuring an adequate level of consciousness, assessment of attention provides fundamental information as to whether evaluation of other cognitive domains, such as intelligence, memory, or language, will be valid. Further, because the ability to focus and maintain attention is highly sensitive to many acute and ongoing conditions (e.g., alcohol withdrawal, intoxication, delirium), a stable, chronic process may be affected less than will a recent or changing one. At the most basic level, this domain measures the patient's ability to attend to incoming information without being distracted. Examples of simple attentional tasks include digit repetition or visual tapping span, requiring forward or backward sequencing of auditory or visual stimuli.

Sustained attention, known as *vigilance or continuous performance*, is another type of attention. An area of cognitive assessment which shows great promise for practitioners who work with attention deficit hyperactive disorder (ADHD) children and adults is continuous performance testing for sustained attention (e.g., Conners Continuous Performance Test and Test of Variables of Attention). Continuous performance tests are most often computer administered, and generally exist in either visual or auditory formats. In the visual modality, the child (or adult) is asked to sit before a computer screen and to respond to one type of stimulus while suppressing responses to another. The tests go on for several minutes, and the boring nature of the task tends to elicit omissions and variable response times from individuals

with attentional deficits. While only limited success has been achieved with these tests as diagnostic instruments for ADHD, they are quite successful in measuring the effectiveness of psychostimulant medication on individuals known to have ADHD. As such, an assessment using these tests can allow the psychiatrist to avoid the use of costly and potentially risky psychostimulant medications among patients who are unresponsive to its effects. These tests are also widely used by neuropsychologists to assess the attentional abilities of brain-injured patients.

Learning and Memory

Compromise of memory is the most common patient complaint and referral question for neuropsychological testing. Milder memory problems, or problems with visual memory, may not be readily apparent on screening tasks such as the MMSE. Since memory is not a static or unitary process, careful assessment can help to characterize variations in performance, which can have diagnostic value. Patients who have anterograde amnesia, or faulty learning of new material or events after the onset of their disorder, have more difficulty consolidating their learning experiences into longer storage. Retrograde amnesia, or the inability to retrieve remote memories, is less prominent in organic memory loss, especially if the onset is sudden, as in head injury. However, certain chronic conditions and disease processes, such as Korsakoff's syndrome and Alzheimer's disease, may produce a more dense retrograde amnesia. Memory is often evaluated in the mental status examination by assessing orientation, current events, and recall of words or objects. Although screening is sometimes adequate to determine the presence of a gross dementia, full neuropsychological evaluation can detect whether the difficulty is with encoding, storage, or retrieval mechanisms, and whether the impairment is associated more with one modality than another (e.g., verbal or visual).

The most widely used global memory test is the Wechsler Memory Scale (WMS), now undergoing its most recent revision, which will result in the WMS–IV. These tests yield memory quotients similar to IQ scores (expected mean is 100; standard deviation is 15). It provides for evaluation of immediate memory, delayed memory, and working memory skills, in both visual and verbal modalities.

Language

Testing for aphasia is a necessary part of diagnosis and treatment planning in some developmental and learning disabilities, progressive disorders (e.g., dementia and tumor), or recovery from an acute injury such as stroke or head injury. Impairment of language on a gross level is often more noticeable because of the frequent need for clear communication. However, subtle language deficits can go undetected in informal conversation and occasionally in more formal assessment. At the very least, language screening should include tasks to measure quality of spontaneous speech, naming, comprehension, repetition, reading, writing, calculation, and left–right orientation. Naming, the most sensitive element of most underlying language disturbances, is often measured through confrontational naming tasks such as the Boston Naming Test, a 60-item test of picture identification. Well-studied aphasia screening batteries include the Boston Diagnostic Aphasia Examination and the Western Aphasia Battery. If the neuropsychological assessment confirms the presence of aphasia, a speech language pathology evaluation may be required to plan detailed treatment.

Executive Functioning

Executive functioning refers to cognition and personality skills that are integrative in nature, allowing the person to attend to salient stimuli while disregarding others, maintain situational awareness, plan, reason hypothetically, solve problems, self-monitor demands and emotional reactions; in short, executive function is composed of all meta-cognitive and emotional processes that serve to help the person adapt to the environment or reach an overarching goal. Though many of these functions are partly, if not primarily, subserved by the frontal lobes, their complex nature generally requires the entire brain working in concert for maximal success; thus the descriptive term *integrative functions* is also often used. Neuropsychological functioning under the rubric of executive tasks includes abstraction, problem solving, set generation and sequencing, ability to maintain or terminate behaviors, and ability to plan and organize. These functions are mediated by the frontal lobes. Personality characteristics having to do with judgment, social appropriateness, inhibition versus impulsivity, and motivation are also at least partially related to frontal

activity. The most famous example of an organically driven personality change is that of Phineas Gage, a railroad worker in the 1880s, who sustained a traumatic injury to the frontal lobes when a tamping iron was blown through his head. This formerly docile, responsible worker became irascible, foul-mouthed, and disinhibited. As his reckless and menacing behavior continued, his coworkers described him as "no longer Gage".

Specific tasks that are frequently used to study the integrity of the frontal systems include the Wisconsin Card Sorting Test. This procedure provides an index of how well the examinee can formulate hypotheses and solve problems. Cards are matched by principles that are not stated directly, and the patient must shift cognitive sets as the rules for sorting change without forewarning. Other good measures of executive functioning include Controlled Oral Word Fluency, which requires verbal set generation (e.g., words beginning with certain letters), the Category Test (concept formation), and the Trail Making Test (measuring visual shifting and sequencing).

Visuospatial Functioning

Visuospatial functioning measures both the patient's ability to function within his or her environment with regard to recognition of objects and his or her construction and perception of spatial relations. Such abilities are important in daily activities that require the patient to recognize faces and remember geographic location and spatial orientation and in procedural learning tasks such as driving a car. Since patients with progressive neurologic disorders, such as Alzheimer's disease, and patients with right-hemisphere strokes, are particularly susceptible to deficits in this area, careful testing will be able to determine whether the patient is likely to encounter problems in getting lost or living independently. Figure copying, clock drawing, visual organization of parts to whole, facial recognition, and map orientation are samples of tasks used to assess this domain.

Malingering in Neuropsychological Assessment

The accuracy of neuropsychological assessment techniques is largely dependent upon the effort and/or truthfulness of the examinee. Malingering (*see also*

Malingering: Forensic Evaluations), or faking, neurocognitive problems is a key consideration in performing forensic neuropsychological assessments. It is estimated that approximately 30–50% of individuals undergoing forensic neuropsychological assessment intentionally underperform on cognitive testing, or otherwise seek to magnify their symptoms. Even young children have been shown in research studies to be able to successfully mislead skilled clinicians. The prospect that one out of every two or three medicolegal patients is feigning or exaggerating is a sobering one.

Patients often malinger physical disorders, pain, psychosis, posttraumatic stress disorder, severe depression, panic disorder, seizures, and memory deficits, to name a few feigned presentations. Disorders that are episodically manifested, such as panic attacks or seizures, represent a unique challenge to the clinician because of the relative lack of power of the mental status examination. In our experience, memory deficits are often feigned, presumably because it seems to many patients that loss of memory would be easy to both describe and feign on examination, though these expectations are, in fact, inaccurate.

The most powerful tool the clinician has in identifying malingered disorders is thorough knowledge of, and experience with, the disorder in question. It is a challenge for most patients to learn what symptoms to report to feign a given disorder, and an even greater challenge to convincingly produce facsimiles of symptoms upon mental status examination. For this reason, referrals to rule out malingering should preferably be sent to clinicians who are very experienced with the disorder in question. The patient suspected of feigning schizophrenia should be referred to a specialist in psychotic disorders, and the apparently head-injured patient to a clinician with extensive experience with patients who have experienced mild, moderate, and severe head injuries.

Detection of Malingered Deficits

Many patients present with malingered memory or reasoning deficits. Intellectual, neuropsychological, and other cognitive tests can be easily compromised by poor effort, and often such lack of effort is intentional. Without formal testing for malingering, low test scores or apparent dementia on mental status

examination may inaccurately result in classifications of patients as demented or mentally retarded.

Cognitive malingering tests utilize several different strategies to detect feigned cognitive problems, and fortunately knowledge of these strategies does not always subvert the tests, even in clever and well-informed patients. One set of tests utilizes floor effect tests, that is, tests that appear to be difficult but, in fact, are nearly always successfully performed even by individuals with moderate cognitive impairment. The malingering patient often scores well below the expected level as compared to genuinely impaired patients, thereby allowing a probabilistic determination of malingering to be made.

Forced choice tests are another strategy, often combined with the strategy above. These tests utilize the fact that forcing the patient to choose between two dichotomous responses, one correct and the other incorrect, results in a known expected value if the patient has no ability in that area at all: 50%. If a patient scores significantly worse than he or she would by flipping a coin, then strong evidence of malingering is produced. In that circumstance, the only credible explanation is that the patient must have known the right answer, since the wrong one was so often chosen. When failed, these tests provide the strongest evidence of malingering. The technique is also adaptable to a wide variety of possibly malingered conditions, e.g., blindness, tactual imperception, and deafness. Unfortunately, very few malingers fail forced choice tests, presumably recognizing that a higher level of performance would be the norm even for a severely impaired individual.

An example of a widely used test that combines both forced choice and floor effect features is the Test of Memory Malingering (TOMM). This test is composed of 50 pictures, which are shown to the patient in repeated trials. The patient is tested by being given a dichotomous choice between each correct picture and a foil. The patient's absolute score yields a classification of likelihood of malingering. If the patient goes on to score below chance levels, a precise probability rating can be assigned demonstrating the certainty level of malingering beyond any reasonable question.

Other cognitive malingering tests utilize known principles of learning or test-taking to identify unusual patterns of test performance. For example, even individuals with severe memory impairment tend to respond with significantly more correct answers when they are given recognition choices. Another principle is that, on average, the patient should score better on easier items than on more difficult ones, and that once a patient's level of ability has been exceeded, further answers should have no greater accuracy than chance. These and other atypical performance patterns offer the neuropsychologist further tools to identify malingering examinees.

The Minnesota Multiphasic Personality Inventory-2 (MMPI-2) is a widely used self-report personality inventory that contains a number of validity scales useful in identifying the individual malingering neuropsychological problems. These scales include the Infrequency Scale or F scale, the Infrequency–Psychopathology Scale or $F(p)$ scale, the Infrequency Back Scale or Fb scale, the F minus K Index, the sum of obvious – subtle differences, the Dissimulation-Revised Scale, and the Fake Bad Scale. These scales, and combinations thereof, have been shown to successfully identify individuals feigning psychiatric and neuropsychological dysfunction. The latter scale, the Fake Bad Scale, appears to have especial utility among persons alleging acquired physical debility and/or neurocognitive dysfunction.

Thus, the forensic neuropsychological assessment is not complete without an adequate assessment for malingering behavior. The assessment should include psychometric techniques for identifying underperformance and symptom exaggeration, as well as careful analysis of the examinee's presentation for indications of inconsistency. Such indications include notable discrepancies between test performances and observed abilities, discrepancies between claimed deficits and observed or reported functional activities, discrepancies between self-reported symptoms and known patterns of brain functioning, and discrepancies between self-reported deficiencies and symptoms reported by reliable collateral informants.

In sum, neuropsychological assessment, the application of standardized cognitive measurement techniques to brain–behavior relationships, has proved a useful and often determinative source of information in individuals with neurodevelopmental disorders and acquired brain dysfunction. Its validity and usefulness has been recognized by other disciplines and by the legal system. Neuropsychological assessment is a valuable resource, particularly in situations involving forensic questions about an individual's mental abilities, the nature/degree of neurocognitive injury, and one's neurobehavioral prognosis.

References

[1] American Psychological Association (1989). Division 40: definition of a clinical neuropsychologist, *The Clinical Neuropsychologist* **3**.

[2] National Academy of Neuropsychology (2001). *Definition of a Clinical Neuropsychologist: Official Position of the National Academy of Neuropsychology*. http://www.nanonline.org/PostitionPageLinks/Pages/DefinitionofaNeuropsychologist.aspx.

[3] American Academy of Neurology (1996). Assessment: neuropsychological testing of adults: considerations for neurologists, *Neurology* **47**, 592–599.

[4] Strauss, E., Sherman, E.M.S. & Spreen, O. (2006). *A Compendium of Neuropsychological Tests: Administration, Norms, and Commentary*, 3rd Edition, Oxford University Press.

[5] Reitan, R. & Wolfson, D. (1993). *The Halstead-Reitan Neuropsychological Test Battery: Theory and Clinical Application*, Neuropsychology Press.

[6] Heaton, R.K., Miller, S.W., Taylor, M.J. & Grant, I. (2004). *Revised Comprehensive Norms for an Expanded Halstead-Reitan Battery: Demographically Adjusted Neuropsychological Norms for African American and Caucasian Adults*, Psychological Assessment Resources.

Further Reading

American Academy of Clinical Neuropsychology (2007). American Academy of Clinical Neuropsychology (AACN) practice guidelines for neuropsychological assessment and consultation, *The Clinical Neuropsychologist* **21**, 209–231.

National Academy of Neuropsychology (2003). *Independent and Court-ordered Forensic Neuropsychological Examinations: Official Statement of the National Academy of Neuropsychology*. http://www.nanonline.org/PostitionPageLinks/Pages/Independent.aspx.)

JAMES S. WALKER

Neuropsychological Assessment: Child

Introduction

Child neuropsychological (NP) assessment involves the application of psychometric test methods in the evaluation of brain abnormalities in children. It shares many of the same goals and principles involved in the NP assessment of adults (*see* **Neuropsychological Assessment**). However, there are many important differences. Developmentalists argue that a child should never be viewed as simply a scaled-down version of an adult. Likewise, an appropriate assessment of brain–behavior relationships in children cannot be based simply on scaled-down versions of assessment methods designed for use with adults. Not only do children differ in terms of the types of brain insult commonly experienced, they also differ with respect to the specificity of behavioral effects manifested, the pattern and course of (re)acquisition after injury, the modifying effects of ongoing developmental change, and the extent to which deficits sometimes can be "silent" until later developmental periods.

There have been a number of books devoted exclusively to the methods and unique issues involved in the NP assessment of children (e.g., [1, 2]). The focus of this article is admittedly selective and begins with a discussion of what *is* NP assessment and how it differs from other related diagnostic methods. Next, there will be an overview of different clinical applications and major test methods and approaches currently available. That will set the stage for a discussion of some key conceptual and practical issues in this area.

Contrast to Other Assessments

What defines a NP assessment and distinguishes it from simply an assessment of a child's mental abilities? In other words, how does it differ from a general psychological assessment?

Many of the standard instruments available for assessing children's abilities, such as the Wechsler Intelligence Scale for Children-Fourth Edition (WISC-IV; [3]), can be used quite effectively in evaluating a child's NP functioning. This is especially true for younger children (up to about 5 or 6 years) for whom decrements in general intelligence are often among the chief manifestations of early childhood brain injury [4]. *Sensitivity to brain dysfunction* is certainly a necessary qualification for a test to be considered a NP measure. This is an empirical issue, based on whether and to what extent performance on the test allows a valid differentiation of normal children and those suffering from one or another type of brain abnormality.

However, most tests used in a general psychological assessment were never developed from a NP perspective, nor were they designed to facilitate various types of inferences regarding a child's NP functioning. For example, different patterns of performance on the WISC-IV may be suggestive of left versus right hemispheric brain dysfunction, but the test was not constructed in a way that readily lends itself to that interpretation. Similarly, although qualitative observations during test performance on the WISC-IV may offer insights regarding a child's executive functioning, it was not designed to isolate this important area of NP functioning. Although virtually any measure of a child's abilities can be used in making NP inferences, some measures are better than others in revealing specific aspects of NP functioning. Thus, another essential feature of NP assessment is that it *facilitates the conceptualization of a child's performance in terms of brain–behavior relationships.* Sensitivity to brain damage is not enough. A test must also be constructed and validated in a manner that permits inferences regarding specific areas of NP functioning.

The NP assessment also should be based on a sufficiently broad appraisal of a child's functioning. The interest is not simply on the child's language abilities, memory, or inhibitory controls – taken separately – but instead on the child's overall performance as reflected in a *functional profile*. This is why a proper assessment typically involves a battery of tests to assure sufficient breadth and depth of coverage. This will be discussed further later on in the section dealing with current approaches to assessment.

To recap, a NP assessment of a child produces a *functional profile derived from a battery of tests sensitive to brain dysfunction and organized in a manner that facilitates inferences regarding brain–behavior relationships.*

What about distinguishing a child NP assessment from other diagnostic methods evaluating neurological abnormalities in children? Specifically, how is it different from a pediatric neurological exam (PNE)? The precise features vary across practitioners, but a PNE typically consists of a review of the child's development, clinical history and presenting complaints as well as a direct examination of areas such as station and gait, basic motor and sensory-perceptual functions, cranial nerves, and reflex integrity. The findings of the exam often are used to judge whether other neurodiagnostic methods should be pursued.

It also includes at least a brief mental status exam (assessing such things as comprehension, naming skills, immediate recall, and so forth) although this is typically rather basic and informal. The child NP assessment, by contrast, is designed to provide a far more in-depth and standardized evaluation of mental processes. Accordingly, it would be more sensitive to neurological conditions having an impact on higher mental functioning. Indeed, this is why suspicious findings on the PNE often may prompt the physician to refer the child for a formal NP assessment. An important distinguishing feature also has to do with the *standardized* nature of the NP assessment – even as it pertains to the evaluation of areas of lower functioning such as motor and sensory-perceptual abilities. In a standardized test or procedure, the components of the exam are administered and scored in a strictly defined manner and evaluated according to specific norms. This permits the measurement of more subtle variations – as, for example, mild decrements in fine-motor speed or control. With this, the NP assessment sometimes may be sensitive to milder or earlier functional changes accompanying a disease process.

The NP assessment can be further differentiated from other neurodiagnostic methods such as brain imaging. Whereas computed tomography (CT) or magnetic resonance imaging (MRI) may identify and localize an underlying brain injury, the NP assessment would instead be used to help specify the particular functional deficit(s) associated with it. Each set of methods occupy opposite ends of a *structural–functional assessment continuum*, with tools such as CT and standard MRI focusing on brain *structure* whereas the NP assessment deals with brain *function*. An abnormal MRI finding may lead to an expectation of a particular functional impairment (as, for example, indications of an injury involving the left temporal lobe suggesting that the child's verbal comprehension and memory may be affected), although this is only an educated inference needing confirmation by actual functional assessment. The reverse is also true – namely, that a particular pattern of performance on NP testing may suggest a particular type or localization of a brain injury, although that too is only an inference based on current knowledge of brain–behavior relationships. In some cases, the findings may diverge, as when abnormalities on NP assessment are not accompanied by abnormalities on brain imaging and *vice versa*. This may occur in cases

with milder injuries, or where the NP finding may relate to other organic variations (such as abnormal blood flow or metabolism) rather than to structural deviations, *per se* [5]. A comprehensive evaluation of the brain injured child often requires an integrated and multimethod approach incorporating both structural and functional assessments.

Applications

Child NP assessment may be used in a broad range of clinical applications. These include: (i) aiding in the detection of brain dysfunction, (ii) providing a specification of the neurobehavioral effects of a known brain injury, (iii) helping to identify specific underlying dimensions of dysfunction in particular handicaps, (iv) using assessment data to help formulate effective treatment strategies, (v) helping to assess the child's prognosis and risk for certain developmental outcomes, and (vi) conducting follow-up assessments of functional change over the course of development and in response to particular interventions [6]. The relative importance of these different applications depends, in part, on the particular clinical population under consideration. Broadly speaking, there are four different but overlapping clinical populations to whom NP assessment may be applied. These include children with: neurological disorders, systemic illness, psychiatric disorders, and learning disabilities.

Children with *neurological disorders* comprise a very broad and varied category. The possible conditions are many, and include children with genetic disorders affecting the brain (e.g., Turner's syndrome), structural abnormalities (e.g., agenesis of the corpus callosum, hydrocephalus), traumatic injuries, epilepsy, and a variety of neuropathological processes such as anoxic episodes, encephalitis, toxic encephalopathy (e.g., carbon monoxide or lead poisoning), metabolic disorders, demyelinating diseases, neuromuscular disorders, brain tumors, and, more rarely in children, cerebral vascular accidents. The NP assessment may serve to identify functional impairments which, taken together with other appropriate evaluations, may lead to the diagnosis of a particular neurological condition. For example, NP findings pointing to a decline in a child's cognitive functioning may prompt a broader neurological work-up that ultimately leads to the diagnosis of a degenerative disorder, such as metachromatic leukodystrophy – a progressive demyelinating disease of the brain. Or, the presence of localizing signs on NP assessment may prompt a more thorough exploration of a specific seizure focus in a child with epilepsy. This could have implications for possible neurosurgical intervention in the child with intractable seizures. However, there is a very important point to emphasize here. In neither of these examples is the NP assessment *diagnostic* of the condition in question; rather the findings may be part of a broader series of evaluations from which a diagnosis is ultimately made. A particular set or pattern of results on NP assessment may correlate with, but, taken by themselves, should never be considered to be diagnostic of these or other neurological conditions.

Besides the issue of detection, an NP assessment may be used to obtain a detailed appraisal of *what* aspects of mental or behavioral functioning have been affected by a known or suspected neurological condition. This was explained before in contrasting what is unique about NP assessment in comparison to other methods used in evaluating the brain-disordered child. The NP assessment is needed to determine what aspects of functioning have been *impaired or spared* as a result of neurological conditions such as epilepsy, congenital abnormalities, toxic states, and so forth.

An area of intensive NP investigation, and one of particular interest within a forensic context, has to do with traumatic brain injury (TBI) in children. The interested reader may wish to refer to one of the published works devoted exclusively to the topic (e.g., [7]). Briefly, some of the key issues in this area have to do with conducting a thorough assessment that is sensitive to the affected areas of functioning, establishing a preinjury baseline (which is especially problematic in younger children) against which current deficits may be compared, and determining not only recovery but possible longer-range developmental impact – especially in terms of delayed effects or deficits that may be "silent" until challenged more as the child grows older. These are among the issues that contribute to the evaluation of TBI and other acquired conditions often being more complicated in children than in adults (more on this later).

Another broad population or category for general application has to do with children having *systemic illness*. This category consists of children having one or more pediatric diseases or conditions, not primarily neurological in nature, which can have a *potentially* adverse impact on central nervous system (CNS) functioning. Examples would include neonatal complications associated with prematurity or very low birth weight, defects in specific organ systems (congenital heart disease, pulmonary or renal dysfunction), infections, metabolic disorders, autoimmune disorders, and cancer. Here too the interested reader is referred to *volumes* dealing thoroughly with the topic (e.g., [8, 9]). What is import to appreciate is that the NP assessment in this general category has become a growing area of need. Advances in medical care over the past several decades have brought about a dramatic increase in the survival of children with serious illnesses. However, with the decrease in mortality has come a corresponding increase in morbidity – as the conditions (or their treatments) sometimes will have an adverse impact on the developing brain and the child's later functioning. The effects can be subtle, and manifested sometimes in the form of low-grade problems with attention or learning. There clearly is a need for careful follow-up in which the NP assessment can play an important role.

Children with *psychiatric disorders* make up another group for whom the NP assessment can be important. This may be viewed from two perspectives. First, children with brain dysfunction are at higher risk for the development (or exacerbation) of a psychiatric disorder. In some cases the relationship may be direct, as when a frontal lobe injury may give rise to impulsive behavior problems. In other cases the relationship is more indirect, whereby brain dysfunction may set the stage for other factors to come into play which, themselves, act to produce or aggravate an emotional or behavioral disturbance [10]. For example, an underlying brain injury may give rise to one or more learning disabilities which may render the child more likely to encounter frustration or failure in school. This, in turn, may result in any of a variety secondary problems ranging from anxiety, depression or social withdrawal to defiance and other acting-out behaviors. Early identification of the functional deficits and behavioral risks in the brain-impaired child can be an important step in limiting the development or progression of a psychiatric disorder.

The other perspective with respect to psychiatric disorders has to do with examining the disorders, themselves, in terms of possible underlying neurobiological and NP abnormalities. Whether or not there is a history of known brain injury or neurological disorder in the case of an individual child, there is rapidly growing evidence that disorders such as autism, attention-deficit/hyperactivity disorder (ADHD), childhood schizophrenia and other psychotic disorders, as well as certain forms of depression and anxiety disorders are each associated with abnormalities in underlying neural mechanisms and NP functioning. For many children with ADHD, for example, disordered frontal-striatal functioning appears to play a key role in the deficits in behavioral inhibition and task persistence commonly seen. Such a perspective has an important bearing on how the condition is approached both in assessment and treatment planning. The interested reader is referred *Tramontana* and associates [11] for a more complete discussion dealing with the neuropsychology of child psychopathology.

Children with *learning disabilities* comprise yet another important population or category for application of NP assessment. Here the interest is not so much on identifying whether or not the child is brain impaired. Nor is there necessarily a question that the child is experiencing a significant handicap in academic learning – whether it has to do with reading, math, writing, and so forth. Indeed, the assessment often may begin with there already being ample documentation that the child is struggling in one or more of these areas. Rather, the emphasis is on using the NP assessment to better understand how and why the learning process may be breaking down. For example, reading can be impeded by any of a variety of underlying problems, including deficits in phonological processing, visual pattern recognition, phoneme-grapheme association, segmentation and sequencing, grammatical awareness, as well as verbal comprehension and memory. The breadth of coverage typically involved in the NP assessment may serve to highlight deficits in relevant underlying component skills. Also, a NP perspective can integrate isolated findings into coherent patterns relevant to brain-based models of learning disabilities. This, in turn, can help to distinguish different patterns or *subtypes* of learning disability having different implications for prognosis and intervention. Here too there are volumes dealing specifically with this topic to which the interested reader may wish to refer (e.g., [12]).

Methods and Approaches

There are a variety of different approaches to child NP assessment. A *fixed-battery* approach is one that aims to provide a comprehensive assessment of brain function using an invariant set of validated test procedures. The composition of the battery is not tailored to the presenting characteristics of the individual child or to the specific clinical questions to be addressed. Rather, the emphasis is on administering a well-defined set of designated tests. It is assumed that individual variability is captured reasonably well as long as the battery is constructed in a fashion that covers a broad range of functioning. An important advantage of this approach is that it provides a standard data base on which different clinical groups can be compared.

Probably the most commonly known example of a fixed-battery approach is the Halstead–Reitan neuropsychological battery (HRNB; see [13]). There are two different versions of the battery for children depending on the age of the child (5–8 years and 9–14). These methods, along with supplemental tests commonly used, were the dominant approach to child NP assessment for decades. Golden [14] introduced a children's revision of a then newly developed NP battery for adults, the Luria-Nebraska Neuropsychological Battery, extending it downward for children ranging from 8 to 12 years of age Luria–Nebraska Neuropsychological Battery-Children's Revision (LNNB-CR). A detailed description and review of these batteries is beyond the scope of this article. These can be found elsewhere [6, 15].

One of the chief limitations of both batteries is that neither was originally developed with children in mind. Areas such as language processing or memory and new learning – areas highly pertinent in the evaluation of children – receive little coverage in the basic HRNB. The same can be said with respect to the area of executive functioning and the LNNB-CR. Neither battery provides an assessment of a key domain such as attention. Thus, more than simply distinguishing brain damaged and normal children (which each battery can do about equally well), an important goal of NP assessment should be to describe how a child is functioning in key domains such as these (more on this in a moment).

At the other extreme are various *flexible approaches* to NP assessment. In *qualitative approaches,* the examiner is less concerned with using methods to quantify the extent of deficits. Instead the emphasis is on determining *how* an individual passes or fails a particular task. Here, for example, the examiner would follow-up with informal inquiries or tasks that may clarify the faulty retrieval strategies that the child used in failing to recall an item correctly. On the basis of this, the examiner may then branch out and select other tasks to gain an evolving picture of what is wrong. *Process-oriented approaches* represent a hybrid of quantitative and qualitative methods. An example is the *Boston Process Approach* [16] that draws selectively from a core set of standardized tests for a quantified overview of general functioning. Depending on the initial results, and guided by clinical hypothesis-testing, the examiner uses various "satellite" tests, including improvised procedures, in order to pinpoint the precise nature of the individual's deficits. Thus, although there are shared components, much of the assessment varies from patient to patient. Another hybrid approach is reflected in the NEPSY-II, (from NEuroPSYological Investigation for Children), which combines a core assessment along with a flexible assessment of selective areas of interest [17]. All of the components of the exam, including those dealing with selective processes, are on the basis of psychometric test scores.

Most neuropsychologists are probably not purists with respect to one approach or set of methods. Whether implicitly or explicitly, many tend to adopt an *eclectic approach* to the NP assessment. Any of a variety of available tests may be selected to quantify the extent of deficit in various areas of functioning. There usually is at least an implicit outline of the relevant functions and abilities to be assessed routinely. The psychometric properties of the tests (adequacy of norms, validated discrimination of brain dysfunction), as well as how well they complement each other in a test battery, are important factors guiding test selection. Qualitative analysis and other flexible approaches may be used to add richness and individualization to the examination, although most neuropsychologists would view these as supplemental rather than primary aspects of the exam.

Table 1 provides an outline of *key domains* for child NP assessment. It is based both on robust factors derived from statistical studies of fixed test batteries as well as a consideration, on conceptual grounds, of key areas that a comprehensive assessment of a child ought to include [6]. In general, the evaluation should include specific measures spanning the following areas: motor functioning, sensory-perceptual abilities, language and spatial processes, attention, memory and new learning, and executive functioning. Also,

Table 1   Key domains in child neuropsychological assessment[a]

Motor control
Sensory-perceptual abilities
Language
Spatial organization
Attention
Memory
Executive functions

[a] A comprehensive evaluation also would include an assessment of intelligence, academic achievement, and behavioral adjustment

whether performed by the neuropsychologist or made available from another source, the evaluation should incorporate findings from tests of general intelligence, academic achievement, as well as measures of behavioral adjustment and personality functioning.

The foregoing has to do with the breadth or scope of the NP assessment. It defines a *horizontal analysis* that is fixed or invariant with respect to the key domains to be assessed. The particular tests used would depend, in part, on the age of the child. They would also depend on the extent to which there are concerns regarding specific areas or subcomponents of functioning on the basis of the history or referral questions concerning the child. Thus, within each domain, there would be a more in-depth or *vertical analysis* of specific areas for which there would be a flexible selection of appropriately normed and validated tests. Table 2 illustrates such an assessment framework. As an example, the domain of language is broken down into subcomponents from which one or more areas might be assessed. The more relevant the domain is in the case of the individual child or population studied, the more thoroughly it would be assessed.

Lastly, Table 3 provides examples of specific tests corresponding to each of the key assessment domains noted above. The listing is only a limited sampling of the possible tests available. There is a helpful volume providing a compendium of these and other NP tests by Strauss *et al.* [18].

Conceptual and Practical Issues

Applying a developmental perspective in child NP assessment means more than simply assuring that the tests and measures are appropriate for the age of the

Table 2   Neuropsychological assessment framework

D1	D2	Language	D4	D5	...	Dx
SD1	SD1	Phonology	SD1	SD1		SD1
SD2	SD2	Repetition	SD2	SD2		SD2
SD3	SD3	Semantics	SD3	SD3		SD3
.	.	Comprehension	.	.		.
.	.	Naming	.	.		.
.	.	Formulation	.	.		.
SDy	SDy	Pragmatics	SDy	SDy		SDxy

D, domain; SD, subdomain

Table 3   Examples of test procedures

Domain	Function assessed
Motor control	
Finger Oscillation Test	Fine-motor speed
Grooved Pegboard	Manual dexterity
Sensory-perceptual	
Tactile Finger Recognition	Simple tactile discrimination
Fingertip Number Writing	Complex tactile perception
Seashore Rhythm Test	Auditory pattern recognition
Picture Completion	Visual closure
Language	
Peabody Picture Vocabulary Test	Word comprehension
Expressive Vocabulary Test	Confrontation naming
Token Test	Listening comprehension
Verbal Fluency	Controlled word association
Spatial	
Embedded Figures Test	Visual-spatial organization
Developmental Test of Visual-motor Integration	Visuoconstructive ability
Tactual Performance Test	Tactile-spatial organization/learning
Attention	
Continuous Performance Test	Vigilance and sustained attention
Trail Making Test	Rapid focusing/sequencing
Memory	
Digit Span	Verbal working memory
Benton Visual Retention Test	Visual reproduction
California Verbal Learning Test	List learning
Wide Range Assessment of Memory and Learning	General memory
Executive functioning	
Category Test	Conceptual reasoning
Wisconsin Card Sorting Test	Flexible problem-solving

child being assessed. It involves understanding how brain functions develop normally as well as under various pathological conditions. A child not only grows more competent with age, but also develops new and more efficient ways of completing tasks and solving problems. An injury or other brain abnormality seldom results in the obliteration of a function or ability. Rather, there often is some recovery of function or compensatory development, although the net effect may be that the function is executed less efficiently than would be true for a normal child of the same age and background. A proper evaluation of a child's NP assessment must be guided by an understanding of concepts such as these.

There are many factors that can obscure or complicate the assessment of brain–behavior relationships in children. These include: (i) problems specifying the precise time of onset for various forms of brain pathology, (ii) the absence of a referential baseline of premorbid functioning in cases of early brain damage, (iii) the sometimes blurred distinction between neurodevelopmental anomalies and normal variations in the rate or pattern of acquisition of function, (iv) the extent to which deficits can sometimes be delayed or "silent" until later developmental periods, (v) the interacting effects of various nonneurological attributes within the child that may serve to compound or mitigate the effects of brain dysfunction, and (vi) the impact of environmental factors, including the family, in shaping the child's outcomes [6]. Although factors similar to these can play a role in the evaluation of adults, they generally are more prominent and complex in the case of the child.

There are practical issues as well. It is well known that an important challenge in working with children in this area has to do with maintaining behavioral compliance and sustained attention for what can be a fairly lengthy assessment. Also, the younger child may be unable to provide a reliable report of deficits and the circumstances in which they are problematic. Reports of parents and teachers often are crucial in providing accounts of the child's abilities outside of the testing situation. On the other hand, feigned impairments on the NP assessment are fairly uncommon in younger children, although distortions of one kind or another may invalidate the history and presenting complaints reported by parents. A careful appraisal of possible parental bias or embellishment in their report of the child's symptoms must be an important part of the overall assessment, especially in cases where litigation is involved.

Age-related constraints on the NP assessment are especially problematic in the evaluation of children during the first 3 or 4 years of life. The limited response repertoire of infants and toddlers, together with the degree to which their performance is state-dependent, place major constraints on formal NP assessment. This is why the bulk of practice in child neuropsychology has dealt mainly with children 5 years of age and older. (See [19], for a thorough discussion of the NP assessment in early childhood.)

In a limited sense, however, the careful application of a NP perspective in the evaluation of standard developmental testing of very young children **is** a NP assessment – as long as it is embedded within a conceptual framework of developmental brain–behavior relationships as discussed above. Areas of potential developmental risk can be identified, on the basis of both known/suspected CNS insults coupled with direct observations of the child, which can then be highlighted for further, more formal NP assessment once the child reaches about 5 years of age.

Finally, there are unique challenges that arise in the evaluation of special populations. Included here are children with handicapping conditions such as sensory loss (blind and hearing impaired), physical deformities, motor disabilities, and language impairment. It is important to appreciate the impact of the handicap on the child's general functioning and adjustment. At the same time, special care must be taken to assure that the handicap does not overshadow and distort the picture of the child's functioning in nonimpaired areas. This is an area that calls upon specific skills, experience, and ingenuity on the part of the examiner. The same is true for working effectively with non-English speaking children and those with other cultural differences.

The foregoing provided a general overview of child NP assessment. Hopefully, with it, the reader has gained an understanding of how to conceptualize and contrast this type of assessment in comparison to other related evaluation methods for children. Major applications were discussed and there was a delineation of the various approaches and methods currently available in the field. Lastly, various conceptual and practical issues were highlighted – including the critical importance of a development framework in conducting and evaluating the child NP assessment, as well as the special challenges that present when evaluating various subgroups of children. The coverage was selective, but nonetheless should have given a general idea of the defining characteristics and current status of this field.

References

[1]   Baron, I.S. (2004). *Neuropsychological Evaluation of the Child*, Oxford University Press, New York.

[2]   Tramontana, M.G. & Hooper, S.R. (1988a). *Assessment Issues in Child Neuropsychology*, Plenum Press, New York.

[3]   Wechsler, D. (2003). *Wechsler Intelligence Scale for Children – (WISC-IV)*, 4th Edition Psychological Corporation, Harcourt Assessment, San Antonio.

[4]   Boll, T.J. & Barth, J.T. (1981). Neuropsychology of brain damage in children, in *Handbook of Clinical Neuropsychology*, S.B. Filskov & T.J. Boll, eds, John & Sons Wiley, New York, pp. 418–452.

[5]   Hillary, F.G. & DeLuca, J. (2007). *Functional Neuroimaging in Clinical Populations*, Guilford Press, New York.

[6]   Tramontana, M.G. & Hooper, S.R. (1988b). Child neuropsychological assessment: overview and current status, in *Assessment Issues in Child Neuropsychology*, M.G. Tramontana & S.R. Hooper, eds, Plenum Press, New York, pp. 3–38.

[7]   Granacher, R.P. (2003). *Traumatic Brain Injury: Methods for Clinical and Forensic Neuropsychiatric Assessment*, CRC Press, New York.

[8]   Hynd, G.W. & Willis, W.G. (1988). *Pediatric Neuropsychology*, Grune and Stratton, New York.

[9]   Yeates, K.O., Ris, M.D. & Taylor, H.G. (2000). *Pediatric Neuropsychology: Research, Theory, and Practice*, Guilford Press, New York.

[10] Tramontana, M.G. (1983). Neuropsychological evaluation of children and adolescents with psychopathological disorders, in *Foundations of Clinical Neuropsychology*, C.J. Golden & P.J. Vincente, eds, Plenum Press, New York, pp. 309–340.

[11] Tramontana, M.G., Hooper, S.R., Watts-English, T., Ellison, T. & Bethea, T.C. (2008). Neuropsychology of child psychopathology, in *Handbook of Clinical Child Neuropsychology*, C.R. Reynolds & E. Fletcher-Janzen, eds, 3rd Edition, Springer Press, New York.

[12] Fletcher, J.M., Lyon, G.R., Fuchs, L.S. & Barnes, M.A. (2007). *Learning Disabilities: From Identification to Intervention*, Guilford Press, New York.

[13] Reitan, R.M. & Davison, L.A. (1974). *Clinical Neuropsychology: Current Status and Applications*, John Wiley & Sons, New York.

[14] Golden, C.J. (1981). The Luria-Nebraska Children's battery: theory and formulation, in *Neuropsychological Assessment and the School-age Child: Issues and Perspectives*, G.W. Hynd & J.E. Obrzut, eds, Grune and Stratton, New York, pp. 277–302.

[15] Reynolds, C.R. & Fletcher-Janzen, E. (eds) (2008). *Handbook of Clinical Child Neuropsychology*, 3rd Edition, Plenum Press, New York.

[16] Milberg, W.P., Hebben, N. & Kaplan, E. (1986). The Boston process approach to neuropsychological assessment, in *Neuropsychological Assessment of Neuropsychiatric Disorders*, I. Grant & K.M. Adams, eds, Oxford University Press, New York, pp. 65–86.

[17] Korkman, M., Kirk, U. & Kemp, S. (2007). *NEPSY*, 2nd Edition Psychological Corporation, Harcourt Assessment, San Antonio.

[18] Strauss, E., Sherman, E.M.S. & Spreen, O. (2006). *A Compendium of Neuropsychological Tests: Administration, Norms, and Commentary*, 3rd Edition, Oxford University Press, New York.

[19] Aylward, G.P. (1988). Infant and early childhood assessment, in *Assessment Issues in Child Neuropsychology*, M.G. Tramontana & S.R. Hooper, eds, Plenum Press, New York, pp. 225–248.

MICHAEL G. TRAMONTANA

Neuropsychological Assessment: Head Injury *see* Head Injury: Neuropsychological Assessment

Northwest Juvenile Project

The Northwestern Juvenile Project (NJP) is the first large-scale, prospective longitudinal study of alcohol, drug, and mental (ADM) disorders in juvenile detainees. The NJP is funded by a consortium of nine federal agencies and five private foundations. The sample includes a diverse sample of 1829 youth, aged 10–18 years at baseline, who were arrested and detained between 1995 and 1998 in Cook County (Chicago metropolitan area), Illinois. Initially funded to examine the ADM disorder service needs and service use of juvenile detainees, the aims of the NJP have expanded to include an examination of (i) changes in ADM disorders and the comorbidity of disorders over time; (ii) patterns of mental health service use over time; and (iii) pathways and patterns of drug use, violence, and risk behaviors for human immunodeficiency virus (HIV)/acquired immune deficiency syndrome (AIDS) and other sexually transmitted infections (STIs) over time. The NJP tracks and reinterviews these youth wherever they are living, whether they are back in their communities or incarcerated. The NJP also obtains records cross-validating self-reported data on criminal justice involvement, and mental health and substance use service utilization from 16 correctional and service agencies.

Background to the Northwestern Juvenile Project

Reports issued by the Surgeon General [1] and the President's New Freedom Commission on Mental Health [2, 3] note that the mental health needs of juvenile detainees are largely underserved. Under the Eighth Amendment (barring cruel and unusual punishment) and the Fourteenth Amendment (right to substantive due process for youths in the juvenile justice system) of the US Constitution, juvenile detainees with serious mental disorders have a right to receive needed treatment as part of the state's obligation to provide needed medical care. Providing appropriate services, however, requires accurate and reliable data on the prevalence of mental disorders among juvenile detainees. Data are necessary for planning how to best utilize the finite resources of the juvenile justice and community mental health systems to meet the mental health needs of detained youth.

Despite the importance of epidemiological data on the mental health and substance abuse needs of juvenile detainees, the juvenile justice system has not had comprehensive, accurate, and reliable data upon which to guide policy decisions. Although a number of studies have examined the mental health and substance abuse needs of detained youth, estimates of rates across studies are discrepant. For example, estimates of the prevalence of affective disorder vary from 5% [4] to 72%; [5] substance use disorders vary from 20% [6] to 88%; [5] and psychosis varies from 16% [5] to 45% [6].

The variability in rates may result from discrepancies in the methods of prior studies in the following areas:

Sample Composition

The composition of samples substantially varied across prior studies. The racial and ethnic compositions of the samples in many of these studies are not representative of the national juvenile justice population; some studies did not even report the racial or ethnic composition of the sample. Females, an increasing proportion of juvenile detainees, were excluded entirely from some investigations.

Small Size

Because of the difficulties associated with the study of detained youth, many studies had small samples. Small samples make it difficult for studies to generate reliable rates, especially for more severe mental disorders with low base rates in the general population (i.e., 1–4%). Many of the studies sampled too few subjects to generate reliable rates even for the more common mental disorders [7]. Most studies did not have enough participants in key demographic subgroups to compare participants by gender, race and ethnicity, or age.

Measurement

Some studies relied on nonstandard or untested instruments; others failed to consider impaired functioning or reported data on only one category of disorder (e.g., substance use disorders, anxiety disorders, and personality disorders) rather than a spectrum of disorders. Even when multiple disorders were assessed, most of the studies did not examine patterns of comorbidity between mental and substance use disorders.

The Northwestern Juvenile Project

The NJP was designed to overcome the methodological limitations of prior studies. The NJP has three interrelated goals:

1. To assess how ADM disorders develop over time among detained youth.

The NJP assesses persistence and change in mental and substance use disorders (including remission and recurrence) patterns of comorbid disorders, and associated functional impairments and outcomes during critical points of development: adolescence, emerging adulthood, and young adulthood.

2. To investigate barriers, pathways, and patterns of service use.

The NJP assesses if and when youth who *need* services *receive* them and from which sectors: corrections, child welfare, education, general health, mental health, and informal services. The NJP can also evaluate how patterns of service use are associated with longitudinal outcomes.

3. To determine pathways and patterns of drug use, violence, and risk behaviors for and prevalence of HIV and other STIs.

The NJP examines the development of these risk behaviors among our subjects, focusing on gender differences, racial/ethnic differences, the antecedents of these risky behaviors, and how these behaviors are interrelated. The NJP will also provide the first estimate of the prevalence and incidence of HIV and other STIs in this population.

Methods

The sample, longitudinal design, and assessments used in the NJP address many of the limitations of prior studies of detained youth.

Sample

Participants in the NJP were a randomly selected sample of male and female youth who were arrested and subsequently detained at the Cook County Juvenile Temporary Detention Center (CCJTDC) between November 20, 1995 and June 14, 1998. As part of the study design, selected strata were oversampled to obtain enough data within key subgroups. The sample was stratified based on the following variables: age (10–13 years or ≥ 14 years), gender, race/ethnicity (African-American, non-Hispanic white, and Hispanic), and legal status (processed as a juvenile or an adult). Sample weights were used in statistical analyses so that the findings reflect CCJTDC's population rather than the stratified sample. The sample provides several advantages over prior studies, including:

1. Large sample size.

The final sample includes 1829 participants, a sample size large enough to allow for reliable estimates of uncommon disorders, comorbidity of disorders, and high-risk behaviors.

2. A large subsample of females.

Because females were oversampled, the NJP has a large enough subsample of females (657 females; 35.9% of the sample) to examine differences by gender, as well as differences among females on other key variables. Studying females is critical because females make up increasing proportions of juvenile arrestees (24%), juvenile detainees (19%),

adult arrestees (22%), and adult detainees (21%) [8–11].

3. Racial/ethnic diversity.

The stratification of the sample also provides the NJP with adequate participants to examine racial/ethnic diversity within the sample, including 1005 African-Americans (54.9%), 524 Hispanics (28.7%), 296 non-Hispanic whites (16.2%), and four from other racial/ethnic groups (0.2%).

4. Wide age range.

The age range of the sample is 10–18 years old (mean, 14.9 years) at baseline. Youth aged 10–13 were oversampled to provide adequate numbers to examine age differences.

5. Diversity of criminal behavior.

Because the NJP sampled participants from *all* newly arrested youth entering detention, it represents a variety of youngsters who are sent to detention centers. In contrast, other studies focus on specific subpopulations of juvenile detainees, such as serious and violent offenders (i.e., those adjudicated (convicted) of a felony, misdemeanor weapons offense, or misdemeanor sexual assault).

6. Youth processed as adults.

The sample of the NJP includes youth that are automatically transferred to the adult system for processing. These youth are excluded from the jurisdiction of juvenile court based on their type of offense, criminal history, and/or age.

Longitudinal Design

Although cross-sectional studies can be useful to ascertain basic epidemiologic data, a developmental epidemiologic approach requires prospective longitudinal studies [12]. Longitudinal studies allows researchers to (i) examine the antecedents of disorders and other behavioral problems within a temporal context, thereby providing the basis for understanding causal mechanisms [13]; (ii) reveal pathways, changes *within* individuals, variation *among* individuals, and, most important, *sequences* in the development of disorders and other problem behaviors; and (iii) examine age-dependent change, independent of disorder [12, 13].

The NJP is currently funded to collect 9 waves of data spanning 14 years. The longitudinal design allows for the examination of detailed data on mental disorders, substance use patterns, criminal behavior (including violence), use of mental health and other health services, and HIV/AIDS risk behaviors across three critical developmental periods: adolescence (ages 10–18 years), emerging adulthood (ages 18–25 years), and young adulthood (ages 25–30 years). All participants are tracked until located, and subsequently interviewed wherever they are found. Records cross-validating self-reported data (e.g., on arrests, incarceration history, health, and service use) are also obtained from 16 correctional and community service agencies.

Measurement

The NJP employs standardized diagnostic instruments that are sensitive to the varying developmental stage of our participants. The Diagnostic Interview Schedule (DISC) version 2.3 (based on revised third edition of the Diagnostic and Statistical Manual for Mental Disorders (DSM)) [14, 15], the most recent English and Spanish version then available, was used for the baseline assessments. Diagnostic assessments were changed in accordance with changes in participants' age and improvements in diagnostic technology. For subsequent interviews, the NJP administered version 4.0 of the DISC (based on *DSM-IV*), modified by its authors for use with young adults. The Diagnostic Interview Schedule, version IV (DIS-IV) (based on *DSM-IV*) was used to assess disorders not assessed, or not adequately assessed by the DISC 4.0, including substance use disorders, schizophrenia, cognitive impairment, and antisocial personality disorder (APD) [16]. Most of the samples aged 18 years or older in 2002, at which time the NJP stopped using diagnostic tools designed for children and adolescents and began administering the World Mental Health – Composite International Diagnostic Interview (WMH-CIDI). The WMH-CIDI assesses suicidality and the following *DSM-IV* disorders: depression, mania, panic, generalized anxiety, and posttraumatic stress [17]. The WMH-CIDI represents the state-of-the-art in structured diagnostic interviews, building on earlier versions of the CIDI (World Health Organization (CIDI version 2.1); University of Michigan (UM-CIDI); and Munich, Germany (M-CIDI)) and the DIS-IV [17]. The NJP continues to use the National Institute of Mental Health DIS-IV to assess (i) APD, because it is not included

in the WMH-CIDI 2000; (ii) substance use disorders, because the WMH-CIDI 2000 classified drugs into "other" categories rather than identifying specific drugs abused; and (iii) schizophrenia, because the WMH-CIDI 2000 only screens for psychosis.

In addition to the assessment of mental disorders, the NJP assesses the use of mental health services, risk behaviors for HIV/AIDS and other STIs, and a variety of risk and protective factors:

- cognitive and behavioral risk factors for HIV/AIDS and other STIs (self-efficacy, perception of risk, behavioral information and skills, HIV/AIDS knowledge, normative support for HIV prevention, and attitudes and beliefs about HIV prevention);
- functional and cognitive impairments;
- adverse life events, victimization, trauma exposure, and experiences of loss and death;
- criminal and violent activity;
- adult social role performance (education, employment, finances, residential stability, living situation, and parenting);
- physical health;
- mortality (including the cause of death);
- quality of life;
- general attitudes and beliefs (self-esteem, self-efficacy, attitudes toward deviance, stages of change, religiosity, and future orientation);
- characteristics of the family of origin;
- marital and intimate relationships;
- deviant associations;
- social network and support;
- acculturation; and
- neighborhood and community characteristics.

Overview of Published Findings from the NJP

Published data from the NJP have been cited in the Surgeon General's Report on Children's Mental Health and is used by national advocacy groups and in reports to Congress. Analyses of data from the NJP are ongoing. To date, articles have been published in *Archives of General Psychiatry, American Journal of Public Health, Journal of the American Academy of Child and Adolescent Psychiatry, Journal of Consulting and Clinical Psychology, Pediatrics*, and *Psychiatric Services*. The following is a brief summary of key findings.

- **Prevalence of mental disorders.**

Almost three-quarters of females and two-thirds of males had one or more mental disorders. Substance use disorders, the most common type of disorder, affected over 50% of males and 46% of females. Females had significantly higher odds than males of having any disorder. Non-Hispanic whites had significantly higher odds than the African-Americans or Hispanics of having any disorder [18]. Nearly 93% of participants reported 1 or more traumas; 11% met criteria for post-traumatic stress disorder in the past year [19].

- **Comorbidity of ADM disorders.**

Comorbidity was common. Significantly more females (57%) than males (46%) had comorbid mental disorders. Participants with major mental disorder (i.e., major depression, mania, and psychosis) were significantly more likely to have a substance use disorder than those without major mental disorders [20]. Log-linear and latent class models were used to empirically identify the most common combinations of alcohol, marijuana, and other drug use disorders. Over 21% had 2 or more substance use disorders. The most prevalent combination was alcohol and marijuana. Four of the five participants with an alcohol disorder also had one or more drug use disorders [21].

- **Substance use.**

Self-reported drug use had a high level of veracity for the use of cannabis; among detainees with positive urinalysis results, 88% reported use in the past six months. Combining self-report and urinalysis reveals a *minimum* prevalence of 85% for any illicit drug use in the past 6 months [22].

- **Prevalence of HIV/AIDS risk behaviors.**

Baseline HIV/AIDS risk behavior data were collected from 800 participants when funding for this component became available. HIV/AIDS risk behaviors were prevalent, irrespective of gender, race/ethnicity, or age; 95% engaged in three or more risk behaviors, and over 60% engaged in 10 or more risk behaviors. All specific risk behaviors were more prevalent in our sample than the general population. Significantly more African-Americans than non-Hispanic whites had *sexual* risk behaviors; significantly more non-Hispanic whites than the African-Americans had *drug* risk behaviors [23].

- **Substance use disorder, major mental disorder, and HIV/AIDS risk behaviors.**

Substance use disorder significantly increased the odds of engaging in HIV/AIDS risk behaviors. Among youth who had comorbid major mental and substance use disorders, 58% engaged in unprotected sexual activity while drunk or high, compared to only 7% of youth with a major mental disorder but no comorbid substance use disorder. Among the youth with a substance use disorder, more than 63% engaged in 5 or more sexual risk behaviors [24].

- **Development and persistence of HIV/AIDS risk behaviors.**

The development of HIV/AIDS risk behaviors among participants between their baseline and three-year follow-up interviews was examined. Among males, high-risk sexual behaviors were significantly more prevalent at the follow-up than at baseline. Significantly more females engaged in other sexual behaviors at the follow-up than at baseline, including trading sex and drugs and recent unprotected vaginal sex. Patterns of development of HIV/AIDS risk behaviors differed by gender and race/ethnicity. More males than females developed sexual risk behaviors; more females than males developed drug risk behaviors. Significantly more non-Hispanic whites and Hispanics than African-Americans developed drug risk behaviors [25].

- **Development of antisocial personality disorder.**

On the basis of a subsample of 1112 detained youth who were adults at the time of the 3-year follow-up interview, nearly one-fifth of the male juvenile detainees later developed APD. Significantly more males than females developed APD; no differences were found by race/ethnicity. Conduct disorder (CD) diagnosis and the number of CD symptoms were significantly associated with developing modified-APD (M-APD; APD without the CD requirement). *Post hoc* analyses, however, suggested a threshold effect: participants with five or more CD symptoms were significantly more likely to develop M-APD than participants with fewer than five symptoms. Analysis also indicated that several other disorders were significantly associated with the development of M-APD, including dysthymia, alcohol use disorder, or generalized anxiety disorder. Although some disorders were strong predictors of APD, none were useful for identifying which youth would later develop M-APD [26].

- **Detecting and treating mental disorder.**

Institutional records on the provision of mental health services by the detention center and public health system were examined for up to 6 months after intake to detention. Among detainees who had major mental disorders and associated functional impairments, only 15% were treated in the detention center and even less (8%) received treatment in the community. Significantly more females than males with major mental disorders were identified and treated for mental disorders. Detection of need for mental health treatment and undergoing treatment were predicted, in part, by clinical, demographic, and legal variables. Specifically, the odds of being detected or treated was greater among the youth with a major mental disorder, treatment history, or suicidality reported at intake, and lower among racial/ethnic minorities, males, older detainees, and detainees transferred to adult court for legal processing [27].

- **Mortality.**

Seventy-seven participants (4%) died since the study began. Mortality rates of the 65 (4%) who died before March 2004 were analyzed; 96% of these youth died from homicide or legal intervention (e.g., killed by police). Standardized mortality is more than *4 times* the general population rates. Mortality among females is nearly *8 times* the general population rates. African-American males have the highest mortality; yet, they have the lowest mortality *ratio* because their mortality in the general population is high [28].

Conclusions

A substantial number of youth are involved in the juvenile justice system. Approximately two million youth are arrested each year and over 100 000 juveniles are in custody on any given day [29]. The public health and justice systems must have accurate and reliable data from which to guide public policy for youth entering the justice system. The NJP provides data that are critical to improving the outcomes of one of our nation's most needful population of youth.

References

[1] US Department of Health and Human Services (2000). *Report of the Surgeon General's Conference on Children's Mental Health: A National Action Agenda*, US Government Printing Office, Washington, D.C.

[2] The President's New Freedom Commission on Mental Health (2003). *Achieving the Promise: Transforming Mental Health Care in America* (Final Report), Report No: SMA-03-3832, Department of Health and Human Services, Rockville, MD.

[3] Hogan, M.F. (2003). New freedom commission report: the president's new freedom commission: recommendations to transform mental health care in America, *Psychiatric Services (Washington, D.C)* **54**, 1467–1474.

[4] McCabe, K.M., Lansing, A.E., Garland, A. & Hough, R. (2002). Gender differences in psychopathology, functional impairment, and familial risk factors among adjudicated delinquents, *Journal of the American Academy of Child and Adolescent Psychiatry* **41**, 860–867.

[5] Timmons-Mitchell, J., Brown, C., Schulz, S.C., Webster, S.E., Underwood, L.A. & Semple, W.E. (1997). Comparing the mental health needs of female and male incarcerated juvenile delinquents, *Behavioral Sciences and the Law* **15**, 195–202.

[6] Atkins, D.L., Pumariega, A.J., Rogers, K., Montgomery, L., Nybro, C., Jeffers, G. & Sease, F. (1999). Mental health and incarcerated youth, I: prevalence and nature of psychopathology, *Journal of Child and Family Studies* **8**, 193–204.

[7] Cohen, J. (1988). *Statistical Power Analysis for the Behavioral Sciences*, 2nd Edition, Lawrence Earlbaum Associates, Hillsdale.

[8] Snyder, H.N. (2005). *Juvenile Arrests 2003*, August. Report No.: NCJ209735, Office of Juvenile Justice and Delinquency Prevention, Washington, D.C.

[9] Sickmund, M., Sladky, T.J. & Kang, W. (2005). *Census of Juveniles in Residential Placement Databook*. Available from: http://www.ojjdp.ncjrs.org/ojstatbb/cjrp/, [cited 2007 March 1].

[10] Greenfeld, L.A. & Snell, T. (1999). *Women Offenders*, Report No.: NCJ 175688, US Department of Justice, Washington, D.C.

[11] US Department of Justice (2001). *Correctional Populations in the United States, 1998*, Report No: NCJ 192929, US Department of Justice, Washington, D.C.

[12] Angold, A. & Costello, E.J. (1991). Developing a developmental epidemiology, in *Rochester Symposium on Developmental Psychopathology*, D. Cicchetti & S.L. Toth, eds, University of Rochester Press, Rochester, pp. 75–96.

[13] Kessler, R.C. (1995). Epidemiology of psychiatric comorbidity, in *Textbook in Psychiatric Epidemiology*, M.T. Tsuang, M. Tohen & G.E.P. Zahner, eds, Wiley-Liss, New York, pp. 179–197.

[14] Shaffer, D., Fisher, P., Dulcan, M.K. & Davies, M. (1996). The NIMH diagnostic interview schedule for children version 2.3 (DISC-2.3): description, acceptability, prevalence rates, and performance in the MECA study, *Journal of the American Academy of Child and Adolescent Psychiatry* **35**, 865–877.

[15] Bravo, M., Woodbury-Farina, M., Canino, G.J. & Rubio-Stipec, M. (1993). The Spanish translation and cultural adaptation of the diagnostic interview schedule for

children (DISC) in puerto rico, *Culture, Medicine and Psychiatry* **17**, 329–344.

[16] Shaffer, D., Fisher, P., Lucas, C.P., Dulcan, M.K. & Schwab-Stone, M.E. (2000). NIMH diagnostic interview schedule for children version IV (NIMH DISC-IV): description, differences from previous versions, and reliability of some common diagnoses, *Journal of the American Academy of Child and Adolescent Psychiatry* **39**, 28–38.

[17] Kessler, R.C. & Üstün, T.B. (2004). The World Mental Health (WMH) survey initiative version of the World Health Organization (WHO) Composite International Diagnostic Interview (CIDI), *International Jounral of Methods in Psychiatric Research* **13**, 93–121.

[18] Teplin, L.A., Abram, K.M., McClelland, G.M., Dulcan, M.K. & Mericle, A.A. (2002). Psychiatric disorders in youth in juvenile detention, *Archives of General Psychiatry* **59**, 1133–1143.

[19] Abram, K.M., Teplin, L.A., Charles, D.R., Longworth, S.L., McClelland, G.M. & Dulcan, M.K. (2004). Posttraumatic stress disorder and trauma in youth in juvenile detention, *Archives of General Psychiatry* **661**, 403–410.

[20] Abram, K.M., Teplin, L.A., McClelland, G.M. & Dulcan, M.K. (2003). Comorbid psychiatric disorders in youth in juvenile detention, *Archives of General Psychiatry* **60**, 1097–1108.

[21] McClelland, G.M., Elkington, K.S., Teplin, L.A. & Abram, K.M. (2004). Multiple substance use disorders in juvenile detainees, *Journal of the American Academy of Child and Adolescent Psychiatry* **43**, 1215–1224.

[22] McClelland, G.M., Teplin, L.A. & Abram, K.M. (2004). *Detection and Prevalence of Substance Use Among Juvenile Detainees*, June. Report No.: NCJ 203934, Office of Juvenile Justice and Delinquency Prevention, Washington, D.C.

[23] Teplin, L.A., Mericle, A.A., McClelland, G.M. & Abram, K.M. (2003). HIV and AIDS risk behaviors in juvenile detainees: implications for public health policy, *American Journal of Public Health* **93**, 906–912.

[24] Teplin, L.A., Elkington, K.S., McClelland, G.M., Mericle, A.A. & Washburn, J.J. (2005). Major mental disorders, substance use disorders, comorbidity, and HIV-AIDS risk behaviors in juvenile detainees, *Psychiatric Services (Washington, DC)* **56**, 823–828.

[25] Romero, E.G., Teplin, L.A., McClelland, G.M., Abram, K.M., Welty, L.J. & Washburn, J.J. (2007). A longitudinal study of the prevalence, development and persistence of HIV/sexually transmitted infection risk behaviors in delinquent youth: implications for health care in the community, *Pediatrics* **119**, e1126–e1141.

[26] Washburn, J.J., Romero, E.G., Welty, L.J., Abram, K.M., Teplin, L.A., McClelland, G.M. & Paskar, L.D. (2007). Development of antisocial personality disorder in detained youth: the predictive value of mental disorders, *Journal of Consulting and Clinical Psychology* **75**, 221–231.

[27] Teplin, L.A., Abram, K.M., McClelland, G.M., Washburn, J.J. & Pikus, A.K. (2005). Detecting mental disorder in juvenile detainees: who receives services, *American Journal of Public Health* **95**, 1773–1780.

[28] Teplin, L.A., McClelland, G.M., Abram, K.M. & Mileusnic, D. (2005). Early violent death among delinquent youth: a prospective longitudinal study, *Pediatrics* **115**, 1586–1593.

[29] Sickmund, M. (2004). *Juveniles in Corrections. Report*, Report No.: NCJ 202855, Office of Juvenile Justice and Delinquency Prevention, Washington, D.C.

Jason J. Washburn, Linda A. Teplin and Karen M. Abram

Nuclear Forensics

Introduction

Nuclear forensics (nuclear forensic science/nuclear forensic analysis) is the branch of science that seeks to examine the nature, use, and origin of nuclear (fissile) and radioactive (nonfissile) materials. Nuclear forensic analysis produces a characteristic "signature" for the material and therefore may provide major evidence for nuclear attribution. It is most often applied to investigations involving the malevolent use of nuclear or radioactive materials and is of assistance in determining adherence to international safeguards against illicit trafficking [1].

Nuclear forensic analysis aims to provide legally admissible evidence that could lead to prosecution of the offenders involved with trafficking of the illicit material. Thus, it assists law enforcement agencies in the fight against illicit trafficking in nuclear and radioactive material in order to minimize the likelihood of such materials being used by terrorists as weapons in the form of radiological or nuclear (R or N) agents. Together with specific chemical and biological (C and B) agents, they form part of the CBRN agents, sometimes also called *weapons of mass destruction* (WMD). CBRN is a commonly used acronym which refers to chemical, biological, radiological or nuclear weapons that can be used to kill or injure large numbers of people, damage infrastructure, damage the economy or damage the environment in general (*see also* **Chemical, Biological, Radiological, and Nuclear Investigations**; **Biological Agents**; **Chemical Warfare Agents** and **Bomb Scene Management**).

Nuclear attribution is the process of identifying sources of an interdicted nuclear or radioactive material in order to determine its origin, intended or original use; the routes of transfer between the point where legitimate control over the material was lost and the point where the material was intercepted; and the perpetrators responsible for the illicit dealings with the material [1].

A nuclear forensic investigation is conducted in conjunction with traditional forensic examinations of the illicit material. Such examinations might include analysis of explosive residues, biological samples, documents, ballistics, hairs, pollens, fibers, and other associated physical evidence.

The desired outcome of the nuclear forensic analysis is the appropriate prosecution of offenders in a court of law. Therefore, implementation of scientifically defensible sampling and analytical methods and the need to strictly observe chain of custody requirements are essential.

Radiological and Nuclear Agents

Examples of fissile and nonfissile radioactive materials that might be of interest in illegal trafficking are listed in Table 1. The classification of the radioactive materials (sources) follows the five categories as defined by the International Atomic Energy Agency (IAEA) [2]. Apart from nuclear materials, the radioactive sources in Radioactive source Categories 1, 2, and 3 are of specific concern. This is due to both, their high activities and their ubiquity. Devices containing sources such as caesium-137, cobalt-60, or americium-241 are used heavily in industrial and medical establishments worldwide, with access to the materials often poorly controlled. Depending on their nature and the radiation characteristics, terrorists may use such materials in the form of an improvised nuclear device (IND), a radiological dispersion device (RDD; e.g., a "dirty bomb"), or a radiological emission device (RED).

An IND is a crude nuclear weapon constructed from material such as weapons-grade uranium (20–90% U-235) or plutonium. Its explosion would have similarly disastrous consequences, although

most likely on a smaller scale, than a modern, dedicated nuclear weapon. The high degree of technical expertise and the cost of building a functional IND make this scenario less likely to occur.

A possible alternative to the construction of an IND is the acquisition of a nuclear weapon through the black market or from rogue nations, or *via* theft from the arsenal of a vulnerable nuclear-weapon state. Nuclear weapons, depending on the yield, have the potential to destroy entire cities. Their impact would be physically, psychologically, and economically devastating.

An RDD disperses radioactive material into the environment, resulting in radioactive contamination of an area. Perhaps the most well-known form of the RDD is the "dirty bomb", in which a conventional high explosive is combined with a radioactive material. Alternatively, specific installations (such as a nuclear reactor, nuclear fuel manufacturing or reprocessing plant, and a radiation source manufacturing plant or a radioactive waste disposal facility) could be targeted as a means of releasing radioactive material and causing contamination of the environment. The extent of radioactive contamination would depend on the size of the explosion, weather conditions, the nature of the affected environment, and the amount, type, and form of radioactive materials involved.

An RED is a high-activity radioactive source that emits energy in the form of highly penetrating gamma or neutron radiation under concealment in a frequented public place. Unlike an IND or RDD, a RED is not designed to cause destruction and/or radioactive contamination of an area, but is aimed at exposing people to high levels of radiation. The existence of the device may not be realized until radiation exposure symptoms are observed among the affected individuals or the perpetrators make the existence of the device publicly known. The detrimental health impact of such a device on the exposed would vary, depending on the total dose received by an individual and is influenced by the duration of their exposure, the activity of the source, and the type and the energy of the radiation emitted from the source. Exposure to high doses of radiation, of the order of sieverts (i.e., hundreds of rems), would cause serious adverse health effects within a short time, and could lead to death [4].

The severity of consequences associated with the use of a device and the probability that a device will

Table 1 Categories of nuclear and other radioactive material[a]

Category	Type of material or device	Radioactive components
Unirradiated direct-use nuclear material	High enriched uranium (HEU)	>20% U-235
	Plutonium and mixed U-Pu oxides (MOX)	<80% Pu-238
	U-233	Separated isotope
Irradiated direct-use nuclear material	Irradiated nuclear fuel material	In irradiated nuclear fuel elements or in spent fuel reprocessing solutions
Alternative nuclear material	Americium-241	Separated element or present in irradiated nuclear material, in separated plutonium, or in mixtures of uranium and plutonium
	Neptunium-237	
Indirect use nuclear material	Depleted uranium (DU)	<0.7% U-235
	Natural uranium (NU)	0.7% U-235
	Low enriched uranium(LEU)	>0.7% U-235 and<20% U-235 (typically 3–5%) U-235
	Plutonium (Pu-238)	>80% Pu-238
	Thorium	Th-232
Radioactive source Category 1	Radioisotope thermoelectric generators	Pu-238, Cm-244 and Sr-90
	Irradiators/sterilizers	Co-60 and Cs-137
	Teletherapy source	Co-60 and Cs-137
Radioactive source Category 2	Industrial gamma radiography sources	I-192[b]
	High/medium dose rate brachytherapy sources	Co-60 and Cs-137
Radioactive source Category 3	Fixed industrial gauges	Co-60, Cs-137, and Am-241
	Well logging gauges	
Radioactive source Category 4	Low dose rate brachytherapy sources	Co-60, Cs-137, and Am-241
	Thickness/fill level gauges	
	Portable gauges (e.g., moisture, density)	
	Bone densitometers	
	Static eliminators	
Radioactive source Category 5	Eye plaques, permanent implants	Sr-90[b]
	X-ray fluorescence devices	Fe-55[b]
	Electron capture devices	Ni-63[b]
	Mössbauer spectrometers	Co-57[b]
	Positron emission tomographs	Ge-68[b]
	Medical diagnostic sources	Short-lived radioisotopes, e.g., I-131
	Fire detectors	Am-241 and Pu-238

[a] Reproduced with permission from Ref. 3. © IAEA, 2006.
[b] Information added by the authors.

be used is directly linked to the type of the device (Figure 1).

The most detrimental consequences would result from the use of a technologically sophisticated device, such as an illegally obtained nuclear weapon or the use of an IND. However, the difficulties associated with procuring a nuclear weapon or constructing an IND markedly diminishes their probability of being used. Perpetrators would likely favor the use of a device that is less complicated

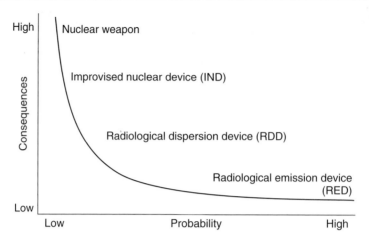

Figure 1 Relationship between the probability of the use of a given device and the detrimental consequences of its use. [Figure adapted from [5]]

and/or easier to procure, such as an RDD or a RED.

Nuclear Forensic Analysis

Nuclear forensic analysis involves physical characterization and subsequent forensic interpretation of nuclear or radioactive material [1, 3].

Characterization of the nuclear or radioactive material aims to determine the chemical and physical signature of a sample of the intercepted illicit material. A number of analytical tools may be utilized to determine the signature of the material being investigated. As in traditional forensic analysis, selection of a particular analytical method is often determined by the results obtained in the consecutive stages of sample analysis. These analytical methods can be grouped into three categories: bulk analysis tools, imaging tools, and microanalysis tools [3, 6].

Bulk analysis tools enable the determination of the elemental and isotopic composition of the material, including the presence and concentrations of trace constituents. They include chemical assays, high-resolution gamma spectrometry (HRGS), radiochemistry and radiation counting techniques, X-ray fluorescence (XRF) and X-ray diffraction (XRD) analysis, inductively coupled plasma–mass spectrometry (ICP–MS), thermal ionization mass spectrometry (TIMS), gas chromatography–mass spectrometry (GC–MS), and glow discharge–mass spectrometry (GD–MS).

Imaging tools are used to document the physical characteristics of the material such as size, shape, and topography. In addition, imaging tools allow the determination of the chemical composition across the material, such as identifying whether the sample is homo- or heterogeneous. Imaging methodologies include the use of visual inspection and photography, optical microscopy, scanning electron microscopy (SEM), and transmission electron microscopy (TEM).

Microanalysis tools are used to quantify individual constituents of heterogeneous samples *via* determination of elemental and isotopic composition. Examples of microanalysis tools include ICP–MS, TIMS, XRD, secondary ion mass spectrometry (SIMS), scanning electron microanalysis with energy dispersive sensor (SEM/EDS) or scanning electron microanalysis with wavelength dispersive sensor (SEM/WDS), and infrared (IR) spectrometry.

After the material has been characterized, the process of forensic interpretation begins. It involves matching analytical data to existing information about the origin of similar materials and the methods used in the production and processing of this material. In addition, potential similarities with previously investigated cases of illicit materials are examined. High-quality national and international databases of reference information, in addition to improved information sharing between nuclear forensic laboratories worldwide, promote a high degree of successful investigations.

Nuclear attribution is the culmination of the analysis and interpretation of nuclear and traditional forensic evidence. It is divided into two key areas: source attribution and route attribution [1]. Source attribution considers data on the investigated material, including physical characteristics and origin, in addition to the analysis of packaging and other collateral items, the point where the material was diverted from a legitimate pathway, and the potential for further supply of such material.

Route attribution focuses on the potential involvement of a black market trafficking network, the identities of traffickers, the throughput capability of the illicit network, the frequency of shipments, and the likely end-user applications.

To date, nuclear forensic analysis has been applied to investigate illicit dealings with nuclear or radioactive material with the potential for terrorist use [1, 7]. It also has been successfully applied to investigations of a criminal (nonterrorist) or an accidental nature. An example of the former is the 2006 political assassination of Alexander Litvinenko in London, United Kingdom, by targeted radiation poisoning with polonium-210 [8]. An example of the latter is the 1992 "Cold Fusion" experiment-related explosion in an electrochemistry laboratory at Menlo Park in California [1].

International Collaboration in Nuclear Forensic Science

Commencing in late 1980s, the nuclear forensic discipline has become established in an international arena as a primary technological tool employed to investigate intercepted smuggled or illicitly traded nuclear and radioactive material for the purpose of attribution. This has been possible due to an early international collaboration of nuclear forensic scientists, conducted predominantly within the framework of the 1996 chartered International Technical Working Group (ITWG) on combating nuclear smuggling and its subset, the 2004 chartered association of the International Nuclear Forensic Laboratories (INFL) [6, 9].

References

[1] Moody, K.J., Hutcheon, I.D. & Grant, P.M. (2005). *Nuclear Forensic Analysis*, Taylor & Francis, Boca Raton

(Note: this is currently the primary textbook and a reference publication in the field of the Nuclear Forensic Analysis).

[2] IAEA (2005). *Categorization of Radioactive Sources (Safety Guide), IAEA Safety Standard Series No. RS-G.1.9*, International Atomic Energy Agency, Vienna.

[3] IAEA (2006). *Nuclear Forensics Support, IAEA Nuclear Security Series No.2*, International Atomic Energy Agency, Vienna.

[4] Bevelacqua, J.J. (2004). *Basic Health Physics*, Wiley-Vch Verlag, Weinheim.

[5] Wilber, K.T. (2003). *Overview of Radiological/Nuclear Devices and Response*, JUSTNET Justice Technology Information Network, National Law Enforcement and Corrections Technology Centre, Rockville (accessed 8 Feb 2008) www.nlectc.org/training/nij2003/wilber.pdf.

[6] Mayer, K., Wallenius, M. & Ray, I. (2005). Nuclear forensics – a methodology providing clues on the origin of illicitly trafficked nuclear materials, *Analyst* **130**, 433–441.

[7] Wallenius, M., Mayer, K. & Ray, I. (2006). Nuclear forensic investigations: two case studies, *Forensic Science International* **156**(1), 55–62.

[8] Harrison, J., Leggett, R., Lloyd, D., Phipps, A. & Scott, B. (2007). Polonium-210 as a poison, *Journal of Radiological Protection* **27**, 17–40.

[9] Lawrence Livermore National Laboratory (2007). *Identifying the Sources of Stolen Nuclear Materials*, LLNL Science & Technology Review January/February 2007, 12–18.

J. GEORGE KOPERSKI AND SERENA F. ABBONDANTE

Nuclear Investigations *see* Chemical, Biological, Radiological, and Nuclear Investigations

Number Restoration *see* Serial Number Restoration: Firearm

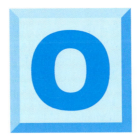

O

Obliterations in Documents: Detection of *see* Alterations:

Erasures and Obliterations of Documents

Odontology

Crime Scene and Recovery of Remains

Often the activity of an odontologist begins at the scene of crime, or where a body is found. All data useful for identification of an unidentified corpse or of an offender are therefore directly gathered by whoever has the knowledge to collect useful dental information. When dealing with charred (Figure 1), badly preserved, skeletonized bodies, some dental features, very important for individualization, could become very fragile or could be displaced from the mouth. During the recovery of a corpse, it should be mandatory to protect the oral area so as to preserve all useful information and to avoid the loss of teeth, bone fragments, or prosthetic devices. The oral region is therefore protected from any loss of data by using a fixative spray or means of mechanical protection; the scene is then accurately inspected to find any useful dental element or fragment (sometimes partially or totally charred).

In other crime scene scenarios, the odontologist may be useful for finding useful evidence that may help identify an offender by his lip prints or by his bitemarks on objects or food.

The Biological Profile

Teeth can provide useful information for biological profile reconstruction (*see* **Anthropology**), which is briefly summarized here.

Species

Knowledge of dental anatomy, when intact teeth are found, allows for an easy species attribution to

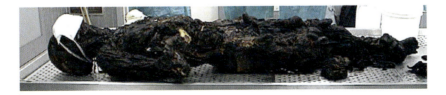

Figure 1   Surgical mask used to protect the oral region during corpse transportation

a trained eye (Figure 2) [1, 2]. When macroscopic morphology is not sufficient for a sure attribution of species or when studying small dental fragments, microscopic analysis of the teeth can sometimes solve the problem.

Microscopic observation of tooth enamel in fact can show the typical keyhole shape of the human enamel prisms.

Sex

The lack of reliable differences between sexes renders this approach redundant for sex determination for forensic purposes; so anthropological or genetic methods, through the extraction of genetic material from the pulp chamber, are to be preferred.

Race

Teeth can provide some indication about racial affiliation. Some characteristics are for example more frequent in Negroid subjects (as the presence of a diasthema between upper central incisors or an evident prognathism), in Mongoloid subjects (shovel-shaped teeth) (Figure 3) or in Caucasoids (Carabelli's cusp) [1, 2].

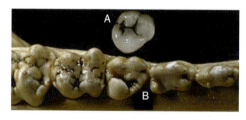

Figure 2   The very similar shape of a third human upper molar (A) and pig premolar (B)

These dental features are not sufficient, however, for a definite race determination, and only add information to the study of the entire skeleton.

Age

Starting from intrauterine life till about 21 years of age (when complete maturation of the third molar occurs) teeth are a reliable indicator of biological age, correlated to chronological age [1–4]. The age of a fetus can be evaluated via odontological methods studying the mineralization of the cusps visible in a radiograph of the mandible (Figure 4).

Up to about 14 years of age, simple observation of the number of primary and permanent teeth allows for age estimation with a growing error starting from about three months (when aging subjects of a few months of age) to a maximum of 36 months (when aging subjects of about 14 years of age). By studying the maturation of teeth apices, it is possible to age subjects till about 21 years of age. Once dental development has ended it is possible to estimate the age of an adult via continuous tooth modification. Dental abrasion is usually used to estimate the age of ancient populations, but is not considered a valuable indicator for forensic purposes anymore. Other dental modifications such as root transparency, root reabsorption, migration of the periodontal junction, continuous apposition of dentin, and cementum are studied, categorized and measured to estimate adult subject age (Figure 5). Root transparency seems to be the variable most closely linked to aging.

There are also some more complex dental methods for estimating age, such as cementum annulation count, the quantification of aspartic acid in teeth or of artificial radiocarbon.

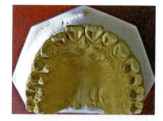

Figure 3   Palatal view of upper dental arch where shovel-shaped incisors are evident

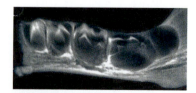

Figure 4   Mineralization of dental cusps in a radiograph of a fetus mandible. The presence of the cusps of the two deciduous molars denotes a fetal age of 38 weeks

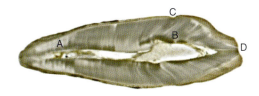

Figure 5 Canine transilluminated section in which some features correlated to chronological age are visible: (A) root transparency, (B) apposition of dentin, (C) periodontal junction degeneration, and (D) occlusal abrasion

Aging the Living

Since teeth are a reliable indicator of chronological age, they are used to evaluate the age of individuals without valid documents, often to verify if they reached a specific age (for instance 14, 16, or 18). It is thus possible to establish with which probability a subject reached 18 years of age by studying the development of the third molar, to evaluate the age of a young subject via the ratio between the open apices and the length of the crowns or the age of an adult by observing the ratio between the area of a pulp chamber and the entire tooth.

A final remark should be made, before proceeding to the more common applications of forensic odontology (positive identification and bitemark analysis) concerning a frequently used sign in cases of suspected infanticide – the neonatal line. This is a defect in enamel (or dentine) formation occurring at birth which, in the case of enamel, shows up as a thin dense line visible microscopically which separates prenatal from postnatal enamel. The neonatal line is related to the physiological and temporary interruption of the continuous deposition of dentine and enamel and is an indicator of survival of a newborn for some hours after birth (when the body is decomposed and other markers of survival cannot be searched on soft tissue). Therefore, if the neonatal line is noticed on the dental cusps of a newborn skeleton this suggest that the baby was born alive and survived for some hours.

Positive Identification

Odontological identification is the restitution of identity to a decomposed, skeletonized, charred, or heavily traumatized corpse via oral and dental features [2–6]. Identification is probably the main activity of the odontologist as unidentified bodies are a reality in every country: giving back a name to a corpse is important for every culture either for moral, religious, criminal, or civil reasons. Teeth are the most resistant part of the human body, they are particular to each individual due to anatomical, pathological, and therapeutic features; they also are the only human skeletal/calcified part visible during the life of a subject; these considerations make teeth a good individualization tool. Some cultural modification as color alteration, nontherapeutic morphology modification, setting of stones or jewels in enamel, and nontherapeutic crowns, can provide information about a subject, sometimes these are geographical variants. Some habits or occupations (wind instrument players, pipe smokers, carpenters, or tailors who use teeth to hold metal objects) can leave distinctive marks making individualization much easier. Odontological individualization is based on the comparison between antemortem (AM) data (information about a missing person) and postmortem (PM) data (observation made on an unidentified corpse).

Antemortem Data

Odontological AM data include all information regarding teeth and the contiguous tissues, pertaining to a missing person who is believed to correspond to an unidentified corpse. In most industrialized countries such information is quite easy to find as most citizens have been visited at least once by a dentist who probably kept his or her patient's radiographs, casts or pictures. Precious individualization information can be found in dental files, in orthopantomographs (OPGs) in which it is possible to see all the teeth, in periapical radiographs with a better resolution than OPGs that allow the observation of even the smallest peculiarities, in lateral and anteroposterior skull radiographs which can show dental features (Figure 6), in every radiograph in which a part of the mouth is visible, in clinical pictures (often taken by dentists to document their works) and in normal portraits which show the teeth of the photographed subject.

All antemortem data are summarized in special forms (for instance the INTERPOL DVI form) devised to standardize data collection, to make the matching process between a missing person and an unidentified body easier, to avoid misunderstanding due to the use of different teeth nomenclatures or different scientific vocabularies.

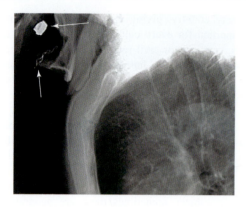

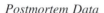

Figure 6 In this antemortem radiograph of a missing person, it is possible to see (white arrows) dental treatment useful for a positive individualization. It is thus possible to perform a positive odontological individualization starting from nondental radiographs

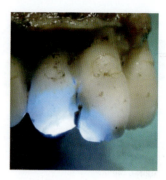

Figure 7 Aesthetic fillings can be hard to find, especially if of good quality and if teeth are not perfectly clean. A UV light can enhance the shape of this kind of restoration

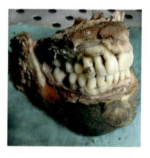

Figure 8 Maxillary bones and mandible after resection. Postmortem examination can be carried out accurately only if every dental surface is visible

Postmortem Data

Odontological PM data includes all information gathered from an unidentified corpse and inserted into special forms similar to those used for AM-data collection. As unidentified bodies are usually charred, decomposed, skeletonized, or traumatized, oral structures can become very fragile and oral examination should be considered unrepeatable; therefore it is advisable to record and take pictures of every step of the examination procedures (especially if the case will be brought in a court of law). An elementary kit to perform a PM oral examination should include: oral mirrors, probes, scalpel, saws, brushes, sponges, ultraviolet light (to better detect aesthetic restorations) (Figure 7), a camera, radiographic instrumentation, and cast materials.

To collect all dental elements and dental works that could be displaced from the oral cavity a first inspection of the entire body could be necessary; some useful elements for individualization are often found in the pharynx, trachea, and esophagus or even in the bag used to carry the corpse. Especially in case of charred or mummified bodies, mouth opening could be a difficult operation. Temporomandibular joint disarticulation and removal of the entire mandible can be a solution; a quick way is to perform three cuts, using a "stryker" type saw, parallel to the occlusal plane: one passing through the nasal spine to remove the maxillary bone and two passing through the vertical parts of the mandible to remove the jaw (Figure 8).

Before taking the jaws from the body the type of occlusion should be recorded. Which teeth are present and which are not is then recorded (dental formula); if missing teeth are noticed it is important to chronologically place their loss by studying the bone remodeling process. Any kind of anomaly (in shape, size, and position) is recorded as well as the presence, type and location of every kind of oral disease. Very often dental individualization is based on the comparison of therapeutic features because they are usually well described in dental antemortem files (Figure 9). For each dental work, one must therefore carefully describe the type, location, and the applied technique and technology. Postmortem examination is then completed by taking dental impressions and radiographs.

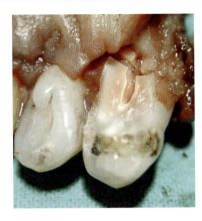

Figure 9 It is possible to detect the presence of a filling even if lost. In this example the shape of the cavity on the broken premolar and the dark stain suggest the presence of an amalgam filling probably lost because of the trauma

Matching Process

During individualization processes all AM and PM data collected in the forms are compared to discover compatibility or incompatibility between a missing person and an unidentified body. Positive identification is commonly achieved via radiographic comparison, which nowadays is usually computer aided. In a radiographic comparison, for even the smallest anatomical, pathological, and therapeutic features, antemortem and postmortem radiographs are placed side by side, superimposed and eventually measured and quantified to establish if they come from the same subject (Figure 10).

Postmortem radiographs should be taken with the same technique and with the same projection used for the antemortem ones so that the results are reliable.

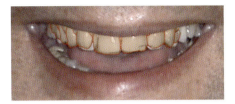

Figure 11 Postmortem dental profile superimposed to the picture of a missing person

Dental Superimposition

When dealing with missing persons who do not have clinical data dental superimposition is frequently a reliable identification technique (Figure 11) [5]. It is based on the superimposition of the teeth visible in a picture of a missing person to the dental cast of an unidentified corpse so as to study any incompatibility and correspondence.

Palatal Rugae

Palatal rugae are mucosal ridges on the hard part of the palate. They are morphologically peculiar in each individual and do not change shape for a long time during the life of an individual. When a superior dental impression is taken the palatal rugae configuration is recorded and then transferred onto the cast. All these characteristics make palatal rugae a suitable tool for individualization even with the limitation of being a soft tissue (think of modifications due to dehydration, decomposition, and carbonization). Morphological comparison of palatal rugae is usually performed by superimposition of scanned antemortem casts (provided by the missing person's dentist) and

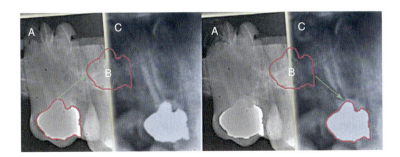

Figure 10 Postmortem radiograph (A) compared to antemortem radiograph (C). Filling postmortem outline (B) is superimposed to the antemortem one to increase comparison reliability

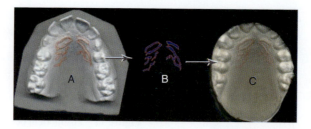

Figure 12 Antemortem (A) palatal rugae pattern (B) superimposed to postmortem cast (C). In this example of a positive identification case, more than 20 years had passed between the antemortem and the postmortem casts

of scanned postmortem casts of the corpse's palate (Figure 12).

Mass Disasters

The contribution of odontology in the identification of the victims of a mass disaster is often decisive. Subjects identified with odontological methods are often more than 80% of the victims [2, 3, 6, 7]. Therefore forensic odontologists should always be included in antemortem and postmortem identification teams. Identification methods applied in case of mass disaster are the same as those used in cases of a single unidentified body; special care is to be taken with respect to logistics, to the organization of the team work, and to the precise compilation of ante and postmortem forms.

Bitemark Analysis

A forensically useful bitemark is a physical alteration or a lesion showing some characteristic of the dental arches that produced it [3, 2, 8, 9]. Bitemarks can be found on a crime scene on objects or food, on the skin of a corpse or of an assaulted subject and can be used to identify who provoked them. The comparison between the dental status of a defendant and the bitemark is almost always done by a computer aided image superimposition: the occlusal pattern of the defendant's dental arches is superimposed to the bitemark image so as to analyze the similarity of the two patterns. Bitemarks are frequently found in sexual assault and the typical locations are arms, breasts, legs, and genitalia. The lesion is usually elliptic, with a central ecchymosis, and with tooth marks on its perimeter (Figure 13).

It is important to study a bitemark as soon as possible either on a living subject (because of

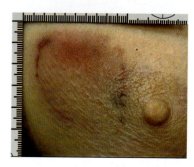

Figure 13 Typical elliptic bitemark found on the breast of a corpse: note the teeth pattern on its perimeter, the ecchymosis, and the presence of the American Board of Forensic Odontology (ABFO) ruler

morphological changes due to tissue healing), or on a corpse (to avoid postmortem alterations). First of all DNA swabs must be taken from the lesion as the aggressor could have left some genetic material on the skin. Then photographs are shot taking care to use a metric scale and to avoid any possible deformation or distortion (Figure 13). It is possible to produce a cast of the lesion by using dental impression materials (e.g., polyvinylsiloxane). The lesion can be excised from the corpse and if transilluminated can better show some important peculiarities. If the lesion is in a place which can be reached by the dentition of the victim it could be necessary to take his or her dental impression in order to exclude a self-inflicted bite. Some bitemarks can hardly be associated with a human bite because of the low-pressure applied (only a round ecchymosis is visible) (Figure 14), because of excessive pressure (tissue amputation), or if multiple, because bites are superimposed or partial or because they have been inflicted on a portion of skin which has an excessive curvature. Some objects with a tubular section can leave on the skin a mark that could erroneously be associated with the action of human dental arches.

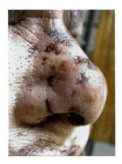

Figure 14 Multiple bitemarks on a curved surface: it could be difficult to compare the dental pattern to a defendant's dental arch or even to associate this kind of lesions to a human bitemark

The defendant is usually subjected to a dental visit: missing teeth are recorded as well as any pathology, dental fracture, abnormal tooth position, rotation, or inclination; a dental cast is then produced from accurate impression materials so as to record even the smallest enamel peculiarity.

References

[1] Hillson, S. (1996). *Dental Anthropology*, Cambridge University Press, Cambridge.
[2] Stimson, P.G. & Mertz, C.A. (1997). *Forensic Dentistry*, CRC Press, Boca Raton.
[3] Bowers, C.M. & Bell, G. (1995). *Manual of Forensic Odontology*, American Board of Forensic Odontology.
[4] Whittaker, J. & MacDondal, D.G. (1989). *Color Atlas of Forensic Dentistry (Wolfe Medical Atlases)*, Mosby International Press.
[5] Clark, D. (1992). *Practical Forensic Odontology*, Butterworth Heinemann, London.
[6] Bowers, M.C. (2004). *Forensic Dental Evidence: An Investigator's Handbook*, Elsevier Academic Press.
[7] Cattaneo, C., De Angelis, D. & Grandi, M. (2006). *Mass Disasters in Forensic Anthropology and Medicine: Complementary Sciences From Recovery to Cause of Death*, A. Schmitt, E. Cunha & J. Pinheiro, eds, Humana Press, New York.
[8] Bowers, C.M. & Johansen, R. (2000). *Digital Analysis of Bitemark Evidence*, Academic Press.
[9] Dorion, R.J. (2005). *Bitemark Evidence*, Marcel Dekkeer, New York.

CRISTINA CATTANEO AND DANILO DE ANGELIS

Older Adults in Court *see* Elderly in Court

Opioids

Introduction

Natural and synthetic morphine derivatives possessing morphinelike actions are known as *opioids*. These include common drugs such as morphine, heroin, codeine, etc. and are collectively known as *opioids*. Other terms used to describe these drugs include narcotic analgesics and opiates.

After cannabis and stimulants, the most widely used illicit drugs are opioids. Legitimate opioids, such as morphine, codeine, oxycodone, and hydrocodone, are being consumed at an increasing rate. According to the International Narcotic Control Board, approximately 50 countries have increased their consumption of opioid analgesics by more than 100% during the last decade [1]. The increase is particularly evident in Europe and North America.

Globally, it is estimated that 16 million people take opioids, including 11 million who use heroin. In many countries, the majority of heavy drug users seeking treatment are primarily addicted to heroin; however, it is of increasing concern that legitimate opioids, such as oxycodone and methadone, are being diverted for illegal use.

The use of heroin is common in Asia (54%), Europe (25%), America (14%), and Oceania (6%) [1]. Evidence from national surveys and other data sources suggests that the prevalence of the use of heroin in general populations is relatively low (ranging from 0.2 to 2%). According to the USA 2005 National Survey on Drug Use and Health survey, 379 000 persons (0.2%) reported using heroin in the past year. It was estimated in the year 2000 that there were between 40 000 and 100 000 heroin users in Australia [2] comparable to Britain and other countries in Europe.

The worldwide production of heroin has more than doubled or even tripled since 1985. Scientific reports published by the United Nations Drug

Control Program [1] showed that there was a global increase in the production, transportation, and consumption of opioids, throughout the 1990s; however, in the last 5 years, the production of opium has steadily decreased. World events including the political changes in Afghanistan, the world's largest producer of heroin, led to significant decline in the supply and subsequent demand of the drug. In the golden triangle consisting of Laos, Myanmar, and Thailand, production has fallen by 85% from 1998 to 2006 [1]. Recent reports suggest that production is reaching the high levels of the 1990s.

The use of heroin, in particular, is causing widespread health and social problems in many countries. In Europe, heroin injectors who regularly consume large amounts of different drugs face a risk of death, which may be 20–30 times higher than non-drug users in the same age range. Since heroin is commonly used by injection, the health risks including that of human immunodeficiency virus (HIV) and hepatitis transmission are substantial.

The primary use of legal opioids is for the relief of pain. Depending on the severity of pain, different opioids can be used to diminish or relieve pain. Severe pain can be treated using fentanyl, hydromorphone, methadone, morphine, oxycodone, tramadol, and pethidine, while mild-to-moderate pain can be treated with codeine, dihydrocodeine, and dextropropoxyphene. Other opioids are used to induce or supplement anesthesia, such as fentanyl and the fentanyl analogues alfentanil, remifentanil, etc.

Some opioids (codeine, dihydrocodeine, and, to a lesser extent, pholcodine) can also be used as cough suppressants (antitussives). Methadone, buprenorphine, naltrexone, and naloxone can be used for the treatment of addiction to opioids.

Opioids can also be mixed with other pharmaceuticals (nonopioid drugs) to enhance analgesia (e.g., analgesic-antipyretic preparations and use with some phenothiazines). A summary of selected opioids and their uses are given in Table 1.

There are substantial region-to-region differences in the availability and usage of opioids. For example in 2004, the United States accounted for more than 99% of the global consumption of hydrocodone.

Sources of Opioids

Morphine and codeine are naturally occurring alkaloids extracted from the milky juice and stalks of the opium poppy, *Papaver somniferum*. The content of morphine in these plants can vary from as little as 5% to as high as 25%. Codeine is usually found in much smaller amounts (~0.2%) and the content of other naturally occurring opioids, such as thebaine (~0.1 – 0.3%), narcotine (~0.3%), narceine (~4 – 10%), and papaverine (~1%), can also vary depending upon the quality and origin of the plant [3]. Many semisynthetic opioid derivatives are made by relatively simple modifications of the morphine or thebaine molecule, e.g., heroin (diacetylmorphine) is a semisynthetic opioid produced from the acetylation of morphine. Other semisynthetic drugs produced from morphine or thebaine molecules include hydromorphone, oxycodone, and naloxone (Figure 1).

Pharmacology of Opioids

Effects on the Central Nervous System

Opioids exert their diverse pharmacological effects by binding to opioid receptors that are distributed in distinct patterns throughout the central nervous system (CNS) and peripheral nervous system. The major therapeutic use of opioids is the modulation or reduction in pain. When an opioid is administered therapeutically to patients suffering from pain, the sensation of pain is reduced and their distress becomes less intense. However, when an opioid is given to normal drug-free individuals, nausea and vomiting are more common symptoms along with drowsiness, lethargy, and a reduced physical activity. Patients may experience euphoria, and at increased doses side effects become more severe along with muscular rigidity and respiratory depression. Higher doses far in excess of those required to produce analgesia may lead to convulsions [3].

Respiratory Depression

Most opioids depress the respiratory center. The depression is a dose-dependent effect, which can be fatal. Opioids act to reduce the responsiveness of the brain stem respiratory centers to increased concentrations of arterial carbon dioxide. The subsequent effect of increasing concentrations of hydrogen ions as a result of dissociation of carbonic acid lowers blood pH that directly affects the pontine and medullary centers involved in regulating respiratory function.

Table 1   Selected opioids, the action at drug receptor, typical dose, half-life, and indication for use

Drug	Receptor action	Dose (mg)[a]	$T_{1/2}$ (h)[b]	Indication for use[c]
Naturally occurring				
Morphine	Agonist	5–20	2–3	Analgesia, moderate-to-severe pain, postoperative pain control
Codeine	Agonist	30–60	2–4	Analgesia, moderate-to-severe pain, cough suppressant
Semisynthetic				
Heroin	Agonist	5–10	0.03–0.05	Analgesia, moderate-to-severe pain, not available for therapeutic use
Hydromorphone	Agonist	2–4	1.5–4	Acute pain, chronic cancer pain
Naloxone	Antagonist	0.4–2	1–2	Used to reverse effects of opioids, such as heroin
Oxycodone	Agonist	5–20	4–5	Analgesia, relief of chronic pain
Synthetic				
Buprenorphine	Partial agonist	–	2–3	Analgesia, maintenance drug used to treat heroin dependence
Fentanyl	Agonist	0.05–0.2	1–6	Analgesia, strong pain, used in anesthesia as adjuvant
Methadone	Agonist	5–100	10–25	Analgesia, relief of chronic pain, maintenance drug used to treat heroin dependence
Pethidine	Agonist	50–100	3–10	Analgesia
Propoxyphene	Agonist	50–150	8–24	Analgesia
Tramadol	Agonist	50–400	4–8	Analgesia

[a] Common recommended therapeutic dose given orally
[b] Time for blood concentration to halve
[c] Most common medical applications

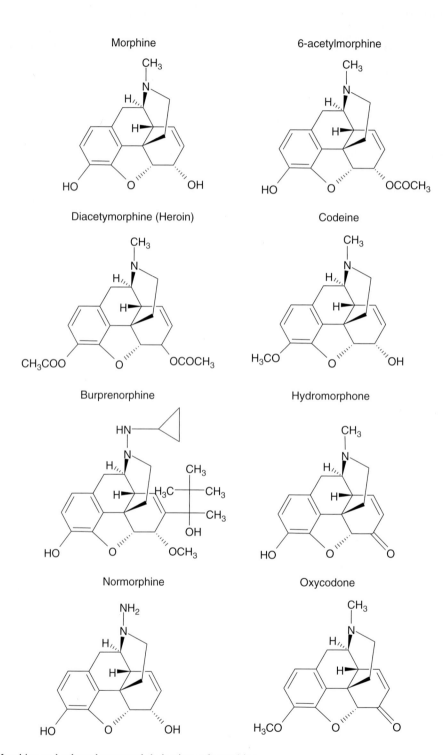

Figure 1   Morphine and selected structural derivatives of morphine

This has the effect of reducing the rate of breathing and with toxic amounts of morphine the rate may fall to 3 or 4 breaths per min instead of 12–16. Codeine is much less toxic than morphine and even in large doses does not appear to have the strong CNS depression characteristics of morphine.

Suppression of Cough Reflex

Opioids depress the cough reflex by a direct effect on the cough center in the medulla. There seems to be no relationship between the analgesic, respiratory-depressant action of opioids, and cough suppression; however, some opioids are more effective in depressing the cough reflex than others. Codeine and, to a greater extent, pholcodine are more effective than morphine in depressing the cough reflex [4, 5].

Nausea and Vomiting

Nausea and vomiting occur as a result of opioids affecting the chemoreceptor trigger zone in the brain. These effects are common initially but usually disappear with repeated administration. All clinically useful opioids produce some degree of nausea and vomiting [3]. Antiemetic drugs such as haloperidol and prochlorperazine are commonly used to treat vomiting in clinical situations. Metoclopramide is often useful if nausea and vomiting persist [5].

Effects on the Gastrointestinal Tract

Opioids cause varying effects on the gastrointestinal tract depending on the dose and the drug species. For example, morphine causes a marked increase in tone and a reduced motility, resulting in constipation, while codeine is less constipating than morphine and may be used to relieve abdominal pain. The emptying of gastric contents can also be delayed, which can further retard the absorption of drugs, a property shared by most opioids [3].

Tolerance and Dependence

Tolerance is a condition whereby after repeated administration, a given dose of a drug produces a decreased effect and increasingly larger doses must be taken to obtain the pharmacological effects observed with the original dose.

It is the level of tolerance that is of particular importance in heroin addicts. When the use of opioid becomes more regular, the intensity of response diminishes from one injection to the next. To produce the same response or as before, the dose of the drug has to be increased. Thus, in the course of days or weeks, tolerance may build up until many times a lethal dose can eventually be tolerated.

In humans, for example, an initial dose of 100–200 mg of morphine would be sufficient to cause profound sedation, respiratory depression, anoxia, and death; however, tolerant subjects can handle this and more. Tolerance diminishes rapidly (few days) after withdrawal so that a previously tolerated dose may prove fatal [4]. Tolerance to other opioids can also occur depending on the potency of the drug.

Dependence is a condition that has developed as a result of repeated drug administration and/or abuse. It is characterized by an overwhelming need to continue taking the drug, or one with a similar pharmacological property. Opioid analgesics, such as heroin, are abused for their euphoriant effects and dependence develops rapidly with regular use. Prolonged administration of heroin or morphine in a clinical environment is less likely to produce dependence as a result of therapeutic use and the dose of the drug can be reduced as the underlying pain decreases [6].

The abrupt withdrawal of opioids from persons physically dependent on them precipitates a withdrawal syndrome, the severity of which depends on the individual, the drug used, the size and frequency of the dose, and the duration of drug use. Opioid analgesics with some antagonist activity, such as buprenorphine, butorphanol, or pentazocine, may also precipitate withdrawal symptoms in patients who are dependent on opioid narcotics.

The onset and duration of withdrawal symptoms also vary according to the duration of action of the specific drug. Withdrawal symptoms may be terminated by a suitable dose of morphine or another opioid. Methadone is currently the most widely used pharmacotherapeutic agent for maintenance treatment of heroin addicts [7]. Methadone is effective in the suppression of withdrawal symptoms and in the reduction or elimination of an addict's compulsion to take heroin. The major objective of the methadone maintenance program is to achieve long-lasting stabilization of the user's drug dependence by providing methadone indefinitely in doses large enough to produce a level of cross-tolerance that is sufficient to diminish the effects of ordinary doses of heroin.

Serious Adverse Effects/Toxic Reactions

Overuse of opioids can lead to depression of the CNS, slowing down breathing that may result in postural asphyxia or cardiorespiratory arrest. Intravenous drug abuse of heroin can lead to a number of other life-threatening side effects and/or complications. These can include neurological disorders, low blood pressure, swelling of the brain, stroke, death of vascular tissue, i.e., necrotizing angiitis, and nerve damage.

Intravenous drug users show a high susceptibility to infections and other diseases due to the suppression of their immune systems. The manifestation of infectious diseases in intravenous drug users plays a critical role in life-threatening complications for addicts. The factors below contribute to their diminished immune function. Factors such as needle sharing, unsafe sexual practices, under nourishment, poor hygiene, devastation of skin barrier, and the injection of unfamiliar substances into the body all increase the risk of acquired immune deficiency syndrome (AIDS), viral hepatitis, pneumonia, and tuberculosis. Infectious complications as a result of all these factors include endocarditis and septicemia, viral hepatitis, liver cirrhosis, meningitis, and tetanus [8].

Disposition of Opioids

Absorption and Metabolism

The extent of absorption depends on the type of opioid and the route of administration. When given orally, some opioids, particularly morphine and heroin, are removed from the portal circulation very efficiently by the liver and are metabolized extensively so that the amount reaching the systemic circulation is considerably less than the amount absorbed into the portal vein. This effect is known as *first-pass metabolism*. As a consequence the available dose is only a proportion of the dose taken. Oral administration of morphine is one-sixth as effective as parenteral administration. In contrast, codeine is well absorbed and quite active when given orally. In fact, codeine

is approximately two-thirds as effective orally as parenterally [9]. Other opioids that are well absorbed orally include oxycodone and pethidine (meperidine).

Some opioids are also available as sustained release preparations (i.e., slow or controlled release). This means that a patient suffering from chronic pain may only have to take a tablet once or twice per day, which results in stable blood concentrations as a consequence of the drug's more predictable pharmacokinetics. Methadone and oxycodone rectal suppositories are useful alternatives to oral sustained release morphine preparations.

Opioids undergo extensive metabolism in humans. There are three main biotransformation pathways that have been established for the metabolism of opioids: hydrolysis, glucuronidation, and oxidation.

For example, following intravenous injection, heroin is rapidly converted (within seconds) to 6-acetylmorphine (6-AM), which is subsequently hydrolyzed (within minutes) to morphine. The conversion of heroin to 6-AM occurs both as a result of enzymes and spontaneous hydrolysis [10].

The majority of opioid metabolism in humans occurs in the liver through a process called *glucuronidation*; this occurs mainly in the liver and to a lesser extent in the intestine and kidneys [11, 12]. For example, morphine is conjugated primarily to morphine-3-glucuronide (M3G) and to a lesser extent the biologically active morphine-6-glucuronide (M6G) (Figure 2).

Excretion

Most opioids are excreted in the urine usually within the first 24 h following administration. The concentrations of conjugated metabolites usually exceed those of the parent drug and can be present for longer periods of time [13]. As with most pharmacokinetic parameters, there is great individual variation in the elimination half-life. This value is greatly prolonged in renal failure resulting in drug accumulation. Some opioids with long half-lives such as methadone can accumulate in tissues. Such accumulation can be toxic or even fatal if doses are not appropriately administered and the drug not given enough time to be cleared by the body. This can lead to prolonged respiratory depression and pronounced enterohepatic recirculation (excretion into the gastrointestinal system through bile followed by reabsorption) [14].

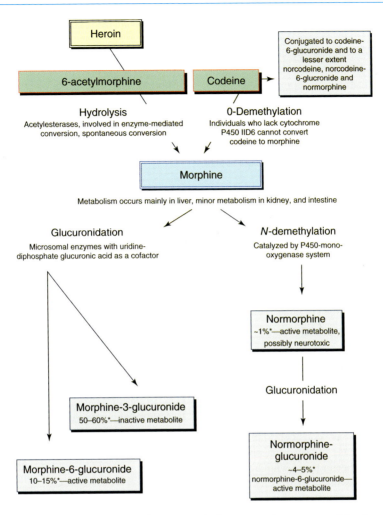

Figure 2   Fate of heroin, morphine, and codeine in humans (*urinary excretion, percent of dose)

Death from the Use of Opioid

The mechanism of death in opioid users is often uncertain, but it is likely to be multifactorial. For example, the use of heroin results in a wide range of adverse effects due to a variety of pharmacological and physiological responses to heroin, hypersensitivity reactions to the cutting agents or contaminants, and diseases associated with intravenous use. The largest numbers of deaths have been attributed to an acute reaction, whereby death occurs shortly after injection [15, 16]. Three overdose syndromes are recognized: death from profound respiratory depression, death from arrhythmia and cardiac arrest, and death as a consequence of severe pulmonary edema [17].

Death may also occur indirectly as a complication of unconsciousness. This is caused by a nonfatal dose, leading to airways obstruction in a setting of diminished respiratory function. Respiratory disease can also reduce the ability of person to tolerate a dose of opioid.

Fentanyl, methadone, oxycodone, hydrocodone, and morphine are the most common legal opioids known to cause death if misused [18].

Drug Interactions

Drugs such as alcohol, barbiturates, and benzodiazepines enhance the depressant effects of opioids on the CNS [19].

Opioid users frequently take benzodiazepines, e.g., diazepam, nitrazepam, etc., to reduce anxiety and to minimize the unpleasantness of any withdrawal symptoms. Drug combinations are therefore potentially serious complications in opioid users, particularly for heroin users. Data from a review of deaths in Victoria [20] show that benzodiazepines were the most prevalent drug group (~55%) and alcohol was present in ~30% of all heroin-related deaths. Amphetamines were also present in many cases (~13%) (*see also* **Benzodiazepines**).

Drugs such as the sedating antihistamines can prolong morphine metabolism, leading to increased respiratory depression. Phenothiazines, including promethazine and chlorpromazine, are also known to potentiate the effects of opioids by interfering with the metabolism of morphine [21].

One of the problems confounding the forensic toxicologist and pathologist is the relevance and interpretation of drug concentrations in different specimens following the use of opioids.

Interpretation of Toxicological Data; Difficulties for the Expert

The interpretation of postmortem tissue results is dependent upon number of considerations. These include chronic or acute use of the drug; concentrations of drug may be higher in those who are regular users, allowing some assessment of toxicity.

The route of administration is also important. Oral ingestion of opioids means that some of the efficacy of the dose is removed by the liver before the drug enters the blood stream (first-pass metabolism).

Another factor that will affect the interpretation of toxicology results includes the incidence of disease, i.e., AIDS, hepatitis, etc., presence of liver and kidney dysfunction as well as other immunological suppressive diseases that may affect metabolism and excretion of opioids and their metabolites. The accumulation of opioids may result in adverse effects and even death. Concurrent natural disease may predispose individuals to cardiovascular collapse and even unpredictable responses such as convulsions[3].

The presence of other drugs, the possibility of antagonism for one drug by another, and more often the additive or synergistic effects produced by the interaction of two or more depressant drugs must all be considered.

Tissue distribution and redistribution of opioids and its metabolites are also important in assessing postmortem contributions of opioids to adverse effects and death. The statistical data on body distribution and redistribution studies from fatalities associated with heroin, morphine, and other opioids use are invaluable in the evaluation of future toxicological findings (*see* **Postmortem Toxicology: Artifacts**).

Methods of Analysis

Initial Testing

Most clinical and forensic laboratories test for the presence of the class of opioids in the initial phase of their investigations. These immunoassays are effective for the more common opioids, such as morphine, codeine, and heroin metabolites. This technique using commercial kits enables all members of the class to be detected; however, owing to their differing immunoreactivities, the sensitivity to different opioids and their metabolites will vary, and for some may be quite poor. This applies particularly to the more synthetic opioids, e.g., oxycodone, buprenorphine, and methadone. Hence, more specific immunoassays are required to detect these drugs.

Initial tests are commonly conducted in urine since the concentration of the opioids or its metabolite is often much higher than blood. However, immunoassays designed for blood/plasma, or even oral fluid, are commercially available. An example of this is the enzyme-linked immunosorbent assay (ELISA).

When a class test is positive, further (confirmation) tests are required to detect the specific opioid (or its metabolite) that is causing this positive response (*see* **Toxicology: Initial Testing**).

Confirmation Testing

The definitive confirmation method in forensic toxicology is mass spectrometry. This can be gas chromatography/mass spectrometry (GC-MS) or liquid chromatography/mass spectrometry (LC-MS). liquid chromatography/tandem mass spectrometry (LC-MS/MS) or tandem LC-MS methods are now dominating the measurement for this class of drugs due to its very high sensitivity and specificity and require very little or no chemical modification to permit chromatographic analysis.

Depending on the specimen, the metabolic pathway of the target opioid (or metabolite) will vary. When determining heroin, most if not all of the drug is metabolized to 6-AM and ultimately morphine, which are the main target metabolites, whereas for buprenorphine, the parent drug and metabolite norbuprenorphine are measured.

References

[1] International Narcotics Control Board, United Nations (2007). *Annual Report International Narcotics Control Board 2006*.

[2] Hall, W.D., Ross, J.E., Lynskey, M.T., Law, M.G. & Degenhardt, L.J. (2000). How many dependent heroin users are there in Australia? *The Medical Journal of Australia* **173**(10), 528–531.

[3] Jaffe, J.H. & Martin, W.R. (1985). *Goodman and Gilman's The Pharmacological Basis of Therapeutics*, 7th Edition, A.G. Gilman *et al.*, eds, Macmillan, New York, pp. 495–531.

[4] Rang, H.P. (1987). in *Pharmacology*, 2nd Edition, H.P. Rang & M.M. Dale, eds, Churchill Livingstone, Edinburgh, pp. 547–567.

[5] Badewitz-Dodd, L.H. (1994). *The MIMS Annual*, Australian Edition, Intercontinental Medical Statistics (Australasia), Crows Nest, pp. 302–333.

[6] Victorian Drug Usage Advisory Committee. Analgesic Guidelines Sub-Committee (1988). *Analgesic Guidelines*, [Prepared by the Analgesic Guidelines Sub-Committee Victorian Drug Usage Advisory Committee], 1st Edition, Victorian Medical Postgraduate Foundation, Toorak, on behalf of the Victorian Drug Usage Advisory Committee.

[7] Peachey, J.E. (1986). The role of drugs in the treatment of opioid addicts, *The Medical Journal of Australia* **145**(8), 395–399.

[8] Janssen, W., Trubner, K. & Puschel, K. (1989). Death caused by drug addiction: a review of the experiences in Hamburg and the situation in the Federal Republic of Germany in comparison with the literature, *Forensic Science International* **43**(3), 223–237.

[9] Reynolds, J.E.F. (1999). *Martindale: the Complete Drug Reference*, 30th Edition, Pharmaceutical Press, London, pp. 1065–1098.

[10] Yonemitsu, K. & Pounder, D.J. (1992). Postmortem toxico-kinetics of co-proxamol, *International Journal of Legal Medicine* **104**(6), 347–353.

[11] Regnard, C.F. & Twycross, R.G. (1984). Metabolism of narcotics, *British Medical Journal (Clinical Research Ed)* **288**(6420), 860.

[12] McQuay, H.J., Moore, R.A., Hand, C.W. & Sear, J.W. (1987). Potency of oral morphine, *Lancet* **2**(8573), 1458–1459.

[13] Schneider, J.J., Ravenscroft, P.J., Cavenagh, J.D., Brown, A.M. & Bradley, J.P. (1992). Plasma morphine-3-glucuronide, morphine-6-glucuronide and morphine concentrations in patients receiving long-term epidural morphine, *British Journal of Clinical Pharmacology* **34**(5), 431–433.

[14] Hanks, G.W., Hoskin, P.J., Aherne, G.W., Chapman, D., Turner, P. & Poulain, P. (1988). Enterohepatic circulation of morphine, *Lancet* **1**(8583), 469.

[15] Helpern, M. (1972). Fatalities from narcotic addiction in New York City. Incidence, circumstances, and pathologic findings, *Human Pathology* **3**(1), 13–21.

[16] Baden, M. (1993). Investigations of death from drug abuse, in *Spitz and Fisher's Medicolegal Investigation of Death: Guidelines for the Application of Pathology to Crime Investigation*, 3rd Edition, W.U. Spitz, ed, with a foreword by R. Clark, C.C. Thomas, Springfield, pp. 527–555.

[17] Cotran, R.S., Kumar, V. & Robbins, S.L. (1989). *Robbins and Cotran Pathologic Basis of Disease*, 4th Edition, V. Kumar, A.K. Abbas & N. Fausto, eds, with illustrations by J.A. Perkins, Saunders, Philadelphia, pp. 497–498.

[18] Stout, P.R. & Farrell, L.J. (2002). Opioids – effects on human performance and behavior, *Forensic Science Review* **15**, 29.

[19] Iwamoto, E.T., Fudala, P.J. & Mundy, W.R. (1987). *Toxicology of CNS Depressants*, I.K. Ho, ed, CRC Press, Boca Raton, pp. 145–196.

[20] Gerostamoulos, J., Staikos, V. & Drummer, O.H. (2001). Heroin-related deaths in Victoria: a review of cases for 1997 and 1998, *Drug and Alcohol Dependence* **61**(2), 123–127.

[21] Keeri-Szanto, M. (1974). The mode of action of promethazine in potentiating narcotic drugs, *British Journal of Anaesthesia* **46**(12), 918–924.

DIMITRI GEROSTAMOULOS

Oral Fluid Toxicology

Introduction

Over the last few decades, oral fluid has been evaluated as a diagnostic aid in medicine for determining oral and systemic disease markers as well as for monitoring the presence of numerous drugs, narcotics, and hormones. The easy, rapid, and noninvasive nature of collection and the relationship between oral fluid and plasma levels make oral fluid a valuable clinical tool and an alternative specimen where blood sampling could be difficult to perform e.g., in children, in those with poor venous access, and in anxious subjects. Furthermore, it may provide a cost-effective approach for the screening of large populations. However, unlike plasma, the composition of oral fluid varies widely both intra- and interindividually. The result of any oral fluid analysis is influenced by many different factors, including the sampling protocol, which must be performed under standardized conditions.

Oral fluid analysis for drugs was first used almost 30 years ago for the purpose of therapeutic drug monitoring. At that time, it was already known that it is possible to predict the free fraction of a circulating drug by analysis of the corresponding oral fluid sample. Since abuse of drugs is now a widespread problem across society, its negative impact on performance and safety cannot be overstated. New strategies for drug testing should offer an effective solution to persistent problems such as the potential for sample adulteration and substitution and concerns over issues of individual privacy. These have resulted in the use of oral fluid for drugs of abuse testing in the workplace. Other areas of interest include testing of intoxicated drivers, monitoring illicit drug use in drug treatment, and oral fluid testing for drug detection in schools and in transportation and insurance industries. This article discusses developments in the field of collection devices, pharmacokinetics of common drugs of abuse in oral fluid, and recent technological advances and guidelines that increase the actual use of oral fluid testing in a legal context and its acceptance by the criminal justice system. Oral fluid testing is a reliable, new technology that overcomes many of the problems of older methods for drug detection.

Physiology of Oral Fluid

Oral fluid originates from three pairs of major salivary glands (parotid, submandibularis, and sublingualis) (Figure 1), a great number of minor salivary glands, the oral mucosa, and gingival crevices. The mixture of gingival crevicular fluid and mucosal transudate is referred to in the literature as "saliva", "whole saliva", and "oral fluid". In addition to these fluids, oral fluid contains a certain amount of cell-debris arising from the epithelial cells of the mouth, together with food residues. Water is the major constituent (99%). Other components include mineral salts, proteins such as mucins (lipoproteins related to lubrification), and enzymes for digestion. The total protein concentration is less than 1% of that of plasma, but almost all of the organic compounds of plasma may be detected in oral fluid in trace amounts. The most important functions of oral fluid are as follows: (i) to moisten the mucous membranes of the upper aerodigestive tract in order to facilitate speech and solubilize food to ease swallowing; (ii) maintenance of oral health by controlling the bacterial flora of the mouth, and establishing defense and killing mechanisms; and (iii) to supply enzymes for food digestion, hormones, and other pharmacologically active compounds.

The detailed morphology of salivary glands has been reviewed by several authors [1–3]. The glandular tissue comprises acinar or tubular cells, specialized groups of cells arranged as endpieces surrounding a small central lumen. A narrow intercalated duct leads from the secretory endpieces to the striated ducts, which in turn drain into the secretory ducts to form a single main secretory duct that drains into the oral cavity.

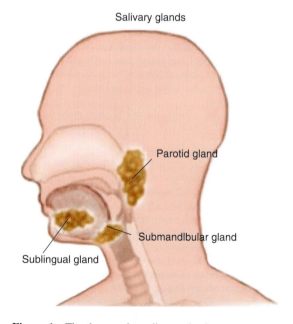

Figure 1   The three major salivary glands

Saliva contains the usual electrolytes of the body fluids. The formation of a primary saliva, isotonic compared to plasma, is situated in the endpieces of the salivary glands, and depends on the active transport of one or more of the principal ions (Na^+, Cl^-, K^+, and HCO_3^-) from the interstitial fluid to the acinar cells and the lumen. Water enters the lumen by osmosis. As this initial fluid moves down the ductal system of the salivary gland, both an active reabsorption of Na^+ and an active secretion of K^+ occur. The resulting saliva becomes increasingly hypotonic in the ductal system, the osmolality depending on the salivary flow (Figure 2). Generally, as the salivary flow increases, higher concentrations of Na^+ and Cl^-, and lower concentrations of K^+ are obtained in the final saliva. The excretion patterns of HCO_3^- are extremely variable among different glands. Usually, the bicarbonate concentration increases when the salivary flow increases, resulting in a higher salivary

pH. The resting pH is about 6.8. Increasing the salivary flow results in a higher osmolality and a pH that approaches the pH of plasma or even slightly higher [4].

Under healthy conditions, adults approximately produce 500–1500 ml oral fluid per day. Salivary secretion is a reflex response controlled by both parasympathetic and sympathetic nerves. In addition, the fluids secreted by the various glands are considerably different from each other. The glandula parotis produces a serous fluid i.e., devoid of mucin, the glandula submandibularis a sero-mucous secrete, while the glandula sublingualis secretes a mucous saliva. Moreover, every type of salivary gland is stimulated to another degree by different stimuli, thus contributing differently to the total salivary production. Several factors are important such as the moment of the day (circadian rhythm), sex, age, nutritional or emotional state, and the type of the

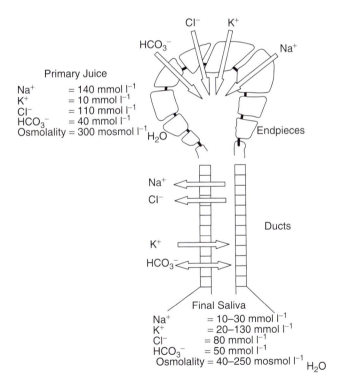

Figure 2 Hypothetical model of electrolyte transport to explain the two-stage formation of saliva. The isotonic primary fluid is produced in the secretory endpieces and is postulated to be either Cl^- rich or HCO_3^- rich. As the primary fluid passes down the gland duct system, Na^+ and Cl^- are reabsorbed while K^+ is secreted actively at somewhat lower rates. The result is the formation of a hypotonic final saliva, usually poor in NaCl and rich in $KHCO_3$ [Reproduced with permission from Ref. 4. © Central Police University Press, 1999.]

salivation stimulus [5]. Taste and olfactory stimuli, mechanical stimulation (chewing), pain, pregnancy-related hormonal changes, aggression, and sympathomimetic and parasympathomimetic drugs increase the salivary flow rate. Menopause-related hormonal changes, stress, antiadrenergic, and anticholinergic drugs decrease the salivary flow rate. An overview of the influence of different therapeutic drugs on salivation has been published recently by Aps and Martens [5]. For example, a typical β-adrenergic drug causes a viscous, protein and mucin rich, secrete. This type of saliva has a foamy appearance, while the volume produced is rather low. The cholinergic (parasympathetic) drug pilocarpine can be used, in some limited cases, to help patients complaining of dry mouth. Variations in salivary flow can also be affected, reversibly or irreversibly, by numerous physiological and pathological factors. This is the major difference between oral fluid and serum, in which the concentrations of the various components can only vary between narrow border values.

Mechanisms of Drug Transfer in Oral Fluid

Salivary glands have a high blood flow. Before any drug circulating in plasma can be discharged into the salivary duct, it must pass through the capillary wall, the basal membrane, and the membrane of the glandular epithelial cells, which is the rate-determining step. Different mechanisms are thought to occur: passive diffusion through the membrane, active processes against a concentration gradient, and filtration through pores in the membrane. Passive diffusion is by far the most common mechanism of drug transport, and is limited to nonprotein bound, nonionized molecules, with a molecular weight of less than 500 Da and a certain degree of lipophilicity. Oral fluid contains predominantly the parent drug because of the higher lipid solubility and, therefore, higher potential for passive diffusion.

In addition to the physicochemical properties of the drug (pK_a, lipid solubility, molecular weight, and spatial configuration) and the degree of plasma protein binding, this transport process is influenced by the pH of both media. Mathematical models have been developed for prediction of the saliva-to-plasma (S/P) drug concentration ratios for both acidic and basic drugs [6]. Especially for drugs with a pK_a

close to the pH of saliva e.g., cocaine and most opiates, the degree of ionization changes drastically with small changes in pH, which is reflected in the S/P ratio. Calculated S/P ratios assuming a resting pH of 6.8 have been listed for a large number of substances [7]. The influence of salivary pH on the S/P ratio of many drugs is perhaps the reason why experimentally determined S/P ratios are different from the theoretical values. This phenomenon is also directly associated with the importance of the salivary flow and the collection protocol (with or without stimulation). Since only nonionized drugs can cross biological membranes and the pH of saliva is usually lower than the plasma pH (7.4), basic drugs usually concentrate in oral fluid due to ion-trapping. As such, oral fluid concentrations are much higher for these drugs than the corresponding plasma concentration [8–10]. In addition, in a controlled study with 3,4-methylenedioxy-N-methylamphetamine (MDMA), salivary pH appeared to be lowered by the actual intake of the drug itself, which explained to some extent the high S/P ratios observed, exceeding by far the theoretical calculated value [8, 11].

In contrast, there is very little partitioning of Δ^9-tetrahydrocannabinol (THC), the active ingredient of cannabis, between plasma and oral fluid. Since THC is a weak acid with a pK_a of about 9.5 and substantially plasma protein-bound, the calculated S/P ratio is 0.1. In practice, it has been demonstrated that shortly after drug use by smoking, oral ingestion, or nasal insufflation (e.g., heroin, methamphetamine, marijuana, and cocaine), contamination of the oral cavity can lead to dramatically elevated oral fluid concentrations of the parent drug, clearly inflated relative to concomitant blood levels. Only after a period of 2 h the oral fluid levels more approximately reflect blood levels. For THC, similarity in time profiles between oral fluid and plasma occur. This is possibly due to reserves of THC deposited in the oral mucosa that are leached out with time [12].

Collection of Oral Fluid

Any potential application for oral fluid testing needs a thorough understanding of the chosen collection method in order to interpret test results. In addition, the choice of a collection protocol should not only depend on the ease-of-use, but also the analytical considerations have to be taken into account. Common methods of oral fluid collection are spitting, draining, suction, and collection on various types of absorbent swabs.

Since drug concentrations can be decreased when increasing the salivary flow, it might be advantageous to collect oral fluid without stimulation. Spitting itself is usually a sufficient stimulus to elicit a flow but the sample volume is often insufficient and the intra- and intersubject variability is large. Moreover, it is not a well-accepted and hygienic procedure for donor and acceptor and it is time-consuming in subjects suffering from dry mouth caused by stress, smoking, and the use of amphetamines and other psychotropic drugs that pharmacologically reduce salivation. In these circumstances, the flow can be stimulated mechanically (by placing paraffin wax, Teflon™, rubber bands, or chewing gum in the mouth) or chemically (lemon drops or citric acid crystals) to obtain a cleaner, more abundant specimen. A mechanical stimulus stimulates a flow of approximately $1-3\,ml\,min^{-1}$; citric acid stimulation may produce flows from 5 to $10\,ml\,min^{-1}$. It is also suggested that stimulation might decrease the intersubject variability [13]. Stimulation of salivary flow is not without drawbacks though. Different studies have confirmed that stimulation of oral fluid (citric acid) reduces drug concentration [10, 14–16]: two- to threefold for codeine and methamphetamine and fivefold for cocaine. These changes are attributed to a dilution effect by the increased output of oral fluid as well as a possible pH effect.

To allow the use of oral fluid testing for drug screening of large populations, a variety of devices have been marketed over the years. They promote an easy, quick, and reproducible collection and a cleaner specimen that is more suitable for analysis. As a general rule, they consist of a sorbent material that becomes saturated in the mouth of the donor, and after removal, the oral fluid is recovered by centrifugation or by applying pressure. Commercial devices include Omni-Sal® (Cozart Biosciences Ltd., Abingdon, UK), Salivette® (Sarstedt AG, Rommelsdorf, Germany), Intercept® (OraSure Technologies, Bethlehem, PA, USA), Finger Collector® (Avitar Technologies, Inc, Canton, MA, USA), ORALscreen™ (Avitar Technologies, Inc,), and Quantisal™ (Immunalysis Corporation, Pomona, CA, USA). Significant differences are reported in percent recovery from the sorbent material for various drugs and a large variability in the ultimately measured oral fluid concentrations [16]. For some devices, e.g., the Quantisal device, excellent recoveries were obtained [17], whereas for other devices, e.g., Salivette, a substantial sequestration on the cotton roll could be observed [18–20]. A typical example is the observation that THC remains bound to the sampling device and that an organic solvent is needed to release it [21–23]. A modification of the sampling procedure for the Intercept® collector (Figure 3), consisting of the addition of 2 ml of methanol to the elution buffer, resulted in complete recovery of THC over a large concentration range [22]. In addition, various pretreatment methods of the spitted samples can lead to significant differences in concentrations between collection protocols [23, 24]. The most recent study on this topic studied the recovery using three different collection devices supplied by Cozart, Immunalysis, and Microgenics [25]. Drugs studied were THC, benzodiazepines, methamphetamine, and morphine. Of the three systems studied, only the Cozart product gave acceptable recovery of THC from drug-spiked oral fluid.

Significant differences in analyte stability were observed for some compounds, e.g., THC and 6-AM (6-acetylmorphine), depending on the storage conditions and the sampling device used [16, 26–28]. In general, the presence of a stabilizing buffer guarantees the stability of the analytes for longer periods of time. The addition of buffer results in difficulties in estimating the actual volume of oral fluid collected [16, 25, 29]. It has been shown that for the Intercept® device, reliable quantitative results can still be obtained when applying a gravimetric

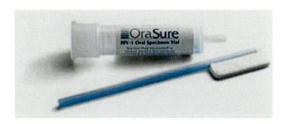

Figure 3 Example of an oral fluid collection device: Intercept®. After gently wiping the collector pad between gum and cheek for approximately 2 min (as a kind of toothbrush), the device is placed in the supplied vial, which contains a stabilizing buffer solution, and sealed. After centrifugation in the laboratory, the recovered fluid can be transferred and analyzed

determination of the amount of oral fluid [19]. An additional problem is that, even when using a collection device, the amount of oral fluid collected can be inadequate for analysis [20].

Pharmacokinetics and Interpretation

A large number of key publications contain valuable concentration kinetics data for oral fluid after controlled administration of the substance to volunteers. An excellent review on the pharmacokinetics of drugs in oral fluid has been recently published by Drummer [30].

Analytical Procedures

A comprehensive review of the analytical methods from 2000 to 2006 for the analysis of drugs of abuse in oral fluid, has recently been submitted [31]. A correct procedure for forensic toxicological analysis involves two different methods. In general, after application of an immunoanalysis technique, a chromatographic method is performed: the first allows for a preliminary monitoring of a large number of samples in a reduced period of time, while the second step provides the required specificity for confirmation. For oral fluid, the amount of matrix collected is smaller when compared to urine and blood and the target range of concentrations is generally lower than in the corresponding urine sample.

The assays routinely used for screening of blood and hair, have a high sensitivity and cross-reactivity for the parent drug and are therefore also advantageous for the analysis of drugs in oral fluid. Several microtiter plate enzyme immunoassays (EIA) have been evaluated for the screening of oral fluid specimens; they only need a limited amount of specimen [25, 28, 29, 32–41]. Erroneous quantitative results might be caused by eating or drinking shortly before sampling or by the collection technique itself, e.g., interference of citric acid or the cotton roll [12, 16]. Commercially available EIA kits are designed for use with specific collection devices. However, it was shown that the application of certain EIA kits was not restricted to the use with one single type of collection method through the validation of sensitive and specific assays [25, 39–41].

As for the confirmation analysis, oral fluid can be extracted and analyzed in the same manner as

other biological fluids, such as blood. Although gas chromatography (tandem) mass spectrometry GC-MS(MS) is regarded as the standard technique for drug testing in oral fluid [21, 42], the use of liquid chromatography (tandem) mass spectrometry (LC-MS(MS)) for the analysis of this sample matrix has steadily increased [43–50]. Analytical sensitivity is a significant concern when conducting oral fluid drug testing. Decreased salivary secretion is a side effect of many drugs including stimulants yielding small volumes of oral fluid available for analysis. In addition, metabolite concentrations can be lower than parent drug concentrations, further elevating sensitivity concerns [30].

As oral fluid contains considerably less proteins and lipids compared to blood or plasma, it was suggested that this allows an easier and faster analysis [51]. However, in view of the higher protein, amino acid, and especially mucin content of oral fluid relative to the urine matrix [52], the development of fast and easy sample preparation methods could be hampered [51, 53]. In addition to the endogenous substances present in oral fluid, specific collection devices mostly include a preservation buffer containing other compounds such as stabilizing salts, nonionic surfactants, and antibacterial agents. Their presence can significantly impact precision and accuracy of subsequent LC-MS-MS measurements through a phenomenon called *ion suppression* or *ion enhancement* [54].

Cannabinoids

Cannabis is the collective term for the psychoactive substances of the *Cannabis sativa* plant and one of the most frequently used illicit drugs in the Western world. THC (Figure 4), the primary psychoactive analyte, is found in the plant's flowering or fruity tops, leaves, and resin. Cannabis is usually smoked but can also be ingested in preparations such as tea and cake. The composition of the cannabinoids in oral fluid samples remains a topic of interest for several research groups. For several years, the only compounds detected in oral fluid after smoking of cannabis were THC, cannabidiol, and cannabinol. As mentioned above, THC has a calculated *S/P* ratio of approximately 0.1 [7]. The Substance Abuse and Mental Health Service Administration (SAMHSA) proposes a screening cutoff of 4 ng ml^{-1} for THC as the target analyte for the initial screen and 4 ng ml^{-1}

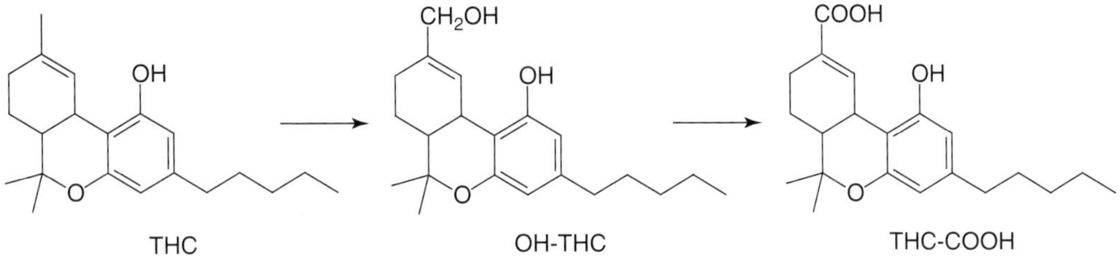

Figure 4   Major metabolic route for Δ^9-tetrahydrocannabinol (THC)

of THC in the confirmation analysis [55]. However, a recently published document by Standards Australia refers to target concentrations of 25 and 10 ng ml^{-1} for screening and confirmation analysis, respectively [56] (Table 1).

Since 2000, five studies investigating the pharmacokinetics of THC in this matrix have been published [12, 48, 57–59]. Substantial differences in THC levels were observed depending on the sampling method. In the studies by Niedbala *et al.* and Laloup *et al.*, oral fluid samples from volunteers having smoked a "joint" were collected with the Intercept® device

and analyzed using GC-MS/MS (limit of quantification (LOQ): 0.2–0.25 ng ml^{-1}) or LC-MS/MS (LOQ: 0.1 ng ml^{-1}) [48, 57–59]. Average peak concentrations ranged from 31 to 596 ng ml^{-1} 15–20 min after smoking. Interestingly, doubling the THC dose and removal of tobacco did not result in a significant increase in the observed THC concentrations in oral fluid. A typical concentration profile for the detection of THC in these oral fluid samples is shown in Figure 5.

Collection of oral fluid by spitting after citric acid stimulation yielded much higher THC concentrations

Table 1   Cutoff concentrations (ng ml^{-1}) for screening and confirmation for each drug in undiluted oral fluid[a]

Drug	SAMHSA[b]		Australian standard[c]	
	Initial test	Confirmatory test	Initial test	Confirmatory test
Cocaine	20		50	
Cocaine		8		25
BE		8		25
EME		–		25
Opiates	40		50	
Morphine		40		25
Codeine		40		25
6-AM		4		10
Amphetamines	50		50	
Amphetamine		50		25
Methamphetamine		50		25
MDMA		50		25
MDA		50		25
MDEA		50		–
Cannabis	4		25	
THC		4		10

[a]Reproduced with permission from Reference [56]. © Standards Australia, 2006
[b]SAMHSA-proposed cutoff concentrations for workplace drug testing (Draft 4) [55]
[c]Approved target concentrations by Standards Australia for the detection and quantification of drugs in oral fluid, intended for workplace, medico-legal and court-directed issues [56]

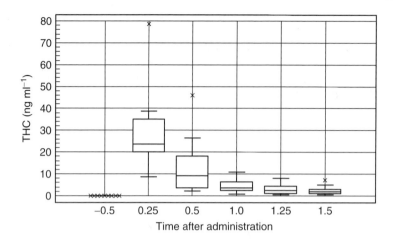

Figure 5 Box- and whisker plots of THC levels in preserved oral fluid samples from nine healthy volunteers following smoking of a single marijuana cigarette. Oral fluid samples were taken with Intercept® 0.5 h prior to smoking and at 0.25, 0.5, 1, 1.25, and 1.5 h after smoking. Concentrations plotted on the Y-axis are expressed as ng ml^{-1}. The central box represents the values from the lower to upper quartile (25–75 percentile). The middle line represents the median. The horizontal line extends from the minimum to the maximum value, excluding "outside" (not present) and "far out" values (cross marker) that are displayed as separate points [Reproduced from Ref. 48. © Elsevier, 2005.]

relative to the former collection method [12]. As discussed previously, this is probably due to the fact that THC was only partially recovered from the Intercept® sampling device [22]. In citric acid stimulated oral fluid, peak concentrations of 864 and 4167 ng ml^{-1} were observed 0.2 h after smoking of a 'joint' containing 1.75% (15.8 mg) and 3.55% (33.8 mg) THC, respectively. In addition, a close relationship between oral fluid and plasma concentrations of THC was observed, possibly due to reserves of THC deposited in the oral mucosa that is leached out with time. This was confirmed in a study by Ramaekers *et al.* [60], where a strong and linear relation between THC in serum and oral fluid was obtained after single doses of 250 and 500 µg kg^{-1} THC by smoking.

Irrespective of the collection method, the concentrations of THC in oral fluid appear to decline in a biphasic manner. After cannabis administration, peak concentrations observed in the first oral fluid specimen are attributed to initial contamination of oral fluid during smoking. The elevated THC concentrations in oral fluid due to this initial direct contamination dissipate rapidly (within 30 min) followed by a second phase of decline of oral fluid-sequestered THC in a similar manner as plasma THC. Estimates of the initial half-life of THC show a mean value of 21 min. Estimates of the terminal half-life of

THC show a mean of 122 min [59]. Oral fluid concentrations generally declined below 1 ng ml^{-1} after 12–16 h.

After the oral consumption of 20–25 mg THC in the form of brownies, much lower peak oral fluid concentrations of about 4 ng ml^{-1} at 1–2 h were observed [57]. Concentrations declined rapidly and were below the limit of detection (LOD) of the GC-MS/MS by 16 h.

One additional issue in the use of oral fluid for drug screening is the possibility of passive contamination. Indeed, two recent studies demonstrated the presence of detectable THC concentrations in oral fluid from volunteers exposed passively to cannabis smoke in an unventilated room (area 36 m^2) [59] or van (15.3 m^2) [58]. Concentrations ranged from 7 to 26 ng ml^{-1} (mean 13 ng ml^{-1}) and from 4.5 to 7.5 ng ml^{-1} (mean 6.2 ng ml^{-1}), respectively. THC concentrations declined rapidly and became negative within 30–45 min. However, oral fluid collector devices exposed to circulating air inside the van but not to oral fluid were also highly contaminated with THC. Further analysis revealed that, when the subjects were removed from the space where passive exposure occurred prior to sample collection, the THC concentrations in oral fluid specimens were only minimal (0.0–1.2 ng ml^{-1}). Considering a SAMHSA cutoff of 4.0 ng ml^{-1}, passively exposed subjects are considered to be negative by avoiding the environmental contamination.

Moore *et al.* and Day *et al.* recently demonstrated the presence of the principal urinary metabolite, 11-nor-9-carboxy-Δ^9-tetrahydrocannabinol (THC-COOH) in the oral fluid matrix [61, 62]. To approach the required sensitivity, oral fluid samples were analyzed using GC-MS/MS [61] or two-dimensional GC-MS [62]. Day *et al.* reported an LOQ of 10 pg ml^{-1} and concentrations up to 240 pg ml^{-1} present in the oral fluid specimens, previously identified as positive for THC. In a study involving a frequent marijuana user, THC-COOH could be detected in all samples collected at 15 min until 8 h after smoking (range 51–134 pg ml^{-1}) [62]. Interestingly, the last sample was the highest in concentration, which suggests that the increase may be reflective of deposition of this metabolite in blood. Therefore, THC-COOH could be a potential long-term marker of marijuana use since it is unlikely to come from oral contamination as is the case for parent THC. In another report of these authors, the same GC/GC-MS method was used to study the contribution of THC-COOH to enzyme-linked immunosorbent assay (ELISA) commonly used for oral fluid screening [63]. They have shown that the inclusion of this metabolite in the confirmation profile for cannabinoids in oral fluid increases the confirmation rate of the immunoassay result by at least 9.7% and minimizes the argument for passive contamination of the oral cavity.

Amphetamines

Amphetamine, methamphetamine, and the designer amphetamines are synthetic stimulants, with similarities to some naturally occurring weak stimulants such as ephedrine and pseudoephedrine (*Ephedra* species). The β-phenylisopropylamine backbone is the structural basis for many of the sympathomimetic amines. Substitutions on the nitrogen and the ring system account for most of the structural variations and differences in stimulating and euphoric effects. MDMA ('ecstasy') is increasingly used for its desired feelings of emotional closeness and sensory pleasure in the context of large, all-night dance parties where the drug is regarded as safe by the party visitors, and where multiple doses are consumed during the night [64, 65]. The calculated theoretical *S/P* ratios for amphetamine, methamphetamine, and MDMA are 2.2, 4.0, and 3.9, respectively [66]. However, the experimental values obtained always exceeded the theoretical value, possibly due to the effect of the salivary pH as discussed previously.

Proposed SAMHSA screening cutoff values are 50 ng ml^{-1} for *d*-methamphetamine as the target analyte and confirmation cutoff values are 50 ng ml^{-1} for amphetamine, methamphetamine, MDMA, MDA (3,4-methylenedioxy-*N*-amphetamine), and MDEA (3,4-methylenedioxy-*N*-ethylamphetamine). In addition, when methamphetamine is present in the specimen, it must also contain amphetamine at a concentration $\geq$ LOD. Standards Australia established similar screening cutoff values; however, the confirmation cutoffs were lowered to 25 ng ml^{-1} for amphetamine, methamphetamine, MDMA, and MDA (Table 1). In two controlled studies [8, 9] where healthy volunteers were administered a single dose of MDMA, the patterns of oral fluid and plasma MDMA concentration–time profiles agreed well. However, the intersubject variability was substantially higher for oral fluid [8, 9]. Peak MDMA concentrations of 1728–6510 ng ml^{-1} at 1.5 h after administration of 100 mg MDMA were observed, declining to a mean concentration of 126 ng ml^{-1} at 24 h [8]. A lower mean peak concentration of 1215 $\pm$ 944 ng ml^{-1} was noted by Samyn *et al.* 2 h after administration of 75 mg MDMA [9]. Levels of MDMA averaged 526 $\pm$ 372 ng ml^{-1} at 5 h after administration. Oral fluid samples were collected by spitting, without any kind of stimulation, and the salivary pH was determined for MDMA users and control subjects in one study [8]. MDMA levels exceeded the plasma concentrations by, on average, a 10-fold at peak concentrations declining to a lower more constant value (4–7) after 5–24 h. MDA, the metabolite of MDMA, was also present in these oral fluid samples, with concentrations representing about 4–5% of the concentration of oral fluid MDMA, as was also observed for plasma in this study [8].

One study documents the presence of MDMA and MDA in oral fluid samples collected with the Intercept® device [54]. Specimens were collected 1.5 and 5.5 h after the administration of a single dose of 75 or 100 mg MDMA. Analysis using LC-MS/MS (LOQ: 2.0 ng ml^{-1}) revealed a median MDMA concentration of 448 and 316 ng ml^{-1} after 1.5 and 5.5 h, respectively, in the preserved oral fluid samples. The corresponding MDA concentrations remained quite low, with a median concentration of 7.7 and 16.5 ng ml^{-1} respectively.

There is only one recent report dealing with methamphetamine and amphetamine pharmacokinetics in oral fluid after a controlled administration of methamphetamine [10]. Oral fluid specimens were collected using citric acid candy stimulation or Salivette® cotton swabs treated with or without citric acid after a single 10- or 20-mg dose of sustained release methamphetamine. Significant higher concentrations were obtained in oral fluid samples collected with neutral cotton swabs in comparison with those obtained from citric acid-treated swabs and after citric acid candy stimulation. Following citric acid candy stimulation, mean peak methamphetamine concentrations were 106 ± 25 and 192 ± 121 ng ml^{-1}, respectively, occurring 4–8 h and 2–12 h postdose. All citric acid candy stimulated oral fluid specimens collected at 24 h after drug administration were above the LOQ of the GC-MS method for methamphetamine (2.5 ng ml^{-1}). When using the SAMHSA-proposed cutoff values, only one of 13 individuals tested positive 24 h after a single methamphetamine dose. Oral fluid methamphetamine concentrations were double than those observed in plasma. However, a considerable within- and between-subject variability contributed to the poor observed correlation between plasma and oral fluid methamphetamine concentrations. Amphetamine, as the metabolite of methamphetamine, was not always detected in oral fluid specimens following administration of methamphetamine. When present, concentrations were about one-tenth that of methamphetamine.

Cocaine

Cocaine is an alkaloid obtained by extraction of the leaves of *Erythroxylon coca*, a plant that grows at 1000–2000 m elevations in the Andean mountains under warm tropical conditions. Cocaine has been used by the Peruvian Indians for centuries for the well being and increased endurance it produces after chewing the leaves of the plant. In the late nineteenth century, it was used medically as an anesthetic. It was not until the late 1960s that the recreational use of cocaine became a significant social problem in the Western world, especially in the US [67–69]. Cocaine is sold on the street in two forms: the hydrochloride (HCl) salt and the free base form "crack". Street purity ranges from 1 to over 90%, with cocaine HCl mainly used for intravenous injection and nasal insufflation, and the free base used for smoking (volatilization with a glass pipe and heat).

The metabolism of cocaine has been thoroughly studied (Figure 6) [67, 70, 71]. The main primary metabolites of cocaine are benzoylecgonine (BE), formed by chemical hydrolysis and enzymatic hydrolysis by a liver methylesterase, and ecgonine methyl ester (EME), formed by enzymatic hydrolysis by liver carboxylesterases and plasma butyrylcholinesterase. Both inactive metabolites are further metabolized to ecgonine [72]. Norcocaine is a minor metabolite in humans.

Cocaine is a highly lipophilic, basic drug and has a pK_a of 8.6. The theoretical *S/P* ratio calculated

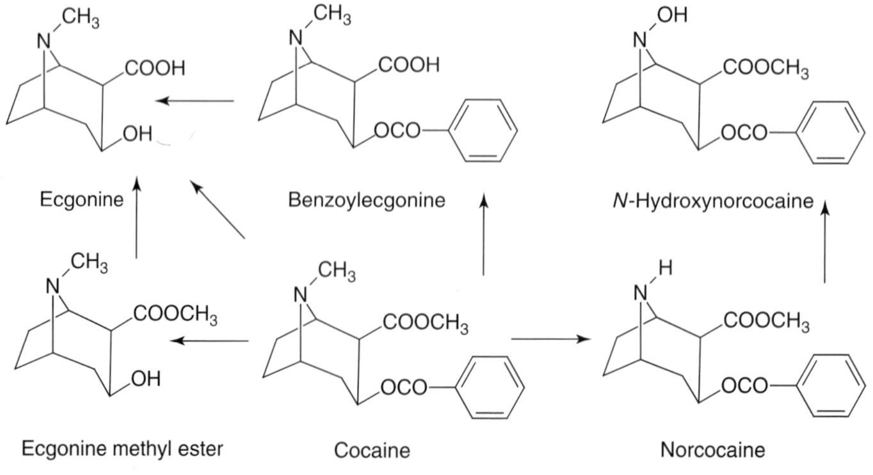

Figure 6 Main metabolic pathways of cocaine

for a salivary pH of 6.8 is 3.8 [7]. When assuming a pH in the range of 6.8–7.8 (depending on the nature of stimulation), *S/P* ratios of 3.82–0.44 were calculated. SAMHSA-proposed oral fluid cutoff values are 20 ng ml^{-1} for cocaine metabolites for screening assays and 8 ng ml^{-1} for cocaine or BE in confirmation analyses. Higher cutoff concentrations for cocaine and metabolites of 50 and 25 ng ml^{-1} for screening and confirmation, respectively, were adopted by the Australian standard (Table 1).

The Cone group published the most complete study on cocaine excretion in saliva in 1997 [73]. Cocaine appeared in saliva rapidly following different administration routes. Contamination of the oral cavity after smoking and sniffing was variable but significant during the first hours after administration of a single low dose of cocaine, resulting in high *S/P* ratios. BE and EME usually appeared in oral fluid between 0.08 and 1 h after administration. Typically, cocaine concentrations exceeded metabolite concentrations over the first 2 h, rapidly declining, sometimes below metabolite concentrations within 4–6 h. Anhydroecgonine methylester (AEME) is a pyrolysis product that also appears in oral fluid in high concentrations; it can be used as a marker of cocaine smoking.

Following repeated oral cocaine administration, the obtained pharmacokinetic parameters were generally comparable to those reported from acute dosing studies [74].

A study on the disposition and elimination of cocaine in self-reported users of cocaine (0.1–2 g smoked cocaine daily) showed cocaine oral fluid concentrations on average 2.4-fold higher than those found in plasma [75]. These findings suggest a prolonged elimination of cocaine in active street users than in occasional users, though the half-life of its main metabolite BE remains similar.

Opiates

The opiates are a large family of drugs with a mechanism of action and pharmacological activities related to morphine. Potent opiates such as morphine are particularly important in medicine due to their ability to relieve moderate to severe pain. Codeine is one of the most widely used opiates, and is easily available in some countries in low dose over-the-counter preparations with weak analgesic properties and as a cough suppressant. A number of synthetic opiates have been developed that resemble morphine when viewed as a 3D image on the receptor, although at first glance they do appear quite different.

Heroin is widely available as an illicit drug, and is produced in clandestine laboratories by synthetic acetylation of morphine from crude extracts of the exudates from the opium poppy (*Papaver somniferum*). Heroin is more lipophilic and crosses the blood–brain barrier more rapidly than morphine resulting in more intense euphoric effects. Heroin is injected intravenously (usual dose 10–15 mg), snorted or inhaled (by smoking the free base or inhaling the vapors of heated powder). Intravenous injection of heroin is common and is the fastest way to deliver the drug to the brain. Peak heroin plasma concentrations are obtained within 2 min, and are no longer detectable after 30 min. Heroin is almost immediately metabolized to 6-AM, which is detectable at 1 min and peaks at 5 min and which is rapidly transformed to morphine (Figure 7).

Heroin has a pK_a of 7.6, which results in variable *S/P* ratios, highly depending on the salivary pH. Morphine is less lipid soluble than heroin. It has a pK_a of 8.1 and is for about 65% bound to plasma proteins. The theoretical *S/P* ratio, assuming a salivary pH of 6.8, is 1.22. Since codeine has a pK_a of 8.2 and is only bound to plasma proteins to a minor extent, it has a higher theoretical *S/P* ratio of 3.32.

As for cocaine, heroin, and its metabolites 6-AM and morphine are detected in oral fluid after administration of heroin by different routes; concentrations are depending on the route of administration and on the salivary pH. For opiates, their levels in oral fluid appear to mimic blood levels suggesting that comparable results between these matrices can be achieved [76, 77]. The proposed SAMHSA cutoffs are 40 ng ml^{-1} for screening and confirmation, except for 6-AM, for which a 10-fold lower confirmation cutoff value was suggested. Laboratories are also permitted to initial test all specimens for 6-AM using a 4 ng ml^{-1} cutoff. Standards Australia recommends a screening target concentrations of 50 ng ml^{-1} with confirmation at 25 ng ml^{-1} for morphine and codeine and 10 ng ml^{-1} for 6-AM (Table 1).

The number of studies concerning heroin are limited. Heroin is detected within minutes in oral fluid following nasal insufflation (snorting). A 12-mg

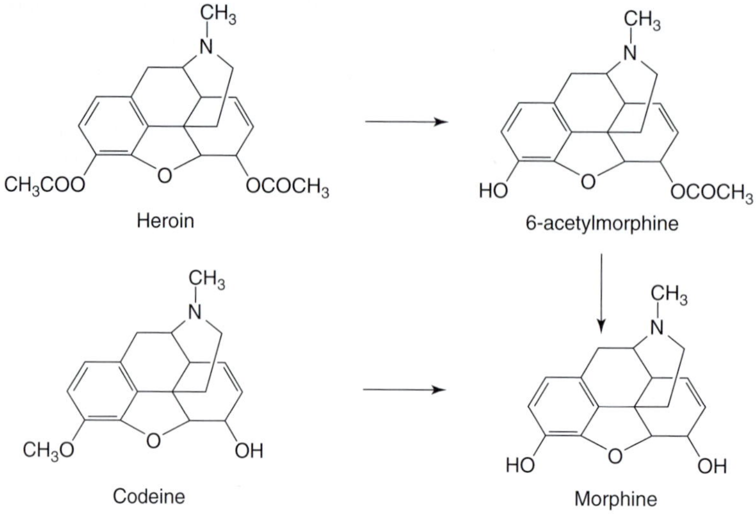

Figure 7   Major metabolic route for heroin

dose resulted in a peak heroin concentration of $300\,ng\,ml^{-1}$ in oral fluid and it was detectable for about 1 h (LOD: $1.0\,ng\,ml^{-1}$). 6-AM and morphine were rapidly detected in oral fluid peaking at 60 and $25\,ng\,ml^{-1}$ at 10 and 60 min, respectively [78]. Two subjects given 2.6–10.5 mg smoked doses revealed peak concentrations of heroin greater than $3000\,ng\,ml^{-1}$, but less than $10\,ng\,ml^{-1}$ beyond 60–120 min. Much lower peak concentrations were detected after i.v. injection of heroin: up to $30\,ng\,ml^{-1}$ after 3–12 mg doses. The mean S/P ratio was approximately 1 [76].

Intramuscular morphine sulfate at doses of 10 and 20 mg resulted in a peak concentration of 11 and $38\,ng\,ml^{-1}$ in two subjects, respectively, using a stimulated collection process [79]. At 24 h, concentrations were barely detectable.

Codeine presence in oral fluid has been studied in four studies [15, 37, 80, 81]. Screening/confirmation cutoffs of 20/20 [80] and $30/40\,ng\,ml^{-1}$ [37] have been proposed based on two studies with volunteers given 60 and 120 mg codeine.

Substantially different pharmacokinetic parameters were obtained for codeine with different collection methods [15]. After stimulation with citric acid, mean peak concentrations of $556 \pm 301, 639 \pm 64$, and $1599 \pm 241\,ng\,ml^{-1}$ were observed following 30 mg liquid codeine phosphate and 60 and 120 mg codeine sulfate capsules, respectively

[15, 81]. Although a high intra- and intersubject variability was observed, the time course of codeine concentration in oral fluid was similar to that seen in plasma [81]. Generally, codeine concentrations were higher in oral fluid than in plasma and codeine could be detected 5–9 h longer in oral fluid than in plasma when the LOQ of the GC-MS method ($2.5\,ng\,ml^{-1}$) was used as cutoff value. Norcodeine was also detected in small amounts in oral fluid.

Dihydrocodeine is a weak narcotic analgesic and used as an antitussive [82]. Following a single 60-mg dose, peak oral fluid concentrations ranged from 423 to $1421\,ng\,ml^{-1}$, reached 2–4 h after dose. The concentrations of this compound in oral fluid samples from 20 chronic users (0.4–2.7 g daily) within 24 h after the last dose ranged up to $66\,154\,ng\,ml^{-1}$. Samples were collected with the Salivette®. Dihydrocodeine was detectable until about 24 h after the last use with an LOD of $5\,ng\,ml^{-1}$.

Finally, one study was conducted to determine the concentrations of morphine in oral fluid and urine following the consumption of commercially available poppy seeds [83]. Oral fluid samples from volunteers who ingested in addition to one poppy seed bagel as many possible poppy seeds as possible (amounts ranging from 9.82 to 20.82 g), tested positive up to 1 h after ingestion with a concentration greater than the proposed SAMHSA confirmation cutoff for morphine.

Benzodiazepines

The benzodiazepines are a large class of prescribed drugs, used widely for different medical conditions such as the treatment of insomnia (mostly short-acting analogues), the treatment of anxiety-related conditions (mostly longer acting analogues), as muscle relaxants, and as anticonvulsants [84–86]. Some of them are abused, either by themselves or in combination with other drugs, particularly the narcotic analgesics (opiates). Their ability to suppress withdrawal symptoms and to boost the effects of heroin have made them a favored drug type among the drug-using population [87, 88]. They are also abused by cocaine users to increase the seizure threshold [84].

The benzodiazepine structure is based on the diazepine ring fused to benzene, with the nitrogens usually in the 1,4 positions. Substitution leads to varying degrees of metabolic stability, pharmacological potency, and lipid solubility (Figure 8). The 7-nitro substituted 1,4-benzodiazepines, such as flunitrazepam, are often abused. Somewhat newer analogues are based on the diazolo- and triazolo-ring types and include alprazolam and triazolam, very potent benzodiazepines requiring much lower doses. Zolpidem is an imidazopyridine derivative, with a chemical structure unrelated to benzodiazepines.

In general, *S/P* ratios below 1 are expected due to the extensive plasma protein binding of benzodiazepines.

Until now, five recent studies have examined the presence of benzodiazepines in oral fluid. Samyn *et al.* reported peak concentrations of flunitrazepam (0.29–0.58 ng ml^{-1}) and its metabolite 7-aminoflunitrazepam (0.94–3.05 ng ml^{-1}) at 1–4.5 h following the administration of 1 mg flunitrazepam to four subjects [89]. Owing to the extremely low concentrations of flunitrazepam and its metabolite in oral fluid, GC-MS in chemical ionization mode was used (LOQ: 0.10 and 0.15 ng ml^{-1}, respectively). Sodium fluoride preservative was required to detect flunitrazepam in the oral fluid specimens. These authors proposed a cutoff value of approximately 0.25 ng ml^{-1} of 7-aminoflunitrazepam in oral fluid to detect use of flunitrazepam within the last 6 h.

Following the ingestion of a single oral dose of 2.5 mg lorazepam to one volunteer, a peak concentration of 18 ng ml^{-1} was observed in oral fluid after 15 min of intake. Oral fluid samples were still positive for this compound after 8 h (0.3 ng ml^{-1}) [90].

Peak concentrations of midazolam in oral fluid samples following a single 2 mg bolus of the drug to three patients ranged from 1.42 to 13.98 ng ml^{-1} after 10–40 h [20]. However, substantially higher concentrations of midazolam in these specimens were obtained after continuous infusion of the drug.

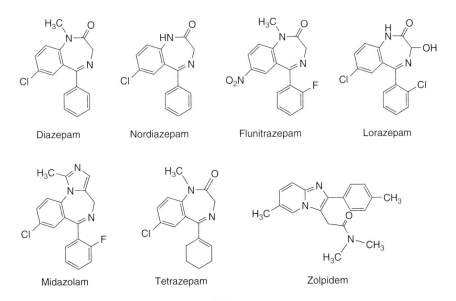

Figure 8 Structures of selected benzodiazepines and zolpidem

Oral administration of a single 50-mg dose of tetrazepam to one volunteer produced a peak concentration of $6.6\,ng\,ml^{-1}$ after 150 min, which is approximately the time of peak plasma concentration [91]. Oral fluid tested positive for tetrazepam over 8.6 h with an LOQ of the LC-MS/MS method of $0.03\,ng\,ml^{-1}$.

After oral administration of 10 mg zolpidem to two subjects, peak concentrations of this drug were obtained after 150 min ($53.5\,ng\,ml^{-1}$) and 180 min ($75.7\,ng\,ml^{-1}$), respectively [92]. Oral fluid still tested positive for zolpidem at 8 h ($9-15\,ng\,ml^{-1}$).

As suggested, an *S/P* ratio lower than 1 was obtained for the studied benzodiazepines [90–92].

Applications

Oral fluid drug testing has been used as an alternative matrix to blood and urine in clinical and forensic toxicology [93]. Owing to its particular advantages, interest in the use of oral fluid testing for drugs in the workplace [29, 94] and at the roadside [23, 95–97] is increasing rapidly. The use of oral fluid in drug treatment facilities [98] and for therapeutic drug monitoring [99–101] has also been reported.

Workplace Drug Testing

It is clear that laboratory-based analytical methods to measure drugs in oral fluid are robust and well developed. Many published studies have examined the known or potential rate of error of these tests (sensitivity, specificity, positive predictive value, negative predictive value, overall accuracy). There is certainly an acceptance of the accuracy and reliability of oral fluid testing within the scientific community. Unfortunately, there are no formal laboratory certification programs yet established for drug testing in oral fluid [102]. In April 2004, SAMHSA has published in the Federal Register a Proposed Rule for incorporating oral fluid in its federal workplace drug-testing program. This was followed recently by an Australian standard that is also intended for workplace drug testing (Table 1). In the United Kingdom, the UK Workplace Drug-testing forum is currently working on guidelines for oral fluid specimen analy-sis. However, to date, no published document is available. Alltrix, the largest specialist oral fluid drug-testing laboratory in Europe is using its own cutoff levels, which are based on the levels proposed by the manufacturer of the immunoassays (OraSure Technologies) for the screening assays (Clarke, J. Altrix Healthcare, *Personal Communication*, January 2007). All samples are collected using the Intercept® device.

The results of the first large-scale database on oral fluid testing in private industry were published by Cone *et al.* [29]. A total of 77 000 specimens were screened by the Intercept® immunoassay at manufacturer's recommended cutoff values for five drug categories (marijuana, cocaine, opiates, phencyclidine, and amphetamines). Presumptive positive specimens were confirmed by GC-MS. An overall positive rate of 5.06% was noted. The confirmed positive specimens consisted primarily of THC and cocaine (85.75%). In comparison to the corresponding urine samples, the prevalence of positives for cocaine and amphetamines was approximately 60% higher in oral fluid. Of the 48 morphine-positive specimens, 32 specimens were also positive for 6-AM. Considering the short detection window for this unique metabolite in urine (approximately 3.3 h following single dose administration of heroin), it is concluded that oral fluid is superior to urine in the confirmation of recent use of heroin [29, 103]. After a single administration of THC by inhalation, there was a substantially higher rate of detection of positive oral fluid specimens over the first 8 h in comparison to the corresponding urine testing [57]. This unique characteristic is of great importance when one considers the short time course of marijuana's effect on performance. In general, oral fluid is considered as the only other body fluid revealing recent drug use and therefore related to possible impairment, whereas urine testing is clearly more useful to detect past use of the drug.

Both SAMHSA and Standards Australia have also established guidelines for the collection and storage of specimens. For SAMHSA, the suggested minimum amount of specimen to be collected is 2 ml, which can be divided into 1.5 ml for the primary specimen and 0.5 ml for retesting. SAMHSA is presently recommending oral fluid sampling by spitting into a neat tube, whereas for Standards Australia specimens either collected by spitting or through the use of a device are accepted. However, to overcome the problems of adsorption of certain drugs to the devices (as discussed previously), each manufacturer is required to document recovery of all target analytes from the devices. In addition, some oral fluid specimen collection schemes involve collection on an absorbent swab with subsequent transfer into a buffer, an issue that can cause difficulties for the interpretation of quantitative results. Another problem is that many devices cause either a mechanical or chemical stimulation of oral fluid flow. As already discussed above, this process affects the pH of oral fluid, and therefore the concentrations of drugs and metabolites in the oral fluid sample.

Owing to a lack of resolution of several of the above mentioned important research questions, SAMHSA has proposed a conservative approach to the addition of oral fluid testing to the different drug-testing matrices. In its proposed rules, SAMHSA noted that less is known about the pharmacokinetics and disposition of drugs in oral fluid as compared to urine. However, several authors have investigated these pharmacokinetics, and, therefore, it is important to note that although it may not be possible to answer some of these questions definitively, qualified experts may nonetheless be able to provide sufficient information to assist in its decision-making. The new SAMHSA guidelines also recommend collecting urine specimens simultaneously with oral fluid, because of the potential of passive contamination for THC, as discussed previously. However, the recent demonstration by Moore *et al.* and Day *et al.* of the presence of THC-COOH in the oral fluid matrix may eliminate the necessity of the additional urine sampling [61, 62].

Substance Abuse Monitoring

Drug testing of patients in treatment is generally practiced to provide objective assessment of patients' progress. Many treatment programs require individuals to detoxify from the offending drug(s) and remain drug-free throughout treatment. Other programs utilize substitution therapy in which the patient is switched from an illicit drug, e.g., heroin, to an acceptable substitute, e.g., methadone or buprenorphine, which is administered by treatment personnel. In most of the programs, patients' progress is monitored by urinalysis. However, interest in oral fluid as an alternative drug-testing tool has grown in this area. Oral fluid testing appears to be a good indicator of the validity and reliability of drug user's self-report data [101].

Dihydrocodeine, codeine, morphine, 6-AM, heroin, cocaine, BE, methadone, amphetamine, MDA, MDMA, MDEA were measured by GC-MS in oral fluid of donors being monitored in a drug misuse treatment program as part of the investigators' effort to evaluate the Cozart® RapiScan screening device and the Cozart® Microplate EIA [33–36, 104].

The concordance of oral fluid and urine opiate results for participants in drug withdrawal therapy was assessed [105]. Oral fluid specimens were collected with a Clin Rep® device from Recipe and analyzed by GC-MS for dihydrocodeine, codeine, 6-AM, and morphine. The authors found a good correlation between opiate results in both matrices, in specimens collected every 2–4 days over a 3-month period. They concluded that oral fluid was appropriate for analysis of drugs of abuse. Niedbala *et al.* [28] collected oral fluid and urine specimens from known opiate abusers in a drug treatment center and found an agreement of more than 90%, applying a cutoff of 10 ng ml^{-1} for one or more opiates in the collected oral fluid and a 2000 ng ml^{-1} cutoff for interpretation of the urine results. This was confirmed by Bennett *et al.* [98] comparing the accuracy of on-site testing of oral fluid with urine on-site testing in 157 drug-dependant persons and concluded that oral fluid testing is as accurate as urinalysis in detecting the presence of opiates and methadone.

Recently, Dams *et al.* [106] analyzed oral fluid specimens from 16 pregnant opiate-dependent women. Specimens were collected with the Salivette® oral fluid collection device. 6-AM, heroin, and morphine were the major opiates detected with median concentrations of 5.2, 2.3, and 7.5 ng ml^{-1}, respectively. Detection of 6-AM and/or heroin in 84% of positive oral fluid specimens proved heroin usage, rather than licit codeine or morphine, or ingestion of opiate-containing foodstuffs. In contrast, only 37 urine specimens collected the same day in the same subjects as the oral fluid samples were positive at a 300 ng ml^{-1} cutoff concentration of opiates in urine. Cocaine and BE had median concentrations of 6.4 and 3.4 ng ml^{-1}. The major analytes identified were cocaine and BE, detected in approximately 98% of all cocaine positive specimens. In contrast, only 22 urine specimens were positive for cocaine metabolites at a 300 ng ml^{-1} cutoff. These authors conclude that oral fluid is a promising alternative matrix to monitor opiate and cocaine use in drug-testing programs.

Acetylcodeine has also been reported as a marker of illicit heroin abuse in oral fluid samples [107]. A significant correlation was found between this new marker and 6-AM ($r = 0.95$) in samples collected from patients attending a substance abuse clinic.

Oral fluid has also been examined as an alternative matrix for the therapeutic monitoring of methadone [108, 109]. A poor correlation between oral fluid and serum was obtained when considering total methadone concentrations [108]. However, a good correlation was found between both matrices when the enantiomeric ratios of methadone were taken into account. Methadone and its major metabolite, 2-ethylidene-1,5-dimethyl-3,3-diphenylpyrrolidine (EDDP), were examined in oral fluid and plasma as a function of salivary pH [110]. Oral fluid methadone ranged from 120 to 3460 ng ml^{-1} with *S/P* ratios from 0.6 to 7.2. For EDDP the ranges were 40–100 ng ml^{-1} for oral fluid, with an *S/P* ratio of 0.2–1.8. An inverse correlation was found between the methadone concentration and the oral fluid pH.

Roadside Drug Testing

While there is only limited knowledge of the prevalence of drugs other than alcohol in road traffic, it appears that drugged driving is a significant problem worldwide [111–113]. Since the late 1990s, several western countries have, in analogy to alcohol, introduced *per se* legislation for driving under the influence of drugs (DUID). The policy is in whole or in part based on the detection of any amount of illicit drug in blood or urine of the driver. However, a positive urine test is by no means an indication that the subject was "under the influence" at the time of sampling. The presence of certain illicit drugs or their metabolites in urine of potentially impaired drivers is merely evidence of relatively recent exposure, except for certain drugs such as cannabis. The urinary metabolite of THC can be detected in urine for days, or even weeks, after the last use in regular users. When the drug is detected in blood, there is a higher probability that the subject is experiencing pharmacological effects at the time of sampling. A recently published controlled study has approached the relatively obscure relation between THC concentration in serum and driver impairment [60]. It was concluded that a serum THC concentration of 2–5 ng ml^{-1} was associated to the limit for impairment in performance tests measuring skills related to driving.

Oral fluid is probably the only other body fluid that might parallel blood in some regards and therefore may be related to behavioral performance [4, 114]. Using receiver operating characteristic (ROC) analysis of data from 139 individuals suspected of driving under the influence of cannabis, Laloup et al. [115] calculated an optimal cutoff value of 1.2 ng ml^{-1} THC in preserved oral fluid to predict a positive plasma result (LOQ 0.5 ng ml^{-1}) (sensitivity: 94.7% and specificity: 92.0%). Several studies have shown that a reasonably good correlation can be found between the presence or absence of drugs in oral fluid and in blood [8, 23, 116, 117]. Moreover, oral fluid appears to be superior to urine in correlating with serum analytical data and impairment symptoms of drivers under the influence of drugs of abuse [95]. Epidemiological data from drivers (randomly stopped) and accident-involved drivers, respectively, have been collected by analysis of oral fluid samples in the context of the European project IMMORTAL (Impaired Motorists, Methods of Roadside Testing, and Assessment for Licensing) [97, 118].

Since many years, police officers involved in road safety have expressed the need for a rapid and reliable drug test that can be applied at the roadside. The on-site urine drug tests and the first generation of the oral fluid tests were thoroughly evaluated in the DG VII EC project ROSITA (Roadside Testing Assessment) [112]. At that time, three on-site tests for oral fluid screening were available: Drugwipe® (Securetec, Germany), RapiScan® (Cozart Bioscience, UK), and Oralscreen® (Avitar, US). A clear majority of the participants preferred oral fluid as the matrix of choice for on-site testing. The possibility of collecting oral fluid by nonmedical personnel and without the need for special facilities (i.e., sanitary van) was a distinct advantage. However, police officers and researchers encountered problems related to insufficient sample volume, the viscosity of the samples and insufficient sensitivity of the analytical methods. The on-site oral fluid screenings, particularly for testing of THC, required significant improvement [96].

As has been mentioned earlier in this article, steady progress has been made in the last five years in the field of sample collection and laboratory-based immunoassays and confirmation techniques. Most of the newer generation on-site devices offer the possibility to collect enough sample volume (sometimes diluted with buffer) that can be used for confirmation analysis in the laboratory. In 2002, a compilation of the analytical advantages and test performances of out-of-lab drug-testing devices was published [119]. Several authors have compared the use of some of these on-site devices with laboratory results, including Cozart® RapiScan [37, 38, 104, 120–122], Drugwipe® [23, 123, 124], Toxiquick® [125], Dräger® DrugTest [115], Oratect® [126], and Oraline® [127]. However, the absence of internationally accepted cutoff values for oral fluid hampers the comparison of on-site test results with chromatographic results.

In an evaluation of six on-site test devices using spiked oral fluid samples [128, 129], it appeared that theoretical cutoff values for a specific analyte are considerably different across devices. The ability to accurately and reliably detect cocaine and amphetamine was dependent on the individual device. Most devices performed well for the detection of methamphetamine and opiates, but all performed poorly for the detection of THC. Two reasons appear to be apparent: (i) the devices target the wrong analyte (THC-COOH instead of THC) and (ii) the cutoff concentrations are too high considering the low concentrations of THC generally present in oral fluid.

In late 2003, the Rosita-2 project was started, involving six European countries and five US states [111]. Nine devices were evaluated: American Biomedica Oralstat, Branan Medical Oratect, Cozart Bioscience RapiScan (only in the United States), Dräger/Orasure DrugTest/Uplink, Lifepoint Impact, Securetec Drugwipe, Sun Biomedical Oraline, Ultimed Salivascreen, and Varian OraLab. For six devices, the number of failed test runs exceeded 25%, and their evaluation was stopped. During the study, two devices were withdrawn from the market: the Dräger DrugTest and Lifepoint Impact. At the end of the study, based on the analytical evaluation (comparison to reference methods in oral fluid and/or blood), no device was considered reliable enough to be recommended for roadside screening of drivers. The sensitivity of the on-site screening devices for cannabis and benzodiazepines needs to be improved dramatically. For example, the performance of the Dräger DrugTest to screen for THC in oral fluid was evaluated using oral fluid and plasma as reference samples [115]. Whereas the specificity of the test was high (93–100%), a sensitivity of only 50% was calculated, indicating a high number of false-negative test results. Despite these drawbacks, in a

few countries, legislation was passed that allows the potential use of oral fluid as a matrix for screening or confirmation [96].

In the state of Victoria in Australia, legislation introduced in December 2003 allows police to perform random roadside oral fluid testing for cannabis, methamphetamine, and MDMA [130]. Police officers use the Drugwipe II® device (Securetec) to do the initial screening by wiping the tongue, when the driver is still in his car. If this test shows a positive result, for cannabis, methamphetamine, or MDMA, an oral fluid sample is requested so the police can do an immediate screening on-site with the Cozart RapiScan system for the same drug classes. When this second test is positive for either drug, the oral fluid sample is confirmed in the laboratory for amphetamines and THC using predefined cutoff values, and the driver can take the split sample with him. From the 13 176 drug tests performed at the roadside, 313 positive cases were selected for GC-MS analysis (2.4%). A high number of positive methamphetamine ($n = 269$; median: $1136\,\text{ng ml}^{-1}$) and MDMA ($n = 118$; median: $2724\,\text{ng ml}^{-1}$) findings are reported, and a relatively low number of THC positives ($n = 87$; median: $81\,\text{ng ml}^{-1}$) [131]. It would be interesting to analyze the data further with respect to THC levels in those cases where both oral fluid tests were positive for THC, and to know the prevalence of THC-only positives. Based on the results of Rosita-2, the relatively good performance of the test devices to pick up amphetamines should reflect in a high number of methamphetamine positive tests and the low sensitivity to detect THC in oral fluid, should lead to a serious underestimation of the number of cannabis positives. However, the aim of this type of random roadside drug testing is to have a deterrent effect on drugged drivers and ultimately decrease the accident risk. One major risk is the possibility that drivers will realize that they often test negative after having used cannabis.

Conclusion

Oral fluid appears to sufficiently meet the requirements to be added to workplace drug-testing laboratory-based programs. There are adequate methods available for screening and confirmation in the laboratory and the relevant drugs and metabolites have been identified. External proficiency testing is being developed and cutoff concentrations have been proposed by scientific organizations. Appropriate certification of laboratories worldwide and introduction of legal provisions in several countries is the next step. In different environments such as drug treatment facilities, oral fluid has become an interesting alternative matrix for drug testing. Advantages of oral fluid testing include noninvasive sample collection, and the ability to collect the sample under observation reducing the opportunity for adulteration. The potential to estimate circulating drug concentrations and therefore closely associated to 'being under the influence', make it the matrix of choice for police officers and law enforcement agencies for screening of intoxicated drivers. However, the search for an on-site screening method that can provide acceptable accuracies for the detection of cannabinoids in oral fluid remains a major hurdle. Additional considerations that have received attention are the variability in the volume of sample collected and the drug recovery from the many different specimen collection systems on the market.

References

[1]   Mandel, I.D. (1993). A contemporary view of salivary research, *Critical Reviews in Oral Biology and Medicine* **4**, 599.

[2]   Veerman, E.C.I., van den Keijbus, P.A.M., Vissink, A. & van Nieuw Amerongen, A. (1996). Human glandular salivas: their separate collection and analysis, *European Journal of Oral Sciences* **104**, 346.

[3]   Young, J.A. & Van Lennep, E.W. (1978). *The Morphology of Salivary Glands*. Academic Press, London.

[4]   Samyn, N., Verstraete, A., van Haeren, C. & Kintz, P. (1999). Analysis of drugs of abuse in saliva, *Forensic Science Review* **11**, 1.

[5]   Aps, J.K. & Martens, L.C. (2005). Review: the physiology of saliva and transfer of drugs into saliva, *Forensic Science International* **150**, 119.

[6]   Mucklow, J.C., Bending, M.R., Kahn, G.C. & Dollery, C.T. (1978). Drug concentration in saliva, *Clinical Pharmacology and Therapeutics* **24**, 563.

[7]   Idowu, O.R. & Caddy, B. (1982). A review of the use of saliva in the forensic detection of drugs and other chemicals, *Journal of the Forensic Science Society* **22**, 123.

[8]   Navarro, M., Pichini, S., Farre, M., Ortuno, J., Roset, P.N., Segura, J. & de la, T.R. (2001). Usefulness of saliva for measurement of 3,4-methylenedioxymethamphetamine and its metabolites: correlation with plasma drug concentrations and effect of salivary pH, *Clinical Chemistry* **47**, 1788.

[9]   Samyn, N., De Boeck, G., Wood, M., Lamers, C.T., de Waard, D., Brookhuis, K.A., Verstraete, A.G. & Riedel, W.J. (2002). Plasma, oral fluid and sweat wipe ecstasy concentrations in controlled and real life conditions, *Forensic Science International* **128**, 90.

[10]   Schepers, R.J., Oyler, J.M., Joseph Jr, R.E., Cone, E.J., Moolchan, E.T. & Huestis, M.A. (2003). Methamphetamine and amphetamine pharmacokinetics in oral fluid and plasma after controlled oral methamphetamine administration to human volunteers, *Clinical Chemistry* **49**, 121.

[11]   Pichini, S. (2005). *Distribution of 3,4-methylenedioxymethamphetamine (MDMA) in Non Conventional Matrices and its Applications in Clinical Toxicology*. Doctoral Thesis, Universitat Autonoma de Barcelona, Spain.

[12]   Huestis, M.A. & Cone, E.J. (2004). Relationship of delta 9-tetrahydrocannabinol concentrations in oral fluid and plasma after controlled administration of smoked cannabis, *Journal of Analytical Toxicology* **28**, 394.

[13]   Choo, R.E. & Huestis, M.A. (2004). Oral fluid as a diagnostic tool, *Clinical Chemistry and Laboratory Medicine* **42**, 1273.

[14]   Kato, K., Hillsgrove, M., Weinhold, L., Gorelick, D.A., Darwin, W.D. & Cone, E.J. (1993). Cocaine and metabolite excretion in saliva under stimulated and nonstimulated conditions, *Journal of Analytical Toxicology* **17**, 338.

[15]   O'Neal, C.L., Crouch, D.J., Rollins, D.E. & Fatah, A.A. (2000). The effects of collection methods on oral fluid codeine concentrations, *Journal of Analytical Toxicology* **24**, 536.

[16]   Crouch, D.J. (2005). Oral fluid collection: the neglected variable in oral fluid testing, *Forensic Science International* **150**, 165.

[17]   Quintela, O., Crouch, D.J. & Andrenyak, D.M. (2006). Recovery of drugs of abuse from the Immunalysis Quantisal oral fluid collection device, *Journal of Analytical Toxicology* **30**, 614.

[18]   Campora, P., Bermejo, A.M., Tabernero, M.J. & Fernandez, P. (2003). Quantitation of cocaine and its major metabolites in human saliva using gas chromatography-positive chemical ionization-mass spectrometry (GC-PCI-MS), *Journal of Analytical Toxicology* **27**, 270.

[19]   Campora, P., Bermejo, A.M., Tabernero, M.J. & Fernandez, P. (2006). Use of gas chromatography/mass spectrometry with positive chemical ionization for the determination of opiates in human oral fluid, *Rapid Communications in Mass Spectrometry* **20**, 1288.

[20]   Quintela, O., Cruz, A., Concheiro, M., de Castro, A. & Lopez-Rivadulla, M. (2004). A sensitive, rapid and specific determination of midazolam in human plasma and saliva by liquid chromatography/electrospray mass spectrometry, *Rapid Communications in Mass Spectrometry* **18**, 2976.

[21]   Gunnar, T., Ariniemi, K. & Lillsunde, P. (2005). Validated toxicological determination of 30 drugs of

abuse as optimized derivatives in oral fluid by long column fast gas chromatography/electron impact mass spectrometry, *Journal of Mass Spectrometry* **40**, 739.

[22]   Kauert, G.F., Iwersen-Bergmann, S. & Toennes, S.W. (2006). Assay of delta9-tetrahydrocannabinol (THC) in oral fluid-evaluation of the OraSure oral specimen collection device, *Journal of Analytical Toxicology* **30**, 274.

[23]   Samyn, N., De Boeck, G. & Verstraete, A.G. (2002). The use of oral fluid and sweat wipes for the detection of drugs of abuse in drivers, *Journal of Forensic Sciences* **47**, 1380.

[24]   Teixeira, H., Proenca, P., Verstraete, A., Corte-Real, F. & Vieira, D.N. (2005). Analysis of delta9-tetrahydrocannabinol in oral fluid samples using solid-phase extraction and high-performance liquid chromatography-electrospray ionization mass spectrometry, *Forensic Science International* **150**, 205.

[25]   Dickson, S., Park, A., Nolan, S., Kenworthy, S., Nicholson, C., Midgley, J., Pinfold, R. & Hampton, S. (2006). The recovery of illicit drugs from oral fluid sampling devices, *Forensic Science International* **165**, 78.

[26]   Concheiro, M., de Castro, A., Quintela, O., Lopez-Rivadulla, M. & Cruz, A. (2005). Determination of MDMA, MDA, MDEA and MBDB in oral fluid using high performance liquid chromatography with native fluorescence detection, *Forensic Science International* **150**, 221.

[27]   Moore, C., Vincent, M., Rana, S., Coulter, C., Agrawal, A. & Soares, J. (2006). Stability of delta(9)-tetrahydrocannabinol (THC) in oral fluid using the Quantisal™ collection device, *Forensic Science International* **164**, 126.

[28]   Niedbala, R.S., Kardos, K., Waga, J., Fritch, D., Yeager, L., Doddamane, S. & Schoener, E. (2001). Laboratory analysis of remotely collected oral fluid specimens for opiates by immunoassay, *Journal of Analytical Toxicology* **25**, 310.

[29]   Cone, E.J., Presley, L., Lehrer, M., Seiter, W., Smith, M., Kardos, K.W., Fritch, D., Salamone, S. & Niedbala, R.S. (2002). Oral fluid testing for drugs of abuse: positive prevalence rates by Intercept immuno-assay screening and GC-MS-MS confirmation and suggested cutoff concentrations, *Journal of Analytical Toxicology* **26**, 541.

[30]   Drummer, O.H. (2005). Review: pharmacokinetics of illicit drugs in oral fluid, *Forensic Science International* **150**, 133.

[31]   Laloup, M., De Boeck, G. & Samyn, N. Unconventional samples and alternative matrices, in *Handbook of Analytical Separations*, M.J. Bogusz, ed, Elsevier, Amsterdam, Vol. 2, (2008).

[32]   Clarke, J. & Wilson, J.F. (2005). Proficiency testing (external quality assessment) of drug detection in oral fluid, *Forensic Science International* **150**, 161.

[33]   Cooper, G., Wilson, L., Reid, C., Baldwin, D., Hand, C. & Spiehler, V. (2005). Comparison of GC-MS and EIA results for the analysis of methadone in oral fluid, *Journal of Forensic Sciences* **50**, 928.

[34]   Cooper, G., Wilson, L., Reid, C., Hand, C. & Spiehler, V. (2006). Validation of the Cozart((R)) amphetamine microplate EIA for the analysis of amphetamines in oral fluid, *Forensic Science International* **159**, 104.

[35]   Cooper, G., Wilson, L., Reid, C., Baldwin, D., Hand, C. & Spiehler, V. (2005). Validation of the Cozart microplate EIA for analysis of opiates in oral fluid, *Forensic Science International* **154**, 240.

[36]   Cooper, G., Wilson, L., Reid, C., Baldwin, D., Hand, C. & Spieher, V. (2004). Validation of the Cozart microplate EIA for cocaine and metabolites in oral fluid, *Journal of Analytical Toxicology* **28**, 498.

[37]   Kacinko, S.L., Barnes, A.J., Kim, I., Moolchan, E.T., Wilson, L., Cooper, G.A., Reid, C., Baldwin, D., Hand, C.W. & Huestis, M.A. (2004). Performance characteristics of the Cozart RapiScan Oral Fluid Drug Testing System for opiates in comparison to ELISA and GC/MS following controlled codeine administration, *Forensic Science International* **141**, 41.

[38]   Kolbrich, E.A., Kim, I., Barnes, A.J., Moolchan, E.T., Wilson, L., Cooper, G.A., Reid, C., Baldwin, D., Hand, C.W. & Huestis, M.A. (2003). Cozart RapiScan Oral Fluid Drug Testing System: an evaluation of sensitivity, specificity, and efficiency for cocaine detection compared with ELISA and GC-MS following controlled cocaine administration, *Journal of Analytical Toxicology* **27**, 407.

[39]   Laloup, M., Tilman, G., Maes, V., De Boeck, G., Wallemacq, P., Ramaekers, J. & Samyn, N. (2005). Validation of an ELISA-based screening assay for the detection of amphetamine, MDMA and MDA in blood and oral fluid, *Forensic Science International* **153**, 29.

[40]   Niedbala, R.S., Kardos, K., Fries, T., Cannon, A. & Davis, A. (2001). Immunoassay for detection of cocaine/metabolites in oral fluids, *Journal of Analytical Toxicology* **25**, 62.

[41]   Kim, I., Barnes, A.J., Schepers, R., Moolchan, E.T., Wilson, L., Cooper, G., Reid, C., Hand, C. & Huestis, M.A. (2003). Sensitivity and specificity of the Cozart microplate EIA cocaine oral fluid at proposed screening and confirmation cutoffs, *Clinical Chemistry* **49**, 1498.

[42]   Cognard, E., Bouchonnet, S. & Staub, C. (2006). Validation of a gas chromatography-ion trap tandem mass spectrometry for simultaneous analyse of cocaine and its metabolites in saliva, *Journal of Pharmaceutical and Biomedical Analysis* **41**, 925.

[43]   Oiestad, E.L., Johansen, U. & Christophersen, S. (2006). Drug screening of preserved oral fluid by liquid chromatography-tandem mass spectrometry, *Clinical Chemistry* **53**, 300–309.

[44]   Clauwaert, K., Decaestecker, T., Mortier, K., Lambert, W., Deforce, D., Van Peteghem, C. & Van Bocxlaer, J. (2004). The determination of cocaine, benzoylecgonine, and cocaethylene in small-volume oral

fluid samples by liquid chromatography-quadrupole-time-of-flight mass spectrometry, *Journal of Analytical Toxicology* 28, 655.

[45] Concheiro, M., de Castro, A., Quintela, O., Cruz, A. & Lopez-Rivadulla, M. (2004). Development and validation of a method for the quantitation of delta9tetrahydrocannabinol in oral fluid by liquid chromatography electrospray-mass-spectrometry, *Journal of Chromatography. B, Analytical Technologies in the Biomedical and Life Sciences* 810, 319.

[46] Dams, R., Murphy, C.M., Choo, R.E., Lambert, W.E., De Leenheer, A.P. & Huestis, M.A. (2003). LC-atmospheric pressure chemical ionization-MS/ MS analysis of multiple illicit drugs, methadone, and their metabolites in oral fluid following protein precipitation, *Analytical Chemistry* 75, 798.

[47] Kintz, P., Villain, M., Concheiro, M. & Cirimele, V. (2005). Screening and confirmatory method for benzodiazepines and hypnotics in oral fluid by LC-MS/MS, *Forensic Science International* 150, 213.

[48] Laloup, M., Ramirez Fernandez, M.M., Wood, M., De Boeck, G., Henquet, C., Maes, V. & Samyn, N. (2005). Quantitative analysis of delta9-tetrahydrocannabinol in preserved oral fluid by liquid chromatography-tandem mass spectrometry, *Journal of Chromatography A* 1082, 15.

[49] Mortier, K.A., Maudens, K.E., Lambert, W.E., Clauwaert, K.M., Van Bocxlaer, J.F., Deforce, D.L., Van Peteghem, C.H. & De Leenheer, A.P. (2002). Simultaneous, quantitative determination of opiates, amphetamines, cocaine and benzoylecgonine in oral fluid by liquid chromatography quadrupole-time-of-flight mass spectrometry, *Journal of Chromatography. B, Analytical Technologies in the Biomedical and Life Sciences* 779, 321.

[50] Wood, M., De Boeck, G., Samyn, N., Morris, M., Cooper, D.P., Maes, R.A. & de Bruijn, E.A. (2003). Development of a rapid and sensitive method for the quantitation of amphetamines in human plasma and oral fluid by LC-MS-MS, *Journal of Analytical Toxicology* 27, 78.

[51] Mortier, K.A., Clauwaert, K.M., Lambert, W.E., Van Bocxlaer, J.F., Van den Eeckhout, E.G., Van Peteghem, C.H. & De Leenheer, A.P. (2001). Pitfalls associated with liquid chromatography/electrospray tandem mass spectrometry in quantitative bioanalysis of drugs of abuse in saliva, *Rapid Communications in Mass Spectrometry* 15, 1773.

[52] Kidwell, D.A., Holland, J.C. & Athanaselis, S. (1998). Testing for drugs of abuse in saliva and sweat, *Journal of Chromatography. B, Biomedical Sciences and Applications* 713, 111.

[53] Dams, R., Huestis, M.A., Lambert, W.E. & Murphy, C.M. (2003). Matrix effect in bio-analysis of illicit drugs with LC-MS/MS: influence of ionization type, sample preparation, and biofluid, *Journal of the American Society for Mass Spectrometry* 14, 1290.

[54] Wood, M., Laloup, M., Ramirez Fernandez, M.M., Jenkins, K.M., Young, M.S., Ramaekers, J.G., De Boeck, G. & Samyn, N. (2005). Quantitative analysis of multiple illicit drugs in preserved oral fluid by solid-phase extraction and liquid chromatography-tandem mass spectrometry, *Forensic Science International* 150, 227.

[55] Department of Health and Human Services Substance Abuse and Mental Health Services Administration (2004). *Proposed Revisions to Mandatory Guidelines for Federal Workplace Drug Testing Programs*, Vol. 69, FR 19673.

[56] Standards Australia *Australian Standard® – Procedures for Specimen Collection and the Detection and Quantitation of Drugs in Oral Fluid*, AS4760-2006, available from www.standards.org.au.

[57] Niedbala, R.S., Kardos, K.W., Fritch, D.F., Kardos, S., Fries, T., Waga, J., Robb, J. & Cone, E.J. (2001). Detection of marijuana use by oral fluid and urine analysis following single-dose administration of smoked and oral marijuana, *Journal of Analytical Toxicology* 25, 289.

[58] Niedbala, R.S., Kardos, K.W., Fritch, D.F., Kunsman, K.P., Blum, K.A., Newland, G.A., Waga, J., Kurtz, L., Bronsgeest, M. & Cone, E.J. (2005). Passive cannabis smoke exposure and oral fluid testing. II. Two studies of extreme cannabis smoke exposure in a motor vehicle, *Journal of Analytical Toxicology* 29, 607.

[59] Niedbala, S., Kardos, K., Salamone, S., Fritch, D., Bronsgeest, M. & Cone, E.J. (2004). Passive cannabis smoke exposure and oral fluid testing, *Journal of Analytical Toxicology* 28, 546.

[60] Ramaekers, J.G., Moeller, M.R., van Ruitenbeek, P., Theunissen, E.L., Schneider, E. & Kauert, G. (2006). Cognition and motor control as a function of delta9-THC concentration in serum and oral fluid: limits of impairment, *Drug and Alcohol Dependence* 85, 114.

[61] Day, D., Kuntz, D.J., Feldman, M. & Presley, L. (2006). Detection of THCA in oral fluid by GC-MS-MS, *Journal of Analytical Toxicology* 30, 645.

[62] Moore, C., Coulter, C., Rana, S., Vincent, M. & Soares, J. (2006). Analytical procedure for the determination of the marijuana metabolite 11-nor-delta9-tetrahydrocannabinol-9-carboxylic acid in oral fluid specimens, *Journal of Analytical Toxicology* 30, 409.

[63] Moore, C., Ross, W., Coulter, C., Adams, L., Rana, S., Vincent, M. & Soares, J. (2006). Detection of the marijuana metabolite 11-nor-delta9-tetrahydrocannabinol-9-carboxylic acid in oral fluid specimens and its contribution to positive results in screening assays, *Journal of Analytical Toxicology* 30, 413.

[64] Banken, J.A. (2004). Drug abuse trends among youth in the United States, *Annals of the New York Academy of Sciences* 1025, 465.

[65] Degenhardt, L., Copeland, J. & Dillon, P. (2005). Recent trends in the use of "club drugs": an Australian review, *Substance Use and Misuse* 40, 1241.

[66] de la Torre, R., Farre, M., Navarro, M., Pacifici, R., Zuccaro, P. & Pichini, S. (2004). Clinical pharmacokinetics of amfetamine and related substances: monitoring in conventional and non-conventional matrices, *Clinical Pharmacokinetics* **43**, 157.

[67] Baselt, R.C. (ed) (2000). *Disposition of Toxic Drugs and Chemicals in Man*, Chemical Toxicology Institute, Foster City.

[68] Benowitz, N.L. (1993). Clinical pharmacology and toxicology of cocaine, *Pharmacology and Toxicology* **72**, 3.

[69] Isenschmid, D.S. (2002). Cocaine – effects on human behavior and performance, *Forensic Science Review* **14**, 133.

[70] Brzezinski, M.R., Abraham, T.L., Stone, C.L., Dean, R.A. & Bosron, W.F. (1994). Purification and characterization of a human liver cocaine carboxylesterase that catalyzes the production of benzoylecgonine and the formation of cocaethylene from alcohol and cocaine, *Biochemical Pharmacology* **48**, 1747.

[71] Inaba, T., Stewart, D.J. & Kalow, W. (1978). Metabolism of cocaine in man, *Clinical Pharmacology and Therapeutics* **23**, 547.

[72] Blaho, K., Logan, B., Winbery, S., Park, L. & Schwilke, E. (2000). Blood cocaine and metabolite concentrations, clinical findings, and outcome of patients presenting to an ED, *The American Journal of Emergency Medicine* **18**, 593.

[73] Cone, E.J., Oyler, J. & Darwin, W.D. (1997). Cocaine disposition in saliva following intravenous, intranasal, and smoked administration, *Journal of Analytical Toxicology* **21**, 465.

[74] Jufer, R.A., Wstadik, A., Walsh, S.L., Levine, B.S. & Cone, E.J. (2000). Elimination of cocaine and metabolites in plasma, saliva, and urine following repeated oral administration to human volunteers, *Journal of Analytical Toxicology* **24**, 467.

[75] Moolchan, E.T., Cone, E.J., Wstadik, A., Huestis, M.A. & Preston, K.L. (2000). Cocaine and metabolite elimination patterns in chronic cocaine users during cessation: plasma and saliva analysis, *Journal of Analytical Toxicology* **24**, 458.

[76] Jenkins, A.J., Oyler, J.M. & Cone, E.J. (1995). Comparison of heroin and cocaine concentrations in saliva with concentrations in blood and plasma, *Journal of Analytical Toxicology* **19**, 359.

[77] O'Neal, C.L., Crouch, D.J., Rollins, D.E., Fatah, A. & Cheever, M.L. (1999). Correlation of saliva codeine concentrations with plasma concentrations after oral codeine administration, *Journal of Analytical Toxicology* **23**, 452.

[78] Wang, W.L., Darwin, W.D. & Cone, E.J. (1994). Simultaneous assay of cocaine, heroin and metabolites in hair, plasma, saliva and urine by gas chromatography-mass spectrometry, *Journal of Chromatography. B, Biomedical Applications* **660**, 279.

[79] Cone, E.J. (1990). Testing human hair for drugs of abuse. I. Individual dose and time profiles of morphine and codeine in plasma, saliva, urine, and beard compared to drug-induced effects on pupils and behavior, *Journal of Analytical Toxicology* **14**, 1.

[80] Barnes, A.J., Kim, I., Schepers, R., Moolchan, E.T., Wilson, L., Cooper, G., Reid, C., Hand, C. & Huestis, M.A. (2003). Sensitivity, specificity, and efficiency in detecting opiates in oral fluid with the Cozart Opiate Microplate EIA and GC-MS following controlled codeine administration, *Journal of Analytical Toxicology* **27**, 402.

[81] Kim, I., Barnes, A.J., Oyler, J.M., Schepers, R., Joseph Jr, R.E., Cone, E.J., Lafko, D., Moolchan, E.T. & Huestis, M.A. (2002). Plasma and oral fluid pharmacokinetics and pharmacodynamics after oral codeine administration, *Clinical Chemistry* **48**, 1486.

[82] Skopp, G., Potsch, L., Klinder, K., Richter, B., Aderjan, R. & Mattern, R. (2001). Saliva testing after single and chronic administration of dihydrocodeine, *International Journal of Legal Medicine* **114**, 133.

[83] Rohrig, T.P. & Moore, C. (2003). The determination of morphine in urine and oral fluid following ingestion of poppy seeds, *Journal of Analytical Toxicology* **27**, 449.

[84] Drummer, O.H. (ed) (2001). Benzodiazepines, in *The Forensic Pharmacology of Drugs of Abuse*, Arnold, London, pp. 103–175.

[85] Greenblatt, D.J. (1992). Pharmacology of benzodiazepine hypnotics, *The Journal of Clinical Psychiatry* **53**, 7.

[86] Shader, R.I. & Greenblatt, D.J. (1993). Use of benzodiaepines in anxiety disorders, *The New England Journal of Medicine* **328**, 1398.

[87] Barnas, C., Rossmann, M., Roessler, H., Riemer, Y. & Fleischhacker, W.W. (1992). Benzodiazepines and other psychotropic drugs abused by patients in a methadone maintenance program: familiarity and preference, *Journal of Clinical Psychopharmacology* **12**, 397.

[88] San, L., Tato, J., Torrens, M., Castillo, C., Farre, M. & Cami, J. (1993). Flunitrazepam consumption among heroin addicts admitted for in-patient detoxification, *Drug and Alcohol Dependence* **32**, 281.

[89] Samyn, N., De Boeck, G., Cirimele, V., Verstraete, A. & Kintz, P. (2002). Detection of flunitrazepam and 7-aminoflunitrazepam in oral fluid after controlled administration of rohypnol, *Journal of Analytical Toxicology* **26**, 211.

[90] Kintz, P., Villain, M., Cirimele, V., Pepin, G. & Ludes, B. (2004). Windows of detection of lorazepam in urine, oral fluid and hair, with a special focus on drug-facilitated crimes, *Forensic Science International* **145**, 131.

[91] Concheiro, M., Villain, M., Bouchet, S., Ludes, B., Lopez-Rivadulla, M. & Kintz, P. (2005). Windows of detection of tetrazepam in urine, oral fluid, beard, and hair, with a special focus on drug-facilitated crimes, *Therapeutic Drug Monitoring* **27**, 565.

[92]   Kintz, P., Villain, M. & Ludes, B. (2004). Testing for zolpidem in oral fluid by liquid chromatography-tandem mass spectrometry, *Journal of Chromatography. B, Analytical Technologies in the Biomedical and Life Sciences* **811**, 59.

[93]   Kintz, P. & Samyn, N. (2002). Use of alternative specimens: drugs of abuse in saliva and doping agents in hair, *Therapeutic Drug Monitoring* **24**, 239.

[94]   Caplan, Y.H. & Goldberger, B.A. (2001). Alternative specimens for workplace drug testing, *Journal of Analytical Toxicology* **25**, 396.

[95]   Toennes, S.W., Kauert, G.F., Steinmeyer, S. & Moeller, M.R. (2005). Driving under the influence of drugs – evaluation of analytical data of drugs in oral fluid, serum and urine, and correlation with impairment symptoms, *Forensic Science International* **152**, 149.

[96]   Verstraete, A.G. (2005). Oral fluid testing for driving under the influence of drugs: history, recent progress and remaining challenges, *Forensic Science International* **150**, 143.

[97]   Wylie, F.M., Torrance, H., Seymour, A., Buttress, S. & Oliver, J.S. (2005). Drugs in oral fluid Part II. Investigation of drugs in drivers, *Forensic Science International* **150**, 199.

[98]   Bennett, G.A., Davies, E. & Thomas, P. (2003). Is oral fluid analysis as accurate as urinalysis in detecting drug use in a treatment setting? *Drug and Alcohol Dependence* **72**, 265.

[99]   Lintz, W., Beier, H. & Gerloff, J. (1999). Bioavailability of tramadol after i.m. injection in comparison to i.v. infusion, *International Journal of Clinical Pharmacology and Therapeutics* **37**, 175.

[100]   Moolchan, E.T., Umbricht, A. & Epstein, D. (2001). Therapeutic drug monitoring in methadone maintenance: choosing a matrix, *Journal of Addictive Diseases: The Official Journal of the ASAM, American Society of Addiction Medicine* **20**, 55.

[101]   Neale, J. & Robertson, M. (2003). Comparisons of self-report data and oral fluid testing in detecting drug use amongst new treatment clients, *Drug and Alcohol Dependence* **71**, 57.

[102]   Kadehjian, L. (2005). Legal issues in oral fluid testing, *Forensic Science International* **150**, 151.

[103]   Presley, L., Lehrer, M., Seiter, W., Hahn, D., Rowland, B., Smith, M., Kardos, K.W., Fritch, D., Salamone, S., Niedbala, R.S. & Cone, E.J. (2003). High prevalence of 6-acetylmorphine in morphine-positive oral fluid specimens, *Forensic Science International* **133**, 22.

[104]   Cooper, G., Wilson, L., Reid, C., Main, L. & Hand, C. (2005). Evaluation of the Cozart RapiScan drug test system for opiates and cocaine in oral fluid, *Forensic Science International* **150**, 239.

[105]   Speckl, I.M., Hallbach, J., Guder, W.G., Meyer, L.V. & Zilker, T. (1999). Opiate detection in saliva and urine – a prospective comparison by gas chromatography-mass spectrometry, *Journal of Toxicology. Clinical Toxicology* **37**, 441.

[106]   Dams, R., Choo, R.E., Lambert, W.E., Jones, H. & Huestis, M.A. (2007). Oral fluid as an alternative matrix to monitor opiate and cocaine use in substance-abuse treatment patients, *Drug and Alcohol Dependence*, **87**, 258–267.

[107]   Phillips, S.G. & Allen, K.R. (2006). Acetylcodeine as a marker of illicit heroin abuse in oral fluid samples, *Journal of Analytical Toxicology* **30**, 370.

[108]   Ortelli, D., Rudaz, S., Chevalley, A.F., Mino, A., Deglon, J.J., Balant, L. & Veuthey, J.L. (2000). Enantioselective analysis of methadone in saliva by liquid chromatography-mass spectrometry, *Journal of Chromatography A* **871**, 163.

[109]   Rosas, M.E., Preston, K.L., Epstein, D.H., Moolchan, E.T. & Wainer, I.W. (2003). Quantitative determination of the enantiomers of methadone and its metabolite (EDDP) in human saliva by enantioselective liquid chromatography with mass spectrometric detection, *Journal of Chromatography. B, Analytical Technologies in the Biomedical and Life Sciences* **796**, 355.

[110]   Bermejo, A.M., Lucas, A.C. & Tabernero, M.J. (2000). Saliva/plasma ratio of methadone and EDDP, *Journal of Analytical Toxicology* **24**, 70.

[111]   Verstraete, A.G. & Raes, E.E. (eds) (2006). *Rosita-2 Project. Final Report*, Academia Press, Gent.

[112]   Verstraete, A.G. (ed) (2001). *Rosita: Roadside Testing Assessment*, Rosita Consortium, Gent.

[113]   Walsh, J.M., de Gier, J.J., Christopherson, A.S. & Verstraete, A.G. (2004). Drugs and driving, *Traffic Injury Prevention* **5**, 241.

[114]   Verstraete, A.G. (2004). Detection times of drugs of abuse in blood, urine, and oral fluid, *Therapeutic Drug Monitoring* **26**, 200.

[115]   Laloup, M., Ramirez Fernandez, M.M., Wood, M., De Boeck, G., Maes, V. & Samyn, N. (2006). Correlation of delta9-tetrahydrocannabinol concentrations determined by LC-MS-MS in oral fluid and plasma from impaired drivers and evaluation of the on-site Dräger DrugTest®, *Forensic Science International* **161**, 175.

[116]   Toennes, S.W., Steinmeyer, S., Maurer, H.J., Moeller, M.R. & Kauert, G.F. (2005). Screening for drugs of abuse in oral fluid–correlation of analysis results with serum in forensic cases, *Journal of Analytical Toxicology* **29**, 22.

[117]   Verstraete, A.G. & Puddu, M. (2001). Evaluation of different roadside drug tests, in *Rosita: Roadside Testing Assessment*, A.G. Verstraete, ed, Rosita Consortium, Gent, pp. 167–232.

[118]   Bernhoft, I.M., Steentoft, A., Johansen, S.S., Klitgaard, N.A., Larsen, L.B. & Hansen, L.B. (2005). Drugs in injured drivers in Denmark, *Forensic Science International* **150**, 181.

[119]   Jenkins, A.J. & Goldberger, B.A. (eds) (2002). *On-site Drug Testing*, Humana Press, Totawa.

[120]   Jehanli, A., Brannan, S., Moore, L. & Spiehler, V.R. (2001). Blind trials of an onsite saliva drug test for

marijuana and opiates, *Journal of Forensic Sciences* **46**, 1214.

[121] Moore, L., Wicks, J., Spiehler, V. & Holgate, R. (2001). Gas chromatography-mass spectrometry confirmation of Cozart RapiScan saliva methadone and opiates tests, *Journal of Analytical Toxicology* **25**, 520.

[122] De Giovanni, N., Fucci, N., Chiarotti, M. & Scarlata, S. (2002). Cozart Rapiscan system: our experience with saliva tests, *Journal of Chromatography. B, Analytical Technologies in the Biomedical and Life Sciences* **773**, 1.

[123] Kintz, P., Bernhard, W., Villain, M., Gasser, M., Aebi, B. & Cirimele, V. (2005). Detection of cannabis use in drivers with the drugwipe device and by GC-MS after Intercept device collection, *Journal of Analytical Toxicology* **29**, 724.

[124] Samyn, N. & van Haeren, C. (2000). On-site testing of saliva and sweat with Drugwipe and determination of concentrations of drugs of abuse in saliva, plasma and urine of suspected users, *International Journal of Legal Medicine* **113**, 150.

[125] Biermann, T., Schwarze, B., Zedler, B. & Betz, P. (2004). On-site testing of illicit drugs: the use of the drug-testing device "Toxiquick", *Forensic Science International* **143**, 21.

[126] Wong, R.C., Tran, M. & Tung, J.K. (2005). Oral fluid drug tests: effects of adulterants and foodstuffs, *Forensic Science International* **150**, 175.

[127] Cirimele, V., Villain, M., Mura, P., Bernard, M. & Kintz, P. (2006). Oral fluid testing for cannabis: on-site OraLine IV s.a.t. device versus GC/MS, *Forensic Science International* **161**, 180.

[128] Crouch, D.J., Walsh, J.M., Flegel, R., Cangianelli, L., Baudys, J. & Atkins, R. (2005). An evaluation of selected oral fluid point-of-collection drug-testing devices, *Journal of Analytical Toxicology* **29**, 244.

[129] Walsh, J.M., Flegel, R., Crouch, D.J., Cangianelli, L. & Baudys, J. (2003). An evaluation of rapid point-of-collection oral fluid drug-testing devices, *Journal of Analytical Toxicology* **27**, 429.

[130] Parliament of Victoria (2003). Road Safety (drug driving) act 2003, 111/2003.

[131] Drummer, O.H., Gerostamoulos, D. & Chu, M. (2006). Drugs in oral fluid in randomly selected drivers. *Presented at the 44th TIAFT meeting*, August 26th-September 1st 2006, Ljubljana.

Related Articles

Amphetamine

Benzodiazepines

Confirmation Testing: Toxicology

Cannabis

Cocaine

Drug-Impaired Driving

Opioids

Toxicology: Initial Testing

LALOUP MARLEEN, SAMYN NELE AND DE BOECK GERT

Outpatient Commitment *see* Civil Commitment

Outreach: Mental Health *see* Disaster Mental Health

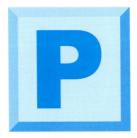

Packaging and Transport

General Issues

Anticontamination and Continuity Measures

Where an investigation involves more than one scene (a location, vehicle, or subject), no person should recover or package items from more than one of them. All subjects, victims and suspects, should be kept apart and transported in different vehicles using different officers.

Whenever possible, packaging material should be taken to the location where evidence is found and packaged *in situ*. Vital evidence may be lost if evidence is transported to a different location for packaging. Every item of evidence must be packaged separately in a sealed container, bag or box. The package must be sealed with tape to prevent tampering with the evidence. While normal adhesive tape is permissible in some countries, some jurisdictions disapprove of the practice and require tamperproof evidence tape be used to seal evidence.

Staples, pins, and paperclips must *never* be used to seal forensic packaging or attach evidence vouchers to the packaging. They will puncture the packaging and it could be alleged that cross contamination of hair, fibers, microscopic pieces of glass and paint could have occurred through any holes caused.

While contamination and cross contamination have always been issues for any evidence types in forensic science, the increasing sensitivity of DNA profiling have made anticontamination measures even more important.

Storage and Transport

All storage of exhibits must be in secure facilities. The basic requirements for exhibit storage are a secure store or locker, depending on the size of agency. If secured by key, there should only be one available to personnel and agencies should have protocols governing entry and documentation of such entry. If entry is by keypad or swipe card, this must be linked to a computer that records entry and exit.

A suitable freezer and refrigerator are also required for biological and other exhibits and access should be *via* a secure exhibit storage facility.

Some larger crime labs and agencies have adopted the use of radiofrequency identification (RFID) tags to track the location of exhibits.

Items from one subject (suspect or victim) or scene must *never* be stored or transported in the same box or large paper sack containing items from any other subject or the scene they are suspected of involvement in. This will prevent any accidental cross contamination.

Packaging of Exhibits

Clothing, Footwear, Bedding, and Similar Items

Dry items, such as clothing, bedding and footwear, should be placed in separate paper bags. These bags are also referred to as *Kraft* bags in some areas. The top of the bag should be folded over about 1 in. (2.5 cm) and then folded over the same distance again. The bag should then be completely sealed, using 2-in. (5 cm) wide adhesive tape or, if not acceptable in the jurisdiction, an approved tape. Where protocols dictate, it may be necessary to sign across the seal, half on the tape and half on the bag. Where bags have no chain of custody details printed on them, the relevant evidence voucher (*see* **Crime Scene Documentation**) should then be attached using an approved tape. Where the item is too large to fit in standard paper bags, it should be carefully wrapped in one or more sheets of brown paper, fully sealed to prevent contamination of the item. As an extra preventative measure, a second layer of wrapping may be employed.

In the United Kingdom, advice from forensic laboratories is that dry items must *never* be placed in polyethylene bags as it is possible that a buildup of moisture could degrade any biological or trace evidence. However, advice in other countries may vary and it may be permissible to ensure items are completely dry before placing them in polyethylene bags.

Wet or Damp Items

With the exception of footwear, damp or wet items recovered from scenes or subjects should be placed in individual polyethylene bags. Items of footwear must *never* be placed in polyethylene bags as they will become moldy.

Wherever possible, polyethylene bags with self tamperproof seals should be used as a normal adhesive tape will lose adhesion and compromise the integrity of the exhibit.

Never seal or store damp or wet items in polyethylene bags without freezing at the earliest opportunity. Frozen items must not be allowed to thaw during transportation to the laboratory. When folding, personnel should avoid folding the item in such a manner that could affect bloodstain patterns.

Where facilities, such as forensic drying rooms and cabinets are available, the items should be air dried prior to being repackaged as per the guidelines for dry items. The air-drying process should not include heating to accelerate the drying time. The items should be hung separately and a large sheet of paper placed below to collect any debris that may fall off during the drying process.

The polyethylene bag should then be packaged and labeled as an exhibit.

Where no forensic drying cabinets are available, extreme care should be taken when choosing a drying location. Careful consideration should be given to the possibility of infection from the person shedding the blood, not only to prevent any accidental contamination or interference with the evidence but also where the item is bloodstained.

When dry, the items should be carefully moved using appropriate anticontamination and protective measures. The item should be carefully folded as necessary and placed in a paper bag and sealed and labeled accordingly. If the item is bloodstained, in addition to protective clothing and gloves, personnel dealing with the clothing should wear a protective mask and goggles to prevent any possible infection from airborne dried blood particles.

The sheet of paper placed below the item should be packaged separately and treated as a new exhibit. The clothing, polyethylene bag, and paper sheet should all be sent to the laboratory for examination. In this way, all debris that may have detached from the exhibit can be examined if necessary.

Weapons, Tools, and Miscellaneous Items

There are many flat-pack forensic boxes of many different sizes available. They vary from small boxes through some similar to pizza boxes to others capable of containing a rifle or possibly a baseball bat.

Weapons and tools should be placed a suitable flat-pack cardboard box. Ensure that adhering debris is protected by paper folded around the tip and shaft. The implement should then be tied securely in place with string to prevent movement. This is achieved by piercing holes in the box close to the item and threading string through them. The knots should be on the inside of the box, to prevent accidental or deliberate interference and the holes created to thread the string through must be sealed with an approved tape. The box should be fully sealed around the edges, with an approved tape. Where protocols dictate, each piece of tape should be signed, half on the tape and half on the box to prevent any allegations of tampering. Some evidence boxes come with a card insert with a grid of prepunched holes, to allow items to be secured without the need to pierce the box.

The relevant evidence voucher (*see* **Crime Scene Documentation**) should then be attached using an approved tape.

The box should always be stored and transported flat, with the securing string to the bottom. The box should be labeled to indicate which way up the box should remain and also if it contains a sharp object and any health hazards such as bodily fluids.

Wherever possible, rigid knife tubes should be used to package knives and other sharp instruments. These are two plastic tubes, open at one end, which fit inside each other by means of a spiral groove and hold the item in position at either end. The tube is then sealed in the same way as a box and an evidence voucher attached.

Firearms should be made safe by an authorized officer, under the supervision of crime scene investigators (CSIs). Where protocols dictate, an appropriate certificate should be attached to the outside of the exhibit. A suitable box should be used, sealed, and labeled as above. Ammunition and magazines should be packaged separately.

A magazine should be packaged in a box as above. Dependent on local protocols, ammunition may need to be removed from the magazine or chamber of a revolver. It is good practice to mark a revolver to show the relative position of the chambers at the time of recovery.

Ammunition, either projectiles or shell casings, spent or otherwise, should be packaged in small plastic pots padded with tissue paper to prevent damage. The pots should be individually sealed and the appropriate evidence voucher attached.

A recent suggestion for the packaging of spent shell casings is to insert a dry swab into the open end and place the casing in a plastic urine pot. Those pots with a conical base mean that only the smallest part of the rim is in contact with anything. The swab is then broken at the lip of the pot allowing the casing to be held in position. This method prevents possible damage to the casing and any fingerprints on it.

Footwear Impressions

Where a footwear or tire impression has been cast, they too are placed in a cardboard box. The cast is placed soil side up in the box. The soil should not be removed as this provides a sample from exactly where the offender stood or the vehicle was driven. The cast is tied into the box, sealed, and labeled as above.

If a footwear impression in dust has been recovered using an electrostatic lifting apparatus (ESLA),

it is also packaged in a box. The foil is placed black side up in the box and taped into position in each corner. If the impression was recovered from a movable object, such as paper strewn across the floor, this too is taped into a box. The boxes should be sealed and labeled as above.

Glass Exemplars

Whenever glass has been broken at a crime scene, *exemplars*, also known as *control samples*, should be taken and packaged in a cardboard box. The box should be sealed and labeled as above.

Storage. Store all the above "right way up" in a dry exhibit store.

Transport. No special requirements other than keep "right way up".

Dry Miscellaneous Traces

Paint flakes, exemplars or unknown source, powders or other debris, should be placed in folded paper, druggists' wraps. The wrap should then be sealed in a polyethylene bag, and the appropriate evidence voucher completed and attached.

Damp or Wet Miscellaneous Traces

Items such as oils and greases should be submitted in the original container if available. If not, they should be recovered into a suitable container, sealed in a polyethylene bag and the appropriate evidence voucher completed and attached.

Storage. Store all the above "right way up" in a dry exhibit store.

Transport. No special requirements other than keep "right way up".

Fiber Tapings

Each recovered taping should be sealed in a polyethylene bag and the appropriate evidence voucher completed and attached.

Storage. They should be stored in a dry environment.

Transport.   No special requirements.

Accelerants or Volatile Substances

Liquid Samples – Packaging and Storage.   These must be packaged in a nylon bag, tied, and sealed at the top with a swan neck. This bag should then be placed in a polyethylene bag, again tied and sealed with a swan neck. An evidence voucher must be attached using string (*see* **Crime Scene Documentation**). Do *not* use an approved tape to attach an evidence voucher to the packaging. Containers with rubber or plastic seals and plastic vials should *not* be used. They should be stored in a dry environment, isolated from other items.

Transport.   When transporting, the sample bags should be placed in a rigid outer container, and suitably padded to prevent impact damage.

Clothing.   Clothing should be searched prior to submission. It should be loosely packaged in a nylon bag, tied, and sealed at the top with a swan neck. This is achieved by twisting the top of the bag tightly until a long "spout" is made. This is then tied around itself and then the knot is tied with string to secure it. No form of adhesive tape should be used to secure the knot. This bag should then be placed in a polyethylene bag, again tied, and sealed with a swan neck. An evidence voucher must be attached using string (*see* **Crime Scene Documentation**). Do *not* use any type of adhesive tape to attach an evidence voucher to the packaging. They should be stored in a dry environment, isolated from other items.

Transport.   When transporting, the sample bags should be placed in a rigid outer container, and suitably padded to prevent impact damage.

Fragile Items from Fire Scenes.   Fragile items should be packed in a sealed sturdy box or tin.

Transport.   The items should be carefully transported. They should be transported personally to the laboratory.

Accelerant Samples from Fire Scenes.   These must be packaged in a nylon bag, tied, and sealed at the top with a swan neck. This bag should then be placed in a polyethylene bag, again tied and sealed with a swan neck. An evidence voucher must be attached using string (*see* **Crime Scene Documentation**). Do *not* use an adhesive tape to attach an evidence voucher to the packaging. Leave a quantity of air above the sample, often known as a *headspace*. Unused glass jars with well-fitting caps can be substituted for nylon bags.

Where methylated spirits are suspected, a glass bottle with a well-fitting cap should be used. Double wrapping in nylon bags may be used as an alternative.

Samples should be submitted as soon as possible.

In some cases, items suspected of containing accelerants will have sharp or broken edges or protrusions. Any sharp items should be placed in a rigid box, sealed in a nylon bag. The packaging should be marked to clearly indicate that a sharp item is contained within.

Biological Samples

Swabs.   Swabs as an evidence type are the most complex as regards packaging. What is accepted practice in some jurisdictions is frowned upon in others. Reference must be made to local protocols.

In many US states, swabs are air dried. They may be placed into sample envelopes to dry prior to submission. Some jurisdictions use a small box with an insert designed to allow the swab to be held in position away from the box and air dried in that. The box is sealed and the details documented on an evidence voucher.

In some jurisdictions worldwide, swabs from subjects and also crime scenes are frozen as soon as possible and submitted frozen. In others, swabs from subjects are frozen but scene stains are air dried.

In England and Wales, where the majority of swabs are frozen, standard medical swabs are used for crime scenes, including victims and suspects. They are sealed in the tube provided, placed in a polyethylene bag and the appropriate evidence voucher attached.

Cigarette Ends.   They can be placed in individual polyethylene bags, envelopes or paper bags, sealed, and the evidence voucher attached. If dry they are stored in a dry environment. If wet they are frozen.

Storage.   Frozen samples should remain frozen. Air-dried samples should be stored in a dry environment.

Transport. Frozen samples should remain frozen in transit. Air-dried samples should remain in a dry environment.

Condoms. Condoms should be knotted to prevent the loss of any liquid inside. They should be placed in a rigid plastic pot. The pot should be placed in a polyethylene bag, sealed, and the appropriate evidence voucher attached. The exhibit should be frozen as soon as possible and remain frozen in storage and transit.

ALLAN MATHIESON SCOTT

Paint

Introduction

Paint can be defined as a coating applied to a surface to provide decorative, protective, or other properties. In the context of forensic trace evidence, paint can be encountered in a range of situations, from traffic accidents and criminal damage, through burglaries and art fraud, to murder and terrorist activity.

"Essentially, a paint consists of a pigment dispersed in a resinous binder, reduced to an acceptable application viscosity with solvent. One or more additives may be incorporated to modify one or more of the paint's film properties, application, or storage characteristics [1]."

Paint is a common material in everyday life: buildings, vehicles, furniture, tools, and even fashion accessories can be painted. However, each of these uses is different; there are very many colors and shades of paint available; the composition of paints can vary widely; each additional layer of paint adds to a paint flake's individuality. Traces of paint can be transferred from one item to another, or to a person in contact with a painted item, and this can have major forensic significance.

Forensic Aspects

The forensic characterization of a paint usually involves microscopic examination allied to some chemical analysis of the organic and/or inorganic components.

Forensic paint analyses and comparisons are typically distinguished by a small sample size that precludes the application of many standard industrial paint analysis procedures or protocols. The forensic paint examiner must address concerns, such as the issues of a case or investigation, sample size, complexity and condition, environmental effects, and collection methods. These factors require that the forensic paint examiner choose test methods, sample preparation schemes, test sequence, and degree of sample alteration and consumption that are appropriate for each specific case.

Forensic science is concerned with generating information, which can be used to support or refute propositions made within the legal context, principally in courts of law. It is important at the outset, therefore, to identify the nature of the customer's proposition and any reasonable alternatives in some detail, to enable the correct approach to be followed to obtain all the relevant data.

Paint investigations are mostly requested in relation to incidents where cars have been involved (e.g., hit and run accidents, a raid on a bank where a car has been used to crash through a window, or a murder where a body has been carried in a car) or to incidents where paint has been transferred to or from a tool or another painted object (e.g., burglaries or assaults).

Normally, the request will be to determine if there is a link between a microtrace of paint found on one object/person and another painted object. In hit and run cases, the request may be to determine from paint microtraces which model of car, and from what year, has been involved in the incident.

Two stages can be distinguished in many investigations:

- In the *investigative stage,* the customer is interested in clues which help him to determine which avenues of investigation appear to be most fruitful. Speed of the response is normally more important in this phase than the strength of evidence.
- In the *evidential stage,* a suspect has been found and procedures have been started to determine if the suspect should be prosecuted in court. In this phase, strength of the evidence is normally more important than the speed of response.

During the paint investigation, the emphasis of the request may shift from speed of response to strength of evidence. Normally, from the request it can be deduced what the current phase of the investigation is and what the priorities of the customer are [2].

In the majority of cases involving paint, the requirement is for the laboratory to compare samples of paint to see if they could have a common origin. This will mean the application of a range of techniques from low-power microscopy to more specialized analytical methods.

Other cases require that the paint samples submitted to the laboratory are examined to assist an investigation where there is as yet no comparison sample. Such cases include traffic accidents where automotive paint databases are searched for paint matching traces recovered from an injured person's clothing to help identify the vehicle involved.

Paint Composition

In the past, it was easy to define paint. Paint in its simplest form was composed of four main types of ingredient described as follows:

1. Resin (also referred to as *polymer* or *binder*)
This is essentially the "glue" that binds the pigments and additives in place and dries to a solid "film". The polymeric binder (or resin) provides the continuous matrix for the paint film and gives the paint its adhesive quality, durability, flexibility, and chemical resistance. Sometimes a modifying resin is also used with the primary resin.

2. Pigment
Finely divided particles, which are dispersed throughout the liquid paint and give the dried paint film: color, opacity (hiding power), film reinforcement and functionality, gloss, and permeability.

3. Solvent
The solvent is the volatile portion, which is used to provide application-related properties including flow and dry time. Often this "solvent" is primarily water. Several "solvents" may be used in a coating. Upon drying of the paint film, the solvent is evaporated and eventually lost. Proper drying of the paint film is essential to achieve desired film properties.

4. Additives
Additional components, which lend added properties to the finished film and/or make application and manufacturing easier. They also contribute to gloss, viscosity, and other properties.

Today, with the advent of high technology, paint is still essentially as described above; however, certain types of coatings – such as most powder coatings – are 100% solid and do not contain solvent [3].

Paint Application

Different paints can be applied to surfaces by several means: for example, by brush and roller, by manual or robotic spraying, by dipping or as a powder coat [4].

Architectural or domestic paints are most often applied by *brush,* at least in the case of the paint types submitted for forensic examination. Manual application will typically lead to more variation in thickness and in homogeneity than more controlled industrial application procedures. This may mean that a greater number of control or known samples will need to be taken from the surface to ensure that the examiner has a representative sample for comparison.

Other decorative finishes featuring paint can also be found on items like furniture, or on products like fire extinguishers and domestic appliances, but these are encountered less frequently in case work.

Where paint is *sprayed*, either from an aerosol can or using a compressed air or pump paint sprayer, layer thickness and homogeneity may also vary. There may also be a contribution from paint that was previously sprayed using the same equipment (for example, traces of mica or aluminum particles from an "effect" paint carried into a solid paint). Stray paint droplets ("overspray") can drift during spraying onto nearby surfaces, which are not being painted, resulting in microscopic droplets of a different color on the surface, which individualize the paint further.

Robotic application, for example, in the motor industry, gives very reproducible results, with even layers of a consistent thickness. On a continuous production line, the color of the applied paint can change to meet the requirements of the product: the undercoat color of cars can change to suit the topcoat color, and during the change there may be a variation from the front to the back of a single vehicle.

Dipping a vehicle body into an electrostatic paint bath is a technique, which allows paint to penetrate into cavities that would otherwise be inaccessible, and is used for applying anticorrosion paint. Again, the results are consistent in terms of layer thickness and anticorrosion coatings may be very thin.

New technologies and environmental, health, and economic considerations have meant that water-borne paints, paint with less solvent, and powder coating (where no solvent is present) have become more common. The phasing-out of pigments like lead chromate was also a feature of paint development in the late twentieth century.

Transfer Mechanisms

Dry paint is normally transferred by direct contact. As paint is designed to bind strongly to a substrate, unless the paint is old and flaking, it will require some force to remove it. Scene of crime examiners will be familiar with the difficulty of removing samples from surfaces like automobiles. For this reason, paint may not transfer unless sufficient force is involved. In a minor traffic accident where there is a glancing blow at a shallow angle, only a smear of paint may be transferred, or none may be transferred at all. If a more severe impact occurs, one or more layers may be transferred, in one or both directions. There may also be smearing and mixing of the layers, indicating impact. The more layers transferred, the stronger the evidential value.

In a burglary, where a window is forced open with a tool such as a jemmy or pry bar, paint may be transferred from the window to the tool and from the tool to the window, while there may also be other evidence types like toolmark impressions, fingerprints, fibers, or DNA involved [5, 6].

Transferred smears of paint can indicate forceful contact, as in a collision between two cars, but the examiner should be cautious in arriving at a conclusion as to the color of the offending vehicle based only on smears of paint. Paint smeared thinly onto a light colored surface can appear a lighter color than the paint from which it came and the reverse may be true with paint smeared onto a dark surface. With effect paints or paints with a clear topcoat, if only the top layer (the *clearcoat*) is smeared, it may appear white, though it is usually colorless.

Wet paint can be transferred by direct contact with a painted surface, by splashing or spraying. A vandal painting or spraying graffiti could get paint splashes or droplets on their shoes, skin, or clothing; an intruder's clothing in contact with a newly painted surface could transfer paint to the clothing.

Loose paint particles can flake from a surface and be recovered at a scene. If this is a possibility, the examiner should consider whether there might be physical matches (also called *physical fits* or *fracture matches*) between pieces of recovered paint and a painted item. The author has encountered a case where a white-painted metal bar was used to break into motor cars. Flakes of paint were left inside one of the cars. Some of this recovered paint was found to fit precisely back onto the metal bar so as to show that it had come from this item.

On a larger scale, pieces of automobile body filler left at accident scenes can also provide scope for physical matches as well as for paint layer examination.

Persistence

In contrast with glass, there has been little published on the persistence of transferred paint. Published clothing surveys for paint describe work by Lau *et al.* [7] and Pearson *et al.* [8].

Other Paints

Other types of paint may be encountered from time to time. One such paint is anticlimb paint, which is designed to remain slippery and not to dry, to deter burglars or intruders from climbing on buildings. These paints may have additional components added as markers in the paint to help identify offenders when caught.

French scientists have studied the paint from weapons rockets to try to identify the types of rockets used in terrorist attacks [9].

Layer Structure

It is a combination of the layers and colors, which give paint flakes their individuality. It is easier to discriminate colored paints microscopically than black or white paints because they have a range of shades of color. The greater the number of layers, the more distinctive the paint will be. If a paint has many layers, the examiner may decide that no further examination is needed, other than microscopy, as the paint is already sufficiently characterized. This is more likely to be the case with an architectural paint, particularly from an old building, but it could also apply to a vehicle that has been repaired and repainted. Laboratory policy and an examiner's own judgment will determine whether chemical analysis, in addition to microscopic comparison, is required.

Where fewer layers are present, the examination should include some analysis of the paint. In most forensic laboratories, this means that Fourier transform infrared (FTIR) spectroscopy follows comparison microscopy. The availability of other instrumentation, the judgment of the examiner and laboratory policy will again provide guidance as to the tests conducted on a sample.

Paint Recovery

Paint flakes may have been recovered by a scene of crime examiner and submitted to the laboratory, or an item may have to be examined in the laboratory to recover paint from it. Paint traces can be very small ($<1\,\mathrm{mm}^2$) so that appropriate anticontamination measures must be adopted throughout the examination.

The combination of a searching microscope and a fine forceps will allow even very small paint flakes to be recovered. This method will also allow the precise location of recovered flakes to be recorded, unlike brushing or shaking where the paint could have come from any part of an item or garment.

Paint may be recovered from tools or clothing under a searching microscope (magnification of $10\times$ to $100\times$ or so) or loose flakes can be recovered from clothing by brushing the surface or shaking the garment over a large sheet of paper or a special collection receptacle (e.g., a stainless steel funnel. See Figure 1).

Although the collection of paint at scenes using adhesive tape can be convenient for scene of crime examiners, the submission of paint flakes on tape lifts is not recommended as it can be difficult to remove the paint from the adhesive and the presence of adhesive traces can cause difficulties in interpreting infrared spectra. The best method is to remove the paint down to the underlying surface with a clean scalpel blade and place the paint flakes in a suitable

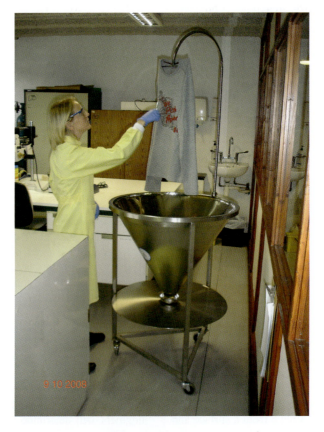

Figure 1 Brushing paint from clothing into a stainless steel funnel

container like a self-seal (e.g., Ziploc) plastic bag, which can be labeled.

Laboratory Examination.   A possible stage-wise scheme for comparison of paint samples is shown below. The aim is to discriminate the paints using the techniques available. If at any stage significant differences are noted the examination may be stopped and the paints reported as different.

> Sample description
> Examine physical characteristics: potential physical match?
> Evaluate sample for analytical approach: sufficient quantity? sequence of tests?
> Comparison microscopy
> FTIR analysis of selected layer(s)
> Additional analysis: e.g., elemental analysis (scanning electron microscopy with energy-dispersive X-ray spectrometry (SEM–EDX); X-ray fluorescence spectroscopy (XRF)), fluorescence microscopy, pyrolysis gas chromatography–mass spectrometry (PGC–MS), and microspectrophotometry (MSP).

Microscopic Examination

Following the recovery of any paint, the first examination step is normally comparison microscopy (See Figure 2).

The human eye is capable of distinguishing over 100 000 different colors [10] and microscopy is an extremely powerful tool for the paint examiner. The subsequent laboratory analysis will depend on the instruments available.

Samples of control (*known or "K"*) and transferred (*questioned or "Q"*) paint are mounted on microscope slides and placed on the stages of a comparison microscope. The top and bottom surfaces of a paint flake can be viewed at a magnification of $250\times$ using incident light. Cross sections of the paints can be prepared and mounted on the same slides as the surface samples.

If multiple layers are present they can be recorded in notes, diagrammatically or photographically. Layers of similar colors (e.g., shades of white) may be examined using UV light: any fluorescence may help discriminate the layers.

Cross sections of multilayer paint flakes can be prepared using a microtome, with or without embedding, or by the technique of "thin peels" where the edge of the flake is shaved with a scalpel blade to remove a sample containing all the layers.

"Effect" paints can contain aluminum flakes, mica (for a pearlescent appearance) or other particulate components. A feature of metallic paints is the form of the aluminum flakes, which should be noted; these can be rounded ("dollar") or with indented edges ("cornflake"). Effect paints may have one or both types of aluminum, with or without mica, or interference pigments (for example, mica coated with metallic oxides) to give color, which varies with coating thickness, illumination angle, or viewing angle.

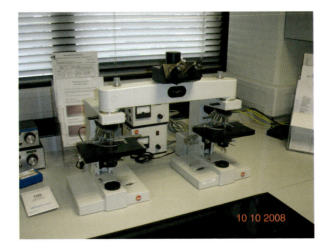

Figure 2   FT-IR microscope and bench

Other microscopic examinations (involving polarized light microscopy, cathodoluminescence, or high-power microscopy) can also be used to characterize paint components.

Analysis

Following microscopy, the normal procedure is for an analytical scheme, which allows both the organic and inorganic components of a paint to be examined,which can cope with small samples, and which,

as far as possible, uses nondestructive techniques [11].

Fourier Transform Infrared (FTIR) Spectroscopy. Most modern forensic laboratories use FTIR spectroscopy to analyze paint flakes, which are indistinguishable by comparison microscopy. This technique has the advantage of being fast, nondestructive, requiring little sample preparation and, when the microscope attachment is used, being able to cope with small sample sizes (See Figures 3 and 4).

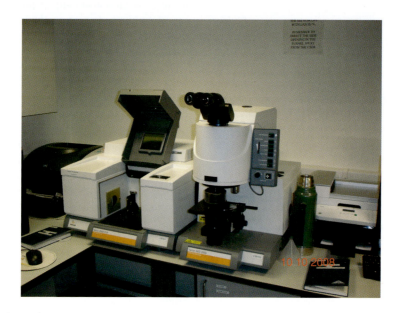

Figure 3   Comparison microscope

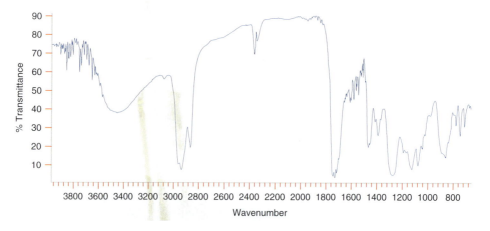

Figure 4   Infrared spectrum of paint

The mercury cadmium telluride (MCT) detector currently fitted to many FTIR microscopes has a wave number range from 4000 to 650 cm^{-1}, allowing the organic and some inorganic components to be detected. Wide-band MCT detectors are also available, providing a range of 4000–450 cm^{-1} but with lower sensitivity.

FTIR microscopes generally have an FTIR bench associated with the microscope, with a deuterated triglycine sulfate (DTGS) detector. If sufficient sample is available it may be possible to use this detector, giving a range of 4000–200 cm^{-1}, allowing the examiner to obtain more information about the inorganic components of the paint. This may be particularly useful when looking at vehicle undercoats.

Infrared (IR) spectroscopy deals with the infrared region of the electromagnetic spectrum. It covers a range of techniques, the most common being a form of absorption spectroscopy. It can be used to identify compounds or investigate sample composition. Infrared spectroscopy exploits the fact that molecules have specific frequencies at which they rotate or vibrate corresponding to discrete energy levels (vibrational modes).

The infrared spectrum of a sample is collected by passing a beam of infrared light through the sample. Examination of the transmitted light reveals how much energy was absorbed at each wavelength. This can be done with a monochromatic beam, which changes in wavelength over time, or by using a Fourier transform instrument to measure all wavelengths at once (FTIR). From this, a transmittance or absorbance spectrum can be produced, showing at which IR wavelengths the sample absorbs. Analysis of these absorption characteristics reveals details about the molecular structure of the sample. Current models of instrument are normally Fourier-transform infra red spectrometers which can collect a spectrum in seconds rather than minutes required for an older grating instrument. A further refinement, the addition of a microscope, means that very small samples can be analyzed with little sample preparation. Spectra can be presented in either transmittance or absorbance mode.

A detailed account of this technique is given by Beveridge *et al.* [12].

Elemental Analysis

Further information on a paint can be obtained by elemental analysis. Because of the small size and the condition of the samples typically encountered in forensic science laboratories, the examiner may be limited in what tests can be performed.

SEM–EDX is a technique used quite widely in forensic laboratories for elemental analysis. The technique is nondestructive and can cope with small samples. Some sample preparation is normally required (usually mounting and coating with carbon to make the surface conductive), but if a paint flake has been embedded and cross sectioned, only a very small additional amount is required for SEM.

If a low-vacuum or environmental SEM is available, no sample preparation may be needed [13, 14].

XRF and micro-XRF are techniques, which may also be applied to obtain elemental information. These require no sample coating but require larger samples than SEM.

SEM and XRF analysis can be done as a comparative test (semiquantitatively) or quantitatively by using either standards of known elemental composition or using the instrument's software to calculate percentage composition.

The scanning electron microscope is widely used as an analytical tool in forensic laboratories. The main advantage of this instrument is that multidimensional information may be gathered: chemical visualization by means of back-scattered electrons (BSE) and X-ray mapping, topographical information, detection of secondary electrons (SE), and qualitative and quantitative elemental composition collected by the energy-dispersive spectrometer (EDS). It is a nondestructive technique requiring some sample preparation but can be applied to samples of <1 mm^2.

XRF is the emission of characteristic "secondary" (or fluorescent) X-rays from a material that has been excited by bombarding with high-energy X-rays or γ rays. The phenomenon is widely used for elemental analysis. Instruments can either use energy-dispersive X-ray (EDS or EDX) or wavelength dispersive X-ray (WDX) detectors. Little sample preparation is required and both qualitative and quantitative analysis can be performed.

Pyrolysis Gas Chromatography. PGC, usually coupled with PGC–MS, can be used to analyze organic material such as paint, plastic, or rubber. Although it is a destructive technique, it can be used on quite small samples. If suitable databases are available, it can also be used as an investigative tool to identify unknown samples such as flakes of car paint or plastic at an accident scene.

Some work has also been done on characterizing automotive clearcoats and coatings on plastic headlight lenses using PGC–MS.

Without the mass spectrometer, however, PGC alone may add little additional information because of the difficulty in identifying peaks in a chromatogram with certainty [15].

PGC–MS or PyGC–MS is a method of chemical analysis in which the sample is heated to decomposition (pyrolysis) to produce smaller molecules that are separated by GC and detected using MS. Although it is a destructive technique, it is useful in identifying and comparing polymeric materials like plastics, rubber, or individual layers of paint.

Microspectrophotometry. Microspectrophotometry using visible light and ultraviolet light (UV-MSP) can also be used as a comparative technique to provide objective information about whether two paints can be distinguished on the basis of their color. The MSP can produce a graphical printout of the color spectrum or can process the results into tristimulus values or color coordinates.

In certain situations, two paints may be visually indistinguishable even though the color has been achieved in different ways (e.g., by using different pigments). This phenomenon (metamerism) may be identified by MSP.

Though MSP is often used for fibers, it can also be used with paint using transmitted or incident light. Transmitted light is preferred as it eliminates any problems associated with sample preparation, surface features and illumination angle, although the thickness of the cross sections from paints being compared must be the same.

For color measurement and comparison, paint sections of approximately 3-μm thickness are prepared, while for the examination of UV-absorbers in clearcoats, thicker sections (20 μm) are required [16–18].

Hand-held spectrophotometers are available for objective color measurement. While they may have applications in collecting data for inclusion in databases, their use in the laboratory is limited because of their inability to measure the small samples (<3-mm diameter) usually seen in casework.

MSP is the technique used to measure the color spectrum of a microscopic sample. Depending on the type of sample it can be operated in the transmission mode (e.g., for fibers) or the reflectance mode (for opaque samples). Some instruments can also measure in the ultraviolet range.

Raman spectroscopy

Raman spectroscopy is a vibrational spectroscopy technique that is becoming more common in forensic laboratories. Raman spectrometers are becoming smaller, less costly, and more user-friendly. Raman spectroscopy can provide complementary information to that provided by infrared spectroscopy and can be useful in comparing and identifying pigments, extenders, and other components [19].

Raman spectroscopy is used to study vibrational, rotational, and other low-frequency modes in a system. It relies on inelastic scattering (Raman scattering) of monochromatic light, usually from a laser in the visible, near infrared, or near ultraviolet range. Infrared spectroscopy yields similar, but complementary information. In the past, photomultiplier tubes were the detectors of choice for dispersive Raman setups, which resulted in long acquisition times. Modern Fourier Transform Raman instruments have shorter acquisition times. In paint examination, Raman spectroscopy is a useful technique for analyzing pigments.

Other Analytical Techniques

Some laboratories may have other instruments available to them, which can be used for paint analysis. One example is *inductively coupled plasma mass spectrometry* (ICP-MS), possibly with laser ablation (LA-ICP-MS). Although it is a destructive technique, the amount of sample consumed in analysis is very small, and it can provide information on the elemental composition of paints, though currently it is more usually associated with glass analysis. These instruments are becoming smaller and more affordable and should become more common in forensic laboratories in the future [20].

Another analytical method being developed is *laser-induced breakdown spectroscopy* (LIBS), which may, in the future, provide a fast and relatively inexpensive alternative to LA-ICP-MS [21].

Investigative Examination

Most of the techniques and procedures referred to above relate principally to a comparison of a recovered sample of paint with a control or reference sample.

Cases also arise where only a recovered paint sample is submitted and the examiner is requested to establish its origin or provide the investigator with some other information to assist the enquiry.

Cases of this type include the identification of automotive paint to establish what type of vehicle it came from. Much work has been done in this area by expert paint working groups and databases of automotive paints from Europe, North America, Japan, and other countries have been built up over the years.

It may be possible to identify the source of a flake of automotive paint recovered from the clothing of a traffic accident victim by examining the color, layer structure, and chemical composition of the recovered paint layers. At best, the make, model, year, and manufacturing plant could be identified. In other cases, useful information on the source can still be provided to the investigator; for example, the likely manufacturer of the vehicle, the approximate age and the range of models to which this particular paint was applied.

These results depend on having the full original layer structure present. If the vehicle has been repainted or if only certain layers are present, the information available will be reduced, or it may not be possible to provide any useful information at all.

Both the European Network of Forensic Science Institutes (ENFSI) European Collection of Automobile Paints (EUCAP) [22] and Scientific Working Group on Materials Analysis (SWGMAT) Paint Data Query (PDQ) [12] search procedures can provide information on automotive paint. It should be remembered that not all car paints are in the databases and certain categories of paint (e.g., commercial vehicles and motorcycles) are not currently included.

Significance and Reporting

Following laboratory examination, the examiner's next step is to report the results. One approach to assessing the significance of results is to review the information available before starting any laboratory work. The examiner may need to make some enquiries as to what happened, what the prosecution and defense positions are, whether all relevant material has been submitted, etc. The examiner may then develop an examination plan and also formulate a set of expectations and alternative propositions. For example, the examiner may decide that, in a certain set of circumstances, there should be transfer of a large amount of multilayer paint between two items. If the result of the examination shows this to be the case, then the evidence supports this particular version of events; if the results do not match the expectations, then the results may favor an alternative version of events, perhaps favoring the defense hypothesis; in some situations, the results may not be clear-cut and may add nothing to the existing knowledge about what really happened. This approach will depend on whether the legal system in the particular jurisdiction will allow it.

Reporting results should be done in a descriptive, factual way, bearing in mind that the reader is unlikely to have scientific training and – if the evidence is presented in court – those hearing the evidence presented may not have the written version in front of them but may have to rely on hearing the oral evidence only.

There have been publications on assessing the significance of paint evidence using Bayes' Theorem and work on this aspect of reporting physical evidence is continuing [23–25].

In order to assess the significance of a result, it may be necessary to refer to collections of paint color frequency data or national vehicle populations, or information may have to be collected to address specific issues in particular cases.

In general, the higher the number of layers present in a paint flake, the more individual a paint will be, and the more significance will be attached to a positive result. Two-way transfer of paint flakes (e.g., between two vehicles or between a tool and a point of entry) will be more significant than one-way transfer, but the assessment of the significance becomes more complex because the two-way transfers are not independent events. Further discussion on this area is beyond the scope of this article.

Reporting paint results from clothing will require knowledge of transfer and persistence studies, to reflect the prevalence of paint flakes on the clothing of relevant populations. Studies by Lau et al. [7] and Pearson et al. [8], for example, have documented the frequency of finding paint flakes and glass on clothing from dry cleaners and on students' clothing, and are valuable starting points.

Further Information

An excellent source of up-to-date information on forensic examination of paint is the Best Practice Guidelines produced by forensic expert groups such as the ENFSI Paint and Glass Working Group or its North American equivalent, the SWGMAT Paint Group. Details of these can be found on the ENFSI

and Federal Bureau of Investigation (FBI) web sites www.enfsi.eu and www.fbi.gov.

In addition to these expert working groups, Interpol organize a triennial International Forensic Science Symposium. Part of this meeting is a review of all relevant papers published in the preceding three years, which is a very valuable resource on current work. Further information can be found on the Interpol web site www.interpol.int.

Periodic reviews of the current literature are also published in the scientific journals (for example, Ryland et al. [26]).

Case Histories

Green River Murders. In 1982, five women were murdered and left in or near the Green River, Washington, USA. Over the next several years, more bodies were found in the same area. In many cases, months or even years had passed since the victim's disappearance, and all that was found were skeletal remains. Eventually, 49 victims were listed as victims of the Green River Killer. The murders remained unsolved for nearly two decades.

In 1987, police took saliva samples and other evidence from a man called Gary Ridgway but did not find anything that linked him to the murders.

By 1991, the killings stopped and the case was dormant. Then in 2001, with DNA testing technology becoming more widespread, police began reexamining some of the evidence they had collected during the 1980s. They discovered a DNA match between Ridgway and semen taken from four of the victims.

Police arrested Ridgway and charged him with murder. He appeared to have been absent or off duty from work on every known occasion when a victim had disappeared.

His attorney planned to make the argument that the DNA evidence proved nothing more than that he had been a customer of the women. Prosecutors were hesitant about basing their case nearly exclusively on the DNA evidence. Police turned to forensic scientist Skip Palenik in an effort to find additional evidence to link Ridgway with the victims.

Ridgway had a job painting trucks during the time when the murders occurred. Paint samples had been collected from his car, clothes, and work locker and also from the victims. Several thousand small paint samples associated with Ridgway were analyzed by FTIR microscopy. When Palenik found a sample with a matching infrared spectrum, he examined it using high magnification polarized light microscopy to identify the pigment, and X-ray spectroscopy to determine the elemental composition. While there were a number of initial spectral matches, none of the samples held up all the way through the analysis process.

"I had completed my assignment but I had a hunch that there was a lot more to this aspect of the case than met the eye," Palenik said. "I asked the prosecutors to provide me with Ridgway's and the victims' clothing so I could take a much closer look."

Palenik used reusable cassette-type filters connected to a vacuum cleaner, and collected particles with sizes in the $20-100$-μm range, only about one hundredth the size of the particles he had examined in the first phase of his analysis. Spray painting guns, such as those used by Ridgway in his job, generate tiny spheres of paint in the micron range that are so light they float in the air rather than fastening themselves to the object being painted.

Palenik collected tiny particles and then, viewing them through a powerful optical microscope, picked them out with tungsten needles and placed them on microscope slides for analysis.

The fact that no further sample preparation was required for IR microscopy was essential because it would have been difficult or impossible with samples this small. It was possible to generate usable IR spectra from particles as small as $10\,\mu\text{m} \times 10\,\mu\text{m}$.

Palenik said, "As the Green River investigation demonstrates, the smaller the particle you can analyze the better chance you have to solve the case. This investigation also illustrates another important advantage of this instrument. It can save huge amounts of time by automating the process of checking a sample against a reference library."

He found hundreds of these tiny spheres in many colors on the clothes of six of the victims, including two that had been linked to Ridgway by DNA evidence. Most of the samples were of Imron paint, a very rare type that was used extensively in the paint shop where Ridgway worked at Kenworth Trucks. Working with Dupont, who manufactured the paint, he was able to tie the samples to paint that Ridgway had been using around the time of the murders.

On the basis of this evidence, prosecutors charged Ridgway with further murders. In November 2003,

shortly before the trial was to begin, Ridgway confessed to murdering 48 women. He said that these were only the ones he could remember out of a total that he estimated at 70.

Ridgway's attorney was quoted in the press as saying that the paint evidence was crucial in his client's change of heart. "When this paint business came up, here you have something other than DNA – it's a particular paint you can link to Gary – and you start saying 'Well, here are seven dead women and they all can be linked to Gary one way or another,' Savage said." "What are the odds of that happening by accident?" [27].

Murder of Lord Mountbatten. In Europe, paint has also provided crucial evidence in high profile court cases. One of the first major cases in which the Irish Forensic Science Laboratory in Dublin was involved was the murder in 1979 of Lord Mountbatten, a cousin of Britain's Queen Elizabeth II, by the illegal Irish Republican Army (IRA).

He was going fishing in his green, wooden boat, *Shadow V*, when an explosion ripped through the vessel, killing him and three others and badly injuring three more.

That morning, before the explosion, two men were stopped by a police checkpoint more than $100\,\text{km}$ away and questioned. One denied putting any bomb on the boat – but at this stage there had been no explosion and the police did not know what he was talking about. The second man, Thomas McMahon, was a known IRA man and explosives expert.

When news came of the explosion on Lord Mountbatten's boat, the two suspects were detained and their clothing and samples from their car were taken.

At the laboratory, flakes of two-layer green paint were recovered from McMahon's jacket and boots and from the passenger seat of the men's car. This paint matched the green paint recovered from the bodies and taken from the boat.

In addition, grains of sand and traces of nitroglycerin recovered from the suspects added to the trace evidence in the case against them. McMahon was convicted of murder and sentenced to life imprisonment [28].

Graffiti. Graffiti is a widespread phenomenon arising, for example, from simple vandalism or from the actions of racist or activist groups. The financial cost of removal can be substantial and it is treated very seriously by transport police.

Allegation of criminal damage involving one suspect and two submitted control scrapings from a control box at the side of a London underground station.

A suspect was arrested running from a scene where the spraying of graffiti had been witnessed. A hooded top, seized soon after arrest, was submitted to the laboratory and microscopically examined. It was found to have a moderate concentration of paint balls on the outside surface, the majority of which were located on the front of the right sleeve and cuff. Both control paints were red and were optically indistinguishable from each other, but were chemically different when tested using FTIR. Red paint was the only color found on the surface of the hooded top. When tested microscopically, this red paint was indistinguishable from both of the red control paint samples. Both the control paints and these recovered paint balls contained red and brown particles when examined with transmitted, polarized light and did not fluoresce when observed under light passed through blue and ultraviolet filters. The recovered paint was indistinguishable from one of the submitted controls when analyzed by FTIR. The finding of red paint, indistinguishable from one of the submitted control samples on a hooded top, was deemed to provide *moderately strong scientific support* for the proposition that the wearer of the top had been in the vicinity of this graffiti while it was being sprayed [29].

References

[1]   Woodbridge, R. (1991). *Principles of Paint Formulation*, Taylor and Francis.
[2]   EUROPEAN PAINT GROUP (2006). *Guidelines for Best Practice in Forensic Paint Examination*, ENFSI.
[3]   Brezinski, DR (1994). *SciQuest Paint Tutorial CD*, Consolidated Research, Kingsford, MI, USA, Vol. 1.
[4]   Bentley, J. (2001). Composition, manufacture and use of paint, (Ch 7), *Forensic Examination of Glass and Paint*, B. Caddy, ed, Taylor and Francis, New York, London, pp. 123–141.
[5]   Buzzini, P., Massonnet, G., Birrer, S., Egli, N., Mazzella, W.D. & Fortini, A. (2005). Survey of crowbar and household paints in burglary cases – population studies, transfer and interpretation, *Forensic Science International* **152**, 221–234.
[6]   Buzzini, P., Massonnet, G. & Mizrahi, S. (2003). Interpretation of household paint transfer: a burglary case

[7]   Lau, L., Callowhill, B.C., Conners, N., Foster, K., Gorvers, R.J., Ohashi, K.N., Sumner, A.M. & Wong, H. (1997). The frequency of occurrence of paint and glass on the clothing of high school students, *Journal of Canadian Society of Forensic Science* **30**, 233–240.
[8]   Pearson, E.F., May, R.W. & Dabbs, M.D.G. (1971). Glass and paint fragments found in men's outer clothing, *Journal of Forensic Sciences* **16**, 283–300.
[9]   Helstroffer, S., Espanet, B. & Milet, S. (2003). Class identification of rockets types by paint analysis. A new way? *Forensic Science International* **136**(Suppl 1), 353–354.
[10]   Boynton, R.M. (1979). *Human Color Vision*, Holt, Rheinhart and Winston, New York.
[11]   ASTM E1610-02 (2008). *Standard Guide for Forensic Paint Analysis and Comparison*, American Society for Testing & Materials, Philadelphia.
[12]   Beveridge, A., Fung, T. & MacDougall, D. (2001). Use of infrared spectroscopy for the characterization of paint fragments (Ch. 10), in *Forensic Examination of Glass and Paint*, B. Caddy, ed, Taylor and Francis, New York, London, pp. 183–241.
[13]   Henson, M.L. & Jergovich, T.A. (2001). Scanning electron microscopy and energy dispersive X-ray spectrometry (SEM/EDS) for the forensic examination of paints and coatings (Ch 11), in *Forensic Examination of Glass and Paint*, B. Caddy, ed, Taylor and Francis, New York, London, pp. 243–272.
[14]   ENFSI (2007). *ENFSI Best Practice Guide: SEM/EDS and Paint Analysis*, ENFSI.
[15]   Challinor, J.M. (2001). Pyrolysis techniques for the characterization and discrimination of paint (Ch 9), in *Forensic Examination of Glass and Paint*, B. Caddy, ed, Taylor and Francis, New York, London, pp. 165–183.
[16]   ENFSI (2007). *ENFSI Standard Guide for Microspectrophotometry and Colour Measurement in Forensic Paint Analysis*, ENFSI.
[17]   Stoecklein, W. (2001). The role of colour and microscopic techniques for the characterization of paint fragments (Ch 8), in *Forensic Examination of Glass and Paint*, B. Caddy, ed, Taylor and Francis, New York, London, pp. 143–163.
[18]   Cousins, D.R. (1989). The use of microspectrophotometry in the examination of paints, *Forensic Science Review* **1**, 141.
[19]   Buzzini, P., Massonnet, G. & Monard-Sermier, F. (2006). The micro Raman analysis of paint evidence in criminalistics: case studies, *Journal of Raman Spectroscopy* **37**(9), 922–931.
[20]   Hobbs, A.L. & Almirall, J.R. (2003). Trace elemental analysis of automotive paints by laser ablation inductively-coupled plasma mass spectrometry, *Analytical and Bioanalytical Chemistry* **376**, 1265.
[21]   Almirall, JR., Umpierrez, U., Castro, W., Gornushkin, I. & Winefordner, J. (2005). *Forensic elemental analysis*

of materials by laser induced breakdown spectroscopy (LIBS), Proc SPIE, v. 5778, pp. 657–666.

[22] Piotrowski, G. (1999). European collection of automotive paints (EUCAP), *Problems of Forensic Sciences* **V224**, 19.

[23] Willis, S., McCullough, J. & McDermott, S. (2001). The interpretation of paint evidence, (Ch 12), in *Forensic Examination of Glass and Paint*, B., Caddy, ed, Taylor and Francis, New York, London, pp. 273–287.

[24] Seccombe, A.L. (2001). *Discrimination and Evidential Value of Vehicle Paint in Forensic Casework*, Master of Science thesis, University of Auckland, New Zealand.

[25] Edmondstone, G., Hellmann, J., Legate, K., Vardy, G.L. & Lindsay, E. (2004). An assessment of the evidential value of automotive paint comparisons, *Canadian Society of Forensic Science* **37**, 147.

[26] Ryland, S.G., Jergovich, T.A. & Kirkbride, K.P. (2006). Current trends in forensic paint examination, *Forensic Science Review* **18**, 97.

[27] Moving IR spectroscopy down to the micron level puts serial killer behind bars, Perkin Elmer case study, (2005.

[28] O'Connor, N. (2001). *Cracking Crime*, O'Brien Press, Dublin.

[29] Marsh, L. (2007). Some call it art: case studies investigating the spraying of illegal graffiti in the UK, *NIJ/FBI Trace Evidence Symposium*, Clearwater Beach, August 2007, http://projects.nfstc.org/trace/.

JOHN MCCULLOUGH

Paint: Interpretation

Introduction

Paint may be used as an investigative or an evaluative tool. Here, the focus is on interpretation, which is fundamental for paint and other transfer evidence (*see* **Paint**). When comparing two paint samples with a given analytical sequence, two main outcomes are possible. They are the following:

- The two samples can be differentiated.
- The two samples are not differentiated, they are analytically indistinguishable.
- There is a physical fit (rare).

In the first scenario, given that the reference paint is representative of the source material, a common origin can be excluded. In the second

scenario, the examinations reveal a concordance in properties, but are these properties common or rare?

The authors believe that the forensic scientist is in the best position to give an opinion on the value of this concordance. In general, paint interpretation is based on the frequency of occurrence of the measured characteristics. Very common paint types have less evidential value than very rare paints. An estimate of the frequency of occurrence of the different characteristics measured for each paint type would be an invaluable tool.

Even if the literature on paint interpretation is rather sparse in comparison to other trace evidence like fibers or glass, there are surveys or information that can help the scientist to evaluate the strength of evidence. The main ones are the following:

Frequency figures:
- population studies and frequency distribution;
- information on batch variations; and
- databases/reference collections.

Others:
- expert opinion;
- paint found at random on clothing and surveys on paint traces;
- transfer and persistence; and
- a likelihood ratio approach.

Paint experts also rely on data concerning the discrimination power of the technique, or the sequence of techniques, used to present their findings. The discriminating power is calculated according to the formula from [1] and is usually mentioned in population studies.

Automotive Paints

Introduction

In the automotive industry, the application of the different paint layers to the metallic automotive body follows several steps. The process stages for original equipment manufacturer (OEM) paints can be simplified as follows [2]:

- *Metal pretreatment*: degreasing, passivation, phosphatage layer.
- *Electro dip coating*: application of the primer layer by electro deposition.

Table 1 Automotive paints, population studies

Authors	Countries	Number of samples	Methods	Number of nondifferentiated pairs
Gothard [3]	Australia	500	Optical: color, layer sequence Chemical tests Analytical: infrared spectroscopy, emission spectrography, pyrolysis GC	2
Ryland and Kopec [4]	USA	200	Optical: color, layer sequence Chemical tests Analytical: infrared spectroscopy, emission spectrography, pyrolysis GC, X-ray fluorescence, NAA	0
Gothard and maynard [5]	Australia	500	Optical: color, layer sequence Chemical tests Analytical: infrared spectroscopy, pyrolysis GC	3
Massonnet [6]	Switzerland	124 Gray metallic	Optical: color, layer sequence Analytical: infrared spectroscopy, MSP	4
Reeza Alwi and Kuppuswamy [7]	Malaysia	100	Optical: color, layer sequence	0
Edmonstone *et al.* [8]	Canada	260	Optical: color Analytical: infrared spectroscopy	2 (1 with the analysis of all layers)

- *Fillers*: application of the primer surface layer.
- *Finish or topcoat*: usually applied in one layer for solid paints and in two layers for metallic or effect finishes (first the effect layer is applied then a clearcoat).

Other original layers can be added to this sequence like protection against chipping by stone, sealing layer, or other extra layer to increase the quality of the final product. During this process, nonoriginal or repair layers can also be added at any step if paint defects are observed.

Automotive paint traces are mostly found in road accident and are transferred to the recipient surface when contact occurs. Paint can be transferred to vehicles, pedestrians, or fixed objects. Paint may be the only evidence in hit-and-run cases. Paint smears or fragments may also be found on objects or bodies transported in cars.

Population Studies

Several authors published comprehensive studies concerning the differentiation of paints collected at random on vehicles in different countries [3–8]. A summary of these surveys is presented in Table 1. These researches provide details on the distribution of automotive paints using a chosen analytical sequence.

Some general conclusions may be drawn from these population studies as follows:

- Optical examinations alone are very discriminating. According to Ryland and Kopec [4], 87% of their sample set is discriminated on the basis of color and layer sequence.
- All the authors agree that the layer sequence is the most significant point of comparison. Figure 1 shows the frequency distributions of the paint samples according to their number of layers in the different surveys. Gothard [3] states that "a large number of layers agreeing with regards to color, thickness, and layer sequence can be taken as proof of common origin without further examination". According to Ryland and Kopec [4] "... the probability of two paint chips originating from different sources is extremely remote

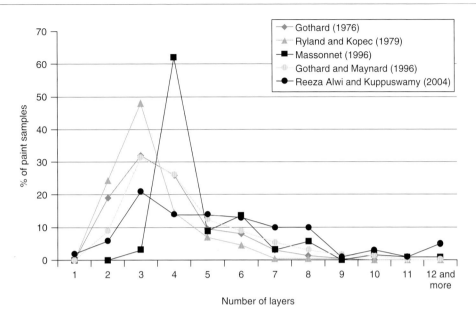

Figure 1   Frequency distribution of the paint samples in the different surveys according to their number of layers

when they have numerous layers (six or more) consistent in color, tint, type of finish, and layer thickness".

- When a complete sequence of analysis (optical and analytical) is applied, non-OEM or refinished paints are easily differentiated. The number of nondifferentiated pairs is low (between zero and four) and these samples are all OEM paints belonging to vehicles of the same make, model, color, and approximate year of production.

- Edmonstone *et al.* [8] compared the topcoat only (microscopy and chemical composition). Only two sample pairs were indistinguishable: they belonged to vehicles of the same make, model, and production plant. The first pair belonged to vehicles from 1995 and 1997, and the second pair had been produced the same year (1989). When all layers where compared and analyzed using FTIR, samples from the first pair were distinguished, and the second pair remained nondifferentiated.

Globally, these surveys show that if two paints with numerous nonoriginal layers are indistinguishable using a state-of-the-art analytical sequence, there are generally few doubts that they have a common origin [2].

Vehicle Topcoat Colors: Frequency Distribution

Several authors worked on the frequency distribution of vehicles' topcoat color [9–14]. Vehicles in circulation were counted according mainly to their topcoat color, but sometimes also considering their make, model, or year of production.

The main outcomes of these surveys are the following:

- Color categories chosen by the authors are more detailed than the one used in the official statistics and can include the difference between effect and solid paints. The frequencies obtained are lower than in the official register. The most common color group depends on the country considered and has a frequency of occurrence between 20 and 25%.

- When combining detailed color group and car make, the most common combination has a frequency of occurrence of less than 5% (between 3.2 and 4.8% depending on the survey). Thus, the occurrence of vehicle from particular make and color on the road can be considered from a statistical point of view as an unusual event.

- Globally, there is a rather good accordance between the data observed (color and make) and the corresponding numbers in the official statistics of vehicles in a given country or geographic area.

Tippett [9] counted the number of cars from a specific make and color in 100 groups of 100 cars. Two car makes were chosen, one being the most common (10.8%, frequency of occurrence) and the other one being rare (1%). He found that the data obtained follow a Poisson distribution and thus that they can be statistically predicted. With this model, it is possible to predict the number of times a particular colored model is seen on the road in a given time frame depending on the density of traffic.

McDermott *et al.* [14] collected and used the data obtained in a likelihood ratio framework for the interpretation of automotive paint evidence.

Batch Variations

The conclusion that was drawn from population studies is that if two multilayer paint systems are nondifferentiated with a complete sequence of analyses, they are original OEM paints from vehicle of the same make and model and approximate year of production.

The next question is, are we able to distinguished OEM paints or, according to Stoecklein and Palenik [15]. "In how many vehicles produced by one manufacturer and painted in the same color, can the paint be distinguished?"

Different batches from three of the most frequent colors applied to vehicles produced between 1989 and 1994 were analyzed by [15]. Their conclusions are that by using a broad spectrum of analytical techniques (microscopy, fourier transform infrared spectroscopy (FTIR), Microspectrophotometry (MSP), Raman, and pyrolysis gas chromatography mass spectrometry (Py-GC-MS)), it is possible to discriminate between OEM topcoat of different batches. Within one batch only a limited number of automobiles can be coated. After being in use, only few of these cars have coatings, which still show the same physical and chemical features. Therefore, one can assume that by analyzing OEM paints, the expected weight of the evidence will be strong or very strong [15].

To evaluate the correspondence of OEM multilayer paint systems, the following facts must be considered [2]:

- One batch of paint (topcoat) can be used to paint 8–3,500 vehicles.

- About 40% of the cars are locally repainted at the production plant.
- Change in batches can also occur for the other layers.
- In circulation, paints are differently affected by weathering and can be repainted after damage.

When using a comprehensive range of methods, in particular quantitative analysis instead of only qualitative, it is possible to differentiate between batches as well as between different conditions of weathering [15, 16]. Thus, the number of vehicles on the street with exactly the same OEM layer sequence is very low. Stoecklein [2] concludes that "there is very little likelihood of a second vehicle, with an identical characteristic profile of its coating material, being on the street at the time of the accident, in the vicinity of the scene of crime. The evidential value of such result is to be regarded as very high".

Databases/Reference Collections

Two main databases of automotive paints are available to police forces. Paint data query (PDQ) is mainly used in Canada and in the United States [17, 18]. The European collection of automotive paint (EUCAP) is used by the European laboratories [2]. Japanese police forces also have their own database for Asian cars. These collections are continuously updated.

The aim of these databases is to provide information to the police about cars (make, model, color, and production years) based on the analysis of paint traces found in hit-and-run accidents. Infrared spectra of thousands of samples are recorded for each different paint layer.

These databases can also provide information concerning the commonness/rarity of different paint types. For example, a clearcoat based on acrylic melamine and styrene will be present on several different vehicles and thus will have a rather low evidential value. On the other hand, a very special paint corresponding to only one vehicle will have a higher evidential value. Care should, however, be taken as the frequency distributions obtained in such databases do not represent the population of vehicles in circulation in a specific country but the variations observed between the different car make and color present in the database.

More generally, there should be reference collections available for each of the techniques used in

Table 2 Conclusions used by paint examiners for paint exchange scenarios [21]. Reprint with permission of Thomson Publishing Service

Scenario	Conclusion (%)				
	Slight support	Support	Strong support	Very strong support	Conclusive
A	**77.4**	19.4	1.6	1.6	0
B	15.3	**64.5**	15.3	4.8	0
C	4.0	**68.5**	23.4	4.0	0
D	0.8	8.9	**51.6**	34.7	4.0
E	0.8	21.8	**57.3**	19.4	0.8
F	0.8	8.1	35.5	**46.8**	8.9
G	0.8	19.4	**44.4**	31.5	4.0
H	0.8	1.6	10.5	**51.6**	35.5

A, one layer transferred in one direction;
B, one layer transferred in each direction;
C, multilayer manufacturer's finish transferred in one direction;
D, multilayer manufacturer's finish transferred in each direction;
E, multilayer manufacturer's finish transferred in one direction and one layer transferred in the other direction;
F, multilayer nonmanufacturer's finish transferred in one direction and one layer transferred in the other direction;
G, multilayer nonmanufacturer's finish transferred in one direction;
H, multilayer nonmanufacturer's finish transferred in each direction.

the different laboratories. A few surveys can also be found in the literature. For example, using Raman spectroscopy it was determined that 59% of the 27 light red automotive paint samples analyzed contain a specific red pigment (CI PR254). As this pigment is very commonly used in red paints, the evidential value of such finding will be low. On the other hand, a very rare combination of pigments will have a higher evidential value [19].

Expert Opinion

McDermott and Willis [20] circulated a questionnaire to 235 paint examiners. Different hypothetical automotive paint transfer scenarios were presented and the respondents were requested to use a scale of conclusions ranging from slight support to conclusive. Table 2 illustrates the hypothetical transfer scenarios and the answer given by the paint experts [21].

This survey gives an insight into the value placed on such evidence by forensic scientists working in the field of paint analysis. This survey globally shows that a multilayer repaint system has more evidential value than a multilayer OEM paint system and that a multilayer paint has more evidential value than a single layer paint. Scientists also give more evidential value to cross transfer compared to a single direction transfer if the same type of paint is considered [20].

Household Paints

Introduction

Paints covering surfaces other than vehicles are commonly called *household paints* [21]. The interpretation of this kind of paint evidence is quite different from the interpretation of vehicle paint. Vehicle paint follows a definite sequence of color, number, and thickness of layers, which are specified by the manufacturer. Household paint is more often encountered in single layer, but is considered to provide strong evidence due to the large range of paints available.

Household paint traces encountered in forensic cases can originate from buildings (architectural paints), tools, spray cans, etc. In a burglary, paint traces can be transferred on the tool used to force a door, and if the tool is covered by a paint layer, paint particles from the tool can be possibly found on the door. In graffiti case, the paint can be compared with a reference spray can, but microscopic wet aerosol paint droplets can be transferred on the clothes and on the hands of the offender and could provide highly significant evidence. In these two examples, three kinds of paints (building, tools, spray) and four kinds of supports (door, tool, clothes, hands) are encountered. To evaluate the evidential value of these paint traces, the forensic expert will need information about the frequency of the analytical characteristics of the type of paint encountered, and about the frequency of pounding randomly paint traces on the kind of support on which the traces were found.

Population Studies

Several authors have studied the discriminating power of an analytical sequence on different populations of household samples [22–29]. Table 3 shows a summary of these surveys.

These researches show that certain binder types are more commonly encountered. They also demonstrate the high potential of common analytical sequences to discriminate between household paint samples, even for samples of the same color and binder type.

Table 3   Household paints, population studies

Authors	Samples	Methods	Commonest binders/ extenders combinations		Number of subgroups (maximum number of items per group)	Discriminating power of the whole sequence
Tippett et al. [22]	200 paint samples from buildings	Microscopy	–			0.999
		Solvent tests Spectrography Py-GC-MS				
May and Porter [23]	31 household gloss paints (11 white, 10 red and 10 green)	Microscopy	ALK	80%	8 (3)	0.93 (white)
		Emission spectrography	ALK + PUR	10%	10 (1)	1 (red)
		Solvent tests	ALK + fire retardant	10%	10 (1)	1 (green)
		FTIR X-ray diffraction Py-GC-MS Py-FTIR				
Laing et al. [24]	169 household gloss paints (divided in 12 color categories)	Microscopy	–			0.89 to 1
		MSP				
Castle et al. [25]	100 case-openers	MSP	ALK	61%	–	–
		Py-GC-MS	ALK + STY	8%		
			EPOXY	8%		
			ALK + VINYL TOL	6%		
			ACR	6%		
Buzzini and Masson-net [26]	40 green spray paints	FTIR	ALK OPH + NCL	28%	31 (6)	0.98
		Raman	ACR	23%		
			ALK OPH + BaSO$_4$	15%		

(*continued overleaf*)

Table 3   (*continued*)

Authors	Samples	Methods	Commonest binders/ extenders combinations		Number of subgroups (maximum number of items per group)	Discriminating power of the whole sequence
Govaert and Bernard [27]	51 red spray paints	Microscopy	ALK + NCL	45%	37 (4)	0.988
		FTIR	ALK	24%		
		X-ray fluorescence				
Buzzini *et al.* [28]	41 blue crowbars	FTIR	ALK OPH + NCL	71%		
			ALK OPH + CaCO$_3$	17%		
			ALK OPH	7%		
Gosse *et al.* [29]	38 black spray paints	FTIR	ALK OPH +NCL	42%	34 (2)	0.994
		X-ray fluorescence	ALK OPH	21%		
		Py-GC-MS	ACR	13%		
			ALK OPH +NCL + STY	11%		
Gosse *et al.* [29]	38 black spray paints	FTIR	ALK OPH +NCL	42%	34 (2)	0.994
		X-ray fluorescence	ALK OPH	21%		
		Py-GC-MS	ACR	13%		
			ALK OPH +NCL + STY	11%		

ACR, acrylic; ALK, alkyd; ALK OPH, orthophthalic alkyd; NCL, nitrocellulose; PUR, polyurethane; STY, styrene; VINYL TOL, vinyl toluene

For example, all the red spray paints analyzed by [27] are alkyd based, but these samples can be classified into 37 different groups. The discriminating power of this sequence (microscopy, FTIR, and X-Ray fluorescence) is 0.988.

Batch Variations

As for vehicle paints, if two household paints are indistinguishable, the question of batch to batch variation is asked. Could this paint trace come from any other batch of the same brand, or is it possible to exclude other batches and to link the trace to a given batch?

Inkster *et al.* [32] compared 14 batches of the same architectural acrylic white paint by microscopy, microspectrophotometry, FTIR, micro-XRF and Py-GC-MS. Only one batch could be differentiated from the other. In this study, only qualitative analysis was used. On the other hand, [33] observed significant differences between two pairs of batches, using statistical analysis of the results by principal component analysis (PCA). These results suggest the high potential of chemometric tools or semiquantitative analysis to differentiate between closely related spectra.

Databases/Reference Collections

Databases for household paint are less developed than for vehicle paints. However, some specific databases exist. For example, the European database of spray paint contains the infrared spectrum of 209 spray paints. This database can be used to identify an unknown spray paint trace, but also to evaluate the frequency of the infrared characteristics of a given spray paint. The French database of black spray contains the infrared spectrum of 38 black spray paints with information about the Py-GC-MS results [29].

Each laboratory has the opportunity to create their own databases, for example, containing traces found in caseworks or various reference samples.

Paint Found at Random on Clothing and Surveys on Paint Abrasion Traces

Introduction

When paint cannot be unambiguously attributed to criminal activity, it is then necessary to assess if it could be present as background. Population studies demonstrate the potential of analytical methods, but cannot be used to evaluate the frequency of paint traces found on different kind of supports. To do so, it is necessary to collect and analyze traces, and not control samples. Indeed, background paint may not have the same origin (i.e., vehicle, household, tools) as samples. These backgrounds or so-called random paint studies are more complicated to carry out, because of the difficulty of pinding samples and the time needed to collect and count them. These

studies often contain information about the frequency of the color, the size, and number of layers of the traces. Analytical results are less often available.

Paint Found at Random on Clothing

The two available studies about paint found at random on clothing show contradictory results. Lau *et al.* [31] found that on the majority of searched items no paint traces are recovered. If traces are recovered, it is rare to find more than one fragment. On the other hand, in the study of [30] four or more fragments are recovered on 80% of the items. This difference, also observed for glass, as the authors looked at both paint and glass sample, could be explained by the size of the fragments: for 52% of the recovered fragments by [30] the size is less than 0.3 mm. Lau *et al.* [31] indicate that the majority of the recovered paint fragments were smaller than 1×1 mm, but no information is available about the minimum size considered. In addition, it must be noted that Pearson *et al.* looked at particles recovered in pockets and cuffs, where one might expect to find more particles, because of longer retention time. Table 4 shows a summary of the main results obtained in both studies.

Table 4 Paint fragments found at random on clothing

Authors	Items searched	Commonest colors of paint traces		Number of paint fragments on each item
Pearson *et al.* [30]	100 suits	Red	29%	0 : 3%
		Green	23%	1 : 8%
		Cream	14%	2 : 3%
		Blue	12%	3 : 6%
				4 and more : 80%
Lau *et al.* [31]	216 upper body garments	Yellow	31%	0 : 86%
		Pink	18%	1 : 12%
		Red	15%	2 : 1%
				3 : 1%
	213 lower body garments	Yellow	32%	0 : 88%
		Pink	22%	1 : 10%
		White	8%	2 : 2%
				3 : 0.5%
	164 pairs of footwear	White	27%	0 : 77%
		Red	21%	1 : 10%
		Black	15%	2 : 4%
		Yellow	13%	3 : 2%
				4 and more : 5%

Table 5 Survey of abrasion paint traces

Authors	Items searched	Commonest colors of paint traces		Number of types of paint traces on each item
McDermott et al. [14]	1000 vehicles	–		0 : 91% one and more : 9%
Ranzi et al. [34]	147 foreign traces found on damaged cars	Gray	26%	–
		Red	22%	
		Blue	17%	
		Green	6%	
		White	6%	
		Yellow	6%	
		Black	5%	
Buzzini et al. [28]	207 crowbars	White	61%	0 : 34%
		Red	18%	1 : 50%
		Green	7%	2 : 13%
		Brown	5%	3 : 2%
				4 : 1%

Surveys on Paint Traces

Studies on paint found on clothing concern paint fragments, which have to be differentiated from paint abrasion traces. A few studies on paint abrasion traces are available for cars [14] and tools [28, 34], see Table 5.

Transfer and Persistence

Again, when paint cannot be unambiguously attributed to criminal activity, knowledge of transfer and persistence phenomena becomes important to assess the value of paint traces.[a] The expert should be able to evaluate if the quantity of paint recovered is consistent with the alleged contact. However, transfer experiments are difficult to perform, especially with vehicle paints. For this reason, the number of studies involving transfer experiments is low.

Generally, a strong contact is necessary to remove paint from its support (metal, wood, etc.). This can be caused by an impact or an abrasion. The quantity of paint transferred depends on the force applied, the condition of the paint, the duration of the contact, and the nature of the object in contact with the paint.

This concerns dry paint, but sometimes wet paint could be transferred, for example, in cases involving spray paint, where wet paint could be transferred on the hands and on the clothing of the suspect [21]. Moreover, the persistence of wet paint is expected to be very good, because after drying the paint is strongly attached to the recipient.

Krausher [35] studied the transfer of droplets of paint to clothing during the use of aerosol paint. The density of droplets on the clothing of a sprayer is high, especially in areas exposed to the paint cloud. The size of the paint droplets is generally about 10–40 microns. Owing to their small size, the persistence of the paint droplets is lower than that for large wet paint transfer. The droplets are easily removed from the surface by washing. Marin et al. [36] have also studied the transfer of paint droplet from spray paint and obtained quite similar results.

Buzzini et al. [28] studied the cross transfer of paint between a crowbar and a painted wooden surface. In every simulated contact, a reciprocal transfer of paint was observed. A correlation between the quantity of household paint transferred in one direction and the quantity of tool paint transferred in the other direction was observed.

A Likelihood Ratio Approach Within a Hierarchy of Propositions

Bayes theorem shows how the evidence influences the probabilities associated with two alternative hypotheses. Three different levels of hypothesis can be considered: source level, activity level, and offense level [37]. For example, in a case where paint traces are recovered on a tool and compared with the paint of a forced door, the hypothesis could be as follows:

Source level

H_p: the traces found on the tool come from the paint of the forced door;
H_d: the traces found on the tool do not come from the paint of the forced door and are present as background.

Activity level

H_p: the tool has been used to force the door;
H_d: another tool has been used to force the door.

Offense level

In most cases, the information to consider is neither known by the forensic scientist (e.g., modus operandi of the suspect), nor in his/her field of expertise. It is therefore very rare for paint specialists to assess likelihood ratios at the offense level, such as follows:

H_p: the suspect has forced the door using that tool;
H_d: the suspect has not forced the door.

The assessment of the source level depends on analytical information obtained during examination [38]. The frequency of the analytical characteristics of the evidence is the important factor of the likelihood ratio. This frequency is evaluated in a given population. The choice of the relevant population is crucial, because a wrong population could drastically change the value of the frequency. In transfer evidence, the relevant population is often traces found on a given support. For example, in the case of paint traces recovered on a tool, the relevant population could be paint traces recovered on a population of tools seized by the police on suspects. Paint traces studies give the appropriate information to the evaluation of the frequency. However, the number of population studies

of paint traces is quite low and in some cases the corresponding trace population study is not available. In this situation, general population studies could be used. Generally, the role of the expert is to make an inventory of all the information found in the literature, and to estimate the frequency of the paint trace on the basis of these studies.

The assessment of the activity level is more complex. In addition to the frequency parameter, transfer and background parameters have to be taken into account. Transfer parameters concern the probability that paint traces were transferred to the given support, persist, and are recovered. Compared to glass or fiber evidence, the phenomenon of paint transfer is not fully understood, especially the transfer of vehicle paint. Background parameter concerns the probability of finding such a paint trace at random on this given support. Background parameter could be estimated on the basis of population studies of traces.

The number of studies about Bayesian interpretation of paint evidence is limited. McDermott *et al.* [14] and Willis *et al.* [21] calculated the likelihood ratio for various transfer scenarios for automotive paints and [28] used the Bayesian approach to evaluate the value of a cross transfer of paint between a tool and a forced door.

Conclusion

The ability of the expert to estimate the frequency of a specific paint type will rely mainly on experience and familiarity with the relevant literature as well as on access to representative databases. Other information like paint found at random or other expert opinion is also a great help to the interpretation of some cases.

Background data are available in the literature to help the scientist to assess the evidential value of his/her paint examination (automotive and household). Databases are very important to provide frequency of occurrence on different paint categories. If possible, these databases should be local to take into account the population of paint in a given geographic area. More work is needed principally on traces population studies and on paint interpretation using a likelihood ratio approach.

End Notes

a. If the paint is unambiguously attributed to the criminal activity, the probability of the evidence being transferred, having persisted and being recovered, is one under the prosecution's proposition (i.e. Vehicle A*** hit vehicle B). The probability of the evidence given the defense proposition (i.e.Vehicle A*** did not hit vehicle B) is the frequency of the observed characteristics in the suspect population. It is certain that the evidence is not background.

References

[1]   Smalldon, K. & Moffat, A. (1973). The calculation of discriminating power for a series of correlated attributes, *Journal of the Forensic Science Society* **13**, 291–295.

[2]   Stoecklein, W. (1992). Die Verkehrunfallflucht: Kriminaltechnische Möglichkeiten der Aufklärung am Beispiel Autolack, *Schriftenreihe der Polizei-Führungsakademie* **1**, 36–59.

[3]   Gothard, J.A. (1976). Evaluation of automobile paint flakes as evidence, *Journal of Forensic Sciences* **21**, 636–641.

[4]   Ryland, S.G. & Kopec, R.J. (1979). The evidential value of automobile paint chips, *Journal of Forensic Sciences* **24**, 140–147.

[5]   Gothard, J. & Maynard, P. (1996). Evidential value of automotive paint, *Proceedings 13th International Symposium of the ANZFSS*, Sydney.

[6]   Massonnet, G. (1996). *Les peintures automobiles en criminalistique*, PhD thesis, University of Lausanne, Law faculty and School of forensic sciences, Switzerland.

[7]   Reeza, A.A. & Kuppuswamy, R. (2004). Studies on the layer structure of paint flakes collected from motor vehicles in Kuala Lumpur, Malaysia, *Journal of Forensic Identification* **54**, 645–652.

[8]   Edmondstone, G., Hellman, J., Legate, K., Vardy, G.L. & Lindsay, E. (2004). An assessment of the evidential value of automotive paint comparisons, *Canadian Society of Forensic Science Journal* **37**, 147–153.

[9]   Tippett, C.F. (1964). Car distribution statistics and the hit-and-run driver, *Medicine, Science and the Law* **4**, 91–97.

[10]   Ryland, S.G., Kopec, R.J. & Somerville, P.N. (1981). The evidential value of automobile paint. Part II: frequency of occurrence of topcoat colors, *Journal of Forensic Sciences* **26**, 64–74.

[11]   Buckle, J., Fung, T. & Ohashi, K. (1987). Automotive topcoat colours: occurrence frequencies in Canada, *Canadian Society of Forensic Science Journal* **204**, 45–56.

[12]   Volpé, G.G., Stone, H.S., Rioux, J.M. & Murphy, K.J. (1988). Vehicle topcoat colour and manufacturer: frequency distribution and evidential significance, *Canadian Society of Forensic Science Journal* **21**, 11–18.

[13]   Stone, H.S., Murphy, K.J., Rioux, J.M. & Stuart, A.W. (1991). Vehicle topcoat colour and manufacturer: frequency distribution and evidential significance, part II, *Canadian Society of Forensic Science Journal* **24**, 175–185.

[14]   McDermott, S.D., Willis, S.M. & McCullough, J.P. (1999). The evidential value of paint. Part II: a Bayesian approach, *Journal of Forensic Sciences* **44**, 263–269.

[15]   Stoecklein, W. & Palenik, C. (1998). Forensic analysis of automotive paints: evidential value and the batch problem, *Proceeding of the 4th European Paint Group Meeting*, Paris.

[16]   Stoecklein, W. & Fujiwara, H. (1999). The examination of UV-absorbers in 2-coat metallic and non-metallic automotive paints, *Science and Justice* **39**, 188–195.

[17]   Cartwright, N. & Rodgers, P. (1976). A proposed data base for the identification of automotive paint, *Canadian Society of Forensic Science Journal* **9**, 145–154.

[18]   Cartwright, N., Cartwright, L., Norman, E., Cameron, R., MacDougall, D. & Clark, W. (1982). A computerized system for the identification of suspect vehicles involved in hit and run accidents, *Canadian Society of Forensic Science Journal* **15**, 105–115.

[19]   Massonnet, G. & Stoecklein, W. (1999). Identification of organic pigments in coatings: application to red automotive topcoats. Part III: Raman spectroscopy (NIR FT-Raman), *Science and Justice* **39**, 181–187.

[20]   McDermott, S.D. & Willis, S.M. (1997). A survey of the evidential value of paint transfer evidence, *Journal of Forensic Sciences* **42**, 1012–1018.

[21]   Willis, S., McCullough, J. & McDermott, S. (2001). The interpretation of paint evidence, in *Forensic Examination of Glass and Paint*, B. Caddy, ed, Taylor and Francis, London and New York, pp. 273–287.

[22]   Tippett, C.F., Emerson, V.J., Fereday, M.J., Lawton, F., Richardson, A., Jones, L.T. & Lampert, S.M. (1968). The evidential value of the comparison of paint flakes from sources other than vehicles, *Journal of the Forensic Science Society* **8**, 61–65.

[23]   May, R.W. & Porter, J. (1975). An evaluation of common methods of paint analysis, *Journal of Forensic Science Society* **15**, 137–146.

[24]   Laing, D.K., Dudley, R.J., Home, J.M. & Isaacs, M.D.J. (1982). The discrimination of small fragments of household gloss paint by microspectrophotometry, *Forensic Science International* **20**, 191–200.

[25]   Castle, D.A., Curry, C.J. & Russell, L.W. (1984). A survey of case-openers, *Forensic Science International* **24**, 285–294.

[26]   Buzzini, P. & Massonnet, G. (2004). A market study of green spray paints by Fourier transform infrared (FTIR) and Raman spectroscopy, *Science and Justice* **44**(3), 123–131.

[27]   Govaert, F. & Bernard, M. (2004). Discriminating red spray paints by optical microscopy, Fourier transform infrared spectroscopy and X-ray fluorescence, *Forensic Science International* **140**, 61–70.

[28] Buzzini, P., Massonnet, G., Birrer, S., Egli, N.M., Mazzella, W. & Fortini, A. (2005). Survey of crowbar and household paints in burglary cases – population studies, transfer and interpretation, *Forensic Science International* **152**, 221–234.

[29] Gosse, R., Milet, S. & Espanet, B. (2005). Discrimination of Black Spray Paints, *Proceedings of the European Paint and Glass Group Meeting*, Berlin.

[30] Pearson, E.F., May, R.W. & Dabbs, M.D.G. (1971). Glass and paint fragments found in men's outer clothing – report of a survey, *Journal of Forensic Sciences* **16**(3), 283–300.

[31] Lau, L., Beveridge, A.D., Callowhill, B.C., Conners, N., Foster, K., Groves, R.J., Sumner, A.M. & Wong, H. (1997). The frequency of occurence of paint and glass on the clothing of high school students, *Canadian Society of Forensic Science Journal* **30**(4), 233–240.

[32] Inkster, J., Maynard, P., Roux, C. & Fergusson, B. (2006). Intrasample vs intersample variability in architectural paint, *Fourth European Academy of Forensic Science Meeting*, Helsinki.

[33] Bell, S.E., Fido, L.A., Speers, J. & Armstrong, W.J. (2005). Rapid forensic analysis and identification of "lilac" architectural finishes using Raman spectroscopy, *Applied Spectroscopy* **59**(1), 100–108.

[34] Ranzi, R., Antonetti, G., Buzzini, P. & Massonnet, G. (2004). Population study of foreign traces recovered on bodies of damaged cars, *Proceedings of the 10th European Paint and Glass Group Meeting*, Prague.

[35] Krausher, C.D.J. (1994). Characteristics of aerosol paint transfer and dispersal, *Canadian Society of Forensic Science Journal* **27**(3), 125–142.

[36] Marin, D., Berger, N., Buzzini, P. & Massonnet, G. (2004). Transfer, detection and in situ Raman analysis of spray paint traces on clothes, *Proceedings of the 10th European Paint and Glass Group Meeting*, Prague.

[37] Cook, R., Evett, I.W., Jackson, G., Jones, P.J. & Lambert, J.A. (1998). A hierarchy of propositions: deciding which level to address in casework, *Science and Justice* **38**(4), 231–239.

[38] Aitken, C.G.G. & Taroni, F. (2004). *Statistics and the Evaluation of Evidence for Forensic Scientists*, John Wiley & Sons, Chichester.

GENEVIÈVE MASSONNET AND FLORENCE MONNARD

Palmprints *see* Friction Ridge Examination (Fingerprints): Interpretation of

Palynology

Introduction

One of the newer techniques now being used more frequently is forensic palynology: the collection and examination of pollen and spores associated with crime scenes, other types of illegal activities, or terrorism. The value of using pollen and spores (collectively called *palynomorphs*) as forensic tools relies on four important aspects.

First, many types of pollen and spore-producing plants disperse vast quantities of these palynomorphs into the air that are carried by air currents and eventually fall to the ground in a thin coating called the *pollen rain*. In some regions, the amount of pollen and spores dispersed is so great that exposed land and water surfaces turn yellow from the pollen rain. Although not a precise measurement of the surrounding vegetation, and thus by inference the climate of the area, the pollen rain in each region of the world is nevertheless a snapshot of that area and becomes a "pollen print" that can be used to assist in identifying the region.

Second, pollen and spores are microscopic in size, invisible to the naked eye, and can become trapped on almost any type of surface. This means that at any geographical location, pollen or spores from plants in that region, or more specifically, the pollen and spores from a specific crime scene can become evidence that will link a suspect or some object with the region or crime scene.

Third, there are nearly one-half million different plant species that produce either pollen or spores. Fortunately, each of these species produces pollen or spores that can be identified as coming from the parent plant; however, often differences in the pollen and spores of closely related species or even related genera may appear so similar that precise identification can only be achieved through detailed studies using the resolution capabilities of a scanning electron microscope (SEM) or transmission electron microscope (TEM).

Fourth, most pollen and spores are highly resistant to destruction or decay. This means that pollen and spore evidence from a region or crime scene can remain intact for years, hundreds of years, or even thousands and millions of years. This means that if crime scene evidence is handled correctly and stored safely, years or decades later the trapped pollen and spores can still be recovered and used to assist investigators.

Even though the first reported use of pollen to help solve a crime occurred nearly 50 years ago, very few attempts to use this forensic tool occurred in the meantime, and even then the number of times it was used has been rare. Only recently, during this century, the number of applications and attempts to use pollen and spore evidence for forensic use has been increasing. As the number of times that pollen and spores are successfully used as evidence in forensic cases increases, so does the range of its potential applications. Recently solved criminal cases demonstrate that the forensic use of pollen and spores can be applied to cases of forgery, production and distribution of illegal drugs, assaults, robbery, rapes, homicide, genocide, terrorism, arson, hit and run crimes, counterfeiting of currency, identifying the origin of fake prescription drugs such as Viagra, and various other types of criminal activity. Pollen and spore evidence has been used to resolve a variety of civil cases involving forged documents, fake antiques, authentication of paintings by master artists, removal of artifacts from historic or archaeological sites, illegal poaching of animals or fish, and cases involving illegal pollution of the environment [1].

Successful use of pollen and spores in forensic applications may depend on the palynologist's knowledge and experience. One must know and understand the plant ecology and plant communities in and around the crime scene area or the region where pollen samples were collected. A sound understanding of palynology including knowledge of the production, dispersal patterns, preservation potential, and identification of pollen and spores is essential to understand and interpret the expected total palynomorph assemblage recovered in forensic samples. As with most types of forensic evidence timing is critical. The sooner the palynologist is called to investigate a crime scene, the more likely will be the potential value of the collected samples. Because pollen and spores are small, light, easily recycled, and present in abundant amounts in the atmosphere, a crime scene can quickly become contaminated by recycled palynomorphs accidentally carried into the area on the clothing or shoes of crime scene investigators, deposited out of the atmosphere, or from other noncrime scene sources if the forensic pollen sample collection is delayed or collected improperly. Under ideal circumstances, and with proper and timely collection of forensic pollen samples, one might even be able to determine the season of the year when a crime was committed and occasionally how long ago a crime was committed. Much of that information pertains to knowing the pollination cycles of various plants and being able to check for the presence of cytoplasm and the innermost wall of pollen grains, called the *intine*, which is composed of cellulose and degrades fairly rapidly after pollen grains are dispersed [2].

Pollen Types

Some of the most useful types of pollen and spores for forensics are the wind-pollinated types. This group includes the spore-producing plants such as fungi, ferns, and mosses as well as a wide range of pollen types produced by the gymnosperms (nonflowering seed-bearing plants such as pines, cedars, and spruce), and a significant number of angiosperms (flowering seed-bearing plants such as aspen, elms, and chestnuts). Because wind pollination is an inefficient method of dispersal, these plants must produce vast quantities of pollen or spores that are usually lightweight and are aerodynamically designed to travel easily in air currents. The enormity of pollen production in many of the wind-pollinated (anemophilous) plants is exemplified by statistics such as the following: a single shoot of marijuana (*Cannabis*) produces about 500 million pollen grains, one dock (*Rumex*) plant produces about 400 million pollen grains, a single panicle of sorghum (*Sorghum*) disperses 100 million pollen grains, and just one male strobilus on a branch of a lodgepole pine (*Pinus contorta*) produces over 600 000 pollen grains. In addition to these examples, many of the other wind-pollinated plants such as ragweed, grasses, some species of eucalyptus, oaks, hickory, walnut, birch, alder, and elms produce between 10 000 and 100 000 pollen grains per anther (the part of a flower that produces and contains pollen and is usually borne on a stalk). Other anemophilous plants, some of which are low pollen producers, still produce more than 10 times the amount of pollen per anther and flower than almost all species of insect-pollinated plants. The amounts of pollen dispersed annually by the wind-pollinated plants is so vast that their pollen can be found in almost every environment in the world and the distribution of those pollen types in the pollen rain (total pollen deposited annually at any given location) of each region gives each locale its own pollen print. As such, these pollen types are the most common ones found in the fossil pollen record of a region and are also the most common types found in forensic pollen samples [3].

Some flowering plants live completely submerged in water, release their pollen underwater, and then rely on the pollen to float to the surface or ride water currents in an effort to accomplish fertilization. This method of transport, like the wind, is an inefficient method of pollination; therefore, like wind-pollinated plants, submerged plants produce high levels of pollen. These types of pollen could be found on the clothing, in the lungs, or possibly in the stomach of individuals who drown or were thrown into lakes or streams after being killed. Nevertheless, these types of pollen are often of little potential value for forensic work because they decay very easily and are difficult to recover without accidentally destroying them in the process.

The largest group of flowering plants is the insect or animal-pollinated types (entomophilous). This group depends on the transport of their pollen grains from the anther (male portion) of one flower to the stigma (female portion) of another by some type of insect (bee, wasp, beetle, moth, mosquito, and ant) or by some type of animal (hummingbirds, lizards, nectar-feeding bats, or other small mammals). The pollen grains produced by these entomophilous plants are generally ornate, have a surface covered with sticky lipids and waxes so that they attach easily to insects and mammal hairs, and most of these pollen types have a strong, thick outer wall (exine) that protects them from abrasion during transport and from rapid changes in humidity [4].

Because of the pollination efficiency of entomophilous plants, pollen productivity per anther and flower is much less than that in wind-pollinated plants. In maples (*Acer*), for example, each anther often contains no more than 1000 pollen grains and in flax flowers (*Linum*) each anther may contain as few as 100 pollen grains. In spite of the low pollen production in most entomophilous plants, they can often provide some of the most useful forensic clues. Because these pollen types are often large and heavy, and have a sticky surface, they are rarely cast adrift in wind currents and thus are rarely found in the normal pollen rain of a region. This means that it

would be extremely rare to find these types of pollen grains in the natural deposits of an area and thus they would rarely be an important type found in a region's pollen print. These attributes are both good and bad. They are good because if any of these types of pollen grains are found on objects at a crime scene or in another type of forensic sample, it generally means that the object or sample came in direct contact with the flowers or perhaps the leaves of the parent plant. This becomes an advantage because it often means that one can confidently conclude that an item or person was associated with a crime scene or some other specific locale where those parent plants and pollen types are found. It also provides a high degree of confidence that the pollen in the forensic sample belongs with the sample and that the pollen was not an atmospheric "contaminant". The downside of entomophilous pollen types is that so little pollen is produced by each plant that the chances of those pollen grains being transferred from the plant to some foreign object or person is often reduced.

Interpretation of Pollen Data

Understanding the rules that govern pollen production and dispersion are essential factors, which must be considered before evaluating forensic samples. Other important factors that will affect forensic pollen samples include how rapidly different types of pollen and spores settle out of the atmosphere (sinking speed), how well various types of pollen and spores remain preserved once they are deposited, and what types of clues indicate that pollen grains may have been recycled after they were deposited.

How rapidly airborne pollen and spores sink to the surface will determines how much and which species of pollen and spores will actually becomes part of the pollen rain and thus the pollen print of a given locale or region [5]. For example, marijuana, alder, juniper, and birch pollen are very small and very light pollen grains that have a sinking speed of about 1 or $2 \, \text{cm} \, \text{s}^{-1}$. This means that finding a few of these pollen grains in a forensic sample does not necessarily mean these plants are actually growing at the sampling spot. Instead, it might mean that the pollen resulted from long distance transport from sources many miles away. Before being able to determine this possibility, one would need to calculate how much pollen from these airborne types occurred in a forensic sample, how strong and from which direction the prevailing winds are in the sampled region, and what the total pollen concentration value (amount of total pollen deposited and subsequently preserved in one unit of deposit such as pollen per cubic centimeter or pollen per gram) is for the pollen rain of the sampled region. On the other hand, if one were to find anemophilous pollen types such as maize (*Zea mays*), wheat (*Triticum*) spruce (*Picea*), Douglas fir (*Pseudotsuga*), or fir (*Abies*) pollen in a forensic sample, it generally means that either someone may have carried those pollen grains to the sample site or those source plants were growing very close to the sampled area. The reason one could make that assumption is because the sinking speeds for these pollen types are very fast causing them to fall to the surface at a rate of $6-12\,\mathrm{cm\,s^{-1}}$, which is 4–6 times faster than the lighter ones. Each pollen type has its own sinking speed, which will cause it to be dispersed either very close to the parent plant or scattered over a wide area. In addition to sinking speeds, pollen grains of different sizes and mass will be more or less subject to be scoured out of the air currents when they are hit by raindrops or when they hit objects of various sizes, such as twigs, leaves, or various manmade objects. All of these factors must be carefully calculated for each locale in order to determine the potential, or expected, composition of the pollen rain in a given region. Once those data have been determined, then the pollen print for that region can be used for comparison against forensic samples that are suspected to have come from the same region. Depending upon how well the comparison of pollen spectra match, the palynologist may conclude that there is, or is not, a valid relationship between both samples. One way this is done is by using the likelihood ratio, which is based on using Bayes' theorem and considers how well the pollen spectra match and what are the probabilities of finding similar pollen assemblages in other locations [6].

Pollen degradation can also become an important factor in some types of samples. Pollen samples that might be only days or weeks old usually do not suffer much pollen destruction; however, pollen samples associated with buried objects or buried bodies might become degraded or in some cases completely destroyed by a variety of conditions. However, the potential of pollen destruction caused by germination is not a factor. When examining forensic pollen samples associated with buried objects, the palynologist must consider how much, and which types, of pollen or spores may have been destroyed. Depending upon a variety of conditions, the total pollen and spore spectrum of a sample might be altered due to the differential pollen preservation and degradation. Those potential changes in the overall pollen spectrum of a sample must be considered when trying to interpret the overall pollen assemblage for a sample [7].

Some of the important factors, which will affect pollen and spores and can, cause the total loss of certain taxa include the degrading effects caused by microbial activity, high soil pH and Eh (oxidation/reduction potential as judged by whether on not it is an oxygen rich or oxygen poor environment) that can cause mechanical breakdown of soils, various types of soil movement such as solifluction (a type of mass wasting where waterlogged sediments slowly move downslope over impermeable material), frequent changes in the level of soil moisture, and the inherent strength and durability of the pollen grain's outer wall. A number of previous studies have demonstrated that some very durable types such the spores of ferns and lycopods and the pollen from grasses, pigweed, amaranths, composites, oaks, and pine often remain preserved even in fairly harsh environments where most other pollen and spore types are totally destroyed by oxidization or have become so broken and degraded that they are no longer recognizable. Being able to recognize the levels and types of pollen grain and spore damage and destruction in forensic samples are critical aspects that must be recognized and understood before trying to interpret the overall pollen data. Although a few deposited pollen grains might occasionally burst open or rarely a spore might germinate, these potential problems are not of major concern.

Pollen recycling is another aspect that one must recognize when examining pollen samples. Understanding the vegetational environments where recycling occurs and being able to recognize the severity of recycling become important interpretive clues when examining pollen samples. Sometimes ancient fossil pollen and spores will erode from deposits thousands or millions of years old and will be recycled into contemporary samples. Such recycling might prove extremely useful because different fossil pollen or spore types tend to be deposited, and later eroded out from different aged sediments. An example of this type of clue became the key evidence leading to the conviction of a murder suspect who could be placed at the crime scene because of a unique, 20-million-year old Miocene-age hickory pollen grain that eroded out of a sediment outcrop, became recycled, and then got trapped as part of the dirt (*see* **Soil: Forensic Analysis**) in the tread of the suspect's boots [8]. In some cases, such as this example, the recycled fossil pollen provided the precise clue needed for identifying the exact location where the crime was committed and where the victim's body was buried. In other cases, recycled pollen from fairly recent deposits might combine with modern pollen in ways that might mislead some palynologists into making an incorrect interpretation.

Depending upon what types of sediments have yielded recycled pollen grains and depending on how badly the contemporary fossil pollen has been degraded, those recycled pollen types may, or may not be easily separated from the actual modern pollen rain at a given locale. If the recycled pollen grains cannot be distinguished from the modern pollen rain, the addition of recycled pollen may mask the true identity of an actual locale by producing a combined pollen spectrum quite different from the expected pollen print for that locale. Nevertheless, most skilled forensic palynologists with years of experience would not mistake most types of recycled pollen for contemporary pollen deposited by the local pollen rain.

There are several techniques palynologists have used to try to correctly identify fossilized recycled pollen in modern pollen samples. O'Rourke [9] tried to separate recently deposited pollen from recycled pollen by staining them with basic fuchsine. She found that the different layers in a pollen wall stain differently depending on their molecular structure. Modern pollen, she found, still contained the innermost cellulose layer in the pollen wall called the *intine*, which stained a light pink as opposed to the outer layers in the pollen wall that stained dark red. During her subsequent study of the pollen spectra from modern samples, she considered only the pollen still containing an intine as being part of the normal pollen rain; all other pollen grains that stained dark red were considered to be recycled pollen. That technique is useful in some situations but not others. For example; the destruction of a fresh pollen grain's cytoplasm and intine layer can occur very rapidly in warm and moist environments where oxidation rates are rapid. In cold and dry regions fresh pollen grains are slower to lose their cytoplasm and intine. Unless one knows for certain what environmental conditions

exist and how rapidly fresh pollen lose these aspects, this technique should be considered fairly unreliable. Likewise, the degree to which a pollen grain's wall will absorb stain, such as basic fuchsine or Safranin-O, and thus will appear as being lighter or darker depends on a number of factors including the thickness or the pollen wall, the percentage of the pollen wall that is composed of cellulose and protein molecules, and the amount of sporopollenin (a very durable substance composed of long-chains of carbon-based molecules that are similar to structure to carotenoids) present. Sporopollenin is a group of highly resistant organic molecules that are unique to various types of palynomorphs, including pollen and spores. In pollen and spores this molecule does not absorb stain but forms a latticework in the pollen and spore walls that help gives them shape, durability, and structure. As pollen and spores slowly degrade, the cellulose and protein molecules in the walls break down into compounds that no longer absorb stains. Eventually, degraded pollen and spores have very little cellulose and protein left and yet may maintain their shape due to the durable sporopollenin latticework remaining in their walls. When pollen and spores reach this point of degradation most will become very lightly stained or almost completely transparent even when immersed in pure stain. Because different pollen and spore taxa have different wall thicknesses and different proportions of cellulose, protein, and sporopollenin molecules in their outer walls, staining alone is not a reliable indicator of recycling. Different degrees of staining often reflect different levels of decay and recycling, but those differences might also reflect the innate differences found in the outer walls of various taxa of pollen or spores (Figure 1).

Another technique sometimes used to try to identify recycled or reworked pollen from modern examples is fluorescence microscopy [10]. The theory behind using both staining and fluorescence is the belief that recycled pollen and spores have different depositional histories than recently released pollen assemblage and thus will make the recycled grains appear as being different. What makes fluorescence perhaps a more useful technique for determining recycled pollen and spores is that pollen, spores, and other types of organic materials in different stages of preservation, or in different stages of carbonization, will emit light of varying intensity and wavelengths [11]. These differences can be detected under

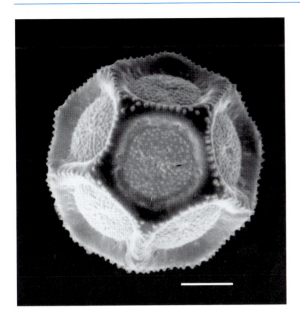

Figure 1 This is an SEM micrograph of *Alternanthera philoxeroides* (K. von Martius) A. Grisebach. This plant is in the Amaranthaceae plant family and the common name is alligator weed. The bar scale is 5 μm long [Courtesy of Gretchen D. Jones, Ph.D., & Ester F. Wilson, USDA-ARS, APMRU.]

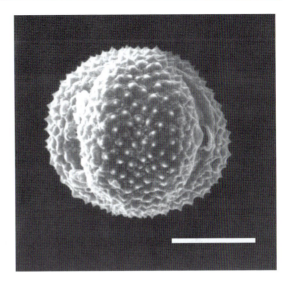

Figure 2 This is an SEM micrograph of *Artemisia californica* (Less). This plant is in the Arteraceae plant family and the common name is California sagebrush. The bar scale is 10 μm long [Courtesy of Gretchen D. Jones, Ph.D., & Ester F. Wilson, USDA-ARS, APMRU.]

ultraviolet light during fluorescence studies because those differences will give various pollen and spores different color hues.

Although differential staining and fluorescence microscopy has proven useful for some types of pollen studies, neither has helped us very much in forensic applications, thus there are reservations concerning their applicability in most forensic pollen work. In a laboratory experiment we conducted we "spiked" 18 000-year-old peat sediments collected from a subarctic environment with modern pollen from tropical plant taxa. Those combined samples were then processed using standard laboratory techniques for pollen recovery. After staining the recovered pollen and spores with Safranin-O, we found that only a few (less than 10%) of the added tropical pollen grains could be recognized strictly by differences in either staining or their fluorescence. In a similar study conducted in Arizona by Shellhorn *et al.* [12] they found that fluorescence microscopy did not help them separate modern surface pollen taxa from fossil pollen types known to be recycled from 20 000-year old deposits of the Wilcox Playa.

In forensic work we have found that a better guide to recycling seems to be the overall condition of the individual pollen grains and spores in a sample. Pollen samples recovered from crime scene locations in deserts, steppes, and semiarid regions where vegetation is usually minimal and where high winds are frequent, usually contain a wide variety of examples of degraded pollen and spores. The degrading process from those regions often produces grass pollen that is cracked, broken, crumpled, or shredded; pine and other types of bisaccate (conifer pollen types with a pair of air bladders to help keep them aloft after dispersion) pollen grains that usually have one or both bladders detached or broken and often are reduced to broken fragments of the main body of the pollen grain; and broken or fragmented parts of fragile pollen types such as the polyads (groups of individual pollen grains united into one large grain) of acacia (*Acacia*), and the inaperturate (pollen grains that lack any type of aperture) pollen grains produced by sedges (Cyperaceae), popular (*Populus*), cypress (*Cupressus*), and junipers (*Juniperus*) (Figures 1–10). The overall species composition of a pollen sample, the specific pollen types and the condition of the pollen in a sample can usually provide essential

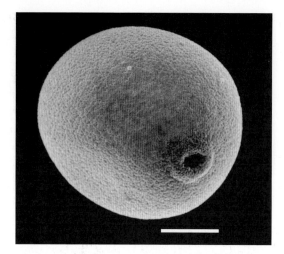

Figure 3 This is an SEM micrograph of *Arundinaria gigantea* (T. Walter) G. H. Muhlenberg. This plant is in the Poaceae plant family and the common name is giant southern cane. The bar scale is 10 μm long [Courtesy of Gretchen D. Jones, Ph.D., & Ester F. Wilson, USDA-ARS, APMRU.]

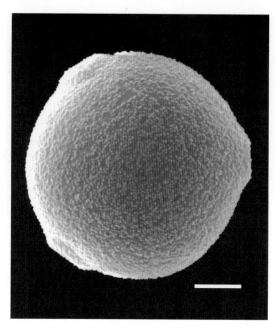

Figure 4 This is an SEM micrograph of *Cannabis sativa* (C. Linnaeus). This plant is in the Cannabaceae plant family and the common name is marijuana. The bar scale is 5 μm long [Courtesy of Gretchen D. Jones, Ph.D., & Ester F. Wilson, USDA-ARS, APMRU.]

clues about the ecology of a region where the sample originated as well as the degree and frequency of the recycling process. Once familiar with the types of potential degradation and overall appearance of pollen spectra from various types of environments, one can almost immediately determine, within broad parameters, whether the sample comes from an arid, semiarid, temperate, tropical, or arctic type of environment.

Collection and Extraction of Forensic Pollen Samples

Collection and extraction of forensic pollen and spore assemblages must be done with great care. If possible, the palynologist should be given access to a crime scene before other investigators arrive and begin collecting their samples. As a forensic specialist I realize that nearly "everyone" working a crime scene believes that they must be the first to visit the area. Nevertheless, the pollen and spore composition of the crime scene is extremely fragile and can easily be inadvertently altered, removed, or contaminated by the action of other forensic and crime scene investigators who also arrive to complete their own investigations. In addition, the use of

improper collection techniques and/or accidental contamination of collected materials may render a sample useless for forensic pollen use and will provide a basis for the dismissal of forensic pollen evidence in court (*see* **Error Rates in Forensic Methods**). Whenever possible, forensic pollen samples should be collected by a trained forensic palynologist or someone immanently familiar with proper collection protocol. This type of training generally comes from working with established professional forensic palynologists or gaining the basics from attending short courses on proper collection procedures. Collection by these types of specialists will ensure that the samples are collected correctly, that they remain contamination-free through all stages of storage, and that the samples will be processed and analyzed correctly. When forensic palynologists are present, others members of the crime scene investigation team should follow prescribed protocol to ensure that all forensic pollen samples are collected properly and that the samples remain contamination-free. In all cases, as with other forensic samples, it is essential to keep detailed and accurate records and pictures

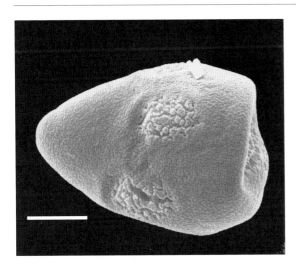

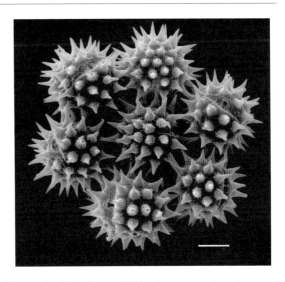

Figure 5 This is an SEM micrograph of *Carex microdonta* (J. Torrey & W. J. Hooker). This plant is in the Cyperaceae plant family and the common name is little-toothed Caric-sedge. The bar scale is 10 μm long [Courtesy of Gretchen D. Jones, Ph.D., & Ester F. Wilson, USDA-ARS, APMRU.]

Figure 7 This is an SEM micrograph of a cluster of seven pollen grains stuck together of *Helianthus annuus* (C. Linnaeus). These are in the Asteraceae plant family and the common name is common sunflower. The bar scale is 10 μm long [Courtesy of Gretchen D. Jones, Ph.D., & Ester F. Wilson, USDA-ARS, APMRU.]

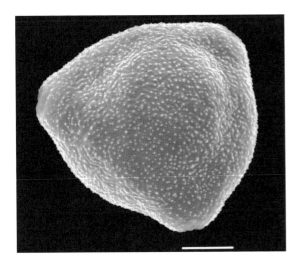

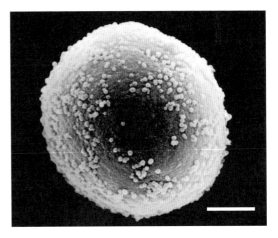

Figure 6 This is an SEM micrograph of *Corylus americana* (Walter). This plant is in the Corylaceae plant family and the common name is American hazelnut. The bar scale is 5 μm long [Courtesy of Gretchen D. Jones, Ph.D., & Ester F. Wilson, USDA-ARS, APMRU.]

Figure 8 This is an SEM micrograph of *Juniperus virginiana* (C. Linnaeus). This plant is in the Cupressaceae plant family and the common name is Virginia red cedar. The bar scale is 5 μm long [Courtesy of Gretchen D. Jones, Ph.D., & Ester F. Wilson, USDA-ARS, APMRU.]

of how and where each sample was collected, what happened to each sample from the time of collection until it is analyzed, and the security of all pollen evidence until reports are written or statements are

presented in court. If any hint of contamination, either natural or unintentional can be implied or proven, then doubt can be cast upon the resulting interpretations. Herein lays one of the greatest problems facing

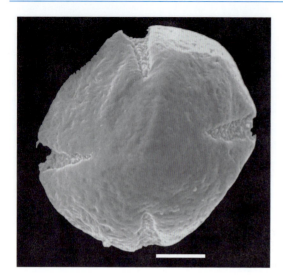

Figure 9 This is an SEM micrograph of *Melia azedarach* (C. Linnaeus). This plant is in the Meliaceae plant family and the common name is Chinaberry tree. The bar scale is 10 μm long [Courtesy of Gretchen D. Jones, Ph.D., & Ester F. Wilson, USDA-ARS, APMRU.]

forensic palynology. Because there are so few forensic palynologists, most crime scene pollen samples are collected by other people. Although most forensic personnel and other crime scene investigators can be trained to collect samples using proper protocol, and even though a crime scene photographer might take ample photographs, there are still other, subtle observations that only a trained forensic palynologist might notice as being important. Often the composition of the plant associations at and near the crime scene (*see* **Botany**), damage to individual plants, or evidence that someone brushed against a bush, or the presence of some exotic or unusual outcrop nearby each might become a vital clue when trying to understand and interpret the collected forensic pollen evidence from the crime scene or match pollen evidence collected from some suspect at a later time. These are reasons why, under ideal circumstances, the forensic palynologist should be present and should collect the samples.

An essential part of any forensic pollen investigation is the collection of control (also called *comparator*) samples. Control samples are samples of surface dirt, dust, fibers, or other materials at, near, or directly associated with a crime scene. The control samples are essential for any forensic pollen study because their pollen spectra provide a "baseline" of pollen information about the "expected pollen assemblage" from a specific object or the pollen print from a given

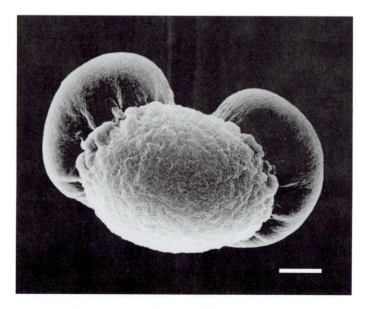

Figure 10 This is an SEM micrograph of *Pinus echinata* (P. Miller). This plant is in the Pinaceae plant family and the common name is short-leaf pine. The bar scale is 10 μm long [Courtesy of Gretchen D. Jones, Ph.D., & Ester F. Wilson, USDA-ARS, APMRU.]

crime scene or locale. Once the baseline of expected pollen data are determined from the various control samples, then the pollen recovered from a suspect or from forensic specimens thought to be associated with the object or crime scene can be compared against the control data to see if both match. One example involved a pollen control sample consisting of surface dirt collected from the ground where a sexual attack occurred. A forensic pollen study of the woman's soiled clothing matched the pollen types found in the control sample, confirming that she had been attacked at that location and had struggled with her assailant. Later, a suspect was identified and a search warrant revealed a soiled shirt and pants containing a pollen spectrum matching the control sample collected from the location where the sexual attack occurred. The pollen evidence alone did not confirm the suspect's guilt, but it did confirm he had been at that precise location, which was an area he said he had never visited.

Knowing how many control samples to collect from the scene of a crime is difficult. The more control samples one collects, and examines, the more pollen information one has about the locale where a crime was committed. Because the pollen spectrum in each control sample may vary slightly in reference to pollen types and percentages of each type, their combined spectra offer a potential range of pollen variation that can be expected for the actual crime scene. These types of data make matching the pollen results found on objects or suspects thought to be associated with a crime scene either convincing or obviously not similar. Not having enough or not having adequate control samples from a crime scene prevent a forensic palynologist from knowing what pollen types, and in what percentages, he or she should "expect" to find at the crime scene location. Without that knowledge, it becomes difficult to argue either for or against the confirmed association of the pollen assemblage found on a suspect's shoes, or car, or clothing, with the pollen types found at the actual crime scene.

Often a forensic palynologist has only a very small amount of material available for analysis. A few examples that I have examined in the past include the dust collected from the top of a table, a tissue wipe of the surface of a sandal, a piece of crumpled wire from some type of electrical device, a piece of electrical tape 3 cm long, one shoelace, a tiny piece of torn tissue no larger than a postage stamp, a sticky tape of dust collected from the dash of an vehicle, small tuffs of human hair from a body, the remains of a few bugs caught on the windscreen of a car, moths, honeybees, and a few pollen grains vacuumed from an item of clothing. Sometimes, when I have been fortunate, I could examine pollen trapped in a few specks of dirt trapped in the tread of a shoe or dirt caught in the carpet of a car. Once, the pollen recovered in the tiny bits of "fuzz" trapped in the bottom of the pockets of a pair of corduroy pants helped solve a murder case. There is almost no limit to what types of samples one can collect for potential use in forensic pollen studies. Nevertheless, often these types of samples create two major challenges for the forensic palynologist. First, there will rarely be enough material in a sample to try different extraction techniques. Second, there is rarely enough material to conduct a second test if something goes wrong during the initial pollen extraction and recovery process (e.g., centrifuge tube breaks, a beaker spills, a sample is dropped or accidentally mixed, a microscope slide breaks, etc.). For these reasons, the pollen extraction and recovery process must be conducted with the utmost care. In addition, in an effort to remove and concentrate the durable pollen and spores in forensic samples, it is generally necessary to destroy all of the nonpollen components. This means a sample's matrix will not be available later for other types of forensic testing. Studies of the DNA, trace elements, hairs and fibers present, or particles of dirt and sand in a forensic pollen sample must be conducted before pollen extraction occurs. Such studies, however, must be completed carefully and must not increase the risk of potential pollen contamination

Almost anything can be tested for forensic pollen. Dirt and dust trapped in almost any object often contain pollen and spores from the locale where the object originated. The following case illustrates this point. In New Zealand a man robbed a store and escaped on a motorcycle. Police gave chase and almost caught the thief, but at the last minute the thief abandoned his motorcycle and ran up a muddy hill and escaped into a wooded area. The next day a man reported that his motorcycle had been stolen the day before. When the claimant arrived to recover his motorcycle, the police realized he closely resembled the suspected thief. Armed with a search warrant, the police recovered a pair of muddy boots owned by the suspect. When asked about the mud, the suspect said that the mud came from the farm where he worked and denied that he has ever been in the area where his motorcycle had been abandoned. A forensic palynologist collected a series of control soil samples from areas on the farm where the suspect worked and examined them to obtain a pollen print of the farm region. Next, the palynologist collected a series of control soil samples from the muddy hill where the motorcycle had been abandoned and examined them for their pollen contents. Finally, after examining the pollen trapped in the mud on the suspect's boots, the palynologist could confidently say that the pollen assemblage matched the pollen print from the muddy hill, and not those of the control samples from the farm. This type of forensic sample discrimination between two or more different locales is one of the common ways in which pollen evidence is being used to aid in criminal investigations (*see* **Soil: Forensic Analysis**).

Almost any item of clothing becomes an ideal trap for pollen. Clothing made from wool, linen, and cotton are among the best pollen traps, while garments made of leather, nylon, rayon, and other types of materials often make good potential pollen traps. In a murder case from Australia a man killed his girlfriend and then drove her car 50 km to a remote coastal park where he then hid her body under some wattle (*Acacia*) brushes that had been planted to stabilize coastal dunes. After returning home he parked her car at her home and then thoroughly washed his clothing. Later, when he became a suspect, police collected items of his clothing and gave them to a forensic palynologist to examine. In spite of the suspect's attempt to thoroughly wash and clean his clothing, a few pollen grains from two different species of wattle bushes remained trapped on his clothing. Although one species of wattle plants were quite common in that region of Australia, the second species was not native and was imported to help stabilize coastal dunes. The imported species occurred only in the coastal park region but grew close to other native species of wattles. The trapped pollen from both species of wattle bushes had already been found in the victim's car and now both were also found on the suspect's clothing. Eventually, it emerged that the suspect had driven his estranged wife's car to the coastal crime scene where he hid her body under wattle bushes and also brushed against other species of native wattle bushes growing in the car parking area near the coast. Although the pollen evidence alone did not provide

proof that the suspect was the murderer, it did place him and his wife's car at the crime scene. In spite of his vigorous denial that he had not used his wife's car and had never visited to the coastal park, the pollen evidence placed him at the crime scene and helped to convict the suspect [13].

In a recent murder case, a young teenage girl, believed to be hitch hiking or a runaway, was killed in 1979 and left abandoned in a field with no identification. Her fingerprints were not on file and she was killed before DNA studies became routine in forensic work. Her identity remains a mystery even today and the murderer is still at large. However, nearly 30 years after her death, her clothing was thoroughly examined for traces of pollen and spores. Time had not degraded any of the pollen and spore evidence and wisely all of her clothing had been sealed in sterile containers and stored in a contamination-free environment for decades. On the basis of the forensic pollen studies in 2006, her identity could not be determined, but the pollen assemblage found in the pockets of her clothing and the inner lining of her jacket strongly suggested that she had very recently visited or had lived in a region more than 2000 miles west of the place where she was murdered. Among the pollen evidence recovered from her clothing were pollen grains from she oaks (*Casuarina*), which is a tree native to Australia and now grows only in restricted coastal areas of frost-free southern California and in similar regions in Southern Florida. These trees have never grown in New York because of winter freezes. In addition, it is highly improbable that even a single pollen grain from a she oak tree could have traveled 2000 miles from its source to the region of New York where the body was discovered. Other pollen from inside the murdered girl's pockets included species of spruce and birch that are common in the mountain flora of California, but do not grow in the region of New York where the body was discovered.

At the time of her death, authorities believed she was a local girl and thus searched only for missing person cases in the immediate vicinity of the crime scene. What made this case (one of the author's) interesting was how a rare combination of pollen can convincingly point to the victim's direct association with a distant region on the West Coast of the United States even though she had been murdered near the East Coast. This case also illustrates that if forensic samples are stored properly, decades later they can still reveal their pollen evidence [14]. At the time of this writing authorities are now searching the missing person records for the West Coast of the United States for the years of the late 1970s and early 1980s.

Vehicle air filters can also become good sources of forensic pollen evidence. Pollen evidence from vehicle air filters have been used to reconstruct the regions where the vehicle had traveled. A case from the 1980s, that illustrates this point occurred on the island of Oahu in Hawaii. A stolen van was used in a bank robbery in Honolulu and then abandoned only a few miles away. A forensic pollen study of the air filter in the van contained not only pollen types typically found in the city of Honolulu, but also unusual tropical pollen and spore types found only in the nearby Koolau Mountains in the center of the island of Oahu. Using the forensic pollen and spore evidence as intelligence information rather than direct evidence, Honolulu police began interviewing residents in the Koolau Mountain region. A grocery store worker remembered the van visiting his store on several occasions and later seeing the van parked near a small cabin in the area. That information led to the capture of the bank robbers who were hiding in the cabin until they could safely leave the island.

Human and other types of animal hair are ideal pollen traps for pollen from given locales [15]. Therefore, when a person or animal travels to another region and their hair is examined fairly soon after arrival, the analysis of the pollen still trapped in the hair would provide a pollen print of the previous, not the current location. This type of use for pollen data was applied to a murder case in Texas where it was hoped that forensic pollen studies of hair samples would provide a key to where five murdered women had lived. Hair samples collected from the five bodies of the unidentified women found buried in a series of shallow graves were examined for pollen in hopes that it might provide a clue as to where the women had lived before being murdered. Soil samples collected from the graves and from the surface soil in nearby areas of the pine forest provided the control samples and the "expected" pollen prints from that region. The recovered pollen assemblages from the women' hair were then compared to the pollen prints of the crime scene to find major pollen differences. As in the case with the murdered teenage girl, it was hoped that the forensic pollen samples might provide suggestions regarding where each of the women may have lived before

being killed. Authorities hoped that such information could help them search in the appropriate geographical regions for the identity of the missing women. Unfortunately, the recovered forensic pollen samples from the women's hair closely matched the pollen prints of the crime scene. This led to the suggestion that either the hair samples had become so contaminated by local pollen from the pine forest and from the soils in the grave site that it obscured any original potential pollen present, or perhaps all of the women came from areas of East Texas. Many areas in East Texas have pine forests and each area produces a fairly similar pollen print making it difficult to distinguish them apart. As of this time, those answers have not yet been resolved.

Like human hair, animal hairs are also excellent pollen traps. In New Zealand a rustler stole 300 sheep from a ranch and weeks later tried to sell them at a livestock auction. Although the sheep had no markings on them, the auctioneer became suspicious because he knew the seller was selling more sheep than the pastureland on his small ranch could support. The police were called in and they impounded the sheep. The original owner believed they "might" be his sheep, but had no proof so the police sheared a small patch of wool from the backs of several impounded sheep and sent them to a forensic palynologist for study. Control pollen samples were collected from sheep in both areas and also the surface soils in various locations on both the seller's and original owner's pasturelands. The pollen prints from each control sample was compared with the pollen assemblage recovered from the sheep's wool, which closely matched the control samples from the original owner's pasturelands. The thief complained that the pollen trapped in the sheep's wool had no relationship to pollen found in the surface soils of the two pastures. Countering this argument, the palynologist pointed out two important facts. First, the natural pollen rain in both regions would deposit airborne pollen on any surface in the pastures including the backs of sheep, the ground, or on the surface of several ponds and thus the pollen prints would indeed be similar. Second, there was a much different vegetational assemblage in and around each of the two pastures, which therefore produced very different types of pollen prints, as was noted in the pollen profiles of the various control samples. Thus, the pollen evidence proved critical in showing a clear discrimination between the expected pollen rain and pollen prints of each of the two different pasturelands. As a result, the sheep were returned to the original owner and the rustler was convicted and sent to prison [16].

A shipment of 500 g of cocaine hydrochloride was seized in New York City. A portion was sent to a forensic palynologist for analysis. In similar situations, previous examinations of illegal marijuana (*Cannabis*) seized in New Zealand had revealed two important clues. First, the pollen print recovered from the seized sample contained not only marijuana pollen but it also contained many pollen types indicating the plants had been grown in Asia and not at any location in New Zealand. Second, pollen studies of marijuana samples seized in different drug raids carried out in widely dispersed regions of New Zealand revealed that all the samples contained very similar pollen spectra. This indicated that the illegal marijuana seized in all the raids came from the same, large imported shipment originating in Asia. It also suggested that the marijuana was being distributed through a single distribution network. A similar type of reconstruction was attempted for the seized cocaine from New York. After processing the sample, the recovered pollen assemblage provided three important clues about the cocaine. First, some of the trapped pollen came from tropical plants that typically grow in regions of Bolivia and Colombia where coca plants are grown commercially. Those pollen types linked the origins of the cocaine to those regions of tropical South America. A second group of pollen grains recovered from the cocaine came from subalpine conifers including Canada hemlock (*Tsuga canadensis*) and jack pines (*Pinus banksiana*). These two species of conifers do not normally grow in the same habitat, but both are found growing together in only limited regions of Eastern Canada and the Northeastern US. Therefore, the occurrence of pollen from both of these conifer types in the same sample suggests the cocaine was smuggled into North America someplace in Eastern Canada or the Northeastern United States. Once in North America, the cocaine was apparently opened, and exposed to airborne pollen types while it was being "cut" with powered sugar to increase its value. If that had occurred in any other region, then both conifer pollen types would not have been present in the same cocaine sample. Finally, the remaining pollen found in the cocaine came from weeds and plants (composites, grasses, birch, goosefoot and pigweed, etc.) commonly found growing in vacant lots in the urban slums of New York City. It is suspected that when the cocaine reached New York City it was again opened and cut further before being packaged for distribution on the street. It was during that time that the cocaine was again exposed to airborne pollen, which then became trapped in the sample [17].

A European manufacturing company shipped a number of crates filled with expensive machinery to a company in Asia. The ship carrying the cargo stopped at a number of ports between Europe and its final destination in Asia. When the crates were opened at their destination in Asia, the machinery was gone and had been replaced by bags of soil of approximately the same weight. Since the ship had stopped at a number of ports it was unknown where the machinery had been stolen and replaced with dirt. An analysis of the dirt revealed a wide variety of pollen and spores that closely matched the pollen composition found in soil samples collected from the port area in Capetown, South Africa. Although the pollen analysis did not solve the question of who stole the machinery, it did suggest that the switch had occurred in Capetown, which was one of the more than a dozen potential ports where the theft could have occurred. Thus, the pollen identified the location and therefore narrowed the search for the missing machinery to only one location between the ship's departure in Europe and final arrival in Asia [16].

Pollen evidence has also been useful in helping to resolve details about events in the past (*see* **Length Measurement**; **Archaeology**; **Mass Grave Investigation**. In a recent example, a mass grave containing the remains of 32 young males was discovered in 1994, in Magdeburg, Germany. An examination of the bodies revealed that they had been shot, but the unanswered question was who did it. Bits of clothing and other evidence found with the bodies did not provide conclusive proof about who killed them. Two possibilities emerged. Some believed they were partisans who were captured and killed by the Nazi Gestapo in the spring of 1945 before the area was overrun by advancing Soviet troops. Others believed the Soviet Secret Police captured and then killed a number of Russian soldiers who refused to kill local German citizens who rioted in late summer of 1953 against Soviet rule. The nasal cavities of seven skulls were rinsed and the material was examined for trapped pollen. The pollen analysis revealed high amounts of pollen from plants that pollinate in the late summer, not plants that are spring pollinators. Comparisons of pollen types found in the dirt at the burial site confirmed that high levels of pollen from late summer blooming plants found in the nasal cavities must have been inhaled just prior to death and had not come from pollen in the dirt of the burial site. Thus, the pollen study confirmed that the victims probably died in late June or July, not during the spring and therefore were probably Russian soldiers killed by the Soviet Secret Police in the late summer of 1953 [18].

Summary

Although the use and application of forensic pollen studies are relatively new in many areas of the world, there is growing evidence that its use has a bright future. As more and more crime enforcement agencies become aware of the potential value of forensic pollen work, the need for trained personnel in the field will increase and will provide the emphasis needed to encourage the establishment of training centers for these specialists. Some countries and some law enforcement agencies are already aware of the value of pollen studies as a forensic technique and therefore conduct these studies routinely. In other countries pollen evidence is rarely collected at crime scenes and there appears to be little interest in using pollen for its potential forensic value. Perhaps one way to draw attention to this underutilized forensic tool is to briefly outline some of the important ways in which pollen evidence has already proven useful in helping to solve criminal and civil cases. Some of the crimes that pollen evidence has already helped to solve include instances involving homicide, terrorism, genocide, bombings, forgery, theft, rape, arson, counterfeiting, manufacturing and distribution of illegal drugs, assault, cases of hit and run, poaching, and identity theft.

Potentially, pollen evidence could be used to help resolve a wide range of circumstances associated with crime scene investigations. For example, pollen evidence could help relate a suspect to the scene of a crime, confirm that some item was associated with a crime scene or that some item left at a crime scene belonged to some suspect. Other types of information derived from pollen evidence might include proving or disproving a suspect's alibi, it might help narrow down a list of potential suspects to only one or two

individuals, it might help track the travel route of some item or suspect, or provide the geographical source of some item. In other circumstances, pollen evidence has proven useful in helping authorities find human remains and clandestine graves, determined the season or sometimes even the general time of death, and confirmed the illegal poaching of wild animals or the adulteration of commercial foods.

References

[1]   Mildenhall, D., Wiltshire, P.E. & Bryant, V.M. (2006). Forensic palynology: why do it and how it works, *Forensic Science International* **163**, 163–172.

[2]   Milne, L.A., Bryant, V.M., Mildenhall, D.C. & Coyle, H.M. eds, (2005). Forensic palynology, in *Forensic Botany. Principles and Applications to Criminal Casework*, CRC Press LLC, Boca Raton, FL, pp. 217–252.

[3]   Faegri, K., Kaland, P.E., Krzywinski, K., Faegri, K. & Iversen, J. eds (1989). *Textbook of Pollen Analysis*, 4th Edition, John Wiley and Sons, Chichester, p. 328.

[4]   Woodhouse, R.P. (1935). *Pollen Grains*, McGraw Hill, New York, p. 574.

[5]   Jackson, S.T. & Lyford, M.E. (1999). Pollen dispersal models in Quaternary plant ecology: assumptions, parameters, and prescriptions, *The Botanical Review* **65**(1), 39–75.

[6]   Horrocks, M. & Walsh, K.A. (1998). Forensic palynology: assessing the value of the evidence, *Review of Palaeobotany and Palynology* **103**, 69–74.

[7]   Wiltshire, P.E. (2006). Consideration of some taphonomic variables of relevance to forensic palynological investigations in the United Kingdom, *Forensic Science International* **163**, 173–182.

[8]   Erdtman, G. (1969). *Handbook of Palynology*, Hafner Publishing Co., New York, p. 486.

[9]   O'Rourke, M. (1990). Pollen reentrainment:contributions to the pollen rain in an arid environment, *Grana* **29**, 147–152.

[10]   Traverse, A. (2007). *Paleopalynology*, 2nd Edition, Springer, Dordrecht, p. 814.

[11]   Hunt, C.O., Rushworth, G. & Dykes, A.P. (2007). UV-fluorescence microscopy and the coherence of pollen assemblages in environmental archaeology and Quaternary geology, *Journal of Archaeological Science* **34**, 562–571.

[12]   Shellhorn, S.J., Hull, H.M., & Martin, P.S. (1964). Detection of fresh and fossil pollen with fluorochromes, *Nature* **202**, 315–316.

[13]   Milne, L.A. (2005). *A Grain of Truth: How Pollen Brought a Murderer to Justice*, Reed New Holland, Sydney, p. 175.

[14]   Associated Press (2006). http://www.iht.com/articles/ap/2006/10/03/america/NA_GEN_US_Cold_Case_Pollen.php.

[15] Wiltshire, P.E. (2006a). Hair as a source of forensic evidence in murder investigations, *Forensic Science International* **163**, 241–248.

[16] Bryant, V.M. & Mildenhall, D.C. (1998). Forensic palynology: a new way to catch crooks, in *New Developments in Palynomorph Sampling, Extraction and Analysis*, *American Association of Stratigraphic Palynologists, Contributions Series*, V.M. Bryant & J.H. Wrenn, eds, American Association of Stratigraphic Palynologists, Foundation, Dallas, Vol. 33, pp. 145–155.

[17] Stanley, E.A. (1992). Application of palynology to establish the provenance and travel history of illicit drugs, *Microscope* **40**, 149–152.

[18] Szibor, R., Schubert, C., Schöning, R., Kruse, D. & Wendt, U. (1998). Pollen analysis reveals murder season, *Nature* **395**(6701), 449–450.

VAUGHN M. BRYANT

Paper Analysis

Introduction

Writing and printing papers are largely composed of bleached botanical fiber and mineral fillers to which can be added fluorescent whitening agents (FWAs) to enhance the whiteness of the paper or organic dyes to make papers of different colors. The purpose of the fiber is to form a bright contrasting flat surface to which darker inks, pigments, and toners can be applied. Fillers (usually in the form of finely ground calcium carbonate or various mineral clays) are also added to increase sheet opacity and improve the printing or writing surface. Modern printing papers (and much less commonly writing papers) may also have a coating, comprising calcium carbonate and/or clay, and/or titanium dioxide mixed with an organic polymer binder on one, or more frequently both sides of the sheet.

This article deals mainly with A4 and A3 copy papers, bond papers, and standard US Letter "A" paper, as these papers are now the most common hardcopy medium for commercial, legal, and personal communication. The principles, practices, and tools discussed below can be applied to all samples of paper, paperboard, ("cardboard" in common parlance) and fiber-based packaging materials.

Ever since monetary, commercial, and legal transactions have been committed to paper they have been subject to fabrication and fraud. Sometimes spurious documents remain in currency undetected but at other times, for various reasons, they fall under suspicion. A few examples among many are the fabrication of whole documents which are backdated, fabrication of company documents, minutes and receipts, fabrication of wills, fabrication of certificates and academic qualifications, and the manufacture of spurious historical documents.

Often fraudulent documents are exposed by discrepancies or inconsistencies in their written content (i.e., structure of signatures, dates appended, poorly composed letterheads, logos, etc.) and sometimes by the chemistry of the inks, pigments, and toners employed in their manufacture. For instance, the printing technologies with which the ink is applied, or the chemistry of the ink or toner itself can demonstrate that the document in question is either inconsistent with the purported date, or the period in which an undated document is represented to have been written or printed. These areas fall within the realm of the document examiner, ink and printing expert, and forensic chemist.

Another useful technique in exposing fraud is the field of "paper and fiber analysis" in which the paper on which the document is written can be characterized and differentiated from properly validated samples. Paper properties, both physical and botanical, although outwardly similar in appearance to the layman, can be, and often are, distinctly individual to a particular hemisphere, country, company, and even papermaking machine.

In the course of any investigation, the paper is first characterized for a range of physical properties which include basis weight or mass per unit area (commonly called *grammage* in countries using the metric system of measurement), caliper (or apparent thickness), sheet density, filler content, filler type, paper chemistry, direction of cut, etc. After these initial tests are completed, a small but representative portion of the paper can be mechanically broken down and dispersed into a dilute aqueous suspension of individual fibers. A few milliliters of this dilute suspension is placed on a standard microscope slide, dried, stained, and then examined under low magnification ($\times 40$ or $\times 100$) to determine paper or fiber "furnish". Fiber furnish is basically the particular combination of pulp types, or the "pulp recipe", a papermaker, or individual paper mill uses to create a particular grade of paper.

"Fiber furnish analysis" can be a powerful tool. In essence, it is the identification of the various pulp types found in a particular sheet of paper and the determination of the ratio in which they occur. The technique can be further refined by identifying the various plant species from which the fibers derive. This latter identification, in combination with the other factors, is very useful in determining the possible origin (or, conversely, rendering that it came from a particular country or source highly improbable) with regard to hemisphere and region, and sometimes even country, company, and mill, depending on the depth of industrial knowledge of the forensic analyst. As in most aspects of forensic analysis, great care should be exercised when drawing conclusions and some common pitfalls will be detailed later.

Even if the origin of a sample of paper cannot be established, it is often just as important to determine whether the paper used in a document is consistent with similar material emanating from the same government body, public company, or private premises at the time the document was alleged to have been produced. Also, if there is a belief that a particular page has subsequently been appended to the front or back, or inserted within the body of a document, the page in question can be analyzed and compared with those adjoining. Paper examination can also be useful in such circumstances when, for example, narrowing down possible origins of a ransom note. If the paper on which the note is written is of an unusual type, and it cannot be differentiated from the remains of an open ream or loose sheets found at the suspect's premises, these findings could add weight to circumstantial evidence against the suspect.

It is fortunate for forensic science that technology and manufacturing processes are in a constant state of flux as commercial companies are either trying to improve their product or make changes to it to maintain a competitive edge. These changes, and knowledge of when they were made, are an invaluable tool in determining the legitimacy or otherwise of certain articles. The same is true within the paper industry and knowing the manufacturing history within various geographic regions, countries, and companies within these countries, is of great advantage to the forensic examiner.

To an industry outsider, however, it is almost a matter of impossibility to keep track of all these

changes so it is very useful for the analyst to maintain strong links with the key personnel within a country or locality's paper industry. It is also important for the paper analyst to regularly examine locally produced, "off the shelf" paper products in order to keep familiar with these changes. When purchasing photocopy or bond papers for examination, it is always useful to retain the ream wrapper (outer packaging) as it also contains much useful information together with a dozen or so sheets of the content as a growing archive. Apart from obvious general information such as country of origin, company, brand, grade, grammage, etc., wrappers often carry a discretely positioned inkjet printed company code that can inform the manufacturer when, and at what mill and on what machine, the paper was manufactured.

Most paper companies retain a history of when various manufacturing changes take place and, for their own protection, usually retain (often for many years) a swatch of "out-turn" paper sheets sampled from every commercial machine roll of paper produced. In the case of criminal investigations, most companies will willingly assist in providing samples for comparison with police evidence.

As a considerable quantity of paper is traded internationally and individual grades from a single paper machine can be packaged in a dozen, or more ream wraps for large volume purchasers (so-called home brand papers) the archive kept by each analyst can become very valuable in determining that a particular sheet of paper could have been produced, for example, in an Indonesian paper mill and purchased at a large retail office stationary chain in the United States in a given year. A year later the same US stationary chain might well be purchasing its "home brand" copy paper from a mill in China, or Thailand, or Finland, depending on the market price fluctuations.

Some Notes of Papermaking and Paper Testing

Paper is made by a formula of raw materials, set by individual paper mills, depending on the desired performance qualities required in the end product. The inclusion of certain raw materials is also governed by availability and price. As already stated, paper is largely composed of botanical fiber, be it softwood (gymnosperm) fiber, hardwood (angiosperm) fiber, Gramineae fiber (grass fiber such as that derived from cereal straw, sugar cane, or bamboo), or other plant materials such as cotton, cotton linter fiber, or (rarely) fiber extracted from more exotic sources, such as the paper mulberry tree. The common factor between the vast majority of botanical fibers used in the papermaking process is that they are derived from the modified cell walls of elongated structural cells (i.e., fibers). Adventitiously, smaller quantities of other nonfibrous types of plant cells, such as vessel cells and ray cells will also be included with the fibers. Broadly speaking, all plant cells used in papermaking are largely composed of cellulose. In the living plant (and in some types of paper), these cellulose structures are impregnated with, and tightly bonded to adjoining cells with two organic bipolymers known as *hemicellulose* and *lignin*.

Fibers are extracted or freed (prepared) from the plant matrix by various chemical and mechanical means. These processes, particularly the chemical processes, are designed to liberate individual fibers from the plant material by dissolving or making soluble the lignin component that bonds the cellulose and hemicellulose materials together. Chemical pulps, as the name implies, are prepared by "cooking" the raw plant material in a chemical cocktail (usually weak acids or strong alkalis) at elevated temperature and pressure to facilitate the transformation of lignin into water-soluble products that can be separated from the fibers by washing. Often 50% or more of the original plant material is lost during this procedure but a very strong and flexible fiber, ideal for later use in writing and printing papers, is produced. In the case of most printing and writing papers (excluding newsprint and many cheaper magazine and catalog papers – see below) the freed fiber or pulp has to be further chemically treated by bleaching to remove the last traces of lignin giving the desired whiteness.

In contrast, heat in combination with various mechanical processes is also employed by the paper industry to separate the fibers from the wood matrix. These "thermomechanical" processes leave most of the lignin *in situ* around and within the fiber. The lignin can be made almost colorless in a second processing stage using oxidizing chemicals, such as hydrogen peroxide, however, this change is not permanent and the paper will start to show the yellow–brown color of unoxidized lignin after a period of days to months depending on the conditions of storage. Therefore, pulps produced via these latter thermomechanical methods are usually not used in

high-quality writing or printing papers, but form the basis of many ephemeral products, such as newspaper and cheaper magazines and leaflet/catalog grade papers as they tend to form a weak sheet and "yellow" rapidly in sunlight. The main advantage of such papers is their lower cost of production stemming from the fact that almost twice the quantity of mechanical grade paper can be made from each tonne of wood, compared to chemical or "wood-free" papers. The most prevalent of these pulping processes, and their importance to the paper and fiber analyst, will be gone into more detail later. Combinations of smaller amounts of chemical processing with heat and mechanical energy are also used to produce the so-called chemimechanical and chemithermomechanical pulps and papers.

Physical Properties of Paper

As already mentioned, when characterizing a sheet of paper, it is not only the composition of the sheet that is important but also the paper's physical properties. For evidence to hold up in a legal enquiry, it must be demonstrated that, as far as physically possible, the paper from a document has been tested scientifically, and according to the accepted standard test methods. Like most other manufacturing industries, the paper industry globally has a recognized system of standard pulp and paper test methods that are overseen and continually reviewed by a number of industry-related organizations; a selection of these being the Scandinavian Pulp and Paper Association (SCAN), the US Technical Association of the Pulp and Paper Industry (TAPPI), and the Australian Pulp and Paper Industry Technical Association (APPITA). Many of these methods refer back to fundamental ISO standard methods.

Industry methods usually specify the minimum number of tests and the minimum area or number of sheets from which these tests must be taken (e.g., for grammage of photocopy paper, 10 individual measurements must be derived from 10 individual A4 sheets selected from specified positions throughout the ream). A common handicap for the paper and fiber analyst, however, is that there is usually only a very limited amount of sample to work with (often a single page) and the police or investigating body are often loathe to let it out of their hands, leave alone have part of it irretrievably destroyed for the purposes of testing. In these cases, the analyst can only stick to the standard as close as possible, taking note of where deviations from the method occur, and the reasons why, for later inclusion in their report. Physical test results derived from limited sample should be treated as indicative only.

Further information in this article is presented in three sections; Some Basic Paper Properties, Fiber Analysis Using Light Microscopy & Fibre Sources for the Paper Industry.

Some Basic Paper Properties

For standard test methods for measuring the physical and chemical properties of paper and paperboard samples, readers are recommended to contact the national standard setting organizations in their respective countries. For convenience, some standards specified by TAPPI (North America) are provided in the Reference Section at the end of this article.

Moisture Absorbent Properties of Paper/Paper Conditioning Prior to Testing

One important property of paper is its moisture content. All commonly encountered paper sheets absorb between 5 and 12% of moisture from air depending on the ambient relative humidity and an equilibrium exists between water absorbed and the vapor in the atmosphere in contact with the paper, so water is an integral part of the sheet [1].

The amount of moisture a paper carries can significantly affect properties such as sheet weight, thickness, tensile and tearing strength, and optical properties such as brightness and opacity. Therefore, for results generated by one laboratory, to be comparable with those generated by another, paper and paperboard products are tested under strictly controlled atmospheric conditions. The International Organization for Standardization (ISO) standard environmental conditions for paper testing are as follows: relative humidity $50 \pm 2\%$ and temperature $23 \pm 1\,^{\circ}\text{C}$.

Most paper strength properties show hysteresis behavior with respect to moisture content, so it is important that papers are dried in an atmosphere at 25% relative humidity at $25\,^{\circ}\text{C}$ before being allowed to equilibrate under the atmospheric conditions specified by ISO prior to testing. "Conditioning" as this equilibrium is called, usually takes 24 h and sometimes longer if the paper or board sample is coated, exceptionally compact or thick.

Anisotropic Properties of Paper

Commercially made papers are anisotropic materials, meaning that almost all physical properties differ depending on the direction in which the measurement is made within the plane of the sheet. Papermakers often refer to paper as having a "grain" that will generally run along the longer axis of the rectangular sheet (long grain) or less commonly along the perpendicular shorter axis of the sheet (short grain).

The anisotropy of the sheet results from the process by which paper is manufactured. A dilute suspension of pulp fibers in water together with any mineral filler particles and chemical such as sizing agents, filler retention aids, and FWAs are dewatered on a revolving fine mesh forming fabric (commonly called a *wire*) moving at speeds that can range from $100\,\text{m}\,\text{min}^{-1}$ on machines making heavier basis weight paperboards to $2000\,\text{m}\,\text{min}^{-1}$ for lighter weight papers, such as newsprint. The continuous wire rotates around two drive metal cylinders that rotate about an axis that runs from the back of the machine to the front – the so-called cross direction (CD) of the machine. The axis that is perpendicular to the CD that runs longitudinally parallel to the length of the machine is called the *machine direction* (MD) – this is the direction in which the paper is formed. The fluid dynamics that applies to the fiber suspension as it impacts the forming fabric causes the majority of the fibers to align in the "MD". Some directional-dependant paper properties are tensile strength (greater in the MD), stretch (greater in the CD), tearing strength (greater is the CD), and paper stiffness (greater in the MD).

When reels of office papers are slit and cut into A4 or quarto sheets, the long direction of the sheet is usually aligned in the MD. Occasionally, however, certain photocopy and bond papers are found where the MD of the paper is orientated across the short dimension of the A4 sheet. "Direction of cut" is usually decided on the basis of which cut will minimize the "trim" (paper that must be deliberately cut from the front and back edges of the machine reel in order to guarantee an acceptably straight smooth edge on every sheet). Given that the cross directional width of the forming fabric (the "deckle width") is fixed at the time the machine is built, the minimum trim wasted will be achieved when either the MD or the CD dimension of the cut sheet is an integral factor of the trim width of the machine. "Direction of cut" is sometimes useful in distinguishing a sheet made on one machine from a very similar sheet made on another machine (perhaps in a different mill) with a different deckle width.

For the sake of completeness, it should be noted that the remaining axis of the paper sheet that is orthogonal to both the MD and the CD is referred to as the *Z direction* (ZD).

Paper has many physical properties that are routinely measured by the manufacturer against either internal specifications or those specified by the mill's customers. The suite of tests is chosen depending on the ultimate end use. For the purpose of characterizing photocopy, bond and security papers, the forensic scientist would initially be interested in the following:

- sheet dimensions (metric, American or Imperial);
- grammage (basis weight);
- caliper (thickness);
- sheet density (calculated from sheet dimensions, grammage, and caliper);
- basic paper chemistry (is the sheet acid sized with a pH between 3.5 and 4.5, neutral sized with a pH between 6 and 6.5 or "alkaline" sized with a pH between 7.0 and 7.5 – "permanent paper")
- filler content and type;
- ISO brightness, opacity, and CIE color coordinates (L* a* and b*); and
- fluorescent properties under UV light (FWA content).

Photocopy and Bond Paper – Standard Paper Dimensions

The nominal dimensions of an A4 sheet are 297 mm × 210 mm *(L × W)* and an A3 sheet, 420 mm × 297 mm. These dimensions are governed by the ratio 1 : $\sqrt{2}$ or 1 : 1.414 such that sheets of diminishing sizes in the A series (and the B series) decrease by 50% in area in going from A1 to A2 and from A3 to A4, so there is zero wastage when the paper is cut to standard sizes.

Using this principle, two A5 sheets cut from a "long grain" A4 sheet will be 210 mm long × 148.5 mm wide and will be "cross grain". To elaborate on this discussion is beyond the scope of this article but an excellent explanation titled "International standard paper sizes" is given at the Internet site http://www.cl.cam.ac.uk/~mgk25/iso-paper.html. The purpose of discussing sheet

dimensions here is to state that, for various reasons, sheets are not always cut exactly to these dimensions, and because a typical writing paper can expand and contract by up to 4% in the CD and 1.5% in the MD as the moisture content goes from 12 to 5%, the length and width of the conditioned sheet must be accurately remeasured after conditioning.

Grammage (Basis Weight)

In countries using the metric system of measurement, a basic property of paper is "grammage" or the weight of the sheet in grams per square meter (gsm). General use photocopy paper is usually manufactured to a grammage specification of 80 gsm but cheaper A4 "draft papers" are often made to lighter grammages (e.g., 65 and 70 gsm). Higher quality specialty printing and bond papers can have specific grammages in the 90–120 gsm range [2].

Continental North America runs to a different system. The dimensions of a standard US Letter "A" Paper (commonly used in North American homes and offices) is 11 in. × 8.5 in. or 280 mm × 216 mm. The basis weight of US Letter paper can range from 16 lb to 24 pounds (lb).[a] An explanation of the American paper basis weight system is also given at the above quoted website but a simpler explanation can be found under "Weights & Sizes of Paper" at http://www.inkjetart.com/weight.html.

Calculation of Paper Grammage for an A4 sheet – An Example.   Area of an A4 sheet = 62 370 mm² (i.e., length by width in millimeters, assuming the dimensions of the conditioned sheet are 210 mm × 297 mm). This is equivalent to 0.06237 m².

Factor (No. of A4 sheets per square meter) = 1 m²/0.06237 m² = 16.03

For this example, the conditioned weight of a single A4 page was found to be 4.97 g.

Therefore 4.97 g × 16.03 = 79.7 gsm.

Some notes on Grammage.   Grammage with regard to copy and bond paper will not give the forensic investigator much information in itself as all paper manufacturers strive to produce paper within a certain grammage specification (e.g., copy paper with a nominal grammage of 80 gsm may have a product/manufacturing specification "Aim" grammage of 79.5 gsm with an "upper control limit" of 80.7 gsm and a "lower control limit" of 78.5 gsm. Often manufacturers will endeavor to run the machine in the lower portion of the product range but keep within specification. A small saving in raw materials over each production run can result in large cost savings annually. Copy and bond paper is sold by area, not by weight – each ream containing normally 500 sheets (31.2 m^2 of paper), but sometimes 750 or 1000 sheets in "economy reams". On modern paper machines, grammage between sheets should not vary by >2%.

The importance of grammage is in the later calculation of sheet density. Every paper machine is unique. Despite, in this instance, copy paper being made to a nominal grammage of 80 gsm, depending on the pulp type, the amount of mechanical work done to the pulp (refining), filler content, calendering, and other machine parameters, thickness, and sheet density may vary significantly. If the authenticity of a page from a particular document is under suspicion, and its caliper and density differ significantly from measurements on other pages in the document, the discrepancy often warrants further investigation.

Sheet Thickness – Single or Bulking Thickness

Often a document examiner has only the document at hand to examine and, as already mentioned, the document may constitute a single sheet or even a fragment of a single sheet. Bulking thickness, determined on a stack of 10 sheets, is the preferred method when sufficient sample is available. Determination of thickness on a single sheet should be treated as a sighter measurement only. Determination of thickness, like grammage, should be done on fully conditioned sheets. Single sheet thickness or caliper is measured using a specialized "dead weight" paper micrometer fitted with a wide diameter foot (16 mm) to compensate for the paper's inherent surface variability. The dead-weight pressure between the two measuring platens must be 100 kPa ± 10. The weighted foot should rest on the paper's surface for at least 2 s and no greater than 5 s before a reading is taken. For writing and printing papers, as with most other papers, thickness is recorded in micrometers. Readings should be evenly spaced over the CD of the sheet as this is the direction of greater variability. "Apparent thickness" is what is actually measured, not true average thickness (refer to *TAPPI test method*) [3].

Apparent Sheet Density

Sheet or paper density can be determined by calculation using the grammage and thickness data obtained. Paper density is usually quoted as kilogram per cubic meter. There are many different ways to calculate the sheet density. One format is given below.

Consider a stack of sheets cut into squares measuring 1 m × 1 m. If the sheets are neatly stacked one atop another until they reach a height of 1 m they would take up a volume of 1 m^3.

Calculation. Each sheet being a meter square would weigh 79.7 g or 0.0797 kg. (see previous calculation). For the purpose of this example, 20 individual thickness measurements for the sample gave an average caliper of 104 μm.

The apparent volume of each sheet is therefore $1 \times 1 \times 0.00104$ m^3.

Therefore apparent density = mass per unit apparent volume = 0.0797 kg/0.00104 m^3 = 766.3 kg m^{-3}

Wire and Felt Marks

One final and potentially useful characteristic for confirming that two samples of paper came from the same ream when all the other analyses point to this being highly likely is the characterization of the subtle indentations left on the surface of many office, printing and writing papers by the forming fabric (or "machine wire"), and/or the drying felts on the paper machine. These markings can be made visible by very low angle illumination (typically 5–°10) and image capture using a low magnification (typically × 10) microscope, followed by contrast enhancement using image analysis software.

If a fast Fourier transform is performed on the enhanced image, and then all sections of the transformed pattern are deleted and the pattern "reverse transformed", a useful image of the particular weave pattern used in making the forming fabric is often obtained. If the weave pattern obtained from the evidentiary document (e.g., a ransom note) is identical to the weave pattern from samples of paper taken from the suspect's home, or office, and all other features of the sample are identical, this is fairly strong evidence that the paper sheets are from the same ream.

If, alternatively, the weave patterns are not identical, caution must be exercised. Nonidentity of the weave patterns does not necessarily mean that the sheets are not from the same ream as five to six different machine rolls (made at different times on the same machine when the machine was "clothed" using forming fabrics of different weaves) may have been cut simultaneously to produce the ream of cut sheets. In a case where the first sheet from the ream gives a different pattern, it would be necessary to examine up to six sequential sheets from the ream in order to determine whether all the rolls that were sliced and cut to produce the ream have the same nonidentical weave pattern. In the event that all the six weave patterns from the sequential sheets taken from the ream are identical, but different to the evidentiary sample, then it can be concluded that the evidentiary sample is not from that source. The way in which common A4 (or US Letter) sheets are cut and compiled into reams involves cutting and sheeting between four and six machine rolls simultaneously in the same sequence.

To take a specific example, if mill personnel had taken six machine rolls from the reel store of which five rolls were made between October and December when the machine was clothed with a forming fabric with the weave pattern "A" and one roll was made in, say, January (following a holiday maintenance shut when the old forming fabric was replaced with a new forming fabric having a weave pattern "B"), then the sheets in the ream when subjected to image analysis above would show the sequence . . . A,A,B,A,A,A,A,A,B,A,A,A,A,A,B,A,A, . . . and so on, repeating this pattern with one sheet of pattern B separated by five sheets of pattern A down through the ream. If the identity of the mill that produced the paper is known and accessible, consultation with the mill staff will be a useful way of confirming how the reams from that mill are normally made up and whether or not there were changes made to the machine fabrics during the period in question.

An Introduction to Paper Chemistry

Major chemical properties of paper are also important in characterizing samples of paper. One of the quickest and simplest chemical tests is the pH of the sizing agent used when the paper was manufactured. A "pH pen" (a felt-tipped pen filled with an aqueous solution of pH indicator dye, phenol red) will produce a yellow spot on older "acid sized" papers and a violet spot on more modern "alkaline sized" sheets (i.e., 7.0–7.5 pH). Although convenient, the results of this simple test can be difficult to interpret if the paper has

been sized with a modified "neutral" rosin size with a pH between 6.0 and 6.5 when a grayish color results. More certain data is obtained using TAPPI methods T509 and T435, or American Society for Testing and Materials ASTM D778.

Most commercial office, printing and writing grade papers contain mineral fillers in quantities up to 25% of the mass of the paper. Most alkaline sized papers (paper sized with the synthetic chemicals alkyl ketene dimer (AKD) or alkenyl succinyl anhydride (ASA)) will usually contain calcium carbonate as a filler, whereas the most common filler in acid sized (using emulsions made from natural softwood rosin soaps precipitated onto the fibers using aluminum sulfate) and neutral sized (using chemically modified rosin soaps and aluminum sulfate) papers is kaolin. Talc, calcium sulfate, barium sulfate, and titanium dioxide are also used as fillers but much less commonly. Paper made from de-inked recycled fiber will usually contain a mixture of many mineral pigments.

If the paper contains calcium carbonate, bubbles of carbon dioxide will form if a drop of dilute hydrochloric acid is placed on the surface. The amount of calcium carbonate present can be determined by ashing a portion of the sheet in a muffle furnace at $520°C$ and taking note of the weight of the ash obtained. The same sample is then further heated to $925°C$ to drive off carbon dioxide after which it is again weighed. The calculation of how much carbonate (as equivalent $CaCO_3$) was present in the original sample can be determined by simple stoichiometry. The mineral content of the residual ash can then be further analyzed using electron dispersive spectroscopy. Access to a scanning electron microscope can be invaluable in fully characterizing papers.

The presence of fluorescent whitening agents (FWAs), less correctly called *optical brightening agents* (OBAs) can be established by examining the paper sample under a UV light source in the 350–390 nm wavelength range. The paper will fluoresce if FWA's have been used during manufacture. More definitive results can be obtained by measuring ISO Brightness using one of the many light and colour measuring instruments now available. This is achieved by measuring the paper's brightness with the UV filter absent, and then present, in the incident light beam. By subtracting the former value from the latter, a measure of fluorescence can be obtained.

Most office papers also contain cooked starch to impart strength to the surface of the sheet. Spreading a few drops of dilute iodine solution in aqueous potassium iodide on the surface will confirm the presence of starch by the appearance of a characteristic but transient blue-black color.

Fiber Analysis Using Light Microscopy

Fiber Analysis

As previously mentioned, "fiber analysis" is the technique of breaking down a representative portion of a sheet of paper into its individual fibrous and nonfibrous cellular components, dispersing the resultant dilute suspension on a microscope slide and then drying and staining the fiber for microscopic analysis [4–9].

The cellular components are examined from two perspectives; firstly, to determine pulp types (and the proportion of each type in the total furnish) and secondly, the identification of the various wood or nonwood species represented in the furnish. Species from which the fibers derive can be identified by their morphology (i.e., shape and structure) and pulp types can be determined by the way individual fibers react to, or take up, chemical stain. The reaction to a particular stain is very much influenced by the chemical processes employed in producing or treating the raw plant material to produce the particular papermaking pulp.

It is impossible to cover the subject of fiber analysis in detail within this article but a full and broad understanding of the techniques can be gained from the above listed the standard methods sighted in the Reference Section. Distinguishing fibers from different trees, for example, is not a skill that can be picked up immediately and it often takes many years of gaining experience examining fibers from well-documented sources before a fiber analyst can feel fully competent in his or her abilities.

The fiber analyst's main tool is a binocular compound light microscope fitted with a mechanical stage and Abbe condenser capable of making observations at ×40, ×100, and ×400. Higher magnification is of no advantage. One eyepiece should be fitted with a crosshair. A multistation tally counter, similar to that used to count blood cells, is also required.

Briefly, in the course of an analysis, the investigator would prepare two or more representative slides.

After staining and the application of a cover slip, a few minutes should be allowed before observing to allow let the stain develop. It is recommended that the investigator first scan the slide at ×40 to gain a general feel for the pulp types and species represented. Only then should they increase the magnification to ×100 to make a formal analysis.

The analysis would start by the investigator moving to the top left or right hand corner of the cover slip, and moving vertically down the slide – by means of moving the mechanical stage – record each fiber passed over by the crosshair, taking note of its pulp type and whether it is a softwood, hardwood, or nonwood fiber. Each fiber and its pulp category must be immediately registered on the multistation tally counter and the traverse continued. When the investigator reaches the bottom of the cover slip the slide should be moved a few mm across and the traverse continued in the opposite direction until the cover slip has been fully examined. This process is continued until at least 800 fibers are counted. During or after the count, the individual species encountered should be noted for later inclusion in the investigator's report, if relevant. Sometimes, in species identification, ×400 is used to clarify species by allowing closer examination of microstructure (e.g., hardwood vessel elements or softwood crossray pitting).

Fiber or Pulp Weighting

It will be obvious to the observer that not all fiber types are the same with regard to length and cross-sectional area and, if the proportion of each fiber type is to be reported as a weighted percent of the total, a weight factor must be applied. A list of generic weight factors for various pulp types and species is given in the right hand column of Table 1 – but it is recommended that each fiber analyst further refine these factors by calibrating their own observations against manufactured "dummy" furnish samples of known composition. It is also recommended that the analyst regularly cross-check their observations against those of other analysts. Between trained analysts, the weighted results obtained for each fiber type should not vary by more then 3%.

An example of a typical fiber analysis report compiled by the author is given in Figure 1. In this particular instant, the report pertains to a customer complaint where the printing company thought they were using paper from a local manufacturer but

Table 1 Stain reaction and weight factor for various fiber types

Pulp type	Norval–Wilson stain resultant color	Graff C stain resultant color	Fiber weighting
Unbleached chemical hardwood (kraft and soda pulp)	Dark or navy blue through to pink	Dark or navy blue through to pink	0.4
Bleached chemical hardwood (kraft and soda pulp)	Dark or navy blue through to pink	Dark or navy blue through to pink	0.4
Unbleached sulfite softwood pulp	Light brown	Usually yellow	1.0
Bleached sulfite softwood pulp	Lavender	Purplish blue	0.9
Unbleached kraft softwood pulp	Brown	Yellow to brownish yellow	1.0
Bleached kraft softwood pulp	Bluish gray	Blue to gray	0.9
Semichemical hardwood pulp	Khaki green to yellow brown	Brownish orange	0.6
Thermomechanical softwood pulp	Golden yellow	Bright yellow	1.7
Bleached chemi-thermomechanical softwood pulp	Copper brown	–	1.6
Cereal straw	Green to blue	Greenish yellow to greenish blue	0.4
Rag/linen/cotton	Pink	Red to pink	1.0
Jute/manila	–	Yellow orange	0.6
Esparto	–	Blue	0.5

were actually using an imported grade. Details of the various parties involved have been changed in order to maintain commercial confidentiality. An example of how fiber is weighted and calculated as a percent of the total is shown in the table included in the Figure 1 report. The reader will also note that the weight factors used by the analyst differ from the generic weight factors. These have been refined through trial and error to correlate with the author's own observations.

Fiber Sources for the Paper Industry

Common fiber sources used in the paper industry are categorized as wood fibers and nonwood fibers.

Wood Fibers – Two Types. *Gymnosperms (i.e., Wood Fibers from Coniferous (Cone Bearing) Trees).* Some examples of families of coniferous trees used commercially are pine, fir, spruce, cedar, larch, and hemlock. Conifers are often referred to as *softwoods.* Softwoods produce "long-fibered" pulp and are ideal where high tearing strength is required in the paper (e.g., paper sacks and bags). Addition of small percentages of long-fiber pulps also provide wet strength to office, printing, and writing papers (that are made mainly from short hardwood fibers (see below)) so

that manufacture and converting operations can be carried out at higher line speeds. Depending on the species, average fiber length can range from 2 to 7 mm but most species fall within the 2–4 mm range with a wide distribution of lengths present within almost all the samples of fiber. Softwood fibers are called *tracheids.* Their function is to provide both mechanical support and the conduction of fluids.

Angiosperms (Flowering Plants). Angiosperms produce flowers and fruit and have a more complex and specialized vascular structure within their woody tissue. In the case of trees, angiosperms include both deciduous and evergreen examples. Angiosperm trees are generally referred to as *hardwoods* because of the normally higher density of their woody tissue compared to woods derived from most gymnosperm trees. Some examples of angiosperm tree families are elm, maple, alder, birch, poplar, eucalyptus, acacia, dipterocarps, and other tropical hardwoods.

Hardwoods produce "short-fiber" pulps. Average fiber length ranges from 0.7–1.5 mm depending on the species, with again a wide distribution of lengths being present in almost all samples observed. Hardwood fibers have a narrow diameter (typically 10–50 µm), compared with softwoods fibers and lack pits in their walls. Hardwood fibers (referred to as

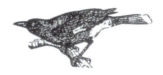

CURRAWONG PAPER TEST LABORATORIES
Test Report

1st November 2007

To:	Mr. Kevin Kraft	Austral Paper Co. 6 Ream Road Papercut, Victoria, Australia, 3999
From:	John Murphy	Currawong Paper Test Laboratories
cc:	Mr. Peter Parchment	Austral Paper Co.

Subject: Fibre Analysis Report
Emporium Sales Catalogue

An Emporium Pre-Christmas Sale brochure (valid from Wednesday Dec. 8th until Sunday Dec. 19th, 2007) which manifested unacceptable levels of print mottle has been subjected to examination by optical microscopy in order to determine whether the paper on which it was printed is Australian product, or otherwise. The results of this investigation are given below.

Fiber Class	Chemical Hardwood*	Chemical Softwood#	Semi-Chem. Hardwood$	Mechanical Softwood**	Total
Fiber Count	12	328	444	61	845
Factor	×0.33	×1.0	×0.6	×1.8	
Weighted Factor	4	328	266	110	708
%	<1 (Trace)	46	38	16	~100

* Chemical Hardwood Component – Birch (Exclusively)
\# Chemical Softwood Component – Scot's pine (in the majority) & Norway Spruce (in the minority).
$ Semi-chem. Hardwood Component – Aspen (Exclusively)
** Mechanical Softwood Component (TMP) – Norway Spruce

Fibre Analysis according to AS/NZS 1301-451rp using Norval-Wilson stain.
Date analysed – 31.10.2007

Conclusion: The paper used to produce this brochure <u>is not</u> Australian made. The mix of species noted in the paper's furnish point strongly towards a European origin.

John Murphy
<u>Research Scientist – Currawong Paper Test Laboratories</u>

Figure 1   A typical fiber analysis report recommercial claim

libriform fibers) are ideal for producing printing and writing papers as they form a very flat, uniform, smooth surface.

Nonwoods (Angiosperms that Include Grasses and Shrubby Plants). The stems from wheat, rice, sugar cane, bamboo, papyrus, kenaf, sisal, jute, hemp, flax and the bolls, and the seed coat (linters) from cotton are all used to make paper in countries that lack adequate forest resources.

For the purposes of papermaking, nonwood fibers can be broadly broken down into "bast fibers" (from the outer tissues of the stems of sisal, jute, hemp, and flax plants) and Graminaceae (grass) fibers. Graminaceous fibers can be further broken down into cereal straw fibers (e.g., wheat, oats, and rice) and noncereal stems (e.g., reed, bamboo, and sugarcane (bagasse)).

Cotton, collected from the cotton boll and seedpod coverings of the cotton plant, falls into a category of its own. Cotton as a papermaking fiber is very much in decline, except for use in specialty writing papers, surgical tissues, and laboratory filter papers.

An excellent resource for the fiber analyst is a publication from the *Springer Series in Wood Science* titled *Fiber Atlas, Identification of Papermaking Fibers* by Marja-Sisko Ilvessalo-Pfäffli ([10]/ISBN 3-540-55392-4). This publication gives a thorough description of fiber morphology for species identification.

Common Pulp Types

The four most common pulp types employed in the paper industry today are chemical hardwood pulp (kraft or sulfite pulping process), chemical softwood pulp (kraft or sulfite pulping process), semichemical hardwood pulp (pulping processes using mechanical and heat energy with small quantities of chemicals), and thermomechanical softwood pulp (pulping processes using a combination of heat and mechanical energy and no chemicals (other than water)).

Other pulp types less commonly used in developed countries in recent years are "soda pulp" (chemical) and "groundwood" (mechanical).

1. Kraft process (also known as the *sulfate process*). Woodchips are cooked using NaOH and Na_2S in water at $170°C$ and 8 atm. This process takes place in alkaline conditions and produces very strong pulps used for both packaging and writing papers (kraft is German for strength). Extensive chemical processing is followed by minimal mechanical processing. If the pulp is going to be used to produce photocopy/printing/writing papers pulping is followed by a multistage bleaching process that can be based on chlorine, chlorine dioxide (elemental chlorine free (ECF)), or ozone and hydrogen peroxide (totally chlorine free (TCF)) that dissolve the last traces of brown-colored lignin.

2. In sulfite cooking the "cooking liquor" a mixture of water, calcium, or magnesium bisulfite (referred to as *combined SO$_2$*) and free SO_2 in excess. The excess SO_2 reacts with water to form sulfurous acid and therefore the cooking is acidic in nature. This process is also conducted at $170°C$ and pressure in excess of 8 atm and produces a very light-colored pulp with high opacity that is relatively low in strength compared to kraft pulp. Extensive chemical processing is followed by minimal mechanical processing. If the pulp is going to be used to produce photocopy, printing, or writing papers, it is followed by a similar multistage bleaching process to that used to bleach kraft pulps.

3. The semichemical method involves treatment of woodchips with lower quantities of either sodium sulfite (at pH 7–9) or sodium hydroxide at pH 12 followed by considerable mechanical processing. Cheaper to produce than full chemical pulps, bleached chemi-thermomechanical hardwood pulps (BCTMP) are sometimes added to lower quality writing papers to increase opacity and bulk.

4. To make thermomechanical pulps (TMP) softwood chips are pretreated with steam and then broken down into fiber by extensive mechanical processing. Comparatively the pulp is low cost to produce and is used in ephemeral products such as newspapers, magazines, junk mail, low cost paper back books, and writing pads. TMP has comparatively low-strength properties and readily yellows when exposed to sunlight and other light sources containing UV wavelengths.

5. Soda pulp is produced by cooking wood chips using sodium hydroxide in water as the sole chemical agent. As with sulfate and sulfite pulps, lignin removal is achieved at elevated temperatures and pressures.

6. Groundwood pulping is achieved by pressing whole logs against a heavily burred rotating grindstone.

Fiber Staining

The most common microscopy stain used for plant fiber identification is Norval–Wilson stain. Another useful stain is Graff C. Norval–Wilson and Graff C stain termed as *differential* stains. They are capable of staining different classes of fiber with different diagnostic colors depending on the chemical or mechanical processes utilized to produce them as shown in Table 1.

Softwood Identification

As stated earlier, softwood fibers are called *tracheids* and provide both mechanical support for a plant and also act as a conduit for the conduction of fluids to all the living parts of the plant. Fluids are transferred from fiber to fiber via "pits" in the tracheid wall. These pits act as valves to prevent the flow of liquids reversing. Basically there are two types of pitting. "Bordered pits", which convey fluid from tracheid to tracheid in an axial direction, and "crossray" pits, which convey fluids throughout the plant in a transverse direction. The structure of crossray pitting is particularly useful in identifying the species. "Spiral thickenings" can also help to identify species, as in the case of the commonly utilized softwood fiber from the Douglas fir (*Pseudotsuga menziesii*). See *Fiber Atlas, Identification of Papermaking Fibers,* referred to in section 2.3, or a similar publication.

Hardwood Identification

Hardwoods, and in fact all angiosperms, use fibers for structural support and use an auxiliary specialized vascular system for the conduction of fluids. These conduits, called *vessels*, are made up of smaller units or "vessel elements" which act in a similar fashion to man-made water conduit pipes laid end to end. These vessel elements are separated during the pulping process but remain mixed with the fibers in the pulp after the pulping and bleaching process. Fortunately for the fiber microscopist, vessel elements have very distinctive morphology depending on genus, and can be readily utilized to identify the various species of angiosperm present in a paper's furnish. See *Fiber Atlas, Identification of Papermaking Fibers* referred to in **Fiber Sources for the Paper Industry** section, or similar publication.

Comments on Indigenous and Exotic Species

Tree and other plant species can help identify the continent and sometimes country of origin of a paper sample. This, however, is becoming increasingly more difficult as plantations of various exotic species are becoming evermore prominent in paper-producing countries far from the regions in which they occur as natives. For example Spain, Portugal, South Africa, South America (and now, Southeast Asia) grow substantial plantation stands of eucalyptus for papermaking. This genus was once only indigenous to Australia and parts of New Guinea. One species, *Eucalyptus deglupta* is also native to the Celebes and the Philippines. It is worth noting that some species that were formerly classified within the genus *Eucalyptus* have recently been separated into a new genus, *Corymbia* by taxonomists, while retaining their specific names. *Corymbia maculate maculate* (spotted gum) and *Corymbia maculate citriodera* (lemon-scented gum) are the only two Corymbia species that may rarely find their way into commercially produced papers and neither species is cultivated in plantations as a papermaking resource.

The Monterey pine (*Pinus radiata*), originally native to a very confined region of the west coast of the United States, is now grown widely in Australia, New Zealand, South Africa, South America, and countries surrounding the Mediterranean. Outside its country of origin, it is a very fast growing tree and an ideal wood pulp resource. The same is true for Douglas fir, which can be found in plantation in Britain, Portugal, central Europe, and New Zealand.

Further Notes on Fiber Furnish

Identification of paper can sometimes be further refined by measuring the proportion, or percent, of different fiber types in a paper furnish (provided the paper manufacturing specifications are known). An example is given below.

Although bleached hardwood is the ideal raw material for the manufacture of photocopy paper, paper manufacturers in the southern hemisphere and tropics add a small portion of bleached softwood to improve wet strength and speed of manufacture, and to also add dry strength for converting and cutting process (i.e., roll to ream). Until recent decades, there was insufficient capacity for producing bleached softwood fiber in the southern hemisphere (although Brazil, Chile, and New Zealand now have substantial output) and in countries such as Australia, for instance, that still import all their bleached softwood requirements, this material is an expensive impost. Most bleached softwood pulp arriving in Australia comes directly from New Zealand, Canada, and the United States but ever-increasing amounts are sourced from other regions such as Brazil and Chile depending on quality, availability, and price. As the imported softwood pulp is comparatively expensive, machine operators try to keep this component of the furnish down to 10 or 15% of the total fiber furnish (for an 80 gsm sheet). Indonesia, on more modern paper machines, can run with softwood concentrations as low as 1–3%. Information such as this can be very useful to the fiber analyst in identifying likely country of origin.

Recycled Fiber

A point of caution when examining paper furnish is to be certain that the paper does not contain recycled de-inked bleached fiber as this will greatly obscure the country of origin and could cause the analyst to reach quite misleading conclusions. To determine whether a paper contains recycled fiber or only virgin stock, it is good practice to first examine the intact sheet under ×10 magnification using a stereo (binocular) microscope to pick up any signs of debris on the surface. The debris could be in the form of ink particles, toner particles, unbleached fiber or minute globules of adhesives (called *stickies*). Valid conclusions from such an examination will be made increasingly difficult if the sample has become soiled or dirty during the suspected or alleged criminal activity.

Acknowledgment

The author would like to gratefully acknowledge the assistance, guidance, and technical input of Dr Warwick D. Raverty, CSIRO Forest Biosciences, Bayview Avenue Clayton Victoria 3168, Australia.

End Notes

[a.] Approximate conversion from lbs (pounds per 100 square feet of paper) to gsm:

- 16 lb ~ 60.2 gsm
- 18 lb ~ 67.9 gsm
- 20 lb ~ 75.2 gsm
- 24 lb ~ 90.3 gsm.

References

[1] TAPPI Method T402 2003. *Standard Conditioning & Testing Atmospheres for Paper, Board & Pulp Handsheets and Related Product.*
[2] TAPPI Method T410 2002. *Grammage of Paper & Paperboard – Weight per Unit Area.*
[3] TAPPI Method T411 2005. *Thickness (Caliper) of Paper, Paperboard & Combined Board.*
[4] ISO Method 9184/1-3 1990. *Paper, Board & Pulps – Fiber Furnish Analysis.*
[5] ISO Method 9184/2 1990. *Paper, Board & Pulps – Fiber Furnish Analysis Part 2: Staining Guide.*
[6] TAPPI Method T401 2003. *Fiber Analysis of Paper & Paperboard.*
[7] TAPPI Method T263 2002. *Identification of Wood & Fibers from Conifers.*
[8] TAPPI Method T259 2005. *Species Identification of Nonwood Plant Fibers.*
[9] ASTM D1030 1999. *Standard Test Method for Fiber Analysis of Paper & Paperboard.*
[10] Ilvessalo-Pfäffli, M.-S. (1995). *Fiber Atlas, Identification of Papermaking Fibers Springer Series in Wood Science,* ISBN 3-540-55392-4.

Further Reading

McDonald, R.G. & Franklin, J.N. (eds) (1969). *The Pulping of Wood,* McGraw Hill Book Company, Vol. 1, Library of Congress Catalog Card Number 68-20994.
Browning, B.L. (1977). *Analysis of Paper',* 2nd Edition, Marcel Dekker, New York, 1977 ISBN 0-8247-6408-0.

JOHN P. MURPHY

Paraphilia *see* Sex Offenders: Treatment of

Parental Alienation

History of Parental Alienation

In the context of divorce, the pathological alignment of a parent and a child resulting in the child's rejection of the alienated parent was originally described by Wallerstein and Kelly (1977, 1980). Gardner (1987) [3] later introduced the term, *parental alienation syndrome*, to describe a diagnosable disorder occurring in the context of separation and divorce. Although Gardner contributed a good deal by describing the features of parental alienation, his work has been criticized because of his use of the word, "syndrome". Almost all mental health professionals who work with children of divorce agree that the phenomenon occurs, that is, children of high-conflict divorces sometimes gravitate to one side of the conflict and view that parent as totally good and the other parent as totally bad, all without a good cause. However, many professionals who work in this area do not refer to this phenomenon as a syndrome. Thus far, parental alienation syndrome or disorder has not been adopted into the *Diagnostic and Statistical Manual of Mental Disorders*. Most professionals in the family law setting – including judges, lawyers, and custody evaluators – simply refer to *parental alienation* and do not use the term, *parental alienation syndrome*.

Role of the Evaluator

Often the family law court is faced with a situation where a child is rejecting a parent. Sometimes the child is refusing to spend time with the parent, and sometimes the child is alleging that the parent is emotionally, physically, or sexually abusive. The rejection could be mild ("I just don't want to spend a lot of time with him.") or sizable ("I never want to see him again.")

There are three main reasons for a child's rejection of a parent: (i) The accused parent is indeed abusive and the child's rejection is appropriate and understandable. This is *not* considered parental alienation. (ii) The aligned parent (or another person) is responsible for the child's rejection of the other parent. This may result in parental alienation. (iii) The child is rejecting the alienated parent for the child's own inappropriate reason, despite the efforts of the nonalienated parent to support the relationship between the child and the alienated parent. This may also be called *parental alienation*.

Faced with the situation of a child who is rejecting a parent, the reason for the rejection may be obvious to the court. For example, the hated parent may have a long history of abusing the child, documented by child protective service investigations and/or admissions of abuse by the parent. At other times, the court may be convinced that the aligned parent is responsible for the parental alienation, for example, if there is clear proof to that effect. In these cases – when the cause of the child's rejection is obvious to the court – the court may not order an expert to evaluate the family for parental alienation. The court will base its conclusions and orders on these certain, proved reasons for the rejection.

Much of the time, however, the court is not certain. The aligned parent's argument that the alienated parent is abusive is persuasive, as is the alienated parent's assertion that the aligned parent is behind the alienation. The court may decide that an evaluator should interview the child, in the hope that the result of the interview will provide enough information to resolve the issue. The child interviewer often will inform the court about the content of the interview and provide an opinion regarding the believability of the child's statements. Sometimes, the court believes that the issues are too complex for a child interview to elucidate the truth and orders a full custody evaluation.

In some jurisdictions, there are other possibilities for the court to secure the truth. In Los Angeles, for example, the court can order a limited or "solution-focused evaluation". This involves a court evaluator's speaking to both parents and the child individually, observing the parent–child relationships, interviewing collaterals, and reviewing records, all in the short time frame of one morning. In the afternoon, the evaluator testifies to his or her opinion.

Occasionally, the alienated parent and attorney believe that they can persuade the judge by retaining an expert to opine after performing a limited investigation. For example, the expert would review records, interview collaterals, or interview the alienated parent and then, based on this limited information, render an opinion. Sometimes, the expert's opinions are helpful for clarifying the issue, despite the opposing side's argument that the retained expert's opinion is biased.

Experts performing these tasks need to limit their opinions as they have not performed an entire custody evaluation (*see* **Visitation Rights**).

Aligned Parents' Contributions to Parental Alienation

An aligned parent's behaviors may have contributed to the child's stance of refusing visitation. The aligned parent may have repeatedly expressed extremely negative views to the child such as, "She never wanted you", "He is a horrible mean man", or "He is an adulterer and caused the divorce"! Alternatively, the aligned parent's criticism may not be so overt. The criticism may merely contain innuendos that the alienated parent is dangerous: "Call me immediately if he tries to hurt you."

The aligned parent may contribute in other ways to the child's refusal of the alienated parent. For example, the aligned parent may tell the child that the other parent did not call, when the parent had. The aligned parent might discard letters from the other parent to the child. The aligned parent may not inform the alienated parent about school events important to the child, such as back-to-school nights and school performances. The rejected parent's parenting and personality flaws may be exaggerated and continuously discussed with the child. The aligned parent may praise the child ("That's right. Stand up for yourself.") when the child criticizes the other parent, and scorn the child when the child compliments the rejected parent ("You don't know what you're talking about. He's not smart at all.").

Sometimes the parent may cause the child's alienation from the other parent, but has not done so on purpose. For instance, the mother may be an anxious person who is unaware that she is communicating her anxiety to the child. She may start crying or be noticeably worried when the child leaves for visitation, but insist that the child should go and "have a good time". Similarly, a child may be so concerned about the depressed parent that the child feels that he or she needs to provide emotional support to that parent instead of going on the visitation with the other parent. The continuous drumbeat of negative statements, whether direct or indirect, and actions by whatever method may cause the child to adopt the aligned parent's negative feelings and reject the other parent.

Child's Contribution to Parental Alienation

Despite a parent's best efforts to support the other parent's relationship with the child, sometimes the child alienates an otherwise appropriate parent for no good reason.

Oppositional Child

The child may be oppositional and defiant and reject the parent who does not succumb to the child's demands. He or she may choose the parent who is least restrictive and vehemently reject the rule-setting parent.

Worried Child

The child may be worried after the departure and loss of the nonresidential parent, so the child becomes fearful that he or she is also going to lose the remaining residential parent as well. As a result, the child experiences an attachment to the residential parent that is greatly exaggerated, and fears separation from that parent.

Stubborn Child

Although the child has a good attachment to both parents, the child may be very upset that they have separated and divorced. That is, the child is upset (for example, sad, angry, resentful, worried) about the situation and doesn't want to participate in the process. The child expresses his or her feelings by objecting vehemently and stubbornly to the visitation, even though ordinarily he or she enjoys being with the other parent.

Child Escaping Conflict

Finally, there is a common psychological mechanism – cognitive dissonance – through which the child's affections can become extremely polarized. Specifically, the child's intense like of one parent and dislike of the other becomes his or her way of resolving the psychological tension that he or she experiences. For example, if the mother and father have been actively and visibly fighting with each other, the child would experience cognitive dissonance when trying to have affection for both of them at the same time. The child is unable to reconcile two dissonant thoughts, "My mother is right" and "My father is right". The dissonance creates a tension in the child's mind, which is resolved by believing that he or she loves one parent and hates the other.

Other Alienators' Contributions to Parental Alienation

At times, the alienating party is a person other than one of the parents. That is, despite one parent's actively supporting the relationship between the other parent and the child, another person is actively indoctrinating the child against the other parent. The alienator could be a grandparent, stepparent, girlfriend, boyfriend, or even a sibling. The reasons for the alienation are diverse: a grandparent may be seeking revenge against the parent who left his or her child; a stepparent may be worried that the child will see the parent as a "real parent" and the stepparent as some unimportant figure; or perhaps a sibling may be trying to punish the parent who "caused" the divorce.

Court Orders for Treatment of Parental Alienation

Family court orders for a fractured parent/child relationship should match the reason for the relationship problems.

If the parent is truly abusive and the child's rejection is justified, the family court may order the parent to participate in parenting classes or enact other orders aimed at rehabilitating the abusive parent. The court will likely order any visitation to be monitored until the parent shows that he or she will behave appropriately. Therapy for the child should include the following components: supporting the child for having been abused ("What a difficult thing that you went through. You did not deserve to be abused."); teaching the child how to stay safe in the presence of the parent ("If he ever hits you again, call me immediately."); and education ("Not all authority figures are abusive."). Conjoint therapy involving the child and the abusive parent may help them reestablishing a healthy and mutually satisfying relationship.

If an alienating parent is found to be a source for the child's rejection of an appropriate parent, the court's approach varies. If the alienation is severe,

the court may order that the child's time with the alienating parent be limited and monitored. If the child is refusing to live with the alienated parent and the court fears that the child may run away or hurt the alienated parent, the court may order the child to live with a third party until therapy corrects the situation. At times, in extreme circumstances (suicidality, running away, poor school performance, or delinquent behavior), the court may order that the child be placed in a residential facility.

In cases where the alienation is not very severe, the court may order therapy without removing the child from the alienating parent's custody. The ordered therapy may include "reunification therapy". The role of the therapist is to aid in building a better relationship with the alienated parent ("Tell me about a good time you had with your father."). Occasionally, the reunification therapist may choose to bring the alienating parent into therapy. The alienating parent may also be ordered into individual therapy. The individual therapy for the alienating parent should include education about the damaging effects of parental alienation on the child and the consequences of alienating behavior within the legal system ("The judge will never allow unmonitored visitation if you continue criticizing the mother in front of the child."). The therapist should monitor for alienating behavior and express praise when the alienating behavior is improving ("I spoke to the monitor and she says that you are doing a great job at not criticizing the father in front of the child."). The therapist should also express disappointment if the alienating behavior continues ("The letter you wrote your child stating 'your dad is a jerk' was inappropriate. I know you can do better."). The individual therapist should speak with the conjoint therapist and with others, so that alienating behavior can be promptly addressed. Both the conjoint therapist and the individual therapist may be asked to provide updates to the court regarding progress so that custody and visitation orders can be modified. An individual therapist for the child may be ordered by the court as well.

If the child is alienating a parent even though the favored parent is supporting the alienated parent's relationship, the focus of the therapy should be to stop this oppositional behavior. The child should be confronted with his manipulative ways and told that the behavior should stop. He should not be rewarded for refusing visitation; he should be disciplined. If the child cannot be forced to have visitation, his privileges should be withdrawn. Behavior such as making false allegations should be similarly punished. The individual and conjoint therapists may be ordered to accomplish these treatment goals. Residential treatment may be ordered in special circumstances.

One of the important treatment goals in circumstances of alienation is for the child to learn proper conflict management skills. Prior to terminating therapy, the child should experience that it is unacceptable to lie, vilify, and reject those with who they are in conflict, especially loved ones.

References

[1] Bernet, W. & Ash, D. (2007). *Children of Divorce: A Practical Guide for Parents, Therapists, Attorneys, and Judges*, 2nd Edition, Kreiger, Malabar.

[2] Garrity, C.B. & Baris, M.A. (1994). *Caught in the Middle: Protecting the Children of High-Conflict Divorce*, Lexington Books, New York.

[3] Gardner, R. (1992). *The Parental Alienation Syndrome*. Creative Therapeutics, Cresskill.

[4] Gardner, R. (2001). *Therapeutic Interventions for Children with Parental Alienation Syndrome*. Creative Therapeutics, Cresskill.

[5] Gardner, R., Sauber, S.R. & Lorandos, D. (2006). *The International Handbook of Parental Alienation Syndrome: Conceptual, Clinical and Legal Considerations*, Charles C. Thomas, Springfield.

JOSEPH KENAN AND WILLIAM BERNET

Parental Rights and Prerogatives

Introduction: Parent, Child, and State

Parental possession and exercise of rights concerning their children must be understood in context. The rights of parents, the rights of children, and the interests of the state form a triangle. Laws affecting the parent–child relationship reflect the three legs of this triangle. The sources of such laws include the United States Constitution and the legislative, executive, and judicial branches of the federal and of state governments. Traditionally the states, as opposed to the federal government, are the primary source of law concerning families and there is considerable variation in statutes, regulations, and case law (court decisions) among states. Therefore, a forensic expert should not assume that, for example, laws defining sexual abuse or a parental duty to provide health care are exactly the same in every state; rather, the expert should take steps to inform him or herself about the law of the state where the expert is asked to work. Experts should also be aware that a state constitution may provide parents or children with rights beyond those guaranteed under the federal constitution, and that these rights will be enforced by that state's courts.

The parent–child relationship itself is the source of both parental rights and duties. A parent has the right to custody and companionship of his or her child – and a corresponding duty to provide the child with care and support. Generally, under the United States (federal) Constitution, a parent has a fundamental right to raise a child as the parent sees fit. The parent may exercise rights and prerogatives (and the law will defer to the parent) up to the point where there is actual harm or a substantial risk of harm to the child. At that point the state can intervene and impose restrictions upon the parent and child relationship.[a]

Thus, for example, the state can make education compulsory for children between certain ages (typically 6 to 16). It can enforce this requirement by prosecuting at criminal law parents who do not send their child to school. It can also act through the juvenile justice system against children of school age who are truant – whether or not the parent knows of or condones the truancy. However, the parent has a constitutional right to choose for the child's education a public or private school, or alternative types of education such as homeschooling.[b] The child does not have the legal right to choose how or where he or she will be educated. However, the state's interest in educating children and the child's interest in being educated are enforced by state curriculum and record-keeping regulations, which nonpublic schools, including homeschools, must satisfy.[c]

Similarly, parents have the right to give or deny their children permission to engage in paid labor. However, the state has power to limit the types of work, hours, and conditions under which children can be employed.[d] And although traditionally parents were entitled to their children's wages, state and federal laws now impose trustee obligations on parents of child entertainers, athletes, models, etc. to manage and preserve the earnings for the benefit of the child.[e]

Parents have a "privilege" to use "reasonable, nonexcessive force" to discipline their children, including using physical restraint and corporal punishment. "Privilege" means that the parent has a right to do something to the child (confinement, infliction of pain) that would be otherwise be unlawful. The parent may delegate the privilege to a third party (a baby-sitter, a private school teacher) but cannot authorize any action that would exceed the scope of parent's own privilege. The privilege only applies to "reasonable, nonexcessive force". The state can act to prosecute criminally a person whose punishment of the child exceeds the scope of that privilege, can find the child abused under dependency court protection, or permit the minor through a legal representative to sue the person at civil law (in tort) for battery.[f]

The state's authority to do all this derives from two sources: the police power and the state's role as *parens patriae*. Under police power, the state can act to protect the child from harm and to protect the community from danger caused by the parent and possibly the child: for example, through criminal laws against child abuse and the juvenile justice system for children who commit acts that would be crimes if the minors were adults. *Parens patriae* means the state is acting as a parent. Under this source of authority, the state can use law to encourage and help parents carry out their duties of care and support, and to provide for and protect children whose parents are unable or unwilling to do so. Citing the special vulnerability of minors, states invoke *parens patriae* to justify individual laws such as special curfews for minors,[g] as well as dependency court jurisdiction over abused, neglected, or abandoned children.[h]

Juvenile Justice System

Juvenile justice courts generally have jurisdiction over three categories of children: those who have committed offenses which would be crimes if committed by adults (delinquents); those who have committed offenses that were against the law only because of the status of being a child (status offenders); and those who have been abandoned, abused, or neglected by their parents or guardians (dependent or neglected children). The juvenile justice system is a civil rather than a criminal one, and uses a distinctive terminology reflecting its original nonpunitive, rehabilitative

purpose.[i] In the adult criminal justice system, the state files charges alleging that the defendant committed a crime; the case title reads "State (or Commonwealth) versus Name, Defendant". By contrast, in a juvenile delinquency, status offense, or dependency case, the state files a petition "in the matter of [first name and initial], a minor". The subject of the petition is referred to as *the minor*, rather than *the defendant*, and the petition contains not "charges" but reasons why the minor should be taken under the court's jurisdiction: the minor is a delinquent, the minor is a status offender, the minor is dependent or neglected. The court does not find the minor "guilty" or "not guilty" in delinquency or status offender cases, but rather sustains or denies the petition for jurisdiction. The hearing at which the court does this is called *an adjudication* rather than a trial. If the petition is sustained (that is, the court finds jurisdiction over the minor), the next step is "disposition" rather than "sentencing" of the minor. If the petition is denied, the case is dismissed. Similarly, in dependency cases the court does not find the minor's parent or parents "guilty" of abuse or neglect – rather it does or does not find the minor to be abused, neglected, or dependent. Only if the court sustains the dependency petition can it proceed to disposition and impose restrictions on the parent–child relationship up to and including termination of parental rights.

Delinquency

Under state codes, "delinquent" acts generally include the full range of behaviors considered criminal for adults, from minor crimes (misdemeanors) such as petty theft or disturbing the peace, to major crimes (felonies) such as robbery, rape, and murder.

The US Supreme Court has ruled that children who are the subject of delinquency petitions have the fifth amendment constitutional right against self-incrimination (also known as *the right to remain silent*) and the sixth amendment right to the assistance of an attorney (at state expense if the child is indigent)[j] Moreover, the state has to prove each element of the alleged delinquency beyond a reasonable doubt – the same standard of proof required in adult criminal cases.[k]

Minors alleged to be delinquent have most of the same rights to due process as are provided to adults in criminal proceedings, with two exceptions. Minors do not have the right to bail, nor the right to a jury trial.[l]

Dispositions in delinquency cases may range from "home on probation" to placement in "boot camps" or "group homes" to confinement in secure state youth facilities barely distinguishable from adult prisons. In most states, the maximum age for persons over whom the juvenile court has jurisdiction is 18 years. The age of jurisdiction refers to the age of the juvenile at the time the offense was committed. In the great majority of delinquency cases, the disposition imposed will end when the minor turns 18. However, for extremely serious offenses (such as murder) a juvenile may remain under the court's authority until age 21 or even 25, serving the years after age 18 in the adult prison system.[m]

Every state's juvenile justice system provides for some minors to be tried in adult court. Some state laws permit the district attorney to file charges directly in adult court when minors above a stated age are accused of a serious crime. Most states begin the case in juvenile court and hold a "fitness" or "waiver" hearing to determine whether the minor should be tried as an adult. "Fitness" refers to the minor's fitness to remain in the juvenile justice system: 'waiver' to the procedure under which the juvenile court waives jurisdiction over the minor in favor of transfer to the adult criminal court. Minimum age at which a minor can be transferred to or tried in the adult criminal court varies from state to state (from 10 to 16 years).[n] An adjudication of guilt in adult court exposes the minor to the same penalties for crime established by statute for adults, with the sole exception of the death penalty. The United States Supreme Court has declared it unconstitutional to execute an individual for a crime committed before his or her 18th birthday.[o]

In delinquency cases, parents' rights are minimal. The minor, not the parent, is the subject of the proceeding and his or her rights are those at stake. The minor, not the parent, has the right to assert or waive the 5th amendment right to remain silent, the amendment right to counsel, and the minor alone can choose to waive trial and enter a plea.[p] State laws typically give the parent a right to notice that a delinquency petition has been filed concerning the child, and the right to be present at critical stages of the case, such as a detention hearing or adjudication. However, the parent is not a party in the delinquency case and does not have a right to be heard by the court. The state can call the parent as a witness against the minor, however, and if the parent refuses to testify, the court can impose contempt penalties.

Because the *minor* has a constitutional right to counsel in a delinquency case, one will be provided at public expense if he or she cannot afford one. Of course, a parent may hire a private attorney to represent the child's interests; but whether private or public defender, ethically the attorney is bound to follow the minor client's instructions and serve the client's interests. The parent can urge the child to follow a particular course of action (for example, enter a guilty plea), but the attorney's advice to the minor client must be independent of the parent's wishes. Neither the parent nor the attorney can waive the minor's constitutional rights. Moreover, the attorney cannot reveal attorney–client communications to the parent, and with good reason. In the great majority of states, there is no parent–child privilege, so the parent can be forced to disclose confidential communications made by the child.[q]

Status Offenses

Depending upon the particular state code, "status offenses" may include behaviors such as truancy from school, running away from home, being habitually disobedient or "beyond the control of parents", or violating a local curfew law. These behaviors may be combined under a single label such as "children in need of supervision (CHINS)", "juveniles in need of supervision (JINS)", or "persons in need of supervision (PINS)".

States vary in the degree of procedural protections provided to minors who are the subject of status offender petitions.[r] Since status offenses are not "crimes", children in these proceedings may not be entitled to the 5th amendment right against self-incrimination. The US Supreme Court has not yet ruled on this matter. Under most state laws, children in status offense cases have the right to notice of the allegations against them, the right to a hearing, and right to the assistance of counsel. The standard of proof is only *preponderance of evidence*: that is, to take jurisdiction over the minor the judge need only find it *more likely than not* that the allegations have been proved. Federal and state laws prohibit "secure confinement" (placement in a locked facility such as a juvenile hall) of status offenders except in cases where a minor has been held in contempt for violation of a valid court order.[s]

Parents are likely to have greater involvement in status offense cases. The parent may have contacted the police or the juvenile court asking for help in controlling a child who is habitually disobedient or "incorrigible". In such a case, the parent will likely be the state's primary, if not sole, witness at the adjudication hearing. If the petition is sustained, the judge will try to order a disposition that will reinforce parental authority (often probation with specific conditions that the minor must obey her parents, avoid certain "bad influence" peers, submit to drug tests, etc.). If the minor violates these conditions, the parent can notify the court and the state can file contempt charges as discussed above.

However, the state is not required to file a petition just because the parent wants state reinforcement of his or her authority. The probation officer or prosecuting attorney may decide, rather than filing a petition, to refer the parent and child to family counseling or other services on a voluntary basis. Similarly, the state can file status offense petitions for truancy and curfew violations regardless of the parent's wishes, and may take action against a parent who has condoned the child's unlawful behavior. Once the court has sustained the petition, it can order the disposition it believes is best for the child, even if the parent opposes it.[t] If the court orders placement of a status offender in a foster home, group residence, or other out-of-home program, the parents may be required to pay the costs, as part of their duty to support their child.

Dependency Cases

Every state provides for protective action to be taken where a child is abused, neglected, abandoned by parents or guardians or otherwise "dependent" upon the state.[u] In some states, the "dependency" cases will be heard by the juvenile court: in others by the family court that also hears cases of divorce and child custody. Unlike family law custody cases, however, dependency proceedings are not conflicts between two private parties; rather, the state petitions the court to take jurisdiction over a child as "dependent" because of the acts or failure to act of parents or guardians.[v]

The degree of state intervention into the parent–child relationship through the dependency court can vary greatly. It may be temporary, as when life-saving surgery for a child is authorized by the court over parental objection yet care and custody of the child are returned to the parents immediately after the medical procedure.[w] It may last for months, as one or both parents try to regain custody of the child through compliance with a "reunification plan" designed to remove or alleviate the conditions that caused harm or put the child at risk.[x] It may be permanent, as where all parental rights are terminated, severing the legal relationship between parent and child. (Termination means total parental loss of rights to custody, visitation, and communication. The child becomes eligible for adoption by new parents, or for permanent placement with a legal guardian or foster family where adoption is not possible or appropriate.)[y]

Under the 14th Amendment to the United States Constitution, parents whose rights to care and custody are at risk in dependency proceedings must receive due process of law. Parents are entitled to notice of the allegations supporting the dependency petition and have the right to appear and be heard at the detention hearing (to decide where the child should live pending adjudication), the adjudication, the disposition hearing, and any hearings to review the status of the case. A dependency petition can be sustained at adjudication on a mere preponderance of evidence, because taking jurisdiction over the child is only a temporary deprivation of parental custody. Parental rights cannot be *terminated* without a finding based on clear and convincing evidence.[z] Nevertheless, the United States Supreme Court ruled that indigent parents are not always entitled to the assistance of counsel at public expense before termination of their rights: judges should consider parents' request for court-appointed free counsel on a case-by-case basis.[aa] In practice, most states do provide counsel for indigent parents in cases where termination is proposed.[bb]

The minors who are alleged to be "dependent" have an interest in reunification with their parent or guardian if this is possible without "detriment" or serious harm. If reunification is not possible, however, the child has an interest in permanent placement with legal guardians or adoptive parents who can and will provide appropriate care. Thus both the attorney representing the petitioner state and the attorney(s) for the parent(s) will argue that their client's proposed action also will benefit the child! The dependency court has the power to appoint counsel for the minor, however, and this is increasingly becoming routine.[cc] As in delinquency cases, a minor's attorney, whether paid by the state or retained privately, is ethically required to represent the minor's interests. When the minor is old enough to consult with the attorney and reason out a position, the attorney must inform the court of the minor's wishes. When the minor is too young to do this (in some cases the minor can be an infant), the attorney must act as a *guardian ad litem* and recommend to the court what the attorney believes is in the minor's best interests.[dd] Therefore, minor's counsel may support parents' position or the state's recommendation – or advocate a different disposition from that proposed by either of the other parties.

End Notes

[a.] It is cardinal with us that the custody, care and nurture of the child resides first in the parents, whose primary function and freedom include preparation for obligations the state can neither supply nor hinder … And it is in recognition of this that [cited] decisions have respected the private realm of family life which the state cannot enter. But the family itself is not beyond regulation in the public interest …" *Prince v. Massachusetts*, 321 U.S. 158 (1944).

[b.] Parents Authority over the Education of Their Children: *Pierce v. Society of Sisters*, 268 U.S. 510 (1925) (establishing "the parent's authority to provide religious and secular schooling and the child's right to receive it, as against the state's requirement of attendance at public school").

[c.] Child's wishes not considered: *Wisconsin v. Yoder*, 406 U.S. 205 (1972) (holding that state compulsory education law is unconstitutional as requiring Amish parents to send their children to school for 2 years of high school … without regard to the wishes of the child).

[d.] State enforcement of child labor laws: *Prince v. Massachusetts*, 321 U.S. 158 (1944) (upholding enforcement of child labor law to prohibit 9 year old Jehovah's Witness from distributing religious publication on street).

[e.] For example, California Family Code Section 6750 authorizes the superior court to approve or disapprove minors' contracts "for the provision of artistic or creative services". Based on the "Coogan Law" first enacted in 1939, California Family Code Sections 6752 and 6753 require a portion of the minors'

earnings to be set aside in trust until the minor reaches the age of majority (18).

[f.] Corporal punishment of children: Philip Jr, G. (1990). *Spare the Child: The Religious Roots of Punishment and the Psychological Impact of Physical Abuse*, Alfred Knopf.

[g.] Constitutionality of curfew laws for minors: Katherine, H.F. (1995). Children, curfews and the constitution, *Washington University Law Quarterly* **73**, 1315.

[h.] State power to establish dependency court system: Institute of Judicial Administration and the American Bar Association (IJA/ABA) (1977). Standards Relating to Child Abuse and Neglect.

[i.] History of juvenile court: Douglas, E.A. (2003). *A Very Special Place in Life: The History of Juvenile Justice in Missouri*, Missouri Juvenile Justice Association.

[j.] Due process rights of minors in delinquency cases: *In re Gault*, 387 U.S. 1 (1967) (children in delinquency proceedings are entitled to due process protections under the 14th Amendment to the Constitution, including the 5th amendment rights against self-incrimination, and the right to counsel).

[k.] Standard of proof in delinquency cases: *In re Winship*, 397 U.S. 358 (1970) (each and every element of the state's case in delinquency proceeding must be proved beyond a reasonable doubt).

[l.] No right to jury trial or to bail: *McKeiver v. Pennsylvania*, 403 U.S. 528 (1971) (the due process clause of the 14th Amendment does not assure the right to a jury trial in the adjudicative stage of a delinquency proceeding). *Schall v. Martin*, 467 U.S. 253 (1984) ("pre-adjudication" detention in locked juvenile facility of minors charged with delinquency did not violate their right to due process).

[m.] Juvenile court dispositions: Edward, H. (1996). *No Matter how Loud I Shout: A Year in the Life of Juvenile Court*.

[n.] Waiver laws and practices: Howard, S. & Melissa, S. (1995) *Juvenile Offenders and Victims. A National Report*, pp. 85–89, 154–156.

[o.] No death penalty for offense committed before age 18:
Roper v. Simmons, 543 U.S. 551 (2005).

[p.] Minor exercises own rights:
Katherine, H.F (1996). The Ethics of empowerment: rethinking the role of lawyers in interviewing and counseling the child client, *Fordham Law Review* **64**, 1655.

q. Role of attorney for minor in juvenile delinquency cases:

Institute of Judicial Administration and American Bar Association (IJA/ABA), Standards Related to Counsel for Private Parties (1976).

Jan C.C. (1980). Ethical issues in representing juvenile clients: a review of the IJA-ABA standards on representing private parties, *New Mexico Law Review* **10**, 255.

r. Due process rights afford status offenders:

Erin, M.S. (1992). In a child's best interests: juvenile status offenders deserve procedural due process, *Law and Inequality Journal* **10**(253).

s. Use of the contempt power to confine status offenders:

Jan, C. & Nancy, W. (1981). Incarcerating Status Offenders: Attempts to Circumvent the Juvenile Justice and Delinquency Prevention Act, *Harvard Civil Rights-Civil Liberties Law Review* **16**, 41.

t. Status Offender dispositions:

Status Offenders National Council of Juvenile and Family Court Judges (1990). A new approach to runaway, truant, substance abusing and beyond control children, *Juvenile and Family Court Journal* **41**, 5.

u. Definitions of dependency:

American Bar Association and National Council of Juvenile and Family Court Judges (1995). Resource Guidelines: Improving Court Practice in Child Abuse and Neglect Cases.

v. Distinction between dependency and family law cases:

Leonard, P.E. (1987)The relationship of family and juvenile courts in child abuse cases, *Santa Clara Law Review* **27**, 244–245.

w. Temporary authorization of medical procedures:

Joseph, G. (1977). Medical care for the child at risk: on state supervision of parental autonomy, *Yale Law Journal* **86**, 645. For a discussion of the balance between affording parents the right to limit medical attention to spiritual care *versus* homicide, see Commonwealth v. Twitchell, 617 N.E.2d 609 (Mass. 1993).

x. Reunification efforts:

Robert F.K (2000). Family preservation and reunification in child protection cases: effectives, best practices and implications for legal representation, judicial practice and public policy, *Family Law Quarterly* **34**, 359.

y. Susan, V.M. (2000). Extending non-exclusive parenting and the right to protection for older foster children: creating third options in permanency planning, *Buffalo Law Review* **49**, 835.

z. Preponderance standard for jurisdiction: clear and convincing standard for termination of parental rights: *Santosky v. Kramer*, 455 U.S. 745 (1982).

aa. Indigent parent not entitled to court-appointed counsel in every dependency matter; judge must decide on case-by-case basis:

Lassiter v. Dept. of Social Services, 452 U.S. 18 (1981).

bb. Parent's lawyer in child abuse cases:

Bruce, A.B. (1996). Ethical issues in representation of parents in child welfare cases, *Fordham Law Review* **64**, 1621.

cc. Martin, G. (2006). How children's lawyers serve state interests, *Nevada Law Journal* **6**, 805.

dd. Role of counsel for minor in dependency court:

Special Issue (1996). Ethical issues in the representation of children, *Fordham Law Review* **64**, 1281.

Ann, M.H., The Child's Attorney (1993, American Bar Association).

Related Articles

Children: as Defendants

Parental Alienation

JAN COSTELLO, JOSEPH KENAN, AND
CHRISTOPHER THOMPSON

Parenting: Assessment of Capacity

Child maltreatment (abuse and neglect) is a serious problem that often surfaces with reports of suspected abuse being made to Child Protective Services (CPS) or law enforcement. In cases where serious maltreatment has occurred or where risk cannot be contained, children may be removed from the home by court order and placed in custody of the state. In such cases, there is often involvement of psychologists along with other professionals providing information to the courts about the individuals in the family, their intervention needs, whether maltreatment likely occurred, and suggested ways to deal with risk factors.

In the United States, only in the past 40–50 years have there been national laws regarding the maltreatment of children and widespread state mandated reporting laws. Some of the first interventions for protection of children in this country were offshoots of efforts to control cruelty to animals [1, 2]. The hesitancy to establish state authority in this area was based on notions that children were possessions, that children were undeveloped morally and must be strongly disciplined in order to attain civility, and that family matters were best left to families to work out internally. It was only in the mid-nineteenth century that children came to be regarded as more than chattel, and it was as late as the seventeenth century before parents were prohibited from killing their children. Even then, they were not required to provide basic necessities for their offsprings [3, 4].

A paper by Kempe, a physician, in 1962 introduced the term *battered child syndrome* and urged physicians to inquire about etiology of broken bones, bruises, and soft tissue damage when children were presented for medical care [5]. Kempe's one-year study had found that 39% of the identified battered children suffered permanent brain damage or death. State mandatory reporting laws for physicians followed publication of the paper, and other professionals were later included. In line with this rising awareness of abuse, in1974, the Child Abuse Prevention and Treatment Act, the first national legislation directly addressing child maltreatment, was passed and defined abuse and neglect as the physical or mental injury, sexual abuse or exploitation, negligent treatment, or maltreatment of a child under the age of 18, or the age specified by the child protection law of the state in question, by a person who was responsible for the child's welfare. This federal law required states to adopt similar definitions in order to get child welfare funds [6]. Government reports indicated in 2004 more than 872000 children and youth were found to have been abused or neglected on the basis of investigation of an estimated 3 million referrals. For 1387 children, the maltreatment was fatal. Another half million had been removed and were living in foster care; of these, 117463 would not ever return to parents but were awaiting adoption by someone else [7].

Maltreatment Effects

Physical Effects

Efforts to study the effects of maltreatment on children are made more difficult because of the frequent co-occurrence of other aversive factors, such as family stress, dysfunctional patterns of family interaction, parental psychopathology, child psychopathology, and chaotic home environment. In addition, the age at which abuse or neglect occurs seems to make a difference in sequelae for children [8]. For instance, younger children are at more risk for death from their injuries than are older children because of greater vulnerability to physical damage, lack of ability to seek medical care for themselves, and lack of ability to inform others about risk factors [9].

Even when death does not occur, results can be very tragic as in cases of shaken baby or trauma to the head. Acceleration, deceleration, and twisting of the brain within the cranial vault, produced by shaking or throwing the child, can lead to life threatening emergencies such as hemorrhage and brain swelling [10]. These conditions can result in mental retardation, speech and language delay, and learning disorders. Some research shows significantly lower cognitive skills in abused children even when there is no evidence of head trauma. Some of these deficits may be attributed to physical neglect, malnutrition, or exposure to toxic substances and other factors, which complicate efforts to identify the particular effects of physical abuse [11].

Psychological Effects

Physically abused children have been found to show increased noncompliance, more aggression, deficits in social skills and peer relationships, less empathic tendencies, and worse adjustment to school compared to control groups [8]. Condi [12] listed several factors found to be associated with physical abuse of younger children: developmental delay, anxious attachment to parents, withdrawal or apathy, and hyperarousal. Older children with abuse history have been found to have more problems with social cognition, self-esteem, conduct problems, and substance abuse. Some studies have found over one-third of physically abused children meet criteria for posttraumatic stress disorder (PTSD) with about 10% meeting the criteria as long as 2 years after initial diagnosis [13].

Diagnosis of PTSD is also often justified when children have been sexually abused, and more than one-third continue to meet the criteria for the diagnosis as adults. These children and their grown-up fellow survivors are more likely than their peers to be depressed and to attempt suicide, to have sexual behavior problems, and to engage in self-mutilation [14]. Fortunately, even with the harsh sequelae for some survivors, literature reviews indicate that from 25 to 40% of sexually abused children do not show psychological symptoms in the short term. Of those having initial symptoms, more than half later show improvement [15].

Children who have been neglected show increased behavior problems, aggression, and school maladjustment. In childhood, they are often anxiously attached to parent figures with some studies showing up to two-thirds of neglected one-year olds lacking secure attachment. They often become angry and unaffectionate but highly dependent on caregivers; they tend to lack persistence, to be noncompliant and negativistic, and to be more unpopular than nonneglected peers. They are at greater risk than peers for academic failure and for dropping out of school [16].

Protective Factors

Several protective factors associated with less severe sequelae from sexual abuse were reported by Berlinger and Elliott [14] and include: less serious and less frequent or single occurrences of abuse; perpetrator not a central person in child's life; child informing parent who was then protective and supportive; child having a close bond with supportive parent; child having stable and mature family with limited dysfunctional patterns; child not being subject to lengthy court testimony or repeated interviews; and child being provided stress inoculation and support if facing testimony. In a study of 369 sexually abused children, Conte and Schuerman [17] found the one variable with the greatest predictive power for impact on the child was a poorly functioning family.

For maltreatment in general, research in the field suggests the long-term effects of abuse are ameliorated by the child having a loving, supportive adult who provides a distinct model of a caring child–adult relationship and offers the child a positive way to form a self-concept. Another factor found to be predictive of less harmful adjustment is successful participation in psychotherapy to enhance emotional stability and maturity as well as to facilitate the integration of the maltreatment into a coherent view of self (rather than becoming dissociative or fragmented) [18, 19]. In addition to these environmental or situational factors, internal factors such as flexible coping style (suggestive of emotional maturity), resistance to self-blame, at least average cognitive abilities, self-confidence, and active coping have been found to be helpful [14, 20].

Factors Associated with Maltreatment

Theories of Causation

As the problem of maltreatment has come to be seen as more complex, the models of explanation have likewise shifted from single causes to more multifactorial models which take into account potentiating and protective factors as well as complex interactional factors (information processing, stress management, developmental stage of the child, environmental factors, and interpersonal skills). A critical decision in development of a theory of causation (and its application for treatment approaches) is whether to see abuse and normal parenting as dichotomous or as points on a continuum. Those who hold a dichotomous view see parental maltreatment as the result of permanent "defect" (mental retardation and character disorder) while those who see a continuum of behavior patterns tend to look for parenting "deficiencies" (amenable to change) or "disruption" (changeable social or interpersonal forces interfering with appropriate parenting on a situational basis). A blended approach sees "differences" or mismatches between parent and child (needs, abilities, temperaments, and interactions) which to some degree can be ameliorated. The position one takes regarding the nature of maltreatment shapes the approach to evaluation and intervention [21].

Sociobiological Model. Child abuse is not limited only to humans, and studies show similarities of factors for human and nonhuman parents. A study covering 12 years of records for monkeys kept in a primate lab at the University of Colorado found abuse involving 28% of the infants; abuse was defined as physical abuse or neglect resulting in a medical problem. Of the abused infants, 62% died. Data supported hypotheses that abuse resulted from learned aggression (intergenerational transmission of parenting patterns), aberrations of attachment, social alienation, and overcrowding. The fact that causative factors are similar to those for humans but incidence rates are different in this colony compared to statistics with human studies suggests factors such as cognitive beliefs and/or social norms may function in a protective manner [22].

Belsky [23] pointed out that from a biological perspective, interests of parent and child are not always the same and may even be in direct conflict for success even if not for survival. This may be particularly evident in situations of limited resources (such as poverty or single-parent household) coupled with excessive demands or competition (large families, unplanned pregnancies, ill or handicapped children). This biological/evolutionary model may also explain the higher occurrence of maltreatment of stepchildren or by young mothers (who are more capable of bearing additional children than are older mothers) or on young children (who are not reproductively mature and thus more expendable).

Intergenerational Transmission.   This explanatory model is largely based on the recognition that abused children when grown-up are more likely to be abusive to their children than are parents who were not abused or neglected in childhood. But review of research finds intergenerational transmission rates of about $30 \pm 5\%$ meaning that two-thirds of abused children do not grow up to be abusive (at least during the brief windows of time on which research studies focus) [23, 24]. These figures are compared with self-reported figures obtained in epidemiological studies in which incidence rates in the general population are about 1% [25].

Information Processing Theory.   Crittenden [26] presented a cognitive model with four elements which are involved in decisions and ultimately lead to behavior. These elements are perception (affected by biases); interpretation (affected by schemas and attributions); response selection (limited by repertoire and influenced by expectations); and implementation of behavior (affected by available resources and hierarchy of conflicting demands). Parents who become neglectful or abusive may be influenced by thinking errors, such as bias against a child, filters which block out or minimize significant positive information, faulty attributions such as parental helplessness

or meanness of the child, or role reversing choices based on expecting children to be responsible for the wellbeing of parents.

Other elaborations on this model have been provided by Dix [27] and Azar [21, 28]. Azar's model posits that in the situation of a parent with bad schema for understanding child behavior combined with high risk personality factors (poor empathy, low flexibility, high distress, impulsivity), the abuse unfolds in four stages: (i) parent has unrealistic standard; (ii) child fails to meet standard; (iii) parent misattributes negative intent to the child or blames self when intervention does not change child's behavior; and (iv) parent overreacts and punishes excessively.

Presented below are factors which have been found across reviews of research in the field of child maltreatment. Most of the literature relates to neglect or physical abuse rather than sexual abuse although these categories are by no means mutually exclusive. However, there are also some significant differences between sexual abuse and other forms of maltreatment. For instance, although females (mothers) more often than males are identified with physical abuse or neglect, males by far outnumber females as reported perpetrators of sexual abuse. Also, physical abuse and neglect are almost always perpetrated by parent or other primary care giver while only about one-third of sexual abuse perpetration is by parent or primary care giver [17]. Sexual abuse has other unique dynamics as well such as family enmeshment and deviant sexual arousal patterns or practices of offenders [29].

Contextual Factors Associated with Maltreatment

Many specific contextual factors have been found to be predictive of abuse or neglect [16, 23,30]. For instance, poverty and scarcity of resources have consistently been predictive of higher rates of neglect and physical abuse. Living in a neighborhood with poor social fabric, no community pride, poorly organized resources, or an atmosphere of violence and aggression increases likelihood of maltreatment. Belsky [23] noted that cultures in which corporal punishment was rare had low rates of abuse. Chaotic home environment, occurrence of domestic violence, social isolation of the family, or presence of physically or emotionally demanding child care situations tend to increase risk of abuse.

Parental Factors Associated with Maltreatment

Identified parent factors are more numerous than contextual factors. Some are biological in nature (young age of parents and strongly aroused physical reactivity to stressful stimuli), whereas others are psychological. The neurotic triad of depression, anxiety, and hostility increases risk. Epidemiological studies [25] have found depressed parents have four times the risk for being abusive as nondepressed parents although Belsky [23] stated the association is curvilinear for abuse (greatest for moderate levels of depression) and linear for neglect (greatest for highest levels of depression). Maltreating parents also tend to be impulsive and to have poor self-esteem and low ego strength. The Minnesota Mother–Child Project, which followed at-risk first-time mothers, found emotional stability was the greatest single predictor of good caretaking *versus* maltreatment [31].

Behavioral patterns of parents differentiate maltreating from nonabusive parents. The maltreating individuals tend to be strict disciplinarians (abuse group) or inconsistent (abuse and neglect groups). They tend to use physical punishment or coercive discipline in preference to other forms of guidance and thereby place themselves at greater risk; if they are also more physiologically reactive and psychologically distressed, physical punishment can get out of hand and quickly become violent aggression. They are less effective at managing problems with children. They tend to be less responsive to needs and emotions of children, to have fewer play items for children in the home, and to engage in less communication and physical interaction with their children. Substance abuse is a strong predictor which was found in epidemiological studies to increase risk for neglect fourfold [25]. They tend to isolate themselves, to be more transient than nonabusers, and to remove themselves from social supports that are available to them.

Cognitive factors differentiating maltreating and other parents include more emotion-based than reason-based problem solving. The maltreating parents have less cognitive flexibility and more rigid thinking even though attention, distractibility, and verbal fluency are not found to be significantly different. These parents often have a negative attitude toward their children and tend to see negative behaviors of children as internally caused and stable, whereas positive behaviors are seen as externally caused (perhaps attributed to the parent) but not stable [13]. As a result, abusive parents tend to develop a negative, adversarial schema that leads to misinterpretation; neutral or ambiguous behaviors are seen as examples of misbehavior or even malice on the part of the children. Neglectful parents also have a negative schema but tend to believe that relationships will not be fulfilling. Finally, the internal model for parenting behaviors is often a deficient one as many maltreating parents have themselves been reared by neglectful or abusive parents [23, 30].

Treatment Interventions with Parents

Funding from the Child Abuse and Prevention Treatment Act of 1974 [6] led to many well-developed intervention projects, which were then evaluated in efforts to discover what was effective. Daro [32] reviewed results from 19 demonstration projects and found relapse rates ranging from 20% (sexual abuse) to 66% (neglect). She noted family therapy, individual problem-solving training, and group therapy tended to be associated with more successful results. She also reported on 89 programs involving over 3200 families [33], which found the best outcomes were associated with intensive services initially and a long maintenance period. Better results were also found with use of lay services (volunteers in the homes of target families) and use of groups for the parents (group therapy and classes). Interventions shorter than six months or longer than 18 months were less likely to show progress. Results suggested intervention should be comprehensive in addressing concrete (housing and medical services) and interpersonal needs (social support and faulty interaction patterns), but the most effectively spent money was for prevention.

Other research [34] found in reviewing control study research that a multifaceted, behavioral approach was most effective in reducing posttreatment relapse rates (10% in treated *vs.* 21% in control groups); but also found brief treatment did not work well. Home-based services with practical skills training and with family therapy showed vastly better rates for children remaining in home at one-year follow-up (74% with such services *vs.* 45% without). One example (Project 12-Ways) of this intensive, comprehensive model has been well described by Lutzker [35–37].

Legal Context for Considering Parenting Evaluations

The legal context for most child protection matters is domestic court or family court although criminal courts may become involved where evidence of maltreatment is sufficient to lead to an indictment and criminal prosecution. Domestic courts are not constitutionally established but arise from English common law where chauncery courts or common courts addressed marital disputes and matters concerning children. Although hesitant to become involved in matters of the family until there is breakdown of the family unit and/or harm to a child, the courts have a significant societal interest to take action when natural parent and child bonds are no longer sufficiently effective to assure the best interests of the child are being addressed by the family [3].

Even though parents are under statutory obligation to provide basic needs (physical, medical, and educational), they are mostly free to make decisions about residence, family structure, discipline, religious practices, social activities, financial arrangements, and even educational choices as long as basic needs are addressed and peace and order accomplished. Balanced against this deference to parents and privacy of the family are legal precepts recognizing the rights of children (protection of their best interests in disputed matters) and the obligation of the state to intervene when children need protection. This intervention is based on the concept of *parens patriae*, which regards the state as the protector of those citizens unable to care for themselves [38]. With origins in Roman law incorporated into English common law in the eleventh century, the concept extends the state's interest into the family and other matters when children (or disabled individuals) are unable to be guardians of their own interests.

Below are some of the legal cases from US courts, which help define the balance of interests in child-dependency cases.

Griswold v. State of Connecticutt (1965) [39]: prohibited undue government intrusion into "zone of privacy for family implied by Bill of Rights and 14th Amendment".

Parham v. J.L. & J.R. (1979) [40]: allowed parents to maintain substantial role in decision making for child unless abuse, neglect, or evidence contradicting assumption of parent acting in best interest of child.

Ingraham v. Wright (1977) [41]: corporal punishment not cruel and unusual for child; 8th Amendment protection only for convicted citizens and does not apply to children.

Deshaney v. Winnebago County Department of Social Services (1989) [42]: state is not liable for failure to protect child from injury by parents; 14th Amendment designed to protect citizens from state, not insure state protects individuals from each other.

Santosky v. Kramer (1982) [43]: threshold for permanent removal of children must be clear and convincing evidence of abuse; due process must be afforded to parent.

South Carolina Department of Social Services v. the Father and the Mother; In the Interest of the Child (1988) [44]: court affirmed religious freedom for beliefs but regulation of behavior by laws in case where parents claimed religious right for corporal punishment which left bruises on child.

State v. Evans (1992) [45]: unmarried father not living in home guilty of criminal neglect when child died of malnutrition; father did not assure child received care.

In re Glenn G. (1992) [46]: mother neglectful for failing to protect children from abusing, battering father.

E.C. v. District of Columbia (1991) [47] and *Egly v. Blackford County Department of Public Welfare* (1992) [48]: mental illness or mental retardation alone not grounds for termination of parental rights but effects on child and ability to handle needs of child must be considered.

In *Matter of Joshua O.* (1996) [49]: state must present clear and convincing evidence parent is currently and will remain incapable of caring for child if seeking termination of parental rights.

Assessment Issues

Psychologists and other mental health professionals often are asked to become involved in assessment tasks in cases where child maltreatment has occurred or is deemed to be a significant risk. Evaluators are asked to provide information about risk factors and prognosis for change, risks and benefits for parent–child contact or reunification, services needed, and ability to use services if provided. Reports may be used for treatment planning, case planning, or termination of parental rights suits. Because these cases are always either court cases or have the potential to become such, evaluators are admonished to approach them carefully as the reports may have lasting effects on the lives of the people involved [12, 50]. These evaluations blend elements of clinical assessments and forensic evaluations and are conceptually related most closely to custody evaluations [4, 51]. The following discussion includes the literature from child custody evaluations because of this close relationship and because more research has been conducted on custody evaluations than on care and protection evaluations.

Factors to be Considered in Parenting Evaluations

Lack of Definition of Parenting. Evaluators seeking to conduct assessments within this area of high scrutiny where there is high likelihood of reports being used in an adversarial legal context are handicapped by lack of universal standards or behavioral criteria regarding minimal parenting practices. In addition, there is scarcity of appropriate tools for assessment of parenting skills. In a context of cultural pluralism and social class differences, evaluators provide information so that decisions can be made about "good enough" parenting, a concept arising from a British pediatrician-turned-psychoanalyst, D.W. Winnicott. Winnicott believed that child resilience made up for a host of parental limitations and mistakes.

Conceptual Approach. Grisso [52] proposed a model, which has become well accepted for exploration of various capacities and resulting reports in forensic matters. He suggested five components. "Functional" assessment explores a person's skills and deficits and often uses clinical as well as specialized forensic assessment instruments; it measures what a person is able to do. The "causal" component explains why these deficits occur; sometimes there is a connection between the deficits and a mental health condition. Thirdly, the "interactive" component, too often neglected in forensic reports, applies the functional limitations to the particular forensic context; it states or predicts what a person is specifically able or not able to do in terms of expected behavior in a particular required task. The other two components, "judgmental" and "dispositional", belong not to the evaluator but to the decision maker to determine if the person's abilities are adequate for the task and

how the case proceeds. Such an approach to parenting evaluations does not stop with description of skills and deficits of the parent but relates these factors to specific effects the parent's behavior has or is likely to have on the particular child [4].

Common Elements of Parenting. Hoghughi's conceptual model has been used to simplify the myriad of parenting tasks to three elements: care, control, and development. Care refers to provision of physical needs as well as emotional factors; control refers to guidance and discipline; and development refers to those resources and conditions necessary for a child to mature according to developmental milestones. In order for parents to be successful with these tasks, they must have knowledge, motivation, resources, and opportunity (access) [53]. Another simplification has resulted in a model of two basic tasks: protection and care of the child for the purpose of socialization. The parent must know the child and attend to limits and discipline [54].

Factors Associated with Adequate and Inadequate Parenting. White [50] proposed flexibility as the hallmark of good parenting and suggested it was evident in the sustained pursuit of provision of the child's needs through accommodation to the changing environment and the changing child. Some factors which researchers have found to be identified with adequate or good parenting include being supportive and responsive or 'joining' the child, providing instruction and guidance, providing nurture and showing affection through talk and touch, having clear boundaries between parent and child, and maintaining a mutual positive emotional attachment. In contrast, features that have been associated with inadequate parenting or maltreatment include being controlling or power oriented with the child, being hostile or rejecting, being unresponsive or detached, using inconsistent or physical discipline, having high stress and poor coping skills, being emotionally immature or impulsive, having unrealistic expectations of the child, having substance abuse problems, and having poor frustration tolerance or hyperarousal tendencies [2, 55, 56].

Structuring the Assessment and Report

Guidelines. Guidelines provided by the American Psychological Association (APA) offer help in conducting parenting assessments [57]. Principles of good practice begin by letting the referral question direct the scope of the evaluation, which then develops through the use of multiple methods to gain multiple sources of information. The parent must be informed of the nature and purpose of the evaluation and the limitations on confidentiality. The examiner is cautioned not to make inappropriate interpretations of test data and to tie any recommendations to potential welfare for the child in the matter.

Structure.   The assessment process usually involves face to face contact as well as testing, extensive review of records, and use of collateral sources for obtaining information (extended family members, teachers, day care workers, medical personnel, neighbors, and friends). The process usually is structured into three areas: evaluation of the parent, evaluation of the child, and interaction between parent and child [12, 54]. The parent evaluation explores ability of the person to care for self and to care for the child, significant problems (such as substance abuse, mental illness, serious physical limitations, and behavior problems), problem solving and stress management skills, parenting skills and knowledge, access to resources, and empathy or bonding to the child. The child's evaluation includes exploration of progress with developmental milestones and any serious limitations, social and peer relationships, school adjustment, temperament, bonding with the parent, and physical and emotional health.

Observation of parent-child interaction is strongly recommended in this type evaluation although it is not always possible, particularly when termination of parental rights is the case at hand. A report about parent–child interaction should include comments about mutual attachment and boundaries, enmeshment and use of coercion, complementarity or reciprocity of interactions, parental responsiveness, and "goodness of fit" with temperament and needs of the child. Some suggest adding a fourth area for consideration of systemic factors (social context, environmental risk factors, and extended family issues) [50].

Problems Associated with Parenting Evaluations

Difficulties with Testing.   Research published about custody evaluation methods led Brodzinsky [58] to criticize indiscriminate use of tests which results partly because psychologists are trained to test and therefore do it and partly because there is financial incentive to produce billable services. There was also note that clinical tests were developed for other purposes and often lacked research applying to the particular legal issue. Although an aura of science is associated with use of tests, use for purposes unsupported by research is deceptive. Finally, there was criticism of poor interpretation practices and not basing interpretation on clear research.

Others have pointed out a major difficulty involved in testing parents in this type evaluation is the response bias problem or socially desirable responding [59, 60]. Parents, usually wanting to present self in the most favorable light in order to impress the decision makers, will often resort to minimizing any difficulties and exaggerating reports of desirable traits and behaviors. Carr [61] reported base rates of compromised validity in these evaluations ranged from 20 to 60%, discouraged the use of tests without validity scales for measuring such response bias, and strongly discouraged adoption of separate validity norms for parents in this type evaluation. The Minnesota Multiphasic Personality Inventory 2 (MMPI-2), Personality Assessment Inventory (PAI), and Child Abuse Potential Inventory (CAPI) were noted to have good validity scales (*see also* **Psychological Testing**). Two other frequently used tests were noted to have deficiencies in the detection of bias: Parenting Stress Inventory (PSI) which has a poorly discriminative measure for defensiveness and Adult–Adolescent Parenting Inventory (AAPI-2) which has no validity scales. The CAPI has a validity scale specifically designed for use with this population. Whether the positive response bias is the result only of the evaluation context or is representative of an actual personality trait of this type parent is a question raised by the author.

Heilbrun [62] made three other suggestions for use of psychological test instruments in a forensic context. First, the instrument should be commercially available with a manual for administration and scoring and should have been reviewed in major publications. The psychometric properties should show reliability measures of $r \geqslant 0.80$. Finally, the test should produce data relevant to the legal issue or construct. There should be available appropriate research published in peer reviewed journals, which provides validity for using the instrument for the particular purpose of the evaluation. Added to these criteria would be an expectation the assessment instrument could pass Daubert [63] criteria if challenged in court.

Problems Associated with Parent–Child Observation. With a single event of limited duration, it is easy to place too much emphasis on what is briefly observed and to overinterpret the behaviors. The observer, who may be unaware of personal bias, may make inaccurate interpretations of behaviors as well; the parent–child dyad may have particular, unique patterns or rituals as well as subculture patterns of interaction. The observer must also be cautious about assuming the observed interactions are representative of the way the parent and child would normally behave if not in the unique situation which undoubtedly makes them anxious. In addition, the child may feel torn between loyalty to parent and perceived necessary alliance with foster parents and child protection workers who control life for the time being. It should also be noted that play activity interactions do not necessarily represent level of bonding, nor do displays of affection or failures to display affection [50, 59, 64].

There is, in addition, a problem with perceived expertise when none exists. Starr [65] found that untrained undergraduate students were better at identifying parent–child dyads with a history of abuse than were seasoned professionals in a parent–child observation task even though neither group was correct by more than chance. Examiner bias (personal prejudice), confirmatory bias (selective attention to information supporting favored hypothesis and disregard for data challenging it), and overuse of experience-based schemata (expectancy and overconfidence leading to premature conclusions) pose substantial threats to accurate perception and good decision making in these observations.

Suggestions for improving parent–child observations and the usefulness of resulting data have been offered in articles and books [56, 66, 67] Some basic recommendations include informing the participants and preparing them for the interaction in order to minimize anxiety, holding the event in a naturalistic setting and providing ample time for getting comfortable with the task, providing opportunities to observe free play as well as chores or structured activity, and minimizing observer interaction during the exercise. Whenever possible, it is useful to observe the child with another caregiver to get a sense of what is unique about interaction with the parent. It is also highly recommended the observer have a system for observing and recording actual behaviors rather than only making conclusory notes that provide little more

than overall impressions. One tool which helps is the Keys to Interactive Parenting Scale (KIPS), which is provided by its author along with training and certification for its use [68].

Criticisms of Reports. Budd and colleagues [59, 69, 70] have taken the lead in researching parenting evaluations in child maltreatment cases although their work is largely confined to looking at practices in Cook County (Chicago), Illinois. They have noted several limitations of reports in these cases: failure to clarify and/or note in report the referral question; failure to document informed consent and discussion of limitations of confidentiality; failure to address the believability of the results; and failure to comment on limitations of the methods used in the evaluation and the conclusions provided. Oberlander [71] added a criticism that reports (and conclusions) relied heavily on personal clinical experience and prior courtroom experiences of the evaluator and lacked ties to research findings and professional literature. She also noted reports often failed to protect the rights of parents who were potential defendants as cases developed. Jacobsen *et al.* [72] noted that reports failed to address minimal rather than optimal level of parenting and failure to address cultural practices in discussion of parenting abilities and deficits.

Recommended improvements for parenting assessment reports include the following: clarifying the referral question; articulating parental strengths and available resources as well as problems and risks; using valid and reliable assessment tools but taking a conservative approach by acknowledging limitations of assessment tools and current knowledge of outcomes of differing parenting practices; focusing on direct assessment of parenting skills, preferably in a home setting; maintaining open inquiry which continues to pursue and incorporate information from diverse sources; addressing issues of cultural context and potential observer bias and misinterpretations; and provide information for the decision makers rather than addressing ultimate issue question as psychologists (and other evaluators) have no specialized knowledge or training qualifying them for such conclusions [59, 72].

Current Practices in Assessment of Parenting

Most of this information is taken from research conducted about parenting assessment in the context of custody evaluations as there is more published literature about these evaluations. Bow [73] reviewed results of five major published surveys of custody evaluators. These studies were originally published between 1986 and 2004 and covered in excess of 500 evaluators in the United States and Canada. In conducting the evaluations, most time was spent interviewing the parents with testing, review of records, and parent-child observations taking time in descending order. The MMPI-2 and the Millon Clinical Multiaxial Inventory (MCMI) were the most widely used tests with trends across time showing consistent use of Rorschach Inkblots (about 40%), declining use of intelligence tests, and increasing use of Parenting Stress Inventory (PSI) and Parent–Child Relationship Inventory (PCRI).

A more recent survey by Bow [74] of 89 psychologists who conducted custody evaluations (averaging one-third of their practice) indicated the primary use of testing was to rule out presence of psychopathology; other primary uses were assessment of personality functioning and analysis of parental strengths and weaknesses. The MMPI-2, typically used by 91% of the respondents, was the most widely used test instrument followed by the MCMI (typically used by 58%; no version specified) and the PSI (27%). The Personality Assessment Inventory (PAI) was typically used by 18% of the group. The Child Abuse Potential Inventory (CAPI), not designed for use in such evaluations, and PCRI were listed without percentage of use by respondents who as a group failed to have any clear opinion regarding whether these two instruments met Daubert [63] criteria for admissibility in court (*see* **Psychological Testing**).

Budd's report [69] on Illinois parenting evaluations conducted between 1995 and 1997 contained a subset of 124 evaluations likely conducted by psychologists but for a variety of referral questions. Projective personality tests were used in 81% of these evaluations, cognitive tests in 73%, and objective personality tests in 64%. Parenting questionnaires were used in only 4%, and parent–child observation was present in only 17%.

Summary

There are no specific forensic assessment instruments which have been developed for child protection cases, and there is no consensus as to what constitutes minimally adequate parenting, much less how to measure

such a level. The role of the examiner is to collect and interpret data and to present the results to decision makers who combine those results with other factors such as legal standards, case laws, and community mores and practices. General principles of assessment apply such as clarifying. The referral question, informing the examinee of the nature of the evaluation and limits of confidentiality, using appropriate assessment methods and acknowledging limitations of the tools, and use of multiple sources of information with particular attention to written records and collateral source material. Use of clinical personality tests, parenting inventories, and parent–child observation is recommended although there is caution about using clinical assessment instruments for forensic purposes [75].

Other Resources

Professional organizations have published guidelines offering recommendations about conducting assessment in parent–child forensic contexts [57, 76–79]. White [50] has an excellent literature review; she and Otto and Edens [4] offer critical information about specific test instruments. Condie [2, 12], Gould and Martindale [56] and Dyer [80] provide very useful resources for exploring issues of parenting assessment. Finally, Heilbrun [81] presents an example of a report on a forensic parenting evaluation (*see also* **Parental Rights and Prerogatives**; **Visitation Rights**; **Capacity Assessment**; **Psychological Testing**).

References

[1]   Kalichman, S. (1999). *Mandated Reporting of Suspected Child Abuse: Ethics, Law, and Policy*, 2nd Edition, American Psychological Association, Washington, DC.

[2]   Condie, L.O. & Condie, D. (2007). Termination of Parental Rights, in *Forensic Psychology: Emerging Topics and Expanding Roles*, A.M. Goldstein, ed, John Wiley & Sons, Hoboken, pp. 294–330.

[3]   Hess, K. & Brinson, P. (1999). Mediating Domestic Law Issues, in *The Handbook of Forensic Psychology*, A. Hess & I. Weiner, eds, Wiley, New York, pp. 63–103.

[4]   Otto, R. & Edens, J. (2003). Parenting Capacity, in *Evaluating Competencies: Forensic Assessments and Instruments*, 2nd Edition, T. Grisso, ed, Kluwer, New York, pp. 229–307.

[5]   Kempe, C., Silverman, F., Steele, B., Droegemueller, W. & Silver, H. (1962). The battered child

syndrome, *Journal of American Medical Association* **187**, 105–112.

[6] Child Abuse Prevention Act. Pub L No 93–247, US Code 93rd Congress (1974).

[7] Child Welfare League of America (2007). National Fact Sheet Retrieved 10/12/07 From http://www.cwla.org/advocacy/nationalfactsheet07.htm.

[8] Lamphear, V. (1985). The impact of maltreatment on children's psychosocial adjustment: A review of the research, *Child Abuse & Neglect* **9**, 251–263.

[9] American Academy of Pediatrics Committee on Child Abuse and Neglect (1993). Shaken baby syndrome: inflicted cerebral trauma, *Pediatrics*, **92**, 872–875.

[10] Duhaime, A., Alario, A., Lewander, W., Schut, L., Sutton, L., Seidl, T., Nudelman, S., Budenz, D., Hertle, R., Tsiaras, W. & Loporchio, S. (1992). Head injury in very young children: mechanisms, injury types, and ophthalmologic findings in 100 hospital patients younger than 2 years of age, *Pediatrics* **90**, 179–185.

[11] Miller, L. (1999). Child abuse brain injury: clinical, neuropsychological, and forensic considerations, *Journal of Cognitive Rehabilitation* **17**, 10–19.

[12] Condie, L. (2003). *Parenting Evaluations for the Court: Care and Protection Matters*, Kluwer, New York.

[13] Kolko, D. (2002). Child Physical Abuse, in *The APSAC Handbook on Child Maltreatment*, 2nd Edition, J.E.B. Myers, L. Berlinger, J. Briere, T. Hendrix, C. Jenny & T. Reid, eds, Sage, Thousand Oaks, pp. 21–54.

[14] Berlinger, L. & Elliott, D. (2002). Sexual Abuse of Children, in *The APSAC Handbook on Child Maltreatment*, 2nd Edition, J.E.B. Myers, L. Berlinger, J. Briere, T. Hendrix, C. Jenny & T. Reid, eds, Sage, Thousand Oaks, pp. 55–78.

[15] Finkelhor, D. (2002). Introduction, in *The APSAC Handbook on Child Maltreatment*, 2nd Edition, J.E.B. Myers, L. Berlinger, J. Briere, T. Hendrix, C. Jenny & T. Reid, eds, Sage, Thousand Oaks, pp. xi–xvi.

[16] Erickson, M. & England, B. (2002). Child Neglect, in *The APSAC Handbook on Child Maltreatment*, 2nd Edition, J.E.B. Myers, L. Berlinger, J. Briere, T. Hendrix, C. Jenny & T. Reid, eds, Sage, Thousand Oaks, pp. 3–20.

[17] Conte, J. & Schuerman, J. (1987). Factors associated with an increased impact of child sexual abuse, *Child Abuse & Neglect* **11**, 201–211.

[18] Myers, J. (1992). *Legal Issues in Child Abuse and Neglect*, Sage, Newbury Park.

[19] Edgeworth, J. & Carr, A. (2000). Child Abuse, in *What Works for Children and Adolescents? A Critical Review of Psychological Interventions with Children, Adolescents, and Their Families*, A. Carr, ed, Routledge, New York, pp. 17–48.

[20] Garbarino, J., Kostelny, K. & Dubrow, N. (1991). What children can tell us about living in danger, *American Psychologist* **46**, 376–383.

[21] Azar, S., Povilaitis, T., Lauretti, A. & Pouquette, C. (1998). The Current State of Ecological Theories in Intrafamilial Child Maltreatment, in *Handbook of Child Abuse Research and Treatment*, J. Lutzker, ed, Plenum, New York, pp. 3–30.

[22] Caine, N. & Reite, M. (1983). Infant Abuse in Captive Pig-Tailed Macaques: Relevance to Human Child Abuse, in *Child Abuse: The Non-Human Data*, M. Reite & N. Caine, eds, Alan Liss, New York, pp. 19–27.

[23] Belsky, J. (1993). Etiology of child maltreatment a developmental-ecological analysis, *Psychological Bulletin* **114**, 413–434.

[24] Widom, C. (1989). Does violence beget violence? A critical examination of the literature, *Psychological Bulletin* **106**, 3–28.

[25] Chaffin, M., Kelleher, K. & Hollenberg, J. (1996). Onset of physical abuse and neglect: psychiatric, substance abuse, and social risk factors from prospective community data, *Child Abuse & Neglect* **20**, 191–203.

[26] Crittenden, P. (1993). An information processing perspective on the behavior of neglectful parents, *Criminal Justice and Behavior* **20**, 27–48.

[27] Dix, T. (1991). The affective organization of parenting: adaptive and maladaptive processes, *Psychological Bulletin* **110**, 3–25.

[28] Azar, S. (1997). A Cognitive Behavioral Approach to Understanding and Treating Parents Who Physically Abuse Their Children, in *Child Abuse: New Directions in Prevention Across the Lifespan*, A. Wolfe, R. Mc.Mahon & R. Peters, eds, Sage: Thousand Oaks, pp. 79–101.

[29] Friedrich, W. (1990). *Psychotherapy of Sexually Abused Children and Their Families*, Norton, New York.

[30] Milner, J. & Dopke, C. (1997). Child Physical Abuse: Review of Offender Characteristics, in *Child Abuse: New Directions in Prevention Across the Lifespan*, D. Wolfe, R. Mc.Mahon & R. Peters, eds, Sage, Thousand Oaks, pp. 27–54.

[31] Piante, R., England, B. & Erickson, M. (1989). The Antecedents of Maltreatment: Results of the Mother-Child Interaction Research Project, in *Child Maltreatment: Theory and Research on the Causes and Consequences of Child Abuse and Neglect*, D. Cicchetti & V. Carlson, eds, University Press, Cambridge, pp. 203–253.

[32] Daro, D. (1998). *Confronting Child Abuse: Research for Effective Program Design*, Free Press, New York.

[33] Cohn, A. & Daro, D. (1987). Is treatment too late? what ten years of evaluation results tell us, *Child Abuse & Neglect* **11**, 433–442.

[34] Oates, K. & Bross, D. (1995). What have we learned about treating child physical abuse? a literature review of the last decade, *Child Abuse & Neglect* **19**, 463–473.

[35] Lutzker, J. (1984). Project 12-Ways: Treating Child Abuse and Neglect From an Ecobehavioral Perspective, in *Parent Training*, R. Dangel, & R. Polster, eds, Guilford New York, pp. 260–297.

[36] Wesch, D. & Lutzker, J. (1991). A comprehensive 5 year evaluation of Project 12-Ways: an ecological program for treating and preventing child abuse and neglect, *Journal of Family Violence* **6**, 17–35.

[37] Lutzker, J. & Campbell, R. (1994). *Ecobehavioral Family Interventions in Developmental Disabilities*. Brooks/Cole, Pacific Grove.

[38] Garner, B. (ed) (1999). *Black's Law Dictionary*, 7th Edition, West Group, St. Paul.

[39] Griswold v. Connecticutt, 381 U.S. 479 (1965).

[40] Parham v. J.L. and J.R., 422 U.S. 584 (1979).

[41] Ingraham v. Wright, 430 U.S. 651 (1977).

[42] DeShaney v. Winnebago County Department of Social Services, 486 U.S. 549 (1990).

[43] Santosky v. Kramer, 455 U.S. 745 (1982).

[44] South Carolina Department of Social Services v. The Father and the Mother; In the Interest of the Child, 294 S.C. 518, 366 S.E. 2d 40 (App.1988).

[45] State v. Evans, 171 Wis.2d 471, 492 N.W. 2d 141 (1992).

[46] In re Glenn G., 154 Misc. 2d 677, 587 NY.S. 2d 464 (N.Y.Fam.Ct. 1992).

[47] E.C. v. District of Columbia, 589 A. 2d 1245 (D.C.App. 1991).

[48] Egly v. Blackford County Department of Public Welfare, 592 N.E. 2d 1232 (Ind. 1992).

[49] Matter of Joshua O, 641 N.Y.S.2d 475 (1996).

[50] White, A. *Assessment of Parenting Capacity: Literature Review*, NSW Department of Community Services, Ashfield, New South Wales (Australia) Retrievable from http://www.community.nsw.gov.au.

[51] Halikias, W. (1994). Forensic family evaluations: a comprehensive model for professional practice, *Journal of Clinical Psychology* **50**, 951–964.

[52] Grisso, T. (2003). *Evaluating Competencies: Forensic Assessments and Instruments*. 2nd Edition, Kluwer, New York.

[53] Reder P., Duncan S. & Lucey C. (2003). What Principles Guide Parenting Assessments? in *Studies in the Assessment of Parenting* P. Reder, S. Duncan & C. Lucey, eds, Brunner- Routledge, New York, pp. 3–26.

[54] Ayoub C. & Kinscherff R. (2006). Forensic Assessment of Parenting in Child Abuse and Neglect Cases, in *Forensic Mental Health Assessment of Children and Adolescents*, S.N. Sparta & G.P. Koocher, eds, Oxford, New York, pp. 350–335.

[55] Basic Behavioral Science Task Force of the National Advisory Mental Health Council (1996). Basic behavioral science research for mental health: family processes and social networks, *American Psychologist* **51**, 622–630.

[56] Gould, J.W. & Martindale, D.A. (2007). *The Art and Science of Child Custody Evaluations*, Guilford, New York.

[57] Committee on Professional Practice and Standards, American Psychology Association Board of Professional Affairs (1999). Guidelines for psychological evaluations in child protection matters, *American Psychologist* **54**, 586–593.

[58] Brodzinsky, P. (1993). On the use and misuse of psychological testing in child custody evaluations, *Professional Psychology: Research and Practice* **24**, 213–219.

[59] Budd, K.S. & Holdsworth, M.J. (1996). Issues in clinical assessment of minimal parenting competence, *Journal of Clinical Child Psychology* **25**, 2–14.

[60] Andrews, P. & Meyer, R. (2003). Marlowe-Crowne personal desirability scale and short form C: forensic norms, *Journal of Clinical Psychology* **59**, 483–492.

[61] Carr, G.D., Moretti, M.H. & Cue, B.J.M. (2005). Evaluating parenting capacity: validity problems with the MMPI-2, PAI, CAPI, and ratings of child adjustment, *Professional Psychology: Research and Practice* **36**, 188–196.

[62] Heilbrun, K. (1995). Child custody evaluation: critically assessing mental health experts and psychological tests, *Family Law Quarterly* **29**, 63–78.

[63] Daubert v. Merrell Dow Pharmaceutical, Inc., 509 U.S. 579 (1993).

[64] Milchman, M.S. (2000). Mental health experts' common error in assessing bonding in guardianship cases, *The Journal of Psychiatry and Law* **28**, 351–378.

[65] Starr, R. (1987). Clinical judgment of abuse-proneness based on parent-child interactions, *Child Abuse & Neglect* **11**, 87–92.

[66] Martindale, D.A. & Gould, J.W. (2004). The forensic model: ethics and scientific methodology applied to custody evaluation, *Journal of Child Custody* **1**(2), 1–22.

[67] Acklin, M.W. & Cho-Stutler, L. (2006). The science and art of parent-child observation in child custody evaluation, *Journal of Forensic Psychology* **6**, 51–62.

[68] Comfort, M. & Gordon, P.R. (2006). Keys to interactive parenting scale (KIPS): a practical assessment of parenting behavior, *NHSA Dialogue: A Research-to-Practice Journal for the Early Intervention Field* **9**, 22–48.

[69] Budd, K.S., Poindexter, L.M., Felix, E.D. & Naik-Polan, A. (2001). Clinical assessment of parents in child protection cases: an empirical analysis, *Law and Human Behavior* **25**, 93–108.

[70] Budd, K.S., Felix, E.D., Sweet, S.C., Saul, A. & Carleton, R.A. (2006). Evaluating parents in child protection decisions: an innovative court-based clinic model, *Professional Psychology: Research and Practice* **37**, 666–675.

[71] Oberlander, L. (1995). Psychological issues in child sexual abuse evaluations: a survey of forensic mental health professionals, *Child Abuse & Neglect* **19**, 474–489.

[72] Jacobsen, T., Miller, L. & Kirkwood, K. (1997). Assessing parenting competency in individuals with severe mental illness: A comprehensive service, *Journal of Mental Health Administration* **24**, 189–199.

[73] Bow, J.M. (2006). Review of empirical research on child custody practice, *Journal of Child Custody* **3**, 23–50.

[74] Bow, J.M., Gould, J.W., Flens, J.R. & Greenhut, D. (2006). Testing in child custody evaluations – selection, usage, and Daubert admissibility: a survey of psychologists, *Journal of Forensic Psychology Practice* **6**, 17–38.

[75] Archer, R.P. (2006). *Forensic Use of Clinical Assessment Instruments*, Lawrence Erlbaum, Mahwah.

[76] Committee on Ethical Guidelines for Forensic Psychologists (1991). Specialty guidelines for forensic psychologists, *Law and Human Behavior* **15**, 655–665.

[77] American Psychological Association (1994). Guidelines for child custody evaluations in divorce proceedings, *American Psychologist* **49**, 677–680.

[78] Association of Family and Conciliation Courts (2006). *Model Standards of Practice for Child Custody Evaluation*. Retrieved 2/05/06 from http://www.afccnet.org/resources/resources_model_child.asp.

[79] American Psychological Association (2002). Ethical principles of psychologists and code of conduct, *American Psychologist* **57**, 1060–1073.

[80] Dyer, F.J. (1999). *Psychological Consultation in Parental Rights Cases*, Guilford, New York.

[81] Heilbrun, K., Marczuk, G.R. & DeMatto, D. (2002). *Forensic Mental Health Assessment: A Casebook*, Oxford, New York.

PAUL ANDREWS

Parricide *see* Battered Child Syndrome

Particles: Form

Forensic trace evidence includes small fragments of material (particles) that can be used to assist with an investigation into crimes and accidents [1]. Particles are ubiquitous – cosmetics, pollen, fibers, glass, and minerals to name a few. There are usually many thousands of particles virtually on all exposed surfaces. They can originate from distant sources and be transported through air, sea, or the surfaces of animals, including people. Particles adhere to vehicles, tools, clothes, and objects creating a signature of particles with an almost infinite variety. The potential to relate where something was manufactured, where it has been, and who could have been associated with it is sometimes possible with critical examination. Forensic scientists analyze particles using microscopy and instrumental analysis to characterize, identify, and associate materials; to determine provenance, and

link people, places and objects to assist the judicial system (*see* **Microscopy: Light Microscopes**).

Particles with considerable diversity of form can originate from botanical materials, such as pollen, spores, diatoms, seeds, plant hairs, grass including *Cannabis sativa* L., leaves, needles, rootlets, and phytoliths. Botanical materials are cultivated, altered, and consumed by man and animals as food. From Wonder Bread to Wheaties, from the corn in corn dogs, to the seeds in feces, small particles abound in the plant kingdom. Animals also have or produce an array of particles such as hairs, feathers, eggs, skin cells, teeth, scales, and processed body parts. Natural inorganic particles are ubiquitous in a multitude of types from minerals and rocks, microfossils, deposits evaporated from water, and cosmic particles such as micrometeorites and tektites.

Traces formed by the interaction between man and the environment have increased the range of particles. Botanically derived particles can originate from foodstuffs and vomit. Man-made particles can be derived from the breakdown and disintegration of building materials such as concrete and wallboard. Vehicles contribute metals, fibers, paint, polymers, tire rubber, glass, lubricants, and fuel. Clothing materials often shed fibers. Wood and paper products can form chips, dust, and pulp fibers. Man-made particles can be formed from metals, gunshot residue (GSR), explosives, tapes, putties, corrosion, drugs, fertilizers, insecticides, poisons, toxins, and cosmetics. Particles can be composites from multiple sources such as dust, paint chips, chemicals, and combustion products.

Particle size and shape are fundamental properties that can provide important information in identification, comparison, and provenance. The Particle Atlas [2, 3] uses an ingenious six-digit code and binary sum to classify particles in the process of identifying unknowns. There are six basic classification characteristics in the code: transparency, color, isotropy/anisotropy, refractive index, shape (first characteristic), and shape (second characteristic). The system uses either a "0" or a "1" to signify the absence (0) or presence (1) of the six different particle characteristics. Specifically, the fifth and sixth digits are used to describe a particle's shape or form:

1 1 – elongated and flattened (ribbon, blade, and lath)

1 0 – flattened but not elongated (plate or tablet)

0 1 – elongated but not flattened (needle or rod)

0 0 – neither elongated nor flattened (equant particle).

Particles can exist in crystalline or noncrystalline form. The study and characterization of crystals is known as *crystallography*. Solid particles form into one of six "crystal systems". A crystal system is a category of space groups, which characterize symmetry of structures in three dimensions in three directions, having a discrete class of point groups. The six crystal systems are cubic (isometric), hexagonal, tetragonal, orthorhombic, monoclinic, and triclinic. Crystalline particles can form on any scale, from large particles visible to the naked eye, to submicron crystalline particles that can only be examined microscopically. Cubic crystals are in the shape of a perfect cube. The crystallographic axes used in this system are of equal length and are mutually perpendicular, occurring at right angles to one another. A grain of common table salt is a good example of a cubic crystal. Examples of minerals which crystallize in the cubic system are halite, magnetite, and garnet. Minerals of this system tend to produce crystals of equidimensional or equant habit. A crystal form is a collection of equivalent crystal faces related to each other by mineral symmetry [4].

Trace evidence particles are collected and initially examined by stereomicroscopy at low magnification from 4× to 100×. During this screening process, particle form is often the first characteristic that is recognized. Forms, shapes, structures, angles, etc., between things can be obviously different. The same is true in the examination of particles in trace evidence, even on the microscopic scale.

Pollen

The study of pollen, spores, and other acid resistant microscopic plant particles is called *palynology* and is highly useful in paleoecology, paleontology, archaeology, and forensics. Pollen grains are microscopic in size (10–100 μm), occur abundantly in soil and dust on any exposed surface, are resistant to decay, and as different from each other as the plants that produce them. Pollen assemblages found in soil and water bodies at a crime scene often reflect the vegetation and environment of the area. Pollen grains come in a wide variety of shapes, sizes, and surface markings (Figure 1). The pollen grain has three walls

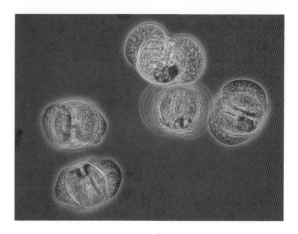

Figure 1   Pollen from *Pinus taeda*, loblolly pine. Phase contrast, original magnification 400×

or layers. The outer wall is most often sculptured, covered with any combination of spines (echinae), pores, ridges (rugulae), or bumps (scabrae) that help in identifying the grain. The middle layer contains the enzymes necessary for plant recognition in pollination. The third layer is a bottom wall and sometimes has columns rising up to the outer wall. Palynologists have classified pollen using two principal morphological features: pori (pores) and colpi (furrows). Pollen grains are divided into groups by the number, position, and shape of their pori and colpi. Pollen grains having only pores are called *porate*, those with only colpi are called *colpate*, and those with both are called *colporate*. The number of pores and colpi is denoted by attaching prefixes such as mono-, si-, terta-, and penta-. Further divisions are made by an examination of the fine structure and patterns observed on the outer layer. Descriptive terminology such as gemmate, pilate, regulate, scabrate, etc., are used [1] (*see* **Palynology**).

Diatoms

Diatoms are unicellular algae that live in any water body, large or small, from fresh to salt and brackish types. A characteristic feature of diatom cells is that they are encased within a unique cell wall made of silica (hydrated silicon dioxide) called a *frustule* or *test* (Figure 2). These frustules show a wide diversity in form, some very beautiful and ornate, usually consisting of two asymmetrical sides. The identification

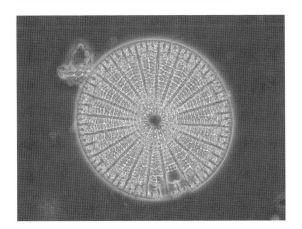

Figure 2 *Arachnoidiscus,* a diatom from San Pedro, California. Phase contrast, original magnification 400×

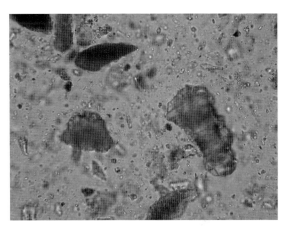

Figure 3 Malachite. An artist's paint pigment, naturally ground. Original magnification 400×

of diatoms is based on the morphology of the test. Two major groups of diatoms are generally recognized: the centric diatoms exhibiting radial symmetry (symmetry about a point) and the pennate diatoms with bilaterally symmetrical (symmetry about a line). Another particle with some similarities to diatoms are radiolarian, single-celled plankton in the kingdom Protista, which secrete silicate exoskeletons. They have lots of spines radiating outward. Seafloor deposits that are formed from radiolarian are called *radiolarian ooze*. This ooze forms a sedimentary rock known as *chert*. Decomposition and decay of diatoms may form diatomaceous earth, which can be mined and processed for use in a variety of products including paint, insulation, abrasives, and filtering agents (*see* **Diatoms**).

Paint Pigment

Paint pigment particles range from ground minerals used since antiquity to processed precipitated types used in the automotive industry. Pigments are often crystalline and tend to influence their external shape. Lead white forms as 1–50 μm hexagonal platelets. Zinc white forms as less than 2-μm rounded particles, many with spiked arms that look like children's jacks using 1000× oil immersion microscopy. Some crystalline pigments are too finely divided to show crystallinity. Titanium dioxide pigment, probably one of the most common, is less than 1 μm in size and is subrounded in shape. A few pigments are noncrystalline glasses and show conchoidal glassy fracture

such as cobalt blue and gamboge. The shape of a particle tells how it was prepared, such as pigment formed by precipitation from a solution or vapor as in zinc oxide. Others are simply ground minerals like quartz, anhydrite, and malachite (Figure 3). The particle size of pigments is usually helpful in distinguishing between synthetic and natural varieties. Synthetic zinc white, titanium oxide, cadmium red, and lamp black are all up to about 1 μm in size. Natural quartz, gypsum, azurite, and ultramarine are much coarser, usually 5–10 μm (*see* **Paint: Interpretation**).

Paint chip particles may show a layer structure in cross section, originating from successive paint applications over time. The layered paint chip may also originate from an automobile having anywhere from three to six original paint layers. Paint chips having embedded reflective glass beads originate from highway fog marker/centerline paint. Still other paint particles may contain remnants of underlying surfaces such as plaster or wood. Microscopic rounded paint beads formed during aerosol deposition via spray painting have been found as associative physical evidence in many homicides including the Green River murders in Washington State.

Mineral and Rock Fragments

Minerals in the size range of fine sand are often examined in forensic soil cases. In the microscopic examination of mineral form, the shape of grains can be described in two categories: thin sections (a mineralogical specimen that has been glued to a microscope slide and ground and polished down to approximately 25 μm, thus allowing examination by transmitted polarized light microscopy) and individual detrital grains mounted in immersion liquids. Grains with well-formed crystal faces are termed *euhedral*. Grains without crystal faces are called *anhedral*. In glassy rocks where crystallization abruptly stops, minerals may show crystallites and microlites [5]. The term *crystal habit* describes the favored growth pattern of the crystals of a mineral. A crystals habit may show little relation to the form of a single, perfect crystal of the same mineral, which would be classified according to crystal system. Crystal habit is often useful in identification. Mineralogists and microchemists use many descriptive terms to describe form such as blocky or equant, tabular, lamellar, flaky, micaceous, elongated, columnar, prismatic, bladed, acicular, platy, scaly, granular, radiating, foliated, felted, and fibrous. Many minerals have certain crystallographic planes where chemical bonding is weaker. These planes of weakness along which a mineral may break are called *cleavage planes*. When a mineral is broken or crushed it may also break along the fracture surfaces, which are unrelated to the mineral's crystal structure. One common crystal observed in soil derived from igneous and metamorphic rocks is zircon. Euhedral zircon crystals, forming in the tetragonal crystal system, are quite distinctive (Figure 4). The surface textures of

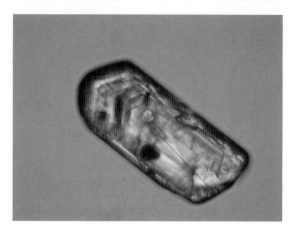

Figure 4   A crystalline zircon crystal. Original magnification 200×

sand grain and microfeatures observed by scanning electron microscopy can be used to link them to specific environments and geologic events (Figure 5) [6] (*see* **Soil: Forensic Analysis**).

Glass

The American Society of Testing Materials (ASTM) describes glass as an inorganic product of fusion that has cooled to a rigid condition without crystallizing [1]. Variables in physical properties of glass include thickness, curvature, manufacture marks, presence of mirror glass, and recognition of finely crushed

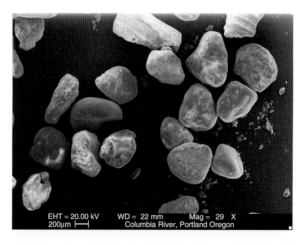

Figure 5   SEM photomicrograph of beach sand along the Columbia River near Portland, Oregon. Original magnification 29×

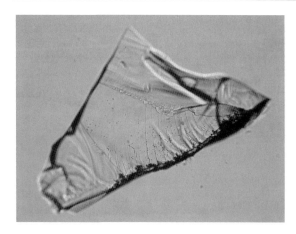

Figure 6 Glass particle showing conchodial fracture. Original magnification 40×

powdered glass originating from impact damage. Glass particles when broken show sharp, jagged edges known as *conchoidal fractures* (Figure 6). Tempered glass particles form "diced" pieces. Glass particles that have been annealed by coming into contact with a hot surface, such as a halogen lamp filament often have a molten smooth, beaded texture. Other glass particles such as pumice that originate from volcanism can show flow banding (Figure 7), glassy beads or glassy coatings on other mineral surfaces. Some glass particles have what are known as *hackle marks* on the edges, which are useful in interpreting the side of the glass where the force was applied when it broke. It have been reported that glass particles recovered as forensic evidence average from 0.35 to 1 mm in size, whereas fragments >5 mm are most likely to be easily lost [7] (*see* **Glass Evidence: Bayesian Approach to**).

Wood

Particles of wood can be identified by their relatively soft, porous, and fibrous texture. If the particle is large enough, the differentiation between softwood and hardwood can be made on the presence or absence of resin canals and vessel elements. The particle may be rough surfaced and torn, suggesting chainsaw wood chips or fine and powdery in form such as sawdust. Some particles may have attached bark and accessory decay particles. Softwood and hardwood fibers found in paper products can be identified microscopically based on fiber anatomy. Softwood fibers, called *tracheids*, are distinguished by bordered pits along their length (Figure 8). Ray cross-field pitting locations have very specific pits that are classified into groups: fenestriform, pinoid, taxodioid, cupressoid, and piceoid, characteristic of softwood species. Hardwood species are identified by

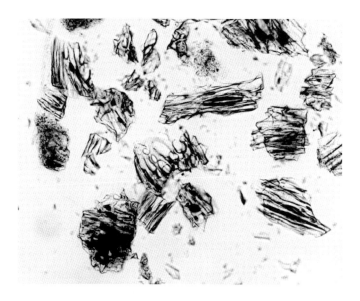

Figure 7 Pumice

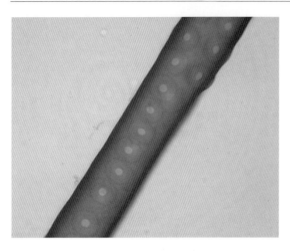

Figure 8 Softwood fiber from *Pinus Ponderosa*, Ponderosa Pine showing bordered pits. Original magnification 200×

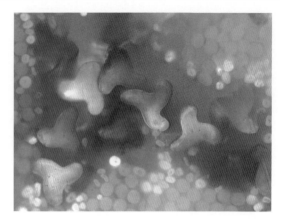

Figure 9 Trilobal nylon fibers encased in cotton backing fibers. Original magnification 200×

their unique water-conducting structures called *vessel elements*. These tube-shaped structures separate out into discrete particles when the wood is pulped (*see* **Wood**).

Fibers

Fibers are often defined as particles having a high length to width ratio. Fibers are classified into groups: manufactured (nylon, polyester, etc.), natural plant (cotton, jute, hemp, etc.), and inorganic (asbestos and glass fibers). Physical characteristics of manufactured fibers include diameter, cross-sectional shape, crimp, striations, and damage. The cross-sectional shape of nonround fibers is often patented and very unique. Many types are extruded through a spinneret, a device having a series of engineered holes that a molten polymer travels through. The fibers leaving the spinneret have a cross-sectional shape matching the holes of the spinneret. Fibers such as nylon can have cross-sectional shapes ranging from round, delta, trilobal, and multichanneled just to name a few (Figure 9). Bicomponent fibers are comprised of two polymers of different chemical and/or physical properties extruded from the same spinneret with both polymers within the same filament. Most commercially available bicomponent fibers are configured in a sheath/core, side by side, or eccentric sheath/core arrangement. Natural plant fibers may be encountered

as the technical fiber (cordage, sacks, mats, etc.) or as individual cells (fabric and paper). Relative cell wall and lumen (canal in central shaft of fiber) thickness, cell length, and presence of surface markings, crystals, and twists are important characteristics to observe [8]. Mineral fibers in the asbestiform group range from chrysotile, having a soft, wavy texture, to the long, straight, inflexible fibers of amosite. Glass fibers can be placed into three catagories: fiberglass (continuous and noncontinuous), mineral wool (rock wool and slag wool having exotic twisty blob-like shapes), and refractory ceramic fibers that have exotic shapes, but are thinner in diameter compared to the others (*see* **Fibers**).

Hairs

Human hairs can be distinguished from other animal hairs by examining features such as the scale pattern, medulla, root, length, and shaft configurations (Figure 10) [5]. Specific terms used to describe human hair shaft form are straight, arced, wavy, curly, twisted, tightly coiled, and crimped. The cross-sectional shape in human hair can vary from rounded, oval, triangular, to flattened. The shaft can appear as buckled, convoluted, undulating, and split, [5]. The somatic origin of human hairs can often be determined by morphology (*see* **Hair: Microscopic Analysis**; **Hair: Animal**).

Many other trace evidence particles can present a variety of forms. Smokeless powder (commonly

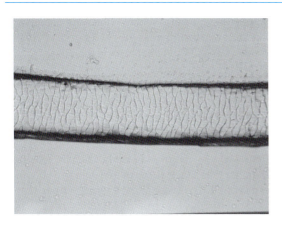

Figure 10 Caucasian head hair showing an imbricate scale pattern typical of man. Original magnification 200×

called *gunpowder*) can be manufactured in ball, flattened ball, disk, and tubular shapes. Databases have been developed, in which these morphological criteria are used to distinguish the different brands. GSR analysis relies on the identification of lead, barium, and antimony residues originating from the primer cap of cartridges. One criterion for identification is the minute (often less than 5 μm), rounded particle form characteristic of GSR.

References

[1] American Society for Testing and Materials (1965). *Standard Definitions of Terms Relating to Glass Products*, ASTM Standards, ASTM, Philadelphia, Part 13, p. 145.

[2] Mahaney, W.C. (2002). *Atlas of Sand Grain Surface Textures and Applications*, Oxford University Press.

[3] McCrone, W.C. & Delly, J.G. (1992). *The Particle Atlas*, 2nd Edition, Vol. 4, Ann Arbor Science.

[4] McCrone, W.C. (1982). The microscopical identification of artists' pigments, *Journal of the International Institute for Conservation* 7(1 & 2), 11–34.

[5] Forensic Science Communications (2005). *Forensic Human Hair Examination Guidelines*, Scientific Working Group on Materials Analysis (SWGMAT).

[6] Heinrich, E.W.M. (1965). *Microscopic Identification of Minerals*, McGraw-Hill.

[7] Almirall, J.R. & Trejos, T. (2006). Advances in the forensic analysis of glass fragments with a focus on refractive index and elemental analysis, *Forensic Science Review* 18(2) 74–95.

[8] Forensic Science Communications (1999). *Forensic Fiber Examination Guidelines*, Scientific Working Group on Materials Analysis (SWGMAT).

Further Reading

Bisbing, R.E. & Schneck, W.M. (2006). Particle analysis in forensic science, *Forensic Science Review* **18**(2) 119–144.

McCrone *McCrone Atlas of Microscopic Particles*, http://www.mccroneatlas.com.

Neese, W.D. (2000). *Introduction to Mineralogy*, Oxford University Press.

WILLIAM SCHNECK

Paternity *see* Missing Persons and Paternity: DNA

Pattern: Fire *see* Fire: Dynamics and Pattern Production

Patty Hearst *see* Stockholm Syndrome

Peak Height: DNA

Peak Height

The height of a peak on an electrophoretogram is measured in relative fluorescent units (rfu) and is a measure of the intensity of light detected by a DNA analyzer as sample is passed through a column. It is roughly proportional to the amount of DNA present, and is expected to be within a certain range of values for standard analyses. For example, using the protocol validated by Applied Biosystems Inc. for the SGM Plus kit, 1–2.5 ng of input DNA will give peaks with heights in the range 150–5000 rfu.

As with any technology for measurement, there is a baseline "noise" that is recorded in the absence of sample, and is related to the sensitivity of the detection machine. There is some debate about the threshold value above which a peak can be declared as a "real" peak that represents a piece of DNA, as opposed to chance occurrence of noise of sufficient intensity to appear as a peak. Different laboratories use different thresholds, decisions that may be based on objective principle, scientific validation, or rule-of-thumb experience.

Two alleles of a heterozygotic locus will give heights that are roughly equal in height, and for the same amount of DNA under the same conditions, a homozygote would produce one peak that is roughly twice the height of the heterozygote peaks. Generally, alleles of smaller size (fewer repeats) (*see also* **Short Tandem Repeats**) amplify better than larger ones and so will have a slightly higher peak. Owing to variation in the analytical chemistry, this correlation is not absolute, but two peaks of a heterozygote are almost always more than 60% in proportion, smaller : larger or larger : smaller, and such peaks are said to be balanced. The loci that have been designed to give smaller (molecule length) PCR products, e.g., D3 *versus* D2 in the SGM Plus kit, will also often produce higher peaks than for the larger loci. This effect may be particularly obvious if the sample of DNA is partially degraded and is due to an increased chance of larger DNA molecules being degraded (and so unavailable for PCR amplification) rather than smaller molecules.

Peak heights may be used to interpret the DNA being analyzed. For example, when two peaks being compared are not above the 60% ratio, this is called peak height imbalance. When imbalance is seen, it is usually an indication that the peaks in question come from DNA that is partly or entirely from different contributing sources, i.e., there is a mixture of contributors. This information is used in conjunction with the number of peaks seen at each locus of a profile to identify the presence of a mixture. When a mixture of DNA sources exists, peaks will be seen that are roughly in proportion to their relative contributing amounts. Where alleles are common to more than one contributor, the rfu for each allele will be added to give a combined higher peak. Looking at the peak heights of a profile at each locus and all loci together, it may be possible to interpret all or part of at least one of the contributors. This is true especially for what are termed major/minor mixtures where there is a much greater proportion of one source compared with another. The major profile will be more completely decipherable than the minor one since some of the minor peaks may be masked by overlapping with peaks from shared alleles of the major profile. Mixtures of DNA in less extreme proportions are much more difficult to interpret objectively, assisted only when there is a reasonable expectation of DNA from one of the sources.

For a discussion of the use of peaks in mixture interpretation, see Gill *et al.* [1] and Clayton *et al.* [2]. Peak values in LCN analysis are discussed in Whitaker *et al.* [3].

References

[1] Gill, P., Sparkes, R., Pinchin, R., Clayton, T., Whitaker, J. & Buckleton, J. (1998). Interpreting simple STR mixtures using allele peak areas, *Forensic Science International* **91**, 41–53.

[2] Clayton, T.M., Whitaker, J.P., Sparkes, R. & Gill, P. (1998). Analysis and interpretation of mixed forensic stains using DNA STR profiling, *Forensic Science International* **91**, 55–70.

[3] Whitaker, J.P., Cotton, E.A. & Gill, P. (2001). A comparison of the characteristics of profiles produced with the AMPFlSTR SGM Plus multiplex system for both standard and low copy number (LCN) STR DNA analysis, *Forensic Science International* **123**, 215–223.

Further Reading

Buckleton, J., Triggs C.M. & Walsh, S.J. (2005). *Forensic DNA Evidence Interpretation*, CRC Press.

Butler, J.M. (2005). *Forensic DNA Typing*, 2nd Edition, Elsevier.

SCOTT BADER

Pedophilia *see* Child Sexual Abuse

Peer Review as Affecting Opinion Evidence

Obtaining the Approval of One's Peers in Science

Peer review is a term that, in scientific, publishing, and other circles, has a number of different meanings. The principal definition, however, describes a method whereby the appropriateness of research project results, as well as of articles, papers, and books based thereon, have been judged as worthy contributions to the scientific or professional field in which they belong. In some academic fields, peer review is referred to as *refereeing* [1–4]. No matter what the process or the end result is, the material under review is a document.

The purposes of peer review are to determine which research proposals will receive grants or monetary support to allow the research to go forth; whether an article of book is worthy to be published; and to evaluate the comparative ranking of researchers, scientists, or academics for advancement, remuneration, professional self-improvement purposes, as well as for comparative ranking among colleagues. Many journals publish guidelines for reviewers and these will usually explain the journal's purpose in using peer review. Not all materials published in peer reviewed journals are actually peer reviewed. For example, letters and correspondence may be peer reviewed in some journals but not in others.

The customary peer review process is applied to matters that include, for example, the dissemination of research results, an article or book on a method or topic. It involves the scrutiny of an impartial panel of several experts (usually two or three) on the same topic with which the research or publication deals. The process takes place prior to, and as a condition of acceptance and publication. Sometimes, peer review occurs by comments in the professional forum (bulletins, publications, or at meetings) made *after* and as a result of a project's publication.

There are many reasons for subjecting a project to an examination by such a panel. Primary among them is to determine whether the methodology followed by the researcher is suitable to support the conclusion. The vast majority of published work is not the final say on a topic, but a contribution to the knowledge in that field.

The possible results of peer review are;

1. outright rejection;
2. suggestions that the paper would be suitable if rewritten with identified problems corrected;
3. accepted with minor amendment; and
4. accepted as is.

Rejection may be for presentational, appropriateness to the readership of the journal, or other reasons not connected with the scientific content.

The end result of peer review does not, ordinarily, carry with it the implication that the approved work came to a correct conclusion, but means, instead, that it is sufficiently worthy of being exposed to the broader professional discipline for judgment, further study, examination, comment, or falsification (**Falsifiability Theory**). This is a frequent source of misunderstanding and even misrepresentation in courts.

In some cases, peer review proceeds anonymously, with reviewers having no prior knowledge of the identity of the authors. This is intended as a protection against bias, although it is sometimes possible to make a good guess at the source just from the content of the article.

Most frequently, the peer review process follows these steps.

Step 1. The project's methodology or an article's conclusions is submitted to a panel of experts, who may or may not know who designed the research project or wrote the article intended for publication and who may also not know who the other reviewers are.

Step 2. The reviewers make comments on the project's worth to a project evaluator or publisher's representative and make a recommendation as to whether the project rests on sound methodological applications of appropriate scientific principles, or whether the conclusions drawn from a research project are deemed to contribute to the body of knowledge and literature in the field. These reviewers recommend approval, rejection, or suggest changes, mandatory, or optional.

Step 3a. If the recommendations of at least two of a panel of three reviewers approve of the project's methodology or the soundness of a paper, it is typically approved for acceptance and/or publication.

Step 3b. If recommendations for changes are made by the reviewers, these comments may be transmitted to the original researcher/author with a request to consider a redesign of the project or a rewrite of the paper. The originator of the project are, most often, not be told who the reviewers were.

The system is not necessarily democratic, with managers of the reviewing process or editors appointed by the publisher retaining the privilege to disregard the opinions of reviewers, appointing new reviewers, or deciding contrary to reviewers' recommendations.

Peer Review in Some Forensic Sciences

In a few forensic disciplines, peer review may have a totally different meaning, one that is more akin to verifying the accuracy of a particular examination result. The scrutiny is provided by having the prior result obtained during an examination of evidence verified by other experts of more advanced or equal stature in the profession.

The purpose of such verification is to determine whether the original conclusion is deemed accurate and trustworthy.[a] The verifier independently retraces the steps of an examiner to see whether the same result is reached by other skilled examiners.

Sometimes, the verifier may not know who the individual is who has reached the original result – a process sometimes referred to as *blind verification.* If the verifier is not aware that an examination was originally done by someone else, the process may be called *double-blind verification.*

Criticism of Peer Review

To accept a publication or a report based on a novel methodology after submission to peer review does not signify the reviewers agree with its conclusions, but rather whether it is deemed worthy to be submitted to the scrutiny of the field. Many studies that have been published are roundly criticized by others even after or as a result of their acceptance or publication.

Others may cause the originators to modify or withdraw their original conclusions as a result of input received from reviewers or from others in the field that have become acquainted with the project.

In the traditional publishing business, the peer review process is also extremely cumbersome and time consuming. Most hard-copy peer reviewed journals work on a schedule involving many months of copy evaluation, submission to reviewers, returning comments to the original researcher, and receiving rewrites or revisions, leading ultimately to approval, copy preparation and publication. By the time publication occurs, the conclusions may already have been altered or, in some cases, shown to be in error.

The Internet is providing an alternative to the traditional peer review process by the existence of blogs, online-only publications, and an almost instantaneous exchange of views on any topic at virtually no cost through interactive science publishing. The Internet also provides a readier tool for identifying plagiarism before publication.

Also, because most novel techniques are developed by pioneers in a field, there is an inherent bias against conclusions reached that may go counter to those of peer reviewers who are considered the "established power structure" in a discipline. These individuals may well have a vested interest in safeguarding their own prior positions on the same topic or the positions which they have spent careers supporting or defending, to prevent them from being replaced by newer approaches. At the other end of the spectrum, some reviewers, in evaluating the worth of a project, may tend to have a bias in favor of conclusions that are in agreement with their own expressed views.

The inefficiency in identifying fraudulent conduct is also seen as a serious drawback of the peer review process. Most professions as well as science publications can offer examples of cases in their own areas wherein researchers who had come to be respected were thereafter exposed as having created fraudulent data or falsified the outcome of research to support their conclusions.

Peer Review in American Law

In American legal circles, the words "peer review" have taken on essentially the first one of the approaches to peer review described herein, as a result of the momentous United States Supreme Court decision in *Daubert v. Merrell Dow Pharmaceuticals* [5] (*see Daubert v. Merrell Dow Pharmaceuticals*), a court opinion that forever changed the legal landscape on how the decision on the admissibility of expert opinion testimony is to be made (**Expert Opinion: United States**).

Peer review, in *Daubert*, came to be lauded as a desirable, though not an essential, factor whereby the soundness of a scientific methodology utilized by particular experts can be judged. As a result, some forensic disciplines that consider peer review as synonymous with "verification of a result obtained in an analysis" have met some resistance in courts in having their conclusions deemed as satisfying a *Daubert*-style of peer review.

Thus, in *United States v. Mitchell*, the court, in examining whether "fingerprint identification" satisfied the peer review factor of *Daubert*, recognized that the type of verification required of latent-print examiners in the analysis, comparison, evaluation and verification ACE-V methodology might "not be peer review in its best form, but, on balance, the peer review factor does favor admissibility" [6]. The overwhelming majority of court decisions of appellate tribunals have reached similar decisions in allowing the "V" in the ACE-V methodology to satisfy the *Daubert* "peer review" factor.[b]

There remain critics of those forensic practices involved in individualization who would like to see the courts reject the admissibility of examination techniques wherein the "scientific" model of peer review is not strictly followed. Defenders of those practices respond that inasmuch as the existence of a peer reviewed literature guarantees neither accuracy nor reliability of an examination result, to impose such a high standard on the verification process in forensic science is probably unwarranted in light of the precise language in the United States Supreme Court's *Daubert* decision itself.[c]

End Notes

[a.] For example: In the Latent Friction Ridge Comparison discipline, verification of the results obtained by one examiner's individualization is required in some circumstances and recommended in others.

See the Scientific Working Group of Friction Ridge Analysis, Study and Technology (SWGFAST), in its guidelines and standards at www.swgfast.org. Several other forensic disciplines use the ACE-V methodology in the comparison sciences, among them forensic document examiners, firearm and toolmark examiners.

[b.] The ACE-V process is described in **Friction Ridge Skin: Comparison and Identification**.

[c.] In *Mitchell, supra* [6] at 244, the court explained: "*Daubert* does not require that a party who proffers expert testimony carry the burden of proving to the judge that the expert's assessment of the situation is correct. As long as the expert's scientific testimony rests on 'good grounds, based on what is known,'" the testimony should be admitted and tested by the adversary system.

References

[1] On peer review generally, Shatz, D. (2004). *Peer Review: A Critical Inquiry*, Rowman & Littlefield, Lanham.
[2] Hames, I. (2007). *Peer Review and Manuscript Management in Scientific Journals: Guidelines for Good Practice*, Black well publishing.
[3] Wagner, E., Godlee, F & Jefferson, T. (2002). *How to Survive Peer Review* BMJ Books, London.
[4] Wiegers, K.E. (2001). *Peer Reviews in Software: A Practical Guide*, Addison-Wesley, Boston.
[5] Daubert v. Merrell Dow Pharmaceuticals, Inc., 509 U.S. 579 (1993).
[6] United States v. Mitchell, 365 F.3d 215, at 239 (3rd Cir. 2004), cert. denied 543 U.S. 974 (2004).

ANDRE MOENSSENS

Pen and Writing Instruments *see* Writing Instruments and Printing Devices

Persistence: Trace *see* Trace Evidence: Transfer, Persistence, and Value

Person Identification *see* Elderly in Court

Personality Testing *see* Psychological Testing

Persuasibility of Children *see* Children: Suggestibility of

Persuasion *see* Deception: Truth Serum

Pharmacodynamics *see* Alcohol: Interaction with Other Drugs

Pharmacogenomics

Introduction

In 1865, Gregor Mendel discovered the basis of inheritance and genetics. Pharmacogenetics and its related science pharmacogenomics emerged as our understanding of genetics advanced, in particular, that certain enzymes coded by the genetic blueprint process both endogenous and exogenous substances (such as drugs). This understanding is likely to develop further in years to come and may even allow personalization of drug treatment – personalized medicine, based on a person's genetic profile [1, 2]. Thus, pharmacogenomics is likely to increasingly contribute to clinical and forensic practices in the future.

Pharmacogenomics has already been useful to optimize treatment of lung cancer by identifying genotypes likely to predispose to toxicity and poor outcome [3]. Patients with homozygous *UGT1A1*28* are more likely to develop neutropenia, whereas patients with *GSTP1 1105 G/A* or *G/G* genotypes may show partial response. Another study identified the combination of five-gene biomarkers (*DUSP6, MMD, STAT1, ER BB3*, and *LCK*) as an independent predictor of relapse-free and overall survival [4].

Pharmacogenomics and pharmacogenetics are currently used interchangeably; however, pharmacogenetics is readily defined as the study of the genetic effect, e.g., single-nucleotide polymorphism (SNP), on an individual's ability to metabolize a drug or other substance, pharmacgenomics is concerned with the whole-genome effect on drug metabolism and efficacy.

The emerging clinical applications of pharmacogenetics/pharmacogenomics may be directly verified by the use (and approval by various regulatory agencies) of genotyping methodologies/platforms, the frequent inclusion of this topic in scientific and clinical meetings, and the availability (in 2007) of a pharmacogenomic survey program offered by the College of American Pathologists.

Pharmacogenomics serves as an "adjunct" to other tests and scientific practices. For example, genotyping can be conducted as an adjunct to the autopsy (molecular autopsy) and complements the current forensic applications such as DNA fingerprinting.

Thus, this article presents pharmacogenomics as a complementing discipline to enhance drug therapy and serve as an adjunct to forensic pathology/toxicology. Forensic applications include an algorithm for the use of pharmacogenomics in forensic pathology/toxicology, with emphasis on interrelationships to circumstances and drug use/abuse history, scene investigation, and autopsy findings.

On the opposite end of the spectrum, the use of molecular/genetic testing in postmortem forensic science has included DNA fingerprinting for identity testing. Recently, pharmacogenomics as molecular autopsy has been used for the assessment of genetic contribution to drug toxicity in postmortem forensic toxicology. In common with the other applications of clinical and scientific findings in forensic science, the findings might add to the understanding of disease mechanisms and optimization of treatment including drug therapy. Thus, the use of pharmacogenomics in forensic toxicology may add to the understanding of drug toxicity due to genetically predisposed impaired drug metabolism, and in so doing thus provide better interpretation and indirectly enabling the emerging personalized medicine.

Principles of Pharmacogenetics/Pharmacogenomics

According to the central dogma of molecular biology, the genetic code of DNA is passed, through transcription, onto *mRNA*. The information in *mRNA* is passed, through translation, in protein synthesis. These proteins may be drug-metabolizing enzymes, transporters, and receptors. As a result, DNA genetic

variations (*see also* **Polymorphism: Genetic**) determine the enzyme activity, transporters, and receptor sensitivity.

For drug-metabolizing enzyme genes, the lack of and the presence of genetic variations results in normal, deficient, or higher enzyme activities. Genetic variations might include SNPs, deletion, duplications, and other variations. The polygenic determinants of drug response are illustrated by Figure 1. By comparing an individual with two wild-type alleles (normal or extensive metabolizer *see also* **Phenotype**) on the left to an individual with two variant alleles (a poor metabolizer) on the right, the genetic variations would result in lower enzymes activity and elevated plasma concentration *versus* time curve (calculated as area under curve, AUC), with corresponding increased toxicity and decreased receptor sensitivity and efficacy. The heterozygous individual in the middle with one variant allele (an

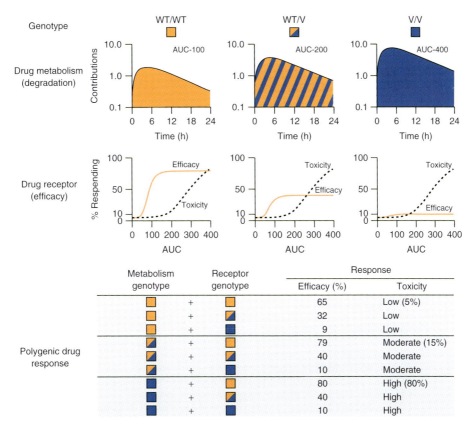

Figure 1 Polygenic determinants of drug response [With permission from publisher of Ref. 5, © Massachusetts Medical Society, 2003.]

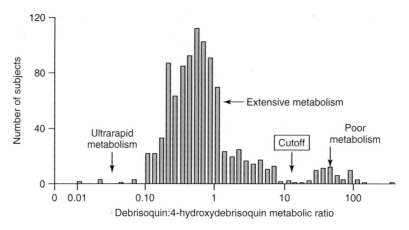

Figure 2   Pharmacogenetics of CYP 2D6 [Reprinted by permission of Macmillan Publishers Ltd: Clinical Pharmacology & Therapeutics [6], ©1992.]

intermediate metabolizer) exhibits AUC, toxicity, and efficacy intermediate between those of the extensive and poor metabolizers. With a possible combination of nine metabolism and receptor genotypes, the therapeutic index (separation of therapeutic and toxic responses) could range from 13 to 0.125.

Further, individuals with multiple copies of the genes are ultrarapid metabolizers (UMs). An example of this is shown in Figure 2, which shows the debrisoquin metabolic ratios (MRs) of these phenotypes [6].

Race and ethnicity can affect the prevalence of "poor" metabolizers, but they are usually relatively uncommon. For example, there are variations in the prevalence of one of the more common P450 enzymes, CYP2D6, in African-Americans and the Chinese. Patients who are genotypically slow metabolizers may, for example, require more

tramadol (analgesic) than other "normal" subjects, possibly explaining the variable response to pain management in some patients.

Genetic variation can also make a person more susceptible to disease [7].

Tests and Methodologies

The majority of the current testing is primarily based on pharmacogenetics (PGx). The top 10 tests in 2005 as assessed by the American Association of clinical Chemists (AACC) are listed in Table 1 (in descending order).

Within the list, CYP and other phase II enzymes (conjugating enzymes) such as uridine diphosphate glucuronosyltransferase 1A1 (UGT1A1) accounted for the majority of drug/substrate metabolism for drugs approved in the United States, about 75%

Table 1   Top 10 pharmacogenomics tests

Abbreviation	Name and function
CYP 2D6	Cytochrome P450 2D6, phase I drug-metabolizing enzyme
TPMT	Thiopurine S-methyltransferase, phase II drug-metabolizing enzyme
CYP 2C9	Cytochrome P450 2C9, phase I drug-metabolizing enzyme
CYP 2C19	Cytochrome P450 2C19, phase I drug-metabolizing enzyme
NAT	N-acetyltransferase, phase II drug-metabolizing enzyme
CYP 3A5	Cytochrome P450 3A5, phase I drug-metabolizing enzyme
UGT1A1	Uridine diphosphate glucuronosyltransferase 1A1, phase II drug-metabolizing enzyme
MDR1	Multidrug resistance (P-glycoprotein), drug protein transporter
CYP 2B6	Cytochrome P450 2B6, phase I drug-metabolizing enzyme
MTHFR	Methylenetetrahydrofolate(CH_2THF) reductase converts CH_2THF to 5-methyltetrahydrofolate

involving CYP 3A4 and cytochrome P450 2D6 (CYP 2D6) enzymes. Testing is complicated since there are more than 160 alterations for *CYP 2D6* genes alone. Assay problems can include allelic drop-out, intra-allelic recombination, the need for specific assays not affected by pseudogenes *CYP 2D7* and *CYP 2D8*, and to address gene conversion of *CYP 2D6* from *CYP 2D7*. Consequently, genetic testing is not yet widespread.

The more common pharmacogenomic tests are readily performed either by home-brew assay or a commercially available test or platform. The approaches included nonamplification, e.g., fluorescent *in situ* hybridization (FISH), target and signal amplification methods including endpoint polymerase chain reaction (PCR) detection, allele-specific primers, length analysis using restriction fragment length polymorphism (RFLP) and oligonucleotide ligation assay (OLA), real-time PCR, signal amplifications, and new methods including solid-phase microarrays and fluorescent-based bead assay (liquid mircoarray). The manufacturers and the status of FDA approvals are listed in Table 2.

Some laboratories performing genotyping have adapted the PCR liquid bead-based detection. The choice of the platform and assays seems to reflect the ease of "home-brew" assay development and the lower cost of the instrument and reagents.

Nevertheless, there are relative advantages and disadvantages of the various testing kits available. These need to be understood before having a test conducted.

Clinical Applications

The clinical applications of pharmacogenomics are classified according to the drug group, specialties, and diseases and include opioids, pain management, nicotine addiction, HIV treatment, immunosuppressants, and thiopurine *S*-methyltransferase (TPMT) for acute lymphoblastic leukemia, and psychiatry. Polymorphisms of the neurotransmitter transporters (serotonin, norepinephrine (noradrenaline), dopamine and P-glycoprotein, and serotonin transporter show little effect on serotonin active antidepressants selective serotonin reuptake inhibitor (SSRI) response, suggesting that the current scientific literature showing transporter genotypes is not yet contributory to predictive therapy [9]. There was evidence to support the use of genotype-based dosing for drug transporters such as P-glycoprotein (ABCB1) and OATP-C (SLC21A6) and other CYP enzyme genes. Other important and emerging areas include cancer, cardiovascular disorders, and hematology (Table 3)

It would be important to recognize the role of therapeutic drug monitoring (TDM) and toxicology

Table 2 Methodologies for pharmacogenetics testing[a]

Method	Company	FDA cleared or approved
Sequencing[b]	Abbott (Abbott Park, IL)	Yes
Real-time PCR	Applied Biosystems (Foster City, CA)	–
PCR arrays	Autogenomics (Carlsbad, CA)	yes
Sequencing[b]	Bayer Healthcare (Tarrytown, NY)	Yes
Pyrosequencing	Biotage AB (Uppsala, Sweden)	–
Real-time PCR	Celera Diagnostics (Alemeda, CA)	–
Real-time, allele-specific PCR	DxS Genotyping (Manchester, UK)	–
PCR	Gentris (Morrisville, NC)	yes
User-developed PCR arrays	Nanogen (San Diego, CA)	–
Nanoparticles	Nanosphere (Northbrook, IL)	yes
PCR arrays	Roche Diagnostics (Indianapolis, IN)	Yes
Invader assay	Thirdwave Technologies (Madison, WI)	Yes
PCR bead-based detection	Tm Biosciences Corp. (Toronto, ON)	–
FISH	Vysis (Des Plaines, IL)[c]	Yes

PCR, polymerase chain reaction; FISH, florescent *in situ* hybridization
[a] Reproduced with permission from Ref. 8. © AACC, 2006
[b] Sequencing for HIV drug resistance
[c] Vysis is now Abbott Molecular Diagnostics

Table 3 Examples of associations between drug response and genetic variants[a]

Drug	Variable clinical effect	Genes with associated variants	Possible mechanism
Azathioprine and mercaptopurine	Bone marrow aplasia	TPMT	Hypofunctional alleles
	Reduced therapeutic effect at standard doses		Wild-type alleles
Some antidepressants and β-blockers	Increase side-effect risk	CYP 2D6	Hypofunctional alleles
	Decreased efficacy		Gene duplication
Omeprazole	*Helicobacter pylori* cure rate	CYP 2C19	Hypofunctional alleles
Irinotecan	Neutropenia	UGT1A1	Decreased expression due to regulatory polymorphism
HIV protease inhibitors	Central nervous system levels	MDR1	Altered P-glycoprotein function
β-Blockers	Blood pressure lowering and heart rate slowing	ADRB1	Altered receptor function or number
Diuretics	Blood pressure lowering	ADD1	Altered cytoskeletal function by adducin variants
Warfarin	Anticoagulation	VKOrC1	Variant haplotypes in regulatory regions leading to variable expression
		CYP 2C9	Coding region variants causing reduced *S*-warfarin clearance
Abacavir	Immunologic reactions	HLA variants	Altered immunologic responses
QT-prolonging antiarrhythmics	Drug-induced arrhythmia	Ion-channel genes	Exposure of subclinical reduction in repolarizing currents by drugs
General anesthetics	Malignant hyperthermia	RYR1	Anesthetic-induced increased release of sarcoplasmic reticulum calcium by mutant channels
Inhaled steroids	Bronchodilation	CHCR1	Unknown
HMG-CoA reductase inhibitors (statins)	Low-density lipoprotein	HMGCR	Altered HMG-CoA reductase activity

[a] Reproduced with permission from Ref. 10. © ACP, 2006

more generally as global phenotypic indexes including contributing pharmacokinetic, pharmacodynamic, drug–drug interaction, and other environmental factors develop. Thus, pharmacogenomic biomarkers might be readily characterized as an adjunct to enable the practice of personalized medicine. To update on these applications, a summary of recent examples would include pharmacogenomics for alcoholism, psychiatric disorders, and opiates (opioids).

Alcohol

Alcoholism is a complex psychiatric disorder with high heritability (50–60%) and with a lifetime prevalence of alcohol dependence of 20% in men and 8% in women in the United States. Alcoholics may be categorized as follows: type 1 – later onset with feelings of anxiety, guilt, and high harm avoidance and type 2 – early age of onset, usually men, manifesting as impulsive and antisocial behavior, and associated with low levels of brain serotonin [11].

Genetic variations of alcohol metabolizing genes affect drinking behavior and hence decrease alcoholism. Genes of neurotransmitter pathways "reward pathway" (serotonin, dopamine, gamma amino-butyric acid (GABA), glutamate, and β-endorphin) and the behavioral stress response system (corticotrophin-releasing factor and neuropeptide Y)

may constitute therapeutic targets. By using the type 1/2 systems, progress is being made to understand the pharmacogenomic response to current pharmacotherapy. Further, alcohol inheritability may be affected by genetic variations for a number of enzymes and other factors such as those affecting cognitive function, stress/anxiety response, and opioid function [12].

Psychiatric Disorders

There are a number of schizophrenia-associated genes associated with affective disorders.

A number of P450 enzymes are involved in metabolizing antipsychotic drugs including CYP 2D6, CYP 1A2, and CYP3A4 (Table 4). Since CYP 1A2 is inducible, individuals with *CYP1A2* variants and some SNP combinations (haplotypes), in the 5′-regulatory regions, may demonstrate variable response [13].

Genetic variability leading to clinically significant changes has been shown for a number of antidepressants and antipsychotic drugs [14–17]. This has led to a lower incidence of adverse effects and has optimized the response to the drug therapy.

Opioids

The best example of an opioid response being affected by genetic variability is codeine [18].

Table 4 CYPs with major roles n the *in vivo* clearance of antipsychotic agents[a]

CYP	Antipsychotic drug	Altered drug substrates and inhibitors that may be used in psychotic patients	Inducers	Numbers of allelic variants
1A2	Clozapine	Omeprazole	Omeprazole	24 plus wild-type (also 9 predicted haplotypes)
	Olanzapine		Cigarette smoke Barbecued meats	
2D6	Risperidone Chlorpromazine Thioridazine	Dextromethorphan Codeine Imipramine Nortriptyline Paroxetine	None	94 plus wild type
3A4	Ziprasidone Quetiapine Aripiprazole Haloperidol	Erythromycin Diltiazem Ciclosporine Ethinyl estradiol	Rifampicin Carbamazepine Phenytoin Dexamethasone	38 plus wild type

[a] Reproduced from Ref. 13. © Pharmaceutical Press, 2006

Codeine is metabolized CYP 2D6 to its active metabolite morphine. UMs may suffer exaggerated and toxic opioidergic effects and poor metabolizers may experience reduced pain relief [19]. Even though P-glycoprotein is an opioid transporter, *ABCB1* genotypes' influence on opioid pharmacodynamics and dosage requirements were highly variable [20].

Forensic Applications

Pharmacogenomics is best treated as an adjunct to forensic pathology (*see also* **Toxicology: Forensic Applications of**), complementing information including autopsy findings, case history including medication, and scene investigation. The term *molecular autopsy* has been used to represent the application of genetic testing to assist the more conventional autopsy examination.

Case review initially assesses the likelihood of a genetic factor explaining a certain event. These factors include the presence of acute or chronic toxicity, autopsy findings (*see also* **Autopsy**), sample collection sites, postmortem intervals, coadministered drugs, case/medical/medication histories, scene investigations, and possible intent. As the case review continues with developing toxicological findings, elevated drug concentrations and identification of known and unknown drug/metabolites that might have interacted are prime criteria for case selection for pharmacogenomics (*see also* **Postmortem Biochemical Examinations** and **Toxicology: Forensic Applications of**). Further, the postmortem intervals are also considered in case selection and in interpretation. Once the case is selected, whole-blood samples are then transferred (*see also* **Toxicology: Analysis**), with chain of custody, for pharmacogenomics testing by the molecular and pharmacogenomics laboratory.

Currently, the testing platform is based on Pyrosequencing™ and include the following: *CYP 2D6*2-*8, CYP 2C9*2*3, CYP 2C19*2-*4, CYP 3A4*1B,* and *CYP 3A5*3.* The forensic applications are illustrated by the opioids (*see also* **Opioids**): methadone, oxycodone, and fentanyl.

UMs will produce larger amounts of morphine from codeine, and this is more likely to cause toxicity as well as increase the likelihood of overdose to breast-feeding infants [21].

Methadone response is affected by the activity of CYP3A4 and CYP2B6 and to a lesser extent CYP 2D6. ABCB1 accounted for minor pharmacokinetic variability. Other studies showed that *CYP* genes did not affect methadone metabolism.

---

*Case History 1. The decedent was a 41-year-old female, 6 month in her pregnancy. She had heart murmur and rheumatoid arthritis treated with methadone. Further, amitriptyline was prescribed for her depression. She celebrated New Year' Eve with her husband. On the following morning, she was found dead in her living room. Scene investigation revealed her ingestion of nine 50-mg tablets of amitriptyline within 17 days and two to three 95-mg dose of methadone. Several years before, she had attempted suicide by drug ingestion. Toxicological analysis of iliac blood showed the following drugs and concentrations in milligrams per liter: methadone, 0.7; amitriptyline, 1.5; nortriptyline, 2.2; diazepam, 0.19; and N-desmethyl diazepam, 0.13. The elevated antidepressant concentrations of iliac, peripheral blood, would not be due to postmortem drug redistribution and more attributable to acute drug ingestion. Molecular autopsy by pharmacogenomics showed that she was homozygous for CYP 2D6*4, corresponding to a poor metabolizer phenotype. This would result in the lack of hydroxylation of methadone, amitriptyline, and nortriptyline, thus resulting in elevated parent drug concentrations. Death certification was as follows: cause, mixed drug toxicity, and manner, accident [22].*

Further, cytochrome P450 2B6 (CYP 2B6) poor metabolizers are more likely to develop QT elongation. In addition, higher doses are needed for individuals with two copies of the wild-type haplotype and lower doses for AGCTT haplotype. Thus, haplotyping may be used to individualize methadone therapy.

Together, the genetic contribution to drug metabolism impairment may be interpreted as a gene dose effect, resulting in more pronounced drug toxicity. Such an effect might be readily demonstrated as a pharmacogenomics converging continuum and is helpful to understand the effect in the living.

Similarly, oxycodone response is affected by the activity of CYP 2D6 isozyme as Case Report 2 illustrates.

Case History 2. A 49-year-old male with a history of alcoholism and chronic lower back pain was prescribed OxyContin™ and Percocet™. He also had depression, posttraumatic stress disorder, and attempted suicide once. The scene investigation revealed only 12 of the 60 oxycodone pills that were obtained from the day before. Last seen by his roommate in the morning, the decedent was found unresponsive later that afternoon. Toxicological analysis of subclavian blood showed methadone, 0.44, mg l⁻¹. Testing showed that he was CYP 2D6*4 homozygous, corresponding to a poor metabolizer phenotype. Autopsy also showed that he had hepatic cirrhosis and atherosclerotic heart disease. Given the short postmortem interval and subclavian blood source, the elevated oxycodone was not due to postmortem drug redistribution but might be due to poor metabolizer phenotype and hepatic cirrhosis, both contributing to impaired drug metabolism. Death was certified as follows: cause of death, oxycodone overdose, and manner of death, accident [23].

Similarly, fentanyl response is affected by the activity of a number of enzyme types as Case Report 3 illustrates.

Other Applications

Pharmacogenomics including proteomic, RNA interference, and other molecular and functional biomarkers are being increasingly used in drug discovery and development as encouraged by governmental agencies and scientific and professional organizations. Pharmacogenomics has been used to enhance patient's safety in therapies with approved drugs. Thus, the use of pharmacogenomics is regarded as an adjunct for optimizing drug therapy and, in forensic pathology/toxicology, for providing a molecular autopsy. Thus, TDM and toxicology would be helpful as global indexes. This would add to the understanding of potential genetic contribution to metabolism of

approved drugs such as methadone and oxycodone, thus enabling and improving the practice of antemortem drug therapy, a tangible benefit for family members of decedents.

Case History 3. A 44-year-old white female complained about her knee pain and was treated with Duragesic™ fentanyl patches. She appeared to be "goofy" and went to bed. She was found dead 24 h later. The decedent was a drug abuser with psychiatric history. Previously, she cut her arm to obtain drugs and also expressed suicidal ideation. Toxicological analysis of subclavian blood showed the following drugs and concentrations in milligrams per liter: fentanyl, 0.019; norfentanyl, 0.008; cyclobenzaprine, 0.16; tramadol, 0.06, diphenhydramine, 0.08; citalopram, 0.22; and olanzapine, positive. The MR of fentanyl/norfentanyl was 2.5. Molecular autopsy by pharmacogenomics showed that she was heterozygous for CYP 3A4*1B and CYP 3A5*3, different from the majority of Caucasians CYP 3A4, WT, and CYP 3A5*3 HM. In this study with limited number of fentanyl cases, the MR of this case is lower than the MRs of majority of the cases with high-fentanyl concentrations. Together, these findings suggested that for the first time, cytochrome P450 3A5 (CYP 3A5) comediated with CYP 3A4 the metabolism of fentanyl to norfentanyl. Death certification for the above case was as follows: cause of death, mixed drug toxicity, and manner of death, accident [24].

The experience may be helpful to apply pharmacogenomics in the possible emerging practice of personalized justice. One such emerging application would be applying pharmacogenomic biomarkers for the interpretation of possible "side effect/behavior/impaired performance" of the drivers arrested in cases involving driving under the influence of drugs (*see also* **Drug-Impaired Driving** and **Behavioral Toxicology**). By using pharmacogenomics, the driver's impaired driving performance may be partially explained on the basis of genetics-predisposed impairment of drug metabolism and therefore accumulation. This might result in driving impairment. Similar to the use of DNA finger-printing in identity testing, applying pharmacogenomics and other molecular biomarkers in the future as adjunct biomarkers in the above context may constitute a rational approach in understanding and the deliberation of the driver's liability, thus offering the possibility of personalized justice.

Further, with the availability of proficiency survey program by the College of American Pathologists in 2007 and quality assurance/control from commercial sources, the clinical adaptations will soon be readily achieved by clinical laboratories. National Academy of Clinical Biochemistry (NACB) guidelines would certainly pave the way. Challenges remain for adequate reimbursement, clinical interpretation, ethical guidelines, and education of the patients and healthcare professionals. Thus, Gregor Mendel's "little trick – long story" would indeed continue in the form of new articles as a result of the human genome project and the rapid advances in molecular biology and pharmacogenomics.

References

[1] Wong, S.H.Y. (2007). Pharmacogenomic and personalized medicine for drug addiction and toxicology – towards personalized justice? *11th Asian Pacific Congress of Clinical Biochemistry*, October 2007, Beijing.

[2] Wong, S.H.Y., Linder, M.W. & Valdes Jr, R. (eds) (2006). *Pharmacogenomics and Proteomics – Enabling the Practice of Personalized Medicine*, AACC Press, Washington, DC, pp. 1–386.

[3] Pillot, G.A., Read, W.L., Hennenfent, K.L., Marsh, S., Gao, F., Viswanathan, A., Cummings, K., McLeod, H.L. & Govindan, R. (2006). A phase II study of irinotecan and carboplatin in advanced non-small cell lung cancer with pharmacogenomic analysis: final report, *Journal of Thoracic Oncology* 1(9), 972–978.

[4] Chen, H.-Y., Yu, S.-L., Chen, C.-H., Chang, G.-C., Chen, C.-Y., Yuan, A., Cheng, C.-L., Wang, C.-H., Terng, H.-J., Kao, S.-F., Chan, W.-K., Li, H.-N., Liu, C.-C., Singh, S., Chen, W.-J., Chen, J.J.W. & Yang, P.-C. (2007). A five-gene signature and clinical outcome in non-small-cell lung cancer, *The New England Journal of Medicine* 356, 11–20.

[5] Evans, W.E. & McLeod, H.L. (2003). Pharmacogenomics – drug disposition, drug targets and side effects, *The New England Journal of Medicine* 348, 538–549.

[6] Bertillsson, L., Lou, Y.Q., Du, Y.-L., Liu, Y., Kuang, T.-Y., Liao, X.-M., Wang, K.Y., Reviriego, J., Iselius, L. & Sjoqvist, F. (1992). Pronounced differences between Chinese and Swedish populations in the polymorphic hydroxylations of debrisoquin and S-mephenytoin, *Clinical Pharmacology and Therapeutics* 51, 388–397.

[7] Paul, N.W. & Fangerau, H. (2006). Why should we bother? Ethical and social issues in individualized medicine, *Current Cancer Drug Targets* 7(12), 1721–1727.

[8] Payne, D. (2006). Pharmacogenetic testing: how to choose a method to analyze genetic changes, *Clinical Laboratory News* 7, 14–16.

[9] Kirchheiner, J., Gründemann, D. & Schömig, E. (2006). Contribution of allelic variations in transporters to the phenotype of drug response, *Journal of Psychopharmacology* 20,(Suppl 4), 27–32.

[10] Roden, D.M., Altman, R.B., Benowitz, N.L., Flockhart, D.A., Giacomini, K.M., Johnson, J.A., Krauss, R.M., McLeod, H.L., Ratain, M.J., Relling, M.V., Ring, H.Z., Shuldiner, A.R., Weinshilboum, R.M. & Weiss, S.T. The Pharmacogenetics Research Network (2006). Pharmacogenomics: challenges and opportunities (review), *Annals of Internal Medicine* 145, 749–757.

[11] Enoch, M.A. (2003). Pharmacogenomics of alcohol response and addiction, *American Journal of Pharmacogenomics* 3(4), 217–232.

[12] Oroszi, G. & Goldman, D. (2004). Alcoholism: genes and mechanisms, *Pharmacogenomics* 5(8), 1037–1048.

[13] Murray, M. (2006). Role of CYP pharmacogenetics and drug-drug interactions in the efficacy and safety of atypical and other antipsychotic agents, *The Journal of Pharmacy and Pharmacology* 58(7), 871–885.

[14] Kirchheiner, J., Brøsen, K., Dahl, M.L., Gram, L.F., Kasper, S., Roots, I., Sjoqvist, F., Spina, E. & Brockmoller, J. (2001). CYP2D6 and CYP2C19 genotype-based dose recommendations for antidepressants: a first step towards subpopulation-specific dosages, *Acta Psychiatrica Scandinavica* 104, 173–192.

[15] Dorado, P., Berecz, R., Peñas-Lledó, E.M., Cáceres, M.C. & Llerena, A. (2006). Clinical implications of CYP2D6 genetic polymorphism during treatment with antipsychotic drugs, *Current Drug Targets* 7(12), 1671–1680.

[16] Lin, Y.-C., Ellingrod, V.L., Bishop, J.R. & Miller, D.D. (2006). The relationship between P-glycoprotein (PGP) polymorphisms and response to olanzapine treatment in schizophrenia, *Therapeutic Drug Monitoring* 28, 668–672.

[17] Baumann, P., Barbe, R., Vabre-Bogdalova, A., Garran, E., Crettol, S. & Eap, C. (2006). Epileptiform seizure after sertraline treatment in an adolescent experiencing obsessive-compulsive disorder and presenting a rare pharmacogenetic status, *Journal of Clinical Psychopharmacology* 26, 679–681.

[18] Kirchheiner, J., Schmidt, H., Tzvetkov, M., Keulen, J.T., Lötsch, J., Roots, I. & Brockmöller, J. (2007). Pharmacokinetics of codeine and its metabolite morphine in ultra-rapid metabolizers due to CYP2D6 duplication, *The Pharmacogenomics Journal* 7(4), 257–265.

[19] Gasche, Y., Daali, Y., Marc Fathi, M., Chiappe, A., Cottini, S., Dayer, P. & Desmeules, J. (2004). Codeine intoxication associated with ultrarapid CYP2D6 metabolism, *The New England Journal of Medicine* **351**, 2827–2831.

[20] Somogyi, A.A., Barratt, D.T. & Coller, J.K. (2007). Pharmacogenetics of opioids, *Clinical Pharmacology and Therapeutics* **81**, 429–444.

[21] Koren, G., Cairns, J., Chitayat, D., Gaedigk, A. & Leeder, S.J. (2006). Pharmacogenetics of morphine poisoning in a breastfed neonate of a codeine-prescribed mother, *Lancet* **368**, 704.

[22] Wong, S.H., Wagner, M.A., Jentzen, J.M., Schur, B.C., Bjerke, J., Gock, S.B. & Chang, C.C. (2003). Pharmcogenomics as an aspect of molecular autopsy for forensic pathology/toxicology: does genotyping CYP2D6 serve as an adjunct for certifying methadone toxicity? *Journal of Forensic Sciences* **48**, 1406–1415.

[23] Jannetto, P.J., Wong, S.H., Gock, S.B., Laleli-Sahin, E., Schur, B.C. & Jentzen, J.M. (2002). Pharmacogenomics as molecular autopsy for postmortem forensic toxicology: genotyping cytochrome P450 2D6 for oxycodone cases, *Journal of Analytical Toxicology* **26**, 438–447.

[24] Jin, M., Gock, S.B., Jannetto, P.J., Jentzen, J.M. & Wong, S.H. (2005). Pharmacogenomics as molecular autopsy for forensic toxicology: genotyping cytochrome P450 3A4*1B and 3A5*3 for 25 fentanyl cases, *Journal of Analytical Toxicology* **29**, 590–598.

Further Reading

Abrahams, E., Ginsburg, G.S. & Silver, M. (2005). The personalized medicine coalition: goals and strategies, *American Journal of Pharmacogenomics* **5**(6), 345–355.

International Human Genome Sequencing Consortium (2001). Initial sequencing and analysis of the human genome, *Nature* **409**, 860–921.

Jicinio, J. & Wong, M.-L. (2002). *Pharmacogenomics*, Wiley-VCH, Weinheim, pp. 1–559.

Linder, M.W., Prough, R.A. & Valdes Jr, R. (1997). Pharmacogenetics: a laboratory tool for optimizing therapeutic efficiency (review), *Clinical Chemistry* **43**(2), 254–266.

Tsai, K.Y., Tsao, H. (2007). Primer on the human genome, *Journal of the American Academy of Dermatology* **56**(5), 719–735.

Venter, J.C., Adams, M.D., Myers, E.W., *et al.* (2001). The sequence of human genome, *Science* **291**, 1304–1351.

Weber, W.W. (1997). *Pharmacogenetics*, Oxford University Press, Oxford, pp. 1–344.

Weinshilboum, R. (2003). Inheritance and drug response, *The New England Journal of Medicine* **348**, 529–537.

http://www.nacb.org/lmpg/LMPG_Pharmacogenetics.pdf. 2007.

STEVEN H. Y. WONG

Pharmacokinetics *see* Alcohol: Interaction with Other Drugs

Phenotype

Introduction

The genomics and bioinformatics era has enabled the recent development of systems and methods for the derivation of human phenotype from the genotyping of crime stain DNA evidence. This is accomplished through an empirical process of inference, either directly through genotypes for the functionally relevant genetic positions (loci) or indirectly through an appreciation of the genetic heritage of the donor. Forensic scientists are accustomed to using DNA sequence polymorphisms as identifiers. On the basis of the frequency of the identifier, we can statistically link individuals with samples associated with criminal investigations. Microsatellites, such as the short tandem repeats (STRs) employed for the Federal Bureau of Investigation (FBI's) combined DNA index system (CODIS) have been most commonly used for this purpose because they are multiallelic. That is to say, they have many alleles (varieties per location, or locus) and so relatively few loci are necessary to produce sequence signatures. Microsatellites are not chosen from the human genome based on their human ancestry or phenotype information, since this type of information would render them more or less powerful as identification tools among different human subpopulations. Thus, they are relatively useless for inferring phenotype. If we find that a suspect or a database entry matches the STR profile, we can extract probative value from the profile, otherwise, we have traditionally employed nongenetic investigative processes designed to produce the suspects necessary to achieve this objective.

For many cases, the investigative process begins with an attempt to ascribe characteristics or features to the perpetrator that can lead to identification. If a human eyewitness were available, we would query the witness about physical appearance – what the suspect was wearing, the suspects "race" and, more specifically, we would obtain estimates and ranges for the basic anthropometric phenotypes such as skin color, eye color, height, etc. In the best-case scenario, we might obtain the basic physical descriptors or features such as those that might be present on a work identification card for the suspect, and, in a suboptimal scenario, we might obtain descriptors that are inaccurate or misleading. Unfortunately, the best-case scenario with human eyewitnesses is rarely achieved; unreliable information is sometimes provided by design (perhaps the witness has a motive to deceive) or by circumstance such as might be the case if the witness observed from afar on a darkly lit street. Assuming that the integrity of the witness is intact, and the witness had a clear view of a suspect, we are still left with fundamental problems created by the subjective nature of the human experience. Human testimony is generally not objective, almost always unstandardized, and never formally quantitative. Physical descriptions provided by one witness may or may not comport with those from another – not necessarily because one is wrong, but because one witness' opinion on what it is to look "dark" or "Asian", for example, may be different from the other. These basic problems translate into a fundamental defect associated with the extraction of phenotype data from human eyewitnesses – namely, that the testimony is not falsifiable, meaning that an investigator cannot verify its accuracy through independent examination. Nonetheless, there is a reason investigators consider themselves lucky to have access to eyewitness testimony. An investigation is much like a classification problem, where one attempts to make the most specific classification possible (the ascription of identity). Given the number of variables, and the fact that the number of incorrect classifications far outnumbers those that are correct (one) the classification problem is complex and we need classification features in order to delimit the likely possibilities. Here, data from witness testimony is analogous to a classification feature, and information theory (e.g., Bayes theorem) teaches us that even suboptimally informative (as opposed to uninformative or misleading) "features" are better than no features at all [1, 2]. Clearly, it would be far better to extract physical information on the donor using empirical techniques that lend themselves to the scientific method – techniques based on the observations of unperturbed nature, producing objective, quantitative and falsifiable data that can be communicated logically to others using standardized terms. It happens that if DNA is available from a crime scene, we now have access to new methods meeting these criteria for the inference of certain aspects of physical appearance (human traits or phenotypes).

The recent completion of the first human genome draft has provided a foundation for the development of empirical processes by which a partial physical portrait of a DNA donor can be constructed. In this article, we discuss certain overt phenotypes that are highly heritable, which are required if we hope to draw connections between DNA sequences and trait values. For example, parents with dark skin tend to have children with similarly dark skin and blue-eyed parents tend not to have brown-eyed offspring, suggesting that if we knew which and how genetic regions controlled or were informative for skin and eye color, we could predict these phenotypes simply through genetic observation. In fact, since most anthropometric (comparative human) phenotypes are determined by inherited gene sequences, much of a crime-scene DNA donor's physical information is imbedded in their DNA – we have only to figure out how to extract it. The inheritance of some phenotypes is relatively simple, and this information can be extracted with the investment of time and money. For others of more complex inheritance, the information is not currently extractable and may never be with existing technology.

There are two basic methods for inferring phenotypes from DNA. If we desire to infer phenotype from DNA using *direct methods*, we need to understand at least the major elements of the genetic architecture of the phenotype – that is, which genes and gene variants (as well as environmental factors) underlie variable expression of the phenotype. These genes are called *phenotypically active loci*, and their variants *phenotypically active variants*. With the direct method, we relate genotypes to specific phenotypes through our understanding of the genetic architecture, or if we do not fully understand the genetic architecture, through an empirical process based on prior experience and the use of databases. Of course, at least some of the genetic architecture must be understood or captured by our databases for the direct method to be possible. Even for "relatively simple" phenotypes, the expression tends to be extraordinarily complex, involving multiple variants per gene, sometimes more than one gene and sometimes even environmental factors. As basic genetics research powered to identify these genes and factors must involve many hundreds, even thousands or tens of thousands of subjects (depending on the phenotype, the number of loci, and their frequency in the relevant populations), arriving at the requisite level of understanding is very expensive and time consuming. As a result, we can so far only use direct methods with a couple of the overt human phenotypes that have so far proven amenable – hair color, iris color and, possibly soon, skin color as well (at least within some human populations).

Another method of inferring phenotype from DNA is based not on any understanding of the genetic architecture of the phenotype, but based on the recognition that expression of the phenotype is correlated with certain elements of human population structure. This is called the *indirect method* of DNA-based phenotype inference. Indirect methods are based on an appreciation of individual genomic ancestry in terms of admixture. We choose the term *admixture*, rather than mixture, because the distribution of ancestry within populations and individuals tends toward amalgamation and the preservation of structure rather than dilutive blending and homogenization (by analogy, the colors yellow and red combining to produce an amalgamation of yellow and red, rather than orange). The correlation between elements of ancestry and phenotype within populations of individuals allow for an inference of the latter on an individual-by-individual basis. If skin color, for example, is systematically and quantitatively darker among individuals with increasing levels of African genetic ancestry, and if we have a good database of individuals of varying African ancestry and their skin color measurements, we can infer the skin color of a crime-scene donor from a precise genomic ancestry estimate of the donor's African admixture. The use of databases makes the process both objective and empirical in that the inference is based strictly on observation (as opposed to based on a model such as a model of the genetic architecture). As we describe, in this article, depending on the phenotype and its distribution among the world's various populations, we can employ the empirical method with reference databases to not only infer trait value but also to do so quantitatively and with predefined levels of confidence (based on the likelihood that the inference is correct). In what follows, we first describe the currently available methods for indirectly inferring phenotype from DNA, then those for direct inference.

We then discuss some of the first cases that have employed these methods with success and close with a brief discussion on the issues associated with the penetration of these new methods into the modern forensics investigative process. Most of our discussion here is necessarily brief and significantly more details can be found in [3] which represents the first text to discuss this topic in depth.

Indirect Method of Phenotype Inference

The indirect method of phenotype inference relies on the empirical process, which itself is driven by observation. With this method, we rely on observations of correlations between phenotypes and ancestry, rather than direct relationships with gene sequences. This focuses our attention to certain phenotypes unevenly distributed among the world's various populations, which arose either because they conferred selective advantage among our ancestors in certain geographical regions or through sampling and genetic drift. Reproductive barriers such as oceans, geographical extremes, and assortative mating helped to solidify a global amalgamation of populations as and after our ancestors expanded out of Africa some 200 000 years ago (reviewed in [4, 5]).

The main phenotypes distributed as a function of genetic ancestry and of interest to the forensic investigator are those that are overt, such as skin color, certain facial features, hair/iris color, stature, etc. To infer them accurately, we thus need an accurate tool with which to measure an individual's ancestry, and we need to measure this ancestry (and phenotype) among large population of individuals. Polymorphism of the Y and mtDNA chromosomes are the gold standard for reconstructing human population histories and measuring the apportionment of genetic diversity among the world's populations (Figure 1), but these chromosomes are uniparental (e.g., the Y is inherited by males from their father, who inherited it from his father, and his father, etc.) and as such, they are of little use to the forensic scientist. For example, from measures of Y chromosome mixes among various worldwide populations, we might note that the distribution of higher eumelanin index values (darker skin colors, Figure 2) is correlated with certain Y-haplogroups such as E that dominates in present-day Africa, or the L of South Asia and that lighter eumelanin index values correlated with those

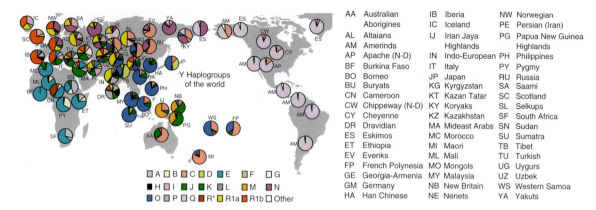

AA	Australian	IB	Iberia	NW	Norwegian
	Aborigines	IC	Iceland	PE	Persian (Iran)
AL	Altaians	IJ	Irian Jaya	PG	Papua New Guinea
AM	Amerinds		Highlands		Highlands
AP	Apache (N-D)	IN	Indo-European	PH	Philippines
BF	Burkina Faso	IT	Italy	PY	Pygmy
BO	Borneo	JP	Japan	RU	Russia
BU	Buryats	KG	Kyrgyzstan	SA	Saami
CN	Cameroon	KT	Kazan Tatar	SC	Scotland
CW	Chippeway (N-D)	KY	Koryaks	SL	Selkups
CY	Cheyenne	KZ	Kazakhstan	SF	South Africa
DR	Dravidian	MA	Mideast Arabs	SN	Sudan
ES	Eskimos	MC	Morocco	SU	Sumatra
ET	Ethiopia	MI	Maori	TB	Tibet
EV	Evenks	MO	Mongols	TU	Turkish
FP	French Polynesia	MY	Malaysia	UG	Uygurs
GE	Georgia-Armenia	NB	New Britain	UZ	Uzbek
GM	Germany	NE	Nenets	WS	Western Samoa
HA	Han Chinese			YA	Yakuts

Figure 1   Global apportionment of Y haplogroup diversity. Pie charts illustrate the proportion of haplogroups as identified in the legend at the bottom. Populations are identified with a two-letter code/defined by the legend to the right [Reproduced with permission from J. D. McDonald. © 2004.]

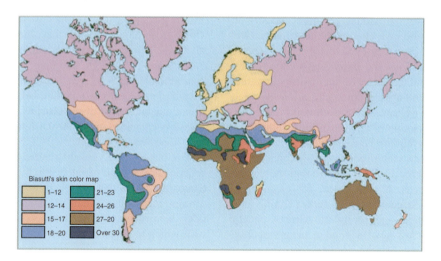

Figure 2   Geographical distribution of skin melanin levels. Higher values correspond to darker colors [Reproduced with permission from Cengage Learning © 2000.]

such as R or I shared among Europeans (compare Figures 1 and 2). Armed with this data, we might predict light European-like skin color for 28% of African Americans based on Y haplogroup sequence alone because no fewer than 28% of African Americans in the United States have a European Y chromosome as a result of recent admixture [6]; [7]; [3]. Indeed, the history of many other populations involves the admixture of those parental populations within which our anthropometric phenotype differences evolved and the ancestry for any one individual is best considered as a unique point along a sliding scale of

admixture among these populations. In the field, we call this "sliding scale" a multidimensional continuum of admixture, based on the graphical methods we use to display the results (Figure 3). Uniparental chromosome polymorphisms are not useful for predicting phenotype because they do not tell us enough about the ancestry of any given individual, which is a complex function of all of the ancestors not just their patrilineal or matrilineal lines.

To indirectly infer a phenotype from the DNA of an individual, we must first have a method by which to quantitatively estimate individual genetic

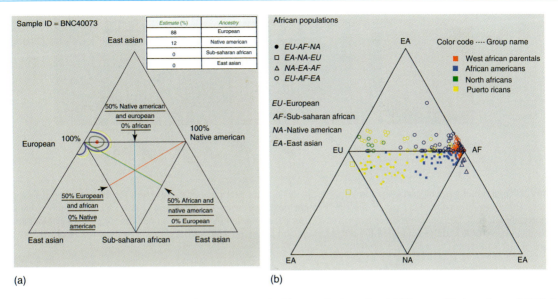

Figure 3 Individual genomic ancestry estimates portrayed with a tetrahedron plot. (a) The most likely estimate (MLE) for an individual is shown with a spot (red) which corresponds to specific percentages shown in the upper right-hand box. The percentages are obtained in four-dimensional space with an algorithm, but can be displayed on a two-dimensional piece of paper using this plot diagram; projecting the MLE spot perpendicularly on the each of the three axes within any of the four subtriangles (arrows) gives the corresponding percentage. The closer the spot is to the triangle vertices (labeled European, sub-Saharan African, East Asian, or Native American), the higher the percentage admixture corresponding to that type of ancestry. (b) Plot of numerous MLEs for individuals of color-coded self-described ancestry (legend upper right) obtained using the 176 AIM panel described in the text. Though continental Africans show predominantly African admixture, this African-American sample shows considerable European admixture and the Puerto Rican sample shows even more

ancestry admixture, contributed by all the ancestors of an individual (e.g., an individual might register with 80% "European" and 20% "African" admixture or some other mix). To do this, we measure ancestry informative markers (AIMs) on all 23 chromosomes of an individual. Secondly, we need to derive our understanding of the relationship between phenotype and ancestry from the same type of data – individual phenotype measurements and individual genomic ancestry admixture estimates. Note that we are therefore working on the level of the individual (within and/or between populations) rather than on the level of the population and so rather than using uniparental polymorphisms we must use AIMs distributed among all 23 chromosomes. Though binning or assigning an individual to a single population (such as "Caucasian") is conceptually easier than estimating the admixture of ancestry, it is not suitable for this purpose for the same reason we cannot use inferences of ancestry from uniparental chromosome polymorphisms. Specifically, we need to know what percentage of an individual's karyotype is derived

from the ancestors of a given population, if we hope to compute the probability that the individual expresses a phenotype that is highly characteristic of that population.

AIMs are polymorphisms showing significant allele frequency differences between human populations. For example, an AIM may come in two "flavors" – a G allele and an A allele, with G rarely found in European or Eurasian populations but commonly found among various African populations. Most AIMs are single nucleotide polymorphisms (SNPs) such as this, with only two alleles, and SNP–AIMs constitute about 0.04% of the 2 million or so SNPs in the human genome. To construct an admixture panel, the most informative AIMs are selected from those that have been databased via the human genome (or similar other) project and the allele frequencies/frequency differentials among our founding parental populations is inferred through analysis of modern-day representative descendants. Using the AIM genotypes of any one individual, we invert the frequency of these alleles in various

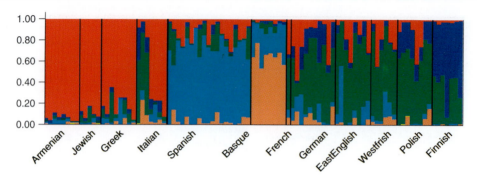

Figure 4 Individual genomic ancestry admixture estimates among Europeans with respect to a five-population European model. The 1346 European AIM panel described in the text was used to generate the data. For each individual, the proportional ancestry derived from these five parental European populations is represented with a bar, using colors coding for each ancestry type and the scaling on the left. Markers and genotype data were derived from the work published by [11] [Reproduced from Ref. 11. © Elsevier, 2007.]

populations in order to calculate the likelihood that the individual's ancestry was derived proportionally from these populations. The likelihood for all possible proportions is calculated, we select the best as the most likely estimate (MLE), and select those within two–tenfold likelihood values fall within the confidence intervals for the MLE (Figure 3a). If the admixture panel is to address the global population, worldwide population models are usually chosen on the basis of hypothesis-free clustering results (e.g., see [9]). One panel that has been well characterized incorporates a four-population model; this panel (developed in the laboratory of the author) was the first to be extensively characterized and applied for forensic cases ([3, 10]; discussed further below). Since individuals derived mainly from the Eurasian continent share one element of ancestry, we can arbitrarily name this element "European" or "Eurasian", and so on for the other three elements. Other more complex global models are possible but whatever the model, the choice of nomenclature is arbitrary, and usually based on either the modern-day origin of the parental representatives or geographical origin of the parental population (estimated from paleoarcheological, linguistics, and/or uniparental chromosome analyses). Mathematical methods allow for an accommodation of uncertainty with regard to the estimation of parental allele frequencies from modern-day representatives, as well as other pertinent variables, and the reader can refer to [3] for more details. For this discussion, here, suffice it to say that whatever the chosen population model, as long as it is based on hypothesis-free clustering

results, an individual's admixture proportions are a function of genetic distance and thus potentially relevant for indirectly predicting phenotype. As of this article, three panels are available to forensic professionals through a company located in Sarasota Florida (DNAPrint genomics, Inc., see www.dnaprint.net or www.ancestrybydna.com) – the aforementioned 176-AIM continental panel (European, African, Indigenous American, and East Asian; [3, 10]), a 320-AIM Eurasian panel (Northern European, Southeastern European, Middle Eastern, and South Asian; [3]) and a 1476-AIM European panel (Figure 4; [3]).

Discerning whether particular elements of individual ancestry are correlated with certain phenotypes is accomplished through databases and regression analyses, where we plot one variable (such as a trait value) against another (such as percent admixture for a given ancestry type) and note whether or not there is a statistical dependence of the former on the latter. Regression analyses have shown correlations for skin eumelanin content and individual African ancestry levels using a 30-AIM ([12], African-American population) and the aforementioned 176-AIM panels ([10], Puerto Rican Afro-Caribbean population; Figure 5). For example, we could conclude from the regression analyses in Figure 5 that an individual with >75% African admixture determined using the 176-AIM panel is most likely to have an M (eumelanin content) value above 40 and an individual with less than 50% African ancestry is most likely to have an M value less than 40. With larger databases, we could provide not only an expected M value by

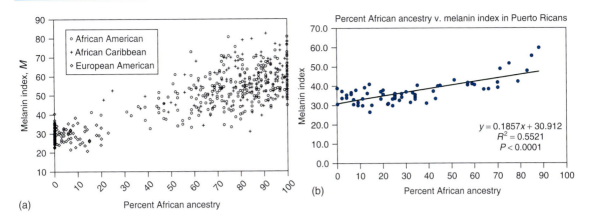

(a)

(b)

Figure 5 Regression of eumelanin value (M) from skin measurement on African individual genomic ancestry estimates in a population of (a) African Americans, European Americans, and Afro-Caribbean samples, obtained using a 30-AIM panel [12] and (b) Puerto Ricans, obtained using the 176-AIM panel described in the text [3, 10]. Each spot represents the point estimate of African admixture for an individual. Higher M values correspond to darker skin colors (higher concentration of eumelanin per unit skin area)

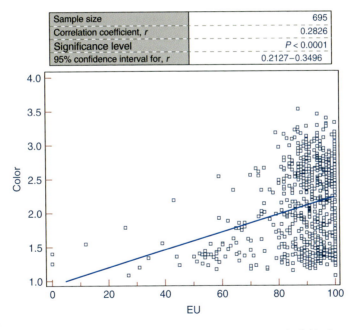

Figure 6 Regression of iris eumelanin scores from digital photographs on European individual genomic ancestry estimates in a population predominantly of self-described "Caucasians". Each spot represents a point estimate of European admixture for an individual. Higher color scores correspond to lighter colors (less eumelanin)

taking an average but we could also quantify the reliability of this value with confidence intervals. A correlation has also been demonstrated between iris color and European ancestry [13]; we can see from Figure 6 that while individuals with high "European"

admixture have light (color > 2.2) and darker iris color (color < 2.2), individuals with substantial non-European admixture (20% or greater) almost always have darker iris colors. Thus, a crime-scene DNA sample determined to have been deposited by an individual with 40% East Asian and 60% European admixture, or 50% African and 50% European admixture can be inferred to have an iris color on the darker end of the range observed in the human population. With larger databases, we could even quantify the likelihood that this type of conclusion is wrong. For example, if we see that the conclusion is true for 999 of 1000 individuals, we could estimate that the conclusion is correct with 99.9% certainty and that only 1 in 1000 such conclusions would be wrong. As of this article, the indirect method can only be used for these two phenotypes but through the construction and use of admixture databases, we may soon learn of others. For example, if we construct an admixture database of individuals, which included the self-described "ethnicity" and a digital photograph for each entry, and then query the database with a particular admixture profile (± a reasonable range), we might get a return of several entries like that shown in Figure 7. From these returns, we could discern whether the individuals are more likely to refer to themselves as belonging to one particular population than another, and how reliable such an inference can be expected to be. Using software biometric tools, we might learn that the average distance between the eyes (for example) is significantly different from that

of a random collection of individuals, or a group of individuals with a different type of admixture profile. Some investigators may be able to use collections of digital photographs corresponding to an admixture profile to mentally compile a composite sketch, though the future promises to provide software for identifying all of the phenotypes statistically characteristic of the profile (compared to randomly specified samples) as well as the ranges of trait values, we can expect algorithms to construct an *in silico* "rendering" of the suspect similar to that provided by a human eyewitness.

A very important point that needs to be highlighted is that if our admixture methods are insensitive or inaccurate, if there are problems with the population model or parental representatives we have built our test on, or if there are glitches with the database software, there will be error. However, assuming that the size of the database is adequate, this error is expected to result in an increase rather than a decrease in entropy of the system [3]. The increase in entropy leads to a loss of information and an inability to recognize correlations in regression analyses (false negatives) rather than an ability to recognize false correlations (false positives). For example, an admixture assay based on only a few AIMs covering only

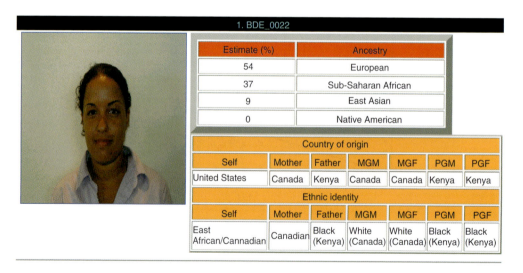

Figure 7 Example of an admixture database entry. Entries in this particular database (www.dnawitness.net) included a digital photograph taken under standardized conditions, country of origin, that of their mother, father, and their maternal grandmother (MGM) and paternal grandmother (PGM) as well as maternal grandfather (MGF) and paternal grandfather (PGF). Similarly, the self-reported "ethnic identity" is provided by each subject. The laboratory that administers this database took the photograph and determined the admixture profile with respect to a global four-population model using the 176-AIM panel discussed in the text. The database had 4700 entries as of August 2007

one chromosome would produce a large standard error in admixture estimates and the imprecise estimates may be so scattered about their true values in a regression plot that the relationship between trait value and ancestry is concealed (e.g., in Figure 5b, imagine the spots so far scattered above and below the line at low as well as high African admixture values that the sum of squared distance to a line indicating no correlation is similar to that for one indicating a good correlation). False positives can only obtain if false positive correlations are produced between phenotypes and elements of ancestry, which equates to the creation of false pattern, but random error that we would expect from a poorly performing assay would, by definition, obfuscate pattern and increase the entropy. It is possible to create false pattern from an assay that produces estimates with biased error, but with admixture/phenotype databases even these tend to result in a decrease rather than an increase in entropy. For example, consider an assay that has a tendency to erroneously estimate low levels of African admixture for South Asians (but not for other "European" populations such as Middle Eastern or Continental Europeans). It might seem that this error could lead to the mistaken conclusion that low levels of African admixture for individuals of primarily European ancestry is correlated with very dark skin color, even though most Continental Europeans with low levels of African admixture exhibit lighter skin colors (e.g., Figure 5). However, note that all of the Europeans would be present in the database, and using the high European/low African profile to query the database would result in a jumble of various light and dark skin color phenotypes rather than the shade that would be observed, were the error not present. Thus, we have an increase in entropy over which we would expect without the error, leading to an inability to make an accurate inference and false negative (type I) error rather than the creation of a false positive. Nonetheless, admixture panels that produce biased estimates are easily identified if they are properly validated and characterized [3]. A properly constructed and validated admixture panel should exhibit single-digit percentage accuracy (total error from statistical imprecision and bias combined). The laboratory of the author operates such a validated admixture/phenotype database ($n = 4700$ samples as of August 2007) and has used it in several homicide cases, but as we discuss later, so far only to indirectly infer skin color and iris color. Finding other phenotypes for which the indirect method will be useful in the future and the development of more advanced data mining and composite sketch software tools will require significantly greater investment.

Direct Method

Though they can be correlated with phenotypes, ancestry and markers of ancestry do not cause phenotypes – genes do. In contrast with the indirect method, the direct method relies on measurements of the actual genes underlying the phenotype of interest. Though far more satisfying in a theoretical sense, since we expect to be able to do a better job of predicting trait value (more accuracy and tighter confidence intervals), the direct method is rarely practicable because it requires an understanding of the dominant aspects of the genetic architecture of a phenotype, and acquiring this understanding is a very expensive and time-consuming endeavor. To date, research on the genetic basis for only human iris color and one aspect of hair color has been productive enough to enable direct phenotyping from DNA. The objective with the direct method is to define polymorphisms associated strongly enough with the phenotype that they are predictive for that phenotype with good sensitivity and specificity. Note that hundreds of good gene/phenotype associations have been described in the literature over the past decade or so (mostly for clinical phenotypes), but few of them are sufficiently strong or detailed enough within each gene to enable "genetic classification". Given the complexity of human phenotypes, useful polymorphisms are likely to be found for phenotypes where expression is controlled by one to a few genes at most, and will almost always be useful in the context of diplotypes (diploid pairs of haplotypes, where a haplotype is a chromosomal string of SNP alleles). Which diplotypes are associated with which trait values would be best determined through an empirical process of database construction and query, as with the indirect method, except we query with diplotypes rather than admixture profiles.

Iris Color

The best example of an effective direct system for inferring a human phenotype is human iris color. Linkage screens and association scans have shown

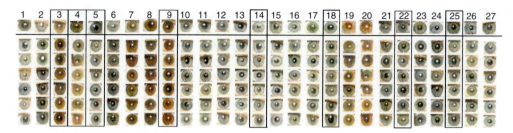

Figure 8   Examples of iris color inference enabled with the 33 marker/iris color database described in the text. Iris color is inferred using the average color exhibited by samples in the database with matching diplotypes and an interval is provided around this point estimate using the range of colors exhibited or a default range, whichever is larger. This inferred range is then used to query the database and all of the irides falling within the range are presented. This typically produces tens or hundreds of irides of similar overall color from a distance (determined by eumelanin content) though of different pattern, depending on the color and database size. Shown here are returns for 27 test subjects. Six representatives of the inferred iris color score range are provided for each of the 27 test irides below the line and the actual color of the test iris is shown above the line

that variable human iris color in humans is primarily determined by polymorphism in the Oculocutaneous Albinism 2 (OCA2) gene [13–15]. OCA2 was first discovered by researchers studying the human albino phenotype as a locus with mutations that affected iris melanin production but not skin melanin production (as well as other mutations that affect both). Recently, [13] built upon earlier reports [14–17] to identify 33 OCA2 SNPs associated with digitally quantified iris color independent from their ancestry information. As it is with many phenotypes (e.g., Figure 5), ancestry was itself correlated with the phenotype (Figure 6) and correcting the associations with respect to population structure was crucial for demonstrating that they were *bona fide* (that is, that the association was with iris color, not an element of population structure that is itself correlated with iris color; [3]). Though each of the 33 SNPs were marginally (independently) associated with iris color, none were very useful on their own as iris color classification features. However, when assembled into diplotypes, the alleles for these 33 SNPs were highly predictive for the overall eumelanin content of the iris; among 1100 diplotypes from individuals of European descent, there existed 96% concordance of iris colors among those samples with the same diplotypes [3, 13]. To predict the iris color of a given sample, this team thus built a database of phenotyped diplotypes, and then queried the database much as we do with the indirect method of phenotyping – though, in this case, with test diplotypes rather than admixture profiles. The return for this query provides an average iris color and range of iris colors as a point estimate and range

of inferred color for the test diplotype. The results were satisfying; a validation sample provided a 96% accuracy rate (the inferred or predicted iris color for the unknown iris fell within the predicted range 96% of the time; Figure 8) and demonstrated that the method was capable of pinpointing the overall eumelanin content of the iris and often the particular shade, though not the pattern of iris pigmentation [13].

Particularly interesting from this work on iris color is what it teaches us to expect for other phenotypes. The predictive power of these SNPs required a consideration within the context of diplotypes. Not only were SNPs unable to provide predictive power on their own, haplotypes were equally insufficient and even diplotypes composed using smaller numbers of SNPs than these 33 (such as hap-tag SNPs) were insufficient to achieve good prediction results [13]. This illustrates the apparent historical and mechanistic complexity of even this relatively simple (predominantly single-gene) phenotype. A by-product of this complexity is the need for a massive database in order to handle most test samples; with so many SNPs part of the equation, the number of diplotypes in the human population is very large and the chances that a test sample from a crime scene would have a match in the database at its current size ($n =$ 1100, Summer, 2007) is about 10%. Nonetheless, the inferences for these 10% are highly accurate and based on this utility, the iris color diplotype database system has been developed as a forensic service by DNAPrint genomics under the trade name Retinome™ (DNAPrint genomics is the laboratory within which the author conducted much of the work described here and throughout this article). So far the method has been applied to several homicide cases; however, due to the currently small size of the database, many detectives desiring to use Retinome™ have been unable to do so because their crime-scene samples did not have a match in the database. For this method of predicting iris color to have more of a broad impact on the investigative process, the size of the database will have to be increased substantially.

In spite of its limitations, the Retinome™ system was the first system for the direct inference of a complex human phenotype. Since its introduction on the lecture circuit in 2004, other OCA2 systems involving additional single nucleotide polymorphisms (SNPs) were described [23], and eventually, a single SNP was discovered in 2008 [24–26] that was so powerfully associated with the light/dark iris color dichotomy that it was posited to represent no less than a founder mutation – an evolutionarily instrumental mutation that not only explains but also represents the historical genesis of the crude light versus dark dichotomy extant throughout the world today. The strength of the association (nearly perfect, with respect to the dichotomy), functional studies with cultured melanocytes, the universality of the association (the C allele associated with lighter colors in individuals from around the world), and the location of the SNP in an important regulatory region of the OCA2 gene all combined to suggest that this hypothesis is indeed true. Although the SNP is only useful for crude predictions (lighter versus darker colors), the founder status of the mutation meant that prediction was suddenly possible for all samples – not merely a small fraction. Indeed, it is likely that some of the previously described SNPs were useful as components of a predictive tool through linkage with this founder mutation. However, others are likely to represent important pieces of the final solution for predicting precise colors and shades with economy and practicality. For example, one of the 33 Retinome™ SNPs (rs1800407) was demonstrated to be a penetrance modifier of the newly discovered founder mutation, and a minimalist set of OCA2 polymorphisms for the "ultimate" in forensics utility (precise color, perhaps pattern as well, for all crime-scene samples) will likely require a composite diplotype system involving the founder mutation and some number of the previously described SNPs in [3] and [23]. This "ultimate" system has not yet been developed, though integration of the founder mutation with those of the Retinome™ system in a newly available forensic service called Retinome™ 2.0 (DNAPrint genomics, Inc., Sarasota, Florida) represents a step toward this goal.

Hair Color

Hair color cannot yet be comprehensively predicted from pigmentation gene genotypes. The iris color polymorphisms just described are not associated with human hair color and association and linkage scans have so far been relatively fruitless in identifying other useful associations ([3]; Zhu G. and Martin N., Queensland Institute of Medical Research, Brisbane AU, personal communication, and T. Frudakis unpublished results). This may be due to the fact that unlike the crudest aspect of iris color – the quantity of eumelanin in the iris – the genetic basis for hair color is a function of significant locus heterogeneity and complex historical origin. However, it appears that red color may be an exception. Valverde et al., [27] was the first to identify MC1R associations with pheomelanogenic red hair color (RHC), and subsequently, several other authors have extended these results to identify what are today called the *RHC* phenotype alleles (all SNPs, Box et al., [28]; Duffy et al., [29]; Smith et al., [30]; Palmer et al., [31]; Box et al., [32]; Bastiaens et al., [33]; Bastiaens et al., [34]; Kennedy et al., [35]; Flanagan et al., [36] and reviewed by Sturm, [37]). The associations are sufficiently strong to enable good predictive power – with odds ratios ranging from 2.3 to over 100 (reviewed in Sturm, 2002; [3]). The United Kingdom's forensic science service (FSS) has condensed the major MC1R red-hair polymorphisms into a 12-marker test that is sold to the forensics community. This test is generally only useful in cases of homozygosity; individuals who are homozygous for any of these mutations, or heterozygous for any two separate mutations (called *compound heterozygotes*) are accurately predicted to be redheaded (accuracy = 96%, from a test with $n = 48$ subjects) and those without a mutation (homozygous wild type) are almost always not redheaded (accuracy = 100%, from a test with $n = 35$ subjects; [18]). Approximately 84% of redheads are detectable by these criteria. Predictive ability is lower in the case of simple heterozygotes (only one mutation present, in the heterozygous state), which is by definition the state in which most of these RHC SNP alleles are expected to be found, in which case 88% are not redheaded while 12% are redheaded ($n = 33$). Indeed, we might expect that each of these mutations will have varying influences on the phenotype depending on the MC1R context within which it is found, and application of diplotype databases as described for iris color may be helpful in teasing more predictive power.

Other Phenotypes

Databases are not yet available for the direct inference of skin color, but this may change soon. [12] and Bonilla *et al.*, [38] used a process called *admixture mapping* to identify variants in the OCA2, MATP, ASIP, and TYR pigmentation genes associated with skin color in a manner that is independent from their ancestry information content. None of these appear to be strong enough to enable accurate prediction, but [19] convincingly described additional variants of the SLC24A5 gene that underlie additional variable skin pigmentation in humans (as well as other vertebrates). Diplotypes involving SNPs in these five genes may be sufficient for accurate inference of skin color within the context of the database systems we have been discussing, though such as database has not yet been constructed. Promising markers for human stature have also been identified in the RUNX2 gene [20] and RANK gene [21], but its unclear whether these two genes are sufficient for predicting this phenotype (especially since environment is likely to play such a role) and RUNX2/RANK variant databases for this phenotype have also not yet been constructed.

Ethical/Procedural Issues and Case Studies. Were the STR profile for each of the world's human inhabitants deposited into an international forensic DNA database, there would be no need to infer phenotype from crime-scene DNA since we would always be able to achieve a database match. Owing to ethical and procedural concerns, this is unlikely to come to pass in the foreseeable future. The ethical issues surrounding the inference of phenotype are extensively covered in [3], but for our purposes here, we can simply note that there is not a fundamental difference between learning about phenotype from human eyewitnesses versus DNA, except when DNA is available, it is more likely to provide reliable and falsifiable information. At some point, ethicists that decry the use of DNA for predicting phenotype as part of the investigative process will have to choose between the rights of DNA donors to remain

anonymous and uncharacterized and the rights of future victims of these donors not to be future victims. Phenotype profiles may cause the inclusion of innocent individuals into suspect pools, which would cause inconvenience to these individuals but not increase the likelihood of a false conviction (their CODIS profile must still match that of the crime-scene sample, the probability of which is not reasonably a function of whether or not they are tested using the current state-of-the-art CODIS assays, and is irrespective of their phenotype). It could be argued that many such individuals would or should become suspects for other reasons – such as a life of crime, proximity to the crime scene and/or relation to the victim – and that information about phenotype merely hones attention to a subset of these individuals. Indeed, many investigators consider these other reasons adequate priors (bases) on their own for defining who is and is not of interest in an investigation and honing attention to a subset of them with DNA-based phenotype information could reduce unnecessary inconvenience for many not fitting the phenotype "profile". Notwithstanding, weighted against the death of innocent victims that could be caused by not applying intelligence provided by DNA-based methods, inconvenience caused to innocent individuals subsequently proven not to match the CODIS profile of a given crime-scene sample pales toward insignificant in comparison. Indeed, we seem to have made the decision to use physical information to shape investigations already – as it pertains to human eyewitness testimony; even with all of its pitfalls, its subjectivity, and poor performance rate, eyewitness testimony currently represents one of the most important cornerstones of the investigative process. The use of DNA-based methods promise only to improve this performance using DNA as an additional and/or alternative source for information, at least for cases where DNA is available. Even so, ethicists have complained that DNA-based phenotyping methods are akin to "racial profiling", but the difference between using physical information gleaned from a crime-scene specimen and "racial profiling" is the application of falsifiable science rather than prejudice. For example, focusing on an individual based on information extracted from a crime scene is an exercise based on evidence and data and the conclusions are falsifiable by other laboratories. In contrast, focusing on an individual based on a belief that individuals of "group X" are more likely to be criminals – lacking specific data derived from a crime scene – is based more on prejudice and subjectivity than the scientific method and generally speaking, such correlations are not adequately powerful in a predictive sense to constitute meaningful priors when determining the likelihood of an individual's involvement in a crime.

The methods described in this article have been applied to numerous criminal investigations. The first application of the indirect method was for the Louisiana Multiagency Homicide Task Force Investigation (Louisiana Serial Killer Case) in the spring of 2003 [3, 22]. Investigators had adequate DNA from various rape/murder scenes throughout the state, but without a CODIS match, they were forced to target their investigation based on two eyewitness accounts that subsequently proved irrelevant to the case. Over a year passed with the task force looking for a "Caucasian" male (not only with standard investigative practices but also with DNA sampling dragnets) until a 73-AIM version of the DNAPrint 176-AIM genomic ancestry panel described in this article (which was also sold under the trade name DNAWITNESS™ as version 2.0) was applied and indicated that the donor was an individual of primarily African ancestry (85%) with a small amount of Indigenous American admixture (15%). In this particular case, the lack of European admixture was used to infer a relatively dark skin shade with respect to the average African-American in the United States (Figure 5a). The investigation was refocused with this data and within a couple of months, the newly refocused investigation lead to an ex-con in the area fitting this profile whose CODIS STR profile was subsequently matched to the crime scene. Were it not for the application of the phenotyping methods, the investigation would have continued on its misdirected path, and others would likely have been raped and murdered [22].

Another murder case in Napa California was initially focused on Hispanic suspects based on an eyewitness account. Napa detectives applied the 176-AIM panel discussed in this article and obtained a continental admixture result that was found from DNAPrint genomics' DNAWITNESS 2.5 database to be consistent with individuals of Continental European as well as Middle Eastern descent – not Hispanic. They then applied the DNAPrint Eurasian panel of 320 AIMs and the RETINOME™ iris color panel described earlier in this article and learned from database searches that the individual was most likely of Northern European ancestry and of light-colored irides. The investigation was focused appropriately, and the perpetrator of the crime in this particular case (who was of Northern European descent with blue eyes) was eventually identified and linked to the crime scene via the CODIS profile. As with human eyewitness data, DNA-based phenotype information does not always result in quick arrests of course, and of the hundred or so investigations that have employed the methods described herein, the majority remain open. However, even for these cases, investigators have saved money and time that would have been spent investigating individuals with phenotypes very different from the crime-scene DNA donor.

To advance the field, the SNP and AIM associations and databases currently available need to be amplified so that an inference for every sample can be obtained, and more research is needed so that additional phenotypes can be considered. In the near future, this may be an uphill battle, at least in the United States. For example, many US grant-funding agencies have not embraced much of the work described in this article – particularly those associated with indirect methods of phenotype inference and it seems most likely that the task of expanding this field will likely to be left to private enterprise or public laboratories outside the United States. Indeed, the work described in this article was funded with private capital, and though commercial demand for the products has not so far economically justified the investment, the work has at least provided some public service and could prove just as useful for other more commercially lucrative areas of research such as in drug development (where constructing a portrait of an ideal patient for a given drug could have a significant impact on the likelihood of clinical trial success). The institutional resistance in the United States toward the type of work discussed in this article is interesting and deserves some thought here. Some argue that the US justice system is not built for efficiency and is biased toward the interests of the accused. If true, this may explain why US budgets for solving crimes are often limited such that US investigators have difficulty funding basic CODIS processing of their crime-scene samples (which should always be done first since identity testing provides probative, not merely presumptive results). For example, backlogs of a year or more and anecdotal reports of rape kits stacked to the ceiling awaiting funding for CODIS processing are not uncommon in the United States. For agencies experiencing such backlogs, budget allocation for phenotyping is likely to remain de-prioritized and until phenotyping methods have had more time to penetrate the field through continued demonstration of utility. Until the problems underlying the CODIS backlogs have been solved, the application of DNA-based phenotyping methods is likely to continue on a case-by-case basis, with emphasis on high-profile cases that investigators are under unusual pressure to quickly solve (such as serial homicide cases).

Acknowledgments

I would like to thank all of the volunteers who provided their informed consent to be part of our forensic databases here at DNAPrint genomics, Inc.

End Notes

[a.] Though, since all loci carry some ancestry information, calculations on the statistical certainty of such a match requires the use of appropriate population databases since they are based on allele frequencies that vary subtly from population to population.

References

[1] Theodoridis, S. & Koutroumbas, K. (1999). *Pattern Recognition*, Academic Press Publishers, London.

[2] Robert, C. (2001). *The Bayesian Choice*, 2nd Edition, Springer-Verlag New York Inc., New York.

[3] Frudakis, T., Terravainen, T. & Thomas, M. (2007). Multilocus OCA2 genotypes specify human iris colors, *Human Genetics*.

[4] Cavalli-Sforza, L. & Bodmer, W. (1999). *The Genetics of Human Populations*, Dover Publications, Mineola, NY.

[5] Jobling, M., Hurles, M. & Tyler-Smith, C. (2004). *Human Evolutionary Genetics. Origins, Peoples and Disease*, Garland publishing, New York, NY.

[6] Lind, J., Hutcheson-Dilks, H., Williams, S., Moore, J., Essex, M., Ruiz-Pesini, E., Wallace, D., Tishkoff, S., O'Brien, S. & Smith, M. (2007). Elevated male European and female African contributions to the genomes of African American individuals, *Human Genetics* **120**(5), 713–722.

[7] Chakraborty, R. (1986). Gene admixture in human populations: models and predictions *Yearbook of Physical Anthropology* **29**, 1–43.

[8] Jurmain, R., Nelson, H., Kilgore, L. & Trevathan, W. (2000). *Introduction to Physical Anthropology*, Wadsworth/Thomson Learning, Belmont, CA.

[9] Rosenberg, N., Pritchard, J., Weber, J., Cann, H., Kidd, K., Zhivotovsky, L. & Feldman, M. (2002). Genetic structure of human populations, *Science* **298**, 2381–2385.

[10] Halder, I., Shriver, M., Thomas, M., Fernandez, J. & Frudakis, T. (2007). A panel of ancestry informative markers for estimating individual biogeographical ancestry and admixture from four continents: utility and applications, *Human Mutation* **29**(5), 648–658.

[11] Bauchet, M., McEvoy, B., Pearson, L., Quillen, E., Sarkisian, T., Hovhannesyan, K., Deka, R., Bradley, D. & Shriver, M. (2007). Measuring European population stratification using microarray genotype data, *American Journal of Human Genetics* In press.

[12] Shriver, M., Parra, E., Dios, S., Bonilla, C., Norton, H., Jovel, C., Pfaff, C., Jones, C., Massac, A., Cameron, N., Baron, A., Jackson, T., Argyropoulos, G., Jin, L., Hoggart, C., McKeigue, P. & Kittles, R. (2003). Skin pigmentation, biogeographical ancestry and admixture mapping, *Human Genetics* **112**(4), 387–399.

[13] Frudakis, T. (2007). *Molecular Photofitting: Predicting Phenotype and Ancestry from DNA*, Elsevier Academic Press Publishers, Burlington, MA.

[14] Zhu, G., Evans, D., Duffy, D., Montgomery, G., Medland, S., Gillespie, N., Ewen, K., Jewell, M., Liew, Y., Hayward, N., Sturm, R., Trent, J. & Martin, N. (2004). A genome scan for eye color in 502 twin families: most variation is due to a QTL on chromosome 15q, *Twin Research* **7**, 197–210.

[15] Frudakis, T., Thomas, M., Gaskin, Z., Venkateswarlu, K., Chandra, S., Ginjupalli, S., Gunturi, S., Natrajan, S., Ponnuswamy, V. & Ponnuswamy, K. (2003). Sequences associated with human iris pigmentation, *Genetics* **165**, 2071–2083.

[16] Rebbeck, T., Kanetsky, P., Walker, A., Holmes, R., Halpern, A., Schuchter, L. *et al.* (2002). P gene as an inherited biomarker of human eye color, *Cancer Epidemiology Biomarkers and Prevention* **11**(8), 782–784.

[17] Sturm, R. & Frudakis, T. (2004). Eye colour: portals into pigmentation genes and ancestry, *Trends in Genetics* **20**(8), 327–332.

[18] Grimes, E., Noake, P., Dixon, L. & Urquhart, A. (2001). Sequence polymorphism in the human melanocortin 1 receptor gene as an indicator of the red hair phenotype, *Forensic Science International* **122**, 124–129.

[19] Lamason, R., Mohideen, M., Mest, J., Wong, A., Norton, H., Aros, M., Jurynec, M., Mao, X., Humphreville, V., Humbert, J., Sinha, S., Moore, J., Jagadeeswaran, P., Zhao, W., Ning, G., Makalowska, I., McKeigue, P., O'donnell, D., Kittles, R., Parra, E., Mangini, N., Grunwald, D., Shriver, M., Canfield, V. & Cheng, K. (2005). SLC24A5, a putative cation exchanger,

affects pigmentation in zebrafish and humans, *Science* **310**(5755), 1782–1786.

[20] Ermakov, S., Malkin, I., Kobyliansky, E. & Livshits, G. (2005). Variation in femoral length is associated with polymorphisms in RUNX2 gene, *Bone* **38**(2), 199–205.

[21] Chen, Y., Xiong, D.H., Yang, T.L., Yang, F., Jiang, H., Zhang, F., Shen, H., Xiao, P., Recker, R.R. & Deng, H.W. (2007). Variations in RANK gene are associated with adult height in Caucasians, *American Journal of Human Biology* **19**(4), 559–565.

[22] Stanley, S. (2006). *An Invisible Man: The Hunt for a Serial Killer Who Got Away with a Decade of Murder*, Berkley Books, New York.

[23] Duffy, D.L., Montgomery, G.W., Chen, W., Zhao, Z.Z., Le, L., James, M.R., Hayward, N.K., Martin, N.G. & Sturm, R.A. (2007). A three-single-nucleotide polymorphism haplotype in intron 1 of OCA2 explains most human eye-color variation, *American Journal of Human Genetics* **80**(2), 241–252.

[24] Eiberg, H., Troelsen, J., Nielsen, M. Mikkelsen M. (2008). Blue eye color in humans may be caused by a perfectly associated founder mutation in a regulatory element located within the HERC2 gene inhibiting OCA2 expression, *Human Genetics* **123**(2), 177–187.

[25] Sturm, R.A., Duffy, D.L., Zhao, Z.Z., Leite, F.P., Stark, M.S., Hayward, N.K. & Martin, N.G., Montgomery, G.W. (2008). A single SNP in an evolutionary conserved region within intron 86 of the HERC2 gene determines human blue-brown eye color, *American Journal of Human Genetics* **82**(2), 424–431.

[26] Kayser, M., Liu, F., Janssens, A.C., Rivadeneira, F., Lao, O., van Duijn, K., Vermeulen, M., Arp, P., Jhamai, M.M., van Ijcken, W.F., den Dunnen, J.T., Heath, S., Zelenika, D., Despriet, D.D., Klaver, C.C., Vingerling, J.R., de Jong, P.T., Hofman, A., Aulchenko, Y.S., Uitterlinden, A.G., Oostra, B.A. & van Duijn, C.M. (2008). Three genome-wide association studies and a linkage analysis identify HERC2 as a human iris color gene, *American Journal of Human Genetics* **82**(2), 411–423.

[27] Valverde, P., Healy, E., Jackson, I., Rees, J., Thody, A. (1995). Variants of the melanocyte-stimulating hormone receptor gene are associated with red hair and fair skin in humans, *Nature Genetics* **11**, 328–330.

[28] Box, N., Wyeth, J., O'Gorman, I., Martin, N. & Sturm, R. (1997). Characterization of melanocyte stimulating hormone variant alleles in twins with red hair, *Humman Molecular Genetics* **6**, 1891–1897.

[29] Duffy, D., Box, N., Chen, W., Palmer, J., Montgomery, G., James, M. *et al.*, (2004). Interactive effects of MC1R and OCA2 on melanoma risk phenotypes, *Human Molecular Genetics* **13**(4), 447–461.

[30] Smith, R., Healy, E., Siddiqui, S., Flanagan, N., Steijlen, P., Rosdahl, I. *et al.*, (1998). Melanocortin 1 receptor variants in an Irish population, *The Journal of Investigative Dermatology* **111**, 119–122.

[31] Palmer, J., Duffy, D., Box, N., Aitken, J., O'Gorman, L., Green, A., *et al.*, (2000). Melanocortin-1 receptor polymorphisms and risk of melanoma: Is the association explained solely by pigmentation phenotype?, *American Journal of Human Genetics* **66**(1), 176–186.

[32] Box, N., Duffy, D., Irving, R., Russell, A., Chen, W., Griffyths, L. *et al.*, (2001). Melanocortin-1 receptor genotype is a risk factor for basal and squamous cell carcinoma, *The Journal of Investigative Dermatology* **116**, 224–229.

[33] Bastiaens, M., ter Huurne, J., Kielich, C., Gruis, N., Westendorp, R., Vermeer, B. *et al.*, (2001a). The melanocortin-1-receptor gene is the major freckle gene, *Human Molecular Genetics* **10**(16), 1701–1708.

[34] Bastiaens, M., ter Huurne, J., Kielich, C., Gruis, N., Wetendorp, R., Vermeer, B. *et al.*, (2001b). Melanocortin-1 receptor gene variants determine the risk of nonmelanoma skin cancer independently of fair skin and red hair, *American Journal Human Genetics* **68**(4), 884–894.

[35] Kennedy, C., ter Huurne, J., Berkhout, M., Gruis, N., Bastiaens, M., Bergman, W. *et al.*, (2001). Melanocortin 1 receptor (MC1R) gene variants are associated with an increased risk for cutaneous melanoma which is largely independent of skin type and hair color, *The Journal of Investigative Dermatology* **117**(2), 294–300.

[36] Flanagan, N., Healy, E., Ray, A., Philips, S., Todd, C., Jackson, I. (2000). Pleitotropic effects of the melanocortin 1 receptor (MC1R) gene on human pigmentation, *Human Molecular Genetics* **9**, 2531–2537.

[37] Sturm, R. (2002). Skin colour and skin cancer – MC1R, the genetic link, *Melanoma Research* **12**(5), 405–416.

[38] Bonilla, C. Parra. E., Pfaff, C., Dios, S., Marshall, J., Hamman, R. *et al.*, (2004). Admixture in the Hispanics of the San Luis Valley, Colorado and its implications for complex trait gene mapping *Annals of Human Genetics* **68**, 139–153.

TONY FRUDAKIS

Phosphatase: Acid *see* Acid Phosphatase

Photography: Length Measurement *see* Length Measurement

Photography: Marks, Impressions, and Documents

Introduction

Photography plays a pivotal role in criminalistics by providing several key functions including nondestructive methods of detection, recording, preservation, and enhancement of physical evidence. Standard operating procedures for most forms of physical evidence require the evidence to be photographed either at the crime scene or in the forensic laboratory. In many cases involving crime scene investigation, the photographs of physical evidence obtained at the scene become the only form in which that evidence exists. The preservation of perishable forms of physical evidence places a higher emphasis on photographic methods to retain the evidence long after the scene has changed or the physical evidence has perished.

Some forms of crime scene photographs also under go a process of comparative analysis made directly from the photographic source. Evidence such as bloodstain patterns, footwear impressions, fingermarks, toolmarks, and tire impressions all require a forensic examination made directly from the images. These photographs become the primary source [1] of the forensic analysis, and the value of the physical evidence is a function of the quality and accuracy of the photographic evidence.

The application of photography certainly covers a broad range of activities and some specific taxonomy needs to be developed when attempting to model photography's purpose in the forensic sciences [2]. This section discusses the central technical aspects of photography when used in criminalistics. Information regarding basic camera operation or techniques for simplistic recording of items found at a crime scene are not provided in this section. It will, however, examine the aspects of photographing evidence that utilize photographs in the analysis of evidence by forensic criminalists. Aspects including accurate recording methods, specialized techniques, and optical enhancement of evidence are discussed.

Currently, photography can be divided into two separate forms: silver halide (film) photography and digital photography. Both the forms of photography are currently practiced in the forensic science domain and are considered the same in this section. The light-sensitive recording mechanisms are the most obvious differences between each technology; however, camera operation remains relatively the same (with some exceptions).

Digital imaging is a different concept that involves using digitized images on a computer platform and a distinction is made between digital photography and digital imaging. Digital photography is the practice of photography using a digital camera, while digital imaging is the processing or alteration of digital images using image editing software programs or the digitization of a photograph using peripheral computer equipment such as a scanner.

The practice of digital photography and digital imaging are naturally implicit. The application of image editing software (i.e., Adobe Photoshop™) is also an integral element within the overall digital photography workflow. It is important to recognize, however, that the improvement capacity of images using image editing software does not substitute for consistent quality photography techniques at the capture stage.

This section presents information regarding the optical enhancement of evidence in three separate components: (i) maintaining the image integrity, (ii) optical enhancement, and (iii) digital imaging enhancement.

Image Integrity

The debate regarding the legitimatization of digital images in law enforcement and forensic science has been an exhaustive process by several law enforcement working parties, committees, and organizations over the years [3–5]. Legal organizations have generally accepted the new technology and have adopted their own forms of operating procedures when using digital photography. Like all modes of physical evidence, continuity of the evidence is a critical component of the management of the evidence integrity. Photography should be not different to any other mode of evidence and sound procedural policy regarding forensic photography practices should be developed and maintained throughout all the forensic organizations. It is, however, not the function of this section to discuss those procedures.

Image integrity also refers to the ability of the image to represent the aspects of the photographic evidence accurately, reliably, and truthfully. The integrity of the photography evidence is a paramount consideration in criminalistics. The following attributes are considered in relation to image integrity for the photography of physical evidence that requires analysis directly from those photographs. More simplistic applications of photography to record the subjects *in situ* may not require such strict technical parameters.

Dimensional Integrity

The reproduction of three-dimensional subjects into accurate two-dimensional photographs is fraught with difficulty by the very nature of this dimensional transition. The need for accurate dimensional representation is, however, a consideration when examining evidence such as fingermarks, footwear impressions, toolmarks, and bloodstain pattern evidence. Conveniently, these evidence forms are mostly represented as two-dimensional (or very close to it) and photography can reproduce a fair representation

in this dimensional exchange (two-dimensions into two-dimensions). Accurate reproduction in this situation is not, however, automatic and requires some technical considerations to exclude the aspects of image distortion. Figure 1 shows four photographs taken of the same subject, a wire frame. It demonstrates how different the same object may be represented in a photograph and the importance of accurate photography. The image in Figure 1(a) has correctly maintained the subject's dimensional integrity, while those in Figure 1(b–d) show keystoning or optical distortion.

Forensic photographs that are used in comparative analysis must maintain the integrity of the subject's dimensional aspects. Images that do not represent the subject's dimensions and shape accurately are considered to be distorted. Image distortion is caused by several visual conditions including: (i) the camera viewpoint in relation to the subject (perspective distortion), (ii) the optical characteristics of the lens (curvilinear distortion), (iii) the dimensional stability of the recording material (film), and (iv) incorrect resizing of images in digital imaging software.

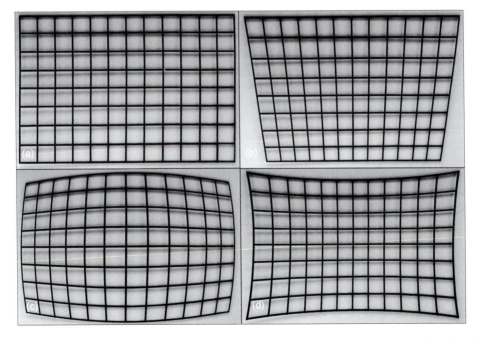

Figure 1 Four photographs of the same object displaying different representations of image dimensional integrity: (a) correctly photographed displaying good image dimensional integrity; (b) image displaying perspective distortion or keystoning; (c) image displaying barrel distortion; and (d) image displaying pincushion distortion

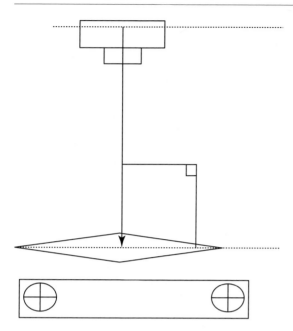

Figure 2   Camera position in relation to the subject. The lens axis is perpendicular to the subject and film planes while the film plane and subject planes are parallel

There are two essential requirements for the successful photography of physical evidence while maintaining the dimensional integrity of the evidence: (i) position the camera correctly to avoid perspective distortion (keystoning) and (ii) always use a distortion-free lens (Hard return). The camera viewpoint must be directly over the subject, which means the lens axis is perpendicular to the subject plane and the camera focal plane and subject plane are parallel [6]. Figure 2 illustrates the camera position in relation to the subject to avoid introducing perspective distortion while maintaining the integrity of the subject's dimensional aspects.

Several lens designs suffer from an optic aberration called *curvilinear distortion* [7], which will also corrupt the integrity of the image dimensional qualities. Curvilinear distortion is often described by the visual result that appears in the image and is referred to as either *barrel distortion* or *pincushion distortion* [8, 9] (see Figure 1). These effects are indicative of their descriptions and are caused by variations of image magnification across the field [1]. Curvilinear distortion can be minimized by using a symmetrical or quasi-symmetrical lens design. Lenses that are significantly asymmetrical in design, such as

telephoto and retrofocus lenses, tend to suffer appreciably from curvilinear distortion [8]. Zoom lens are also prone to distortion aberration and generally display pincushion distortion at longer focal lengths and barrel distortion at shorter focal lengths [8, 10]. Lens designs that are distortion free are called *orthoscopic lenses* [8, 11]. A critical aspect of photographing physical evidence and maintaining the dimensional integrity of the evidence is to select a lens that is free from curvilinear distortion.

Macro lenses are designed for photography at shorter working distances than infinity (∞) or for a magnification range of 0.1–1.0 times [12]. They are also either symmetrical or quasi-symmetrical in design and are considered as highly corrected for curvilinear distortion aberration. All photography of physical evidence that requires a high standard of image dimensional integrity should be taken with a macro lens and never with a telephoto, wide angle retrofocus, or zoom lens. This aspect of forensic photography quality is imperative for evidence such as fingermark impressions, footwear impressions, physical fit evidence, toolmark evidence, and other forms of evidence requiring the examination of photographs. This aspect is naturally not as important for general recording of evidence such as *in situ* images at crime scenes. Zoom lenses are very useful for general crime scene photography but not for more critical forensic photography.

Some digital imaging software provides the facility to correct lens distortion. Even though lens distortion may be corrected using digital imaging software such as Adobe Photoshop™ [13, 14], digital correction of this image artifact should only be applied when it is absolutely necessary and should not replace the standard photography practices that avoid lens distortion. Prevention is better than the cure and it is certainly more preferable to avoid curvilinear distortion by using a lens that is considered as distortion free or orthoscopic in the first instance.

Representation of Scale

The incorporation of linear scales into physical evidence photographs is an essential practice when recording evidence. There are various linear scales available for different types of evidence. Linear scales are used as a reference to the size of the subjects photograph and this reference is used to enlarge the photographs to predetermined magnifications for comparative analysis examination (1 : 1 for footwear impressions, 5 : 1 for fingerprint impressions, etc.). Linear scales are also used to calibrate the scale of digital images when using image analysis applications. Calibration is achieved when the amount of pixels are counted across a known length present in the image. Each pixel then represents a lineal value and several mathematical functions may be applied to the image.

Important considerations when incorporating linear scales include the following: (i) use an appropriate sized scale for the type of evidence photographed, (ii) make sure the scale does not hide the features of the evidence, and (iii) the position of the linear scale must be parallel to the subject and at the same height. Some linear scales also incorporate circular references to detect any perspective distortion that may have resulted from poor photography technique. Digital correction of perspective distortion may also be conducted using Photoshop™ and using the circular references as a standard.

Image Quality

The quality of the image is naturally an important aspect of recording evidence that will undergo further examination and analysis. Image quality for forensic purposes may be defined by several parameters including image sharpness or resolution, detail or clarity, image contrast, color fidelity and dynamic range, and dimensional integrity. Table 1 provides a list of those parameters and also describes what influences these considerations of image quality.

The maintenance of image quality needs to be carefully considered and embedded into the forensic practitioners working practice. Image quality forms a critical basis for forensic photography and is an essential requirement before further optical and digital enhancement techniques may be applied. Digital enhancement is not a correction for poorly executed forensic photography. Evidence enhancement techniques build on the foundation of sound image quality and permit further visualization and the application of forensic evidence.

Table 1 Image quality parameters and their causes

Quality parameter	Cause
Image sharpness and resolution	i) Lens focus ii) Depth of field iii) Camera shake and shutter speeds iv) Quality of optics
Detail and clarity	i) Image sharpness ii) Shadow and highlight detail controlled by camera exposure iii) Lighting technique iv) Color fidelity and tonal range v) Digital workflow
Image contrast	i) Lighting quality ii) Lighting ratios iii) Subject properties (and treatment) iv) Level adjustments (digital photography) or film processing (film photography)
Color fidelity and dynamic range	i) Color temperature balance between lighting and capture source (white balance for digital photography, film, and filter combinations for film photography) ii) Digital photography; color space, bit depth, file applications, and gamma settings iii) Color management and calibration of computer monitor
Image dimensional integrity	i) Camera viewpoint ii) Optics iii) Application of linear scales iv) Resizing digital images

Evidence Enhancement

The most common rationale to enhance physical evidence is to improve the visibility of the evidence. Contrast between the evidence and background can become problematic when evidence is found on items that are of similar color or tonal value. Increasing the difference of brightness values between the evidence and the background provides an increase of contrast. Evidence deposited onto material with complex patterns can also lower the visibility of the evidence and cause problems with interpretation of the evidence. An optical enhancement example is found in the two crime-scene photographs (Figure 3).

The photograph in Figure 3(a) is a bloodstained footwear impression made on a black ceramic tile found at a crime scene. This image displays very little visibility and contrast between the bloodstain impression and the black tile background. Figure 3(b) is the same footwear impression that has undergone chemical and optical enhancement to increase the contrast and improve the visibility of the evidence. The bloodstain footwear impression was first treated with a blood reagent called *Hungarian Red* and photographed using a monochromatic light source of 530 nm. A Wratten 25 barrier filter was attached to the camera lens.

Evidence enhancement may be achieved by using the following methods:

- chemical treatment (development or staining);
- optical enhancement;
- specialized lighting techniques; and
- digital imaging enhancement.

Enhancement may be conducted using a single method or a combination of methods as demonstrated in Figure 3(b). Chemical treatment to enhance or develop physical evidence is a practice that is well established in forensic science. The treatment may independently increase contrast due to chemical staining or it may combine physically with the deposited material and alter the spectral qualities of the material. Optical or photographic enhancement involves various techniques utilizing the optical properties of the evidence material and its relationship to the radiation source and spectral sensitivity

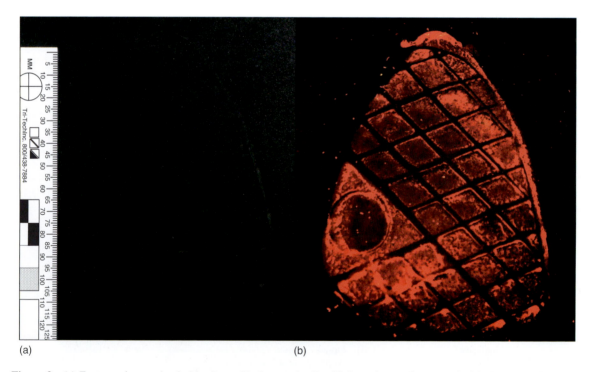

(a)   (b)

Figure 3   (a) Footwear impression in blood on a black ceramic tile. (b) Same impression treated with Hungarian Red and photographed with a 530 nm monochromatic light source and a Wratten 25 barrier filter on the lens of the capture device. Digital imaging enhancement also utilizes digital imaging editing software such as Adobe Photoshop™. Optical and digital imaging enhancement are discussed in the next section.

Optical Enhancement

Chemical treatment of physical evidence (i.e., blood or fingermarks) will either stain the material to increase the contrast or make the material react to a light source of specific spectral output. Details regarding the various chemical treatments are discussed elsewhere in this section, however, the reaction of chemically treated specimens to certain wavelengths of light provides the basis of optical enhancement.

Optical enhancement of physical evidence provides the visualization of latent evidence or provides improved visibility by increasing the contrast between the evidence and its background. There are three essential elements that form the foundation for optical enhancement of physical evidence. These elements include: (i) the specific spectral distribution of the light source illuminating the specimen, (ii) the specimen's response when illuminated by the light source, and (iii) the spectral sensitivity of the capture device (film or digital sensor). Each component requires careful consideration when performing optical enhancement of physical evidence.

Spectral Distribution of Light Sources

The approximate spectral sensitivity range of human vision is between 400 and 700 nm, with higher sensitivity within certain ranges depending on the level of illumination. When light enters the eye and forms an image on the retina, nerve cells called *photoreceptors* [15] convert the light energy into a signal that is translated by the mind. There are two types of photoreceptors within the retina called *rods* and *cones* and these receptors react to different levels of illumination. Malacara [16] suggests there are approximately 100 million rods and 5 million cones. The cone receptors are used for bright light conditions and have a sensitivity peak at 555 nm, while the rod receptors provide vision in low light (night vision) and have a sensitivity peak at 505 nm [16–18].

Most digital cameras capture color by using a color filter array positioned over the camera's sensor.

This array consists of a mosaic of red, green, and blue (RGB) filters known as a *Bayer filter*. The Bayer filter has twice the number of green filters as red or blue to produce color images that relate to the spectral sensitivity of vision [19].

The spectral output of a light source is called its *spectral distribution* and may be measured using a spectrophotometer. Optical enhancement techniques use various different light sources including natural sources such as direct sunlight and open shade, and artificial light sources such as incandescent tungsten, tungsten halogen, electronic flash, xenon arc lamps, and others.

White light containing a mixture of several colors is considered as a polychromatic light source. Polychromatic light is suitable for most general photography applications and essential for color photography. However, optical enhancement techniques often require a light source with a narrow spectrum or monochromatic light sources [20]. Monochromatic light sources are produced by filtering polychromatic light through an optical filter or filters. Lasers are another source of monochromatic light [21].

Specialized forensic lighting equipment such as the Rofin Polilight™ provides monochromatic light for a range of forensic applications including optical enhancement. These units use a high-intensity xeon light source with inbuilt interference filters to produce monochromatic light with bandwidth of ≈40 nm for most settings. The inbuilt interference filters are also tunable by adjusting the angle of the filter in relation to the transmitting light through the filter. A tuning rate of 30 nm may be achieved with a 45° tilt and the shift is always downtuned toward a shorter wavelength. Figure 4 provides details of the spectral distribution of the Polilight on the 590-nm setting. The monochromatic nature of the light output can be seen by the narrow shape of the spectrum.

Spectral Response of Specimen

Optical enhancement operates on the premise that specimens record in a particular way when they are irradiated by specific wavelengths from a monochromatic light source or transmitted through an optical filter over the camera lens. Optical filtering of the illuminating light to produce a monochromatic source isolates the response from the specimen. These effects can be achieved with polychromatic light sources; however, due to the broad nature of polychromatic

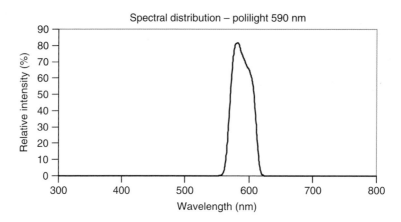

Figure 4   Monochromatic spectra from a Polilight™ forensic light source (setting 590 nm)

lighting, the effects are not seen or are masked by the other wavelengths.

Optical filters placed over the camera lens can also alter the properties of light transmitting through the optical system. Optical filters produce specific spectral responses from the specimen. The application of optical filters on the camera lens allows optical enhancement to be conducted in standard white light conditions, unlike using monochromatic light sources, which will need to be conducted in a darkened room. However, the monochromatic forensic light sources available today provide a narrower spectrum that is difficult to achieve when using a single optical filter over the lens.

Optical enhancement may produce four different conditions or responses from the specimen when illuminated by monochromatic lighting:

- the specimen may *absorb* the light and become darker;
- the specimen may *reflect* the light and become *lighter*;
- the specimen may *transmit* the light and become *transparent*; and
- the specimen may *luminesce* and become *fluorescent*.

These responses to certain wavelengths of monochromatic light may be referred to as *modes of optical enhancement lighting*. These modes may be described as (i) absorption mode, (ii) reflection mode, (iii) transmission mode, and (iv) photoluminescence mode. The purpose of optical

enhancement is to make the specimen visible or introduce greater visibility by enhancing the contrast between the specimen and background. When monochromatic light sources are used in the optical enhancement of evidence, natural color rendition of the specimen is not possible due to the specific spectral range of the light used. Strong color casts are produced when using monochromatic light with color photography and this effect should be avoided because it often appears like a photographic error. Digital images photographed in color should be converted to a grayscale image or the color desaturated to − 100%.

Absorption and Reflection Modes. Absorption and reflection modes are chromatic effects that provide an increase of contrast between the specimen and its background. These modes operate on the principle of selective absorption or selective reflection of a colored specimen when illuminated with a specific monochromatic light source (or transmitted via an optical filter). When a monochromatic light source illuminates a color specimen, the specimen will either darken or become lighter in tone depending on the relationship between the color of the light source and the color of the specimen.

Absorption mode is a method of increasing the contrast between the specimen and the background by darkening the tonal value of the specimen or background. Absorption occurs when a colored specimen is illuminated by a monochromatic light that is an opposite color to that of the specimen [20]. The specimen darkens due to its selective absorption properties

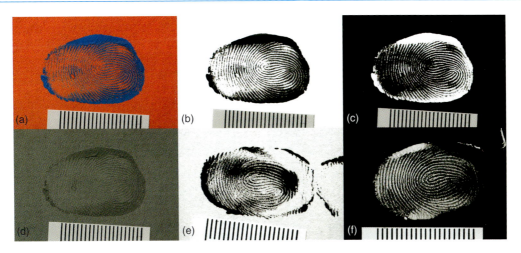

Figure 5   (a) Color image of a fingermark made in cyan-colored paint on a red background. (b) Absorption mode on a red background. (c) Reflective mode on a red background. (d) Grayscale image without enhancement. (e) Absorption mode on white background. (f) Reflective mode on black background

and this mode is most commonly used to increase the contrast.

Reflection mode is also a method of increasing the contrast, however, it lightens the specimen or background by selective reflection. Refection is also a chromatic condition and requires a colored specimen and a monochromatic light source of similar color to the specimen. Figure 5 is a photograph of a fingermark made in cyan colored paint found on a red document. Figure 5(a) is the color image using standard white light (electronic flash), while Figure 5(d) is the same image converted to a grayscale image. Figure 5(b) uses a red monochromatic light (650 nm central bandwidth) and darkens the fingermark due to the absorption of the red illumination. Figure 5(c) uses a blue monochromatic light (450 nm central bandwidth) and lightens the fingermark's tonal value. This series of images also demonstrates an ideal situation for absorption and reflective modes. The color of the background is opposite to that of the specimens. Although this ideal condition is rarely observed in reality, the examples provide an optimum result for this technique.

The general rule for selecting the color of the monochromatic light source for absorption or reflection mode is based on the selective absorption and selective reflection properties of the specimen [20]. It suggests that the color of the light source lightens its own color and darkens its opposing color. Figure 8(a) represents two models of color synthesis

that are regularly used in photography and digital imaging. The two models are "additive" and "subtractive" color synthesis. Additive color synthesis uses primary colors such as red (R), green (G), and blue (B). In an ideal condition, if equal quantities of red, green, and blue light are added together, their combination will produce white light [8]. Hence, RGB primary colors are considered as additive and each color ideally represents one-third of the white light (visual) spectrum. The reproduction of color using the three components of red, green, and blue is called *trichromacy* and relates to the function of color vision known as the *Young* and *Helmholtz theory* [8, 15–17].

The subtractive color synthesis model is based on the subtraction of opposing primary colors (called *complementary*) from white light. Therefore, if green is taken out of white light, the resultant color will be magenta. Magenta light is considered as without the green component of white light due to its subtraction. Primary colors may be subtracted from the white light by using the subtractive color synthesis model comprising of the complementary colors, e.g., cyan (C), magenta (M), and yellow (Y). When an ideal complementary filter (cyan, magenta, or yellow) is placed over a white light source, one-third of the spectrum is subtracted (red, green, or blue) while two-thirds is transmitted. Therefore, subtractive color synthesis is a combination of the two remaining primary colors and makes up two-thirds of the

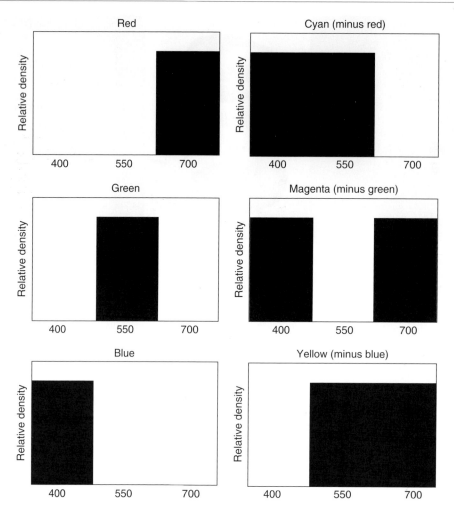

Figure 6 A representation of spectral output from ideal conditions for additive and subtractive color synthesis. The graphs on the left illustrate that each primary color (RGB) produces approximately one-third of the visual spectrum. However, the subtractive model comprising of CMY colors produce two-thirds of the white light spectrum

visual spectrum. Figure 6 illustrates the relationship between additive and subtractive color synthesis models. Each color in the additive color model (RGB) represents one-third of the visual spectrum, while each color in the subtractive model (CMY) make up to two-thirds of the white light.

Additive and subtractive models of color synthesis are also the basis of color film technology and digital imaging color modes [22, 23]. If you examine an image on a color negative film (minus the integral layer which is the amber base color of the film base) you will see that the color image is represented in its negative colors. That is, the reds will

be cyan, greens will be magenta, and blues will be yellow. This effect can also be seen if you invert a color digital image. Figure 7 provides an insight into how these two modes of color synthesis are used in photography. The colors rendered in the inverted or negative image clearly show the relationship between additive and subtractive colors in photography.

Digital imaging also uses the same color modeling with RGB color and CMYK color modes. The "K" is an additional channel and represents black. RGB color is the standard for most digital photography applications, while CMYK is a color space often

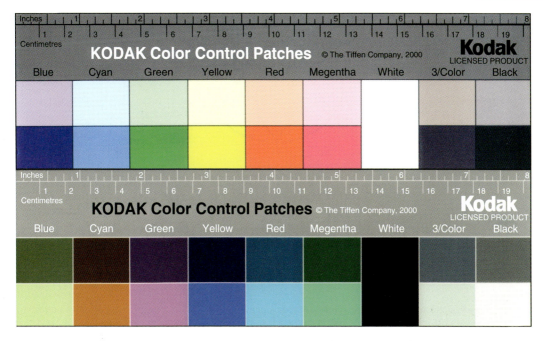

Figure 7 Positive and negative color images displaying the relationship between additive and subtract color synthesis in photography

used for photography used in graphic reproduction (reproduction of images in print media).

Figure 8(a) further displays the relationship between additive and subtractive color models and provides a guide for the selection of monochromatic light for absorption or reflective modes. Each triangle represents a color synthesis model, RGB or additive and CMY (without the K) or subtractive, to produce a color wheel or more appropriately a color star. Colors on the opposing points of the star (e.g., red and cyan) represent opposite colors, while the colors positioned on points next to the additive primary colors are their composites. The opposing colors will provide optimum absorption for specimens and selective monochromatic light sources or optical filters and will darken the specimen. The two adjacent colors next to each opposing color will also darken the specimen.

This diagram forms the basis for absorption mode and the specimens opposing color should be selected as the color of the monochrome light source or optical filter. While absorption mode is usually more effective to enhance contrast than reflective mode, selecting the same color monochrome light source as the color of the specimen will lighten the tonal value of the specimen. Color wheels as

illustrated in Figure 8(a) are for photographic applications and are calculated based on the additive and subtractive models of color synthesis of light [22]. Color wheels that are designed for pigments and used in painting and graphic design are not the same and are not suited for optical enhancement or photography.

The color of the background is also a factor to consider when increasing the contrast using absorption and reflective modes. Neutral backgrounds such as white, gray, or black will display little change when illuminated by monochromatic light due to the achromatic (without color) character of these tones. However, if the background is colored, then the same absorption or reflection principles will occur to the background as it does to the specimen. Backgrounds, which are the opposite color to the specimen, have the potential to produce the highest degree of contrast when applying absorption or reflective modes. White backgrounds also work well with absorption mode because the specimen can be darkened against a light background. Black backgrounds work best with reflective mode by making the specimen lighter to enhance contrast. Figure 5(e) demonstrates the results of absorption mode with a white background, while

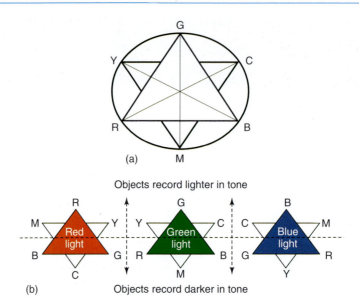

(a)

Objects record lighter in tone

(b)   Objects record darker in tone

Figure 8   (a) Additive and subtractive color synthesis models demonstrating color opposites; (b) Additive and subtractive color synthesis models demonstrating the tonal changes when using monochromatic light sources. The object colors positioned above the horizontal line will record in a lighter tonal value, while the object colors indicated below the line will record darker in tone due to the absorption of the light

Figure 5(f) illustrates the effect of reflection mode on a black background.

As previously mentioned, absorption and reflective modes may also be achieved by using optical filters placed on the camera's lens and photographed using standard white light. This technique has a long history with black and white film photography. Optical filters, known as *contrast filters*, provide a similar effect as monochromatic lighting, except that the effect is influenced and controlled by the transmission properties of the optical filter with white light [24–26]. Filter factors must also be applied to the camera exposure to compensate for the loss of light caused by the absorption of light by the filter. The application of photographic filters may also be achieved digitally with Adobe Photoshop™. Digital imaging enhancement is discussed in the following section.

Transmission Mode.   While an increase of contrast is the objective for absorption and reflective modes of optical enhancement, transmission mode has a different function. The function of transmission mode is to reveal evidence that may be obscured or not visible [27]. It uses the transmission properties of selective wavelengths of light incorporation with the spectral characteristics of the specimen and

the spectral sensitivity of the recording medium. This enhancement mode allows the specific wavelengths of light to transmit through thin specimens of specific spectral qualities and renders the specimen transparent [6, 26–29]. When the specimen becomes transparent, items beneath the specimen can become visible. An example is shown in Figure 9 where the obliterated writing on a document has become visible due to the transparent properties of the ink covering the text.

Photoluminescence Mode.   When specimens possessing certain properties are illuminated by specific wavelengths of monochromatic light, they may absorb the excitation light and then reemit light of a different wavelength. This effect is know as *luminescence* [29, 30]. There are two different results caused by luminescence: (i) fluorescence that emits light at a longer wavelength while the excitation source is illuminating the specimen and (ii) phosphorescence that emits light and continues to do so for a period of time after the excitation source ceases to illuminate the specimen [29, 31, 32]. The material painted onto watch dials that illuminate in the dark is an example of phosphorescence.

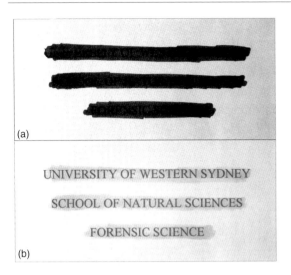

(a)

UNIVERSITY OF WESTERN SYDNEY

SCHOOL OF NATURAL SCIENCES

FORENSIC SCIENCE

(b)

Figure 9 Transmission mode. The ink obliterating the text has become transparent and allowing the visualization of the text beneath the ink

There are also other forms of luminescence such as bioluminescence that is found in several organisms (e.g., glowworms) and chemiluminescence that is caused by a chemical reaction (e.g., luminol) [29]. Bioluminescence and chemiluminescence are caused without the presence of an excitation light source. Lennard and Stoilovic [31] suggest that luminescence caused by the absorption of light is called *photoluminescence* and this type of luminescence is often used in optical enhancement. Bioluminescence, chemiluminescence, and photoluminescence effects can all be photographed; however, due to the low level of light emission, these procedures must be conducted in a darkened environment [29].

Photoluminescence mode enables the specimen to fluoresce and the emitted light from the specimen can be recorded by a camera. Recording specimens using this type of luminescence is also called *fluorescence photography* [29, 32, 33]. This mode requires consideration of all aspects of the optical enhancement triangle including (i) the specific spectral output of the excitation light source, (ii) a photoluminescent response (fluorescence) from the specimen, and (iii) the spectral sensitivity of the recording device (film or digital sensor).

The selection of the specific excitation spectra will depend on the photoluminescent properties of the specimen material. Forensic evidence specimens such as seminal fluid, saliva, and urine fluoresce

naturally when illuminated with certain excitation light sources [30, 33]. This naturally occurring phenomena is referred as *autofluorescence* [1, 29] and optical enhancement may be achieved without chemical treatment in these cases and is nondestructive. Other forms of evidence that do not naturally fluoresce (like blood) may be induced to fluoresce by chemical treatment with a fluorochrome [29]. This process is called the *secondary fluorescence* [1, 29] and treatments such as Rhodamine 6G, Indanedione, Diazofluorenone (DFO), and Hungarian Red are some of the common reagents used in posttreatment for photoluminescence mode [34].

Photoluminescence mode is often an alternative to other optical enhancement methods when the background does not suit the absorption or reflective modes. An example may be found in blood evidence. Absorption mode is generally the preferred method for blood evidence using a monochromatic light source at 415 nm, the maximum absorption of dried blood [33]. However, if the blood evidence is deposited onto a dark background, absorption mode will not provide an increase of contrast. Instead, it will darken the blood against a dark background, resulting in very little contrast. Figure 3(b) provides an example of photoluminescence mode for blood evidence.

Excitation ranges for photoluminescence mode vary depending on the autofluorescent characteristics of the specimen or the reagent used for posttreatment secondary fluorescent photography. Most forensic applications use spectral ranges in the lower order including ultraviolet (UV), violet, blue, and green region wavelengths. The resultant emitting light from photoluminescence mode is always longer in wavelength than the excitation source used. Therefore, most photoluminescence applications provide an emission light within the visual spectrum (400–700 nm). Some document examination applications are the exception where infrared luminescence methods produce an emission source further into the invisible spectrum. This method is generally outside the standard photography range and is conducted using specialized instrumentation called a *video spectral comparator* (VSC).

The emission light source produced by the photoluminescence is usually quite weak in brightness value and as previously mentioned requires photography in a darkened environment. Barrier filters are also applied to the camera lens to improve the contrast

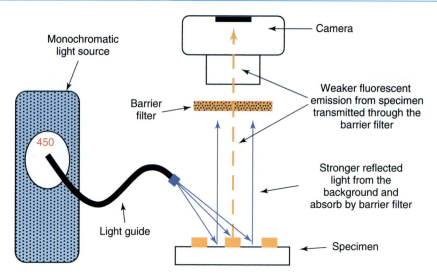

Figure 10   Photoluminescence mode displaying the application of a monochromatic light source, a specimen that fluoresces and a barrier filter over the camera lens

between the specimen and background. The rule for applying barrier filters for photoluminescence mode is to use a filter of the same color as the emission source. This provides maximum transmission of the fluorescence and will also darken any opposing background reflected light. For example, when a blue-colored light source is used to produce an orange-colored fluorescence, an orange barrier filter transmits the orange colored emission and darkens the reflected blue light of the background.

Photoluminescence mode requires the following parameters: (i) an excitation source suitable for the specimen material, (ii) a specimen that provides fluorescence (naturally or induced), (iii) a barrier filter to improve contrast, and (iv) the appropriate spectral sensitivity of the recording device (usually within the visual spectrum). Figure 10 illustrates the requirements of photoluminescence mode. Figure 11 is a fingerprint dusted with a green fluorescent fingerprint powder and photographed using a 540 nm excitation source. Figure 3(b) is a bloody footwear impression treated with Hungarian Red reagent excited by 530 nm excitation source from a Polilight and a Wratten 25 (red) barrier filter on the camera lens.

Spectral Sensitivity of Capture Device

The spectral sensitivity of the recording mechanism (digital sensor or film) is the spectral range that the

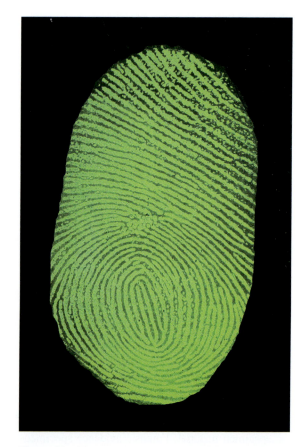

Figure 11   Fingermark using photoluminescence mode

device or material is able to record. Spectral sensitivity is an essential consideration when conducting optical enhancement methods. The recording device must be capable of recording in the spectrum used in the enhancement method.

The spectral sensitivity of film may be examined using wedge spectrograms. Wedge spectrograms are graphs that plot the spectral response of the film. These graphs are produced by exposing film to a dispersed light that has passed through a diffraction grating and then a neutral density wedge, which is placed on the film's surface.

Tripack color films have a spectral sensitivity range within the visual spectrum (400–700 nm). These films are not sensitive in the infrared region and an UV absorption layer is situated before any of the RGB sensitivity layers which prohibits any recording in the UV region. Generally, color films are not used in optical enhancement techniques. They produce a color cast when using monochromatic lighting or using a colored optical filter and are not sensitive outside the visual spectrum.

Film emulsion is the suspension of silver halides in gelatin to form a light sensitive emulsion. It is naturally sensitive only to UV and blue wavelengths and early film remained only sensitivity in these regions. In 1873, Vogel discovered that film emulsions can be made sensitive to blue and green spectra by adding a dye to the emulsion [8]. This process of dye sensitization was later refined and emulsions spectral sensitivity were extended into the red and infrared spectra. Black and white films are regularly used in optical enhancement and are still available in various spectral sensitivities. There are five classes of black and white films with different spectral sensitivity ranges. These classes are as follows:

- blue sensitive – only sensitive to UV and blue wavelengths;
- orthochromatic – sensitive through to the green region;
- panchromatic – sensitive through to red or covering the visual spectrum up to ≈650 nm;
- extended red sensitivity – extends further into the red spectrum up to ≈750 nm; and
- infrared – sensitive into the infrared region up to ≈900 nm.

For a more detailed examination of the film's spectral sensitivity, consult wedge spectrograms for each film type. Film manufactures readily publish this information with the product description.

The spectral sensitivity of digital cameras is more difficult to obtain from most of the camera manufacturers. There are generally three different types of digital sensors, also called *semiconductors*, used in digital cameras:

- charged coupled device (CCD);
- complementary metal oxide semiconductor (CMOS); and
- Foveon.

Single-shot digital cameras using CCD or CMOS sensors use a Bayer filter, which is a mosaic of RGB filters placed over the pixels. Foveon sensors, however, use a system of three different layers of semiconductors stacked together to form a multilayer sensor. These sensors design replicates that of the tripack color film, which consists of three different color sensitive layers (RGB). Each layer is suspended in a silicon wafer and the longer wavelengths are able to penetrate through the previous layer/s [35]. The advantage of Foveon sensors is that they do not require demosaicing interpolation like systems using a Bayer filter and the physical size of the sensor is not divided by each color channel (therefore, increasing sensor resolution).

Digital sensors have spectral sensitivity characteristics like all the light sensitive devices. CCD and CMOS sensor's spectral sensitivity works very differently to that of silver halide film. While film is naturally sensitive to UV and blue light and is made sensitive to other spectral regions using dye sensitization, digital sensors are more sensitive to the infrared (IR) region with very little sensitivity in the blue and UV spectral regions. The lower sensitivity in the blue region is the cause of higher noise levels found in the blue channel. Digital sensors are monochromatic and color is produced by processing of the image using trichromacy (combination of RGB). To improve chromatic aberration effects on the optics, most digital cameras also place an infrared blocking (absorbing) filter over the sensor to limit the spectral sensitivity to the visual spectrum. The spectral sensitivity of digital cameras is therefore a combination of (i) the spectral response of the monochromatic semiconductor, (ii) the absorption properties of the IR blocking filter, and (iii) the transmission properties of the Bayer filter.

Various digital cameras are available for forensic photography. Excluding the standard low-end consumer compact digital cameras, cameras suitable for forensic photography include: standard digital single-lens reflex (SLR) (pro and proconsumer models), digital SLR cameras with the IR blocking filter removed (modified for infrared photography) and scientific-based monochrome digital cameras. These scientific types of digital cameras provide various ranges of spectral sensitivity and generally publish the response data. Standard SLR camera manufacturers rarely publish the spectral sensitivity data and are generally only considered for applications within the visual spectrum (400–700 nm), although some cameras will perform slightly outside this range.

Specialized Lighting Techniques

Photography readily exploits light and its interaction with the surfaces of objects. The term *lighting* is used in photography as a way of describing the "visual effect" that results when this interaction of surfaces and light energy manifests. Some lighting techniques provide aesthetic elements to a photograph, while some others may enhance aspects of the physical evidence. Lighting may provide a visual representation of shape, line, form, subject texture, detail, aerial perspective, and many more visual aspects [35]. The topic of photographic lighting is an expansive consideration and cannot be fully justified in this section of the text. However, four specialized lighting techniques used for the enhancement of physical evidence are discussed in this section, which are as follows:

- axial illumination;
- near-axial illumination;
- diffuse reflection method; and
- oblique lighting.

Axial Illumination

Axial illumination is the light that illuminates the specimen from the camera's optical axis [36]. This form of lighting produces no shadow visible by the camera and is a form of shadowless lighting. Owing to its directionality, it may be used successfully to photograph specimens in cavities when getting light into small crevices is difficult. Axial illumination is used to detect topographical variances found on flat metal surfaces including coins or medals. It is also

a technique that may also be used to photograph untreated fingermarks found on metal or reflective surfaces.

Axial illumination is a similar technique as epi-illumination used in photomicroscopy [18, 36]. This form of illumination is produced by using a collimated (parallel) light source directed onto a thin semitransparent (semisilvered) mirror beam splitter positioned at a 45° to the lens axis [36, 37]. Thin semitransparent mirrors are more suitable than plane glass because the mirror surface increases the illumination efficiency and reduces the double-image effect, which is more visible on plane glass beam splitters. A slight double image results due to the separation between the two surfaces of the beam splitter (front and back). Thicker beam splitters produce a greater shift between each image that makes this artifact more obvious. Other ambient light must also be carefully controlled to avoid extraneous light reflecting off the beam splitter's reflective surfaces. In particular, reflected light transmitting through the beam splitter and illuminating other objects within the room can produce a reflection on the near side of the beam splitter and cause a reflection of the object within the image space. A light absorber such as black velvet cloth should be used to absorb this light (see Figure 12). Figure 12 illustrates the components of axial illumination.

Near-Axial Illumination

Near-axial lighting produces a similar lighting effect as axial illumination. The light source is positioned close to the lens axis [36] producing a light quality that is void of form, texture, and shadow. The intent of near-axial lighting is to illuminate an object or scene evenly. Several portable light sources, including portable flash, may be used to produce this form of illumination. Ring light attachments (see Figure 13) attach to the camera lens and can also produce a diffuse near-axial illumination [36].

Diffuse Reflection Method

When light reflects off a surface, the properties of the surface will affect the type of reflection produced. There are two types of reflected light possible: diffuse reflection and direct reflection [8, 17, 38]. Direct reflection (also referred to as *specular reflection*) results from light reflected off polished surfaces.

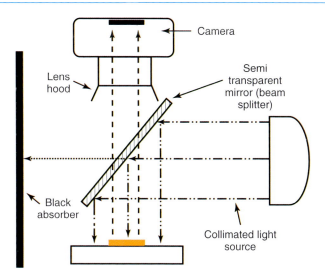

Figure 12 Axial illumination lighting diagram

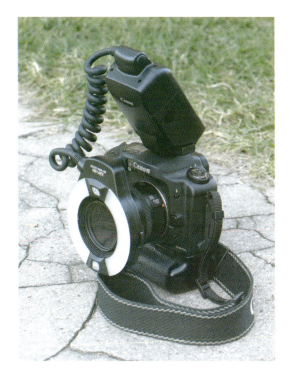

Figure 13 A ring flash attachment on a digital SLR camera used for near-axial illumination

Direct reflection follows the first law of reflection which states that the angle of incidence equals the angle of reflection ($i = r$) [8, 12, 17, 22].

Diffuse reflection is the scattering of reflected light caused by a matt surface. The uneven nature of matt surfaces reflect the incident light in different directions by maintaining the first law of refection ($i = r$). The effect produces reflected light in multiple directions causing a diffuse effect (see Figure 14b). Diffuse reflection may also be considered as partly diffuse or totally diffuse [22]. Totally diffuse reflected light is perfectly diffuse meaning the spread of reflected light forms evenly across the entire surface. Totally diffuse reflections obey Lambert's law and the surface is considered to be a *Lambertian surface* [8, 12, 22].

Diffuse reflection lighting method exploits the outcomes of both direct and diffuse reflection. Figure 15 is a photograph of an untreated (undeveloped) fingermark on a highly polished flat surface, which is a computer hard drive. This subject produces two different surfaces: the highly polished surface of the hard drive and the matt surface of the fatty deposit of the fingermark. When incident light is applied to both surfaces simultaneously, a direct reflection will be produced off the hard drive and a diffuse reflection from the fingermark.

The relationship between the position of the camera lens, the position of the incident light source, and the position of the specimen are all critical aspects of this technique. Their positions are also interrelated and careful consideration is essential. The camera should be positioned perpendicular ($90°$)

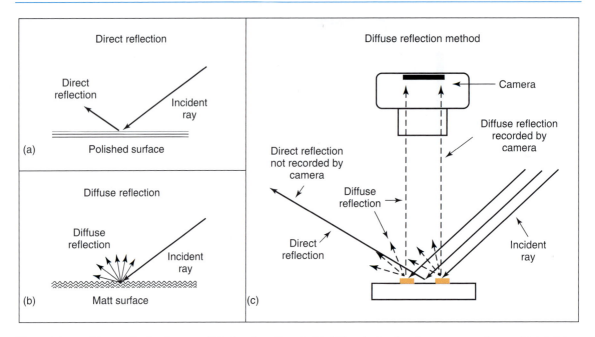

Figure 14   (a) Direct reflection from a polished surface ($i = r$), (b) diffused reflection from a matt surface, and (c) lighting, illustrating diffuse reflection method seen in Figure 15

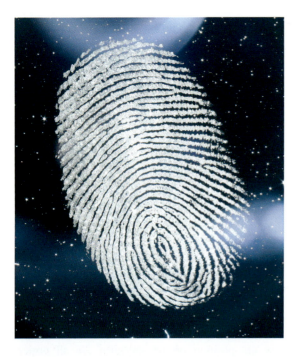

Figure 15   Untreated fingerprint found on a highly polished computer hard drive and photographed using diffuse reflection method

to the subject plane. The incident light source is positioned at $\approx 45°$ angle from the specimen, which will also result in a $\approx 45°$ angle from the lens axis (see Figure 14c). The visualization of the fingermark is achieved due to the differences between the reflected light values from the diffuse light reflected from the fingermark and the direct light from the polished surface. Owing to the law of reflection ($i = r$), $\approx 100\%$ of the direct reflection will reflect away from the camera lens and not record in the camera. This will result in the polished surface having no light entering the camera and producing a dark toned surfaced in the photograph. The diffuse reflection emanating from the fatty deposit of the fingermark will direct some reflected light into the camera lens and record in the photograph. The result is illustrated in Figure 15 whereby the fingermark records a light tone against a dark background. Diffuse reflection method is a simple and effective method of recording fingermarks on polished surfaces without having to treat or develop the mark.

Oblique Lighting

Oblique lighting (also referred to as *side lighting*) is one of the most valuable lighting techniques used

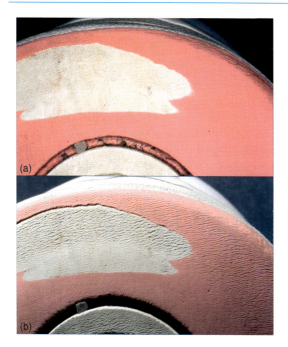

Figure 16 (a) Photograph depicting the heel of a shoe using near-axial illumination (ring flash). (b) Same shoe using oblique lighting. Schallamach patterning becomes more visible with oblique lighting

when photographing mark evidence. Oblique lighting may provide a significant increase in detail and provide the visualization of individual identification characteristics that may be crucial to the examination. Oblique lighting is achieved by positioning the light source at an oblique or low angle to the specimen. The lighting direction runs across the surface of the specimen and essentially increases the local contrast or variations of highlight and shadow on the surface of the specimen. This effect increases the topographic detail and provides further visual information to examine.

Figure 16 provides an example of the differences between oblique and near-axial illumination. The Schallamach patterning found on the heel of a shoe is greatly emphasized by oblique or side lighting. Figure 16(a) was photographed using a near-axial portable flash, while Figure 16(b) uses oblique lighting. Oblique lighting has increased the local contrast on the surface of the heel making the Schallamach pattern more visible.

Digital Imaging Enhancement

Digital enhancement of physical evidence is the application of computer software to make adjustments to digital images of evidence. Digital enhancement provides several similarities to the techniques used in digital photography and optical enhancement. The most significant advantage digital imaging has provided forensic science is its ability to make fine adjustments to image parameters such as contrast, color, sharpness, image noise, and many other adjustments. Items in images can also be quantified by counting, measuring, and making mathematical calculations using image analysis applications. The advantages of digital imaging for forensic science are expansive. This section examines two common practices of digital enhancement using such controls as contrast and the chromatic modification of specimens.

Digital enhancement of physical evidence should not be considered as a process of correcting poorly executed digital photography. Digital enhancement of evidence requires the input of quality digital photography and the enhancement techniques provide further tools for the forensic scientist. Concepts of quality include sharpness, image dimensional integrity, lighting, exposure, and dynamic range.

Digital images record brightness linearly unlike film which responds to light nonlinearly [39]. Film's nonlinear response to light may be seen in the "S"-shaped characteristic curves that plot their exposure and density parameters. Obtaining quality digital images with a higher dynamic range is preferable when performing digital enhancement. Essentially, the more inherent information the digital image contains, the more control image enhancement offers. Best practice suggests digital images should be captured (camera or scanner) using a 16 bit (or a 14 bit for some cameras) and RAW images are better processed using Photoshop processing appliances such as Camera Raw™ than in-camera processed JPEGs.

Compression applications such as the JPEG captured and processed in-camera at an 8 bit offers significant less information and enhancement control. Digital enhancement processing in Photoshop should also be carried out using the 16 bit per channel for improved results [13, 19]. There is a significant difference in pixel depth between 8 and 16 bit per channel modes. The 8 bit per channel provides 256 variations per channel that results in approximately 16 million possibilities for RGB files. While the

16 bit per channel images contain 65 536 variations for each channel and results in billions of color and tonal representation possibilities.

Contrast Adjustment

Digital imaging can provide adjustments to image contrast with significantly more control and ease than more traditional film-based technology. Visualization of evidence is predominately made possible by the contrast between the evidence and its background. Fingermark evidence is a good example and is most reliant on contrast between the friction ridge detail and the substrate background. Like optical enhancement, digital imaging enhancement using contrast adjustments in Photoshop is an effective method of improving the detail and visualization of evidence.

There are various methods in Adobe Photoshop™ that allow contrast adjustment. The most suitable method is using the "curves" function located in the "Image > Adjustments > Curves" menu. In Photoshop versions greater than CS3 the exposure histogram is also embedded into the curve graph. Figure 17 is an example of how curves may adjust to the contrast of the specimen. The image is of a fingermark on a glass window and developed in black

powder. To avoid specular reflections, the fingermark was the photograph using brightfield illumination that combined a small sheet of white Perspex situated behind the fingermark and a portable flash positioned behind the mark was used as the illumination source. The original image displayed high levels of detail but with low contrast and the contrast was enhanced using the "curves" adjustment. The inserts situated in each image provide details of the before and after curve adjustments.

The first graph shows a straight line (curve) diagonally across the graph which represents the linear nature of digital images. The gradient of the curve influences the degree of image contrast. The greater the gradient (more steeper the curve) the less variation there is between certain sections of the shadow and highlight regions resulting in more image contrast. Lowering the gradient (flatter curve) reduces the contrast. The second insert found in Figure 17 shows an increase in the gradient of the curve that has resulted in the increase of contrast. The shadow and highlight regions were also "clipped" slightly which also added to the contrast improvement. Contrast enhancement adjustments using "curves" may be conducted in each channel separately or as an alpha channel indicated as "RGB".

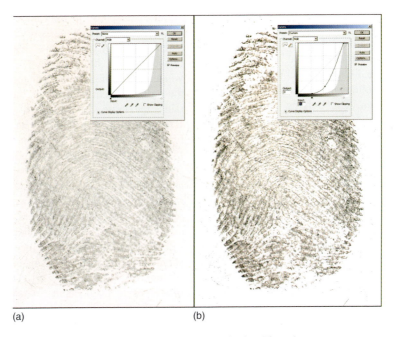

(a)   (b)

Figure 17   Before and after fingermarks when contrast is enhanced using Photoshop curves

Chromatic and Tonal Modification

Adjustments to the spectral response of color may also be modified in digital imaging software in a similar way to optical enhancement techniques. When working with Adobe Photoshop™ there are always several different methods to obtain the same or similar result. Changing the chromatic aspects of specimens can also be achieved using several Photoshop functions; however, the "Black & White" adjustment is most likely the simplest. The "Black & White" adjustment automatically converts the image to a monochrome image while maintaining the file in RGB mode, so that modification of the colors, now tones, can be adjusted. As previously explained, when using optical enhancement techniques using monochromatic lighting or colored optical filters over the camera, the image should be converted to a monochrome image to avoid color casts.

The "Black & White" function can be found on Photoshop versions higher than the CS3 and work on the principles of black and white contrast filters (see optical enhancement). It may be found on the Photoshop menu "Image > Adjustment > Black&White". Like contrast filters used on the camera with monochrome film, the "Black & White" function alters the brightness of tonal values by altering the spectral reflective and absorption properties. Logically, the digital imaging application is altering the spectral response artificially by adjusting the brightness values of each color and its resultant tonal value in monochrome (unlike optical enhancement). The "Black & White" function provides individual darkening or lightening of the following colors; red, green, blue, cyan, magenta, and yellow. These are the colors previously mentioned in the additive and subtractive models. There are three options when operating this function: (i) the custom option which uses slider bars to modify the tonal value of each color, (ii) use preset filters in the drop-down box, and (iii) develop your own presets. The custom function offers more control over the tonal values of each color and is considered more suitable for evidence enhancement. The image must be in RGB mode to operate "Black & White" and it does not operate in grayscale or CMYK modes. As previously mentioned, working with 16 bit per channel images provides a distinctive advantage for this method due the more subtle changes possible between tonal adjustments.

Figure 18 provides and example of how the "Black & White" adjustments function can enhance evidence by selective contrast variations of tones due to their original color. The blue ink of the stamp was lightened by moving the blue slider bar to the right to increase its brightness value. The red ink of the handwriting was darkened slightly by moving the red slider bar left or lowering the brightness value of the red color. The result is a remarkable difference in contrast difference between the blue and red inks and the blue stamp has almost disappeared. The signature can now be examined without the interference of the overlaying blue stamp.

The Black & White function is also useful for removing colored backgrounds that interfere with developed fingermarks. Figure 19 is a ninhydrin

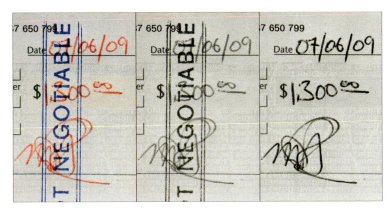

Figure 18 The handwriting on the bank check was written in red ink. The blue stamp has obliterated components of the signature and check amount. The Black & White adjustment has lightened the blue stamp and darkened the writing slightly to increase the contrast between the two inks (stamp and pen)

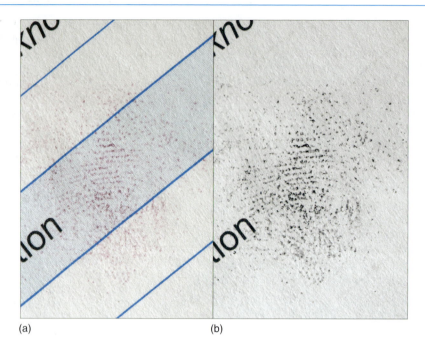

(a)   (b)

Figure 19   (a) Color photograph of a ninhydrin developed fingermark; (b) The same fingermark with the blue lines and blue area of the document removed and the ninhydrin fingermark darkened

developed fingermark on a document with strong blue lines and blocked sections of blue. The blue lines and blue background were removed using the "Black & White" filter application and the magenta color of the ninhydrin print darkened to enhance the contrast between the fingermark and the background. This process takes approximately 20–30 s to complete once the image is loaded into Photoshop™, making it a highly efficient method of evidence enhancement.

References

[1]   Porter, G. (2004). Specialised photography and imaging, in *The Practice of Crime Scene Investigation*, J. Horswell, ed, CRC Press, pp. 139–159.

[2]   Porter, G. (2007). Visual culture in forensic science, *Australian Journal of Forensic Sciences* **39**(2), 81–91.

[3]   House of Lords, Select Committee on Science and Technology (1998). *Digital Images as Evidence: Evidence*, The Stationary Office, London.

[4]   House of Lords, Select Committee on Science and Technology (1998). *Digital Images as Evidence: Report*, The Stationary Office, London.

[5]   SMANZFL (2004). *Australasian Guidelines for Digital Imaging Processes*, Version 2, National Institute of Forensic Science.

[6]   Robinson, E.M. (2007). *Crime Scene Photography*, Academic Press.

[7]   Langford, M. (1998). *Advanced Photography*, 6th Edition, Focal Press.

[8]   Jacobson, R.E., Ray, S.F., Attridge, G.G. & Axford, N.R. (2000). *The Manual of Photography: Photographic and Digital Imaging*, 9th Edition, Focal Press.

[9]   Taylor, J.T. (2005). *The Optics of Photography and Photographic Lenses*, Elibron Classics.

[10] Canon, E.F. (2003). *Lens Works III: The Eyes of EOS*, Canon.

[11] Ray, S.F. (1995). *Applied Photographic Optics*, 2nd Edition, Focal Press.

[12] Ray, S.F. (1992). *The Photographic Lens*, 2nd Edition, Focal Press.

[13] Reis, G. (2007). *Photoshop CS3 for Forensic Professionals: A Complete Digital Imaging Course for Investigators*, Sybex.

[14] Baron, C. (2007). *Adobe Photoshop Forensics: Sleuths, Truths and Fauxtography*, Thompson Course Technology.

[15] Fraser, B., Murphy, C. & Bunting, F. (2005). *Real World Color Management*, 2nd Edition, Peachpit Press.

[16] Malacara, D. (2001). *Color Vision and Colorimetry: Theory and Applications*, Spie Press.

[17] Overheim, R.D. & Wagner, D.L. (1982). *Light and Color*, John Wiley & Sons.

[18] Morton, R.A. (ed) (1984). *Photography for the Scientist*, Academic Press.

[19] Fraser, B. (2007). *Real World Imaging Sharpening With Adobe Photoshop CS2*, Peachpit Press.

[20] Champod, C., Lennard, C., Margot, P. & Stoilovic, M. (2004). *Fingerprints and Other Ridge Skin Impressions*, CRC Press.

[21] Lee, H.C. & Gaensslen, R.E. (eds) (1991). *Advances in Fingerprint Technology*, CRC Press.

[22] Saxby, G. (2002). *The Science of Imaging: An Introduction*, Institute of Physics Publishing.

[23] Mitchell, E.N. (1984). *Photographic Science*, Wiley & Sons.

[24] Langford, M., Fox, A. & Smith, R.S. (2007). *Langford's Basic Photography: The Guide for Serious Photographers*, 8th Edition, Focal Press.

[25] Kodak (1990). *Kodak Photographic Filters Handbook*, Eastman Kodak Company.

[26] Kodak (1976). *Using Photography to Preserve Evidence*, Eastman Kodak Company, Pub. M-2.

[27] McKechnie, M.L., Porter, G. & Langlois, N. (2008). The detection of latent residue tattoo ink pigments in skin using invisible radiation photography, *Australian Journal of Forensic Sciences* **40**(1), 65–72.

[28] Kodak (1980). *Applied Infrared Photography*, Eastman Kodak Company, Pub. M-28.

[29] Kodak (1968). *Ultraviolet and Fluorescence Photography*, Eastman Kodak Company, Pub. M-27.

[30] Vanderberg, N. & van Oorschot, R.A.G. (2006). The use of Polilight® in the detection of seminal fluid, saliva and bloodstain and comparison with conventional chemical-based screening tests, *Journal of Forensic Science* **521**(2), 361–370.

[31] Lennard, C. & Stoilovic, M. (2004). Application of forensic light sources at the crime scene, in *The Practice of Crime Scene Investigation*, J. Horswell, ed, CRC Press, pp. 97–123.

[32] Pountney, H. (1971). *Police Photography*, Elsevier Publishing.

[33] Stoilovic, M. (1991). Detection of semen and blood stains using polilight as a light source, *Forensic Science International* **51**, 289–296.

[34] Lennard, C. (2007). Fingerprint detection: current capabilities, *Australian Journal of Forensic Sciences* **39**(2), 55–71.

[35] Peres, M.R. (ed) (2007). *The Focal Encyclopedia of Photography*, 4th Edition, Focal Press.

[36] Ray, S.F. (1999). *Scientific Photography and Applied Imaging*, Focal Press.

[37] Weiss, S.L. (2009). *Forensic Photography: The Importance of Accuracy*, Pearson Prentice Hall.

[38] Hunter, F., Biver, S. & Fuqua, P. (2007). *Light Science and Magic: An Introduction to Photographic Lighting*, 3rd Edition, Focal Press.

[39] Russ, J.C. (2001). *Forensic Uses of Digital Imaging*, CRC Press.

Glenn Porter

Photography: Scene *see* Crime Scene Photography: US Perspective

Physical Injury *see* Aggression

Plants *see* Botany

Plethysmography *see* Sex Offenders: Treatment of

PMI *see* Human Remains and Identity

Poisons: Detection of Naturally Occurring Poisons

Introduction

A large number of plants produce compounds that may cause serious illness, injury, or even death. Some plants contain toxic compounds in all parts, whereas other plants are poisonous in some parts and edible in others. Examples include potatoes and tomatoes, which contain toxic alkaloids in the green parts of the plant, but these alkaloids are not present in the ripe potato tuber and tomato fruits.

A comprehensive list of toxic plants is not possible because of the large number of poisonous substances. Although many plants contain toxic substances, only a few species cause poisonings in humans. The actual number of cases of plant poisoning is hard to determine. Even the numbers of fatal poisoning by plants is not always very obvious. Severe or even deadly poisonings with plants are relatively rare; the frequencies and the plants involved are regionally different.

A published report of the Poison Information Centre in Chile showed that only 0.43% of the medical consultations from January 1998 to June 2000 were with respect to intoxications with plants or mushrooms [1]. Compared to Chile, the Poison Information Centre of northern Germany reported in 2005 that 12% of medical consultations were related to the use and misuse of plants or plant products. Most of these consultations were due to accidental ingestion of the plant material or the misuse of herbal drugs of abuse [2].

Severe and fatal poisonings by plant materials are very rare.

The Poison Information Center, Mainz, Germany, has recorded 31 severe and fatal poisonings caused by plants from January 1995 to July 2007 [3]. The majority of these cases (55%) were caused by an abuse of plant material; only five cases (16%) were a suicide attempt. A total of 5 of the 31 severe poisonings were recorded as fatal.

A study analyzing the self-poisoning fatalities in rural Sri Lanka from March 2002 to March 2003 has shown that 44 of 198 people died from ingestion of the plant oleander [4]. The higher number of plant poisonings in Sri Lanka compared with other countries may also reflect the availability of drugs or poisons used in suicide attempts.

In Australia, the National Coroners Information Service (NCIS) recorded that 9 persons of 131 400 recorded deaths had died from plant or mushroom poisoning in the period between July 2000 and July 2007 [5]. In general, severe or fatal plant poisonings are not very common and are limited to a small number of poisonous plant species.

Manner of Poisoning with Plants

Unintentional Ingestion of Plants and Plant Material

Unintentional ingestion of plant material not only occurs in children, especially younger ones, but also in adults. It is obvious that the reason for accidental ingestion in different age groups is completely different. Whereas children discover their environment by trying bits of plants that appear attractive to them, adults ingest them accidentally [6].

For children, the attractive parts of plants are mostly fruits and seeds with colorful seed coats. Examples include the fruits of deadly nightshade, which look similar to cherries, and the red seed coats of the yew. In the case of yew, the seed coats are very sweet and are not poisonous, but the seeds inside are very poisonous. Children can also be attracted by fruits that are similar to edible plants. A good example is the fruit of laburnum, which looks like peas or beans.

For adults, the reason for an unintentional ingestion of plant material is usually a mix-up. Poisoning occurs as a result of ingestion of poisonous plant due to confusion. The affected persons are usually looking for alternative sources of food or self-medication with herbal drugs. A common example is the collection of meadow saffron instead of wild garlic. Also the mix-up of mushrooms is very common. Many case reports have shown that the deadliest mushroom is the death cap, which looks similar to edible champignons [7].

Accidental ingestion of plant material is also possible by taking herbal medication that has been either incorrectly prepared or in which the wrong plant material has been used. A common problem is the use of aconitum in traditional Chinese medicine, which can be toxic when prepared incorrectly.

Intended Ingestion of Plant Material

Besides unintentional ingestion of plant materials, plants have always been, and are still, used in homicides and suicide attempts. Historical records show that plant materials have caused the death of many famous personalities. An example is the death of Socrates, which was caused by the application of the plant hemlock [8]. But even today, poisonous plants are used from time to time in homicide cases. However, the suicidal ingestion of natural poisons is more common. In developed countries, drug- or poison-related suicide attempts are mostly in connection with prescriptive drugs. However, case reports describe the use of very poisonous plants like deadly nightshade, aconite, and yew in suicides. These patients are often well educated and know about the toxicity of the plants they use. As an example, one patient was growing aconite in his garden, harvested the root of the plant, and prepared an extract, which he ingested and injected. He had studied literature about the toxicity of this plant and had even shown the literature to an emergency physician [3].

In rural parts of developing countries, suicidal ingestion of plants is far more common due to a lack of availability of prescription drugs [4].

Ingestion of Plant Material Due to an Abuse

The use of plants and plant material for psychoactive effects has been known and recorded for millenniums. The knowledge of the psychoactive effects and the toxic side effects were extensively observed by shamans and other users and has been passed down from generation to generation. In recent years, the use of herbal drugs for their psychoactive properties has become increasingly popular among illicit drug users. The reasons for this increase are diverse. Some of the herbal drugs are not scheduled, and are generally easily accessible, and are sometimes considered to be safe since they are natural.

The assumption of less toxicity is simply not true. Plants often contain pharmacologically highly active compounds. In addition, using hallucinogenic poisonous plants carries the danger of an overdose. The amount of active ingredients in the plant is strongly dependent on geographical and climate conditions. A consumption of two leaves in spring might be hallucinogenic, whereas the consumption of two leaves in autumn may be fatal [6].

Overdoses due to an abuse of plant materials are often described for plants like deadly nightshade [9], datura [10], and kath [11].

Even a nonoverdose situation might cause dangerous behavior. It is well known that the anticholinergic syndrome triggered by atropine or scopolamine causes hallucinations and dry, hot skin. The drug users therefore try to cool down by jumping into water, risking a death by drowning. Hallucinations can also sometimes cause self-inflected injuries. The NCIS (Australia) recorded two cases of death due to self-induced stab wounds under the influence of magic mushrooms [5].

Description of Selected Plants and Fungi

In the following sections toxicologically important plants and some fungi are described in detail. To avoid confusion, scientific names of the plants are

Table 1 List of common names of poisonous plants and their associated botanical names

Common English name	Botanical name
Aconite	*Aconitum napellus*
Angel's Trumpet	*Datura stramonium*
Autumn crocus	*Colchicum autumnale*
Belladonna	*Atropa belladonna*
Castor bean	*Ricinus communis*
Castor oil plant	*Ricinus communis*
Deadly nightshade	*Atropa belladonna*
Death cap	*Amanita phalloides*
Devine cactus	*Lophophora wiliamsii*
Dwale	*Atropa belladonna*
European yew	*Taxus baccata*
Golden chain tree	*Laburnum anagyroides*
Hemlock	*Conium maculatum*
Jimson weed	*Datura stramonium*
Kath	*Catha edulis*
Kava	*Piper methysticum*
Laburnum	*Laburnum anagyroides*
Laurier rose	*Nerium oleander*
Magic mushroom	*Psilocybe mexicana*
Meadow saffron	*Colchicum autumnale*
Mescal button	*Lophophora wiliamsii*
Miraa	*Catha edulis*
Monkshood	*Aconitum napellus*
Naked lady	*Colchicum autumnale*
Oleander	*Nerium oleander*
Peyote	*Lophophora wiliamsii*
Poison hemlock	*Conium maculatum*
Quat	*Catha edulis*
Thornapple	*Datura stramonium*
Wolf's Bane	*Aconitum napellus*
Yaqona	*Piper methysticum*
Yew	*Taxus baccata*

used. The scientific names have the advantage that only one name exists for each plant, whereas the commonly used names may not be unique and can be used for more than one plant. Table 1 translates the most commonly used English names of the plants into their scientific names. In the following sections, selected plants and fungi, which are often involved in plant-related poisonings, are described in monographs. The monographs are listed in alphabetical order of the scientific names of the plants. Figure 1 provides representative photographs of some poisonous plants.

Aconitum Napellus

The herbaceous perennial plant *Aconitum napellus* (Figure 1), known as aconite or monkshood, grows to

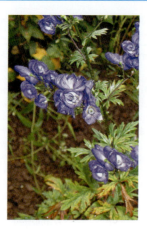

Figure 1   Flower and leaves of *Aconitum napellus*

a height of 1 m, and is native to western and central Europe. The English name "monkshood" is derived from a part of the dark blue flower of *A. napellus* that has the shape of a cylindrical helmet. The toxicity of *A. napellus* is mentioned in Greek mythology, where it is described as the first poisonous plant. In fact, aconite is the most poisonous plant in central Europe due to its alkaloid-like aconitine.

All species of the gender *Aconitum* are highly toxic and have been used for many centuries as arrow poison or common poison in homicides. Roots, leaves, flowers, and seeds are all exceedingly poisonous to man and livestock. The main active alkaloid in plants from the genus *Aconitum* is aconitine [6].

An accidental poisoning due to a mix-up with other nutrient plants is quite unlikely owing to the lack of similarity. Also, children are not attracted by the plant very often. However, aconite is a source of many fatal poisonings described in case reports [12]. The most common causes of a poisoning with plant material of the genus *Aconitum* are either a suicide attempt or an incorrect preparation of the plant in traditional Chinese medicine. Aconite is used in the traditional Chinese medicine [13], and can be freely purchased from herbal shops around the world. An incorrect preparation, or a wrong dosage of the plant material, may produce a fatal dose of the toxic alkaloid.

Amanita Phalloides

Amanita phalloides is a deadly poisonous mushroom, commonly known as *death cap*. This mushroom

appears after periods of rain from late summer to the end of autumn. Death cap originates from Europe, but can be found worldwide. The fungal fruiting body of *A. phalloides* has a convex yellowish or greenish cap, usually 5–15 cm across. The stem is up to 20-cm long. The flesh of the fruiting body is white. With similarities to champignons, parasol mushrooms, and paddy straw mushrooms, this fungus can be confused with other fungi. The toxicity of *A. phalloides* has been extensively studied since the largest number of deadly mushroom poisonings are caused by this species. All parts contain amatoxins and phallotoxins, and the toxin most responsible for the deadly effects is alpha-amanitin [14]. The peptide alpha-amanitin is a very stable compound and even prolonged cooking or maceration with salt does not decrease the toxicity. The toxin acts by inhibition of RNA polymerase II and therefore blocks protein synthesis.

The lethal dose of amanitin is only 0.1 mg kg^{-1}, which means that a medium-sized mushroom can cause the death of a human. Death caps have been reported to have a pleasant taste, and a mix-up cannot be recognized by the taste. The symptoms of a poisoning with *A. phalloides* are initially gastrointestinal in nature. Colicky abdominal pain, vomiting, and watery diarrhea characteristically start approximately 8 h after ingestion. These symptoms resolve in a period of two or three days, giving the false sign of a remission. After a few days, a hepatic and renal failure causes symptoms like jaundice, delirium, seizures, and coma. Death occurs usually 6–16 days after ingestion of the mushroom.

The treatment of a poisoning with death cap includes gastric lavage, activated charcoal, the correction of metabolic acidosis, and an intravenous antidote treatment with silibinin. Silibinin is extracted from blessed milk thistle (*Silibum marianum*) and is supposed to prevent the uptake of amatoxins into liver cells. In some cases, liver transplants have been necessary.

Atropa Belladonna

The perennial plant *Atropa belladonna* (Figure 2) is commonly known as *deadly nightshade*. Other common names such as dwale, death's herb, or witch berry give an impression of its toxicity and use in the middle age. The toxicity and pharmacological effects of the plant are part of the etymology of the botanical name. The genus *Atropa* is named after the goddess

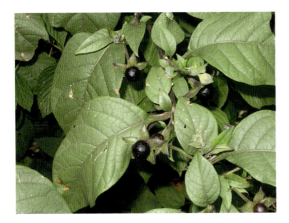

Figure 2   Berry and leaves of *Atropa belladonna*

Atropos, who is known in Greek mythology to cut the life thread. The species name *belladonna* is Italian for beautiful lady and originates from its historical use of the berry juice by women to dilate their pupils [6].

All parts of *A. belladonna* contain toxic tropane alkaloids. Even though the root contains that highest alkaloid concentration, the most dangerous parts, in terms of accidental intoxication, are the berries because of their attractive look and sweet taste. Besides accidental ingestion, poisonings are reported after an abuse of *A. belladonna* due to the hallucinogenic properties of the tropane alkaloids.

The main alkaloids present in *A. belladonna* are l-hyoscyamine and l-scopolamine. Even though only l-hyoscyamine is present in the plant, l-hyoscyamine is converted to a racemic mixture of 50% l-hyoscyamine and d-hyoscyamine. This conversion is either as a result of extraction or release after ingestion. This racemic mixture is called *atropine*.

Atropine acts pharmacologically via blocking acetylcholine receptors of the muscarine subtype. The blockage of these receptors causes symptoms like tachycardia, dilated pupils, decreased gastrointestinal motility, dry hot skin, and dry mouth due to a decreased sweat and saliva production. Apart from these peripheral effects, atropine also affects the central nervous system and causes agitation, disorientation, and hallucinations [15].

Catha Edulis

The evergreen shrub *Catha edulis*, which is native to tropical East Africa and the Arabian Peninsula, is known as *khat* or *qat*. In these countries, the use of khat for therapeutic and recreational purpose has been an integral part of the local culture for centuries. In the second part of the twentieth century, the consumption changed to an uncontrolled abuse and spread throughout other continents. For example, more than 2300 kg of khat was confiscated at Frankfurt Airport (Germany) in 1998 [16]. This new aspect of khat consumption has raised increased concern in international organizations. In 1980, the World Health Organization classified khat as a drug of abuse that is able to produce dependence.

The main psychoactive alkaloids of khat are cathinone and its metabolite cathine, also known as *norpseudoephedrine*. Cathinone was found to have a pharmacological profile closely resembling that of amphetamine. Cathinone acts as a central nervous system stimulant and shows sympathomimetic effects by releasing catecholamines from presynaptic storage sites. Experiments have shown that cathine acts like cathinone, but is less effective. Both substances are controlled substances in many countries due to khat abuse.

Colchicum Autumnale

Colchicum autumnale is a perennial plant that grows from corms. The most common English names are autumn crocus, naked lady, and meadow saffron. These names represent the similarity of the flower to crocuses. However, this similarity is limited to the appearance of the flowers. In contrast to most other plants, the plant flowers in autumn, long after the leaves have died back, and therefore the English name naked lady. The fertilized fruits emerge from the ground with the new leaves appearing the following spring [6].

Colchicine is the main active alkaloid of *Colchicum*. It is present in all parts of the plant, but particularly in the corm, seeds, and flowers. Colchicine inhibits the function of microtubules and therefore acts as a cytotoxic. It also reduces the activity of leukocytes and lymphocytes. This mechanism of action is suspected to be the reason for its success in the treatment of gout. The plant has been used to treat gout for more than 2000 years. Although colchicine has many side effects, it is still recommended as a treatment for acute gout [17].

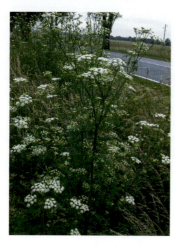

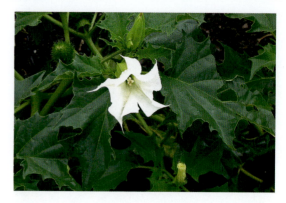

Figure 4 Flower, leaves, and unripe fruit of *Datura strammonium*

Figure 3 Habitus of *Conium maculatum* [Image by Thomas Schoepke – http://www.plant-pictures.com]

Conium Maculatum

The 1.5–2-m tall biennial plant *Conium maculatum* (Figure 3) is known as *hemlock* or *poison hemlock*. The smooth green stem of hemlock is characteristically spotted with purple on the lower half. The leaves are finely divided and the white flowers are small and clustered in umbels. The plant is similar to fennel, parsley, or wild carrot. The root of hemlock, white and fleshy, is often unbranched and shows a similarity to parsnip. The toxicity of hemlock has been known in Greece since 399 BC, as the symptoms of the lethal poisoning of Socrates were described by his pupil Plato. In the middle ages, the medicinal use of hemlock was very limited due to its known high toxicity [8]. *Conium maculatum* is native to Europe but has been introduced and grows as a weed in Asia, North America, and Australia.

All parts of the plant are poisonous. The highest concentrations of the toxic alkaloids are found in unripe seeds, but concentrations vary significantly depending on temperature, moisture, and the season. The main toxic alkaloids of hemlock are coniine and γ-coniceine. The exact mechanism of action of these toxic alkaloids is not known. The primary action is on the central nervous system with symptoms similar to nicotine poisoning. The most common symptoms of hemlock poisoning are problems in movement, dilation of pupils, slow and weak pulse, heavy salivation, and nausea. After a severe poisoning, coma and death from respiratory failure are possible [18].

Datura Stramonium

The annual plant *Datura stramonium* (Figure 4), which is often found in nutrient-rich soils, grows to a height of up to 1 m. This plant of the nightshade family is commonly known as *thornapple*, *Jimsonweed*, or *Angel's Trumpet*. The large flowers of *Datura* are white, erect, and tubular. The tubular shape and its psychoactivity are related to the name Angel's Trumpet. The name thornapple is related to the fruits, which are spiky large green capsules containing numerous black seeds. The plant is distributed generally throughout temperate and subtropical regions. The *Brugmansia* species are similar to *Datura* in botanical appearance and are often cultivated in pots as house plants [6].

All parts of *Datura* and *Brugmansia* are toxic and contain tropane alkaloids. As already described for *A. belladonna*, the main alkaloids are l-hyoscyamine and l-scopolamine. Owing to the presence of these alkaloids, these plants are often abused for their hallucinogenic properties. This increasing misuse has forced a prohibition by law in Florida against planting Angel's Trumpets.

The symptoms of a poisoning as well as the treatment are similar to those described for *A. belladonna*.

Laburnum Anagyroides

Laburnum anagyroides (Figure 5), also known as *laburnum*, grows as a shrub or a small tree. The plant has yellow flowers in pendulous racemes, and therefore it is known in German as "Goldregen", which is often translated as golden rain acacia.

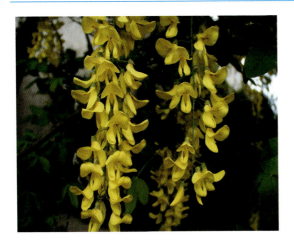

Figure 5 Flower of *Laburnum anagyroides* [Image by Thomas Schoepke – http://www.plant-pictures.com]

Because the plant is attractive and frost tolerant, laburnum is very popular as ornaments in parks and gardens. The fruits are silky hairy pods; the unripe pods are similar to bean or pea pods. The seeds are similar to small beans [6].

All parts of laburnum are toxic and contain quinolizidine alkaloids. The main toxic alkaloid is cytisine, with the highest concentration detected in the ripe seeds and seed pods. Knowing about the toxicity, laburnum has been used in traditional medicine by American Indians, who have consumed the seeds for their emetic effects during rites and magical practices. During the Second World War, the leaves of laburnum were used as a tobacco substitute due to its similar effects. Studies have also shown that cytisine is effective as an aid to smoking cessation [19].

Cytisine binds with a high affinity to nicotinergic acetylcholine receptors. Like nicotine, cytisine acts as a blocking agent on the central nervous system via an overstimulation of these receptors. Owing to the mechanism of action, the symptoms of a poisoning are similar to a nicotine overdose. The central-stimulating effects can cause delirium and convulsions [19]. Death is possible through a respiratory paralysis or failure of the circulatory system. The treatment of a poisoning with laburnum is symptom orientated, with no specific antidote available [6].

Lophophora Williamsii

The small spineless cactus *Lophophora williamsii* is commonly known as *peyote*. This cactus grows extremely slowly and flowers sporadically. It takes in the wild up to 30 years to reach the size of a golf ball and to produce the first flowers. The small pink fruits of peyote are sweet tasting and delicate. The cactus is native to southern United States and Mexico, but is cultivated all over the world.

A recent study has shown prehistoric use of peyote by native North Americans. A radiocarbon study dated dried cacti, so-called mescal buttons, to the time interval 3780–3660 BC. Because in these dated buttons psychotropic alkaloids were present, it was concluded that they were used for their psychoactive effects [20].

The main reason for the psychoactive effects of peyote is due to the presence of the phenethylamine alkaloid mescaline. The effects of peyote and mescaline in humans are well studied. Native peyote cults used the cactus because it produces rich visual hallucinations. These effects were also used in psychiatric studies as a chemically induced model of mental illness. The mechanism of action is similar to that of lysergic acid diethylamide (LSD) or psilocin. These substances act as partial agonists at 5-hydroxytryptamine (5-HT) receptors. Although the acute toxicity of peyote or mescaline is not as high as other herbal alkaloids, fatalities have been described. Owing to the strong hallucinations, fights among drug abusers or self-harm situations are not uncommon.

Nerium Oleander

The evergreen shrub *Nerium oleander* (Figure 6), simply known as *oleander* is native to northern parts of Africa and the Mediterranean region. The scientific name is deduced from their preference to grow near water; Nero is the Greek word for water. The leaves of oleander are thick and leathery, dark green and narrow lanceolate, and up to 20-cm long. The leaves grow typically in pairs or whirls of three. The flowers of oleander are white, pink, or yellow, are up to 5 cm in diameter, and grow in clusters. Even though the flowers of *N. oleander* can be slightly yellow, the so-called yellow oleander is *Thevetia peruviana*. Both oleander and yellow oleander can easily be grown in warm subtropical regions and are extensively used in parks and roadsides worldwide [6].

Both plants are highly toxic and contain cardiac glycosides of the cardenolide type in all parts. The highest glycoside concentrations were detected in the

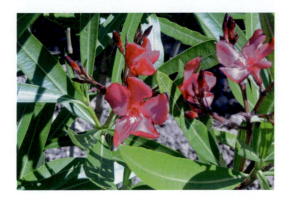

Figure 6   Flower and leaves of *Nerium oleander*

seeds of oleander, and the main glycoside present in these plants is oleandrin. Oleandrin acts like other cardiac (cardiac) glycosides of the cardenolide type by inhibition of the sodium potassium exchange, which causes an increased calcium level in heart cells, which increases contractions of heart muscle cells. An overdose of the cardiac glycosides causes dysrhythmia and a possible heart block. The first scientific study showing the therapeutic usefulness of cardiac glycosides was published in 1785 by Withering [21]. The therapeutic range of the cardiac glycosides is narrow. Many fatal and severe poisonings have been reported after ingestion of oleander or other plants containing cardiac glycosides, such as *Digitalis purpurea* (foxglove), *Adonis vernalis* (pheasant's eye), or *Convallaria majalis* (lily of the valley). The typical symptoms of an overdose with cardiac glycosides are dizziness and vomiting, followed by cardiac arrhythmias [6].

The treatment of an overdose is dependent on the severity of the poisoning. For treatment of severe poisonings, an antibody-based antidote has been developed to specifically remove the glycosides. In case of poisoning with plants or self-prepared extracts, this antidote is unfortunately poorly effective. The antidote removes therapeutically applied pure glycosides, but it is likely that some cardioactive glycosides are not removed [6].

Piper Methysticum

The common English name for the western pacific plant *Piper methysticum* is kava. Other names for the plant are 'awa', used in Hawaii, or 'yaqona', common in Fiji. Kava is an evergreen bush growing up

to 3 min height, with heart-shaped leaves up to 20 cm in length. The plant is closely related to black pepper (*Piper nigra*) and also has a spicy taste. Kava is psychoactive, indicated by the scientific species name *methysticum*, which is Greek for intoxicating. Kava is consumed on many western pacific islands and Australia [6]. Traditionally Kava is prepared by grinding or chewing the rhizome, which is mixed with water or coconut milk. The effects after consumption of kava are talkative and euphoric behavior, anxiolytic effects, sense of well-being, clear thinking, and relaxed muscles. The plant contains a mix of kavalactones and kavapyrones. Extracts of the plant were introduced into modern medicine as a mild anxiolytic. After the report of some deaths due to its medicinal use, kava medicines were banned. Kava-containing medicine causes acute liver failure [22]. The traditional use of kava by Pacific Islanders and by some aboriginal communities is not believed to be associated with liver damage. A recent study has shown that kava feeding in rats does not cause liver damage [23]. Further investigations are necessary to demonstrate the long-term safety of kava preparations.

Psilocybe Species

The small brown mushroom genus *Psilocybe* sp is best known for their psychoactive properties and are therefore called "magic mushrooms". The fruiting bodies of the magic mushrooms are small to medium in size and typically show a brown coloration. Hallucinogenic species of *Psilocybe* can be found in temperate regions throughout the world [24]. The psychoactive species contain as active ingredients psilocin and psilocybin. These compounds are structurally related to serotonin, a neurotransmitter in the central nervous system. Psilocin and psilocybin cause effects like the synthetic drug of abuse LSD. The effects of intoxication with magic mushrooms are mainly hallucination; the acute toxicity of the compounds is low. However, the consumption of these compounds is dangerous. Severe hallucinations can cause self-inflected injuries. Deaths due to self-induced stabbings following consumption of magic mushrooms have been recorded [5]. Two patients died from the wounds after they had stabbed themselves in the chest while under the influence of magic mushrooms.

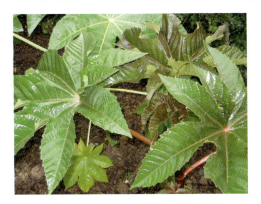

Figure 7   Leaves of *Ricinus communis*

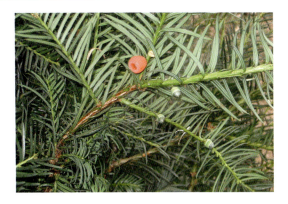

Figure 8   Fruit and leaves of *Taxus baccata*

Ricinus Communis

Ricinus communis (Figure 7), the castor oil plant, is cultivated all over the globe for oil production. The annual bushy shrub is believed to have its origin in tropical Africa, but grows nowadays worldwide. The plant with glossy palmately divided leaves is often used for ornamental purposes in gardens. The fruit of *R. communis* is a soft, spiny capsule with three almost oval seeds, which are the so-called castor beans. The attractive seeds have a hazelnut-like taste and contain 45–55% of fatty oil. The seeds also contain up to 25% protein. The protein fraction contains the highly toxic lectin ricin, which is poisonous via ingestion, inhalation, or injection. Ricin acts via an inhibition of protein synthesis. As a lectin, it binds to glycoproteins, facilitating the entry of the toxin into the cytosol [25].

After ingestion of ricin, the symptoms are nausea and diarrhea. In severe poisonings, liver and renal dysfunction, and possibly death, occurs. After inhalation, coughing and dyspnea can occur. These symptoms can progress to respiratory distress and death. The injection of ricin causes symptoms of general weakness and myalgias. Death is possible due to hypotension and multiorgan failure.

Ricin poisoning is possible by accidental or suicidal eating of the seeds. After oral ingestion of the seeds, the toxicity depends on how well the seeds are chewed. Some factors make the castor beans dangerous, such as their attractive appearance and the stability of ricin toward proteolytic enzymes. The treatment of a poisoning with ricin is recommended to be symptomatic. No specific antidote for ricin poisoning is available [25].

Taxus Baccata

The conifer *Taxus baccata* (Figure 8) is widely known as yew, and is often considered to be the oldest plant in Europe. The age of some yew trees is estimated to be 5000 years. The plant is a small to medium-sized tree, which grows relatively slowly. The leaves of this conifer are dark green and lanceolate, with a length of up to 4 cm. The plant has very characteristic single seed cones surrounded by a bright red colored berrylike structure, called an *aril*. All parts of the plant are highly toxic, except the arils. This enables the cones (including the arils) to be eaten by birds, but the seeds remain undamaged in the bird's droppings. The plant contains pseudoalkaloids of the taxane type. The main compound responsible for the toxicity of the European yew (*T. baccata*) is taxine B [6].

Some taxane-type pseudoalkaloids are also important in the treatment of cancer. In recent years, Taxol®, which contains paclitaxel, has become of particular interest in the treatment of ovarian, breast, and non-small-cell lung cancer. Paclitaxel has been isolated from the Pacific yew, *Taxus brevifolia*. Because of the extensive use of Taxol® and the fact that more than 1000 trees are needed to obtain 1 kg of paclitaxel, pharmaceutical companies have found an alternative source of the drug. A precursor of paclitaxel is isolated from cultivated European yew plants, and paclitaxel is synthesized using this precursor. The mechanism of action of taxanes is an inhibition of cell division by stabilization of the microtubuli. Therefore, these substances have cytotoxic effects.

In the case of an overdose with yew plants, the symptoms are nausea, dizziness, abdominal pain, shallow breathing, and tachycardia. Death can occur as a result of respiratory paralysis, with the heart in diastolic arrest. The treatment of a poisoning with yew is symptomatic, with no specific antidote available [6].

Analytical Methods

Because of the diversity of the toxic compounds in plants and mushrooms, a general laboratory screening procedure is not possible. Therefore, various specific methods for detection have been developed. Table 2 summarizes the major active compounds and the most

Table 2 List of botanical names, the corresponding main toxic compounds, and the common detection of these compounds in biological fluids

Scientific name	Main toxic compound(s)	Common detection in biological fluids
Aconitum napellus	Aconitine	HPLC, LC-MS
Amanita phalloides	Amanitine	Immunoassay, LC-MS
Atropa belladonna	Hyoscyamine, scopolamine	GC-MS, LC-MS
Catha edulis	Cathinone	GC-MS, LC-MS
Colchicum autumnale	Colchicine	HPLC, LC-MS
Conium maculatum	Coniine	GC-MS, LC-MS
Datura stramonium	Hyoscyamine, scopolamine	GC-MS, LC-MS
Laburnum anagyroides	Cytisine	LC-MS
Lophophora wiliamsii	Mescaline	GC-MS, LC-MS
Nerium oleander	Oleandrine	Immunoassay, LC-MS
Piper methysticum	Kavaine	HPLC
Psilocybe mexicana	Psilocin, psilocybin	GC-MS
Ricinus communis	Ricin	Immunoassay
Taxus baccata	Taxine B	LC-MS

common detection methods of the plants described in this article.

Methods for detection of naturally occurring toxic compounds include high-performance liquid chromatography (HPLC), liquid chromatography mass spectrometry (LC-MS), gas chromatography mass spectrometry (GC-MS), and various immunoassay techniques. The use of HPLC is common for detection of compounds like aconitine, colchicines, and the ingredients of kava. Kavalactones and kavapyrones are commonly used for the detection of aconitine and colchicine. The modern and more sensitive LC-MS techniques have been applied to many naturally occurring substances, especially if low concentrations have to be detected. The use of GC-MS techniques is applicable if the substances are thermostable and provides a powerful tool for detection of alkaloids like atropine, cathinone, and mescaline. While GC-MS techniques are useful, LC-MS techniques are preferred for the detection of low concentrations in blood.

The use of immunoassay techniques is possible for some poisonous compounds of herbal origin. It has been shown that the cardiac glycosides of oleander can be detected using an immunoassay technique for cardiac glycosides. This technique is not able to differentiate between the cardiac glycosides. A differentiation is possible using HPLC techniques. Also the detection of ricin is commonly performed using immunoassay techniques, such as radioimmunoassay (RIA) and enzyme-linked immunosorbent assay (ELISA). Owing to the physicochemical properties of the protein ricin, chromatographic techniques are more challenging and cannot at the present time be easily confirmed by conventional chromatographic techniques due to its large molecular size.

Detection methods using immunoassay techniques were also developed for the proof of death cap poisoning. Amanitin can be detected in urine up to 24 h after ingestion by the use of immunoassay techniques.

A postmortem detection of the toxic substances is often challenging. Determination of these is often likely in urine, but for some compounds like colchicine bile is the most useful specimen for postmortem analysis. Some toxins like amanitin are unlikely to be detected in postmortem specimen because death occurs many days after ingestion.

Some substances like psilocin and psilocybin are chemically unstable; hence concentrations need to be interpreted carefully.

See **Toxicology: Initial Testing** for further information on general drug detection techniques.

Summary and Conclusions

Fatal plant and mushroom poisonings are relatively rare. The diversity of poisonous compounds and their widespread occurrence in plants and fungi makes a comprehensive list of dangerous flora impossible. Besides, the majority of fatal cases are limited to a small number of plants and mushrooms. These poisonings can occur either after unintentional or intended ingestion or after abuse for their hallucinogenic effects. While plants and fungi can be dangerous to humans, fatal cases are avoidable. However, the analytical detection of a poisoning from an unknown plant or fungus can be a challenge for toxicologists.

References

[1]   Manriquez, O., Varas, J., Rios, J.C., Concha, F. & Paris, E. (2002). Analysis of 156 cases of plant intoxication received in the Toxicologic Information Center at Catholic University of Chile, *Veterinary and Human Toxicology* **44**(1), 31–32.

[2]   Poison Information Centre Goettingen (2005). *Harmonized Annual Report 2005*.

[3]   Ritter-Weilemann, I. (1995–2007). *Annual Reports*, Poison Information Centre, Mainz.

[4]   Eddleston, M., Gunnell, D., Karunaratne, A., de Silva, D., Sheriff, M.H. & Buckley, N.A. (2005). Epidemiology of intentional self-poisoning in rural Sri Lanka, *The British Journal of Psychiatry* **187**, 583–584.

[5]   Australian National Coroners Information System (NCIS), search conducted in July 2007. www.ncis.org.au.

[6]   Frohne, D. (2005). *Poisonous Plants: A Handbook for Doctors, Pharmacists, Toxicologists, Biologists and Veterinarians/Dietrich Frohne and Hans Jrgen Pfnder*, 2nd Edition, Manson Publishing, London.

[7]   Trim, G.M., Lepp, H., Hall, M.J., McKeown, R.V., McCaughan, G.W., Duggin, G.G. & Le Couteur, D.G. (1999). Poisoning by *Amanita phalloides* ("deathcap") mushrooms in the Australian Capital Territory, *The Medical Journal of Australia* **171**(5), 247–249.

[8]   Daugherty, C.G. (1995). The death of Socrates and the toxicology of hemlock, *Journal of Medical Biography* **3**(3), 178–182.

[9]   Jaspersen-Schib, R., Theus, L., Guirguis-Oeschger, M., Gossweiler, B. & Meier-Abt, P.J. (1996). Serious plant poisonings in Switzerland 1966–1994. Case analysis from the Swiss Toxicology Information Center, *Schweizerische Medizinische Wochenschrift* **126**(25), 1085–1098.

[10] Boumba, V.A., Mitselou, A. & Vougiouklakis, T. (2004). Fatal poisoning from ingestion of *Datura stramonium* seeds, *Veterinary and Human Toxicology* **46**(2), 81–82.

[11] Giannini, A.J. & Castellani, S. (1982). A manic-like psychosis due to khat (*Catha edulis* Forsk.), *Journal of Toxicology. Clinical Toxicology* **19**(5), 455–459.

[12] Elliott, S.P. (2002). A case of fatal poisoning with the aconite plant: quantitative analysis in biological fluid, *Science and Justice* **42**(2), 111–115.

[13] Chan, T.Y., Chan, J.C., Tomlinson, B. & Critchley, J.A. (1993). Chinese herbal medicines revisited: a Hong Kong perspective, *Lancet* **342**(8886–8887), 1532–1534.

[14] Wieland, T. (1967). The toxic peptides of Amanita phalloides, *Fortschritte der Chemie Organischer Naturstoffe* **25**, 214–250.

[15] Rang, H.P. (1987). *Pharmacology*, 2nd Edition, H.P. Rang & M.M. Dale, eds, Churchill Livingstone, Edinburgh, pp. 547–567.

[16] Toennes, S.W., Harder, S., Schramm, M., Niess, C. & Kauert, G.F. (2003). Pharmacokinetics of cathinone, cathine and norephedrine after the chewing of khat leaves, *British Journal of Clinical Pharmacology* **56**(1), 125–130.

[17] (2006). Gout: finally, diagnosis and treatment guidelines. A European task force offers the first recommendations on dealing with this painful arthritic condition, *Health News*, **12**(10), 10–11.

[18] Drummer, O.H., Roberts, A.N., Bedford, P.J., Crump, K.L. & Phelan, M.H. (1995). Three deaths from hemlock poisoning, *The Medical Journal of Australia* **162**(11), 592–593.

[19] Tutka, P. & Zatonski, W. (2006). Cytisine for the treatment of nicotine addiction: from a molecule to therapeutic efficacy, *Pharmacological Reports* **58**(6), 777–798.

[20] El-Seedi, H.R., De Smet, P.A., Beck, O., Possnert, G. & Bruhn, J.G. (2005). Prehistoric peyote use: alkaloid analysis and radiocarbon dating of archaeological specimens of Lophophora from Texas, *Journal of Ethnopharmacology* **101**(1–3), 238–242.

[21] Wade, O.L. (1986). Digoxin 1785–1985. I. Two hundred years of digitalis, *Journal of Clinical and Hospital Pharmacy* **11**(1), 3–9.

[22] (2002). Kava kava may cause irreversible liver damage, *South African Medical Journal* **92**(12), 961.

[23] DiSilvestro, R.A., Zhang, W. & DiSilvestro, D.J. (2007). Kava feeding in rats does not cause liver injury nor enhance galactosamine-induced hepatitis, *Food and Chemical Toxicology* **45**(7), 1293–1300.

[24] Musshoff, F., Madea, B. & Beike, J. (2000). Hallucinogenic mushrooms on the German market – simple

instructions for examination and identification, *Forensic Science International* **113**(1–3), 389–395.

[25] Audi, J., Belson, M., Patel, M., Schier, J. & Oster-loh, J. (2005). Ricin poisoning: a comprehensive review, *Journal of the American Medical Association* **294**(18), 2342–2351.

JOCHEN BEYER

Poisons: Natural *see* Poisons: Detection of Naturally Occurring Poisons

Police Interviews and Interrogations *see* Confessions: Evidentiary Reliability of

Police Use of Force

Traditionally, the hallmarks of policing involve officers responding to criminal and noncriminal calls for police service, detecting and preventing criminal activity, investigating past crimes, and enforcing laws. To carry out these activities, the police have institutional authority to use force. Such authority, power, or legal right comes from rules of law, which recognize that the police must sometimes use coercive action against law-violating citizens to accomplish legal objectives. Because police agency records and published statistics such as the annual figures reported by the Bureau of Justice Statistics consistently show that some citizens are willing to violate the law, use of force by the police remains a central part of their occupation (*see also* **Policing and Critical Incident Teams**).

When the police use force, they have the discretionary power to choose from a range of possible responses available in a given law enforcement activity. Responses can include the police using their presence or show of authority to using deadly force to deal with law-breaking behaviors by citizens. Whenever the police invoke their legal right to use force

against citizens, there are court decisions regarding legal standards for making the right force choice.

Courts in the United States, where the use of force by police is subject to constitutional restraints, generally apply three major legal decisions that clarify standards surrounding the appropriateness of police use of force: *West v. Atkins* [1], *Graham v. Connor* [2], and *Tennessee v. Garner* [3]. Under the umbrella of *West v. Atkins*, the police must act under color of law to be liable for use-of-force actions against citizens that amount to violations of police authority. The police must make objectively reasonable use-of-force choices under the *Graham* rules, which include a balancing test, subjective, objective, hindsight, and totality of circumstances tests. If the police decide to use deadly force against law-violators, then the *Garner* rules highlight three conditions in which deadly force may be reasonable: deadly force is necessary, suspects are dangerous, and the police are able to warn suspects.

Standards Governing Acting Under Color of Law

Before courts consider allegations that the police used wrongful or excessive force against citizens, they make legal determinations on whether the police were acting in their official capacity; that is, whether the police used force while "acting under color of law" whereby they exercised a power or right granted by law [1]. Generally, the use of force by the police against law-violating citizens is a law enforcement activity normally carried out under color of law.

Not all uses of force by the police, however, amount to acts under color of law. The question of official conduct is not always clear especially during off-duty hours, during acts of self-defense that happen in personal circumstances [4], or during acts of force that occur in secondary employment settings such as security venues. When making color of law determinations in these situations, courts weigh heavily the nature of the officer's behavior [5]. They have considered behaviors such as flashing of a badge [6], wearing a police uniform [7], identifying themselves as police officers [4], driving a marked police vehicle [6], or brandishing a department issued weapon [8], in concert with force as acts under color of law. Courts may also consider off-duty police acts within their jurisdiction and on which they file official police reports as behaviors that constitute acting under color of law [9].

Although sometimes the question of official conduct is ambiguous, courts have employed a three-prong test in color of law determinations: public function test, state compulsion test, and nexus test [10, 11]. For example, under the public function test, the court would consider whether an officer's use of force was a state action normally reserved for the police and usually performed by them during their official duties, or a personal action [12]. Making investigatory stops, arrests, or performing searches are uses of force that the police usually carry out under color of law [8, 13].

Under the state compulsion test, the court would determine whether the state or government compelled the officer to use force to enforce a government interest such as arresting a citizen who commits a crime of domestic violence. The central question is whether the use of force was an action required by law or police department policy [7]. Finally, the nexus test would involve the court's consideration of whether the officer's use of force involved conduct closely linked to or associated with the state [14]. For example, the action of an off-duty officer who grabs and arrests a citizen who commits a larceny may constitute state action because there is a sufficiently close nexus between the officer's conduct and the state's regulation of arrest powers.

While courts have employed the police function, state compulsion, and nexus tests in making legal decisions about police uses of force that fall under color of law, they have not used them in a formulaic fashion. Instead, they have considered the totality of circumstances surrounding each particular use of force case when employing them. To hold the police liable for wrongful uses of force that amount to constitutional violations, courts must first find whether they were clothed with official authority.

Standards Governing Objective Reasonableness

Whenever the police use force while acting under color of law, they must ensure that their use-of-force tactics do not violate the constitutional rights of citizens. Police uses of force against free citizens mostly occur in the course of an arrest, investigatory stop, or other seizure. The Fourth Amendment and its "reasonableness" standard is the precise

constitutional right that provides free citizens protection against unreasonable seizures or excessive force by the police. In *Graham v. Connor* [2], the court established five substantive tests for judging the reasonableness of police use of deadly or nondeadly force against citizens: balancing test, subjective test, objective test, hindsight test, and totality of circumstances test.

Using the balancing test, courts weigh the rights of free citizens under the Fourth Amendment against the interests of the government to take action against them. For example, an officer has a legal interest to stop or seize a motorist who travels through a stop sign without stopping. Yet, the motorist has a right to travel freely along the highway without police interference if the officer cannot substantiate a legal interest to carry out the traffic stop.

Where the police establish a legal interest to take action against citizens, the Fourth Amendment recognizes that the interest carries with it the need to use some degree of physical coercion or threat [15]. Built into the application of the balancing test is a principle of proportionality: Is the officer's act of force in the correct relationship to the citizen's violation of law? For example, a suspect disobeys an officer's verbal commands during an arrest. This form of behavior is less severe than is the suspect shooting at the officer. Both suspect behaviors require some degree of force by the officer to handle them and complete the arrest, but at obviously different levels. Therefore, courts balance the amount of force the police use against the amount of force they need to use in a particular situation [16].

When employing the objective test, courts consider whether another well-trained officer under the same set of circumstances would observe and conclude that the use of force by the police was reasonable. It requires a retrospective investigation and opinion by the well-trained officer (or expert) who has special knowledge of issues surrounding police use of force. Both carrying out the investigation and giving an opinion involve seeing through the lens of the officer on scene: what the officer's observations were; what the officer's observations meant; what the officer's experience and situational knowledge were; and what the officer's realty was. The expert weighs heavily the citizen's behavior because it has a large degree of power in influencing the officer's choice of force [17]. In the light of the particular circumstances, the expert conveys to the court whether he or she believes that the officer's choice of force was within the range of objectively reasonable options available because there is no precise formula for determining a single or best force option.

Under *Graham*, the subjective test discounts the personal motivations of the police because they have no value in the court's application of the Fourth Amendment's reasonableness standard. For example, an officer's evil intentions do not raise a Fourth Amendment claim of excessive force when his or her use of force was objectively reasonable. Alternatively, the officer's good intentions do not make an objectively unreasonable use of force constitutional.

Using the hindsight test, courts would not consider every grab or push by the police even if they later seem unnecessary as violations of the Fourth Amendment's protection against unreasonable seizures. Courts make allowances for errors by the police who must at times make split-second decisions about using force in situations that are tense and uncertain, and that evolve rapidly. What gives rise to constitutional violations are more than police acts that amount to mere mistakes. For example, having probable cause to arrest a person but arresting the wrong person, or having a warrant to search a house but carrying it out at the wrong house would not in every case violate the Fourth Amendment's reasonableness standard. The hindsight test takes into account police mistakes and uses the at-the-moment perception of another well-trained officer on scene as the basis for a reasonableness inquiry and not the after-the-fact perception of others.

The last *Graham* test – totality of circumstances – involves evaluating the circumstances of a use of force event. Because the Fourth Amendment's reasonableness standard is not capable of an exact definition, its application requires attention to the totality of circumstances. The central question is whether the totality of circumstances justifies a particular use of force by the police. Circumstances that the police know before and when they use force are relevant in courts' determinations of reasonableness [18].

In *Graham*, the court suggests careful attention to the severity of the crime; whether the suspect poses an immediate threat to the police or others nearby, the suspect attempts to escape police custody, or the suspect fights against arrest. On the face of these circumstances, deciding to use deadly force to shoot a suspect of a felony crime who resists the police and attempts to escape arrest might seem permissible.

The calculus of reasonableness in deadly force cases, however, requires some attention to the *Garner* [3] rules because *Graham v. Connor* is a nondeadly force case.

Standards Governing Deadly Force

The only US Supreme Court decision that deals directly with the use of deadly force by the police is *Tennessee v. Garner* [3]. Under the *Garner* rules, police may use weapons or other use-of-force tactics that amount to deadly force to prevent the escape and make the arrest of fleeing felons under three conditions. First, the police have probable cause to believe that a suspect poses a threat of significant physical harm to them or others: the danger condition. The immediacy of the threat and the dangerousness of it are the cornerstones of this condition. The dangerousness element suggests that suspects who threaten the police or others with weapons "or" suspects who commit crimes where they cause or threaten to cause significant physical harm are dangerous because of their violent or potential violent behavior. Under *Garner*, the "or" aspect of dangerousness suggests that the possession of a weapon or the threat to use one is not necessary to satisfy dangerousness. Courts, however, have considered suspects armed with guns, knives, or flashlights, and suspects who have used a vehicle as a weapon against an officer or have attempted to seize an officer's weapon as dangerous [19–24]. They have recognized murder, bank robbery, and armed robbery as felony crimes that demonstrate dangerous behaviors that justify the use of deadly force [25–27].

The immediacy element of a suspect's physical threat to the police or others suggests that the period during which the threat occurs and the threat actually happens is important. Unfortunately, not all courts measure this period the same. Some may apply an "imminent" yardstick whereby significant physical harm is about to happen such as a suspect pointing a handgun at an officer [28]. Others may use more than a yardstick whereby they consider the "unpredictability" of a dangerous suspect, which is not easily foreseeable and measurable [29]. Nevertheless, courts carefully examine the totality of circumstances in all cases when making determinations about immediacy.

Second, the police may only use deadly force against a dangerous suspect when necessary: the necessary condition. Unless the suspect satisfies the danger condition, deadly force is unnecessary. What is necessary or needed, however, may invite hindsight arguments. For example, in *Plakas v. Drinski* [30], Plakas ran at an officer and tried to use a fireplace poker to kill him. The officer shot and killed Plakas. In this case, the plaintiff argued that the officer had nondeadly force options available and that the officer did not try them. The officer could have used a spray or a police dog to disarm Plakas; deadly force was unnecessary. At both the district and federal court levels, the courts ruled in this case that the officer's force was reasonable. The Fourth Amendment's reasonableness standard does not require police to use less intrusive uses of force. Federal courts have rejected necessary arguments that the police could have used nondeadly force options when deadly force ones were reasonable [31].

Third, the police must warn – where feasible – a suspect of their intention to use deadly force: the warning condition. Unless the suspect satisfies the danger condition, both a warning and deadly force are unnecessary. The use of deadly force may also be unnecessary if a dangerous suspect submits to an arrest after a warning.

Whether the police make decisions to use deadly or nondeadly force options to seize free citizens, their choices must fall within the range of objectively reasonable options available in particular situations. The Fourth Amendment's reasonableness standard is the appropriate test in claims that the police used excessive force in the course of an arrest, an investigatory stop, or other seizures. However, not every police abuse of force occurs under these conditions. An officer who uses excessive force against a prisoner would violate either the Fourteenth Amendment's due process clause or the Eighth Amendment's prohibition against cruel and unusual punishment. It is important then to identify the specific constitutional right that is the precise textual source of an officer's use-of-force conduct [2].

References

[1]   West v. Atkins, 487 U.S. 42 (1988).
[2]   Graham v. Connor, 490 U.S. 386 (1989).
[3]   Tennessee v. Garner, 471 U.S. 1 (1985).
[4]   Huffman v. County of Los Angeles, 147 F.3d 1054, 1058 (9th Cir., 1998).
[5]   Stengel v. Belcher, 522 F.2d 438, 441 (6th Cir., 1975).
[6]   Neuens v. City of Columbus, 303 F.3d 667 (6th Cir., 2002).
[7]   Roe v. Humke, 128 F.3d 1213, 1216 (8th Cir., 1997).
[8]   Abraham v. Raso, 183 F.3d 279, 287 (3d Cir., 1999).
[9]   Kappeler, V.E. (2006). *Critical Issues in Police Civil Liability*, Waveland Press, Illinois.
[10] Ellison v. Garbarino, 48 F.3d 192, 195 (6th Cir., 1995).
[11] Wolotsky v. Huhn, 960 F.2d 1331 (6th Cir., 1992).
[12] Bonsignore v. City of New York, 683 F.2d (2nd Cir., 1982).
[13] Pickrel v. City of Springfield, 45 F.3d 1115 (7th Cir., 1995).
[14] Cooper v. Parrish, 203 F.3d 937, 952 (6th Cir., 2000).
[15] Terry v. Ohio, 392 U.S. 1 (1968).
[16] Flores v. City of Palacios, 381 F.3d 391 (5th Cir., 2004).
[17] Adams, K. (1999). What we know about police use of force, in *Use of Force by Police: Overview of National and Local Data*, J. Travis, J.M. Chaiken & R.J. Kaminski, eds, U.S. Department of Justice, National Institute of Justice and Bureau of Justice Statistics, Washington, DC. pp. 1–14.
[18] Palmquist v. Selvik, 111 F.3d 1332 (7th Cir., 1997).
[19] Butler v. City of Detroit, 386 N.W.2d 645 (Mich. App. 1985).
[20] Ealy v. City of Detroit, 375 N.W.2d 435 (Mich. App. 1985).
[21] Haineze v. Allison, 216 F.3d 1081 (5th Cir., 2000).
[22] Nelson v. County of Wright, 162 F.3d 986 (5th Cir., 1988).
[23] Pittman v. Nelms I.I.I., 87 F.3d 116 (4th Cir., 1996).
[24] Rhiner v. City of Clive, 373 N.W.2d 466 (Iowa, 1985).
[25] Ford v. Childress, 650 F.Supp. 110 (D.C. Ill. 1986).
[26] Ryder v. City of Topeka, 814 F.2d 1412 (10th Cir., 1987).
[27] Trejo v. Wattles, 654 F.Supp. 1143 (D. Colo. 1987).
[28] Boyd v. Baeppler, 215 F.3d 594 (6th Cir., 2000).
[29] Hegarty v. Somerset County, 53 F.3d 1367 (1st Cir., 1995).
[30] Plakas v. Drinski, 19 F.3d 1143 (7th Cir., 1994).
[31] Scott v. Henrich, 39 F.3d 912 (9th Cir., 1994).

FRANK J. GALLO

Policing and Critical Incident Teams

Police calls for service occasionally require the police to resolve high-threat or special-threat situations such as barricaded suspects, hostage situations, drug raids, or warrant services. Although infrequent, these events are significantly different from usual police work that is often less dangerous: They require some degree of special handling. In US law enforcement circles, such special teams have become known by the acronym SWAT, which stands for special weapons and tactics. In other countries, such special teams may be designated by other terms. Since the 1965 Watts riots in Los Angeles, California, the need for SWAT teams (at times called *police paramilitary units, critical incident teams, special response teams*, and other names in the police literature) to deal with special-threat situations that regular officers are traditionally unprepared to handle has become popular among American law enforcement agencies [1].

Police departments of all sizes have working SWAT teams and some are developing them [2, 3]. They most often employ, when available, their SWAT teams to deal with rare high-threat police call outs. Officers who are SWAT members receive special training to work as a team and to use special weapons and force tactics to handle the most dangerous call outs. Because their behaviors involve special uses of force, there are some common risks related to the legal process.

The adequacy of a SWAT team and its training in particular uses of special weaponry, technology, and tactics to confront the most dangerous situations may give rise to a legal action when the team fails to train in the proper use of issued equipment and use of force tactics. When a SWAT team uses force, its choices must be "objectively reasonable." In cases of alleged use of excessive force, criminal and civil liability can attach itself in the form of a team's wrongful actions under Titles 18 and 42 of the US Code respectively. There are legal risks surrounding the intervention of a SWAT team to control and overcome hostage takers where the main concern is the protection of human life and the avoidance of hostage and bystander injuries.

Adequate Training

Police departments that have SWAT teams often call upon them to resolve the most dangerous police–citizen contacts. SWAT teams commonly carry out high-threat warrant services where the police believe that suspects are armed and dangerous. They execute high-threat narcotics search warrants where drug dealers seem likely to defend their drugs and homes using weapons. Sometimes, SWAT team interventions require team members to confront, disarm, and arrest suspects who hold citizen prisoners.

To assist SWAT teams in handling and controlling extreme police callouts, police departments employ their SWAT team members with special weaponry that are not available to regular officers. For example, some police agencies issue high-powered rifles, automatic firearms, diversionary devices, ballistic shields, and chemical munitions [4]. They authorize their SWAT teams to carry out tactical operations that involve the use of special tactics such as warrant, warrantless, or "no-knock" forced building entries. Because police departments arm their SWAT teams with special weapons and tactics to help them to enforce laws and make arrests, they need to train them on their appropriate uses. A failure to train may amount to a "conscious choice" or "deliberate indifference" to the constitutional rights of citizens to be free from unreasonable uses by SWAT teams [5].

Without training, SWAT teams are likely to make mistakes when deploying SWAT such as using diversionary devices to help them to carry out no-knock warrants. It is not reasonable to expect common officers to know the right force option without training [6]. SWAT teams must receive training in specialized tasks they are likely to perform on-the-job [5]. A failure to train them might give rise to a federal cause of action. Community stakeholders could consider police agencies to be deliberately indifferent to the needs of SWAT teams to receive specialized training.

In resolving the responsibility to train, police departments must focus on the adequacy of its training programs to meet the plausible conditions under which its SWAT teams works [5]. Courts suggest that training require officers to make judgments on the use of varying degrees of force [7] and present officers with situations that reflect real-life work conditions [8]. Knowing the prevalence of SWAT team call outs and the unique facts surrounding them can be the basis for making informed training decisions. Use of expert witnesses on the proper application of guidelines enacted by a department often provides the crucial factual information to courts when litigation ensues.

Reasonable and Excessive Force

Free citizens raise a Fourth Amendment claim when they allege that a SWAT team used excessive force against them in a law enforcement capacity (*see also* **Police Use of Force**). The Fourth Amendment prohibits unreasonable searches and seizures. It protects free citizens from the police using excessive force against them. There is no prevailing definition of what is excessive force. The Supreme Court, however, imposed an "objective reasonableness" standard for reviewing claims of excessive force by the police [9]. In such cases and under the *Graham* rules [9], the trier (or judge) or triers (or jury) of facts must first weigh the rights of free citizens under the Fourth Amendment against the interests of the government to take action against them (or balancing test). The Fourth Amendment recognizes that the right to take action against free citizens is associated with the need to use some degree of physical coercion or threat [10]. Second, consider whether a well-trained officer under the same set of circumstances would observe and conclude that the actions by the police were reasonable (or objective test).

Third, discount the subjective motivations of the police because they have no value in a court's appraisal of excessive force (or subjective test). Evil intentions do not raise Fourth Amendment claims when force options were objectively reasonable. Good intentions do not make objectively unreasonable force options constitutional. Fourth, evaluate the circumstances of the police call out. That is, what is the severity of the crime, does the suspect pose an immediate threat to the police or others nearby, and is the person actively resisting or fleeing arrest (or totality of circumstances test). Because the "objective reasonableness" standard is not capable of providing an exact definition, its application requires attention to the totality of circumstances. Only circumstances known to the police before and at the time they use force are relevant [11]. The central question is whether the totality of circumstances justifies a particular use of force by the police.

Fifth, recognize that not every push or shove by the police even if it later seems unnecessary violates the Fourth Amendment (or hindsight test). The standard of "objective reasonableness" makes allowances for errors made by the police who must at times make split-second decisions about force in situations that are tense and uncertain, and that evolve rapidly [12].

Finally, examine carefully at whether the severity of force by the police puts suspects at risk of death "or" serious bodily harm (or deadly force test). Under the *Garner* rules [13], police may deploy weapons or use tactics that amount to deadly force in three conditions. First, if deadly force is necessary to prevent escape (or necessary condition). Second, if the police have probable cause to believe that a suspect poses a significant threat of death "or" serious bodily harm to them "or" others nearby (or dangerous condition). In this condition, the court suggests that suspects who threaten the police or others with weapons and suspects who commit a crime and cause or threaten to cause serious bodily harm are dangerous because of their violent or potential violent behavior. Third, if possible, the police must warn a suspect of their intention to use deadly force against him or her (or warning condition).

Whether SWAT teams use deadly or nondeadly force options against suspects of crimes, allegations of excessive force are possible especially when tactical operations involve the use of SWAT not employed by regular officers. For example, plaintiffs have argued that the uses of certain police tactics such as deploying diversionary devices are excessive. In numerous court cases, however, the courts have suggested that uses of diversionary devices are permissible under the *Graham* rules [9] when the totality of circumstances support their use, when the police use discretion and do not deploy them routinely as a matter of custom, and when the police receive training in their appropriate use [14–16].

A high-risk forced building entry by a SWAT team also raises concern of excessive force. In general, police need consent, exigent circumstances, or an arrest or search warrant to enter buildings. Carrying out a forced building entry will trigger a judicial review of its lawfulness and excessiveness especially when any injuries occur. The more on-scene time a SWAT team has with a police call out such as negotiating with a barricaded suspect, the less the team can rely on exigency to carry out a warrantless entry, search, or seizure. A SWAT team avoids some excessive force liability for using forced building entry tactics when it obtains prior judicial approval.

Questions about excessive force may occur when police regularly execute as a matter of policy or custom warrantless building entries in critical incident situations regardless of the totality of circumstances. For example, in *O'Brien v. City of Grand Rapids* [17], the court held the city liable for a warrantless entry into the home of an armed barricaded suspect with whom the police had contact time for 6-hours. The police here had a custom of executing warrantless building entries in critical incidents regardless of the circumstances.

Sometimes, when police fail to reevaluate prior to entry the circumstances justifying a no-knock warrant, it may be unreasonable or excessive to carry out the warrant. For example, in *United States v. Singer* [18], the court said that if during the period between obtaining a no-knock warrant and executing it the police receive reliable information that exigent or dangerous circumstances no longer exist, the police must reevaluate their plan of entering a home without first knocking and announcing.

In cases of alleged use of excessive force, criminal and civil liability can attach itself in the form of a team's wrongful actions under Title 18 of the US Code section 242 and Title 42 section 1983 respectively. Commonly referred to as *sections 242* and *1983*, police shall not deprive any citizen within their jurisdiction of any rights secured by the Constitution and laws while acting under the color of law. In an action of law (criminal action for deprivation of rights) or redress (civil action for deprivation of rights), police are liable to any persons injured under sections 242 and 1983. Civil liability can also come in the form of specific state statutes that are similar to those of the federal government. For those members of SWAT teams, call outs are at times fraught with certain legal – criminal or civil – problems, dangers, or difficulties.

Hostage and Bystander Injuries

Police have the responsibility to safeguard the well-being of the community. There is the possibility of injuries, however, when tactics to handle dangerous police call outs involve the use of physical force to capture and arrest law violators. Generally, no deprivation of rights occurs when the police use reasonable care, but accidentally shoot hostages or bystanders during police–citizen encounters. For example, in *Green v. Denison* [19], a suspect fired a bullet that shattered glass, which blinded a bystander. An officer fired a bullet that accidentally hit the suspect's girlfriend. Both injured persons sued and claimed that the police had a duty to protect them from harm. The court dismissed the claims and held that police officers are not liable for injuries or damages to the general public that arise from their acting within the scope of their authority or duty. It distinguished duty owed to the public from duty owed to particular persons targeted by the police. Protecting the police or

giving them official immunity from personal liability arising from making discretionary or best judgment decisions allows them to perform their job without distractions.

In *Lee v. Williams* [20], a police deputy unintentionally shot a hostage during a shootout with armed suspects. Postincident litigation brought about a § 1983 civil deprivation of rights claim against the deputy. The court ruled that there was no Fourth Amendment seizure of the hostage because the deputy did not intend to shoot him, but did intend to shoot the armed suspects.

For officers involved in making tactical decisions about handling hostage situations, the courts have established a philosophy of "human life is the main concern." For example, in *Downs v. United States* [21], a Federal Bureau of Investigation (FBI) SWAT team carried out a forceful assault against armed suspects who hijacked an airplane, held passengers as hostages, but released some of them during negotiations. The outcome of the assault approach was the deaths of hostages. The court ruled that the safety of hostages is more important than the arrest of suspects.

There is no constitutional obligation to have specially trained SWAT teams deal with nonnormal police calls for service such as hostage situations [22]. Actions by regular or non-SWAT officers, who generally do not possess the same training, experience, and equipment that SWAT officers posses to handle the most dangerous police call outs, might not automatically result in injuries or police behaviors that would shock the conscious of courts. For SWAT and non-SWAT officers involved in making tough tactical decisions, (*see* **Aggression**) postincident outcomes might involve criminal or civil action for deprivation of rights. Fourth Amendment principles (*see* **Seizures: Behavioral**) are equally applicable (*see* **Threat Assessment: School**) to both SWAT and non-SWAT officers who might injure citizens.

References

[1]   Clark, J.G., Jackson, M.S., Schaefer, P.M. & Sharpe, E.G. (2000). Training SWAT teams: implications for improving tactical units, *Journal of Criminal Justice* **28**, 407–413.

[2]   Kraska, P.B. & Cubellis, L.J. (1997). Militarizing mayberry and beyond: making sense of American paramilitary policing, *Justice Quarterly* **14**, 607–629.

[3] Kraska, P.B. & Kappeler, V.E. (1997). Militarizing American police: the rise and normalization of paramilitary units, *Social Problems* **44**, 1–18.

[4] Williams, J.J. & Westall, D. (2003). SWAT and non-SWAT police officers and the use of force, *Journal of Criminal Justice* **31**, 469–474.

[5] Canton v. Harris, 489 U.S. 378 (1989).

[6] Walker v. City of New York, 974 F.2d 293 (2nd Cir., 1992).

[7] Allen v. Muskogee, 119 F.3d 837 (10th Cir., 1998).

[8] Popow v. Margate, 476 F.Supp. 1237 (D.N.J. 1979).

[9] Graham v. Connor, 490 U.S. 386 (1989).

[10] Terry v. Ohio, 392 U.S. 1 (1968).

[11] Ford v. Childers, 855 F.2d 1271, 1276 (7th Cir., 1988).

[12] Johnson v. Glick, 481 F.2d 1028, 1033 (2nd Cir., 1973).

[13] Tennessee vs. Garner, 471 U.S. 1 (1985).

[14] Commonwealth v. Garner, 423 Mass. 735, 772 N.E.2d 510 (1996).

[15] Langford v. Gates, 43 Cal. 3d 21, 729 P.2d 822 (1987).

[16] United States v. Myers, No. 94-20013-01, 1194 WL 324582 (10th Cir., 1997).

[17] O'Brien v. City of Grand Rapids, 23 F.3d 990, 999 (6th Cir., 1994).

[18] United States v. Singer, 943 F.2d 758, 763 (7th Cir., 1991).

[19] Green v. Denison, 738 S.W.2d 861 (Mo. 1987).

[20] Lee v. Williams, 138 F.Supp.2d 748 (E.D. Va. 2001).

[21] Downs v. United States, 522 F.2d 990 (6th Cir., 1975).

[22] Salas v. Carpenter, 980 F.2d 299, 309–10 (5th Cir., 1992).

Related Articles

Daubert v. Merrell Dow Pharmaceuticals
Police Use of Force

FRANK J. GALLO

Pollen *see* Palynology

Polymorphism: Genetic

Natural genetic variation, within a population, is seen by the existence of more than one type of allele for a locus. Loci with several commonly occurring alleles are useful for profiling purposes because, although some individuals may share the same alleles at a locus, the probability of them sharing the same alleles at all loci reduces dramatically as the number of loci considered increases. For profiling purposes, scientists use loci that comprise sequences with simple tandem repeats (STR) (*see also* **Short Tandem Repeats**). These are regions of DNA that have short sequences of DNA that are repeated as multiple blocks, like carriages of a train. Any one person will have two copies (alleles) of the locus, one from mother and one from father, and each allele will have its own number of STRs. These may be the same (homozygote) or different (heterozygote).

DNA profiling tests the polymorphism, or variation, of the alleles at a set of loci for a sample. For the sake of convenience, the different alleles of any one locus are given a name that is the same as the number of STR contained within the allele's DNA sequence. Thus, a person with profile D3/13,16 is a heterozygote with one allele at D3 that has 13 repeats and a second allele that has 16 repeats.

Polymorphisms in a population have evolved as a result of mutations and the passage of time. In the case of STR, mutations are thought to be due to a low rate of slippage of DNA synthesis of the repeated sequences during the process of making sperm and egg cells. Such mutations are then passed on to a new generation and over time become a measurable proportion of a population. A rule of thumb for a polymorphism is that it occurs in at least 0.05% of a population. Exactly, how common any allele is depends on many factors, including chance, selective breeding, population size, intermingling of populations, and so on. The allele frequencies of a polymorphic locus will remain stable if the population is in Hardy–Weinberg equilibrium (*see also* **Hardy-Weinberg Equilibrium**), but are often different for different populations.

SCOTT BADER

Popper Theory of Falsifiability
see Falsifiability Theory

Postmortem *see* Autopsy

Postal: Going *see* Homicide: Multiple (Behavior)

Postmortem Biochemical Examinations

Introduction

Functional Causes of Death

The diagnosis of *functional causes of death* is, on one hand, based on mostly sparse postmortem findings and, on the other hand, considerably on postmortem biochemical alterations, which frequently originate from illnesses with internal causes and subsequent dysregulations such as diabetes mellitus, alterations of kidney and liver function, and imbalances of water and electrolytes. It is not rare that combinations of such dysregulations with problematic overlappings are seen due to close physiological and biochemical links [1–4] (*see also* **Cardiac and Natural Causes of Sudden Death**; **Natural Causes of Sudden Death: Noncardiac**).

Postmortem Biochemical Estimations and Differences to Clinical Biochemistry

Postmortem biochemical analyses may represent the main clue to the diagnosis of functional causes of death. One of the main problems is to be able to apply clinical biochemical values on postmortem conditions. On one hand, there are big unpredictabilities regarding general postmortem changes in body fluids. On the other hand, biochemical values in postmortem specimen may well represent more or less the results of changes taking place during agony or the early postmortem period. Contrary to clinical biochemical estimations, values obtained postmortem do not necessarily allow conclusions regarding the mechanism of death. Postmortem diagnostic procedures, therefore, require a critical way of looking at them [5].

Obtaining the Appropriate Specimen

Body fluids are usually obtained during postmortem examination. In cases with a limited external examination specimen (e.g., cerebrospinal fluid (CSF), vitreous humor, blood, and urine) can also be taken by cannulation (suboccipital access, puncture of an eyeball, dissection of a femoral vein, and puncture of the urinary bladder). The cranial cavity and the eyeballs provide a relatively good protection of the enclosed body fluids against decomposition effects. After obtaining vitreous humor, the eyeballs should be refilled with water due to cosmetic reasons.

The volume of CSF to be found varies from 50 ml (baby) to 135 ml (adult). A few milliliters are sufficient for the postmortem biochemical analyses and there is usually no problem to get blood-free CSF. Approximately 1–2 ml of vitreous humor can be obtained by the puncture of both eyeballs. Aspiration of small parts of the retina is of no further relevance. Postmortem blood should be taken from the heart and a (peripheral) femoral vein and urine from the bladder immediately after dissection (a few milliliters per specimen) [6].

"Near-Table" Methods

During the postmortem examination, several screening tests with stripes and tablets can be carried out regarding glucose, bilirubin, or acetone. Furthermore, there are a number of electronic test devices on the market, which can be used for screening purposes. These "near-table" methods are useful to confirm or exclude certain differential diagnoses at the time of the autopsy (further information: http://www.roche-diagnostics.com).

Glucose Metabolism and Diabetes Mellitus

General Aspects of Diabetic Coma

Diabetic coma is a life-threatening complication of diabetes mellitus. Owing to a relative or an absolute insulin deficit, there is a typical rise of blood sugar with the possibility of acute complications or damage to blood vessels and nerves after longer duration. Depending on the age group, the incidence of diabetes mellitus varies between 2 and 5%. Causes for coma may be the onset of an unknown diabetes, lack of insulin injections, or increased requirement of

Table 1 Postmortem biochemical values in case of alterations of glucose metabolism

Dysfunction	Parameter	Compartment	Results
Coma (in general)	Sum value[a]	Cerebrospinal fluid	$\sum > 415\,\text{mg dl}^{-1}$[b]
		Vitreous humor	$\sum > 410\,\text{mg dl}^{-1}$[c]
	HbA$_{1c}$	Blood	$>12.1\%$[d]
	Glucose	Urine	$>25\,\text{mg dl}^{-1}$[e]
Ketotic coma	Acetone	Blood, cerebrospinal fluid	$>21\,\text{mg dl}^{-1}$[f]
		Vitreous humor	$>5\,\text{mg l}^{-1}$[f]
		Urine	
Hypoglycemia	Sum value	Cerebrospinal fluid	$\sum < 50\text{--}80\,\text{mg dl}^{-1}$
		Vitreous humor	$\sum < 100\text{--}160\,\text{mg dl}^{-1}$

[a] According to Traub: concentrations of glucose and lactate
[b] Mean value $= 500\text{--}600\,\text{mg dl}^{-1}$
[c] Mean value glucose $= 300\text{--}950\,\text{mg dl}^{-1}$; mean value lactate initially $= 80\text{--}160\,\text{mg dl}^{-1}$, after $20\,\text{h} = 210\text{--}260\,\text{mg dl}^{-1}$
[d] Mean value $= 13\text{--}15\%$, nondiabetics $= 9.15\%$
[e] Most of coma cases $>50\,\text{mg dl}^{-1}$, partly $2000\text{--}4000\,\text{mg dl}^{-1}$
[f] Coma: mean value $= 100\text{--}150\,\text{mg l}^{-1}$

insulin due to acute infections, poor diet, operations, gastrointestinal diseases, or myocardial infarction. Twenty-five percent of all diabetic comas are so-called manifestation comas with previous unknown diabetes. Infections are the most frequent triggers for coma onset (approximately 40% of the cases). The frequency of fatal coma among known diabetics is between 0.5 and 1.5% with a peak in the age group of 40–60 years. The overall lethality from coma varies from 5 to 25% and rises to 70% with coma of longer duration. Lethality of diabetic coma is tenfold in 70-year-old individuals compared to 30-year-old patients. Furthermore, the risk for coma in juveniles is four- to sevenfold higher than in adults [1, 2] (see Table 1).

Types of Diabetic Coma

Typically, diabetes mellitus type I is associated with ketonemic coma, whereas hyperosmolar coma normally results from type II diabetes mellitus. A lack of insulin causes a rise of blood glucose with subsequent loss of fluids and electrolytes. In addition, increased lipolysis is used to compensate the deficit of energy resulting from the inhibition of glucose metabolism leading to increased levels of ketone bodies with metabolic acidosis. The latter may be excessive ($500\text{--}1000\,\text{mg l}^{-1}$ acetone or higher), whereas hyperglycemia remains mostly moderate ($250\text{--}600\,\text{mg dl}^{-1}$). Hyperosmolar coma is more rare (approximately 10–20% of the cases) and associated with relative lack of insulin causing reduced

peripheral utilization of glucose with simultaneous release of glucose from the liver. Low levels of insulin prevent ketosis due to inhibition of lipolysis. Therefore, it is typical to find excessive hyperglycemia (often above $1000\,\text{mg dl}^{-1}$) with lacking or only mild ketosis.

Diabetic coma may lead to fatal outcome via different pathophysiological pathways. There is a cardiovascular type with leading oliguria or a renal type with acute kidney failure. Moreover, there exists pseudoperitonitis type with the symptoms of an acute abdomen. Typical accompanying diseases of fatal diabetic decompensation may be myocardial infarctions, apoplexy, embolism, pneumonia, pancreatitis, pyelonephritis, and a predisposition for lactic acidosis [5].

The most important body fluids for postmortem diagnostic purposes are CSF and vitreous humor using the so-called sum value according to Traub, which provides a combined calculation to compensate postmortem alterations of blood glucose level due to glycolysis, accordingly [7].

Glucose

The hourly metabolic decrease of glucose in CSF is about $10\text{--}15\,\text{mg dl}^{-1}$ but may vary between approximately 5 and $45\,\text{mg dl}^{-1}$. The hourly rate is below $1\,\text{mg dl}^{-1}\,100\,\text{h}$ postmortem. Given normal metabolic conditions, therefore, zero levels are reached after 10–12 h. Longer persisting glucose levels are indicative of antemortem hyperglycemia [8].

The speed of postmortem glycolysis depends on a number of factors, e.g., the temperature and duration of body storage. Postmortem glycolysis is slower in diabetics compared to nondiabetic individuals, whereas obesity accelerates degradation of glucose. Isolated assessment of elevated glucose levels in CSF requires critical reserve (normal range: $ca.$ 50–90 mg dl^{-1}), because multiple other dysregulations may be accompanied by the same symptom as carbon monoxide poisoning, acute cardiac death, brain trauma, strangulation, protracted agony, asphyxia, pneumonia, and pancreatitis. This aspect has also to be taken into account regarding other body fluids [6].

Lactic Acid (Lactate)

The product of postmortem glycolysis is lactate (normal level in CSF $ca.$ 9 mg dl^{-1}). Its concentration increases postmortem with a rate of approximately 10–15 mg dl^{-1} up to the 10th hour after death. After this time, the increasing rates vary considerably. Under differential diagnostic aspects also other disorders may cause hyperlactacidemia, e.g., tumors, respiratory insufficiency, severe chronic inflammations, uremia, especially inflammations of the central nervous system or alcohol-induced with lack of thiamine, physical strain, and alimentary factors (e.g., strict fasting).

Sum Value

This combined method, according to Traub, compensates arithmetically for the postmortem production of lactate from glucose by using a "sum value". It is based on the fact that 1 mol of glucose produces, via glycolysis, two moles of lactate so that the concentrations can be added using milligrams per deciliter. If the "sum value" exceeds 362 mg dl^{-1} in CSF, the probability of fatal diabetic coma is about 89%, if other, e.g., toxicological and morphological, alterations can be excluded. In cases of diabetes mellitus, the "sum value" remains almost stable up to the 200th hour postmortem. If there are nondiabetic causes of death, the "sum value" increases up to the 30th hour postmortem, but remains nearly stable afterwards. Although the formula, according to Traub, has to be used under critical view, the "sum value" may be considered the most important criterion for the diagnosis of fatal diabetic coma. However, the author's research

has revealed that it is more realistic to increase the limit "sum value" in CSF to 415 mg dl^{-1} (upper limit of the 95% confidence interval in cases of cardiac death), with cases of diabetic coma ranging on average between $ca.$ 500 and 600 mg dl^{-1} [9, 10].

Vitreous Humor

The calculation method according to Traub may also be applied on vitreous humor. The glucose level herein is about 50–85% of the serum glucose. Values for postmortem glucose concentrations vary from 20 mg dl^{-1} (nondiabetics) to 90 mg dl^{-1} (known diabetics), but wide variation ranges have to be taken into account. Owing to slower glycolysis in vitreous humor compared to CSF, normal glucose values may be found as long as two days postmortem. In cases of fatal coma, glucose values between $ca.$ 300 and 950 mg dl^{-1} may be found. Lactate values are already around 80–160 mg dl^{-1} in the intramortal period and between 210 and 260 mg dl^{-1} approximately 20 h postmortem. The upper limit value is 410 mg dl^{-1} and if this is exceeded, it can be taken as a strong indication of fatal diabetic coma, given the condition that other possibly competing mechanisms can be excluded. The procedure is said to be applicable until the 10th postmortem day [11–15].

Blood Glucose

Blood sugar levels alone are only of low diagnostic relevance, if at all limited to blood from the femoral veins within the 1st and 2nd hour postmortem in which the level is ca 40–100 mg dl^{-1}. Contrary to this, glucose levels in central blood (right ventricle) may easily reach 1000 mg dl^{-1} and over due to postmortem hepatic glycogenolysis. Normally, postmortem glycolysis (approximately 13 mg dl^{-1} h^{-1}) results in complete metabolization of the blood glucose within 6–8 h. This leads to a corresponding increase of lactate up to 180 mg dl^{-1} after 1 h and $ca.$ 450–680 mg dl^{-1} after 12–24 h. Especially due to postmortem diffusion of serum and its components from surrounding tissues into blood vessels, the "sum value" cannot be used [10].

Hemoglobin A_{1c}

This glycosylated fraction of hemoglobin represents an important parameter regarding a basic diagnosis of diabetes mellitus. Owing to the fact that kinetics of its formation is depending on time and concentrations, HbA_{1c} can be used as a long-term indicator of diabetic conditions (so-called blood sugar memory for *ca.* 120 days). Levels of 6–8% (maximum of 10%) are consistent with a normal glucose metabolism, whereas higher concentrations are indicative of inappropriate metabolic conditions (hyperglycemias in the past). Periods of increased blood sugar have to last 6–8 h minimum to cause significant rises of HbA_{1c} due to its slow reaction kinetics. Furthermore, the prefinal and postmortem drop of the pH value in blood, due to formation of lactate, are likely to result in a reduction of HbA_{1c} because of separation of its unstable component. Blood sugar also decreases rapidly after death. The stable part of hemoglobin A_{1c} makes up approximately 90% of the whole. For example, hyperglycemia around 360 mg dl^{-1} takes around 12 h to cause an increase of HbA_{1c} of 1.3% absolute. In reverse, a reduction of around 5% needs around seven days.

There has been found a positive connection between "sum value", urine glucose concentration, and HbA_{1c} level. This means that there usually is a coincidence of elevated "sum value", high urine glucose, and HbA_{1c}. Hemoglobin A_{1c} has proven to be relatively stable versus autolysis especially in hemolyzed blood and can be measured postmortem in frozen samples and also in samples stored in a normal fridge. It has been revealed that storage at temperatures between +4 and −80 °C does not cause any relevant changes to the HbA_{1c} concentrations. The result is independent from the actual total hemoglobin level because HbA_{1c} is measured as percentage of the current hemoglobin value [16].

Falsely elevated hemoglobin A_{1c} concentrations can be found due to increased HbF levels in cases of thalassemia or advanced renal failure. In principle, HbA_{1c} has proven to be a reliable parameter for the basic diagnosis of diabetes mellitus without being too liable for interferences. It is also possible to measure other glycosylated proteins such as fructosamine, but assessment is rather difficult. The mean levels of HbA_{1c} in cases of diabetes mellitus differ considerably from those in nondiabetic individuals and are around 12.1% in diabetic coma (range: ∼13–15%). However, the lower portion of the range in case of diabetes mellitus may overlap with the upper portions of the range in nondiabetic cases as it has been shown for the "sum value" [17].

Ketone Bodies

The ketotic type of diabetic coma is characterized by an increased level of ketone bodies in blood and other body fluids (acetone and acetylacetate *ca.* 25–35%, β-hydroxyl-butyrate *ca.* 65–75%; normal values for acetylacetate 0.8–2.4 mg l^{-1}, for β-hydroxyl-butyrate 2.5–9.8 mg l^{-1}). Estimation of acetone may easily be carried out in connection with blood alcohol analysis using headspace chromatography. The normal concentrations for free acetone range from 2.3 to 2.5 mg l^{-1} in nondiabetic patients and may reach 23 mg l^{-1} in diabetics. The levels are almost independent from the postmortem interval [2, 5].

The level of acetone in CSF with diabetes mellitus differs considerably from those seen with nondiabetic causes of death, especially in cases of diabetic coma, with an obvious association regarding an elevated "sum value". If other causes can be ruled out, acetone levels exceeding 5 mg l^{-1} are suspicious of diabetes mellitus. Ketotic coma may be associated with levels higher than 100 mg l^{-1}, but ketonemia is rarely seen if the blood glucose concentration is only 200 mg dl^{-1} and below. According to the author's research, acetone levels in ketotic coma exceed 21 mg l^{-1} in most of the cases, with mean values in this group of 100–150 mg l^{-1}. Single cases may show levels of more than 1000 mg l^{-1}. Nondiabetic factors that might cause elevated ketone levels are, e.g., chronic hepatic and renal diseases, pancreatitis, shock, chronic alcoholism and isopropanol poisoning (levels up to 160 mg l^{-1}) as well as protracted fasting (acetone levels may exceed 5000 mg l^{-1}) [18].

Urine

As the fourth column of postmortem diabetes mellitus diagnostics, an examination of urine can reveal important clues. Urine glucose levels higher than 25 mg dl^{-1} (maximum in healthy individuals) may be indicative of diabetes. Diabetic coma is sometimes associated with urine glucose concentrations above a few 1000 mg dl^{-1}, but usually higher than 500 mg dl^{-1}. These excessively high values only show very small overlapping with other cause of death groups, although positive findings for glucose in urine alone are only of lower value. Glucosuria is a rather frequent nonspecific symptom, e.g., due to brain trauma, myocardial infarction, intoxication, apoplexia, and leukemia. Likewise, glucosuria may be absent even in cases of manifest diabetes mellitus caused by diabetic glomerulosclerosis itself or postmortem degradation. Ketone bodies are likely to be found in urine longer than 24 h postmortem. Concentrations exceeding $0.5\,mg\,dl^{-1} = 5\,mg\,l^{-1}$ of free acetone may be indicative of ketotic dysregulation. However, a positive test for ketonuria is not a proof for ketonemia, because the kidneys have a relatively high clearance rate for ketone bodies. Furthermore, there are multiple conditions that might cause considerable ketonemia (see above). Hyperosmolar coma is typically characterized by a lack of ketonemia (approximately 30% of diabetic comas) [1, 2, 5].

Lactic Acidosis

There are some secondary effects of lactic acidosis that might gain special forensic medical relevance. For example, moving potassium to the extracellular space may cause hyperkalemia (see below). Acidosis decreases the reactivity versus catecholamines with a negative-inotrope effect on the heart. Severe acidosis may result in massive reduction of the kidney blood circulation leading to acute renal failure. Diabetic coma can also cause acidosis by production of β-hydroxyl-butyrate and acetylacetate (see above). Lactic acidosis plays an important role, particularly regarding overlapping with postmortem diagnosis of diabetes mellitus. Considerable amounts of lactic acid are being released during shock and hypoxia, due to poor perfusion caused by diabetes mellitus, following renal failure, hepatic diseases, and ethanol/methanol intake, rarely as complication of a treatment with biguanides or due to severe lack of thiamine with chronic increased alcohol intake. The conditions can be exacerbated by chronic renal failure due to reduced excretion of acids and also by an increased loss of bicarbonate resulting from diarrhea and/or vomiting.

The central causal mechanism is an increased concentration of pyruvate from protein catabolism together with a lack of oxygen, so that energy can still be provided by glycolysis. Accumulation of lactate happens more frequently in diabetics than in other patients what is due to disturbances of oxygen supply and alterations of metabolic activities. The clinical picture is characterized by gastrointestinal discomfort, muscular spasms, central nervous disturbances and deep frequent respiration. The severe type of biguanide-induced lactic acidosis shows a lethality rate of over 50%.

Patients suffering from chronic alcoholism represent a special risk group regarding fatal lactic acidosis and ketotic coma as well. There are often only very few and/or nonspecific morphological findings. On one hand, considerable ketonemia may follow acute alcoholization (free acetone from 74 to $400\,mg\,l^{-1}$), but, on the other hand, high "sum values" may also result in this condition. Their range (*ca.* $294-594\,mg\,dl^{-1}$) can also be associated with fatal diabetic coma. Given the precondition that diabetes mellitus and other competing mechanisms can be ruled out, ketotic coma or lactic acidosis has to be considered as a cause of death in such cases. The lower limiting values for the "sum value" are *ca.* $300-400\,mg\,dl^{-1}$, for acetone in blood around $90\,mg\,l^{-1}$ and 6% for HbA_{1c} [19, 20].

Hypoglycemia (Endogenous vs. Exogenous Hyperinsulinism)

Although fatal hypoglycemia appears to be a rather rare event among forensically examined death cases, they might be the source of serious diagnostic problems. Under clinical conditions, hypoglycemia is diagnosed if the blood glucose level lies below $40\,mg\,dl^{-1}$ *or* if the so-called Whipple's triad can be found. It comprises blood glucose level below $45\,mg\,dl^{-1}$, symptoms of hypoglycemia, which disappear under administration of glucose. Multiple circumstances may be responsible for hypoglycemia in individuals with an empty stomach, e.g., insulinomas and other tumors, severe hepatic diseases, uremia and glycogenoses. The initial manifestation of diabetes mellitus may also be accompanied by reactive hypoglycemia as well as alterations of gastric mobility, vegetative instability, or massive alcohol intake with simultaneous lack of food due to inhibition of gluconeogenesis. The autonomous or glucopenia-associated spectrum of symptoms includes hyperorexia, nausea, restlessness, sweating, tachycardia, endocrine neuropsychologic disorder, primitive automatisms, risk of convulsions, and focal signs with apoplectiform symptoms. The final state with somnolence, coma, and central alterations of respiration and circulation until death has forensic medical relevance.

Hypoglycemias due to exogenous causes are mostly seen with an existing diabetes mellitus. Important mechanisms are accidental or intentional overdosage of insulin or sulfonyl-urea derivates with subsequent reactive hypoglycemia. Such a situation may arise from lack of regular alimentation due to intercurrent diseases without changing the doses of antidiabetic drugs. Other possibilities for hypoglycemias can be interferences with drugs which decrease the blood sugar level indirectly or unusual physical strains. However, types of hypoglycemia with a forensic medical impact are those caused by overdosages of antidiabetics.

The so-called factitious hypoglycemia needs special attention. It is caused by (unnecessary) administration of insulin or sulfonyl-urea derivates and can be seen in connection with psychic alterations (e.g., borderline personality disorder) or suicidal intention. It is rare to find a primary criminal background, e.g., cases of homicide. The most important diagnostic criterion of this type of hypoglycemia is that it happens independently from alimentation. Affected persons often have relations to professional health care or are relatives of known diabetics [21].

The calculation procedure regarding a "sum value" can also be used for the diagnosis of hypoglycemia. Consequently, low sum values in CSF in vitreous humor below *ca.* 50–80 mg dl^{-1} or rather 100–160 mg dl^{-1} are strongly indicative of fatal hypoglycemia. This conclusion is particularly supported by simultaneously high insulin levels suggesting that estimation of insulin levels and also of c-peptide postmortem is essential. In case of endogenous secretion, insulin and c-peptide are both found elevated. If there is exogenous hypoglycemia due to administration of insulin, the level of c-peptide will be noted as much lower than normal. Contrary to this, there are usually increases of insulin and c-peptide concentrations following an intake of sulfonyl-urea derivates, but, in diabetic individuals, often rather high insulin levels can be seen without any indication of hypoglycemia. The procedure has also proven to be reliable in cases of suspected hypoglycemia in car drivers [22, 23].

Postmortem estimations of insulin levels can be carried out by radioimmune assay (RIA) and have revealed levels very similar to those of healthy individuals in blood from a femoral vein and also from the heart. Nevertheless, postmortem concentrations of insulin in blood from the right ventricle may be increased to about 10-fold of normal values due to release of insulin after death. Putrefaction may cause problems as well. Furthermore, single estimations have a wide variation and, therefore, cannot be used

as the only criterion for the diagnosis of insulin-based hypoglycemia. Sometimes it is possible and useful to have a proof of suicidal insulin injection by analyses of the tissues close to the injection site. It is a strict rule that the postmortem diagnosis of hypoglycemias must be based on a combined assessment of different criteria and can only be made "per exclusionem". According to this, especially cardiac diseases, cerebral hemorrhages, pulmonary embolism, strangulation/asphyxia, ruptures of vessels and intoxications have to be ruled out. Estimations of insulin should always be carried out in peripheral venous blood or CSF/vitreous humor because diffusion of insulin from the pancreas via the portal vein might take place postmortem. The "sum value" calculated from glucose and lactate levels is of special importance (see above) [24, 25].

Alterations of Liver Function

In case of an advanced stage of *hepatic cirrhosis* from different causes, it is not rare that there develops an alteration of liver metabolism, often resulting in potentially reversible complications, due to retention of neurotoxic substances in blood with decompensation and final *hepatic failure*. Suspicion may arise from the previous medical history, desolate housing conditions, known alcohol abuse, and sometimes the presence of jaundice. Acute deterioration of hepatic insufficiency with a danger of hepatic coma originates from an increased production of ammonia due to a high portion of proteins in the intestinal contents that may be caused by gastrointestinal hemorrhages (especially esophageal varicosis due to alcoholism), protein-rich nutrition, febrile infections with increased protein catabolism and drugs (e.g., benzodiazepines, analgesics). Clinically, the advanced stage is characterized by permanent drowsiness but patients can be woken up, later on hepatic smell, and electroencephalogram (EEG) alterations. This picture leads to coma with unmistakable "foetor hepaticus" and massive EEG changes until fatal outcome with total hepatic failure [1, 2].

The terms *acute hepatic insufficiency* or *endogenous hepatic coma* describe a failure of the liver function *without previously existing chronic liver disease*. Contrary to the chronic hepatic failure, decompensation can occur suddenly without any indications from the medical history. Important morphological findings are dermal and scleral jaundice and, clinically, disturbances of blood coagulation and consciousness (somnolence, coma). It is especially the fulminant type with a duration of less than seven days, which may gain forensic medical relevance. Important causes are viral hepatitis (65%) and hepatotoxic substances (30%) such as medication (Paracetamol), drugs, chemicals (CCl_4), or poisons from mushrooms (Amanita phalloides). This elucidates the importance of accompanying *toxicological analyses.* Potentially fatal complications may be brain edema (80%; most frequent cause of death), gastrointestinal hemorrhages (50%), as well as hypoglycemia and renal failure with electrolyte imbalances.

The typical enzymes of liver metabolism represent important parameters, which can also be examined postmortem, as well as bilirubin. The daily bilirubin production comes to approximately $510\,\mu mol\,l^{-1}$ ($30\,mg\,dl^{-1}$; normal value up to $1.1\,mg\,dl^{-1}$). Hepatic failure is typically associated with an increased level of serum bilirubin causing jaundice if it exceeds $34\,\mu mol\,l^{-1}$ ($2\,mg\,dl^{-1}$). A differentiation between direct bilirubin bound to biglucuronide and nondirect bilirubin bound to albumin is only useful under clinical aspects. *Postmortem bilirubin levels* may well be compared with those obtained antemortem. Differences are only ranging in the area of $0.1\,mg\,dl^{-1}$, especially in death cases showing jaundice. During the postmortem period, there can be seen a slight but steady increase (*ca.* $0.2\,mg\,dl^{-1}$ after 2 h and $0.7\,mg\,dl^{-1}$ after 20 h). Furthermore, there is an increase of *enzymes typical for the liver (GPT glutamate pyruvate transaminase, GGT gamma glutamyl transferase, and AP alkaline phosphatase)* as well as of *ammonia* ($>100\,mg\,dl^{-1}$; normal value below $0.05\,mg\,dl^{-1}$) primarily not only in blood but also in other body fluids (CSF, vitreous humor). However, clinical reference ranges of values can only be used as a basis for assessment. Most of the bilirubin in CSF belongs to the conjugated type, often associated to hypokalemia and hypoglycemia [6].

Disturbances of Kidney Function

Chronic renal failure represents the result of a nonreversible reduction of the function of both kidneys. Important causes are, e.g., diabetes mellitus (nephropathy, *ca.* 35%), hypertension (*ca.* 25%), chronic inflammations (*ca.* 15%) and abuse of analgetics (*ca.* 1%). The chronic reduction of the renal

function can also show acute decompensation leading to unexpected sudden death, which is not an unusual development during diabetic coma. The *compensated chronic phase* showing only a functional reduction of a low degree and the phase of *compensated retention* (azotemia, creatinine levels up to $6\,mg\,dl^{-1}$) are not associated with symptoms of uremia. Preterminal renal failure with creatinine levels above $8\,mg\,dl^{-1}$ plus symptoms of uremia is called *decompensated retention. Terminal renal failure* (uremia) showing creatinine levels over $10\,mg\,dl^{-1}$ is associated with massive symptomatology of uremia. During the phase of *decompensated retention* (preterminal phase), there may be seen edematous changes, cardiac failure, gastroenteritis due to uremia and neuropathy. The *terminal phase* is characterized by acute life-threatening symptoms, such as neuropathy and encephalopathy, overhydration with pulmonary edema, bleeding tendency, coma, and death (see Table 2).

Acute renal failure or acute renal insufficiency represents a mostly *reversible reduction of the renal function* with loss of urine production and increasing retention parameters (urea, creatinine). Fifteen percent of the cases with acute renal failure show polyuria or normuria with an increase of retention values being the only symptom. Without sufficient therapy, e.g., dialysis, acute renal failure mostly has a fatal outcome. Sometimes bilateral necroses of the renal cortex can be seen. There are multiple possible causes for *acute renal failure,* such as alterations of the blood circulation, toxins, medication (antirheumatics, cytostatics, and antibiotics), chemicals (glycols), and inflammatory or vascular processes.

The most critical clinical phase is the third one with polyuria and extensive loss of water/electrolytes and simultaneous increase of urea and creatinine. Fatal complications may occur associated with other organs, e.g., shock lung, cardiac failure and arrhythmia, and cerebral edema with further central nervous complications. The most significant biochemical changes of acute and chronic renal failure are increased levels of urea and creatinine, electrolyte imbalances (often decreased with acute renal failure) and also a reduced concentration of urine [1, 2, 6].

Creatinine

Under postmortem conditions, an increased level of creatinine in CSF and vitreous humor can be indicative of renal failure (normal value $0.6\text{--}1.4\,mg\,dl^{-1}$).

Table 2 Postmortem biochemical values in cases of renal failure (insufficiency)

Dysfunction	Parameter	Clinical values	Compartment	Results
Compensated retention	Creatinine	≤6 mg dl⁻¹		
Preterminal failure (f)		>8 mg dl⁻¹		
Terminal failure		>10 mg dl⁻¹		
RF ruled out			CSF/VH	Creatinine <2.5 mg dl⁻¹
RF possible				2.5–4.0 mg dl⁻¹
RF primary fatal				>4.0 mg dl⁻¹
Normal values (urea–nitrogen)/urea[a]			Blood (heart)	Maximum 179 (83) mg dl⁻¹ (mean value = 102 (47) mg dl⁻¹)
			CSF	Maximum 197 (92) mg dl⁻¹ (mean value = 89 (41) mg dl⁻¹)
Uremia (urea–nitrogen)/urea[a]) dysfunction[b])		(First 13 hpm)	Blood and CSF	>200 mg dl⁻¹ (93)
		CSF/blood (heart) Urea	CSF Creatinine	Blood (heart) Creatinine
RF ruled out		<100 mg dl⁻¹	<2.5 mg dl⁻¹	<3.5 mg dl⁻¹
RF possible		100–200 mg dl⁻¹	2.5–4.0 mg dl⁻¹	3.0–4.5 mg dl⁻¹
RF primary fatal		>200 mg dl⁻¹	>4.0 mg dl⁻¹	>4.5 mg dl⁻¹

RF, renal failure; CSF, cerebrospinal fluid; VH, vitreous humor; pm, postmortem

[a] Urea–nitrogen × 2148 (mg dl⁻¹) = urea (mg dl⁻¹)

[b] Different method of assessment (see text and references)

During the early postmortem interval, the creatinine concentration is rather stable. In healthy individuals, the mean values are 1.6 mg dl⁻¹ (8 h postmortem), 1–2 mg dl⁻¹ (12 h postmortem) and 3–4 mg dl⁻¹ (24 h postmortem). Therefore, reliable assessment is possible for pathological levels if the specimens are obtained during the early postmortem period.

Renal failure can be ruled out if the creatinine level is below 2.5 mg dl⁻¹. It is possible if its concentration ranges between 2.5 and 4.0 mg dl⁻¹ and renal failure is to be considered as the primary cause of death with levels exceeding 4.0 mg dl⁻¹, given CSF being obtained within the first hours postmortem. After death, the normal relation between creatinine levels in serum and CSF remains almost the same.

On one hand, problems may arise from a connection between renal damage and creatinine level. On the other hand, high creatinine values are seen without any or only slight alterations of the kidneys. However, there is also the possibility that advanced kidney damage coincides with levels below 4 mg dl⁻¹. It must be pointed out that disturbances of the circulation and toxicemia may cause creatinine retention but that partial renal function can still be in place during uremia [6].

Urea

In case of renal failure, there exists a close relation between the levels of urea in serum and CSF (normal range: 13.8–34.6 mg dl⁻¹). The urea level in CSF is approximately three fourths of the serum value. However, there have been reported reduced levels in CSF and also slight increases in blood from the femoral veins and also in liquor compared to antemortem values and also independent from the cause of death. If renal diseases can be excluded, such changes may be due to agonal or postmortem effects. Furthermore, there is a rising difference between the concentrations of urea in liquor and blood with the postmortem interval increasing. Often postmortem values are slightly higher compared to intravital estimations. However, this increase is lower if the intravital concentration has been rather high. In case of manifest renal insufficiency, possibly with uremia, there are usually considerable differences to the levels found in healthy individuals.

There is an arithmetical connection between urea–nitrogen and urea, which is as follows: urea–nitrogen $\times 2.148\,(\mathrm{mg\,dl}^{-1}) = \mathrm{urea}\,(\mathrm{mg\,dl}^{-1})$. Urea levels in CSF above $20\,\mathrm{mg\,dl}^{-1}$ ($9.3\,\mathrm{mg\,dl}^{-1}$ urea–nitrogen) are indicative of renal disease, whereas the postmortem "normal values" for blood from the heart is $179\,\mathrm{mg\,dl}^{-1}$ maximum ($83\,\mathrm{mg\,dl}^{-1}$ urea–nitrogen), with a mean value of $102\,\mathrm{mg\,dl}^{-1}$ ($47\,\mathrm{mg\,dl}^{-1}$ urea–nitrogen). The corresponding concentrations in CSF are $197\,\mathrm{mgYdl}^{-1}$ ($92\,\mathrm{mg\,dl}^{-1}$ urea–nitrogen) with a mean value of $89\,\mathrm{mg\,dl}^{-1}$ ($41\,\mathrm{mg\,dl}^{-1}$ urea–nitrogen). Contrary to this, urea levels in CSF and blood from the heart do usually exceed $200\,\mathrm{mg\,dl}^{-1}$ ($93\,\mathrm{mg\,dl}^{-1}$ urea–nitrogen) during the first $13\,\mathrm{h}$ postmortem in the case of uremia from all imaginable causes [26].

Diagnosis

Postmortem estimation of creatinine and urea levels in blood from the heart (left ventricle preferred) and CSF have important relevance regarding the postmortem diagnosis of renal failure. The following ranges of values can be differentiated for a practicable combined diagnostic procedure:

Urea below $100\,\mathrm{mg\,dl}^{-1}$ in CSF/blood, creatinine below $2.5\,\mathrm{mg\,dl}^{-1}$ in liquor and below $3.5\,\mathrm{mg\,dl}^{-1}$ in blood: renal failure can be excluded.

Urea $100–200\,\mathrm{mg\,dl}^{-1}$ in CSF/blood: renal failure possible if there is an additional creatinine level of $2.5–4.0\,\mathrm{mg\,dl}^{-1}$ in liquor and of $3.0–4.5\,\mathrm{m\,gdl}^{-1}$ in blood from the heart. Urea above $200\,\mathrm{mg\,dl}^{-1}$ in CSF or blood: renal failure represents the primary cause of death if creatinine levels in liquor simultaneously exceed 4.0 and $4.5\,\mathrm{mg\,dl}^{-1}$ in blood from the heart [2, 6].

Water- and Electrolyte Imbalances

The regulation of the water and electrolyte balance aims to maintain *isotonia* and *isovolumia* within the intravasal space. Sodium, chloride, and bicarbonate show the highest extracellular concentrations, whereas potassium and phosphoric esters predominate in the intracellular space. Owing to the fact that the relation between extracellular fluid volume and water exchange is much lower in *infants* than in adults, water imbalances may develop much earlier and be life-threatening.

It is not rare that electrolyte imbalances occur due to other diseases such as diabetes mellitus, chronic alcoholism, and nutritive disturbances. There are some types of dysregulations, which can lead to sudden unexpected death and may therefore be of forensic medical relevance. *Isotonic dehydration* is characterized by extracellular loss of sodium and water in isotonic relation, e.g., during the polyuric phase of acute and chronic renal failure, vomiting and diarrhea, pancreatitis and peritonitis, and due to dermal loss (following burn injuries). The main mechanism of *hypotonic dehydration* is salt depletion together with extracellular deficit of water. Delirium and convulsions are typical cerebral symptoms, which have to be considered as causes of sudden death. *Hypertonic dehydration* (with hypernatremia) leads to a deficit of free water in the extracellular and also in the intracellular space and is caused e.g., by a lack of water supply, dermal loss (sweating), and also via the lungs (e.g., hyperventilation from infections and fever), the kidneys (diabetic coma), and the gastrointestinal tract (diarrhea, vomiting). The typical morphology comprises tinting of the skin, sunken eyes, dry surface of the galea and/or dry cutting areas of organs. A biochemical pattern was proposed as diagnostic tool. The so-called dehydration pattern consists of an elevation of sodium $>155\,\mathrm{mmol\,l}^{-1}$, chloride $>135\,\mathrm{mmol\,l}^{-1}$, and urea $>40\,\mathrm{mg\,dl}^{-1}$. Persisting imbalances also result in corresponding alterations within the CSF (osmotic gradient) [27, 28].

Regarding the postmortem diagnosis of *water and electrolyte imbalances,* measurements of the pH is of no value. Estimations of electrolytes in CSF and vitreous humor can only be of limited meaningfulness. On one hand, the pH strongly depends on the state of the body, and, on the other hand, liquor often becomes sanguinolent when it is obtained so that there may be considerable alterations especially to electrolytes. Centrifugation may be of certain help, but cannot remove all components originating from damaged erythrocytes. This is why liquor from the lateral ventricles should be obtained, because after

12–24 h there are no differences to lumbar liquor [29].

Potassium

Disturbances of the potassium balance can gain forensic medical relevance because they have been described to occur not only isolated but also in connection with other diseases and sudden death (acute myocardial failure due to arrhythmias). Particularly, intestinal or renal loss or insulin treatment of diabetic coma are likely to result in *hypokalemia* (<3.6 mmol l^{-1}). The main causes of *hyperkalemia* (>5.0 mmol l^{-1}) are acute renal failure, chronic renal insufficiency, or extensive tissue damages. The main possible complications are disturbances of conduction, ventricular flutter, and fibrillation, which may lead to asystolia (acute danger to life with potassium levels >6.5 mmol l^{-1}) [1, 2, 6].

Estimation of potassium in blood and serum specimens obtained postmortem have proven not to be reliable due to extremely fast and intense potassium release from cytolysis. In CSF, the potassium value can reach up to sevenfold of the normal level within the first 10 h postmortem, but the range of variation is rather wide. The potassium content of liquor is, to a large extent, independent from the serum level and in infants lower than in adults (normal range: *ca.* $2.1–4.6$ mmol l^{-1}). Contrary to this, the increase of the potassium concentration in vitreous humor has been reported to be regular. This can provide certain conclusions regarding the time of death within the first 12 h postmortem. There seem to be no other relevant disturbances from other diseases on the potassium content of vitreous humor except hepatic failure. Furthermore, there do not exist any comprehensible associations between the concentration differences of sodium and potassium, which appear to allow further reliable conclusions [30–34].

Sodium/Chloride

There is an extracellular decrease of *sodium* parallel to an increase of potassium (see above) postmortem. As a general rule, there is a variation of the sodium level within CSF mostly corresponding to the serum concentration (*ca.* $128–157$ mmol l^{-1}), except situations with severe infections of the central nervous system.

Without differentiation regarding the mechanisms of death, sodium levels in CSF and serum are usually found within the normal range, but the variation range differs considerably from intravital values (*ca.* $123–205$ mmol l^{-1}). Although there is a distinct decrease of sodium in CSF and serum after death, its concentration in vitreous humor remains rather stable up to 30 h postmortem, followed by an almost linear decrease in the following 50 h. Sodium levels above 155 mmol l^{-1} and below 130 mmol l^{-1} in adults and larger differences outwith the normal range in children can be indicative of hypernatremia or hyponatremia antemortem. Sodium levels in *fluid obtained from the pericardial sac* show distinct correlation to the postmortem interval, namely, a decrease of approximately 0.4 mmol l^{-1} during the first 85 h after death, but also with a wide range of variation.

The level of *chloride* in CSF is approximately 20% higher compared to serum and shows a range of *ca.* $110–129$ mmol l^{-1} in healthy individuals. The postmortem changes of chloride are comparable to those of sodium (see above), so that there happens also a typical decrease of the chloride concentration in plasma and CSF. The levels of chloride and sodium in vitreous humor appear to be almost "parallel" and remain nearly constant for over 30 h postmortem. However, any close correlations between chloride values and causes of death or time could not be identified postmortem.

Calcium

The homoeostasis of calcium has an important impact onto the neuromuscular conduction. *Hypocalcemia* (total Ca <2.2 mmol l^{-1}, ionized Ca <1.1 mmol l^{-1}) results in pathological reflexes or arrhythmia. Causes of *hypocalcemia* (total Ca >2.7 mmol l^{-1}, ionized Ca >1.3 mmol l^{-1}) are chronic osteolytic or endocrine processes in most of the cases, which may be the reason for sudden unexpected deaths via electrolyte imbalances with arrhythmias, somnolence, and coma.

Under postmortem conditions, the serum calcium concentration is constant for *ca.* 10 h with a slight increase thereafter (normal range in healthy individuals: $1.96–2.60$ mmol l^{-1}). The calcium contents of CSF reflect approximately the serum level of ionized calcium. In vitreous humor, calcium levels are much more stable and there is less influence of agonal and postmortem effects [1, 2].

Diagnosis

Postmortem diagnosis of imbalances of electrolyte and water metabolism cannot be based on isolated single parameters. Assessment must always include a synopsis of different values. Furthermore, the postmortem interval has to be taken into account in each case. Postmortem biochemical analyses regarding electrolyte imbalances are believed to be most successful in cases being characterized by elevations of parameters such as states of dehydration. One main disadvantage are the wide range of variation referred to single analyze results. This requires a combined interpretation of different values with consideration of all morphological and toxicological findings as well as the possibility of combined dysregulations (e.g., kidney and glucose metabolism).

High Excitation and Hypothermia

A state of *high excitation* is characterized by a massive release of catecholamines, especially in situations with mechanical restraints and also in cases of prolonged agony. Such stress situations can be classified by estimation of adrenaline and noradrenaline levels using high performance liquid chromatography (HPLC) in serum, CSF, and vitreous humor. Analyses in different compartments is useful to achieve semi-quantification of the intensity of stress and its impact on the mechanism of death.

Particularly increased noradrenaline levels in CSF and vitreous humor are indicative of a protracted stress reaction. The author's research has revealed massively increased catecholamine concentrations, partly exceeding the normal ranges many times (adrenaline values in vitreous humor and CSF $100-8000 \, \mathrm{ng} \, \mathrm{l}^{-1}$; noradrenaline levels $4000-70\,000$ $\mathrm{ng} \, \mathrm{l}^{-1}$ (normal ranges in serum: adrenaline $20-120$ $\mathrm{ng} \, \mathrm{l}^{-1}$ and noradrenaline $150-170 \, \mathrm{ng} \, \mathrm{l}^{-1}$)). Especially high noradrenaline levels indicate a longer duration of stress [35–37].

Hypothermia can also cause a massive release of catecholamines in the sense of intense stress. The levels are within the ranges of high excitation with the noradrenaline concentrations being considerably higher than those of adrenaline (10- to 32-fold) comparable to cases with prolonged agony. Contrary to this, adrenaline levels often exceed those of noradrenaline in death cases with short agony. Death due to hypothermia results in mean

quotients adrenaline/noradrenaline considerably <1, whereas quotients >1 are typical for short agony (e.g., myocardial infarction, head trauma) being indicative of higher adrenaline levels [38].

Additional analyses of volatile substances (ethanol, methanol, propanol-1, propanol-2, and acetone) usually show elevated acetone concentrations in all compartments being indicative of hypothermia, but basically only in cases that are ethanol-free. Acetone and propanol-2 are then altered equally. If relevant alcoholization is found, both substances can only be found in very low or physiological ranges that is indicative of an antilipolytic effect of ethanol (acetone $>35 \, \mathrm{mg} \, \mathrm{l}^{-1}$ if blood alcohol level is $<10 \, \mathrm{mg} \, \mathrm{dl}^{-1}$ vs. $<5 \, \mathrm{mg} \, \mathrm{l}^{-1}$ if blood alcohol level is $>185 \, \mathrm{mg} \, \mathrm{dl}^{-1}$) [39].

Conclusions and Final View

Regarding the postmortem diagnosis of *fatal diabetic coma*, morphological findings are only of indicative value. Therefore the diagnosis "death due to diabetic coma" always has to be a *synopsis comprising medical history, macromorphology and histology completed by postmortem biochemistry.* Specimens (CSF, vitreous humor, blood, and urine) should be obtained if there is any suspicion on disturbances of the glucose metabolism. Parameters of major relevance are "sum value" and hemoglobin A_{1c}, which are found to be elevated in most cases of fatal coma (above $415 \, \mathrm{mg} \, \mathrm{dl}^{-1}$ and 12.1%, respectively). The level of free acetone usually exceeds $21 \, \mathrm{mg} \, \mathrm{l}^{-1}$ and urine glucose concentration exceeds $500 \, \mathrm{mg} \, \mathrm{dl}^{-1}$. A correct diagnosis always requires a combination of a minimum of three positive values e.g., increased "sum value", hemoglobin A_{1c} positive, and elevated acetone concentration *or* increased "sum value" and several indicative findings within macromorphology and histology (*see also* **Natural Causes of Sudden Death: Noncardiac**).

Under forensic medical aspects, the diagnosis of fatal diabetic coma can only be made *per exclusionem*. Consequently, other mechanisms of death, e.g., intoxications, have to be ruled out. However, overlapping with other causes of death appears to be rather typical and common. Owing to the fact that the whole diagnostic procedure can only be carried out *per exclusionem,* the only area of overlapping causing problems is that with "natural causes of death" because myocardial infarctions or pulmonary embolism may both represent real complications of diabetic coma and can as well cause metabolic decompensation to preexisting diabetes mellitus. Especially in cases with acute myocardial infarctions differentiation may be problematic, but contrary to such acute changes, the situation is different with chronic alterations as e.g., narrowing coronary arteriosclerosis or myocardial scars. With such preconditions, the higher the relevance of positive biochemical findings is, the more intensive they appear to be (very high "sum value" and acetone level, etc.).

Postmortem biochemical examinations can also provide help in cases without morphological causes of death outwith the field of diabetes mellitus so that specimens of body fluids should also be obtained. Often analyses on certain parameters sensibly complement postmortem morphological diagnostics as in cases of liver disease, chronic renal failure, and electrolyte imbalances. Preliminary studies have also been carried out on the usefulness of other body compartments (e.g., synovial fluid) for a range of examinations as well as for further biochemical parameters (e.g., troponin T) [40, 41].

It has to be mentioned that urea levels in blood and CSF are likely to be elevated in case of *chronic kidney disease* and furthermore slightly following death, but this increase has been found to be considerably lower in liquor compared to blood. Postmortem diagnosis of renal insufficiency can be made with urea levels above $200 \, \text{mg} \, \text{dl}^{-1}$ (urea-nitrogen in excess of $93 \, \text{mg} \, \text{dl}^{-1}$). Creatinine concentrations seem to remain widely unaltered in all body fluids postmortem. The most reliable examinations are possible in CSF with a level below $1.6 \, \text{mg} \, \text{dl}^{-1}$, expected to be typical in individuals without kidney disease. However, postmortem biochemistry can only represent one pillar of the procedure to establish the cause of death as such results are unsuitable to be used as the only diagnostic criterion.

Especially, a combined spectrum of postmortem biochemical values is of most relevant meaningfulness, regarding the diagnosis of fatal metabolic disturbances. They may be strongly indicative of chronic or acute mechanisms and diseases, although, of course, no clinical diagnoses based on postmortem findings can be made. *Exclusion of any competitive mechanisms* is of special importance. A final diagnose regarding the cause of death can only be made by the inclusion of medical history, macromorphology, histology findings, postmortem biochemical results, and toxicology and *per exclusionem* only.

References

[1] Kernbach-Wighton, G. (2003). The diagnosis of functional causes of death, in *Practice of Legal Medicine*, B. Madea, ed, Springer, Berlin, Heidelberg, New York, Tokyo, pp. 239–244.

[2] Kernbach-Wighton, G. (2006). Possibilities of postmortem biochemical diagnostics. Starting points, measurement techniques, evaluation and conclusions, *Rechtsmedizin* **16**, 27–36.

[3] Madea, B. & Musshoff, F. (2007). Postmortem biochemistry, *Forensic Science International* **165**, 165–171.

[4] Coe, J.I. (1972). Use of chemical determinations on vitreous humour in forensic pathology, *Journal of Forensic Sciences* **17**, 541–546.

[5] Kernbach, G. & Brinkmann, B. (1983). Postmortem patho-biochemistry used for the diagnosis of fatal diabetic coma as cause of death, *Der Pathologe* **4**, 235–240.

[6] Kernbach-Wighton, G. (2003). Post mortem biochemical examinations, in *Handbook of Forensic Medicine*, Springer, Berlin, Heidelberg, New York, Tokyo, Vol. 1, pp. 1060–1069.

[7] DiMaio, V.J.M., Sturner, W.Q. & Coe, J.I. (1977). Sudden unexpected deaths after the acute onset of diabetes mellitus, *Journal of Forensic Sciences* **22**, 147–151.

[8] Gormsen, H. & Lund, A. (1985). The diagnostic value of postmortem blood glucose determinations in cases of diabetes mellitus, *Forensic Science International* **28**, 103–107.

[9] Traub, F. (1969). Method for the diagnosis of fatal disturbances of glucose metabolism from post mortem findings (diabetes mellitus and hypoglycemia), *Zentralblatt fuer Allgemeine Pathologie* **112**, 390–399.

[10] Kernbach, G., Püschel, K. & Brinkmann, B. (1986). Biochemical measurements of glucose metabolism in relation to cause of death and postmortem effects, *Zeitschrift für Rechtsmedizin* **96**, 199–213.

[11] De Letter, E.A. & Piette, M.H. (1998). Can routinely combined analysis of glucose and lactate in vitreous humour be useful in current forensic practice? *The American Journal of Forensic Medicine and Pathology* **19**, 335–342.

[12] Gagajewski, A., Murakami, M.M., Kloss, J., Edstrom, M., Hillyer, M., Peterson, G.F., Amatuzio, J. & Apple, F.S. (2004). Measurement of chemical analytes in vitreous humour: stability and precision studies, *Journal of Forensic Sciences* **49**, 371–374.

[13] Karlovsek, M.Z. (2004). Diagnostic values of combined glucose and lactate values in cerebrospinal fluid and vitreous humour-our experiences, *Forensic Science International* **146**(suppl 1), 19–23.

[14] Sippel, H. & Möttönen, M. (1982). Combined glucose and lactate values in vitreous humour for post-mortem diagnosis of diabetes mellitus, *Forensic Science International* **19**, 217–222.

[15] Sturner, W.Q., Sullivan, A. & Suzuki, K. (1983). Lactic acid concentrations in vitreous humour: Their use in asphyxial deaths in children, *Journal of Forensic Sciences* **28**, 222–230.

[16] John, W.G., Scott, K.W.M. & Hawkroft, D.M. (1988). Glycated haemoglobin and glycated protein and glucose concentration in necropsy blood samples, *Journal of Clinical Pathology* **41**, 415–418.

[17] Khun, H.M., Robinson, C.A., Brissie, B.M. & Konrad, R.J. (1999). Post mortem diagnosis of unsuspected diabetes mellitus established by determination of decendent's haemoglobin A1c level, *Journal of Forensic Sciences* **44**, 643–646.

[18] Coe, J.I. (1993). Postmortem chemistry update. Emphasis on forensic application, *The American Journal of Forensic Medicine and Pathology* **14**, 91–117.

[19] Brinkmann, B., Fechner, G., Karger, B. & DuChesne, A. (1998). Ketoacidosis and lactic acidosis – frequent cause of death in chronic alcoholics? *International Journal of Legal Medicine* **111**, 115–119.

[20] Osuna, E., Garcia-Villora, A. & Perez-Carceles, M.D. (1999). Vitreous humour fructosamine concentrations in the autopsy diagnosis of diabetes mellitus, *International Journal of Legal Medicine (Tokyo)* **112**, 275–279.

[21] Kernbach-Wighton, G. & Püschel, K. (1998). On the phenomenology of lethal applications of insulin, *Forensic Science International* **93**, 61–73.

[22] Kernbach-Wighton, G., Sprung, R. & Püschel, K. (2001). On the diagnosis of hypoglycaemia in car drivers – including a review of the literature, *Forensic Science International* **115**, 89–94.

[23] Kernbach-Wighton, G. & Püschel, K. (2003). The evidence of carbohydrate metabolism disturbances in traffic delinquents, *Legal Medicine* **5**, 237–239.

[24] Logemann, E., Pollak, S., Khalaf, A.N. & Petersen, K.G. (1993). Postmortem diagnosis of exogenous insulin administration, *Archiv für Kriminologie* **191**, 28–36.

[25] Winston, D.C. (2000). Suicide via insulin overdose in nondiabetics: the New Mexico experience, *The American Journal of Forensic Medicine and Pathology* **21**, 237–240.

[26] Zhu, B.L., Ishikawa, T., Michiue, T., Tanaka, S., Zhao, D., Li, D.R., Quan, L., Oritani, S. & Maeda, H. (2007). Differences in postmortem urea nitrogen, creatinine and uric acid levels between blood and pericardial fluid in acute death, *Legal Medicine (Tokyo)* **9**, 115–122.

[27] Madea, B. (1996). Post mortem diagnosis of water and electrolyte imbalances, *Rechtsmedizin* **6**, 141–146.

[28] Madea, B. & Lachenmeier, D.W. (2005). Postmortem diagnosis of hypertonic dehydration, *Forensic Science International* **155**, 1–6.

[29] Mulla, A., Massey, K.L. & Kalra, J. (2005). Vitreous humour biochemical constituents: evaluation of between-eye differences, *The American Journal of Forensic Medicine and Pathology* **26**, 146–149.

[30] Henßge, C., Knight, B., Krompecher, T., Madea, B. & Nokes, I. (1995). *The Estimation of the Time of Death in the Early Postmortem Period*, Arnold, London.

[31] James, R.A., Hoadley, P.A. & Sampson, B.G. (1997). Determination of postmortem interval by sampling vitreous humour, *The American Journal of Forensic Medicine and Pathology* **18**, 158–162.

[32] Madea, B., Herrmann, N. & Henßge, C. (1990). Precision of estimating the time since death by vitreous potassium – comparison of two different equations, *Forensic Science International* **46**, 277–284.

[33] Madea, B. & Rödig, H. (2006). Time of death dependent criteria in vitreous humour: accuracy of estimating the time since death, *Forensic Science International* **164**, 87–92.

[34] Rognum, T.O., Hauge, S., Oyasaeter, S. & Saugstad, O.D. (1991). A new biochemical method for estimation of postmortem time, *Forensic Science International* **51**, 139–146.

[35] Zhu, B.L., Ishikawa, T., Michiue, T., Li, D.R., Zhao, D., Quan, L., Oritani, S., Bessho, Y. & Maeda, H. (2007). Postmortem serum catecholamine levels in relation to cause of death, *Forensic Science International* **173**, 122–129.

[36] Kernbach-Wighton, G. & Saternus, K.S. (2004). On the post mortem diagnosis of hypothermia, in *Hypothermia. Clinical, Pathomorphological and Forensic Features. Research in Legal Medicine*, M. Oehmichen, ed, Schmidt-Römhild, Lübeck, Vol. 31, pp. 221–229.

[37] Kernbach-Wighton, G. & Saternus, K.S. (2007). Postmortem biochemical estimations in cases of fatal hypothermia (catecholamines and volatiles), *Romanian Journal of Legal Medicine* **15**, 32–38.

[38] Kernbach-Wighton, G., Sprung, R., Kijewski, H. & Saternus, K.S. (2002). Maximum excitement and sudden death, in *Restraints of Excited Persons. Sudden Death in Hospital and Custody. Research in Legal Medicine*, K.S. Saternus & G. Kernbach-Wighton, eds, Schmidt-Römhild, Lübeck, Vol. 28, pp. 55–74.

[39] Kernbach-Wighton, G. & Saternus, K.S. (2006). Post mortem biochemical estimations in cases of lethal high excitation, *Romanian Journal of Legal Medicine* **14**, 251–261.

[40] Zhu, B.L., Ishikawa, T., Michiue, T., Li, D.R., Zhao, D., Oritani, S., Kamikodai, Y., Tsuda, K., Okazaki, S. & Maeda, H. (2006). Postmortem cardiac troponin T levels in the blood and pericardial fluid. Part 1. Analysis with special regard to traumatic causes of death, *Legal Medicine (Tokyo)* **8**, 86–93.

[41] Madea, B., Kreuser, C. & Banaschak, S. (2001). Postmortem biochemical examination of synovial fluid – a preliminary study, *Forensic Science International* **118**, 29–35.

GERHARD KERNBACH-WIGHTON

Postmortem Interval: Anthropology

One of the most difficult tasks for the forensic anthropologist is establishing the postmortem interval (PMI) – i.e., time since death. The determination of PMI on skeletal remains is affected by enormous limitations, which have to do with the great variability in decomposition rates.

Postmortem phenomena (such as putrefaction and other types of decomposition) severely alter markers, which are essential for the evaluation of the PMI (along with identification of the body, interpretation of manner of disposal of the body, and the manner of death, in particular signs of trauma). To correctly and thoroughly read and interpret human remains in this sense, intrinsic factors (pertaining to the body) may not be sufficient and it is becoming increasingly evident that the environment (i.e., extrinsic factors such as plants, pollen, algae, moulds, macrofauna, and microfauna) may be crucial for answering the question of PMI [1–8]. Much of the difficulty in determining the time since death and/or permanence of a body in a specific environment stems from the lack of systematic observations and research on the decomposition modalities in different environments of the human body. Postmortem changes have been dealt with extensively in the literature but are very specific and bear too little an interdisciplinary approach [1–28]. Many physicochemical changes begin to take place in the body immediately or shortly after death and progress in a fairly orderly manner until the body disintegrates. Each change has its own time factor or rate. Unfortunately, these rates of development of postmortem changes are strongly influenced by unpredictable endogenous and environmental factors. Consequently, the longer the PMI, the wider is the range of estimate as to when the death probably occurred. In other words, the longer the PMI, the less precise is the estimate of the time of death. Shortly after death, enzymes that occur naturally in the body begin the degradation processes (autolysis), subsequent decay by bacteria and fungi is purely aerobic and, ideally, leads to the entire skeletonization of the corpse. According to an old rule of thumb, 1 week of putrefaction in air is equivalent to 2 weeks in water, which is equivalent to 8 weeks buried in the soil, given the same environmental temperature. The interval between the time of death and final skeletonization is governed by the environment in which these processes occur, while the processes of degradation on the soil surface, which is biologically highly active, usually reach completion within several weeks, the time required for the decomposition of interred bodies takes between 3 and 12 years under favorable conditions. Under unfavorable conditions, the processes might require up to a hundred or even thousands of years before completion [29–43]. Once severe decay sets in, tools for determining PMI and permanence in a specific environment move from forensic pathology to forensic anthropology and taphonomy (i.e., the study of decaying organisms over time and the effects environmental factors may have on them) and to the multidisciplinarity of other forensic sciences, more or less well known, such as forensic entomology, forensic botany, zoology, hydrology, etc. In fact, forensic entomology is the only one of these disciplines that has been thoroughly investigated, but may not be sufficient. Taphonomy and other disciplines (such as even biomolecular diagenesis) must take their stand in the medicolegal world in order to solve the above-mentioned issues. This means that a multifactorial approach dealing with intrinsic and extrinsic factors must be sought. Very few studies exist in this sense, perhaps, because the world of natural sciences, anthropology, taphonomy, and forensic medicine are still too far apart. Until now, the following steps have been taken. Tenessee's body farm has led to several observations on decomposition processes of human remains in specific environments, but these deal mainly with macroscopic observations, entomological, and chemical ones. As regards human decomposition processes, sporadic case studies exist on this issue, on the surface, in soil, and in water, which, however, only deal mainly with body intrinsic and entomological factors. Even useful chemical aspects still need to be explored. For example, the articulated processes including physical, chemical, biochemical, and microbiological changes occurring during postmortem events have to be held responsible for the onset of odour. Odour, a complex mixture of volatile compounds, is a complicated and difficult attribute to measure. The electronic nose is an instrument that comprises an array of electronic chemical sensors with a partial specificity and an appropriate recognition system capable of recognizing simple or complex odors. Substantial work has been done to

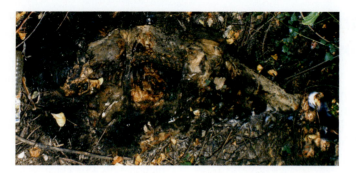

Figure 1   Human remains of a young woman found in a woody area in northern Italy. Much mummified tissue still clings on to the bone surface. Postmortem interval was known to be eight months. Remains were found in spring

apply electronic nose technology for environment and food quality monitoring and evaluation in order to identify, recognize, and discriminate different odors. In food, animal species for human nutrition, spoilage odors as key indicators for fresh or not fresh fish (in conjunction with other factors, such as oxidative changes and growth of microrganisms), and time development of these volatile components in both fish and cereals have been identified. However, no studies are available on the precise identification and possible quantification of odorous molecules from corpses, and this argument at present is the domain of dog conductors, who train dogs to recognize a possible grave localization utilizing their ability to track decomposition odors. The repeatability of cadaver decay in animal models has been treated in an experimental study on the effect of freezing and thawing and on the decomposition of organic matter. Some work has been done for intrinsic changes of the pig body (and some entomology) particularly in forests and in a marine environment, but very few reports combine the data on intrinsic and extrinsic factors. From these few reports, interesting data emerge: the great variability of decomposition and the need to combine decomposition with environmental data. Botany (roots, leaves, and pollen) and zoology (diatoms, plankton, etc.) seem to have a crucial role (Figures 1, 2). The significant contribution of annual growth in woody tissue for PMI estimation has been proven and many have stressed the importance of extrinsic factors – however, the world of combined extrinsic and intrinsic factors still remains uninvestigated.

For the case of skeletonized or partly skeletonized human remains, it is frequently difficult to say whether such remains belong to someone who

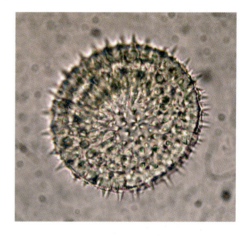

Figure 2   Botanical remains can be of crucial importance. The image shows a grain of pollen in microscopy that denotes the season of deposition on human remains, and therefore a term *antequem non* since death

died 5, 10, 20, or even more years before. Variables dependant on the environment, climate, location, and even animal intervention can seriously modify decomposition rates and preservation of human remains in an unpredictable manner. The exposition to the sun, temperature, climatic rainfall, and wind conditions as well as soil chemical characteristics influence bone surface appearance and may alter PMI estimation.

A rough distinction at times can be made between archaeological and forensic remains. Some scientists claim that it is possible to distinguish among recent bones (less than 10 years), old bones (less than 50 years), and ancient bones according to a more or less dry appearance of the bone. In the past, PMI on bones

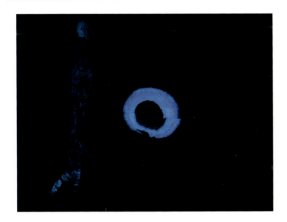

Figure 3   Cross section of a femur with a PMI of 5 years showing a greater degree of fluorescence with UV light

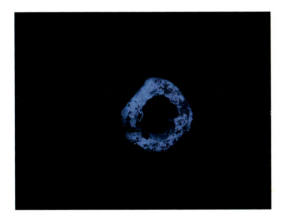

Figure 4   Cross section of a femur with a PMI of 50 years showing a lesser degree of fluorescence with UV light

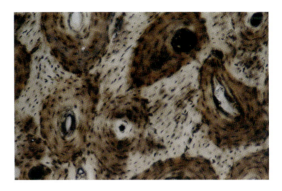

Figure 5   Microscopical aspect (100×) of fresh bone (PMI of several months). The structure of bone is clearly visible

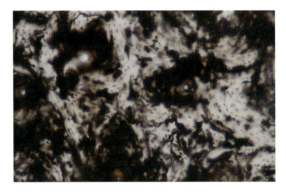

Figure 6   Microscopical aspect (100×) of old bone (PMI of 50 years) that shows severe degradation, destruction of the microscopical structure, and fungal infiltration

has also been estimated according to the quantity of organic material still visible within the bone matrix by illumination with UV light (Figures 3 and 4) or the microscopic appearance of bone (Figures 5 and 6).

These methods, such as the macroscopica appearance, are, however, dependant on too many variables affecting degradation, which may not reflect the actual length of PMI. In other terms, a skeleton with a short PMI may look more degraded, if it was exposed to harsh environmental factors, than a skeleton with a longer PMI with less severe environmental variables. In spite of attempts to standardize fluorescent and microscopic patterns, these tests give no unequivocal classification, and therefore can provide only indicative data on PMI.

This is why in cases of retrieval of skeletal remains, the context becomes fundamental. The botanical analysis of leaves, roots, and seeds on and around the remains, for example, can give a *postquem non* or *antequem non* temporal limit by studying the elements that have colonized the site after the deposition. A PMI indication can also be reached throughout the analysis of clothes and personal belongings found at the site. Entomological study of insects colonizing remains may provide a more accurate indication about the age of deposition; corpses are in fact colonized by different insect populations in accordance with season, climatic conditions, environmental characteristics, and decomposition stage.

Radiochemical tests are another, more expensive, tool by which the anthropologist may try to determine PMI [35–43]. These are based on the decay rates of radioisotopes fixed in bone during life. The use of Carbon-14 provides accurate information about the PMI in case of archeological remains, but its importance in forensic material is reduced because its before period (BP) date refers to the 1950s. Strontium 90 may also be useful; its high atmospheric concentration is due to massive explosions and nuclear weapon pollution that occurred during World War II. Another method benefits from the high levels of artificially introduced Carbon-14 in terrestrial organisms by thermonuclear devices between 1950 and 1963. It is based on the observation that different tissues of the body have a diverse time of development and a diverse turnover rate. Quantifying radiocarbon values in different tissues and placing these values in the bomb-curve, taking care of noting the age of the individual and other factors, allows an estimation of the date of death.

All such methods, however, still need calibration and testing for contamination – and remain exclusive to few laboratories and are quite expensive.

References

[1] Anderson, G.S. & Hobischak, N.R. (2004). Decomposition of carrion in the marine environment in British Columbia, *Canadian International Journal of Legal Medicine* **118**(4), 206–209.

[2] Archer, M.S. (2004). Rainfall and temperature effects on the decomposition rate of exposed neonatal remains, *Science and Justice* **44**(1), 35–41.

[3] Aturaliya, S. & Lukasewycz, A. (1999). Experimental forensic and bioanthropological aspects of soft tissue taphonomy: 1. Factors influencing postmortem tissue desiccation rate, *Journal of Forensic Sciences* **44**(5), 893–896.

[4] Bell, L.S., Skinner, M.F. & Jones, S.J. (1996). The speed of postmortem change to the human skeleton and its taphonomic significance, *Forensic Science International* **82**(2), 129–140.

[5] Boddingtom, A., Garland, A.N. & Janaway, R.C. (1987). *Death, Decay and Reconstruction*, Manchester University Press, Manchester.

[6] Clark, K., Evans, L. & Wall, R. (2006). Growth rates of the blowfly, *Lucilia sericata*, on different body tissues, *Forensic Science International* **156**(2–3), 145–149.

[7] Coe, J.I. (1973). Postmortem chemistry: practical considerations and a review of literature, *Journal of Forensic Sciences* **19**, 13–32.

[8] Courtin, G.M. & Fairgrieve, S.L. (2004). Estimation of postmortem interval (PMI) as revealed through the analysis of annual growth in woody tissue, *Journal of Forensic Sciences* **49**(4), 781–783.

[9] Evans, W.E. (1963). *The Chemistry of Death*, CC Thomas, Springfield.

[10] Galloway, A., Birkby, W., Jones, A.M., Henry, T.E. & Parks, B.O. (1989). Decay rates of human remains in an arid environment, *Journal of Forensic Sciences* **34**(3), 607–616.

[11] Catts, E.P. & Goff, M.L. (1992). Forensic entomology in criminal investigations, *Annual Review of Entomology* **37**, 253–272.

[12] Haglund, W.D. (1988). Contribution of rodents to postmortem artifacts of bone in animal scavenged human skeletons, *Journal of Forensic Sciences* **33**(4), 985–997.

[13] Haglund, W.D. (1993). Disappearance of soft tissue and the disarticulation of human remains from aqueous environments, *Journal of Forensic Sciences* **38**(4), 806–815.

[14] Haglund, W.D. (1997). Dogs and coyotes: post-mortem involvement with human remains, in *The Postmortem Fate of Human Remains*, W.D. Haglund & M.H. Sorg, eds, CRC Press, Boca Raton.

[15] Haglund, W.D. & Reay, D.T. (1993). Problems of recovering partial human remains at different times and locations: concerns for death investigators, *Journal of Forensic Sciences* **38**(1), 69–89.

[16] Haglund, W.D., Reay, D.T. & Swindler, D.R. (1989). Canid scavenging/disarticulation sequence of human remains in the Pacific Northwest, *Journal of Forensic Sciences* **34**(3), 587–606.

[17] Haglund, W.D. & Sorg, M.H. (1997). *The Postmortem Fate of Human Remains*, CRC Press, Boca Raton.

[18] Haglund, W.D. & Sorg, M.H. (2002). *Advances in Forensic Taphonomy*, CRC Press, Boca Raton.

[19] Hobishak, N.R. & Anderson, G.S. (2002). Time of submergence using acquatic invertebrate succession as markers of decompositional change, *Journal of Forensic Sciences* **47**(1), 142–151.

[20] Huntington, T.E., Higley, L.G. & Baxendale, F.P. (2007). Maggot development during morgue storage and its effect on estimating the post-mortem interval, *Journal of Forensic Sciences* **52**(2), 453–458.

[21] Introna, F., Di Vella, G. & Campobasso, C.P. (1999). Determination of postmortem interval from old skeletal remains by image analysis of luminol test results, *Journal of Forensic Sciences* **44**(3), 535–538.

[22] Kahana, T., Almog, J., Levy, J., Schmeltzer, E., Spier, Y. & Hiss, J. (1999). Marine taphonomy: adipocere formation in as eries of bodies recovered from a single shipwreck, *Journal of Forensic Sciences* **44**(5), 897–901.

[23] Lopes de Carvalho, L.M. & Linhares, A.X. (2001). Seasonality of insect succession and pig carcass decomposition in natural forest area in southeastern Brazil, *Journal of Forensic Sciences* **46**(3), 604–608.

[24] Mann, R.M., Bass, W.M. & Meadows, L. (1990). Time since death and decomposition of the human body: variables and observations in case and experimental field studies, *Journal of Forensic Sciences* **35**(1), 103–111.

[25] Micozzi, M.S. (1986). Experimental study of postmortem change under field conditions: effects of freezing, thawing and mechanical injury, *Journal of Forensic Sciences* **31**(3), 953–961.

[26] Micozzi, M.S. (1991). *Postmortem Change in Human and Animal Remains*, Charles C Thomas Publisher, Springfield.

[27] Pollard, A.M. (1997). Dating the time of death, in *Studies in Crime: An Introduction to Forensic Archaeology*, J. Hunter, C. Roberts & A. Martin, eds, BT Batsford, London.

[28] Prieto, J.L., Magana, C. & Ubelaker, D.H. (2004). Interpretation of postmortem change in cadavers in Spain, *Journal of Forensic Sciences* **49**(5), 918–923.

[29] Rodriguez, W.C. & Bass, W.M. (1983). Insect activity and its relationship to decay rates of human cadavers in East Tennessee, *Journal of Forensic Sciences* **28**, 423.

[30] Sledzik, P.S. (1998). Forensic taphonomy: postmortem decomposition and decay, in *Forensic Osteology: Advances in the Identification of Human Remains*, K.J. Reichs, ed, Charles C Thomas Publisher, Springfield.

[31] Sorg, M.H., Dearborn, J.H., Monahan, E., Ryan, H.F., Sweeney, K.G. & David, E. (1997). Forensic taphonomy in marine contexts, in *The Postmortem Fate of Human Remains*, W.D. Haglund & M.H. Sorg, eds, CRC Press.

[32] Spenneman, D.H. & Franke, B. (1995). Decomposition of buried human bodies and associated death scene materials on coral atolls in the tropical Pacific, *Journal of Forensic Sciences* **40**(3), 356–367.

[33] Swift, B., Lauder, I., Black, S. & Norris, J. (2001). An estimation of the post-mortem interval in human skeletal remains: a radionuclide and trace element approach, *Forensic Science International* **117**(1–2), 73–87.

[34] Swift, B. (1998). Dating human skeletal remains: investigating the viability of measuring the equilibrium between ^{210}Po and ^{210}Pb as a means of estimating the post-mortem interval, *Forensic Science International* **98**(1–2), 119–126.

[35] Turner, B. & Wiltshire, P. (1999). Experimental validation of forensic evidence: a study of the decomposition of buried pigs in a heavy clay soil, *Forensic Science International* **101**(2), 113–122.

[36] Ubelaker, D.H. (2001). Artificial radiocarbon as an indicator of recent origin of organic remains in forensic case, *Journal of Forensic Science* **46**(6), 1285–1287.

[37] Vass, A.A., Barshick, S.A. & Sega, G. (2002). *et al.* Decomposition chemistry of human remains: a new methodology for determining the postmortem interval, *Journal of Forensic Sciences* **47**(3), 542–553.

[38] Vass, A.A. (2001). Beyond the grave: understanding human decomposition, *Microbiology Today* **28**, 190–192.

[39] Vass, A.A., Bass, W.M., Wolt, J., Foss, J. & Ammons, J. (1992). Time since death determinations of human cadavers using soil solution, *Journal of Forensic Sciences* **37**(5), 1236–1253.

[40] Vass, A.A., Smith, R.R., Thompson, C.V., Burnett, M.N., Dennis, A., Synstelien, J.A., Dulgerian, N. & Eckenrode, B.A. (2004). Decompositional odor analysis database, *Journal of Forensic Sciences* **49**(4), 760–769.

[41] Verhoff, M.A., Wiesbrock, U.O. & Kreutz, K. (2004). Macroscopic findings for the exclusion of a forensic relevant soil embedded resting period in skeletal remains – an approach based upon literature, *Archiv fur Kriminologie* **213**(1–2), 1–14.

[42] Willey, P. & Heiman, A. (1987). Estimating time since death using plant roots and stems, *Journal of Forensic Sciences* **32**, 1264.

[43] Yoshino, M., Kimijima, T., Miyasaka, S., Sato, H. & Seta, S. (1991). Microscopical study on estimation of time since death in skeletal remains, *Forensic Science International* **49**(2), 143–158.

Related Articles

Anthropology

Botany

Entomology

CRISTINA CATTANEO AND DANIELE GIBELLI

Postmortem Toxicology: Analysis

see Postmortem Toxicology: Laboratory Analysis

Postmortem Toxicology: Artifacts

Introduction

In unnatural, sudden, violent, or unexpected deaths, the investigator often needs evidence whether a foreign compound is present in autopsy material. Moreover, quantification of a drug is necessary to state whether its amount is sufficient to cause, prevent, or be involved directly in the death [1]. The interpretation of an analytical result is often the most difficult aspect of forensic toxicology. It is different from the situation in clinical toxicology, and largely dependent on the type and quality of specimens provided as well as on storage and analytical procedures [2, 3]. Interpretation and evaluation may become more difficult in decomposed or embalmed cases. Nevertheless, in these cases, drug degradation or formation of artifacts is more likely to be expected [4, 5].

Artifacts in forensic postmortem toxicology are substances or drug concentrations present in body fluids or tissues during analysis that do not correspond to the genuine drug or drug level present in the body at the time of death. Because of the immediate history of the treatment of the deceased, the postmortem time period as well as the collection, storage, processing, and analysis of postmortem specimens, these artifacts remain an inherent part of postmortem forensic toxicology. For the analyst, postmortem artifacts may be an intricate and demanding challenge. To avoid errors in the evaluation of an analytical result, it is essential to be aware of and to identify artifacts.

This article illustrates various individual artifacts, explains their origin, and discusses techniques to recognize them and minimize their effects.

Antemortem Factors

In death investigation, quantification of a foreign substance is often necessary to state whether the amount of a particular compound is compatible with fatal poisoning or more in accordance with therapeutic concentrations in the underlying case [6]. In living beings, basic pharmacokinetic concepts and models provide estimates of the quantitative relationship between the dose of a drug and the observed blood or tissue concentration. This field is concerned with drug liberation, absorption, distribution, metabolism, and excretion as well as the relationship of these processes to the intensity and time course of the drug's therapeutic and adverse effects. A large pharmacologic variability can be observed in living individuals. Factors likely to contribute to the individual's response to a drug and to influence the disposition of a drug are given in Table 1 [1, 2].

In acute poisoning, death may usually occur before steady state has been reached, and the arterial blood concentration can be appreciably higher than the venous blood concentration. Studies on arteriovenous differences in drug concentrations during lifetime are rare, most comprehensive data for humans are provided by Chiou [7]. For example, arterial plasma concentrations of amitriptyline were found to be up

Table 1 Factors likely to contribute to pharmacokinetic variability [1, 2]

Different preparations of the drug and clandestine manufacture
Dose, route of administration, and frequency
Pharmacokinetics
Age, gender, race, and genetic disposition
Body weight, exercise, nutrition, condition, and disease state
Genetic variation in drug metabolism
Tolerance
Coadministration of other drugs or alcohol

to fourfold greater than venous concentrations during the absorption/distribution phase. With diazepam and lidocaine, the initial arteriovenous differences were of approximately 2 orders of magnitude and lasted for about 60 min after dosing.

Disease affects the way drugs are absorbed, distributed, metabolized, and excreted. The liver and the kidneys play a central role in the disposition kinetics of most drugs [8]. Patients with renal disease excrete considerably less unchanged drugs than patients with normal renal function. If a drug is only eliminated by hepatic metabolism, however, its clearance should not be markedly altered. This rather simple theory does not apply to all metabolized drugs. For example, patients with impaired renal function may experience severe and prolonged respiratory depression when treated with morphine. Although morphine's metabolism and excretion is not impaired in renal insufficiency, accumulation of morphine-6-glucuronide occurs. There is evidence that morphine-6-glucuronide is an active metabolite [9]. Sulfonurea drugs, such as glibenclamide, are likely to cause significant hypoglycemia due to accumulation of the active metabolite in renal insufficiency [10]. The effects of liver disease on the pharmacokinetics of drugs are unpredictable due to multiple effects that liver disease produces. In alcoholic cirrhosis, the half-life of diazepam is increased about fourfold over control values [11]. An impaired metabolism and changes in the apparent volume of distribution with chlordiazepoxide have also been observed in severe liver disease, but not with oxazepam and lorazepam, whose elimination involves glucuronidation only [12]. Liver dysfunction also affects hepatic blood flow, which is important in the disposition of drugs with a high hepatic extraction ratio [13]. For example, the coefficient of variation for morphine serum concentrations during four consecutive days of stable oral morphine treatment at stable clinical symptoms ranged from 13 to 103% [14]. This day-to-day variation has been attributed to fluctuations in hepatic blood flow [15].

Not only is a high degree of variability routinely found between subjects, but a wide range of blood levels may also be seen in the same subject taking a drug on different occasions. The renal clearance of digoxin is significantly lower during a period of immobilization than during a period of normal physical activity leading to an artifactual increase in digoxin concentration [16]. A large pharmacokinetic variability is consistently observed with drugs that are subject to a substantial presystemic metabolism and/or a high hepatic clearance such as desipramine, where plasma levels differed by 30-fold in patients treated with 25 mg desipramine orally three times a day [17].

Alcohol is a common finding in medicolegal death investigations. Many drugs interact with alcohol, thereby altering the mechanism or effects of the alcohol and the drug involved [18]. Dorian *et al.* [19] have shown that the area under the curve of both amitriptyline and nortriptyline was increased in the presence of ethanol because of a reduction in amitriptyline hepatic clearance.

At present, drug–drug interactions are widely recognized, although the underlying mechanisms are still far from being fully evaluated [20]. A great deal of variability, both pharmacokinetic and pharmacodynamic, has been seen with midazolam in patients on mechanical ventilation in an intensive care unit [21]. The half-life of midazolam ranged from less than 2 to about 10 h. In addition, it was difficult to establish a relationship between consciousness and the concentration of the drug. These differences were associated with the state of the patient and the variety of coadministered drugs. Far less is known about drug–nutrient interactions resulting in therapeutic failure or drug toxicity [22]. For example, the activities of cytochrome P450 (CYP) 3A4, CYP2C9, and CYP1A2 may be increased by use of St. John's Wort, and kava may inhibit CYP1A2, CYP2D6, and CYP3A4 [23]. Carbamazepine causes a loss of biotin, which may lead to poor seizure control, and plays a role in the drug's adverse effects [24].

In drug overdose or critically ill persons, pharmacokinetics of a drug are likely to be very different from the common subjects of pharmacokinetic reports, due to diminished cardiac output, falling blood pressure, decreased tissue perfusion, impaired ventilation, tissue hypoxia, acidosis, dehydration, as well as renal and hepatic failure. With few exceptions, there is little information on this point. Major changes in the clearance and volume of distribution of morphine were found in trauma and burned patients, and sepsis may induce a decrease in the hepatic metabolism of drugs [25].

Also, formation of endogenous compounds may be considered. An elevated blood isopropanol concentration, which is usually attributed to alcohol misuse, can be observed following physical exercise. Isopropanol is also detectable under pathophysiological conditions in diabetes mellitus, and in liver and gastrointestinal diseases. In these cases, the blood acetone concentration is also increased [26]. In ketotic states, isopropanol may function as a shunt regenerating NAD^+, thus contributing to the maintenance of metabolic stability.

Not only analytical results may be biased by clandestine manufacture of drugs, which are frequently impure or adulterated, but substances present with these drugs can also be classified as diluents, adulterants, impurities of manufacture, and impurities of origin. Adulteration may occur by the addition of bulking agents or to fake the pharmacological effect. For example, lidocaine is a common adulterant in cocaine preparations [27]. A comprehensive overview on clandestine drug synthesis including pharmacological activities associated with the analogs and impurities is given by Soine [28].

The presence of tolerance will usually make interpretation of results difficult. Tolerance may result from a decreased efficacy at the receptor site or an increased metabolism due to enzyme induction. The presence of a drug analyte in blood or urine can be used to document recent exposure only. By providing information on exposure to drugs over time, hair analysis may be useful [29]. Although there are still controversies, particularly concerning drug incorporation, the influence of cosmetic treatment, and external contamination, long-term information on an individual's drug use may be accessible through hair analysis [30, 31].

Effects of treatment during resuscitation or hospitalization may produce artifacts. In persons who have undergone emergency medical treatment, the medication given by the emergency physician should be provided, for, even without restoration of the heart action during cardiopulmonary resuscitation, high concentrations of lidocaine in the left cardiac chamber were observed. Obviously, substantial amounts of intubation-related lidocaine had been absorbed by the trachea during cardiac massage [32]. Treatment with intravenous fluids for a period of time before dying often presents interpretative problems in alcohol and drug findings, and blood and tissues may even be devoid of detectable amounts. Devices that automatically deliver medication by the parenteral route can lead to artificially high blood concentrations postmortem [33]. Transdermal patches, e.g., fentanyl containing devices left on the body, will give rise to locally high drug concentrations of the drug [34].

All these factors affect a drug concentration that will be found in the body after death. However, experience has told that there are many additional and even unique aspects of postmortem changes, which are discussed in the following passage.

Changes Occurring after Death

Postmortem Redistribution

Drug concentration is likely to change after death. Early indications that a change does exist are from Curry and Sunshine [35] reporting large differences in the concentrations of barbiturates in blood obtained from different anatomical sites. A comparison of ante- and postmortem drug levels already indicates that postmortem drug concentrations do not necessarily reflect concentrations at the time of death. A study on six cases revealed postmortem blood concentrations as high as, or higher than the antemortem circulating blood concentration [36]. For example, an 11.7-, 3.9-, and 2.6-fold increase could be noticed for dothiepin, amitriptyline, and methadone in postmortem blood. In general, drugs with wide concentration ranges observed in central (c) and peripheral

(p) blood exhibiting a high c/p ratio tended to have a high postmortem/antemortem concentration **Postmortem Toxicology: Interpretation**. In contrast, no significant difference was observed in samples taken at admission and autopsy in heroin fatalities [37]. At present, the attempt to estimate antemortem concentrations from postmortem measurements is prone to considerable error [38–42].

Knowledge on the mechanisms causing artifactual increases or decreases in drug concentration during the postmortem period is still limited. These changes are gathered under the generic term of *postmortem redistribution*. The underlying mechanisms of postmortem redistribution as far as known have been reviewed by Pelissier-Alicot *et al.* [43], Yarema and Becker [44], and references cited therein. The physicochemical and pharmacokinetic properties of a drug are probably favoring factors. Organs such as the gastrointestinal tract, the lungs, the liver, and the myocardium are major sources of postmortem redistribution. Cell and tissue modification during agony, autolysis, and putrefaction are also involved.

Potential factors that have been recognized to govern postmortem redistribution are summarized in Table 2. It appears that drugs that have an apparent volume of distribution $>3\,l\,kg^{-1}$, and are sequestered in tissue and present in extracellular fluid are candidates for postmortem redistribution. Accordingly, amitriptyline exhibited significant postmortem distribution, whereas morphine and its glucuronides indicated only a trend for higher concentrations in heart blood compared with femoral or subclavian blood [37, 45, 46].

Many drugs are sequestered antemortem in organs, and postmortem redistribution may either occur by diffusion through blood vessels or from the lumen of a body cavity toward surrounding organs. The vascular pathway may depend on the blood remaining fluid after death. Investigations on postmortem

Table 2 Major factors governing postmortem drug distribution

Physicochemical and pharmacokinetic properties of the drug	Size, shape, charge, pK_a, partitioning behavior, lipophilicity, volume of distribution, binding to proteins and/or red cells, affinity toward tissues, decreasing or residual metabolic activity during the perimortem and early postmortem time period
Environmental conditions	Initial concentration, pH, orientation of solute flux, temperature, time, blood coagulation and hypostasis, blood movement due to pressure and fluidity changes, position of the corpse, lysosomal enzyme activities, and bacterial invasion

diffusion from gastric residues in a human cadaver model using amitriptyline, paracetamol, and lithium carbonate revealed high concentrations in liver and lungs, whereas diffusion into gallbladder bile, cardiac, and aortic blood was less severe [47]. Diffusion of ethanol from the stomach into blood is not a problem in alcohol analysis. For an intact stomach containing 400 ml of 10% ethanol, contamination of a femoral vein sample was minimal [48]. However, it should be considered that regurgitation of alcohol or drugs from the stomach, esophageal sphincter relaxations, and severe blunt trauma resulting in the rupture of internal organs, especially of the stomach, facilitate postmortem diffusion processes. These circumstances may favor artificially elevated blood concentrations [49, 50].

Drugs accumulated in lungs are rapidly released inducing elevated drug concentrations in thoracic and heart blood samples as well as in liver specimens. These changes were assessed in animal and cadaver models, and were, e.g., also seen in methamphetamine-associated deaths [51]. Redistribution from the lungs seems more intense than redistribution from the gastrointestinal tract due to the large surface of the alveoli, the thin membranes, and the high vascularization. The early rise in dothiepin levels in thoracic blood in a rabbit model reflects postmortem redistribution from the lungs, where the drug was heavily concentrated [52]. Fuke *et al.* [53] observed that torso blood samples showed less toluene after gastric instillation than after tracheal instillation. Also, a higher toluene concentration was present in the left lobe of the liver than in the right with gastric instillation. The pleural and peritoneal fluids are regarded as vehicles for drug exchanges between the lungs and the liver [43].

The redistribution effects from the liver are far more complex, and may occur via the hepatic vessels or directly to adjacent organs, such as the stomach or the gall bladder [39]. Postmortem decreases in concentrations of fluoxetine and norfluoxetine, in both liver and lungs, occurred along with increases in blood concentrations in a dog model [54]. In rats, administered amitriptyline in the liver lobes had high but variable drug concentrations among tissues. Lobes lying closest to the stomach had the highest drug concentrations [55]. In general, a great part of the surface of the left liver lobe being in close contact with the stomach wall will be more involved in postmortem redistribution. Also, it may be difficult to correctly assign the source of hepatic concentrations postmortem [43].

A substantial increase in heart blood could be noticed for drugs, such as calcium channel blockers or cardiac glycosides, which are highly bound to cardiac tissue. In a series of digoxin cases, the drug concentration was invariably higher in heart blood specimens than in peripheral blood samples [56, 57]. The lungs, the liver, and the stomach may serve as further drug sources. A useful compilation of drug concentrations in heart and femoral blood has been published by Dalpe-Scott *et al.* [58].

Variations in postmortem drug concentration largely depend on both the time since death and the site of blood collection. Differences in drug concentrations collected from different anatomical sites have been reported for numerous drugs including imipramine, diphenhydramine and codeine [59], methadone [60, 61], doxepin, clomipramine, barbiturates [39], amitriptyline [45], cimetidine [62], methamphetamine [51], cocaine [63], digoxin [56], zopiclone [64], methylenedioxymethamphetamine, and methylenedioxyamphetamine [65]. A review on site-dependent differences is given by Prouty and Anderson [41] and Baselt [38].

It is evident that postmortem redistribution is governed by the postmortem time interval. Compared to studies on site-dependent differences, only few data on time-dependent differences are available. In a fatal case of dihydrocodeine intoxication, site-to-site differences of the parent drug and major metabolites were very small, probably due to steady state, an apparent volume of distribution of $1.0-1.3 \, \mathrm{l \, kg^{-1}}$ for dihydrocodeine, the fluidity of blood as well as very early postmortem blood sampling [66].

Some case reports have determined that there is little evidence of time-dependent variability, which may be due to delayed sampling. Temporal changes in drug concentrations that have been studied in animal models revealed significant changes to occur already during the early postmortem period [55, 67–70]. The level of dothiepin in cardiac and pulmonary blood samples steadily increased to reach 400% of its original concentration at 8-h postmortem [71]. In a dog model, 2-h postmortem concentrations of fluoxetine and norfluoxetine were 2.2- to 6.0-fold higher than antemortem concentrations, but did not significantly differ from 12-h postmortem concentrations [54]. An overview on drugs in which redistribution is likely to occur or in which postmortem redistribution probably does not occur is provided by Drummer [3], Leikin and Watson [4], and Baselt [38].

Major Changes of the Media and the Analyte Occurring after Death

General Remarks. As indicated in the section "Postmortem Redistribution", body fluids and tissues as well as drugs present in these specimens are subject to fundamental changes during the postmortem time period. Alterations of the media may considerably impact drug analysis. Decomposition of a corpse involves the processes of autolysis and putrefaction. Enzymes naturally present in the body induce autolytic changes; putrefaction is due to destruction by microorganisms. The onset of autolysis is rapid in cells with high concentrations of hydrolytic enzymes, such as the pancreas and the gastric mucosa, and is slower in the cells of the heart and the liver. Being the specimen of choice for detecting, quantifying, and interpreting drug concentrations, a more detailed review of postmortem changes in blood is given.

Postmortem Changes of Blood with Regard to Drug Analysis. Blood is a complex mixture that contains solubilized proteins, dissolved fats, solids, and suspended cells. Serum or plasma is traditionally used in clinical settings because blood affords advanced handling in the laboratory procedures [6]. Drug concentrations provided in literature are usually determined from these fluids. Analytical results obtained from postmortem blood are compared valuably with levels previously reported in therapeutic and toxic conditions [38, 72–74]. However, separation of red blood cells from postmortem blood is usually not possible, and its composition may remarkably differ from a blood sample obtained from a living person.

Changes may already occur during agony [75]. Hypoxia reduces the intracellular pH value, thus inducing an increased accumulation of basic drugs into the cells. Neutral or acidic drugs are less affected. Intracellular acidification and changes in ionic strength lead to a damage to the lysosomal membrane, and, subsequently, to enzymatic digestion of the cell membrane and components. Drugs that are concentrated in the cell are redistributed at this stage into the extracellular compartment. After death had occurred, there is a rapid progress in

postmortem redistribution processes due to disintegration of physiological and anatomical barriers (see the section "Postmortem Redistribution"). Postmortem vascular permeation has been shown in an *in vitro* model using morphine and its glucuronides [76].

In addition to the immediate postmortem dropping of the pH value up to 5.5, a decrease in blood–water content can often be observed [75, 77]. There exist strong variations in the water content of postmortem blood ranging from 59 to 89%. Both hemoconcentration and altered partition behavior affect original drug levels.

As the permeability of all cell membranes increases, hemolysis occurs. In addition to hemolysis seen with most specimens, blood coagulates postmortem, and then becomes liquid again. The effectiveness of these two processes will determine whether postmortem blood is clotted, fluid or partially clotted, and partially fluid [78]. Blood clots distribute unevenly in the body. A few hours after death, hypostasis occurs by sedimentation of blood and serum to the lower parts of the body due to gravitation. As a result, concentration measured for any drug exhibiting unequal distribution between red cells and serum may be biased by blood hypostasis, irregular clotting, and hemolysis.

Average distribution ratios between whole blood and plasma are given for major drugs in Table 3 [61, 79–88]. Further data of blood-to-plasma concentration ratios are provided by Baselt [38] and Iten [89]. For some drugs, varying blood-to-plasma ratios have been observed between individuals. In patients, chlorpromazine erythrocyte concentrations tended to correlate with plasma concentrations, but the erythrocyte/plasma concentration ratio varied from 0.61 to 2.00 among patients [90].

Ratios may not only vary between drugs but also differ between a particular drug and corresponding metabolites. Some caution is advisable using these data. Most of them are derived from *in vitro* partition experiments using systems composed of plasma water, plasma proteins, and erythrocytes. When spiked blood is diluted with autologous plasma water, erythrocytes always discharge the compound overproportionally, compared to plasma proteins [91, 92]. Also, ratios may differ depending on whether the sample had been collected from a living person or a corpse. For example, the plasma-to-whole blood concentration ratios of cannabinoids were found to

Table 3 Blood-to-plasma concentration ratios for some drugs of forensic interest

Drug	Ratio	Reference
Amitriptyline	1.0–1.1	[79]
Nortriptyline	1.5–1.7	
Cocaine	1.00	[80]
Diazepam	0.70	[79]
Oxazepam	1.00	[81]
Ethanol	0.74–0.90	[82]
Methadone	0.75	[83]
	1.00	[61]
Morphine	1.02	[84]
Morphine glucuronides	Dependent on hematocrit	[85]
Δ^9 - Tetrahydrocannabinol	0.55, 0.66	[86, 87]
11-Hydroxy-Δ^9-tetrahydrocannabinol	0.57, 0.58	[86, 87]
11-Nor-9-carboxy-Δ^9-tetrahydrocannabinol	0.62	[88]

be very similar and their individual coefficient of variation to be very low in samples taken from living individuals. However, data obtained postmortem suggest that the distribution of cannabinoids is scattered over a wider range of values compared to those determined in living subjects. Also, cannabinoids favored postmortem "serum", the mean ratio between the blood supernatant and whole blood being 2.4, but only 1.6 in samples collected from living people [88]. Generally, the differences observed between blood or plasma are considered to be less important compared to the changes in concentration that may occur prior to sampling.

Invasion of intestinal flora into tissues and body fluids occurs rapidly after death, especially at ambient or elevated temperatures. Postmortem blood samples taken 6 h after death in patients who had died of causes other than infectious diseases were tested positive for bacteria [93], whereas in a study on heart blood samples collected 85 h after death bacteriologic cultures gave negative results [94]. Microbial enzymes hydrolyze and transform lipids, carbohydrates, and proteins. As a result, the pH value of blood slowly increases again during the postmortem interval [75, 95].

Postmortem Alterations in Drug Concentrations.
Degradation as well as formation of drugs during the postmortem interval as competing processes to postmortem redistribution has been observed. Drugs concentration may change due to chemical and physical degradation, metabolic formation or breakdown (Table 4). Problems also arise from interfering

substances that are endogenously produced during autolysis and putrefactive processes (see the section "Postmortem Redistribution").

Systematic investigations on the time dependence of detectability of drugs or poisons in a putrefying body do not exist. Some case reports revealed that drugs such as morphine or atropine may be identified in specimens from exhumed corpses or from stored tissues many months after death [96]. Comprehensive data on positive drug findings in putrefied bodies had been published by Arnold et al. [97]. For example, phenobarbital, bromazepam, sulpiride, and promethazine could be successfully identified in highly putrefied materials. The interpretative value of these measurements is limited, however.

Recovery of organophosphorous pesticides, such as parathion or malathion, was less successful compared to paraquat, whereas recovery of organochlorine compounds was >72% from putrefactive materials [99, 100]. Stevens [95] studied the stability of 56 drugs and drug-related compounds added to drug-free liver homogenates. Degradation was elevated in samples exposed to fly-borne bacteria. From the results, the following molecular structures are assumed to be prone to putrefactive decomposition: oxygen that is bonded to nitrogen as in nitro groups or N-oxides, sulfur, which forms part of a heterocyclic ring, and aminophenol structures. A variable decomposition rate, which was observed for dothiepin in bacteria-contaminated liver and blood specimens, was suggested to be due to differences in bacterial activity [52].

Table 4 Possible mechanisms operating on drugs postmortem, examples modified according to [98]

Mechanism	Example(s)
Chemical instability	
Hydrolysis	Heroin, cocaine, O-acyl-, and N-glucuronides
Oxidation	Sulfur-containing drugs and morphine
Metabolic instability	
Esterases (endogenous)	Hydrolysis of ester-type drugs
	Hydrolysis of phase-II metabolites
	Reduction, e.g., of nitrobenzodiazepines
	Oxidation, e.g., of thioridazine
Metabolic production	Ethanol, γ-Hydroxybutyrate, carbon monoxide, and cyanide

The possible role of enteric bacteria in the bioconversion of nitrobenzodiazepines was studied in detail by Robertson and Drummer [101]. It is well known, that in deaths involving flunitrazepam, considerably higher concentrations of 7-aminoflunitrazepam than that of the parent compound can be detected in blood [102]. The conversion of the respective 7-aminometabolites of nitrobenzodiazepines by individual bacteria in blood was species dependent. Significantly higher rates were found for obligate anaerobic species than for facultative anaerobic species, and there was little difference among the species for their ability to metabolize nitrazepam, flunitrazepam, or clonazepam. The conversion rate was slowed down by keeping the corpses at $4\,^{\circ}$C. The effect of pH variation on the metabolic activity of different bacterial species was variable.

Postmortem degradation does also concern acid-labile conjugates, such as the ester glucuronides of 11-nor-9-carboxy-Δ^9-tetrahydrocannabinol, propofol, or diflunisal [103, 104] as well as the more stable ether glucuronides [105]. Conversion of morphine glucuronides to free morphine by residual glucuronidase activity or some bacterial enzymes is a most prominent example [106]. The bacteria most likely involved are originating from the gastrointestinal tract. Being the most prominent among them, *Escherichia coli* is an important source of β-glucuronidase activity. Preferential hydrolysis of morphine-3-glucuronide to free morphine by bacterial enzymatic activity was ascertained in *in vitro* experiments, and was shown to depend on storage time, temperature, and initial degree of putrefaction [107].

Bacteria, yeast, and fungi can also produce some compounds in the postmortem blood, the most prominent representative being ethanol. In contrast to drug metabolism, which may persist some time after death, the physiological metabolism of ethanol is assumed to cease at the time of death [108]. A considerable site-dependent variation of the ethanol concentration in blood samples had been observed even in cases where signs of putrefaction could not be noticed [109]. These differences were mainly attributed to death occurring during the absorptive phase where differences between arterial and venous blood exist. Ethanol absorbed from the gastrointestinal tract distributes throughout the body according to the water content of the corresponding tissue or body fluid. The postmortem change in blood alcohol content closely following the change in blood water content, correction for water content has been recommended [110]. In principle, the water content of blood decreases with the time after death. However, there are some exceptions, e.g., drowning experiments with animals indicated a dilution of alcohol in blood [111].

Postmortem changes of ethanol are well documented [112]. The majority of the cases attributed to neoformation did not have significant ethanol concentrations ($<0.07\%$). However, there are a few case reports demonstrating that a significant amount of ethanol up to 0.22% may be produced [113, 114]. The amount of ethanol formed during the postmortem time interval depends on the antemortem conditions, the species of microorganisms present, the availability of substrates, and the storage conditions of the body prior to collection of samples for toxicological analysis **Alcohol: Analysis**. In bodies that were stored refrigerated, even in the presence of microbial species capable to produce ethanol, alcohol formation could not be established within 4–24 h after death [113, 115]. Comprehensive reviews on the variety of organisms capable of producing ethanol and on the microbiology and biochemistry of postmortem ethanol formation are given by Corry and Huckenbeck [116, 117]. Potential substrates are carbohydrates, glucose, lactate, ribose, and amino acids, and glycolysis is thought to be the primary process for ethanol production [116, 118].

For postmortem synthesis of ethanol is difficult to be accurately established, further putrefactive products have been suggested as indicators to differentiate postmortem-formed ethanol from antemortem-ingested ethanol. Along with ethanol, other short chain alcohols, such as 1-propanol, isopropanol, 1-butanol, 2-butanol, isobutanol, and isoamylalcohol, are produced by microorganisms. Methanol is considered not to arise from microbial synthesis. In case reports, *in vitro* and animal studies, most commonly 1-propanol, could be detected [113]. Estimation of the ethanol synthesis based on the 1-propanol or other short chain alcohol levels seems questionable due to their highly variable formation rates as well as for they may derive from ingested alcoholic beverages. Huckenbeck [117] found that different Clostridium and Proteus species produced α- and γ-aminobutyric acid and δ-aminovaleric acid along with ethanol, but a quantitative relationship between postmortem ethanol and putrefactive amino acid production could not be established.

Postmortem cyanide production could give improper estimation of cyanide poisoning from blood analysis. Seto [119] suggested that cyanide is released from methemoglobin cyanide complex by heat denaturation, and diffuses out of the blood vessels via plasma during which it encounters albumin. Also, liberation by superoxide anion radical oxidation of proteins has been assumed. However, these pathways have been judged to be of minor importance compared to cyanide production during storage or as an analytical artifact.

γ-Hydroxybutyrate (GHB) has been widely abused. It is also a naturally occurring compound present in the mammalian central nervous system. Small amounts are formed from γ-aminobutyric acid with subsequent reduction to form GHB again. Besides its premortem production, GHB can be produced as a postmortem artifact [120]. When GHB concentrations are low at a postmortem time interval

of more than a few hours, they may be falsely implicated as a cause of death [121].

Artifacts in Specimens Stored in Formaldehyde or Collected after Embalmment

Sometimes it is necessary to perform analysis on pathologic specimens stored in formaldehyde or on samples that have been collected from an embalmed body. The embalming procedure may have diluted the blood, and/or may have partially or completely removed drugs or poisons present at the time of death from major blood vessels [122]. Embalming fluids are typically based on formaldehyde with final concentrations of 5–20% at acidic or neutral pH values, and may usually also contain alcohols [123]. Formaldehyde is a highly reactive chemical agent, and may mask, alter, or destroy a drug during the fixation or embalming process. Previous studies have demonstrated that formalin can react with various drugs including, e.g., amphetamines [124], barbiturates [125], and benzodiazepines [126] in a time, pH value, and formalin concentration-dependent manner. Most likely, reaction pathways are through hydrolysis and/or methylation via the Eschweiler–Clarke reaction. In addition, body fluids and tissues are difficult to extract due to denaturation.

Results from liver tissue specimens collected from drug-related suicides indicated that some methylation of nortriptyline to amitriptyline had occurred during formalin fixation and storage, but consistent ratios could not be established [122]. In a different study, conversion of nortriptyline to amitriptyline was confirmed [127]. For the formation of amitriptyline was only proportional to the loss of nortriptyline at a pH value of 9.5, it was suggested that the metabolite may be susceptible to degradation in formaldehyde containing solutions at lower pH values. *N*-methylation has also been reported for amphetamine, methamphetamine, and fenfluramine. Disappearance of fenfluramine was higher at elevated formaldehyde concentrations, and an increase in pH directly correlated with the appearance of *N*-methyl fenfluramine [128].

Some drugs appeared to be reasonably stable in formalin. In a study examining chemically fixed tissue specimens of poisoned rabbits, a formalin solution containing 10% formaldehyde (pH 7.4) was found to be most suitable for diazepam- and chlorpromazine-containing tissues for at least 28 days with respect to the recovery of the analytes [129]. Succinylcholine only slowly degraded in embalmed rat tissue samples [130]. It appears that the embalming fluid maintaining acidic conditions contributed to the drug's stability in fixed tissue, whereas succinylcholine is very rapidly hydrolyzed in blood. However, some compounds, such as alprazolam and midazolam, decompose more rapidly under acidic conditions [126].

Stability of volatile substances in formalin-fixed tissues was tested for ethanol, diethyl ether, chloroform, and toluene in a rabbit model by the intravenous route [131]. All volatile compounds were still detectable after a 14-day fixation period. Compared to nonfixed materials, in the fixed tissue samples concentrations had decreased in the following order: ethanol > diethyl ether >> chloroform > toluene.

Leaching of drugs into the fixing/storing solution is evident. In a sildenafil-related death, a comparison of the quantitative values of sildenafil in fixed tissues and those in the same tissues at autopsy revealed a mean decrease of 74%. However, the total recovery from both the fixed tissue and the particular formalin solution was 95% with regard to the original quantity in the same tissue before fixation [132]. Similar observation was reported on the detection and quantification of morphine and strychnine in fixed samples and formalin solutions [133, 134].

Analysis of fixed samples may create problems with regard to the isolation of the analyte and damage of the technical equipment. Iffland *et al.* [135] succeeded in determining carbon monoxide in clots of heart blood collected from an embalmed body following release of carbon monoxide from the sample by nitric acid. Phenobarbital was detected in fixed brain tissue as well as in the formalin solution in a poisoning case using ultraviolet (UV) spectrometry and thin layer chromatography, whereas gas chromatography (GC) was not applicable due to interferences and damage of the column [136].

Acquisition of Specimens

General Considerations

The purpose of sampling is to provide a representative part of the whole that is suitable for analysis and reliable interpretation. Sampling is the most important step in drug analysis because an analytical result will never be better than the sample from which it is derived. Specimens available in postmortem toxicology investigations can be numerous and variable, and may be selected on the basis of the case history, requests, legal aspects, and availability in a given case. So far, a harmonized protocol for sampling in suspected poisoning or drug-related death has not been established [49, 137]. Generally, the specimens routinely collected at autopsy include fluids, such as blood from peripheral sites and heart blood, urine, bile, cerebrospinal fluid, vitreous humor and gastric contents, and organs, particularly liver [49, 138]. The main collection artifact is contamination, but can be reduced by sampling before the autopsy, if appropriate. It is difficult, if not impossible, to acquire quality specimens once autopsy has been completed. An appreciation of how contaminants may be introduced is also important.

Sampling Artifacts

Incorrect Selection and Acquisition of Samples. Samples taken for analysis should always be chosen bearing in mind the disposition of the drug in the body. An incorrect or insufficient sampling will severely affect case investigation **Toxicology: Analysis**. In fatalities requiring quantitative determination, a blood specimen is preferably taken from the femoral vein prior to autopsy, for contamination may be avoided, and this site is less affected by postmortem changes (see the section "Changes Occurring after Death"). If the femoral vein is ligated prior to sampling, the sample is likely to be relatively uncontaminated by blood from the major organs [40]. Cardiac blood is regarded as unsuitable for quantitative analysis of drugs. Diffusion out of the stomach can artificially raise the cardiac blood concentration, and a sample may equally contain blood that has drained from the lungs, the vena cava inferior, the aorta, and the subclavian veins. If a heart blood specimen is sampled through the chest wall, one should be aware that the sample is contaminated with thoracic fluid and gastric contents. Postmortem specimens obtained from patients who have died several days after a drug-related episode are likely to give negative results [2]. It is essential to perform toxicology investigations on specimens obtained on or soon after admission to hospital. In fire victims, blood that is not collected from body regions excluded from severe burning can contain falsely elevated carbon monoxide levels due to diffusion of environmental carbon monoxide and binding to hemoglobin. Relying on a result from a single specimen may be misleading. It is recommended to collect blood from at least two different sites or, if not available, along with other specimens, at least.

Urine is a valuable specimen, because it can easily be tested, and drugs and drug metabolites are usually found in high concentrations **Drug Testing: Urine**. A sample collected during autopsy may be contaminated by blood and should preferably be taken prior to autopsy by puncture of the abdominal wall. A positive identification indicates recent drug use, but does not indicate when or how much drug was ingested. There is little correlation between urine and blood concentrations. If death takes place quickly, urine findings can be negative. Analysis of a specimen may not be a reliable means to reveal ingestion of drugs, e.g., sertraline and norsertraline, which are present in very low concentrations or were not renally cleared [38]. Analysis of a urine specimen may reveal exposure to organophosphate compounds or analysis of toluene, xylene, and trichloroethylene via identification of their major metabolites in cases where blood analysis will fail to detect these compounds [38]. Local anesthetics, e.g., lidocaine, which are used on catheters, are a common finding in urine samples.

Gastric contents are a useful specimen to rapidly discover drug overdose, for oral ingestion is the major administration route of prescribed drugs. The total amount of a drug or poison remaining in the gastric contents is far more important than its concentration. A low absolute amount does not rule out the possibility of an overdose. Also, a low drug concentration in the stomach may arise from passive diffusion from the blood into stomach contents. This phenomenon is frequently observed in drugs being weakly basic in nature [33]. Since the gastric contents can be largely inhomogeneous, the entire specimen should be submitted or mixed before an aliquot is taken. The odor of gastric contents or colored material can potentially point to a specific agent, although, e.g., blue stains may result from parathion or flunitrazepam ingestion.

Bile represents a collection and storage depot for many xenobiotics and corresponding metabolites that have a biliary excretion and are subject to enterohepatic cycling. To avoid contamination of surrounding tissues, the gall bladder should be tied off before removing from the liver. Drug concentrations can be significantly higher in bile than in blood. The mean bile to blood ratios varied from about 1 for acetaminophen and amphetamine to about 2000 for desmethylclobazam. In several cases, a drug could be identified in bile, but was not detectable in blood [139]. A qualitative finding in bile may indicate previous or chronic exposure to a drug or poison.

Cerebrospinal fluid and vitreous humor are aqueous and transparent fluids, which are useful to screen for a variety of drugs [140]. Both cerebrospinal fluid and vitreous humor also contain very little proteins. Therefore, drugs highly bound to proteins or lipophilic in nature tend to be found in lower concentrations in these fluids than in blood [49, 141]. A major limitation to the use of cerebrospinal fluids is the small database of reference values [142], whereas vitreous humor has been used to analyze a larger number of drugs [143–150]. Many studies have stressed the usefulness of vitreous humor for alcohol analysis [151]. However, the wide variation of vitreous humor to blood ethanol ratios must alert when results from vitreous humor are used to estimate the concentration in femoral venous blood [152].

Tissue specimens collected for postmortem toxicology investigations include liver, kidney, lung, brain, skeletal muscle, and adipose tissue [49, 151]. Tissue samples may be useful in cases with an extended postmortem time period and whenever body fluids are not available. Extensive data had been published for liver and kidney, less for brain and lung specimens [38, 153]. Drug concentrations in liver were found to be site dependent (see the section "Postmortem Redistribution"), and sampling from deep within the lobe has been recommended [154]. Concentrations in brain may also significantly vary from one region to another [155]. The within-case variability of drug levels observed in muscle specimens supports the opinion, that drug analysis on skeletal muscle is rather qualitative than quantitative in nature. Muscle specimens had also been considered for alcohol analysis, but the muscle to blood–ethanol concentration was found to depend on the time course of ethanol absorption, distribution, and elimination [156]. A skin specimen or a cube of muscle may support evidence of the route of drug administration [49]. As skin acts as a temporary drug reservoir, the specimen should always be excised together with a random specimen preferably taken from a similar site to act as control [157].

Hair is an ideal specimen for determining, e.g., chronic arsenic and mercury poisoning [158]. Also, numerous drugs and poisons have been detected in hair in recent years (*see* **Hair: Toxicology**) [159, 160]. The amounts deposited in hair are functions of both ingestion/exposure and of the metabolic regimen. Segmentation of the hair can assist in estimating the time of exposure. A decrease in drug concentration in the proximal sections of hair may indicate a decrease in tolerance to the drug. There are many factors that influence drug concentrations in hair: biological factors such as hair structure and pigmentation, individual factors such as drug use, customs culture or race including hair care, environmental factors, and also methodological factors [30]. External uptake of drugs from blood, vomit, or putrefactive fluids leads to artificially elevated drug levels in hair, which will not be fully removed by common wash procedures [31].

Specimen Containers and Preservation. The use of appropriate specimen containers and preservatives can be critical with regard to ultimately identify a substance in an individual specimen. Specimens must be collected in separate, clean containers, which should be filled up to minimize evaporation of volatiles and oxidative losses of drugs.

The best materials to collect and store fluids or tissue specimens are glass containers. Sampling into a glass container is a must, if solvent abuse or an anesthetic death is suspected. Essential are also aluminum foil- or Teflon-lined lids to prevent gas escaping and to minimize drug adsorption. Solid tissue samples may also be placed in nylon bags, which are tightly sealed [138]. Most types of plastic containers are suitable for the collection of tissue specimens in drug-related fatalities. Disposable hard plastic tubes or Nalgene® bottles with screw caps are also recommended for collection of body fluids for breakage of these containers upon freezing had not been observed [161]. The use of evacuated tubes is less desirable, for sample contamination from plasticizers used in their manufacture may occur. For collection tubes containing gel separators, a gross contamination by toluene, 1-butanol, ethyl benzene, and xylene has been reported [162]. Evaluating the container before

routinely collecting specimens in it might reduce production of artifacts.

Obligatory recommendations for specimen preservations do not exist. Specimen preservatives are generally not required for specimens other than blood. In addition to a preserved blood sample, an unpreserved specimen available to the toxicologist is optimal, for preservation strategies depend on the target analytes and are not unique. Fluoride preservation with a final concentration of 1–5% sodium fluoride by weight is recommended for postmortem analyses of alcohol, cocaine, cyanide, and carbon monoxide. Postmortem synthesis of ethanol can be effectively inhibited, whereas hydrolysis of cocaine can only be slowed down by fluoride preservation [163]. A general problem with ester-type drugs is the presence of esterases; as degradation takes place even at $4\,^{\circ}C$, immediate freezing of specimens is recommended [164]. Artificial production of GHB has been observed in blood samples not collected in fluoride-containing tubes [165], and also in specimens collected in citrate buffer [121]. Fluoride preservation must not be used when organophosphorous chemicals are involved. For example, rapid degradation of metrifonate (dichlorvos) was found to be favored by the presence of sodium fluoride, esterases, elevated temperatures, and alkaline condition [166]. Early acidification of the specimen and storage at $-80\,^{\circ}C$ was recommended by Heinig *et al.* [167].

Acidification may also stabilize cocaine or labile conjugates such as N-glycosides [5, 168]. Ascorbic acid may be used as an antioxidant. For example, losses in olanzapine during storage at $4\,^{\circ}C$ may be reduced by the addition of 0.25% ascorbic acid [169]. Apomorphine, like most catechols, is prone to oxidation to quinones, unless ascorbic acid is added as an oxidant [170]. However, the presence of an antioxidant may have reverse effects. During storage reduction of the N-oxide metabolites of chlorpromazine, of samples containing antioxidants, resulting in an increase in the concentration of the parent drug, has been observed [171]. Anticoagulants are not recommended for postmortem blood samples because these additives may also affect drug concentration. Blood concentration of morphine in ethylene diamine tetraacetic acid (EDTA) tubes was 4.8% higher than in heparin tubes [172], which also contain phenolic preservatives such as cresol [171].

Stability During Storage

In clinical chemistry, stability is defined as the capability of sample material to retain the initial value of a measured quantity for a defined period within specific limits when stored under defined conditions. The individual maximal permissible instability is preferably linked to the criteria of analytical imprecision, and is expressed as the critical difference [173]. This procedure allows defining the maximum permissible storage time for an analyte in a particular specimen at a given condition.

In postmortem investigations, such consideration starts at the time of sampling and covers the time until analysis. The presence and extent of alterations since the time of death can only be estimated, part of them even cannot be avoided, and they cannot be undone. Therefore, knowledge on degradation mechanisms in a particular matrix and on resulting breakdown products is important.

A review on poisons, drugs, and heavy metals suspected to be unstable is given by Leikin [4] and Ellenhorn [174]. Unfortunately, the particular biological matrix, which may play a role in the stability of an analyte, has not been considered. For example, in urine, cocaine is chemically stable at a pH of less than 7.0. In blood samples, even acidic conditions do not prevent cocaine to be metabolized by residual esterase activities. Interestingly, cocaethylene seemed to be more stable in postmortem specimens than cocaine. Muscle as well as brain tissues were considered to be the specimen of choice for testing both cocaethylene and cocaine [168]. Valuable information on artifacts is provided by Baselt [38] and Drummer [175]. Comprehensive data on the stability of drugs of abuse in blood were reported by Levine and Smith [176] already in 1989. A recent update was given by Skopp and Pötsch [177]. Data on the stability of drugs in tissues are rare.

In principle, all volatile compounds such as aerosol propellants, anesthetic gases, carbon monoxide, ethanol, and organic solvents are unstable during storage. Losses of up to 25% of blood toluene have been observed in glass tubes stored unopened for 7 days at room temperature, and considerably higher losses were noted in glass tubes with rubber stoppers [178]. There is an artifactual rise in carbon monoxide level in unpreserved blood specimens since bacterial action can result in both the production of carbon monoxide and the denaturation of hemoglobin

[38]. The formation of toxicologically significant concentrations of cyanide in postmortem tissue has been demonstrated, which was attributed, in part, to conversion of thiocyanate to cyanide and breakdown of proteins [179, 180]. Conversely, a significant decrease in blood cyanide concentration has been attributed to mechanisms that include evaporation, thiocyanate formation, and reaction with specimen components [181]. Temperature and cyanide concentration are apparently important factors in these changes [182].

Another important consideration when measuring drugs is the stability of corresponding metabolites. Highly labile metabolites such as sulfate conjugates and N- and acylglucuronides may rapidly be converted back to the unconjugated compound and consequently result in falsely elevated concentrations. Examples are the N-sulfate metabolite of minoxidil, N-glucuronide metabolites of nomifesine, and 11-nor-9-carboxy-Δ^9-tetrahydrocannabinol glucuronide [103].

Some of the degradation mechanisms seen during storage are similar to those observed during autolysis and putrefaction (see the section "Major Changes of the Media and the Analyte Occurring after Death"). Generally, degradation of a drug occurs through hydrolysis, oxidation or reduction processes, and is generally slowed down by decreasing storage temperatures and preservation of the sample (see the section "Specimen Containers and Preservation"). These processes are due to endogenous enzyme activities, e.g., esterases still operating in the sample, chemical reactions or to enzyme activities such as glucuronidase following bacterial invasion during the postmortem interval (see also Table 4) [98].

Experimental investigations on time-dependent changes give information on the reaction type involved in drug degradation [183], and may guide to a more proper estimation of the drug level at the time of sampling. Hydrolysis of ester-type drugs generally exhibited an apparent first-order reaction kinetic, whereas an oxidation can often be described by a second-order reaction kinetic. Investigations on the reaction type involved in the degradation of forensic relevant drugs have already been performed, e.g., for morphine, morphine glucuronides, cocaine, benzoylecgonine, ecgonine methyl ester, lysergic acid diethylamide (LSD), and 11-nor-9-carboxy-Δ^9-tetrahydrocannabinol glucuronide [103, 105, 163, 184].

The mechanisms involved in the breakdown of benzodiazepines are poorly understood. Hydrolysis and reduction are suggested to be involved in their degradation. Degradation of nitrobenzodiazepines occurs very rapidly, whereas other benzodiazepines do not appear to be as unstable [101, 185]. Besides bacteria, major influence factors in the degradation of nitrobenzodiazepines are an increased temperature and the absence of sodium fluoride [186]. Chlordiazepoxide tends to form desoxychlordiazepoxide during storage, and further degrades to nordiazepam, which also represents a metabolite and an artifact in the analysis of the parent drug by GC [187].

Terbutaline was shown to be stable in spiked postmortem blood at room temperature for 7 days. In contrast, a loss of 83% was observed for fenoterol in spiked postmortem blood at the same conditions. Only 7% of the initial concentration was present after 6 months at 4 °C. The instability of fenoterol is most likely a result of the presence of the phenolic group attached to the side-chain nitrogen atom, which is susceptible to oxidation [188].

There is evidence that different degradation mechanisms operate in blood depending on its source, either obtained from living individuals or collected from corpses. An experimental investigation on morphine and its glucuronides in spiked fresh blood and plasma revealed that oxidation primarily affected drug stability, whereas in postmortem samples stored under the same conditions, hydrolysis of morphine glucuronides was assumed to be the predominant reaction [105].

Sometimes, metabolites or breakdown products are far more stable than the parent drug. Complete degradation of furazolidone occurred in muscle tissue stored at 4 °C during 24 h. Even storage in liquid nitrogen did not fully stabilize furazolidone [189] indicating that analysis of a metabolite, which is reasonably stable, may be favored [190]. The poor stability of cocaine, benzoylecgonine, and ecgonine methyl ester is well documented [163, 183, 191]. Alternate analysis for ecgonine representing a rather stable breakdown product may be performed in highly putrefied specimens or specimens stored for long periods of time.

Most drugs or poisons are probably stable in biological materials for months, particularly if frozen and special arrangements may prevent loss of an analyte by degradation (see the section "Specimen Containers and Preservation").

Analytical Artifacts

Although the history of a sample appears to be most relevant to the production of artifacts, analytical artifacts may also be considered during the isolation and identification of an analyte. For most drugs and poisons, a two-stage testing is usually employed, comprising a preliminary screening test followed by confirmatory analysis, which should offer a higher degree of specificity for the analyte than the first test. A gross overview on common methods used in postmortem toxicology investigations has been given by Hearn and Walls [1] as well as by Drummer [3]. There is little to differentiate in analytical procedures used in other forms of forensic toxicology with respect to postmortem toxicology investigations.

Available immunoassays can yield positive results in urine for metabolites from most of the common benzodiazepines, except lorazepam and flunitrazepam [1]. These drugs may not be detected until hydrolyzed [192]. Interaction with putrefactive amines is commonly seen in immunoassays for amphetamine-type drugs [193]. Interactions are not limited to matrix effects or the structural and conformational similarity of compounds. Further information on cross-reactivity and potential mechanisms is given by Richardson [2]. In addition, turbid, highly colored, or opaque specimens can interfere with the detection principle affording an intensive preextraction step.

Chromatography has been the mainstay of drug analysis for many years. Often, a special pretreatment or homogenization according to the specimen's nature and/or a more sophisticated cleanup extraction of putrefied materials is required for all forms of chromatography. Extraction into an organic solvent for partial purification of a biological fluid or a tissue homogenate is still widely used. Lipophilic compounds will be readily extracted by nonpolar solvents. The more polar solvents being partially miscible with water will also remove water-soluble materials. As a result, drug conjugates are also transferred into the organic phase. If phase-II metabolites are subsequently hydrolyzed, this will lead to erroneously high levels of the parent drug [103, 194]. The phenomenon of conjugate instability is most common with labile conjugates such as N- or O-acyl-glucuronides [103, 104].

The chemical properties of a solvent can give rise to chemical reactions of the solvent itself and the insidious breakdown products or stabilizers it may contain. For example, the effect of phosgene in chloroform has been reported as a cause of artifactual formation of carbamate derivatives during extraction of tricyclic antidepressants [195].

The problems associated with solvent extraction can be minimized by using solid-phase extraction. Because of its far greater variability, one must be well informed on the mechanisms of interaction to maintain proper control on the separation. If blood cells are not disrupted or if particles are still present in the sample, flow rates and reproducibility are altered.

The extraction efficiency of a drug or metabolite from a postmortem specimen may be variable from case to case, or even from site to site within the same corpse. It may also be markedly different than from a particular blank specimen used for calibration. The use of stable isotope internal standards may provide a higher degree in the accuracy of the analytical results. Unfortunately, few deuterated standards are commercially available for drugs, metabolites, or artifacts.

It is often necessary to evaporate extracts to reconstitute them into small volumes for transfer to chromatography. The most common routes of sample loss are adsorption onto glassware and volatilization of the drugs, e.g., of amphetamines. Adsorption losses can be prevented, e.g., by silanization of glassware or by including a polar solvent, such as amyl alcohols, as an additive to the extracting solvent or prior to evaporation. The problem of amphetamines' volatilization can be solved by converting them to their nonvolatile hydrochloride salts [6].

Gas chromatography coupled to mass spectrometry (GC/MS) is generally accepted as unequivocal identification for most drugs, and provides best confirmatory information. Also, liquid chromatography coupled to mass spectrometry(LC/MS) is an emerging technique [3]. There are several drawbacks with GC/MS analyses; some of them are included in Table 5.

It is now recognized that determination of major metabolites and degradation products along with the parent drug is essential to avoid misinterpretation of the data due to artifacts [196]. Such a stability-indicating assay is one that can accurately and selectively differentiate the intact drug from its potential decomposition products.

Conclusions

Artifacts must be accepted as an integral part of postmortem toxicology, frequently interfering with a straightforward interpretation of the analytical results.

Reporting all the details of the scene investigation and terminal events as well as of the social and medical history will aid to recognize important issues that may occur during the antemortem phase with respect to postmortem findings.

There is general agreement that drug concentrations are site dependent and tend to change with time, most significant alterations occurring already perimortem or rapidly after death. Heart blood concentrations are often higher than those of peripheral specimens. However, there does not appear to be a way to predict the relationship between drug levels derived from various specimens nor the manner in which the concentrations may change with time. To circumvent the problem of postmortem redistribution, it is recommended that blood be sampled from a peripheral vessel along with at least a second specimen taken from a different site, liver from deep within the right lobe and lung rather from the apex than the base. Tissue samples can be of value to assess the significance of a drug in the death of an individual provided that a sufficiently large database has been established.

Tables of therapeutic, toxic, or fatal ranges or correcting for blood-to-plasma ratio cannot be applied without restrictions. As the exact mechanisms of postmortem redistribution are not fully understood and most likely a combination of several factors, exact estimates of the dose are unreliable.

Postmortem degradation as well as formation of compounds have been observed, and may vary between tissues and body fluids as well as from drug to drug. For example, ethanol may be formed in postmortem blood in variable and nonpredictable amounts. In severely putrefied, embalmed, or formalin-fixed tissue, fundamental changes of both the matrix and the drug should be considered. Complete degradation or even removal of a drug may have occurred.

Table 5 Potential problems with GC/MS analyses[a]

Erroneous identification at a low analyte concentration
Misidentification due to interfering substances
Inadequate information due to similar (barbiturates)
  fragmentation behavior
Production of low mass fragment ions only (tricyclic
  antidepressants)

[a] Reproduced from Ref. 1. © Taylor & Francis Group, 1998

Sampling poses a high risk of contamination and/or production of artifacts. Correct sampling prior to or during autopsy is as essential as is the use of appropriate containers and preservatives including deep freezing. Some drugs or metabolites may undergo further decomposition during storage for several months.

Changes in materials and target analytes often require modifications of routinely applied analytical procedures; the most valuable appears to be a stability-indicating assay.

A thorough cooperation of the pathologist and toxicologist will enable to handle some of the problems addressed above. Some postmortem artifacts will never be resolved, whereas others are amenable to further elucidation from both case reports and experimental studies.

References

[1]   Hearn, W.L. & Walls, H.C. (1998). Introduction to post-mortem toxicology, in *Drug Abuse Handbook*, S.B. Karch, ed, CRC Press, Boca Raton, pp. 863–873.

[2]   Richardson, T. (2000). Pitfalls in forensic toxicology, *Annals of Clinical Biochemistry* **37**, 20–44.

[3]   Drummer, O.H. (2004). Postmortem toxicology of drugs of abuse, *Forensic Science International* **142**, 101–113.

[4]   Leikin, J.B. & Watson, W.A. (2003). Post-mortem toxicology: what the dead can and cannot tell us, *Journal of Toxicology Clinical Toxicology* **41**, 47–56.

[5]   Skopp, G. (2004). Preanalytic aspects in post-mortem toxicology, *Forensic Science International* **142**, 75–100.

[6]   Chamberlain, J. (1995). *Drugs in Biological Fluids*, 2nd Edition, CRC Press, Boca Raton.

[7]   Chiou, W.L. (1989). The phenomenon and rationale of marked dependence of drug concentration on blood sampling site. Implications in pharmacokinetics, pharmacodynamics, toxicology and therapeutics (Part I), *Clinical Pharmacokinetics* **17**, 175–199.

[8]   Gibaldi, M. (1991). *Biopharmaceutics and Clinical Pharmacokinetics*, 4th Edition, Lea & Febiger, Philadelphia.

[9]   Angst, M.S., Buhrer, M. & Lotsch, J. (2000). Insidious intoxication after morphine treatment in renal failure: delayed onset, *Anesthesiology* **92**, 1473–1476.

[10] Harrower, A.D. (1991). Pharmacokinetics of oral anti-hyperglycemic agents in patients with renal failure, *Clinical Pharmacokinetics* **31**, 111–119.

[11] Klotz, U., Avant, G.R., Hoyumpa, A., Schenker, S. & Wilkinson, G.R. (1975). The effects of age and liver disease on the disposition and elimination of diazepam in adult man, *The Journal of Clinical Investigation* **55**, 347–359.

[12] Wilkinson, G.T. (1978). The effects of liver disease and aging on the disposition of diazepam, chlordiazepoxide, oxazepam and lorazepam in man, *Acta Psychiatrica Scandinavica Supplementum* **274**, 56.

[13] Williams, R.L. & Mamelok, R.D. (1980). Hepatic disease and drug pharmacokinetics, *Clinical Pharmacokinetics* **5**, 528–547.

[14] Klepstad, P., Hilton, P., Moen, J., Kaasa, S., Borchgrevink, P.C., Zahlsen, K. & Dale, O. (2004). Day-to-day variations during clinical drug monitoring of morphine, morphine-3-glucuronide and morphine-6-glucuronide serum concentrations in cancer patients. A prospective observational study, *BMC Clinical Pharmacology* **4**, 4–7.

[15] Vermeire, A., Remon, J.P., Rosseel, M.T., Belpaire, F., Devulder, J. & Bogaert, M.G. (1998). Variability of morphine disposition during long-term subcutaneous infusion in terminally ill cancer patients, *European Journal of Clinical Pharmacology* **53**, 325–330.

[16] Wagner, J.G. (1988). Inter- and intrasubject variation of digoxin renal clearance in normal adult males, *Drug Intelligence and Clinical Pharmacy* **22**, 562–567.

[17] Hammer, W., Idestrom, C.M. & Sjöqvist, F. (1967). Chemical control of antidepressant drug therapy, in *Proceedings of the 1st International Symposium on Antidepressant Drugs*, S. Garratini & M.N.G. Dukes, eds, Exerpta Medica, pp. 301–310.

[18] Tanaka, E. (2003). Toxicological interactions involving psychiatric drugs and alcohol: an update, *Journal of Clinical Pharmacy and Therapeutics* **28**, 81–95.

[19] Dorian, P., Sellers, E.M., Reed, K.L., Warsh, J.J., Hamilton, C., Kaplan, H.L. & Fan, T. (1983). Amitriptyline and ethanol: pharmacokinetic and pharmacodynamic interaction, *European Journal of Clinical Pharmacology* **25**, 325–331.

[20] Olkkola, K.T. & Ahonen, J. (2001). Drug interactions, *Current Opinion in Anaesthesiology* **14**, 411–416.

[21] Oldenhof, H., de Jong, M., Steenhoek, A. & Janknegt, R. (1988). Clinical pharmacokinetics of midazolam in intensive care patients, a wide interpatient variability? *Clinical Pharmacology and Therapeutics* **43**, 263–269.

[22] Santos, C.A. & Boullata, J.I. (2005). An approach to evaluating drug-nutrient interactions, *Pharmacotherapy* **25**, 1789–1800.

[23] Boullata, J.I. (2005). Natural health product interactions with medication, *Nutrition in Clinical Practice* **20**, 33–51.

[24] Mock, D.M. & Dyken, M.E. (1997). Biotin catabolism is accelerated in adults receiving long-term therapy with anticonvulsants, *Neurology* **49**, 1444–1447.

[25] Berkenstadt, H., Segal, E., Mayan, H., Almog, S., Rotenberg, M., Perel, A. & Ezra, D. (1999). The pharmacokinetics of morphine and lidocaine in critically ill patients, *Intensive Care Medicine* **25**, 110–112.

[26] Kalapos, M.P. (2003). On the mammalian acetone metabolism: from chemistry to clinical implications, *Biochimica et Biophysica Acta* **1621**, 122–139.

[27] Moriya, F. & Hashimoto, Y. (2000). Determining the state of the deceased during cardiopulmonary resuscitation from tissue distribution patterns of intubation related lidocaine, *Journal of Forensic Sciences* **45**, 846–849.

[28] Soine, W.H. (1986). Clandestine drug synthesis, *Medicinal Research Reviews* **6**, 41–76.

[29] Kintz, P. (2004). Value of hair analysis in postmortem toxicology, *Forensic Science International* **142**, 127–134.

[30] Pötsch, L. & Skopp, G. (2004). Inkorporation von Fremdsubstanzen in Haare, in *Haaranalytik. Technik und Interpretation in Medizin und Recht*, B. Madea & F. Muhoff, eds, Deutscher Ärzteverlag, Köln, pp. 31–98.

[31] Thorspecken, J., Skopp, G. & Pötsch, L. (2004). In vitro contamination of hair by marijuana smoke, *Clinical Chemistry* **50**, 596–602.

[32] Moriya, F. & Hashimoto, Y. (2000). Criteria for judging whether postmortem blood drug concentrations can be used for toxicologic evaluation, *Legal Medicine* **2**, 143–151.

[33] Jones, G.R. (1998). Interpretation of post-mortem drug levels, in *Drug Abuse Handbook*, S.B. Karch, ed, CRC Press, Boca Raton, pp. 970–985.

[34] Larsen, R.H., Nielsen, F., Sorensen, J.A. & Nielsen, J.B. (2003). Dermal penetration of fentanyl: inter- and intraindividual variations, *Pharmacology and Toxicology* **93**, 244–248.

[35] Curry, A.S. & Sunshine, I. (1960). The liver to blood ratio in cases of barbiturate poisoning, *Toxicology and Applied Pharmacology* **2**, 602–606.

[36] Cook, D.S. & Braithwaite, R.A. (2000). Estimating antemortem drug concentrations from postmortem blood samples: the influence of postmortem redistribution, *Journal of Clinical Pathology* **53**, 282–285.

[37] Gerostamoulos, J. & Drummer, O.H. (2000). Postmortem redistribution of morphine and its metabolites, *Journal of Forensic Sciences* **45**, 843–845.

[38] Baselt, R.C. (2004). *Disposition of Toxic Drugs and Chemicals in Man*, 7th Edition, Biomedical Publications, Foster City.

[39] Pounder, D.J. & Jones, G.R. (1990). Post-mortem drug redistribution – a toxicological nightmare, *Forensic Science International* **45**, 253–263.

[40] Pounder, D.J. (1994). The nightmare of postmortem drug changes, in *Legal Medine 1993*, C.H. Wecht, ed, Butterworth Legal Publishers, New Hampshire, pp. 162–191.

[41] Prouty, R.W. & Anderson, W.H. (1990). The forensic implications of site and temporal influences on postmortem blood-drug concentrations, *Journal of Forensic Sciences* **35**, 243–270.

[42] Drummer, O., Forrest, A.R.W., Goldberger, B. & Karch, S.B. (2004). Forensic science in the dock. Postmortem measurements of drug concentration in blood have little meaning, *British Medical Journal* **329**, 636–637.

[43] Pelissier-Alicot, A.L., Gaulier, J.M. & Marquet, P. (2003). Mechanisms underlying post-mortem redistribution of drugs: a review, *Journal of Analytical Toxicology* **27**, 533–544.

[44] Yarema, M.C. & Becker, C.E. (2005). Key concepts in post-mortem drug redistribution, *Clinical Toxicology* **43**, 235–241.

[45] Pounder, D.J., Owen, V. & Quigley, C. (1994). Postmortem changes in blood amitriptyline concentration, *The American Journal of Forensic Medicine and Pathology* **15**, 224–230.

[46] Logan, B.K. & Smirnow, D. (1996). Postmortem distribution and redistribution of morphine in man, *Journal of Forensic Sciences* **41**, 37–46.

[47] Pounder, D.J., Fuke, C., Cox, D.E., Smith, D. & Kuroda, N. (1996). Postmortem diffusion of drugs from gastric residue, *The American Journal of Forensic Medicine and Pathology* **17**, 1–7.

[48] Pounder, D.J. & Smith, D.R.W. (1995). Postmortem diffusion of alcohol from the stomach, *The American Journal of Forensic Medicine and Pathology* **16**, 89–96.

[49] Hepler, B.R. & Isenschmid, D.S. (1998). Specimen selection, collection, preservation, and security, in *Drug Abuse Handbook*, S.B. Karch, ed, CRC Press, Boca Raton, pp. 873–889.

[50] Pounder, D.J. & Yonemitsu, K. (1991). Postmortem absorption of drugs and ethanol from aspirated vomitus – an experimental model, *Forensic Science International* **51**, 189–195.

[51] Mijazaki, T., Kojima, T., Yashiki, M., Wakamoto, H., Iwasaki, Y. & Taniguchi, T. (1993). Site dependence of methamphetamine concentrations in blood samples collected from cadavers of people who had been methamphetamine abusers, *The American Journal of Forensic Medicine and Pathology* **14**, 121–124.

[52] Pounder, D.J., Hartley, A.K. & Watmough, P.J. (1994). Postmortem redistribution and degradation of dothiepin. Human case studies and an animal model, *The American Journal of Forensic Medicine and Pathology* **15**, 231–235.

[53] Fuke, C., Berry, C.L. & Pounder, D.J. (1996). Postmortem diffusion of ingested and aspirated paint thinner, *Forensic Science International* **78**, 100–207.

[54] Pohland, R.C. & Bernhard, N.R. (1997). Postmortem serum and tissue redistribution of fluoxetine and norfluoxetine in dogs following oral administration of fluoxetine hydrochloride (Prozac), *Journal of Forensic Sciences* **42**, 812–816.

[55] Hilberg, T., Bugge, A., Beylich, K.M., Ingum, J., Bjorneboe, A. & Morland, J. (1993). An animal model of postmortem amitriptyline redistribution, *Journal of Forensic Sciences* **38**, 81–90.

[56] Vorpahl, T.E. & Coe, J.I. (1978). Correlation of antemortem and postmortem digoxin levels, *Journal of Forensic Sciences* **23**, 329–334.

[57] Aderjan, R. & Mattern, R. (1980). Zur Wertigkeit post-mortaler Digoxin-Konzentrationen im Blut, *Zeitschrift fur Rechtsmedizin* **86**, 13–20.

[58] Dalpe-Scott, M., Degouffe, M., Garbutt, D. & Drost, M. (1995). A comparison of drug concentrations in post-mortem cardiac and peripheral blood in 320 cases, *Canadian Society of Forensic Science Journal* **28**, 113–121.

[59] Jones, G.R. & Pounder, D.J. (1987). Site dependence of drug concentrations in postmortem blood – a case study, *Journal of Analytical Toxicology* **11**, 186–190.

[60] Levine, B., Wu, S.C., Dixon, A. & Smialek, J.E. (1995). Site dependence of postmortem blood methadone concentrations, *The American Journal of Forensic Medicine and Pathology* **16**, 97–100.

[61] Milroy, C.M. & Forrest, A.R.W. (2000). Methadone deaths: a toxicological analysis, *Journal of Clinical Pathology* **53**, 277–281.

[62] Berg, M.J., Lantz, R.K., Schentag, J.J. & Vern, B.A. (1984). Distribution of cimetidine in postmortem tissue, *Journal of Forensic Sciences* **29**, 147–154.

[63] Hearn, W.L., Keran, E.E., Wie, H. & Hime, G. (1991). Site-dependent postmortem changes in blood cocaine concentrations, *Journal of Forensic Sciences* **36**, 673–684.

[64] Pounder, D.J. & Davies, J.I. (1994). Zopiclone poisoning: tissue distribution and potential for postmortem diffusion, *Forensic Science International* **65**, 177–183.

[65] Elliott, S.P. (2005). Methylenedioxymethamphetamine and methylenedioxyamphetamine concentrations in ante-mortem and post-mortem specimens in fatalities following hospital admission, *Journal of Analytical Toxicology* **29**, 296–300.

[66] Skopp, G., Klinder, K., Pötsch, L., Zimmer, G., Lutz, R., Aderjan, R. & Mattern, R. (1998). Postmortem distribution of dihydrocodeine and metabolites in a fatal case of dihydrocodeine intoxication, *Forensic Science International* **95**, 99–107.

[67] De Letter, E.A., Clauwaert, K.M., Belpaire, F.M., Lambert, W.E., Van Boxclear, J.F. & Piette, M.H.A. (2002). Post-mortem redistribution of 3,4-methylenedioxy methamphetamine (MDMA, "ecstasy") in the rabbit. Part I: experimental approach after in vivo intravenous infusion, *International Journal of Legal Medicine* **116**, 216–224.

[68] De Letter, E.A., Belpaire, F.M., Clauwaert, K.M., Lambert, W.E., Van Boxclear, J.F. & Piette, M.H.A. (2002). Post-mortem redistribution of 3,4-methylenedioxy methamphetamine (MDMA, "ecstasy") in the rabbit. Part II: post-mortem infusion in trachea or stomach, *International Journal of Legal Medicine* **116**, 225–232.

[69] Hilberg, T., Rogde, S. & Morland, H.J. (1999). Post-mortem drug redistribution – human cases related to results in experimental animals, *Journal of Forensic Sciences* **44**, 3–9.

[70] Quatrehomme, G., Bourett, F., Liao, Z. & Ollier, A. (1994). An experimental methodology for the study of postmortem changes in toxic concentrations of drugs, using secobarbital as an example, *Journal of Forensic Sciences* **39**, 1300–1304.

[71] Pounder, D.J., Hartley, A.K. & Watmough, P.J. (1994). Postmortem redistribution and degradation of doth-iepin. Human case studies and an animal model, *The American Journal of Forensic Medicine and Pathology* **15**, 231–235.

[72] Moffat, A.C., Osselton, M.D. & Widdop, B. (eds) (2004). *Clarke's Analysis of Drugs and Poisons*, 3rd Edition, Pharmaceutical Press, London, Vol. 2.

[73] Schulz, M. & Schmoldt, A. (2003). Therapeutic and toxic blood concentrations of more than 800 drugs and other xenobiotics, *Pharmazie* **58**, 447–474.

[74] Winek, C.L., Wahba, W.W., Winek Jr, C.L. & Winek Balzer, T. (2001). Drug and chemical blood-level data 2001, *Forensic Science International* **122**, 107–123.

[75] Schleyer, F. (1958). *Postmortale, klinisch-chemische Diagnostik und Todeszeitbestimmung mit chemischen und physikalischen Methoden*, Thieme, Stuttgart, pp. 39–41.

[76] Skopp, G., Lutz, R., Pötsch, L., Ganßmann, B., Klinder, K., Schmidt, A., Aderjan, R. & Mattern, R. (1997). An in vitro experiment for postmortem vascular per-meation. The passage of morphine and morphine glu-curonides across a vascular wall, *Journal of Forensic Sciences* **42**, 486–491.

[77] Brettel, H.F. (1970). Über Beziehungen zwischen dem Abfall der Blutalkoholkonzentration und dem Wasserverlust des Blutes nach dem Tode, *Blutalkohol* **7**, 54–64.

[78] Thomsen, H. (1998). *Post Mortem Platelets in Blood, Thrombi and Haematomas, Research in Legal Medi-cine*, Schmidt-Römhild, Lübeck, Germany, Vol. 20.

[79] Maguire, K.P., Burrows, G.D., Norman, T.R. & Scog-gins, B.A. (1980). Blood/plasma distribution ratios of psychotropic drugs, *Clinical Chemistry* **26**, 1624–1625.

[80] Jeffcoat, A.R., Perez-Reyes, M., Hill, J.M., Sadler, B.M. & Cook, C.E. (1989). Cocaine disposition in humans after intravenous injection, nasal insufflation (snorting), or smoking, *Drug Metabolism and Disposi-tion* **17**, 153–159.

[81] Shull Jr, H.J., Wilkinson, G.R., Johnson, R. & Schenker, S. (1976). Normal disposition of oxazepam in acute viral hepatitis and cirrhosis, *Annals of Internal Medicine* **84**, 420–425.

[82] Payne, J.P., Hill, D.W. & Wood, D.G.L. (1968). Dis-tribution of ethanol between plasma and erythrocytes in whole blood, *Nature* **217**, 963–964.

[83] Inturrisi, C.E., Colburn, W.A., Kaiko, R.F., Houde, R.W. & Foley, K.M. (1987). Pharmacokinetics and pharmacodynamics of methadone in patients with chronic pain, *Clinical Pharmacy and Therapeutics* **41**, 392–401.

[84] Hand, C.W., Moore, R.A. & Sear, J.W. (1988). Com-parison of whole blood and plasma morphine, *Journal of Analytical Toxicology* **12**, 234–235.

[85] Skopp, G., Pötsch, L., Ganssmann, B., Aderjan, R. & Mattern, R. (1998). A preliminary study on the

distribution of morphine and its glucuronides in the subcompartments of blood, *Journal of Analytical Toxicology* **22**, 261–264.

[86] Widman, M., Agurell, S., Ehrnebo, M. & Jones, G. (1974). Binding of (+)- and (−)-delta-1-tetrahydrocannabinols and (−)-7-hydroxy-delta-1-tetrahydrocannabinol to blood cells and plasma proteins in man, *The Journal of Pharmacy and Pharmacology* **26**, 914–916.

[87] Hanson, V.W., Buonarati, M.H., Baselt, R.C., Wada, N.A., Yep, C., Biasotti, A.A., Reeve, V.C., Wong, A.S. & Orbanowsky, W.M. (1983). Comparison of ^{3}H-and ^{125}I-radioimmunoassay and gas chromatography/mass spectrometry for the determination of Δ^9-tetrahydrocannabinol and cannabinoids in blood and serum, *Journal of Analytical Toxicology* **7**, 96–102.

[88] Giroud, C., Menetrey, A., Augsburger, M., Buclin, T., Sanchez-Mazas, P. & Mangin, P. (2001). Delta(9)-THC, 11-OH-Delta(9)-THC and Delta(9)-THCCOOH plasma or serum to whole blood concentrations distribution ratios in blood samples taken from living and dead people, *Forensic Science International* **123**, 159–164.

[89] Iten, P.X. (1994). *Fahren unter Drogen- oder Medikamenteneinfluss*, Institut für Rechtsmedizin der Universität Zürich, Zürich.

[90] Linnoila, M. & Dorrity, F. (1978). Measurement of plasma and erythrocyte chlorpromazine and N-monodesmethylchlorpromazine levels by gas chromatography with a nitrogen sensitive detector, *Acta Pharmacologica et Toxicologica* **42**, 264–270.

[91] Flanagan, R.J., Amin, A. & Seinen, W. (2003). Effect of post-mortem changes on peripheral and central whole blood and tissue clozapine and norclozapine concentrations in the domestic pig (Sus crofa), *Forensic Science International* **12**, 9–17.

[92] Highley, M.S. & De Bruijn, E.A. (1996). Erythrocytes and the transport of drugs and endogenous compounds, *Pharmaceutical Research* **13**, 186–195.

[93] Morris, J.A., Harrison, L.M. & Partridge, S.M. (2006). Postmortem bacteriology: a re-evaluation, *Journal of Clinical Pathology* **59**, 1–9.

[94] Reinhardt, G., Zink, P. & Legler, F. (1973). Bacteriological findings in cardiac blood of a cadaver, *Beiträge zur Gerichtlichen Medizin* **31**, 311–314.

[95] Stevens, H.M. (1984). The stability of some drugs and poisons in putrefying human liver tissues, *Journal – Forensic Science Society* **24**, 577–589.

[96] Drummer, O.H. (1997). Stability of drugs postmortem: a *review*, *Proceedings of the 35th Annual Meeting of The International Association of Forensic Toxicologists*, Padua, pp. 13–17.

[97] Schmidt, G. (1969). Postmortale Veränderungen von Arzneistoffen und Giften in Organen und Körperflüssigkeiten einschließlich Neubildung von Störsubstanzen, in *Gadamers Lehrbuch der chemischen Toxikologie und Anleitung zur Ausmittelung der Gifte*, R. Preu, ed, Vandenhoeck & Ruprecht, Göttingen, pp. 189–241.

[98] Arnold, D., Naeve, W. & Arnold, W. (1984). Toxikologische Befunderhebungen an Fäulnisleichen, *Zeitschrift für Rechtsmedizin* **93**, 151–164.

[99] Tsunenari, S., Yonemitsu, K., Uchimara, Y. & Kanda, M. (1981). The influence of putrefactive changes on the determination of paraquat in autopsy materials, *Forensic Science International* **17**, 51–56.

[100] Kiyofuji, T. (1970). Studies on the extraction of poisonous substances from cadaveric materials of synthetic organo-pesticides poisoning and effects of postmortem changes on their extraction, *Journal of the Kumamoto Medical Society* **44**, 767–817.

[101] Robertson, M.D. & Drummer, O.H. (1998). Stability of nitrobenzodiazepines in postmortem blood, *Journal of Forensic Sciences* **43**, 5–8.

[102] Drummer, O.H., Syrjanen, M.L. & Cordner, S.M. (1993). Deaths involving the benzodiazepine flunitrazepam, *The American Journal of Forensic Medicine and Pathology* **14**, 238–243.

[103] Skopp, G. & Pötsch, L. (2002). Stability of 11-nor-delta(9)-carboxy-tetrahydrocannabinol glucuronide in plasma and urine assessed by liquid chromatography-tandem mass spectrometry, *Clinical Chemistry* **48**, 301–306.

[104] Shipkova, M., Armstrong, V.W., Oellerich, M. & Wieland, E. (2003). Acyl glucuronide drug metabolites: toxicological and analytical implications, *Therapeutic Drug Monitoring* **25**, 1–16.

[105] Skopp, G., Pötsch, L., Klingmann, A. & Mattern, R. (2001). Stability of morphine, morphine-3-glucuronide, and morphine-6-glucuronide in fresh blood and plasma and postmortem blood samples, *Journal of Analytical Toxicology* **25**, 2–7.

[106] Moriya, F. & Hashimoto, Y. (1997). Distribution of free and conjugated morphine in body tissues in a fatal heroin overdose: Is conjugated morphine stable in postmortem specimens, *Journal of Forensic Sciences* **42**, 736–740.

[107] Carroll, F.T., Marracini, J.V., Lewis, S. & Wright, W. (2000). Morphine-3-d-glucuronide stability in postmortem specimens exposed to bacterial enzymatic hydrolysis, *The American Journal of Forensic Medicine and Pathology* **21**, 323–329.

[108] Felby, S. & Nielsen, E. (1994). The postmortem blood alcohol concentration and the water content, *Blutalkohol* **31**, 24–32.

[109] Iffland, R. & Palm, W. (1979). Untersuchungen zur postmortalen Alkoholverteilung in Butgefäßen und Körperflüssigkeiten, *Blutalkohol* **16**, 81–96.

[110] Brettel, H.F. (1973). Der Korrekturfaktor bei der gaschromatographischen Leichenblutalkoholbestimmung, *Blutalkohol* **10**, 120–124.

[111] Huckenbeck, W. & Bonte, W. (2003). Alkohol, in *Handbuch Gerichtliche Medizin*, B. Madea & B. Brinkmann, eds, Springer Berlin, Heidelberg, New York, pp. 469–485.

[112] Kugelberg F.C., Jones A.W. (2007). Interpreting results of ethanol analysis in postmortem specimens: a review of the literature, *Forensic Science International* **165**, 10–29.

[113] O'Neal, C.L. & Poklis, A. (1996). Postmortem production of ethanol and factors that influence interpretation, *The American Journal of Forensic Medicine and Pathology* **17**, 8–20.

[114] Zumwalt, R.E., Bost, R.O. & Sunshine, I. (1982). Evaluation of ethanol concentrations in decomposed bodies, *Journal of Forensic Science Society* **27**, 549–554.

[115] Hansen, A.C. (1994). Validity of postmortem alcohol determination, *Ugeskrift for Laeger* **156**, 55–57.

[116] Corry, J.E.L. (1978). Possible sources of ethanol ante- and post-mortem: its relation to the biochemistry and microbiology of decomposition, *The Journal of Applied Bacteriology* **44**, 1–56.

[117] Huckenbeck, W. (1999). *Experimentelle Untersuchungen Zum bakteriell induzierten Alkohol- und Aminosäurenstoffwechsel im Blut der menschlichen Leiche*, Habilitationsschrift, Universität Düsseldorf, Germany.

[118] Bogusz, M., Guminska, M. & Markiewicz, J. (1970). Studies on the formation of endogenous ethanol in blood putrefying in vitro, *Journal of Forensic Medicine* **17**, 156–168.

[119] Seto, Y. (1996). Stability and spontaneous production of blood cyanide during heating, *Journal of Forensic Sciences* **41**, 465–468.

[120] Berankova, K., Mutnanska, K. & Balikova, M. (2006). γ-Hydroxybutyric acid stability and formation in blood and urine, *Forensic Science International* **161**, 158–162.

[121] Karch, S.B. (2001). GHB. Club drug or confusing artefact? *The American Journal of Forensic Medicine and Pathology* **22**, 266–269.

[122] Winek, C.L., Zaveri, N.R. & Wahba, W.W. (1993). The study of tricyclic antidepressants in formalin-fixed human liver and formalin solutions, *Forensic Science International* **61**, 175–183.

[123] Gannett, P.M., Daft, J.R., James, D., Rybeck, B., Knopp, J.B. & Tracy, T.S. (2001). In vitro reaction of barbiturates with formaldehyde, *Journal of Analytical Toxicology* **25**, 443–449.

[124] Tirumalai, P.S., Shakleya, D.M., Gannett, P.M., Callery, P.S., Bland, T.M. & Tracy, T.S. (2005). Conversion of methamphetamine to N-methylmethamphetamine in formalin solutions, *Journal of Analytical Toxicology* **29**, 48–53.

[125] Cingolani, M., Cippitelli, M., Froldi, R., Tassoni, G. & Mirtella, D. (2005). Stability of barbiturates in fixed tissues and formalin solutions, *Journal of Analytical Toxicology* **29**, 205–208.

[126] Tracy, T.S., Rybeck, B.F., James, D.G., Knopp, J.B. & Gannett, P.M. (2001). Stability of benzodiazepines in formaldehyde solutions, *Journal of Analytical Toxicology* **25**, 166–173.

[127] Dettling, R.J., Briglia, E.J., Dal Cortivo, L.A. & Bidanset, J.H. (1990). The production of amitriptyline from nortriptyline in formaldehyde-containing solutions, *Journal of Analytical Toxicology* **14**, 325–326.

[128] Gannett, P.M., Hailu, S., Daft, J., James, D., Rybeck, B. & Tracy, T.S. (2001). In vitro reaction of formaldehyde with fenfluramine: conversion to N-methyl fenfluramine, *Journal of Analytical Toxicology* **25**, 88–92.

[129] Nishigami, J., Takayasu, T. & Ohshima, T. (1995). Toxicological analysis of the psychotropic drugs chlorpromazine and diazepam using chemically fixed tissues, *International Journal of Legal Medicine* **107**, 165–170.

[130] Forney Jr, R.B., Carroll, F.T., Nordgren, I.K., Petterson, B.M. & Holmstedt, B. (1982). Extraction, identification and quantitation of succinylcholine in embalmed tissue, *Journal of Analytical Toxicology* **6**, 115–119.

[131] Takayasu, T., Saito, K., Nishigami, J., Ohshima, T. & Nagano, T. (1994). Toxicological analysis of drugs and poisons in formalin-fixed organ tissues, *International Journal of Legal Medicine* **107**, 7–12.

[132] Pagani, S., Mirtella, D., Mencarelli, R., Rodriguez, D. & Cingolani, M. (2005). Postmortem distribution of sildenafil in histological material, *Journal of Analytical Toxicology* **29**, 254–257.

[133] Cingolani, M., Froldi, R., Mencarelli, R., Mirtella, D. & Rodriguez, D. (2001). Detection and quantitation of morphine in fixed tissues and formalin solutions, *Journal of Analytical Toxicology* **25**, 31–34.

[134] Cingolani, M., Froldi, R., Mencarelli, R. & Rodriguez, D. (1999). Analytical detection and quantitation of strychnine in chemically fixed organ tissues, *Journal of Analytical Toxicology* **23**, 219–221.

[135] Iffland, R., Madea, B. & Balling, P. (1988). Diagnose Kohlenmonoxidvergiftung nach Einbalsamierung und Exhumierung, *Archiv fur Kriminologie* **182**, 100–106.

[136] Tsoukali-Papadopoulou, H. (1987). Elucidation of a poisoning case from the analysis of formalin in which brain tissue was preserved, *Forensic Science International* **34**, 63–65.

[137] Brinkmann, B. (1999). Harmonisation of medico-legal autopsy rules, *International Journal of Legal Medicine* **113**, 1–14.

[138] Forrest, A.R.W. (1993). Obtaining samples at post mortem examination for toxicological and biochemical analyses, *Journal of Clinical Pathology* **46**, 292–296.

[139] Vanbinst, R., Koenig, J., Di Fazio, V. & Hassoun, A. (2002). Bile analysis of drugs in postmortem cases, *Forensic Science International* **128**, 35–40.

[140] Maurer, H.H. (1999). Systematic toxicological analysis procedures for acidic drugs and/or metabolites relevant to clinical and forensic toxicology and/or doping control, *Journal of Chromatography. B, Biomedical Sciences and Applications* **733**, 3–25.

[141] Jones, G. (2004). Postmortem toxicology, in *Clarke's Analysis of Drugs and Poisons*, A.C. Moffat, M.D. Osselton & B. Widdop, eds, 3rd Edition, Pharmaceutical Press, London, Chicago, pp. 94–108.

[142] Jenkins, A.J. & Lavins, E.S. (1998). 6-Acetylmorphine detection in postmortem cerebrospinal fluid, *Journal of Analytical Toxicology* **22**, 173–175.

[143] Scott, K.S. & Oliver, J.S. (1999). Vitreous humor as an alternative sample to blood for the supercritical fluid extraction of morphine and 6-acetylmorphine, *Medicine, Science, and the Law* **39**, 77–81.

[144] Ritz, S., Harding, P., Martz, W., Schütz, H.W. & Kaatsch, H.J. (1992). Measurement of digitalis-glycoside levels in ocular tissues: a way to improve postmortem diagnosis of lethal digitalis-glycoside poisoning? I: digoxin, *International Journal of Legal Medicine* **105**, 149–154.

[145] Anastasos, N., McIntyre, I.M., Lynch, M.J. & Drummer, O.H. (2002). Postmortem concentrations of citalopram, *Journal of Forensic Sciences* **47**, 882–884.

[146] Furnari, C., Ottaviano, V., Sachetti, G. & Mancini, M. (2002). A fatal case of cocaine poisoning in a body packer, *Journal of Forensic Sciences* **47**, 208–210.

[147] Decaestecker, T., De Letter, E., Clauwaert, K., Bouche, M.P., Lambert, W., Van Boxclear, J., Piette, M., Van den Eeckhout, E., Van Peteghem, C. & De Leenheer, A. (2001). Fatal 4-MTA intoxication: development of a liquid chromatographic-tandem mass spectrometric assay for multiple matrices, *Journal of Analytical Toxicology* **25**, 705–710.

[148] Gock, S.B., Wong, S.H., Stormo, K.A. & Jentzen, J.M. (1999). Self-intoxication with morphine obtained from an infusion pump, *Journal of Analytical Toxicology* **23**, 130–133.

[149] Wogoman, H., Steinberg, M. & Jenkins, A.J. (1999). Acute intoxication with guaifenesin, diphenhydramine, and chlorpheniramine, *The American Journal of Forensic Medicine and Pathology* **20**, 199–202.

[150] Scott, K.S. & Oliver, J.S. (2001). The use of vitreous humor as an alternative to whole blood for the analysis of benzodiazepines, *Journal of Forensic Sciences* **46**, 694–697.

[151] Caplan, Y.H. & Levine, B. (1990). Vitreous humor in the evaluation of postmortem blood ethanol concentrations, *Journal of Analytical Toxicology* **14**, 305–307.

[152] Jones, A.W. & Holmgren, P. (2001). Uncertainty in estimating blood ethanol concentrations by analysis of vitreous humor, *Journal of Clinical Pathology* **54**, 699–702.

[153] Musshoff, F., Padosch, S., Steinborn, S. & Madea, B. (2004). Fatal blood and tissue concentrations of more than 200 drugs, *Forensic Science International* **142**, 161–210.

[154] Pounder, D.J., Adams, E., Fuke, C. & Langford, A.M. (1996). Site to site variability of postmortem drug concentrations in liver and lung, *Journal of Forensic Sciences* **41**, 927–932.

[155] Merrick, T.C., Felo, J.A. & Jenkins, A.J. (2001). Tissue distribution of olanzapine in a postmortem case, *The American Journal of Forensic Medicine and Pathology* **22**, 270–274.

[156] Garriott, J.C. (1991). Skeletal muscle as an alternative specimen for alcohol and drug analysis, *Journal of Forensic Sciences* **36**, 60–69.

[157] Skopp, G., Potsch, L., Eser, H.P. & Moller, M.R. (1996). Preliminary practical findings on drug monitoring by a transcutaneous collection device, *Journal of Forensic Sciences* **41**, 933–937.

[158] Kijewski, H. (1993). *Die Forensische Bedeutung der Mineralstoffgehalte in menschlichen Kopfhaaren*, Schmidt-Römhild, Köln, pp. 53–95.

[159] Sachs, H. & Kintz, P. (1998). Testing for drugs in hair. Critical review of chromatographic procedures since 1992, *Journal of Chromatography. B, Biomedical Sciences and Applications* **713**, 147–161.

[160] Pragst, F., Rothe, M., Spiegel, K. & Sporkert, F. (1998). Illegal and therapeutic drug concentrations in hair segments – A timetable of drug exposure? *Forensic Science Reviews* **10**, 81–111.

[161] McCurdy, W.C. (1987). Postmortem specimen collection, *Forensic Science International* **35**, 61–65.

[162] Dyne, D., Cocker, J., Streete, P.J. & Flanagan, R.J. (1996). Toluene, 1-butanol, ethylbenzene and xylene from sarstedt monovette serum gel blood collection tubes, *Annals of Clinical Biochemistry* **33**, 355–356.

[163] Klingmann, A., Skopp, G. & Aderjan, R. (2001). Analysis of cocaine, benzoylecgonine, ecgonine methyl ester, and ecgonine by high pressure liquid chromatography-API mass spectrometry and application to a short-term degradation study of cocaine in plasma, *Journal of Analytical Toxicology* **25**, 425–430.

[164] Barrett, D.A., Dyssegaard, A.L.P. & Shaw, P.N. (1992). The effect of temperature and pH on the deacetylation of diamorphine in aqueous solution and in human plasma, *The Journal of Pharmacy and Pharmacology* **44**, 606–608.

[165] Ferrara, S.D., Frison, G., Tdeschi, L. & LeBeau, M. (2001). γ-Hydroxybutyrate (GHB) and related products, in *Drug-Facilitated Sexual Assault*, M.A. LeBeau & A. Mozayani, eds, A Forensic Handbook, Academic Press, San Diego, pp. 107–126.

[166] Moriya, F., Hashimoto, Y. & Kuo, P.L. (1999). Pitfalls when determining tissue distributions of organophosphorus chemicals: sodium fluoride accelerates chemical degradation, *Journal of Analytical Toxicology* **23**, 210–215.

[167] Heinig, R., Zimmer, D., Yeh, S. & Krol, G.J. (2000). Development, validation and application of assays to quantify metrifonate and 2,2-dichlorovinyl dimethylphosphate in human body fluids, *Journal of Chromatography. B* **741**, 257–269.

[168] Moriya, F. & Hashimoto, Y. (1996). The effect of postmortem interval on the concentrations of cocaine and cocaethylene in blood and tissues: an experiment using rats, *Journal of Forensic Sciences* **41**, 129–133.

[169] Olesen, O.V. & Linnet, K. (1998). Determination of olanzapine in serum by high-performance liquid chromatography using ultraviolet detection considering the

easy oxidability of the compound and the presence of other psychotropic drugs, *Journal of Chromatography. B* **714**, 309–315.

[170]   Smith, R.V., Wilcox, R.E. & Humphrey, D.W. (1980). Stability of apomorphine in frozen plasma, *Research Communications in Chemical Pathology and Pharmacology* **27**, 183–186.

[171]   Curry, S.H. & Evans, S. (1976). A note on the assay of chlorpromazine N-oxide and its sulphoxide in plasma and urine, *The Journal of Pharmacy and Pharmacology* **28**, 1467–1468.

[172]   Westerling, D., Bengtsson, D.I., Thysell, C. & Hoglund, P. (1996). The influence of preanalytical factors on concentrations of morphine and metabolites in patients receiving morphine, *Pharmacology and Toxicology* **78**, 82–85.

[173]   Stamm, D. (1982). A new concept for quality control of clinical laboratory investigations in the light of clinical requirements and based on reference method values, *Journal of Clinical Chemistry and Clinical Biochemistry* **20**, 817–824.

[174]   Ellenhorn, M.J. (ed) (1997). Appendix H. The poisoned patients and the laboratory – "the flanagan tables", in *Ellenhorn's Medical Toxicology: Diagnosis and Treatment of Human Poisoning*, 2nd Edition, Williams & Wilkins, Baltimore, pp. 1929–1933.

[175]   Drummer, O.H. (2001). *The Forensic Pharmacology of Drugs of Abuse*, Arnold, London, New York, New Delhi.

[176]   Levine, B. & Smith, M.L. (1990). Stability of drugs of abuse in biological specimens, *Forensic Science Reviews* **2**, 147–157.

[177]   Skopp, G. & Pötsch, L. (2002). Zur präanalytischen Phase chemisch-toxikologischer Untersuchungen. II: Stabilität forensisch relevanter Substanzen in Blut-, Plasma- oder Serumproben – eine Bestandsaufnahme, *Rechtsmedizin* **12**, 195–202.

[178]   Saker, E.G., Eskew, A.E. & Panter, J.W. (1991). Stability of toluene in blood: its forensic relevance, *Journal of Analytical Toxicology* **15**, 246–249.

[179]   Curry, A.S., Price, D.E. & Rutter, R.C. (1967). The production of cyanide in post mortem material, *Acta Pharmacologica et Toxicologica* **25**, 339–344.

[180]   Egekeze, J.O. & Oehme, F.W. (1980). Thiocyanate to cyanide: revisited, *Clinical Toxicology* **16**, 127–128.

[181]   Ballantyne, B., Bright, J.E. & Williams, P. (1974). The post mortem rate of transformation of cyanide, *Forensic Science* **3**, 71–76.

[182]   Ballantyne, B. (1976). Changes in blood cyanide as a function of storage time and temperature, *Journal of Forensic Sciences* **16**, 305–310.

[183]   Giorgi, S.N. & Meeker, J.E. (1995). A 5-year stability study of common illicit drugs in blood, *Journal of Analytical Toxicology* **19**, 392–398.

[184]   Skopp, G., Pötsch, L., Mattern, R. & Aderjan, R. (2002). Short-term stability of lysergic acid diethylamide (LSD), N-desmethyl-LSD, and 2-oxo-3-hydroxy-LSD in urine, assessed by liquid chromatography-tandem mass spectrometry, *Clinical Chemistry* **48**, 1615–1618.

[185]   Robertson, M.D. & Drummer, O.H. (1995). Postmortem drug metabolism by bacteria, *Journal of Forensic Sciences* **40**, 382–386.

[186]   El Mahjoub, A. & Staub, C. (2000). Stability of benzodiazepines in whole blood samples stored at varying temperatures, *Journal of Pharmaceutical and Biomedical Analysis* **23**, 1057–1063.

[187]   Entwhistle, N., Owen, P., Patterson, D.A., Jones, L.V. & Smith, J.A. (1986). The occurrence of chlordiazepoxide degradation products in sudden deaths associated with chlordiazepoxide, *Journal of Forensic Sciences* **26**, 45–54.

[188]   Couper, F.J. & Drummer, O.H. (1999). Postmortem stability and interpretation of beta 2-agonist concentrations, *Journal of Forensic Sciences* **44**, 523–526.

[189]   McCracken, R.J., Blanchflower, W.J., Rowan, C., McCoy, M.A. & Kennedy, D.G. (1995). Determination of furazolidone in porcine tissue using thermospray liquid chromatography-mass spectrometry and a study of the pharmacokinetics and stability of its residues, *The Analyst* **120**, 2347–2351.

[190]   McCracken, R.J., McCoy, M.A. & Kennedy, D.G. (1997). The prevalence and possible causes of bound and extractable residues of the furazolidone metabolite 3-amino-2-oxazolidinone in porcine tissues, *Food Additives and Contaminants* **14**, 287–294.

[191]   Isenschmid, D.S., Levine, B.S. & Caplan, Y.H. (1989). A comprehensive study of the stability of cocaine and its metabolites, *Journal of Analytical Toxicology* **13**, 250–256.

[192]   Meatherall, R.C. & Fraser, A.D. (1998). CEDIA dau: a reformulation, *Journal of Analytical Toxicology* **22**, 270–273.

[193]   Kupiec, T., DeCicco, L., Spiehler, V., Sneed, G. & Kemp, P. (2002). Choice of an ELISA assay for screening post-mortem blood for amphetamine and/or methamphetamine, *Journal of Analytical Toxicology* **26**, 513–518.

[194]   Mauden, M., Skopp, G., Mattern, R. & Aderjan, R. (2000). GC/MS-Bestimmungen von THCCOOH im Serum: Vergleich verschiedener Aufarbeitungsmethoden und Einfluß von THCCOOH-Glucuronid, *Blutalkohol* **37**, 45–53.

[195]   Wester, R., Noonan, P., Markos, C., Bible Jr, R., Aksamit, W. & Hribar, J. (1981). Identification of carbamate derivatives formed during chloroform extraction of tricyclic antidepressants in urine, *Journal of Chromatography* **209**, 463–466.

[196]   Gadkariem, E.A., El-Obeid, H.A., Abounassif, M.A., Ahmed, S.M. & Ibrahim, K.E. (2003). Effects of alkali and simulated gastric and intestinal fluids on danazol stability, *Journal of Pharmaceutical and Biomedical Analysis* **26**, 743–751.

GISELA SKOPP

Postmortem Toxicology: Interpretation

Introduction

The detection of drugs and other substances in biological tissues, such as blood, represents the first stage in the application of toxicology to the forensic sciences. The presence of drug including situations where quantitative data are available requires careful interpretation.

With few exceptions, interpretation requires a thorough understanding of the circumstances of the case and an advanced knowledge of how the substances detected by the analyses interact with the body. Thus, knowledge of both the pharmacokinetics (effect of drug) and the pharmacology of the substance is required and must be carefully related to the known circumstances of the case.

This article provides an overview of the basic pharmacokinetics of drugs and how route of administration and the overall health of the person can influence the interpretation of toxicological results. Several examples are included to illustrate how toxicological data can be misinterpreted.

Other articles in this encyclopedia provide details of the expected effects of substances; see sections on drug classes: alcohol, amphetamines, cocaine, benzodiazepines, and the opioids (opiates). (*See also* **Behavioral Toxicology**).

Basic Pharmacokinetics

To understand the way substances such as drugs are absorbed and the time course of their presence in the body, it is necessary to understand some basic effects of drugs in the body, known as *pharmacokinetics* [1, 2].

The main pharmacokinetic phases can be segregated as follows: absorption, distribution, and elimination.

Absorption

Drugs that are swallowed rely on the release of the drug or other dose form in the stomach or small intestine. This can occur through disintegration of a tablet or through a controlled release of drug from the tablet matrix. Controlled release of drugs is designed to slow the absorption, to (usually) prolong the drug's actions, or sometimes to protect the stomach from potentially harmful drug (i.e., enteric-coated tablets). Except for some acidic drugs (e.g., acetylsalicylic acid), drugs are primarily absorbed in the small intestine and then mainly in the upper sections (jejunum). The delay from swallowing to first appearance of drug in the blood stream can be typically 15–30 min and will occur over many hours.

The time to the maximum blood (or serum) concentration is termed T_{max} (units: time such as hours), while the concentration at this time is termed C_{max} (units: mass per volume, i.e., milligrams per liter).

Many drugs once absorbed (or their subsequent metabolites) can be excreted into the bowel through bile and become reabsorbed further down the gastrointestinal tract. This is known as *enterohepatic recirculation* and can lead to an apparent delay (or even a second peak) in the absorption of drugs. Morphine is a common example in which morphine glucuronide metabolites secreted into bile find their way back into the bowel and are subsequently reabsorbed.

Unabsorbed drug is present in feces and can represent a significant proportion of the administered drug.

A number of pharmaceutical formulations provide a controlled release of drug from a tablet matrix. This is used to control the absorption of drug into the body and provide a longer duration of action of the drug. This is typically used for drugs with short biological actions and has the net result in reducing the need for repeated doses within a 1-day period. For example, morphine and oxycodone can be given twice daily rather than four times daily when formulated into a sustained delivery tablet or capsule.

Distribution

Once the drug is absorbed and has entered the blood stream, it is distributed to all parts of the body. The uptake of drug into tissues and organs will depend on access of drug to all parts of the tissue (e.g., blood supply) and the relative affinity of the drug-to-tissue components. There is considerable variation of drug uptake for different drugs and also between individuals. For some drugs, the affinity of drug to a tissue can be manyfold higher than the blood (e.g., THC in fat and muscle tissue).

The distribution phase is variable but usually requires some hours or days of exposure before some form of steady-state situation is reached.

Elimination

All foreign substances are eventually removed by the body; the rate depends on the drug and its ability to be metabolized (e.g., by liver) and excreted by the kidneys and other organs. Some drugs, e.g. cocaine, are rapidly metabolized to less active compounds and excreted within hours, whereas methamphetamine may only be excreted within days. The metabolism of drugs can be quite complex and often involve multiple pathways. In some cases, metabolites are also biologically active and contribute to the pharmacological response in a person (e.g., methamphetamine is metabolized to the active amphetamine) [3].

The time to halve the blood concentration (following the peak concentration) for methamphetamine can be over 1 day. This time is called *half-life*. This value applies to the terminal elimination phase once the drug has been fully absorbed and distributed to bodily tissues. There is considerable variation in half-lives among individuals, even for the same drug. Half-lives measured before the terminal elimination phase is dominant will generally underestimate the terminal elimination rate.

Some pharmacokinetic data including terminal elimination half-lives for common drugs of abuse are given in Table 1.

The term *clearance* is often used as another measure to quantify the removal of drugs from the body and represents a composite of all forms of drug removal. This includes a combination of kidney excretion, liver metabolism, and other sources of drug removal.

For volatile substances, elimination can also occur through expiration, e.g., alcohol (ethanol), solvents, although this is still a relatively minor source of elimination compared to metabolism and excretion through the kidneys.

Route of Administration and Bioavailability

The proportion of drug available to the body when compared with another route of administration is termed *bioavailability*. This term usually refers to the

Table 1 Typical pharmacokinetic data for some common drugs

Drug	Dose range (mg)[a]	Typical blood concentrations (mg l^{-1})[b]	Half-life (days)[c]
Alprazolam	0.5–4	0.05–0.2	0.3–1
Amphetamine	From 10	0.1–0.2	0.3–1.5
Diazepam	5–40	0.1–0.6	0.8–2
Cocaine	From 25	0.1–0.5	0.6–4
Codeine	8–60	0.1–0.3	0.1–0.2
MDMA	50–150	0.1–0.3	0.4–1
Methadone	5–120	0.1–0.3	0.6–3
Methamphetamine	From 10	0.05–0.2	0.5–1.5
Morphine	From 5	0.1–0.4	0.1–0.4

[a] Usual dose range
[b] Typical blood concentrations following common doses seen in forensic cases
[c] Pharmacokinetic half-life of terminal elimination phase
MDMA, 3,4-methylenedioxymethamphetamine

comparative availability of drugs that are orally taken compared with the same dose given intravenously. Drugs that have a bioavailability of 100% are completely absorbed orally and are not metabolized prior to entering the blood supply. For example, morphine has a bioavailability of 25% when given orally as tablets, meaning that only 25% of morphine is available to the body after oral administration. In total, 75% is either not absorbed or is metabolized prior to entering the blood. When morphine is given by intravenous injection, the bioavailability is 100%. Moreover, the injection has delivered the drug to the blood stream almost instantaneously by passing the absorption phase. Drugs given by intravenous injection will have an immediate intense effect on the person. In abuse situations, such as in the use of heroin, this can precipitate a cardiorespiratory collapse and sudden death [4].

Substances given by other modes of administration, e.g., nasal insufflation (snorting), inhalation (volatile substance abuse), smoking, etc., have different rates of drug absorption.

Single versus Multiple Doses

The pharmacokinetics of drugs do not generally change with repeated doses of drug; however, depending on the time between doses, there can be carryover from previous dose(s). For example, a drug with a half-life of 12 h will need about five times this for the drug to be removed from the body. Hence, the administration of a further dose earlier than 60 h (5 × 12 h) will result in some accumulation of drug from dose to dose. In practice, multiple doses are given at least daily, and sometimes two or three times daily; hence, drugs with half-lives of more than a several hours will result in larger pharmacological responses on repeated dosing [1].

Methadone, a drug related to morphine, is used widely to treat dependency to heroin and other opioids. It has a half-life of about 24 h and when given once daily, the blood concentrations increase substantially over the first 5 days of treatment. This can cause potentially fatal toxicity if the initial doses are too high for the established tolerance to opioids [5]. To avoid this phenomenon, low starting doses are recommended, with daily monitoring for the first week of treatment to ensure optimal safety (and response) for the subject.

The interpretation of blood concentrations in a person on a drug such as methadone is further complicated by the accumulation of drug with repeated doses. Hence, the only way a toxicological result can be properly interpreted is to establish whether the drug was likely to have been taken as one (larger) dose or by repeated (smaller) doses.

Predicting Blood Concentrations

There is considerable variation in the way humans respond to drugs. A standard dose, even when corrected for body weight, will show considerable pharmacokinetic variability from one person to another and will even vary in the same person when the substance is given on separate days. This is because any one of the three processes (absorption, distribution, and elimination) will affect the plasma concentration *versus* time profiles. This difference is increased when the drug is given orally when compared with injection, since variability in absorption also occurs.

Figure 1 illustrates schematically what would be expected of typical person-to-person variability for an orally administered drug when both T_{max} and C_{max} are quite different, and the overall area under the plasma concentration *versus* time profile indicates the amount of drug available to the body.

It is important to understand that each drug has its own pharmacokinetic properties. These include the rate of absorption, the degree of distribution in bodily tissues, and the rate of metabolism and elimination. Standard texts provide details of the relevant pharmacokinetic factors to provide a guide as to the effects of the particular drug [2, 6].

A number of physiological factors can further affect blood concentrations of drugs. These include any disease that alters absorption, distribution, and elimination. The most common diseases are those of the liver and the kidneys, since these are the most important organs involved in the elimination of drugs. Liver is a major organ that metabolizes drugs to (more water soluble) metabolites that are more likely to be excreted by the kidneys [7]. Heart disease, such as congestive heart failure, can also affect drug clearance since blood flow through vital organs is reduced. Advanced age (over 70 year) will usually result in reduced organ function, leading to a reduced ability to process drugs. Older (but otherwise

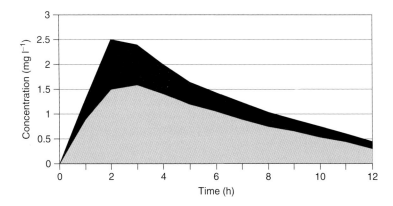

Figure 1 Stylized blood concentration *versus* time profiles showing possible diverse profiles in two different persons given the same dose of drug orally

healthy) persons will often require lower doses for their weight than their much younger counterparts.

The net consequence is that there is substantial variability in blood (and plasma/serum) concentrations for a given dose of substance even if the time of administration is known. In a great proportion of forensic cases, the time of dosage is unknown and in many instances the mode of administration (e.g., oral, intravenous, nasal insufflation, etc.) is usually assumed.

Postmortem Artifacts

In situations involving the interpretation of toxicology results in deceased persons, it is probable that concentrations of drugs (and other substances) would have changed from the time of death [3, 8].

These changes have been described in **Postmortem Toxicology: Artifacts**.

Postcollection Artifacts

Some substances are unstable chemically and can degrade postcollection, particularly, if optimal storage conditions are not maintained. This applies not only to volatile substances such as alcohol but also to nonvolatile substances that are not chemically stable under the storage conditions and, in particular, biological matrix.

These changes have been described in **Postmortem Toxicology: Artifacts**.

Examples

Table 2 summarizes examples of how a particular drug concentration in blood can be differentially interpreted based on the available information.

See **Cocaine**; **Opioids**; **Amphetamine**.

Repeated Use of Drugs

In the case of methamphetamine, where the drug can accumulate with repeated use and produce much greater concentrations than after single doses, it is not possible to infer from a concentration the likely consequence of the drug.

Similarly, with long-acting opiates such as methadone, accumulation occurs from one dose to another, leading to apparent elevated concentrations after some days of use. The interpretation is further compounded by the neuroadaptation that occurs to drugs with repeated use, leading to tolerance of potentially harmful effects [5].

The context of the death is critical to understanding the role, if any, of the drugs detected. For example, a person can die from the effects of using too much cocaine (usually from an adverse effect on the heart), but equally well a person can die from a

Table 2 The effect of circumstances on the interpretation of toxicology results

Drug	Blood concentration $(mg\,l^{-1})^{(a)}$	Circumstances	Likely interpretation[b]
Methamphetamine	0.5	Single oral dose, 2 h postdose	Moderate-to-high doses (<50 mg)
		Several doses over a few days, oral, 2 h postdose	Low-to-moderate doses (~50 mg)
		Single oral dose, 24 h postdose	High dose (>100 mg)
Morphine	0.5 (free)	Single oral dose of morphine, 2 h postdose	Moderate dose, potentially toxic (>50 mg)
		Single intravenous dose of heroin, 2 h postdose	Moderate dose, potentially toxic (>50 mg)
		Multiple oral doses of sustained release morphine (days)	Low-to-moderate doses, likely to be safe (<50 mg doses when given a number of times daily)
Cocaine	0.5	Single oral dose, 1 h postdose	Moderate-to-high doses (<50 mg)
		Single snorted dose, 2 h postdose	Low-to-moderate doses (~50 mg)
		Multiple snorted doses over 4 h	High dose (>100 mg)

[a] Peripheral clinical blood collected without reference to any postcollection artifacts
[b] Doses are only guides and should not be taken literally and will also depend on health and size of person

completely unrelated event such as a fatal shooting or motor vehicle crash and have the same concentration of cocaine (and its metabolites) as the person who died from the effects of cocaine. There is no relationship between the concentration of drug and an outcome for most substances when assessed in isolation.

This lack of relation between blood concentration and response is also seen with other drugs of abuse as well as most prescription drugs.

Natural Disease

As one might expect, the presence of natural disease can complicate the interpretation of drug effects. For example, a person with heart disease, such as an enlarged heart or atherosclerosis (blocked arteries), is more likely to suffer from an adverse reaction to amphetamines than an otherwise healthy person. In fact, the use of chronic amphetamine is linked to the premature development of heart disease itself [9].

Lung disease including infections, such as pneumonia, can increase the harmful effects of opioids by further weakening the ability to withstand compromised respiratory function caused by the opioids themselves (e.g., morphine and heroin).

Multiple Drugs

In most forensic cases, more than one substance is present in the person concerned [3]. When this occurs, it is likely that the combined effects need to be considered. The use of cocaine in a person using an opioid (e.g., heroin) is more dangerous than either drug alone, even though one drug is a stimulant and the other is a depressant.

Commonly, alcohol is seen in the presence of another drug. Unless the concentration of alcohol is toxicologically insignificant ($<0.02\,\mathrm{g}\ 100\,\mathrm{ml}^{-1}$), alcohol will enhance the effects of the other drug(s). Benzodiazepines that are ordinarily relatively safe drugs will be substantially more toxic in the presence of significant amounts of alcohol. Combined drug use is also more likely to lead to behavioral changes. (*See also* **Alcohol**; **Benzodiazepines**; **Behavioral Toxicology**).

Summary

In summary, in a forensic case, a large range of factors affects the interpretation of a drug concentration. It is essential to gather as much information as physically feasible as well as to interpret the information in the context of the case. There is no substitute to proper collection of both medical and forensic evidence.

References

[1] Gibaldi, M. (1991). *Biopharmaceutics and Clinical Pharmacokinetics*, Lea & Febiger, Philadelphia.

[2] Moffat A.C., Osselton W.D. & Widdop B. *Clarke's Isolation and Identification of Drugs*, (2004). The Pharmaceutical Press, London.

[3] Drummer, O.H. & Odell, M. (2001). *The Forensic Pharmacology of Drugs of Abuse*, Arnold, London.

[4] Gerostamoulos, J., Staikos, V. & Drummer, O.H. (2001). Heroin-related deaths in Victoria: a review of cases for 1997 and 1998, *Drug and Alcohol Dependence* **61**, 123–127.

[5] Caplehorn, J.R. & Drummer, O.H. (1999). Mortality associated with New South Wales methadone programs in 1994: lives lost and saved, *The Medical Journal of Australia* **170**, 104–109.

[6] Baselt, R.C. (2004). *Disposition of Toxic Drugs and Chemicals in Man*, Year Book Medical Publishers.

[7] Morgan, D.J. & McLean, A.J. (1995). Clinical pharmacokinetic and pharmacodynamic considerations in patients with liver disease: an update, *Clinical Pharmacokinetics* **29**, 370–391.

[8] Drummer, O.H. (2007). Post-mortem toxicological redistribution, in *Essentials of Autopsy Practice*, G. Rutty, ed, Springer Verlag, London.

[9] Karch, S.B., Stephens, B.G. & Ho, C.H. (1999). Methamphetamine-related deaths in San Francisco: demographic, pathologic, and toxicologic profiles, *Journal of Forensic Science* **44**, 359–368.

OLAF H. DRUMMER AND DIMITRI GEROSTAMOULOS

Postmortem Toxicology: Laboratory Analysis

Introduction

As a major application of forensic toxicology, postmortem toxicology assists pathologists, coroners, and/or judges (in criminal matters) in determining the cause and manner of death. It assists in the assessment of whether injury, toxicity of drug(s) or poison(s) or natural causes (e.g., disease) has any relevance to the death. On the other hand, the circumstance in which the death occurs determines the manner of death, i.e., misadventure, suicide, homicide, etc.

There are several situations that usually require postmortem toxicological analysis:

1. when the direct cause of death is suspected to be drug or poison related;
2. when the cause of death is suspicious or unknown, and investigation is needed to establish cause and/or manner of death (including drug or poison related);
3. when the cause of death is known, toxicological analysis is needed to clarify the manner of death. For instance, in a fatal traffic accident, an investigation is needed to ascertain any influence of alcohol and/or drug(s) on driver;
4. when involvement of drugs or poisons need to be ruled out to support negative pathological findings during autopsies;
5. when detected drugs may give clues as to any underlying disease process, i.e., anticonvulsant drugs, antidiabetic drugs, etc.;
6. when there is a statutory requirement for autopsies and subsequently toxicological examinations are deemed necessary by an authority such as coroners.

The use of postmortem analysis as a crucial evidence in court can be dated back to 1840 when Dr Mattheiu Orfila, a Spanish-born French physician, was asked by the court to investigate a case of Marie LaFarge for the murder of her husband using arsenic, a common poison used in those days [1, 2]. Before Orfila's investigation, toxicological analysis of arsenic was found positive in the food but was not detected in the stomach content of the victim using Marsh test [3]. However, Orfila discovered that the test had been inappropriately performed, and arsenic was later detected in the victim's body. As a consequence, Marie was found guilty of murder.

According to the history of poisons written in an Egyptian manuscript, Ebers Papyrus, approximately 1500 BC, mandrake, hemlock, opium, aconites, and certain metals from the natural sources were known for their poisonous properties and they had been used as weapons or in torture [4]. A poison can be defined as any substance that when taken in a sufficient quantity will cause intoxication or even death. This dose-dependent relationship was first explained by Paracelsus (1493–1541) with the statement "Sola dosis facit venenum" (only dose determines the poison). For instance, even the well-known deadly poison such as cyanide (CN), arsenic, or carbon monoxide may not be harmful if it is inhaled or ingested in a minute quantity. On the other hand, substances as innocuous as drinking water or minerals such as potassium or sodium, if taken in excessive quantity, could induce death. To analyze postmortem samples for a wide variety of potential intoxicants, which are unknown to the toxicologist in most of the cases, is a challenging task.

Specimens for Toxicological Analysis

The collection of specimens in an autopsy is the first and most important step in toxicological examination as the availability of proper biological specimens can maximize the chance of obtaining meaningful analytical findings to assist in determining the cause and manner of death. Since deterioration of specimens increases with postmortem time interval, biological specimens should be collected as soon as practicable after death. Additionally, in most cases, autopsy can only be performed once; the collection of specimens after autopsy is rarely possible.

Unlike in clinical toxicology, where serum/plasma and urine are usually available, the choice of specimens in postmortem toxicological investigation can be extensive and variable. The specimens selected for analysis can vary depending on the case and the information provided to the pathologist during the investigation. Additionally, the instrumentation and methodologies available to the laboratory will also determine what a laboratory can do. Importantly, the specimens obtainable will play a major role, since some specimens may not be available such as urine (if bladder is emptied or because of decomposition) [5, 6]. Generally, the pathologist has the final say on the specimens collected. Prudent facilities will collect a full set of specimens even if not immediately needed since they can be kept and stored if analysis is not immediately required.

The most common specimens used for general toxicological examinations of drugs and poisons in postmortem cases are blood, urine, and vitreous

Table 1 Suggested postmortem specimens to be collected[a]

Type of cases	Specimens collected
General cases	Blood
	Urine
	Vitreous humor
General cases (blood not available)	Cavity fluid (for screening)
	Liver
	Urinary bladder washing (if urine not available)
	Vitreous humor (if any)
Drug- or poison-related cases (suicide cases)	Plus gastric contents
Drug- or poison-related cases (suspicious cases)	Plus gastric content and liver
Gaseous or volatile substances	Plus lung and brain tissue
Heavy metal poisoning	Plus liver, kidney, and hair

[a] Other specimens can also be collected if deemed necessary

humor. When these are not available, tissue samples such as liver, brain, lung, muscle, and bones and body fluids such as bile, pleural effusions, and other specimens (e.g., hair and nails) are all useful in postmortem analysis. Table 1 summarized the specimens recommended, if available, to be collected on the basis of the types of cases.

Blood

Blood is often the specimen of choice for detecting, quantifying, and interpreting drug concentration in postmortem toxicology as most of the literature data are based on their examination in blood [7–10]. Drug concentration in blood is useful for establishing any recent ingestion of the drug in question and to determine the effect of drug on the deceased at the time of death. Blood sample is preferentially taken from peripheral sites such as the femoral (upper leg) or subclavian region rather than from the cardiac region in order to avoid contamination from abdominal fluids and contents, and to reduce artifactual rises in blood concentration due to postmortem redistribution [11]. However, diffusion of drug from urinary bladder to femoral blood can take place if a large amount of urine contains high concentration of the drug [12]. For cases involving hospital treatment before death, clinical specimens obtained soon after admission and immediately before death, whenever appropriate, should also be investigated particularly when poisoning is suspected before admission into hospital (*see* **Postmortem Toxicology: Artifacts**).

If vascular blood cannot be obtained, sampling can be made from the thoracic or the abdominal cavity. However, the composition of these samples will be markedly different from the whole blood and should therefore only be used to qualitatively determine the presence of drugs or poisons. In case of advanced putrefaction, pleural fluid should be collected for screening [6].

Urine

Urine is a convenient specimen for toxicological screening. This is because (i) a relatively high concentration of drugs and their metabolites accumulate in urine and (ii) the drug detection time window in urine is usually longer than that in blood, thereby facilitating detection of any possible exposure to potential drug(s)/poison(s). Immunoassay can be performed directly on urine specimens for the detection of certain drug classes, especially for those commonly abused drugs. However, there is no correlation of urine drug concentration with pharmacological effects because of the time difference between drug absorbed into the bloodstream and drug eliminated into the urine. In addition, in acute drug-related deaths where survival time (probably less than 15 min) is short, drug may not be excreted into the urine. Therefore, when both urine and blood are available, blood cannot be substituted by urine for the screening of drugs and poisons, and if found, the quantitation of drugs or poisons should preferably be performed on blood. Unfortunately, urine cannot be collected in cases due to perimortem voiding or decompositional changes.

Liver

Liver is the major organ for detoxification. Many toxic substances are present in the liver in higher concentrations than in the blood. It is easily collected and can be readily homogenized. Consequently, liver is used to supplement the blood concentration data, or may also be the only specimens available in cases of advanced putrefaction. Usually, the liver from deep within the right lobe is preferred to avoid possibility of gastric diffusion from stomach or from mesenteric circulation [13]. Liver should be finely diced and homogenized in water or a dilute buffer with a minimum water/buffer-to-liver ratio of 1 : 1. The usual method for extraction of biological fluid can be applied to liver homogenate, provided it is properly validated. However, the more complicated matrix present in liver may require additional cleanup to allow better instrumental detection. Unfortunately, the limited toxicological data from the literature limit the ability to interpret liver concentration data [14].

Vitreous Humor

Vitreous humor is the major fluid component of the eye, and is well protected inside the eyeball so that it is less subject to contamination and bacterial action and has little protein content. In conjunction with alcohol levels in blood and/or urine, quantification of alcohol in vitreous humor is useful to assist in distinguishing between alcohol intake before death and postmortem alcohol formation. In addition, this specimen is particularly useful for determining common antidepressants, digoxin, sodium, chloride, glucose, and metabolites related to renal functions (e.g., urea nitrogen, uric acid, and creatinine). Thus, it should be collected whenever possible.

Gastric Contents

As oral ingestion is a major route of drug administration, gastric contents are important to investigate potential poisoning and in case of overdose or acute poisoning, high concentration of drugs or poisons will be detected. In many cases of acute poisoning, undissolved capsules or tablets may be discovered through visual inspection of the contents, allowing relatively simple drug or poison identification. The total amount of a drug or poison present in the gastric contents is more important than its concentration.

When supported by blood and/or tissue findings, a large quantity of the parent drug in the gastric contents as compared to the prescribed dose would indicate drug overdose. Therefore, the total volume of gastric contents should be measured. Recent intake of strong alkali or acids prior to death can easily be determined by pH measurement. In addition, an alkaline pH may also be due to the ingestion of CN and screening test for CN, such as Ferroin test [15], should be considered. The presence of a characteristic odor in gastric content can be a useful indicator for certain toxic substances. Some of the examples are listed in Table 2.

Other Specimens

Sometimes analysis of specimens other than those mentioned may be more appropriate. For instance, bile can be useful for screening of drugs and poisons as a number of drugs, such as morphine, benzodiazepines, and their glucuronide metabolites, ketamine, etc., are present in higher concentrations in bile than in blood. Bile can also be considered as an alternative screening specimen when urine is not available. Lung tissue is particularly useful in the analysis of volatile substances, such as hydrocarbons and other solvents or gases. Brain is useful for the detection of drugs such as antidepressants, narcotics, and halogenated hydrocarbons that act primarily on the central nervous system. In deaths due to chloroform poisoning, a high chloroform concentration can be found in the brain [16]. Kidney is useful in the investigation of heavy metal poisoning. The high concentration of metal deposited in kidney is often associated with structural damage that may be characterized histologically. As the growth rate of hair is approximately $0.6-1.4$ cm per month, it provides a longer drug surveillance window, in a scale of weeks to months, than that of urine and blood. Hair is used

Table 2 Example of characteristic odor in relation to common toxic substances

Odor	Indication
Alcohol	Ethanol
Bitter or burnt almond	Cyanide
Garlic	Organophosphate insecticides
Antiseptic	Chloroxylenol

to evaluate prior exposure to heavy metals, such as arsenic, lead, and mercury, and is now extended to the analysis of a wide range of organic drugs and poisons to provide information on the chronic use or long-term exposure to toxic substances [17].

In case of serious putrefaction, body fluids and tissues including blood, urine, and liver may no longer be available. Under such circumstances, other alternative specimens like muscular tissue, hair, or bone should be considered for toxicology screening but the quantification of drugs and poisons in these samples will be of limited toxicological significance (*see* **Hair: Toxicology**).

Table 3 lists the recommended amount, if available, of specimens taken for analysis and their intended purposes.

All specimens collected should be stored in tightly sealed containers at low temperatures (usually below $4\,^{\circ}C$ for short-term storage during analysis and $-20\,^{\circ}C$ for longer term storage). Except for blood, there is no special preservation required for specimens collected. For blood samples, one of the bottles collected should be preserved by addition of at least 2% w/v of sodium fluoride or equivalent to suppress the postmortem production of alcohol, γ-hydroxybutyrate, CN, and carbon monoxide and

reduces hydrolysis of some drugs, such as cocaine to benzoylecgonine [6, 18].

Additional Information Required Prior to Analysis

Most drug- or poison-related deaths do not present characteristic features pathologically as those found in many disease-oriented deaths, such as cancers. Strategy for postmortem sampling and subsequent analysis should be based on a detailed knowledge about the case in respect of the presence of any foreign substances suspected to be related to the fatality. To facilitate toxicologists in devising the appropriate analytical methods, interdisciplinary discussions between professionals involved in the case (at least between forensic pathologist and toxicologist) prior to commencement of toxicological investigation is recommended. The following information should be provided if available:

1. Evidence(s), such as drug paraphernalia (e.g., syringe), poisons or medications, empty containers, and/or packaging inserts, suspected to be related to drugs or poisons found at the scene

Table 3 Minimum recommended amount of specimens taken for postmortem analysis

Specimen	Where to obtain (amount)	Principal uses
Blood	Peripheral (femoral or subclavian preferred) (2×10 ml)	Useful to confirm recent drug use and concentration, if a drug found, is useful for toxicological interpretation
	Peripheral (preserved using 2% w/v sodium fluoride or equivalent) (at least 2 ml)	Mainly for alcohol and for analysis of some drugs requiring preservation
Urine	(>10 ml)	Useful for broad class of drug screening but may not be useful on timing of drug administered
Liver	Deep within right lobe preferred (>100 g)	Useful solid tissue samples to supplement blood data especially when blood is not available but limited literature data available
Bile	(At least 5 ml or whole gall bladder)	Useful fluid for drug screening especially when urine is not available
Vitreous humor	(All available $\sim$2–5 ml)	Useful in alcohol analysis and, if necessary, some other drugs (e.g., digoxin, glucose, urea nitrogen, uric acid, creatinine, and antipsychotic drugs)
Gastric contents	(All)	Indicative of recent drug administration
Hair	Identify distal and proximal end (>50 mg)	Drug use history provide information of drugs/poisons and metal exposure in scales of months
Lung	(50 g)	For volatile substances (such as H_2S and chloroform poisoning)
Brain	(50 g)	Brain may be useful in infant drug deaths or for volatile poison cases

should be seized as analysis of these items may be valuable for determining the subsequent type of analysis to be performed on the biological specimens. In some cases, household products, such as caustics, solvents, or pesticides, may also provide useful clues. While circumstantial evidence can provide hints, it can never substitute the analysis of body fluids or tissues because substance(s) found at the scene may not necessarily be connected to the death and often other substances are detected that are not obvious from the circumstances.

2. A comprehensive list of medications (especially recent medications prescribed) given to the deceased with relevant medical history should be provided.

3. Any physical abnormalities identified during autopsy may be indicative of intoxication or poisoning and a list of examples is given in Table 4 [6]. In this case, additional analysis targeting for the presence of possible toxic substances may be required.

Analytical Aspects in Postmortem Toxicology

Ingested substances are metabolized, being broken down or transformed into other species before they

Table 4 Useful findings related to toxic substances observable during autopsy

	Possible Indication
Color of skin	
Cherry red to bright red	Carbon monoxide or cyanide
Grayish to brownish	Nitrate, nitrite or aniline
Nasal/oral cavity	
Residues of powder or colored material	Intransal drug use (e.g ketamine, cocaine), ingestion of tablet or capsule residues
Oral cavity/ gastointestinal tract	
White, corrosive staining	Hydrochloric acid
Black-brown, corrosive staining	Sulphuric acid
Glass-like, reddish necrosis	Alkaline agents (e.g. sodium hydroxide)

are excreted. Hence, identification of the original ingested material often involves considerable complications, for example, heroin is first metabolized into 6-acetylmorphine and then to morphine, while Δ^9-tetrahydrocannabinol (THC), an active ingredient in cannabis, is first converted to 11-hydroxy-Δ^9-tetrahydrocannabinol and then to 11-nor-Δ^9-tetrahydrocannabinol-9-carboxylic acid.

In addition, the active constituent in a regular dose ranging from grams or milligrams is diluted to a concentration usually in the range of micrograms or nanograms per milliliter of body fluids or per gram of tissue by way of dispersion throughout the body. The analytical method to be utilized must be capable, both in terms of sensitivity and specificity, of detecting the target substances at low concentrations and in complicated biological matrices (*see* **Postmortem Toxicology: Artifacts**).

Analytical Techniques

There are a wide variety of analytical techniques available for the analysis of toxic substances in biological specimens. The most common techniques used in modern toxicology laboratories include various immunoassays with different detection principles, color tests (e.g., Ferroin for CN, Marsh test for arsenic, etc.), instrumental chromatographic techniques using high-performance liquid chromatography (HPLC) and gas chromatography (GC) coupled with various detectors. To effectively apply chromatographic techniques, an extraction procedure is required to separate the intended drugs/poisons from biological matrices followed by reconstitution in appropriate solvents compatible with the requirements of the intended instrumentation.

Immunoassays. A number of immunoassays intended for antemortem analysis can also be used for postmortem analysis especially when urine is available. Immunoassay is based on the principle that the drug is detected by its ability to displace or block the binding of a fixed amount of labeled drug molecules present in the reagent. The label can be a fluorescent molecule (e.g., fluorescence polarization immunoassay (FPIA)), an enzyme (e.g., cloned enzyme donor immunoassay (CEDIA), enzyme multiplied immunoassay technique (EMIT), and enzyme-linked immunosorbent assay (ELISA)), a radioactive isotope (e.g., radioimmunoassay (RIA)) or other substance that can be detected by means of instrumentation. Some assays can distinguish between bound and free labeled drug in a mixture are known as *homogenous immunoassay*, such as CEDIA, EMIT, and FPIA. For heterogenous immunoassays, such as ELISA and RIA, they require a washing step to separate the bound labeled complex from free labeled reagent prior to analysis. Thus, homogenous immunoassays are easier to be automated and less labor intensive than heterogenous ones. In general, immunoassays are fast, sensitive and, in homogenous immunoassays, direct detection can be achieved without sample purification. It is used for screening of common abused drugs, such as opiates, amphetamines, cocaine, cannabinoids, phencyclidine, and barbiturates. In addition, prescribed drugs, such as propoxyphene and tricyclic antidepressants, can also be screened with the use of specific reagents. For postmortem screening, antibodies having broad drug selectivity within a class of drugs (e.g., sympathomimetic amines) are preferred over those that are sensitive to a specific drug (e.g., methamphetamine) as it allows the screening of drugs within the same class. The sensitivity can be further increased by prior hydrolysis of glucuronide or sulfate conjugates of some drug classes, such as cannabinoids, opiates, and benzodiazepines.

Cutoff values, often applied to workplace drug testing, especially for abused drugs should be used cautiously in postmortem cases since the presence of low drug concentrations can be of forensic significance. In an acute drug-related death, for instance, the drug may not have sufficient time to be excreted into urine before death resulting in a low drug concentration in urine. False positives may occur, either from structurally related drugs or from metabolites of other drugs that are recognized by the antibodies. For instance, phenethylamine, a common putrefactive product from decomposed bodies, can cause a false-positive response to the amphetamines class test when using immunoassays. Cross-reactivity can also be due to chemicals with similar structures to the intended analytes. For example, pholcodine gives rise to a positive response to the opiates reagent of FPIA. Thus, for those samples, which give positive screening results, confirmation tests should be performed, preferably using chromatographic techniques with MS detection.

Extraction Techniques. The usual extraction techniques involve either liquid–liquid extraction (LLE) or solid-phase extraction (SPE).

LLE involves the selective partitioning of the compound of interest into one of two immiscible phases by a judicious choice of extraction solvents. Although there are some developments in SPE techniques, in recent years [19], the traditional LLE technique is still a common extraction method used in postmortem specimens. The method has the advantage of efficient extraction of drugs and poisons present in a wide concentration range and the absence of adsorption loss frequently associated with a solid surface. However, for some postmortem blood or tissues, problems associated with the formation of stable emulsion, variable extraction efficiency and endogenous interferences due to autolysis may occur. To extract acidic and basic/neutral drugs from biological fluids or tissues using LLE, separate extractions using appropriate organic solvent(s) with the addition of acidic and basic buffer, respectively, are required. Various methods using LLE for drug extraction in postmortem specimens show that there is a wide choice of solvents or mixture of solvents with similar extraction efficiency and selectivity [18, 20].

The mechanism of SPE based on the selective partition of one or more components between two phases, one of which is a solid sorbent while the second, mainly a liquid, is more complicated than LLE. Extraction is accomplished by adsorption of the analytes onto the solid sorbent followed by washing with an appropriate solvent to remove the unwanted matrix before eluting the analytes. Compared with LLE, SPE has the advantages of low solvent consumption, provision of cleaner extracts, and ease of automation and high extraction efficiency for certain specific drugs requiring a smaller sample volume. Thus, it provides an excellent alternative to the traditional LLE for the extraction of postmortem samples. Unlike LLE, untreated sample cannot be applied directly onto SPE. Pretreatment procedures, e.g., protein precipitation and centrifugation, may result in a significant loss of analytes due to adsorption or occlusion onto the precipitated constituents. Ion exchange resins have shown to be efficient in the extraction of acidic drugs [21]. On the other hand, mixed-mode SPE, being capable of extracting acidic, basic, and neutral drugs, is suitable for general unknown screening (GUS) [22] (*see* **Toxicology: Initial Testing**).

Chromatographic Techniques. GC and HPLC, coupled with various detectors, are common instrumentations to screen for a wide range of organic toxic substances. A combination of mass spectrometry with either GC or, more recently, HPLC is the definitive technique to establish proof of structure of unknown substances. With the extensive development of commercial MS technology at an affordable cost, gas chromatography mass spectrometry (GC-MS) and high-performance liquid chromatography mass spectrometry (HPLC-MS) (or liquid chromatography mass spectrometry (LC-MS)) become increasingly popular tools employed in toxicological analyses.

GC is one of the most frequently used techniques for separating, identifying, and quantifying a parent drug and its metabolites, other coadministered drugs and endogenous compounds. This technique can be coupled with various detectors from the more universal flame ionization detector (FID) to specific detectors such as electron capture detector (ECD) and nitrogen phosphorus detector (NPD).

FID is useful for the detection of alcohol, other volatile organic compounds and many other organic drugs and poisons. NPD is sensitive to nitrogen- and phosphorus-containing compounds and is useful for the detection of drugs and poisons, such as antidepressants, antipsychotic drugs, benzodiazepines, opiates, cocaine and its metabolites, organophosphorus insecticides, etc. The use of FID and NPD either alone [23–25] or in a combination of both [26] has been shown to be useful for GUS of organic drugs and poisons. ECD is particularly sensitive to halogenated compounds (e.g., chlorinated insecticides), nitriles (e.g., CN) or nitrogen-containing compounds (e.g., benzodiazepines, nifedipine, and zopiclone). Unfortunately, the above detectors can only provide retention time data without any additional information for structural identification. Thus, more sophisticated techniques, such as GC-MS or LC-MS, are recommended for confirmation (*see* **Confirmation Testing: Toxicology**).

The high separation power of capillary GC coupled with a highly selective MS detector has been currently regarded as the "gold standard" in GUS for drugs and poisons. The availability of a well-established and standardized ionization technique (electron impact (EI) at 70 eV) has facilitated the construction of large databases of reference mass spectra for library search and many useful spectral libraries relevant to toxicological screening are now available. However, GC is not suitable for direct analysis of polar compounds although derivatization can partly solve the problem and mass spectral

libraries containing a practically complete coverage of trimethylsilyl (TMS) derivatives are available commercially [27].

HPLC is capable of dealing with the analysis of a wide range of both volatile and nonvolatile compounds. The reversed phase mode column is at present the most common separation method applied in toxicological screening. Unlike GC, derivatization is not necessary for the analysis of polar and thermolabile compounds and this advantage certainly promotes HPLC as a better alternative for compounds not amenable to GC. Detection is often aided by diode-array detectors (DAD), which acquire UV–visible spectra continuously during a chromatographic run and the chromatogram is extracted and plotted at preselected wavelengths. The combined technique of high-performance liquid chromatography diode-array detector (HPLC-DAD) is another suitable technique for GUS of compounds, covering a wide range of polarity, stability, and molecular masses. Since metabolic transformation, in many cases, does not affect the ultraviolet (UV) chromophores of the molecule, one of the added values of this technique in GUS for drugs and poisons is that the low selectivity of DAD facilitates the detection of metabolites. In addition, compounds belonging to the same class with similar chemical structures often display similar absorbance patterns allowing unknown compounds not previously identified are tentatively assigned for further analysis. However, one of the drawbacks of HPLC-DAD is that the resolution of HPLC is usually inferior compared with GC, and UV spectroscopy is less sensitive than that of MS. In addition, for compounds possessing weak UV–visible or without any characteristic UV–visible absorbency, identification using HPLC-DAD is difficult in terms of both sensitivity and specificity.

LC-MS is useful for the analysis of compounds that are not amenable to GC-MS. These compounds include lysergic acid diethylamide (LSD), glucuronide conjugates, such as morphine-3 or 6-glucuronide or for some very potent or large molecules that other techniques are not sufficiently sensitive for detection (e.g., colchicines, cardiac glycosides such as digoxin and digitoxin, β-agonists such as salbutamol and terbutaline) [26].

The most common ionization mode used in LC-MS techniques is atmospheric pressure ionization (API), which mainly comprises of different versions of electrospray ionization (ESI) and atmospheric pressure chemical ionization (APCI) interfaces. With simpler sample preparation, LC-MS is extended to certain analyses originally performed by the less-specific HPLC-DAD or even GC-MS. For these reasons, LC-MS, which combines an almost universal separation process with the most specific and sensitive type of detector, has become a promising alternative approach to GC-MS and HPLC-DAD in toxicological analysis [28–30].

However, there are several drawbacks in the use of LC-MS. First, the ion-suppression effect, especially when operating in the ESI mode, is a well-known problem: signal of the intended analyte is often suppressed because of the presence of coeluting compounds/interferents so that the intended analyte may be underestimated or even overlooked. Thus, the effect of ion suppression on the signal of the intended analyte should be cautiously evaluated before use. If ion suppression does occur, changes in experimental conditions, such as the sample cleanup method, chromatographic conditions relating to the mobile phase, the elution column, and the internal standard, should be considered. Moreover, only certain volatile buffers and mobile phase can be used for LC-MS to be compatible with the MS requirement. Thus, the separation efficiency is often inferior compared with HPLC-DAD although it may not be a problem for tandem MS because separation of analytes can be made in the MS/MS mode.

Systematic Toxicological Analysis

The usual practice in toxicological examination begins with the preliminary identification of alcohol and screening of a wide spectrum of acidic, neutral, and basic organic drugs or poisons. If a toxic substance(s) is detected, confirmatory and, if necessary, quantitative testing has to be performed. In general, a positive identification is achieved using at least two independent analyses and preferably based on different analytical principles. Using GC-MS or LC-MS, confirmation and quantification can be simplified into one single analysis. Quantification of drugs in blood, liver, and gastric content as dictated by the case, provides more meaningful interpretative information. Reference concentrations of many compounds in blood in therapeutic, toxic, and even fatal levels have been published [7–10]. Although limited, useful references are also available for some compounds in liver [14]. It should be noted that while substances found in excretory fluids such as urine or

bile are useful qualitatively, quantification of drugs and poisons in these fluids usually has limited interpretative values.

A comprehensive and systematic analysis for the presence of chemical substances of toxicological significance is termed systematic toxicological analysis (STA). There are thousands of potentially harmful substances ranging from poisonous gases (e.g., carbon monoxide and hydrogen cyanide (HCN), and hydrogen sulfides), food (e.g., ethanol), deadly poisons (e.g., CN salts and arsenic), abused drugs, pesticides, toxins from natural sources, a wide variety of prescribed drugs and even household products, etc. It is impossible to design a single analytical scheme to cover all these substances with distinctly different chemical and physical properties. Screening for a wide scope of drugs and poisons is, however, possible by grouping substances of similar properties for analysis. The most effective strategy includes a series of standard general screening procedures supplemented by as many special methods as required. A combination of immunoassays with chromatographic techniques is usually employed to detect a wide range of substances. Immunoassays detect classes of drugs with similar structures while chromatographic techniques detect large groups of drugs with similar extraction properties, polarity, and detection characteristics.

General toxicological screening usually involves the following tests:

1. alcohol determination;
2. immunoassay screening;
3. GUS of organic drugs and poisons;
4. other specific tests as required such as carboxyhemoglobin, CN, etc.

Table 5 shows the suggested screening tests based on different case nature. Since it is virtually impossible to screen for all toxic substances in every case, a rational selection of case-specific analysis in addition to STA will be necessary. In general, the additional analysis to be conducted is primarily based on the information provided or specific requests made by the relevant parties such as pathologists and the police.

An example of an analytical scheme used for general toxicology screening and scope of analytes likely to be detected is shown in Figure 1.

Alcohol Determination. Alcohol or ethyl alcohol (ethanol) is the most common drug found in

Table 5   Suggested analysis for sample collected[a]

Type of cases	Test conducted	Specimen tested
General cases	Alcohol	Blood, urine, and vitreous humor
	Immunoassay drug screening	Urine
	General organic drugs/poisons screening	Blood (urine)
General cases (blood not available)	Alcohol	Urine and vitreous humor
	Immunoassay drug screening	Urine
	General organic drugs/poisons screening	Liver/cavity fluid
Drug or poison suspected cases	Plus general organic drugs/poisons screening	Gastric content
Fire death	Plus carboxyhemoglobin, cyanide	Blood
Heavy metal poisoning	Plus metal analysis	Blood, kidney, and liver
Gaseous and volatile organic related	Plus sulfide	Blood, lung, and brain
	Plus volatile organic	Blood, lung, and brain

[a] Specific test(s) not covered may be added if deemed appropriate.

postmortem toxicology cases. In particular, ethyl alcohol is one of the leading causes of death by poisoning. In contrast to alcohol determination in living subjects, which is generally more straightforward, analysis of body fluids taken from cadavers is more likely to be contaminated with volatile substances, such as methanol and formaldehyde used in embalming processes, and abnormal metabolic products, such as acetone resulting from fasting or diabetic ketoacidosis. Therefore, techniques for analyzing postmortem alcohol are recommended to allow separation of most, if not all, low-boiling compounds eluting in the same range as ethyl alcohol [31].

Headspace GC coupled with FID is usually the method of choice and it can be used for simultaneous analysis of methanol, acetaldehyde, ethanol, isopropanol, and acetone using either n-butanol or n-propanol as an internal standard. A combination of blood (preferably femoral region), vitreous humor, and urine, if available, should be used for alcohol analysis to aid in the interpretation of the state of absorption and to avoid misinterpretation of blood alcohol concentrations due to diffusion of undigested alcohol from the stomach, and postmortem alcohol production due to bacterial action. The presence of significant amount of alcohol in blood together with the absence of alcohol in urine and vitreous humor cast doubt in the ingestion of alcohol prior to death and is indicative of endogenous alcohol production (*see also* **Alcohol: Analysis**).

Immunoassay Screening.   Screening for drugs by immunoassays in urine is commonly pursued for the main classes of abused drugs (Figure 1), which include amphetamines, benzodiazepines, cannabinoids (metabolite of cannabis), benzoylecgonine (metabolite of cocaine), and opiates (morphine and codeine). The scope for drug screening can be extended to include opioids (e.g., methadone), barbiturates, and tricyclic antidepressants (e.g., amitriptyline/nortriptyline).

As urine is not always available in postmortem cases, screening for drugs and poisons, especially abused drugs, in blood or plasma may be considered and may even be desirable to establish what substances may be affecting the person. Blood, plasma, or even specimens such as bile or liver homogenate can be screened by the urine-based immunoassay test kits, but pretreatment with solvent or protein precipitation are required and validation should be made before use. In addition, techniques intended for analysis of blood, such as RIA and ELISA can be used on postmortem samples, and they tend to be more sensitive than those kits designed for detecting drugs in urine but modified for testing blood. Screening of potent drugs like digoxin or structurally related cardiac glycosides, such as bufadienolides present in Chansu (a remedy from toad venom), can be effectively performed in plasma using a digoxin reagent by various immunoassay techniques [32].

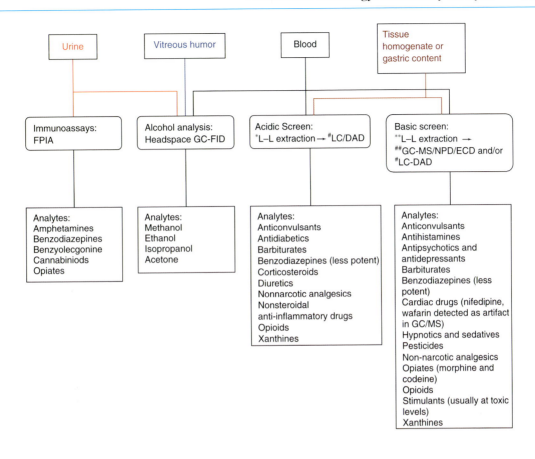

Urine	Vitreous humor	Blood	Tissue homogenate or gastric content
Immunoassays: FPIA	Alcohol analysis: Headspace GC-FID	Acidic Screen: *L–L extraction → #LC/DAD	Basic screen: **L–L extraction → ##GC-MS/NPD/ECD and/or #LC-DAD
Analytes: Amphetamines Benzodiazepines Benzoylecgonine Cannabiniods Opiates	Analytes: Methanol Ethanol Isopropanol Acetone	Analytes: Anticonvulsants Antidiabetics Barbiturates Benzodiazepines (less potent) Corticosteroids Diuretics Nonnarcotic analgesics Nonsteroidal anti-inflammatory drugs Opioids Xanthines	Analytes: Anticonvulsants Antihistamines Antipsychotics and antidepressants Barbiturates Benzodiazepines (less potent) Cardiac drugs (nifedipine, wafarin detected as artifact in GC/MS) Hypnotics and sedatives Pesticides Non-narcotic analgesics Opiates (morphine and codeine) Opioids Stimulants (usually at toxic levels) Xanthines

*Phosphate buffer (pH 1), extracted with diethylether/toluene (1 : 1)

** Bicarbonate buffer (pH 9) extracted with dichloromethane: toluene: isobutyl alcohol (3 : 6 : 1)

#LC-DAD: column: Lichrospher 60 RP-select B (5 μm,125 × 4.0 mm); mobile phase: Triethylamine in phosphate (pH 3)/acetonitrile

##GC-MS/NPD/ECD: column: HP5-MS (30 m × 0.25 mm × 0.25 μm); carrier gas: Helium

Figure 1   An example of general toxicology screening scheme

General Unknown Screening (GUS) for Organic Drugs and Poisons.   As shown in Figure 1, acidic drugs can be extracted by adding an acidic buffer such as phosphate buffer (pH 1) to the samples followed by extraction with toluene: diethyl ether (1 : 1). Other methods, such as protein precipitation of blood with acetonitrile [33] or ammonium chloride salting-out of blood and other tissues with ethyl acetate followed by a washing step with hexane [34] can also be employed for the analysis of acidic and some neutral drugs. Analysis is usually made by HPLC-DAD using a reverse-phase column in conjunction with a mobile phase at acidic pH with gradient elution. Identification is accomplished by automatic library search based on a preinstalled, commercially available, or an in-house developed UV–visible spectral library. The retention times are useful to aid in identification but it should be established in-house using authentic standards according to the type of column and the mobile phase used. Nonnarcotic analgesics (e.g., paracetamol, salicylic acid, mefenamic acid, and sometimes propoxyphene), nonsteroidal anti-inflammatory drugs (e.g., celecoxib, naproxen, and ibuprofen), diuretics (e.g., furosemide and hydrochlorothiazide), anticonvulsants (e.g., carbamazepine, phenobarbital, and phenytoin), antidiabetics (e.g., glicazide), opioids (e.g., methadone), barbiturates (e.g., secobarbital), corticosteroids (e.g., hydrocortisone), the less potent benzodiazepines (e.g., midazolam, diazepam, and sometimes estazolam), and xanthines (e.g., caffeine and theophylline) can be detected using HPLC-DAD after acidic extraction.

Drugs and their metabolites usually have similar UV–visible spectra because metabolic transformations, such as desmethylation and hydroxylation, do not usually affect the chromophores of the drugs. Yet, a drug and its metabolites usually have different retention times (e.g., midazolam and α-hydroxymidazolam, clomipramine, and desmethylclomipramine). Although it may be useful to extend the detection capability to drug metabolites even without the authentic standards, one should exercise caution to avoid misinterpretation when a peak slightly different in retention time and UV–visible spectrum from the parent drug is observed. As many drugs and poisons do not have characteristic UV–visible spectra, retention time becomes the main identification parameter. Thus, whenever standards of parent drugs and/or their metabolites are available, their retention times should be established in-house and their authenticity preferably confirmed by other techniques, such as GC-MS.

Extraction of basic drugs is accomplished by a carbonate buffer (pH 9) followed by extraction with a dichloromethane/toluene/isobutyl alcohol (3 : 6 : 1) mixture. Other combinations of alkaline buffers and extraction solvents such as borate buffer (pH 8.5) extracted with dichloromethane/isopropanol (9 : 1) [35], and using SPE with suitable cleanup procedures compatible with GC analysis [18–20] are also applicable. The use of more than one type of detectors (e.g., NPD and MS) coupled to GC would definitely give a greater coverage of possible drugs and poisons. The extracted sample could be analyzed sequentially by injection into two GCs equipped with different types of detectors or by splitting the effluent of the sample from one GC into two different detectors for simultaneous detection.

Examples of drugs and poisons found in the basic fraction include hypnotics and sedatives (e.g., zopiclone and zolpidem), benzodiazepines (e.g., diazepam, midazolam, estazolam, and bromazepam), antihistamines (e.g., chlorpheniramine, brompheniramine, and promethazine), antipsychotics and antidepressants (e.g., amitriptyline/nortriptyline, cyclobenzaprine, sertraline, clomipramine, and trihexylphenidyl), opiates (e.g., codeine, acetylmorphine, and sometimes monomorphine), opioids (e.g., methadone and meperidine), anticonvulsants (e.g., carbamazepine, phenobarbital, and phenytoin), and pesticides (e.g., melathion, dimethoate, and tetramethylene disulfotetramine). Stimulants such as amphetamines and cocaine may be detected when present at high concentrations. In addition, artifacts due to the presence of certain cardiac drugs such as warfarin and nifedipine may be encountered.

Some basic drugs that are too polar or thermally labile cannot be detected by GC and are not acid extractable for HPLC-DAD analysis. In such case, the basic extract can be analyzed using HPLC-DAD in addition to GC. Typically, the method permits the detection of cardiac drugs (e.g., warfarin, metoprolol, propranolol, dipyridamole, and amiodarone), anti-inflammatory drugs (e.g., ofloxacin), and herbal ingredients (e.g., tetrahydropalmatine).

Alternatively, derivatization prior to GC analysis can increase the volatility and hence thermal stability for those drugs that are not easily detected by GC or GC-MS [36]. Among the available derivatization procedures, trimethylsilylation is the most common method because of its versatility for derivatizing many different functional groups such as hydroxyl, carboxyl, amidic, and some amine groups under relatively mild conditions. Furthermore, the additional mass gain by silylation improves the specificity of the mass spectral information [37]. Typical examples include morphine and sympathomimetic amines. Other derivatized agents such as trifluoroacetylation for basic and neutral drugs, and extractive methylation using methyl iodide or formation of ethereal diazomethane for acidic drugs are also applicable [38, 39].

Some compounds do not exhibit characteristic mass spectra in GC-MS. In this case, unambiguous identification can be difficult if mass spectral matching is solely relied on because many compounds can give seemingly high matching scores. Typical examples include amino-containing compounds with predominant base peaks at m/z 44 ($C_2H_6N^+$) (e.g., amphetamine, methylenedioxyamphetamine MDA), 58 ($C_3H_8N^+$) (e.g., doxepin, cyclobenzaprine), 72 ($C_4H_{10}N^+$) (e.g., methadone, promethazine), or 98

($C_6H_{12}N^+$) (e.g., trihexylphenidyl, thioridazine) and usually associated with very low intensity fragments in the high mass range. If these compounds are well separated chromatographically, they can only be identified on the basis of their differences in retention time. For those substances having similar retention time in GC, however, another technique should be considered for confirmation.

The application of LC-MS to GUS is still not extensive in spite of its versatile analytical capability as well as sensitive and specific detection of a wide range of drugs and poisons. One of the problems is the soft ionization of LC-MS, which produces mass spectra that are not compatible with those generated by EI at standardized 70-eV ionization potential. Hence, the very large libraries of standardized EI spectra of chemicals, drugs, poisons, and their metabolites applicable to GC-MS are not valid for LC-MS. Thus, a totally different strategy for mass spectral identification of compounds is required for LC-MS.

Many efforts have been made to build up large mass spectral database applicable for GUS of compounds of toxicological interest on different types of LC-MS and promising progress has been demonstrated. Identification has been based on single quadrupole, ion trap, triple quadrupole, hybrid linear ion trap, and time of flight (TOF) [28–30]. The hybrid linear ion-trap LC-MS/MS showed promising development for building up a reference MS/MS library for the same type of instrument. This LC-MS/MS technique is unique in that the third quadrupole of the triple quadrupole MS can be operated in either a standard quadrupole MS for multiple reaction monitoring (MRM) experiment or as linear ion trap to produce highly sensitive enhanced product ion (EPI) scan in an information-dependent acquisition (IDA) experiment [40, 41]. The first detection step involves IDA survey scan containing a number of preselected MRM target drugs and metabolites where ions are accumulated and then filtered in the third quadrupole. In case of a signal above a preset intensity threshold is detected for an MRM transition, the EPI scan of the precursor ion is triggered to yield product ion mass spectra at various preselected collision energies. Finally, the resulting EPI mass spectra are then searched against a prebuilt mass spectral library for identification of drugs present in the sample. Alternatively, LC-MS/TOF has provided a novel approach for comprehensive drug

screening. The use of LC-MS/TOF method has the advantages to provide a relatively high mass accuracy (~5 ppm) with reasonable resolution (5000–10 000 full width at half maximum). In this approach, a library is established to contain toxicological relevant compounds that consist of molecular formula and calculated monoisotopic accurate masses. Identification of drugs/metabolites was based on their accurate mass, retention time if a reference material is available, and drug metabolite patterns. Furthermore, the matching of theoretical and measured isotopic patterns of a compound introduces an additional parameter to allow unambiguous identification of compounds present in the sample. This approach allows substance identification even without any reference standards and retention time data [42] (*see* **Confirmation Testing: Toxicology**).

Other Specific Tests

When analysis of specific types of drugs or poisons that are not covered under the general toxicology screening scheme is required, additional tests will have to be performed. Figure 2 shows some of the examples on the analysis of certain specific types of drugs and poisons.

Drug-detection Techniques

Acid Back-Extraction. Although many basic drugs with amine functional groups such as those basic psychotropic drugs and antihistamines can be detected using aforementioned basic screening, an additional acid back-extraction after basic extraction can further improve GC-MS detection by producing a cleaner extract. Examples of psychiatric drugs include tricyclic antidepressants, phenothiazines antipsychotic drugs, tetracyclic antidepressants, butyrophenones, and serotonin reuptake inhibitors. In addition, better detection of other drugs like antiparkinson drugs (e.g., trihexylphenidyl) can also be achieved using this method (Figure 2).

Ketamine, amphetamines, and their analogs can be detected at moderate-to-high level in the basic extract using GC-MS/NPD (Figure 1). To increase the detection sensitivity down to therapeutic or even subtherapeutic levels, a simple acid back-extraction cleanup after basic extraction with diethyl ether (Figure 2) coupled with LC-MS/MS (ion-trap MS) analysis can be considered.

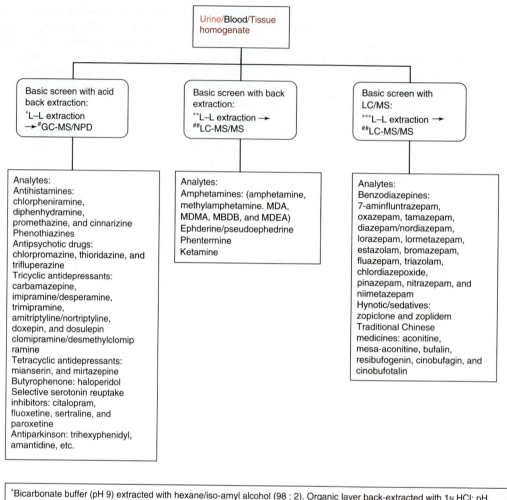

Figure 2   Examples of additional specific drug tests

Basic Extract Analyzed by LC-MS. LC-MS is complementary to the analysis of nonvolatile and thermally labile drugs/poisons that are not amenable to GC or GC-MS. In addition, LC-MS provides a superior sensitivity compared with the HPLC-DAD method, a good example being the LC-MS analysis of benzodiazepines: a structurally diverse class of pharmaceuticals. It is available as prescribed drugs with some of them (e.g., diazepam, midazolam, and nimetazepam) having been widely abused. Benzodiazepines and their metabolites represent one of the most common drug types found in postmortem specimens. While the relatively less potent benzodiazepines (e.g., midazolam and diazepam/nordiazepam) can be screened by the general screening procedures, many potent or thermally unstable benzodiazepines (e.g., lorazepam, triazolam, and oxazepam) cannot be readily detected by standard screening techniques (Figure 1). To cater for a more comprehensive screening of benzodiazepines, the basic fraction from general toxicology screening can be reconstituted into aqueous methanol and subjected to LC-MS analysis (Figure 2). The same extract can also be used for the analysis of a wide range of targeted basic/neutral drugs and poisons including traditional Chinese medicines (e.g., aconitine and mesa-aconitine) and toxic ingredients found in Chan Su (e.g., bufalin, resibufogenin, cinobufagin, and cinobufotalin).

Analysis of Poisoning by Small Molecules. Carbon monoxide (CO), CN, and sulfide are well-known small and highly toxic molecules. Analysis of these molecules should be considered whenever poisoning due to these compounds is suspected.

Carbon Monoxide (CO). Determination of carbon monoxide poisoning will be required when a known source of CO, such as coal gas, burnt charcoal, or automobile exhaust, is located at the scene. On the other hand, it would be of forensic interest to decipher whether a fire victim had died because of CO poisoning, or had already died before the fire broke out. The saturation ratio of carboxyhemoglobin (COHb) in blood is determined by (i) simultaneous spectrophotometric (e.g., CO-Oximeter) measurement of COHb level and total hemoglobin in blood [43] or (ii) analysis of COHb through the release of CO by adding saponin and potassium ferricyanide to blood, followed by catalytic conversion of CO to methane, which is quantified by gas chromatography flame ionization detector (GC-FID) [44]. Analysis of COHb should be made using blood samples; other biological fluids, such as pleural effusion, are not recommended because a considerable amount of postmortem CO can possibly be generated in these samples by bacterial action on hemin [45].

Hydrogen Sulfide (H_2S) and Its Metabolites. Analysis is performed when H_2S poisoning is suspected, usually in industrial accidents, sewers, or ship holds where H_2S poisoning together with oxygen deficiency is suspected. Analysis is mainly based on the detection of H_2S or its metabolite, thiosulfate. Sulfate is also produced due to H_2S

exposure but endogenous levels of sulfate in blood and urine are relatively high making it not an analyte of choice. GC-MS analysis can be performed for the ionized form of H_2S after derivatization using pentafluorobenzyl bromide [46]. The pH of the derivatized mixture is made acidic to suppress the production of sulfide in the blood due to decomposition of sulfur-containing compounds, such as cysteine. A similar derivatization procedure prior to GC-MS method can also be used for the analysis of thiosulfate with the exception that tetradecyldimethylbenzylammonium, a phase-transfer catalyst used in H_2S determination is substituted by ascorbic acid/sodium chloride [46, 47].

Cyanide (CN). Potassium or sodium salts of CN are used in metallurgy and electroplating industries and are relatively easy to obtain. Thus, its involvement in suicide and even homicide is not uncommon in some parts of the world. In addition, incomplete combustion of nitrogen-containing compounds such as urethane at fire scenes can produce HCN as one of the poisonous gases. Thus for fire victims, in addition to measuring the COHb saturation, CN levels in blood should also be determined. Inhalation of HCN or ingestion of CN can be fatal through inhibition of cytochrome oxidase causing cellular anoxia. CN in blood can be determined by automated headspace gas chromatography electron capture detector (GC-ECD). Blood is acidified with sulfuric acid in the presence of silver sulfate to produce HCN, which is diffused into the headspace to react with chlorine produced by chloramine-T to form cyanogen chloride, which is analyzed by GC-ECD [48].

Volatile Analysis. In addition to the analysis of alcohols, determinations of other volatile chemicals including various organic solvents are also of forensic significance. Sudden death due to volatile substance abuse (VSA) is not uncommon particularly for an inexperience user because controlling of dose is often difficult. Solvent from thinners (e.g., toluene and xylene), halogenated solvents (e.g., chloroform and dichloromethane), hydrocarbons (both aliphatic and aromatic) such as gasoline and kerosene, and fuel gas (e.g., butane) are commonly abused substances. Apart from VSA, analysis of volatile substances may also be required in certain circumstances. For instance, chloroform is commonly used for industrial purposes such as solvent and extracting reagents, and death can occur accidentally and sometimes, in homicide cases, with the intent to incapacitate the victims. In addition, analysis for ingredients present in kerosene and gasoline may be useful in fire death cases.

Most volatile substances are stable in blood. The specimens should be stored at low temperature (i.e., less than 4 °C) in tightly sealed glass container, preferably with anticoagulant such as heparin. Analysis of tissues such as brain and lung may prove useful since high concentrations of volatile substances may be detected.

Headspace GC-FID is the method of choice for volatile chemical analysis. If structural identification is required, GC-MS should be employed. The method used for alcohol determinations can be extended for the analysis of other volatile chemicals using same columns (e.g., Elite-BAC1 or BAC-2) with some modification of experimental settings. Examples of compounds that can be analyzed are hexane, dichloromethane, chloroform, hexane, toluene, xylene, diethylether, and ethylacetate. For the analysis of low-boiling hydrocarbons, such as methane, ethane, propane, butane, and pentane, specific columns (e.g., GC-GASPRO) intended for analysis of volatile compounds can be used.

Heavy Metal Analysis.   Although many metals are known to cause toxic effects, only a few are regarded as important toxic hazards: these include arsenic, lead, cadmium, thallium, and mercury. In addition, lithium is a psychiatric drug used for the treatment of manic-depressive disorder. There are many methods available for metal analysis in biological specimens, such as electrochemical, atomic absorption, and flame emission spectrophotometry, inductively coupled plasma coupled with either emission spectroscopy (ICP-AES) or inductively coupled plasma coupled with mass spectrometer (ICP-MS). ICP-MS after digestion of the biological specimens with concentrated mineral acid, such as nitric acid, is recommended. It is because ICP-MS allows a simultaneous screening of both metals and nonmetals as well as selective quantification of a single element with low detection limits. The availability of stable isotopes for most of the metal further enhances the accuracy of metal quantification by isotope dilution method.

Quality Systems and Assay Validation

A proper quality assurance program is an essential element for any analytical laboratory in order to ensure that the results generated are accurate, reliable, and traceable. It is even more important for a forensic toxicology laboratory since the results will be closely scrutinized in the courts of law. A quality manual pertaining all policies and procedures relevant to the reliability and traceability of the analytical results should be clearly written. Criteria affecting the quality of analytical results include the quality of materials used (such as reference standards, reagents, and chemicals), analytical methods adopted such as procedures and instrumentations used and their validity, sampling, and the chain of custody.

All analytical methods used must be properly validated. Suitable internal standards should be used in chromatographic assays, so that any systematic errors affecting the analyte can be compensated for by the internal standard. Compounds with chemical structures similar to the targeted analyte (e.g., deuterated analog) are preferably selected. For a batch of qualitative analyses, a negative control and a control representative of the analytes should be included. Any possible interfering factors that might adversely affect the analysis should be indicated. Quantitative analytical methods must be validated by determining the limit of detection, linearity range, precision, accuracy, and selectivity.

References

[1]   Bertomeu-Sánchez, J.R. & Nieto-Galan, A. (2006). *Chemistry, Medicine And Crime: Mateu J B Orfila (1787–1853) And His Times*, Science History Publications, Sagamore Beach.

[2]   Innes, B. (2000). *Bodies Of Evidence*, Reader Digest.

[3]   Marsh, J. (1836). Account of a method of separating small quantities of arsenic from substances with which it may be mixed, *Edinburgh New Philosophical Journal* **21**, 229–236. The Marsh test is performed by treating the sample with sulfuric acid and arsenic-free zinc in a glass apparatus (such as test tube). The presence of arsenic is indicative by formation of silvery-black deposit on a ceramic bowl holding above the glass apparatus.

[4]   Fenton, J.J. (2002). *Toxicology: A Case-Oriented Approach*, CRC Press, Boca Raton.

[5]   Drummer, O.H. & Odell, M. (2001). *The Forensic Pharmacology of Drugs of Abuse*, Arnold Publishers.

[6]   Skopp, G. (2004). Preanalytical aspects in post-mortem toxicology, *Forensic Science International* **142**(2–3), 75–100.

[7]   Baselt, R. (2004). *Cravey R Disposition of Toxic Drugs and Chemicals in Man*, 7th Edition, Chemical Toxicology Institute, Foster City.

[8] Moffat, A.C., Osselton, M.D., Widdop, B. & Galichet, L.Y. (eds) (2004). *Clarke's Analysis of Drugs and Poisons*, 3rd Edition, Pharmaceutical Press.

[9] TIAFT (The International Association of Forensic Toxicologists), *TIAFT reference blood level list of therapeutic and toxic substances 18-10-2005*, (2005). http://www.tiaft.org/ tmembers/ttvidx.html (Electronic version).

[10] Winek, C.L., Wahba, W.W., Winek Jr, C.L. & Winek, T.W. (2001). Drug and chemical blood-level data 2001, *Forensic Science International* **122**(2–3), 107–123.

[11] Barnhart, F.E., Bonnell, H.J. & Rossum, K.M. (2001). Postmortem drug redistribution, *Forensic Science Reviews* **13**(2), 102–129. Postmortem redistribution (PMR) refers to the change in drug concentrations after death leading to differences in drug concentrations of postmortem blood samples taken from different sites. PMR arises from incomplete distribution of the drugs and/or poisons at the time of death, passive release or from vascular pathway from major organs such as gastrointestinal tract, liver, lungs, and myocardium, and later on cell autolysis and the putrefactive process.

[12] Moriya, F. & Hashimoto, Y. (2001). Post-mortem diffusion of drugs from bladder into femoral venous blood, *Forensic Science International* **123**(2–3), 248–253.

[13] Pounder, D.J., Adams, E., Fuke, C. & Langford, A.M. (1996). Site to site variability of post-mortem drug concentrations in liver and lung, *Journal of Forensic Sciences* **41**(6), 927–932.

[14] Musshoff, F., Padosch, S., Steinborn, S. & Madea, B. (2004). Fatal blood and tissue concentration in more than 200 drugs, *Forensic Science International* **142**(2–3), 161–210.

[15] Schilt, A.A. (1958). Colorimetric determination of cyanide, *Analytical Chemistry* **30**, 1409–1411. Ferroin test is performed by the addition of two drops of Ferroin reagent, 1,10-phenanthroline ferrous sulfate followed by the addition of 2 ml of chloroform. A positive result is characterized by the formation of a purple color in the chloroform (lower) phase.

[16] Gettler, A.O. & Blume, H. (1931). Chloroform in the brain, lungs, and liver, *Archives of Pathology* **11**, 554–560.

[17] Kintz, P. (2004). Value of hair analysis in post-mortem toxicology, *Forensic Science International* **142**, 127–134.

[18] Drummer, O.H. (2002). Gerostamoulos j post-mortem drug analysis: analytical and toxicological aspects, *Therapeutic Drug Monitoring* **24**(2), 199–209.

[19] Franke, J.P. & de Zeeuw, R.A. (1998). Solid-phase extraction procedures in systematic toxicological analysis, *Journal of Chromatography. B, Biomedical Sciences and Applications* **713**(1), 51–59.

[20] Drummer, O.H. (1999). Chromatographic screening techniques in systematic toxicological analysis, *Journal of Chromatography B: Biomedical Sciences and Applications* **733**(1–2), 27–45.

[21] Koves, E.M. (1995). Use of high performance liquid chromatography – diode array detector in forensic toxicology, *Journal of Chromatography. A* **692**(1–2), 103–119.

[22] Chen, X.H., Franke, J.P., Wijsbeek, J. & de Zeeuw, R.A. (1993). Study of lot-to-lot reproducibilities of bond elut certify and clean screen DAU mixed mode solid phase extraction columns in the extraction of drugs in whole blood, *Journal of Chromatography* **617**, 147–151.

[23] Lo, D.S., Chao, T.C., Ng-Ong, S.E., Yao, Y.J. & Koh, T.H. (1997). Acidic and neutral drugs screen in blood with quantitation using microbore high-performance liquid chromatography-diode array detection and capillary gas-chromatography-flame ionization detection, *Forensic Science International* **90**(3), 205–214.

[24] Drummer, O.H., Horomidis, S., Kourtis, S., Syrjanen, M.L. & Tippett, P. (1994). Capillary gas chromatographic drug screen for used in forensic toxicology, *Journal of Analytical Toxicology* **18**(3), 134–138.

[25] Sims, D.N., Felgate, P.D., Felgate, H.E. & Lokan, R.J. (1991). Application of a simple extraction procedure using aqueous ammonia to the analysis of basic drugs in blood by gas chromatography, *Forensic Science International* **49**(1), 33–42.

[26] Huang, Z.P., Chen, X.H., Wijsbeek, J., Franke, J.P. & de Zeeuw, R.A. (1996). An enzymatic digestion and solid phase extraction procedure for the screening for acidic, neutral, and basic drugs in liver using gas chromatography for analysis, *Journal of Analytical Toxicology* **20**(4), 248–254.

[27] Pfleger, K., Maurer, H.H. & Weber, A. (1998). *Mass Spectral Library of Drugs, Pesticides, Poisons and their Metabolites*, 3rd revision, Hewlett Packard, Paol Alto.

[28] Marquet, P. (2002). Progress of liquid chromatography-mass spectrometry in clinical and forensic toxicology, *Therapeutic Drug Monitoring* **24**(2), 255–276.

[29] Van Bocxlaer, J.F., Clauwaert, K.M., Lambert, W.E., Deforce, D.L., Van den Eeckhout, E.G. & de-Leenheer, A.P. (2000). Liquid chromatography-mass spectrometry in forensic toxicology, *Mass Spectrometry Reviews* **19**(4), 165–214.

[30] Maurer, H.H. (2005). Multi-analyte procedures for screening for and quantification of drugs in blood, plasma or serum by liquid-chromatography-single stage or tandem mass spectrometry (LC-MS or LC-MS/MS) relevant to clinical and forensic toxicology, *Clinical Biochemistry* **38**(4), 310–318.

[31] Garriott, J.C. (1996). *Analysis of Alcohol in Post-mortem Specimens of Medicolegal Aspects of Alcohol*, 3rd Edition, J.C. Garriott, eds, Lawyers & Judges Publishing Co., Chapter 6.

[32] Datta, P. & Dasgupta, A. (2002). Effect of Chinese medicines Chan Su and Danshen on EMIT 2000 and Randox digoxin immunoassays: wide variation in digoxin-like immunoreactivity and magnitude of interference in digoxin measurement by different brands of the same product, *Therapeutic Drug Monitoring* **24**(5), 637–644.

[33] Drummer, O.H., Kotsos, A. & McIntyre, I.M. (1993). A class-dependent drug screen in forensic toxicology using diode array detector, *Journal of Analytical Toxicology* **17**(4), 225–229.

[34] Ojanperä, I., Rasanen, I. & Vuori, E. (1991). Automated quantitative screening for acidic and neutral drugs in whole blood by dual column capillary gas chromatography, *Journal of Analytical Toxicology* **15**(4), 204–208.

[35] Bogusz, M. & Erkens, M. (1995). Influence of biologic matrix on chromatographic behavior and detection of acidic, neutral and basic drugs examined by means of a standardized HPLC-DAD system, *Journal of Analytical Toxicology* **19**(1), 49–55.

[36] Hemmersbach, P. & de la Torre, R. (1996). Stimulants, narcotics and beta-blockers: 25 years of development in analytical techniques for doping control, *Journal of Chromatography. B, Biomedical Applications* **687**(1), 221–238.

[37] Segura, J., Venura, R. & Jurado, C. (1998). Derivatization procedures for gas chromatographic-mass spectrometric determination of xenobiotics in biological samples, with special attention to drugs of abuse and doping agents, *Journal of Chromatography. B, Biomedical Applications* **713**(1), 61–90.

[38] Maurer, H.H. & Arlt, J.W. (1998). Detection of 4-hydroxycoumarin anticoagulants and their metabolites in urine as part of a systematic toxicological analysis procedure for acidic drugs and poisons by gas chromatography-mass spectrometry after extractive methylation, *Journal of Chromatography. B, Biomedical Sciences and Applications* **714**(2), 181–195.

[39] Neill, G.P., Davies, N.W. & McLean, S. (1991). Automated screening procedure using gas chromatography-mass spectrometry for identification of drugs after their extraction from biological samples, *Journal of Chromatography* **565**(1–2), 207–224.

[40] Marquet, P., Saint-Marcoux, F., Gamble, T.N. & Leblanc, J.C. (2003). Comparison of a preliminary procedure for the general unknown screening of drugs and toxic compounds using a quadrupole-linear iontrap mass spectrometer with a liquid chromatography-mass spectrometry reference technique, *Journal of Chromatography. B, Analytical Technologies in the Biomedical and Life Sciences* **789**(1), 9–18.

[41] Mueller, C.A., Weinmann, W., Dresen, S., Schreiber, A. & Gergov, M. (2005). Development of a multi-target screening analysis for 301 drugs using a QTrap liquid chromatography/tandem mass spectrometry system and automated library searching, *Rapid Communications in Mass Spectrometry* **19**(10), 1332–1338.

[42] Pelander, A., Ojanpera, I., Laks, S., Rasanen, I. & Vuori, E. (2003). Toxicological screening with formula-based metabolite identification by liquid chromatography/time-of-flight mass spectrometry, *Analytical Chemistry* **75**(21), 5710–5718.

[43] Brehmer, C. & Iten, P.X. (2003). Rapid determination of carboxyhemoglobin in blood by Oximeter., *Forensic Science International* **133**(1–2), 179–181.

[44] Lewis, R.J., Johnson, R.D. & Canfield, D.V. (2004). An accurate method for the determination of carboxyhemoglobin in post-mortem blood using GC-TCD, *Journal of Analytical Toxicology* **28**(1), 59–62.

[45] Kojima, T., Nishiyama, Y., Yashiki, M. & Une, I. (1982). Postmortem formation of carbon monoxide, *Forensic Science International* **19**(3), 243–248.

[46] Kage, S., Ito, S. & Kishida, T. (1998). A fatal case of hydrogen sulfide poisoning in a geothermal power plant, *Journal of Forensic Science* **43**(4), 908–910.

[47] Kage, S., Nagata, T. & Kudo, K. (1991). Determination of thiosulfate in body fluids by GC and GC/MS, *Journal of Analytical Toxicology* **15**(3), 148–150.

[48] Odoul, M., Fouillet, B., Nouri, B., Chambon, R. & Chambon, P. (1994). Specific determination of cyanide in blood by headspace gas chromatography, *Journal of Analytical Toxicology* **18**(4), 205–207.

WING-CHI CHENG

Postmortem Toxicology: Specimens *see* Toxicology: Analysis

Postpartum Psychosis

Introduction

Postpartum psychosis (PPP; also known as *puerperal psychosis*) was perhaps first described by Hippocrates in the fourth century BC. He described an acute onset of confusion, hallucinations, delirium, and insomnia [1, 2]. In 1865, the French physician Marce published his observations and study of perinatal disorders [3]. By the 1800s, symptoms of PPP were believed to be related to lactation, and the term *milk fever* was even used [1]. This "lactational insanity" was the basis for many Infanticide laws across the world. *The Yellow Wallpaper*, a monograph from 1899 [4], though controversial, may illustrate a woman's struggles with PPP.

The time in a woman's life when she is at greatest risk of psychosis or mental illness is in the postpartum period [5]. Fortunately PPP is rare, occurring after approximately 1–2 per thousand births. PPP often has a dramatic presentation, within the first several weeks of childbirth [6], but may begin within just days of giving birth. Early on, symptoms may include sleep disturbance and restlessness. Symptoms may evolve to include either depressed or elevated mood or both, agitation, delusions, hallucinations, and depersonalization. Women may believe they are being persecuted by the baby. Risks may include suicide, child neglect, or infanticide. PPP is considered a true psychiatric emergency, and mothers often require psychiatric hospitalization. Some specialized treatment units allow mothers to be hospitalized with their infants.

The Diagnosis of Postpartum Psychosis

Though cases may begin during pregnancy [2], more often they begin shortly after childbirth. Most cases of PPP begin within a couple weeks of delivery, with an abrupt onset [1, 2, 7]. By this time the mother has most often been discharged home with her fragile infant, rather than remaining in the hospital. Sleep deprivation is a potential trigger [8].

Risk of PPP may be related to hormonal shifts after birth (primarily the drop in estrogen) [7], stressors (such as marital problems), biology (bipolar disorder), and family history – genetic studies are underway [9], and can also be triggered by menstruation or cessation of lactation [2]. Some researchers have reported that the first pregnancy is a risk factor for PPP [2, 10]. Reports of recurrence rates of PPP after further pregnancies range from one in seven to women with bipolar disorder or schizoaffective disorder have a 50% risk of another episode of PPP [7, 11]. However, this rate is modified by prophylactic medication treatment [12]. Delivery complications may also elevate risk [10].

Common symptoms of PPP include symptoms of psychosis, with an impaired concept of reality and fluctuating delirium. Confusion, bizarre delusions (fixed, false beliefs) and behavior, hallucinations (unusual perceptual experiences that can be tactile, olfactory, or visual in addition to auditory), mood lability (ranging from depression to euphoria), and disorganized thinking may occur [1, 13]. For example, a woman might be delusional that she has special powers, that God has chosen her baby to be sacrificed, or that the baby is defective. Because of the lack of insight, suspicion, or conspiracy theories, women may not reveal their symptoms to others.

Among women with PPP, 72–88% have bipolar disorder or schizoaffective disorder, while 12% have schizophrenia [7]. In distinction to PPP, in schizophrenia delusional thinking and hallucinations often have a more gradual onset.

The psychiatric reference book DSM-IV-TR [14] does not list a specific diagnosis for PPP. Some debate exists within the field. According to the DSM-IV-TR, brief psychotic disorder or psychotic disorder not otherwise specified are diagnoses used for PPP, or a woman's symptoms may meet criteria for an affective (mood) episode [14]. Further even, the postpartum period is also defined differently depending on the group defining it; postpartum is 4 weeks according to the DSM-IV-TR, 6 weeks for ICD-10, 3 months in some epidemiological studies, and up to 1 year in some investigations [15].

Comparison with Postpartum Depression and Other Disorders

Postpartum blues or "baby blues" occur in approximately half to three-quarters of mothers [7]. Baby blues are not synonymous with postpartum depression (PPD); they are transient and not as severe. Symptoms usually occur in the first week after giving birth, and are self-limited. Symptoms may include anxiety, mood swings from sadness to irritability, and insomnia.

PPD symptoms are not the same as those of PPP. Approximately 10–15% of mothers experience PPD [3, 7]. Symptoms may occur within a few weeks to a year after giving birth. In PPD, a woman's predominant mood is sad or depressed, and she may lose enjoyment in her activities. Other symptoms may include insomnia, even an inability to sleep when the baby is sleeping. Her appetite may be abnormal. She may be fatigued and have difficulty concentrating. She may lack the interest in caring for her appearance, or even for her baby. She may experience feelings of worthlessness or hopelessness, and may have difficulty bonding with the infant. She may experience suicidal thoughts or thoughts of harming the infant. Symptoms of anxiety often also occur.

Psychiatrists must also differentiate psychotic thoughts and behavior from obsessive thoughts, which are also common in the postpartum [5, 7]. In obsessive compulsive disorder (OCD) or other anxiety disorders, women may experience intrusive thoughts that they have difficulty getting out of their head. These thoughts often represent worries, and the women, in distinction to women with psychosis, are not out of touch with reality. If these women have thoughts or fears, for example of harming someone, they usually realize that these thoughts are not of something that they would ever do and try to avoid the thoughts.

In the evaluation of a postpartum woman with psychiatric symptoms, physicians may consider that the differential diagnosis includes medical problems such as thyroiditis, Late Onset Tay Sachs disease, and vitamin B_{12} deficiency. Laboratory tests, computed tomography (CT) scan, or magnetic resonance imaging (MRI) of the brain may be indicated to rule out alternative organic diagnoses.

Treatment of Postpartum Psychosis

Because of the rapidly evolving and devastatingly severe nature of symptoms, PPP is often a psychiatric emergency. Women with a history of PPP or bipolar disorder have a 100-fold increase in psychiatric hospitalization during the postpartum [1]. In this disorder, treaters will often need to enlist help of family and other support. In some cases, child protective services may need to become involved.

Mood stabilizing medications (such as valproate or lithium) are mainstays of treatment, related to the frequently underlying bipolar disorder. Electroconvulsive therapy (ECT) is another consideration. Though not without risks of its own, ECT may provide for a rapid symptomatic improvement. Atypical antipsychotics such as olanzapine may have a role in the treatment of PPP as well [15]. (These agents are increasingly being used for not only the treatment of psychotic disorders but also of mood disorders.) Typical (older) antipsychotic agents may not lead to remission of symptoms [5]. Side effects of medications, such as sedation, which could impair her ability to respond to her infant, should be considered.

Because of the rarity of PPP, compared to other psychiatric disorders, there are fewer studies regarding evidence-based treatment. PPP is often considered to be a bipolar disorder unless proven otherwise.

Whether the mother is bottle-feeding or breast-feeding is another consideration, as different medications present different potential risks to breast-fed infants. The infant may require monitoring by a pediatrician. Other mothers may prefer to bottle-feed, to avoid any potential risk. With a supportive partner, bottle-feeding at least at night may have the added benefit of allowing the mother with PPP to sleep through the night.

Healthcare providers should educate patients about PPP. Support of families may help alleviate some of the stress associated with PPP [11]. It is important to consider prevention of episodes in future pregnancies/postpartum periods. Women with bipolar disorder are often treated prophylactically, where possible, with lithium or another mood stabilizer [7].

Risks in PPP

Mothers who experienced delusions that the baby is evil or a devil or not truly theirs were more likely to be abusive toward the infant [16]. Mothers with PPP "are at risk of injuring their children through practical incompetence or misguided delusions". [1, p. 106] Women with childbearing-related onset of psychiatric illnesses have reported homicidal ideation more frequently [13]. Risk of suicide is also present in PPP [17].

Neonaticide is specifically the murder of the neonate by the parent in the first 24 h of life [18]. Obviously, as most PPP has not yet begun at the time of birth, but rather has an onset several days to weeks later, there is a lack of relation of PPP to neonaticide in the great majority of cases. However, some cases of neonaticide do involve psychotic mothers [19].

Infanticide is often considered to include the murder of infants less than 1 year of age at the hands of the parent. (However, infanticide is a nonspecific term; in Biblical times, murder of a child at the hand of the state may have been considered infanticide.) Filicide, more precisely, is the murder of a child by the parent. If a woman is suffering from PPP, the physician should consider her risk of harming herself and/or her infant. Though there have been reported cases of infant murder while in the hospital [20], the overwhelming majority of cases occur outside the hospital. In psychiatric studies, mothers who kill their children often have experienced psychosis, suicidality, and depression [21]. Often, alcohol or substance use, limited social support, and a maternal history of abuse are found as well.

The mother's motive for killing her infant or child may fall into any of several categories: *altruistic, acutely psychotic, fatal maltreatment, unwanted child,* or *spouse revenge* [22]. In an altruistic filicide, the mother kills her child out of love. A mother who sees her child suffering from cerebral palsy or leukemia may feel that the loving thing to do is spare the child from suffering. Though difficult to fathom, because of her depressed or psychotic outlook on life, another mother may believe that it is in the child's best interest to go to Heaven, rather than living an awful life on earth. The mother may be suicidal and not wish to leave her child in the hopeless world that she is departing. She may be psychotic, believing that if her child were to live, he or she would be tortured or raped or kidnapped, and may reason that the only humane choice is to kill him.

Alternatively, in an acutely psychotic filicide, the mother kills her child for no comprehensible reason. She may be responding to hallucinated voices commanding her to kill. She may kill in the throes of epilepsy or the confusion of delirium. She may put the baby in the oven instead of the dinner, for no rational reason but borne out of severe confusion and illness.

Fatal maltreatment filicide is the most common type of filicide overall. A child may die because of chronic abuse or chronic neglect. Certainly mothers suffering from psychosis or depression may be abusive, but so may many other mothers who do not have a mental illness. Too, mothers who are severely mentally ill and out of touch with reality may have difficulty providing for their infants' many needs. In an unwanted child filicide, a child who is not desired is killed. In a spouse revenge filicide, the rarest type, a child is killed in order to cause emotional pain in the other parent.

Newborns have a total dependence on their caregivers. If their caregiver is a woman with unidentified PPP, lacking in social support, that is highly concerning. A 4% risk of infanticide has been estimated in untreated PPP [23]. Even if a woman with PPP has support from her social network, if those who care do not understand the risks associated with PPP, there is cause for concern.

Infanticide Laws and Defenses

The British Infanticide Act was initially enacted in 1922, and was reformulated in 1938. The Act allows a woman, still recovering from giving birth, who kills her infant in the first 12 months of life to be charged with infanticide (akin to manslaughter) rather than murder, because "the balance of her mind is disturbed by reason of her not having fully recovered from the effect of giving birth to the child" [24].

Infanticide laws exist in over two dozen other nations, including Canada and Australia [25]. However, the legal criteria for infanticide vary across nations, including in New Zealand the murder of children up to age 10 [26]. In Luxembourg, there is a stricter penalty for child homicide.

However, a causal connectional between mental illness and the crime does not always occur in practice [27]. And, if a psychotic postpartum mother kills her infant and her older child, she could be charged for murder of the older child and infanticide for the killing of the infant. Also, one acutely psychotic mother who killed her 13-month-old baby might not qualify for infanticide though another mother who killed her 11-month-old baby *via* fatal maltreatment borne out of frustration might.

In the United States, there is no such infanticide legislation. The wake of the Andrea Yates child murder case led to proposals for American infanticide legislation [3, 28]. In the United States, the not-guilty-by-reason-of-insanity (NGRI) defense is used in some cases of maternal filicide. Throughout the United States and the world, there are various laws regarding NGRI (*see* **Insanity: Defense**). NGRI laws often include that a mental illness caused an actor not to know her act was wrong, and may include that she was unable to conform her conduct to the requirements of the law.

The diagnosis of PPP may be the mental illness on which the insanity defense is predicated. A woman with PPP and an alternative sense of reality may delusionally believe that she is doing what is right in killing her infant. Another woman may be unable to control her behavior because of manic psychosis. Still another may kill, believing that the hallucinations telling her to do so are from God. However, a mother who fatally abuses her infant may be unlikely to qualify for an NGRI finding because of the aforementioned requirements.

PPP can be difficult to prove in the legal sense – symptoms may have rapid resolution prior to psychiatric evaluation, and there has existed disagreement in the field as well. Psychiatric evaluation may be expedited in cases where PPP is believed to be related to the murder.

Summary

PPP may consist of symptoms including hallucinations, delusions, confusion, insomnia, mood swings, and loss of contact with reality. It must be differentiated from depression, anxiety, and medical disorders. Mothers may decompensate rather rapidly, within several weeks of delivery. Early recognition may be critical. These mothers often merit emergent treatment. Risks may include infant neglect, abuse, infanticide, or maternal suicide. Mothers with PPP who kill their infants may qualify for infanticide or insanity defenses.

References

[1]   Attia, E., Downey J. & Oberman, M. (1999). Postpartum psychoses, in *Postpartum Mood Disorders*, L.J. Miller, ed, American Psychiatric Press, Washington, DC, pp. 99–117.

[2]   Brockington, I. (1996). *Motherhood and Mental Health*, Oxford University Press, Oxford.

[3]   Nelson, K.E. (2004). Postpartum psychosis and women who kill their children: making the punishment fit the crime, *Developments in Mental Health Law* **23**, 23–36.

[4]   Gilman, C.P. (1892). *The Yellow Wallpaper*.

[5]   Wisner, K.L., Gracious, B.L., Piontek, C.M., Peindl, K. & Perel, J.M. (2003). Postpartum disorders: phenomenology, treatment approaches, and relationship to infanticide, in *Infanticide: Psychosocial and Legal Perspectives On Mothers Who Kill*, M.G. Spinelli, ed, APPI, Washington, DC.

[6]   Kendell, R.E., Chalmers, J.C. & Platz, C. (1987). Epidemiology of puerperal psychoses, *British Journal of Psychiatry* **150**, 662–673.

[7]   Sit, D., Rothschild, A.J. & Wisner, K.L. (2006). A review of postpartum psychosis, *Journal of Women's Health* **15**(4), 352–368.

[8]   Sharma, V., Smith, A. & Khan, M. (2004). The relationship between duration of labour, time of delivery, and puerperal psychosis, *Journal of Affective Disorders* **83**(2–3), 215–220.

[9]   Jones, I. & Craddock, N. (2007). Searching for the puerperal trigger: molecular genetic studies of bipolar affective puerperal psychosis, *Psychopharmacology Bulletin* **40**(2), 115–128.

[10]   Blackmore, E.R., Jones, I., Doshi, M., Haque, S., Holder, R., Brockington, I. & Craddock, N. (2006). Obstetric variables associated with bipolar affective puerperal psychosis, *British Journal of Psychiatry* **188**, 32–36.

[11]   Robertson, E. & Lyons, A. (2003). Living with puerperal psychosis: a qualitative analysis, *Psychology and Psychotherapy* **76**(4), 411–431.

[12]   Stewart, D.E., Klompenhouwer, J.L., Kendell, R.E. & van Hulst, A.M. (1991). Prophylactic lithium in puerperal psychosis, *British Journal of Psychiatry* **158**, 393–397.

[13]   Wisner, K., Peindl, K. & Hanusa, B.H. (1994). Symptomatology of affective and psychotic illnesses related to childbearing, *Journal of Affective Disorders* **30**, 77–87.

[14]   American Psychiatric Association (2000). *Diagnostic and Statistical Manual*, Text Revision, 4th Edition, American Psychiatric Association.

[15]   Sharma, V., Smith, A. & Mazmanian, D. (2006). Olanzapine in the prevention of postpartum psychosis and mood episodes in bipolar disorder, *Bipolar Disorders* **8**(4), 400–404.

[16]   Chandra, P.S., Bhargavaraman, R.P., Raghunandan, V.N. & Shaligram, D. (2006). Delusions related to infant and their association with mother-infant interactions in postpartum psychotic disorders, *Archives of Women's Mental Health* **9**(5), 285–288.

[17]   Lindahl, V., Pearson, J.L. & Colpe, L. (2005). Prevalence of suicidality during pregnancy and the postpartum, *Archives of Women's Mental Health* **8**(2), 77–87.

[18]   Resnick, P.J. (1970). Murder of the newborn: a psychiatric review of neonaticide, *American Journal of Psychiatry* **126**, 58–64.

[19]   Putkonen, H., Weizmann-Henelius, G., Collander, J., Santtila, P. & Eronen, M. (2007). Neonaticides may be more preventable and heterogeneous than previously thought-neonaticides in Finland 1980–2000, *Archives of Women's Mental Health* **10**, 15–23.

[20]   Mendlowicz, M.V., da Silva Filho, J.F., Gekker, M., de Moraes, T.M., Rapaport, M.H. & Jean-Louis, F. (2000). Mothers murdering their newborns in the hospital, *General Hospital Psychiatry* **22**(1), 53–55.

[21]   Friedman, S.H., Horwitz, S.M. & Resnick, P.J. (2005). Child murder by mothers: a critical analysis of the current state of knowledge and a research agenda, *American Journal of Psychiatry* **162**, 1578–1587.

[22]   Resnick, P.J. (1969). Child murder by parents: a psychiatric review of filicide, *American Journal of Psychiatry* **126**, 73–82.

[23]   Altshuler, L.L., Hendrick, V. & Cohen, L.S. (1998). Course of mood and anxiety disorders during pregnancy and the postpartum period, *The Journal of Clinical Psychiatry* **59**(Suppl. 2), 29–33.

[24]   Oberman, M. (1996). Mothers who kill: coming to terms with modern American infanticide, *American Criminal Law Review* **34**, 2–109.

[25] Friedman, S.H. & Resnick, P.J. (2007). Child murder by mothers: patterns and prevention, *World Psychiatry* **6**, 137–141.

[26] Dean, P.J. (2004). Child homicide and infanticide in New Zealand, *International Journal of Law and Psychiatry* **27**, 339–348.

[27] d'Orban, P.T. (1979). Women who kill their children, *British Journal of Psychiatry* **134**, 560–571.

[28] Connell, M. (2002). The postpartum psychosis defence and feminism: more or less justice for women? *Case Western Reserve Law Review* **53**, 143.

SUSAN HATTERS-FRIEDMAN

Posttraumatic Stress Disorder

Exposure to psychological trauma is thought to be a risk factor for the development of many mental health disorders including posttraumatic stress disorder (PTSD), acute stress disorder (ASD), other anxiety disorders, depressive disorders, somatic disorders, substance abuse disorders, and psychotic disorders. The specific mental health symptoms that typically become manifest following exposure to trauma appear to vary from culture to culture [1–3] and from era to era, e.g., somatic and psychotic symptoms were much more common in the traumatized World War II (WWII) combatants [4] than they were in traumatized Vietnam combatants [5]. The term *PTSD* was first introduced into the official Western classification of psychiatric disorders in 1980 with the publication of the third edition of the Diagnostic and Statistical Manual for Mental Health Disorders or DSM-III [6]. Prior to 1980, the disorder was referred to by a number of names including soldier's heart in the Civil War, shell shock and traumatic neurosis in WWI, combat fatigue and war neurosis in WWII, and gross stress reaction in the 1970s [7]. PTSD has also been referred to by a number of somewhat pejorative terms to include secondary gain neurosis, compensation neurosis, and litigation neurosis owing to its association with malingering and factitious disorder [8, 9]. Malingering involves the intentional production or substantial exaggeration of physical or psychological symptoms and/or dysfunction in order to secure external incentives, e.g., avoiding work, evading criminal responsibility, and obtaining disability compensation [10]. Factitious disorder also involves intentional feigning or exaggeration of physical or psychological symptoms or dysfunction, but the motivation for doing so is to maintain the sick role, the victim role, or the wounded soldier role rather than obtaining external incentives [10]. Malingering and factitious disorder often coexist; and for the sake of brevity, the term *malingering* henceforth will be used to denote both malingering and factitious disorder.

Six criteria currently define PTSD per the most recent edition of the DSM, the DSM-IV [10]. First, the person must have experienced, witnessed, or have been confronted with a traumatic event that involved an actual or threatened death or serious injury of someone, or involved a threat to the physical integrity of self or others. In addition, the person's emotional response to the traumatic event must have involved intense fear, helplessness, or horror. Second, the person must persistently reexperience the traumatic event in the form of nightmares, intrusive recollections during the waking state, flashbacks (illusions and hallucinations) in which the person feels as if the event were reoccurring, and/or intense psychological distress or physiological reactivity upon exposure to stimuli that resemble an aspect of the traumatic event. Third, the person must persistently avoid stimuli associated with the traumatic event and/or experience a numbing of general responsiveness. Fourth, the person must experience persistent hyperarousal symptoms, e.g., hypervigilance, exaggerated startle reflex, and irritability. Fifth, the person must manifest reexperiencing, avoidance/numbing, and hyperarousal symptoms for more than one month posttrauma. Sixth, the person must manifest clinically significant distress or impairment in social, occupational, or other important areas of functioning. The diagnostic criteria for ASD are very similar to those for PTSD – the major differences being the presence of dissociative symptoms in ASD, but not in PTSD, and the PTSD symptom triad of reexperiencing, hyperarousal, and avoidance/numbing symptoms are experienced for less than one month in ASD, rather than for more than a month as they are in PTSD [10].

A voluminous amount of research has been conducted over the course of the past 25 years on psychological trauma, ASD, and PTSD. One of the more surprising findings is that most individuals in the United States will be exposed to one or more traumatic events in the course of their lifetime – between 68 and 90% depending on the criterion and measurement methods used [11–14]. Perhaps even more surprising is the finding that only a relatively small percentage of those individuals exposed to trauma go on to develop PTSD – between 9 and 14% depending on the stressor criteria and measurement methods used [11–16]. Individuals with certain characteristics have been found to be at greater risk than others to develop PTSD subsequent to trauma – namely, women [17] and individuals with a history of psychiatric disorders as well as individuals with a family history of psychiatric disorders [11–16]. Conversely, individuals with other characteristics appear less likely to develop PTSD subsequent to trauma – namely, men [17] and individuals with good intelligence [5, 15, 18] as well as those individuals with a substantial amount of a personality trait termed *hardiness* [19–22]. Hardy individuals are those who stay committed to life (as opposed to being alienated), who believe in their own ability to control and influence the course of events (as contrasted with a sense of being powerless), and who view negative life events as challenges to be met and overcome (as opposed to view these events as insurmountable threats). Similarly, some individuals respond to traumatic events and PTSD with enhanced mental health, altruism, empathy, spirituality, and prosocial values or what has been termed *posttraumatic growth* [23, 24].

Some types of trauma appear to be more pathogenic than the other types. The most pathogenic appears to be trauma that is repetitive and prolonged (as opposed to a single and brief), man-made (as opposed to natural catastrophes), and particularly gruesome such as is often found in combat, war atrocities, and torture situations [24–27]. Single, brief, and time-limited traumatic events also vary in terms of their pathogenic potential. For example, a situation in which an 18-month-old child is run over in his own driveway by a neighbor and thereafter dies shortly in the arms of his mother is far more likely to provoke PTSD in the neighbor and the mother than the bystanders who are horrified as they witness the tragedy but who have no personal involvement with the child, the mother, or the neighbor [24–27].

Another somewhat surprising finding is that those individuals who develop PTSD subsequent to trauma often spontaneously remit or improve over time without the benefit of formal treatment to the point that they no longer meet the criteria necessary to be diagnosed with PTSD. Estimates vary, but approximately 50% of those with PTSD appears to spontaneously remit within two years posttrauma with the majority of the remission taking place in the first year [5, 12, 16, 28–31]. Those who do not remit spontaneously and who do not remit by way of treatment have an elevated risk to develop other mental health disorders and substance use disorders [11, 12, 14]. Those who do remit are at no greater risk to develop other mental health disorders than those who were never traumatized in the first place [11, 12, 14].

Another important finding is the level of vocational and social dysfunction varies considerably in the PTSD-afflicted individuals. Some individuals function at a high level vocationally and socially, and only experience occasional episodes of acute PTSD symptoms typically provoked by trauma anniversary dates or by severe situational stressors such as the death or serious illness of a loved one. Still others with PTSD are severely and chronically incapacitated emotionally, socially, and vocationally. This usually occurs when the individual has been exposed to a particularly severe trauma or to multiple traumas, has severe psychopathology prior to the trauma, and/or when severe comorbid disorders develop subsequent to the PTSD such as addictions, personality disorders, or psychosis [11–14].

Assessment

Prior to the publication of the DSM-III in 1980 [6], PTSD was frequently misdiagnosed in the form of false negatives (PTSD was present but not diagnosed) simply because it was not recognized as a valid diagnostic entity. Since then, it appears that the frequency of PTSD diagnoses have steadily risen as has the misdiagnosis of PTSD in the form of false positives (PTSD is diagnosed as present when it is not). Described below are some of the errors that are frequently being made today.

Trauma

One of the more common diagnostic errors being made is to equate stressful life events with trauma.

For example, a highly contentious divorce, being fired from a job, being betrayed by a close and trusted family member, or observing a tragic and deadly event unfold on television are often highly distressing and can generate many PTSD-like symptoms; but such events lack the critical element of being personally life-threatening and thus fail to meet one of the essential criteria necessary to diagnose PTSD [27]. For the same reason, being fearful while on sentry duty in a noncombat zone and learning of the deaths of other soldiers killed in a helicopter crash (but not being personally involved with them nor witnessing their deaths) generally does not constitute trauma. Malingers often fabricate traumatic events or they may fabricate their involvement with actual traumatic events. In either case, their stories often have inconsistencies in their retelling, inconsistencies with factual accounts of the traumatic events or in the events leading up to them, and/or implausibilities embedded within their stories [27]. For example, a malinger claiming to have been a sniper in Vietnam could not recall the manufacturer or power of the scope that was mounted on an unlikely weapon he said he employed – a rifle commonly used in Vietnam by infantrymen but generally considered to be inaccurate at long distances.

PTSD Symptoms

Another common error is to diagnose PTSD on the basis of the presence of reexperiencing, hyperarousal, or avoidance/numbing symptoms by themselves [27]. None of these symptoms are unique to PTSD and all can be found in several other mental health disorders to include generalized anxiety disorder, phobia, panic disorder, and substance-induced mood and anxiety disorders. A causal link must be established between this triad of PTSD symptoms and a traumatic stressor before other mental health disorders can be safely ruled out and PTSD diagnosed. To do this, the triad of PTSD symptoms must have first become manifest after trauma exposure has occurred, not before. Most individuals who develop PTSD following trauma exposure will experience the initial onset of the triad of PTSD symptoms within days or weeks of trauma exposure. Occasionally individuals do delay the initial onset of PTSD symptoms for as long as a year or so posttrauma, but reports of delayed onset several years after trauma

exposure should be suspect, particularly if the individual reports his or her mental health to be sound in the intervening period. The triad of PTSD symptoms typically wax and wane in concert with situationally induced stress once the symptoms first become manifest. Reports of severe PTSD symptoms that show little variability across time, stress, and situations should be suspect. Flashbacks wherein an individual with PTSD relives a traumatic experience in a delusional state and out of contact with reality do occur, but they are rare. When flashbacks do occur, they are typically provoked by high levels of situational stress coupled with substance abuse and poor sleep in individuals with a history of severe trauma and severe PTSD symptoms. Reports of frequent, prolonged, and unprovoked flashbacks should be suspect. Reexperiencing symptoms in the form of nightmares, in which the traumatic experiences are veridically recapitulated in the PTSD-afflicted individuals' dreams, are typical. PTSD nightmares usually are accompanied by substantially more body movement than is found in conventional nightmares. PTSD nightmares also normally contain little in the way of fantasy at the outset; although as time progresses, PTSD nightmares may come to incorporate contemporary problems and issues in them as well as some fantastic elements. Conventional nightmares are largely fantastic and contain little in the way of realistic trauma material. Individuals with PTSD typically avoid situations that are connected with, or similar to, the traumatic events. Malingers generally do not avoid such reminders to the same extent. For example, malingers often relish telling war stories and often watch war movies and war footage on the news – things that most individuals with combat-induced PTSD would generally try to avoid. Malingerers tend to over-report or exaggerate the severity and frequency of hyperarousal and reexperiencing symptoms, and they tend to report these symptoms in interviews in an overly dramatic or histrionic fashion. On psychological tests that are sensitive to malingering, malingers tend to endorse obvious PTSD items but not subtle PTSD items; they also tend to endorse extreme but rare PTSD symptoms, and they tend to produce overall "fake-bad" test profiles. For a thorough review of the literature regarding psychological testing and malingering, see the article on forensic matters [32] in the text by Wilson and Keane [27].

Disability

The level of psychological, social, education, and vocational dysfunction related to PTSD varies considerably from one person to the other [27, 32]. Uncomplicated PTSD that is induced by a single, time-limited traumatic event in a mentally healthy adult who has good social support and who resides in a safe and healthy environment generally produces psychological distress in the neurotic (moderate) range along with mild to moderate dysfunction in social/educational/vocational functioning. The level of psychosocial dysfunction tends to markedly increase in those PTSD-afflicted individuals who heavily rely on substances and/or high levels of avoidance to cope with their PTSD symptoms [29, 30]. More psychosocial dysfunction is also generally seen in PTSD-afflicted individuals who have low social support and reside in unsafe, impoverished environments. The most severe psychosocial dysfunction is generally found among those PTSD-afflicted individuals who have substantial pre-existing psychopathology and/or develop such pathology subsequent to the PTSD, e.g., substance abuse disorders, psychotic disorders, and personality disorders. Severe psychosocial dysfunction is also likely to be found in the PTSD-afflicted individuals whose PTSD was induced by prolonged, repetitive, and particularly gruesome trauma, e.g., atrocities, and torture. Psychosocial dysfunction should never be assumed if PTSD is present. It should always be independently assessed across vocational, educational, social, and recreational domains. Malingers tend to exaggerate their psychosocial dysfunction, and they often have marked discrepancies between their capacities for work and play. For example, a malinger claimed high levels of PTSD-related vocational dysfunction yet coached his son's soccer team and routinely hosted social events in his home and in the community for team members and their parents.

Malingering

Few, if any, studies have rigorously examined the prevalence of malingering in either clinical or forensic settings. There are, however, a number of case studies and studies that have employed samples of convenience that have estimated the prevalence to vary from 1% [33] to 50% [34] depending on the

setting and the population being examined. For a review of the literature in this regard, see the article on forensic matters [32] in the text by Wilson and Keane [27]. In most clinical settings, mental health professionals rely almost exclusively on individuals' self-reports to diagnose PTSD that are taken by the way of unstructured interviews or structured interviews such as the Clinician-administered PTSD Scale [35]. Given clinicians' general lack of skepticism and their desire to give clients the benefit of the doubt, many malingerers appear to be able to feign PTSD symptoms and trauma exposure well enough in such interviews to avoid being detected. This generally does not pose a problem provided the prevalence of malingering is low as it is in most clinical settings. However, in a few clinical settings and nearly all forensic settings, malingering is likely to be prevalent. This necessitates taking additional assessment measures to rule maligning out. Such measures usually entail collaborating clients' self-reports of trauma exposure, collaborating their self-reports of PTSD symptoms, and collaborating their self-reports of psychosocial disability by way third party reports, reviews of public and private records (e.g., media accounts, police records, military records, and medical records), and the administration of structured interviews that are sensitive to dissimulation such as the Structured Interview of Reported Symptoms [36] as well as psychological tests that have scales that are sensitive to dissimulation such as the Minnesota Multiphasic Personality Inventory 2 (MMPI2) [37]. Gathering such information usually adds considerable time and expense to the assessment process.

It is generally a good idea to rate individuals in terms of the malingering indicators listed below before diagnosing them with PTSD. The more malingering red flags that are present then the greater the likelihood of malingering. The number of red flags that should trigger efforts to collaborate individuals' self-reports will vary from setting to setting depending on the costs for misdiagnosing PTSD if malingering is overlooked *versus* the costs for conducting the more thorough assessment necessary to rule out malingering. The costs will also be strongly influenced by the relative prevalence rates of PTSD versus malingered PTSD in the population of interest, which are likely to vary from time to time. For instance, malingered PTSD was probably relatively rare in veterans who approached the United States

Department of Veteran Affairs for services throughout the 1980s – about 5% according to one estimate [38]. Thus, the costs of occasionally misdiagnosing PTSD because malingering was overlooked were relatively small then. But clinical observation and some empirical evidence [39–41] now suggest that malingered PTSD is far more common in veterans seeking services from the US Department of Veteran Affairs than it once was. Consequently, the costs of misdiagnosing PTSD because malingering is overlooked are probably substantially greater than they once were. These costs not only include disability compensation being erroneously awarded to malingers but also include the costs of utilizing scarce clinical resources to treat malingers that could be better utilized if these resources were devoted to treating those in greater clinical need.

Malingering (Factitious Disorder) Red Flags

1. Criminal proceedings
Malingering should always be suspected when a diagnosis of PTSD is likely to mitigate an individual's criminal culpability.

2. Disability proceedings
Malingering should always be suspected when a diagnosis of PTSD is likely to result in disability compensation for an individual.

3. History of disability claims
Malingering should always be suspected when an individual has a history of filing disability claims.

4. Antisocial personality disorder
Malingering should always be suspected when an individual has an antisocial personality disorder or antisocial personality traits as evidenced by a long history of significant legal infractions and/or social irresponsibility.

5. Poor work history
Malingering should be suspected when an individual is functioning as a marginal member of society as manifested by a poor work history, no permanent address, a vagabond lifestyle, etc. Severe PTSD or PTSD complicated by severe comorbid disorders can result in a poor work history so it is important to examine an individual's work history prior to the trauma as well as after.

6. Substance abuse disorder
Malingering should be suspected when an individual presents with a substance abuse disorder. Substance abuse disorders sometimes do evolve as a consequence of PTSD so it is important to examine the individual's substance usage before the trauma as well as after.

7. Marked disparities in psychosocial functioning
Malingering should be suspected when an individual claims substantial vocational impairment subsequent to PTSD yet retains the capacity to successfully engage in social and/or recreational activities.

8. Atypical presentational styles
Malingering should be suspected if an individual presents with extreme emotional displays and/or bizarre symptoms when discussing their trauma. At the other extreme, malingering should also be suspected if an individual presents in a bland, matter-of-fact manner when discussing their trauma. Almost all PTSD-afflicted individuals will have some emotional distress and difficulty in discussing their trauma, but it will not be so severe as to disrupt the assessment process nor will it have a histrionic quality to it. Malingerers tend to present themselves as victims and tend to externalize, condemn, and blame others for their misfortune with accompanying anger, whereas individuals with PTSD tend to internalize and perceive themselves as being primarily responsible for their misfortune with accompanying guilt and shame. Malingering should also be suspected when an individual idealizes their life and work prior to the trauma while simultaneously attributing any and all shortcomings they currently have to the trauma and/or PTSD. Malingering should also be suspected when an individual behaves in an evasive, noncooperative, or hostile manner during the assessment. Such presentational styles are atypical of PTSD-afflicted individuals in most assessment settings.

9. Atypical trauma
Malingering should be suspected when traumatic events cannot be independently verified. Malingering should also be suspected when the traumatic events contain one or more implausible elements or when there are significant inconsistencies noted from one retelling of the trauma story to the next. Malingering should also be suspected when severe PTSD is claimed, the individual has no

pre-existing psychopathology, and the trauma is a single, brief, and not a particularly gruesome tragedy.

10. Atypical PTSD symptoms

Malingering should be suspected when an individual reports a number of atypical symptoms or symptom patterns to include: substantial time delays between traumatic events and the initial onset of the PTSD symptom triad, the complete cessation of the PTSD symptoms for substantial periods of time owing to the heavy use of substances, PTSD symptoms that fail to vary in frequency and severity in concert with situational stressors, the presence of rare PTSD symptoms such as flashbacks occurring in the absence of high stress and substance abuse and a history of severe PTSD symptoms, nightmares that contain substantial fantasy and little trauma content, little in the way of avoidance of situational stimuli associated with the traumatic events, the endorsement of obvious PTSD symptoms but not subtle PTSD symptoms on psychological tests as well as overall fake-bad test profiles.

Treatment

Treatment for individuals with PTSD takes a variety of forms depending on the severity and chronicity of the PTSD symptoms, the severity and type of any comorbid disorders that might be present, the characteristics of the community and prevailing mental health service delivery system, and the characteristics of the individuals themselves, e.g., motivation, secondary gain, age, ethnicity, and gender [42, 43]. PTSD that is of recent onset and is uncomplicated by other mental health disorders or problematic environmental circumstances (e.g., homelessness or dangerous environments) generally can be effectively treated on an outpatient basis with antidepressant medications [42, 43] and exposure-based cognitive-behavior therapy [42, 43]. Exposure-based CBT safely exposes PTSD-afflicted individuals to trauma-related stimuli in imagination and/or *in vivo* while simultaneously facilitating the assimilation of their traumatic events into healthy beliefs or cognitive schema regarding themselves and their world [42, 43]. It is also often beneficial to treat PTSD-afflicted individuals' co-occurring situational problems by way of supportive problem-solving while simultaneously treating their

uncomplicated, recent onset PTSD way of antidepressants and CBT – exposure. This is particularly true in the case of soldiers recently returning from a war zone. Nearly all returning soldiers will be struggling with the task of transitioning from the military back into civilian life, with all of its attendant housing, job, education, family, and social support stressors; and some of the soldiers will be struggling with recent onset PTSD symptoms as well. In most cases, the stress of their readjustment issues will aggravate and prolong the PTSD symptoms of those who have them. By reducing the readjustment-related stress, the PTSD symptoms are likely to be lessened and the spontaneous remission process is likely to be strengthened.

Hospitalization for the treatment of PTSD is seldom necessary. With the possible exception of one study [44], most of the evidence suggests that there is little sustained therapeutic benefit from treating chronic PTSD in specialized inpatient PTSD units [45–49]; and such hospitalizations appear to have iatrogenic effects for a significant minority of those who undergo such treatment [44–49]. Treatment of PTSD complicated by severe comorbid disorders is usually dictated by the nature of the comorbid disorders rather than the PTSD *per se* [42, 43]. For example, those with PTSD accompanied by severe depression and significant suicidal risk usually require hospitalization to treat the depression and suicidal threat before beginning treatment for the PTSD. In other cases of chronic, severe, and highly complicated cases of PTSD, it is sometimes best to approach treatment as one would approach an incurable and chronic medical illness. That is, the treatment should focus on palliative care and try to help the individual manage his or her psychiatric symptoms rather than directly focus on the traumatic events and PTSD symptoms in an effort to eliminate them, as would be the case with exposure-based CBT [42, 43].

Summary

In summary, approximately 75% of all adults will be exposed to one or more traumatic events during the course of their lives. About 10% of those exposed to trauma will develop PTSD subsequent to the trauma, and about 50% of those who do develop PTSD will spontaneously remit within two years posttrauma. Those who do not remit are at increased risk to develop additional disorders such as mood disorders and substance abuse disorders. Some individuals are at greater risk to develop PTSD than the others, particularly those with pre-existing psychopathology. Multiple trauma that is gruesome, prolonged, and man-made is more pathogenic than is less repetitive and less gruesome forms of trauma. The psychosocial dysfunction stemming from PTSD varies greatly from person to person depending on the severity of the trauma, the severity of the PTSD symptoms, and the type and severity of the comorbid disorders that are often present. Recent onset PTSD can be effectively treated by way of CBT exposure-based psychotherapy and antidepressant medications on an outpatient basis. The treatment of chronic PTSD in specialized PTSD inpatient units appears to be largely ineffective and possibly harmful for a significant minority of those who undergo it. PTSD appears to be frequently misdiagnosed in the form of false positives today. Malingering should always be suspected in forensic settings. Malingering should also be suspected in clinical settings when a significant number of malingering red flags are present. Collaborating clients' self-reports of trauma, PTSD symptoms, and psychosocial dysfunction are usually required to rule out malingering.

References

[1]   Miller, K., Kulkarni, M. & Kushner, H. (2006). Beyond trauma-focused psychiatric epidemiology: bridging research and practice with war-affected populations, *The American Journal of Orthopsychiatry* **76**, 409–422.

[2]   Kagee, A. & Naidoo, A. (2004). Reconceptualizing the sequela of political torture: limitations of a psychiatric paradigm, *Transcultural Psychiatry* **41**, 46–61.

[3]   Jenkins, J. (1996). Culture, emotion and PTSD, in *Scurfield Ethnocultural Aspects of Post-traumatic Stress Disorder*, A. Marsella, M. Friedman, E. Gerrity & R. Scurfield, eds, American Psychological Association, Washington, DC, pp. 165–182.

[4]   Kardiner, A. (1941). *The Traumatic Neuroses of War*, P.B. Hoeber, New York.

[5]   Kulka, R., Schlenger, W., Fairbanks, J., Hough, R., Jordan, B., Marmar, C. & Weiss, D. (1990). *Trauma and the Vietnam War Generation*, Brunner/Mazel, New York.

[6]   American Psychiatric Association (1980). *Diagnostic and Statistical Manual of Mental Disorders*, 3rd Edition, APA Press, Washington, DC.

[7]   American Psychiatric Association (1968). *Diagnostic and Statistical Manual of Mental Disorders*, 2nd Edition, APA Press, Washington, DC.

[8]   Resnick, P. (1997). Malingering of posttraumatic disorders, in *Clinical Assessment of Malingering and Deception*, R. Rogers, ed, Guilford, New York, pp. 130–152.

[9]   Mendelson, G. (1984). Follow-up studies of personal injury litigants, *International Journal of Law and Psychiatry* **7**, 179–187.

[10]   American Psychiatric Association (1994). *Diagnostic and Statistical Manual of Mental Disorders*, 4th Edition, APA Press, Washington, DC.

[11]   Breslau, N., Kessler, R., Chilcoat, H., Schultz, L., Davis, G. & Andreski, P. (1998). Trauma and posttraumatic stress disorder in the community: the 1966 detroit area survey of trauma, *Archives of General Psychiatry* **55**, 626–632.

[12]   Breslau, N. (2002). Epidemiologic studies of trauma, posttraumatic stress disorder, and other psychiatric disorders, *Canadian Journal of Psychiatry* **47**, 923–929.

[13]   Breslau, N. & Kessler, R. (2001). The stressor criterion in DSM-IV posttraumatic stress disorder: an empirical investigation, *Biological Psychiatry* **50**, 699–704.

[14]   Kessler, R., Sonnega, A., Bromet, E., Hughes, M. & Nelson, C. (1995). Posttraumatic stress disorder in the National Comorbidity Survey, *Archives of General Psychiatry* **52**, 1048–1060.

[15]   Brewin, C., Andrews, B. & Valetine, J. (2000). Meta-analysis of risk factors for posttraumatic stress disorder in trauma-exposed adults, *Journal of Consulting and Clinical Psychology* **68**(5), 748–766.

[16]   McFarlane, A. (1989). The aetiology of post-traumatic morbidity: predisposing, precipitating, and perpetuating factors, *The British Journal of Psychiatry* **154**, 221–228.

[17]   Breslau, N., Davis, G., Andreski, P., Peterson, E. & Schultz, L. (1997). Sex differences in posttraumatic stress disorder, *Archives of General Psychiatry* **54**, 1044–1048.

[18]   McNally, R. & Shin, L. (1995). Association of intelligence with severity of PTSD symptoms in Vietnam combat veterans, *The American Journal of Psychiatry* **156**(6), 936–938.

[19]   Kobasa, S. (1979). Stressful life events, personality and health, *Journal of Personality and Social Psychology* **37**, 1–11.

[20]   Linley, P. (2003). Positive adaptation to trauma: wisdom as both process and outcome, *Journal of Traumatic Stress* **16**, 601–610.

[21]   Bonanno, G. (2004). Loss, trauma, and human resilience, *The American Psychologist* **59**, 20–28.

[22]   Waysman, M., Schwarzwald, J. & Solomon, Z. (2001). Hardiness: an examination of its relationship with positive and negative long term changes following trauma, *Journal of Traumatic Stress* **14**(3), 531–547.

[23]   Linley, P. & Joseph, S. (2004). Positive change following trauma and adversity: a review, *Journal of Traumatic Stress* **17**, 11–21.

[24] Wilson, J. (2006). *The Posttraumatic Self*, Routledge, New York.

[25] Roth, S., Newman, E., Pelcovitz, D., van der Kolk, B. & Mandel, F. (1997). Complex PTSD in victims exposed to sexual and physical abuse, *Journal of Traumatic Stress* **10**(4), 539–555.

[26] Yehuda, R., Southwick, S. & Giller, E. (1992). Exposure to atrocities and severity of chronic posttraumatic stress disorder in Vietnam combat veterans, *American Journal of Psychiatry* **149**(3), 333–336.

[27] Wilson, J. & Keane, T. (2004). *Assessing Psychological Trauma and PTSD*. Guilford, New York.

[28] Green, B. (1994). Psychosocial research in traumatic stress: an update, *Journal of Traumatic Stress* **7**(3), 341–362.

[29] Perkonigg, A., Pfister, H., Stein, M., Hofler, M., Lieb, R., Maercker, A. & Wittchen, H. (2005). Longitudinal course of posttraumatic stress disorder and posttraumatic stress disorder symptoms in a community sample of adolescents and young adults, *American Journal of Psychiatry* **162**, 1320–1327.

[30] Karamustafalioglu, O., Zohar, J., Guveli, M., Gal, G., Bakim, B., Fostick, L., Karamustafalioglu, N. & Sasson, Y. (2006). Natural course of posttraumatic stress disorder: a 20-month prospective study of Turkish earthquake survivors, *The Journal of Clinical Psychiatry* **67**, 882–889.

[31] Shlosberg, A. & Strous, R. (2005). Long-term follow-up of PTSD in Israeli Yom Kippur war veterans, *The Journal of Nervous and Mental Disease* **193**, 693–696.

[32] Wilson, J. & Moran, T. (2004). Forensic/clinical assessment of psychological trauma and PTSD in legal settings, in *Assessing Psychological Trauma and PTSD*, J. Wilson & T. Keane, eds, Guilford, New York, pp. 603–636.

[33] Keiser, H. (1968). *The Traumatic Neurosis*, JB Lippincott Co., Philadelphia.

[34] Miller, H. & Cartlidge, N. (1972). Simulation and malingering after injuries to the brain and spinal cord, *Lancet* **1**, 580–585.

[35] Blake, D., Weathers, F., Nagy, L., Kaloupek, D., Klauminizer, G., Charney, D. & Keane, T. (1990). *Clinician – Administered PTSD Scale*, National Center for PTSD, West Haven.

[36] Rogers, R., Bagby, R. & Dickens, S. (1992). *Structured Interview of Reported Symptoms*, Psychological Assessment Resources, Odessa.

[37] Butcher, J., Dahlstrom, W., Graham, J., Tellegen, A. & Kaemmer, B. (1989). *Minnesota Multiphasic Personality Inventory-2 (MMPI-2): Manual for Administration and Scoring*. University of Minnesota Press, Minneapolis.

[38] Lynn, E. & Belza, M. (1984). Factitious posttraumatic stress disorder, *Hospital and Community Psychiatry* **35**, 697–701.

[39] Frueh, B., Hamner, M., Cahill, S., Gold, P. & Hamlin, K. (2000). Apparent symptom overreporting in combat veterans evaluated for PTSD, *Clinical Psychology Review* **20**(7), 853–885.

[40] Frueh, B., Smith, D. & Barker, S. (1996). Compensation seeking status and psychometric assessment of combat veterans seeking treatment for PTSD, *Journal of Traumatic Stress* **9**(3), 427–439.

[41] Freuh, B., Gold, P. & de Arellano, M. (1997). Symptom overreporting in combat veterans evaluated for PTSD: differentiation on the basis of compensation seeking status, *Journal of Personality Assessment* **68**, 369–384.

[42] Wilson, J., Friedman, M. & Lindy, J. (2001). *Treating Psychological Trauma and PTSD*, Guilford, New York.

[43] American Psychiatric Association (2004). *Practice Guideline for the Treatment of Patients with Acute Stress Disorder and Posttraumatic Stress Disorder*, APA Press, Washington, DC.

[44] Creamer, M., Morris, P., Biddle, D. & Elliott, P. (1999). Treatment outcome in Australian veterans with combat-related PTSD, *Journal of Traumatic Stress* **12**(4), 545–558.

[45] Fontana, A. & Rosenheck, R. (1997). Effectiveness and cost of the inpatient treatment of PTSD, *American Journal of Psychiatry* **154**, 758–765.

[46] Creamer, M., Forbes, M., Biddle, D. & Elliott, P. (2002). Inpatient versus day hospital treatment for chronic, combat-related PTSD, *The Journal of Nervous and Mental Disease* **190**(3), 183–189.

[47] Fontana, A., Rosenheck, R. & Spencer, H. (1993). *The Long Journey Home: The Third Progress Report on Specialized PTSD Programs*, Northwest Program Evaluation Center, Department of Veteran Affairs Medical Center, West Haven.

[48] Johnson, D., Rosenheck, R., Fontana, A., Lubin, H., Charney, D. & Southwick, S. (1996). Outcome of intensive inpatient treatment for combat-related PTSD, *The American Journal of Psychiatry* **153**, 771–777.

[49] Hammarberg, M. & Silver, S. (1994). Outcome of treatment for posttraumatic stress disorder in a primary care unit serving Vietnam veterans, *Journal of Traumatic Stress* **7**(2), 195–216.

Related Articles

Behavioral Science Evidence

Deception: Detection of

Disaster Mental Health

Malingering: Forensic Evaluations

Rape Trauma Syndrome

Recollective Accuracy of Traumatic Memories

Syndromes: Psychological

LARRY D. SMYTH

PowerPlex

Introduction

The ability of polymerase chain reaction (PCR)-based short tandem repeat (STR) multiplexes to successfully analyze human DNA from a diverse range of circumstances is at the cornerstone of forensic DNA science. A contemporary version of these sophisticated systems has been the GenePrint PowerPlex range of multiplex STR systems (Promega Corporation, Madison, WI; Table 1).

These systems originally emerged in 1997 with PowerPlex 1.1 and progressed iteratively towards the current 16-locus PowerPlex®16 autosomal STR multiplex PCR system. The PowerPlex®16 offers extremely high discriminating power due to the combination of 15 STR loci plus the sex marker amelogenin [1, 2]. There is also the PowerPlex Y male-specific STR multiplex [3], which has specific advantages for the analysis of sex-assault cases and population genetic testing. The PowerPlex range of tests has shown its applicability to all forms of human identification casework, including kinship and disaster victim identification cases.

References

[1]   Spreecher, C.J., Krenke, B., Rabbach, D., Hennes, L., Amiott, E., Nassif, N. & Mandrekar, P. (2000). The PowerPlex 16® system: development and validation, in *Proceedings of 11th International Symposium on Human Identification*, Promega Corporation, Madison, WI.
[2]   Krenke, B., Tereba, A., Anderson, S.J., Buel, E., Culhane, S., Finis, C.J., Tomsey, C.S., Zachetti, J.M., Masibay, A., Rabbach, D.R., Amiott, E.A. & Sprecher, C.J. (2002). Validation of a 16-locus fluorescent multiplex system, *Journal of Forensic Sciences* **47**, 773–785.
[3]   Krenke, B.E., Viculis, L., Richard, M.L., Prinz, M., Milne, S.C., Ladd, C., Gross, A.M., Gornall, T., Frappier, J.R., Eisenberg, A.J., Barna, C., Aranda, X.G., Adamowicz, M.S. & Budowle, B. (2005). Validation of male-specific, 12-locus fluorescent short tandem repeat (STR) multiplex, *Forensic Science International* **151**, 111–124.

Related Articles

Microsatellites

Simon J. Walsh

Predecisional Bias: Jury *see* Jury Dynamics

Premenstrual Syndrome

The Medical Perspective

The idea that hormones control a woman's emotional state has been entrenched in populist thinking. For centuries, physicians tried in vein to link the cyclical hormonal pattern of estrogen and progesterone to

Table 1   GenePrint PowerPlex® STR multiplex systems produced for use in forensic DNA profiling

Name	No. of loci	Target loci included
PowerPlex (1.1 and 1.2)	8	TH01, TPOX, CSF1PO, vWA, D16S539, D13S317, D7S820, D5S818
PowerPlex 2.1	9	Penta E, D18S51, D21S11, TH01, D3S1358, FGA, TPOX, D8S1179, vWA.
PowerPlex ES	9	D3S1358, TH01, D21S11, D18S51, vWA, D8S1179, FGA, SE33 (also known as *ACTBP2*), Amelogenin
PowerPlex 16	16	D3S1358, vWA, FGA, TH01, TPOX, CSF1PO, D5S818, D13S317, D7S820, D8S1179, D21S11, D18S51, D16S539, Penta D, Penta E, Amelogenin
PowerPlex Y	12	DYS19, DYS385a, DYS385b, DYS389I, DYS389II, DYS390, DYS391, DYS392, DYS393, DYS437, DYS438, DYS439

premenstrual syndrome (PMS). After all, it seemed so logical. Despite these efforts, medical science was never able to make the connection work. Attempts to treat PMS with hormonal treatments continuously failed. Hysterectomy and oopherectomy rarely afforded significant relief.

The breakthrough came with the discovery of serotonin, a ubiquitous neurotransmitter, now well established to underlie moodiness, anxiety, irritability, and hostility – symptoms commonly seen in PMS. Consequently, on 6 July 2000, fluoxetine became the first food and drug administration (FDA) recognized and approved treatment for the severe form of PMS, known as *premenstrual dysphoric disorder* (PMDD).[a]

So, the answer was not hormones – it was serotonin. Despite an understanding of the chemical etiology, PMS itself is a remarkably common experience and cannot itself be considered abnormal or pathological. Most women who experience PMS have mild or moderate symptoms and are not socially or occupationally impaired by them. However, a small subset of women experience significant impairment and disability in the premenstrual phase. Psychiatry has chosen to define the women suffering from this severe form of PMS as having PMDD. While deemed as an area of interest and research, PMDD is not considered to be a mental illness. It can be classified alternatively as a depressive disorder, not otherwise specified (coded 311); this category includes disorders with depressive features that do not meet the criteria for major depressive disorder. The sensitivity of the political correctness of this issue is obvious. The american psychiatric association (APA) has established diagnostic criteria, which are provided in the box below.

Legal Usage

In the 1980s, two British cases raised PMS as the basis for a diminished capacity defense reducing the quantum of guilt assessed against the accused.[b] First, in November, 1981, Sandie Smith was put on three years' probation after conviction of threatening to kill a police officer and for carrying a knife. She suffered from PMS and had committed almost 30 crimes, including arson, assault, and manslaughter, during the premenstrual period. Smith responded to progesterone therapy, advocated by English gynecologist Dr

Katharine Dalton, to curb PMS. Dalton was a pioneer researcher who used her patients as a source of information for formulating what she and Dr Peter Green, a fellow researcher, named "premenstrual syndrome" in 1953.

Then, that same month Christine English pleaded guilty to manslaughter by reason of diminished responsibility. She drove her car into her lover after an argument that occurred while she was suffering from severe PMS [1]. She was conditionally discharged for 12 months.

One court martial case and an unreported US decision admitted PMS evidence as grounds for a defense. In *United States v. Morton*, the accused was charged with assault with a dangerous weapon, communicating a threat, and unlawfully carrying a concealed weapon. She pled not guilty by reason of insanity due to PMS. Morton had to establish by clear and convincing evidence that her PMS was so severe that she was unable to know and appreciate the consequences of her conduct [2]. The court held that she failed to establish insanity. It is unlikely that any US jurisdiction would allow PMS as an insanity defense.

In *People v. Santos* [3], the defendant testified in a preliminary hearing that she beat her child while in a "blackout" induced by PMS [4]. She was able to get a favorable plea bargain based on diminished capacity. Diminished capacity is an excuse defense that shifts the burden to the prosecution to disprove the excuse beyond a reasonable doubt once evidence of the excuse is admitted.[c] American states that recognize a diminished capacity defense might permit evidence of PMS to be admitted to show diminished capacity [5]. However, several states have abolished the diminished capacity defense.[d] Some states permit a diminished capacity defense murder prosecutions [6], following *United States v. Brawner* [7]. Other states permit a diminished capacity defense when the accused is charged with any crime of specific intent [8]. Federal practice under the 1983 Insanity Defense Reform Act [9] permits expert evidence on diminished capacity. Alaska allows expert testimony on diminished capacity that would permit PMS evidence during the guilt phase of trial.[e]

Diminished capacity must be established by expert opinion evidence that shows that the defendant both suffers from PMS and committed the crime charged while under the influence of PMS. Half the states[f] and the Federal courts follow *Daubert v. Merrell Dow Pharmaceuticals Inc.* [10] and exclude expert opinion evidence if the expert's underlying scientific principles fail to meet a four-part test [11]:

1. Has the theory been tested by other researchers?
2. Has the theory been published?
3. What is the error rate?
4. Is the process generally accepted?

An expert in a *Daubert* jurisdiction must testify that PMS is a mental illness as diagnosed using diagnostic and statistical manuel of mental disorders, fourth edition, Text Revised (DSM-IV and DSM-IV(TR)) and explain the DSM-IV(TR) criteria for PMS (see Box). The expert must state that the diagnosis and criteria for PMS have been published and subject to peer review. She/he must assert the error rate for making the diagnosis of PMS. Finally, the expert should state that the criteria for diagnosing PMS and diminished responsibility are generally accepted (*see* **Expert Opinion: United Kingdom, Canada, and Australia**).

Some states follow the *Frye* rule (*see* **Frye v. United States**) that requires the underlying scientific principles be "generally accepted" before an expert gives an opinion based on those principles [12]. Others have adopted a modified *Frye* rule with modifications using some or all of the *Daubert* factors [13]. In the *Frye* states and mixed states, the expert must testify that psychotherapists generally accept that PMS causes the sufferer to be unaware of the consequences of her action or to distinguish right from wrong.

Expert opinion evidence on PMS should be freely allowed during the sentencing phase of any trial. According to ¶ Section 5K2 of the Federal Sentencing Guidelines, the court may make a downward departure from the statutory maximum sentence for a convicted defendant on the ground of diminished capacity.[g]

Concerns about the use of PMS in the Courtroom

The forensic use of PMS has generated global controversy. Some of the principle arguments are as follows.

- **PMS is yet another sexist "woman as mad" explanation for female criminality**

Historically, deviant women have often been characterized as either "bad" or "mad" since their antisocial behavior conflicted with certain socially defined and desirable female personality traits and roles. Medical theory, from at least the mid 1800s, espoused that women's reproductive organs controlled their minds, bodies, and personalities. Such biological determinism was strongly endorsed and promulgated by psychiatry: in Freud's model of psychoanalysis, sexual temperament was conceived as a function of biology [14].

Accordingly, the nineteenth century doctors and lawyers agreed that menstruation and uterine malfunction could lead a woman to insanity or criminality. As an example, in the 1867 case *United States v. Harris*, attorneys called a psychiatrist and six other physicians who testified that the defendant was "morally insane" at the time of the homicide due to painful dysmenorrhea that led to mental derangement and hysteria. After a brief deliberation, the jury returned a verdict of not guilty by reason of insanity.[h] English courts also recognized some form of mental derangement related to the menstrual cycle as an excuse for criminality before *Harris* [15, 16]. One woman was acquitted of shoplifting in 1845 while two others were acquitted of murder in 1851. All three were found to have acted with temporary insanity due to "suppression of menstruation" [17]. One of these women had murdered her lover who had rejected her. A doctor testified that her wild eyes indicated problems with her uterus [18].

The specifics of the sociomedical theoretical explanations for female deviance shifted with time as the understanding of the female reproductive system evolved from the uterus to ovaries and then to hormones in the 1920s. With the UK cases of Smith and English discussed above, the focus in the early 1980s became PMS and its relationship to female criminality. In part, this undoubtedly reflected the growing interest in studying the female offender and etiology since statistics during the 1970s were reflecting an increasing number of crimes committed by women or, at the least, a higher number of arrests or prosecutions [19].

To some of its detractors, PMS is therefore the latest in a long line of anatomical deterministic theories of female criminality that have prevailed as a substitute for looking at how entrenched gender inequality might contribute to crime. Instead, women's deviance has been linked with the anatomical parts that differentiate them from males and which allow them to fulfill their primary gender role of reproduction.

- **Its usage in court could stigmatize women as a whole and/or affect their equal participation in the public sphere**

There is concern that if PMS is raised as exculpatory grounds, people might generalize from the few and negatively stereotype all women or at the least those who experience any premenstrual symptoms [20]. Sensationalist captions such as "raging hormones", "premenstrual frenzy", and "Dr Jekyll and Ms Hyde" that appeared in British newspapers during the *English* and *Smith* cases can fuel imagery of women as periodically unstable and therefore unsuitable for some employment positions and/or responsibilities.

As with all medical disorders, a whole class of people with similar maladies could be stigmatized. As discussed earlier, the syndrome is fairly common, although only a minute percent manifest the symptoms that can substantially impact on their actions.

- **Its use relies upon acceptance of the legitimacy of PMS and PMDD and advocates/specialists**

All medical practitioners do not share in Dalton's belief in temporary psychosis as a symptom of the most severe PMS cases [21, 22]. The medical literature is confusing in its diversity of opinion concerning the possible connection of PMS to criminal behavior with no universally accepted medical consensus about the correlation of the severe variant with antisocial behavior.

In some countries like Australia where PMS is not raised except very infrequently in sentencing mitigation,[i] it continues to be referred to as *premenstrual tension* (PMT) and lacks acknowledgment as a legitimate medical condition. This is illustrated in a popular news feature story on PMS:

> Despite the popular belief that "it is all in the hormones", there is no convincing evidence that women with severe PMS have different hormonal fluctuations than other women … cause of PMS are still unknown … [23].

A number of female medical practitioners are quoted in the article articulating the view that women who think they have PMS may actually have clinical depression.

Yet to use it successfully a forensic expert is required. With insanity the defense must show that PMS is a disease of the mind and that the sufferer did not know the nature or quality of the act or that it was wrong (McNaughton Rule). Doing so with PMS can be highly problematic.

To raise automatism (a state in which the mind or the will does not accompany physical acts) by arguing that certain women with PMS who go hours without eating produce an excess amount of adrenalin that causes a hypoglycemic state of impaired consciousness requires an expert like Dalton to testify that hypoglycemia can be a symptom of PMS and that the defendant possessed that abnormality.

The defense with diminished responsibility or capacity must show that PMS prevented the accused from having the specific intent (*mens rea*) with hazy thinking, and impairment of self-control, judgment and willpower. Again, proof is problematic. Plus, there are several legal issues since the defense has to show that PMS is an abnormality of the mind (which is difficult since the symptoms of PMS are not even universally accepted), that it arose from an inherent cause, and that it substantially impaired the defendant's mental responsibility [24]. With potentially lengthy sentences, the convicted has the added stigma of mental illness [25].

- **It could be misused and or abused by defendants**

There is concern that PMS might be used as grounds for a defense by *non-bona fide* sufferers – either charlatans and/or women who experience some of the more mild PMS symptoms.

However, the diagnosis of PMDD can be substantiated by a heavy burden of proof, with medical evidence showing a clinically demonstrable physical disorder. A causal connection must be shown between the premenstrual symptom(s) and the criminal act. Additional evidence could include personal diaries, medical records, prior arrest record that could illustrate deviant activity correlation with the individual's premenstrual time of her cycle, and evidence by family and friends of marked premenstrual behavioral changes.

PMDD

APA Diagnostic Criteria [26]

In most menstrual cycles during the past year, symptoms (e.g., markedly depressed mood, marked anxiety, marked affective lability, decreased interest in activities) regularly occurred during the last week of the luteal phase (and remitted within a few days of the onset of menses). These symptoms must be severe enough to markedly interfere with work, school, or usual activities and be entirely absent for at least 1 week post menses.

The essential features are symptoms such as markedly depressed mood, marked anxiety, marked affective lability, and decreased interest in activities. These symptoms have regularly occurred during the last week of the luteal phase in most menstrual cycles during the past year. The symptoms begin to remit within a few days of the onset of menses (the follicular phase) and are always absent in the week following menses.

Five (or more) of the following symptoms must have been present most of the time during the last week of the luteal phase, with at least one of the symptoms being one of the first four:

1) feeling sad, hopeless, or self-deprecating;
2) feeling tense, anxious *or* "on edge";
3) marked lability of mood interspersed with frequent tearfulness;
4) persistent irritability, anger, and increased interpersonal conflicts;
5) decreased interest in usual activities, which may be associated with withdrawal from social relationships;
6) difficulty concentrating;
7) feeling fatigued, lethargic, or lacking in energy;
8) marked changes in appetite, which may be associated with binge eating or craving certain foods;
9) hypersomnia or insomnia;
10) a subjective feeling of being overwhelmed or out of control; and
11) physical symptoms such as breast tenderness or swelling, headaches, or sensations of "bloating" or weight gain, with tightness of fit of clothing, shoes, or rings. There may also be joint or muscle pain. The symptoms may be accompanied by suicidal thoughts.

This pattern of symptoms must have occurred most months for the previous 12 months. The symptoms disappear completely shortly after the onset of menstruation. The most typical pattern seems to be that of dysfunction during the week prior to menses that ends mid-menses. Atypically, some females also have symptoms for a few days around ovulation; a few females with short cycles might, therefore, be symptom free for only 1 *week per cycle*.

Typically, the symptoms are of comparable severity (but not duration) to those of a Major Depressive Episode and must cause an obvious and marked impairment in the ability to function socially or occupationally in the week prior to menses. Impairment in social functioning may be manifested by marital discord and problems with friends and family. It is very important not to confuse long-standing marital or job problems with the dysfunction that occurs only premenstrually. There is a great contrast between the woman's depressed feelings and difficulty in functioning during these days and her mood and capabilities the rest of the month. These symptoms may be superimposed on another disorder but are not merely an exacerbation of the symptoms of another disorder, such as Major Depressive, Panic, or Dysthymic Disorder, or a Personality Disorder. The presence of the cyclical pattern of symptoms must be confirmed by at least 2 consecutive months of prospective daily symptom ratings. Daily symptom ratings must be done by the woman and can also be done by someone with whom she lives. It is important that these diaries be kept on a daily basis rather than composed retrospectively from memory.

Delusions and hallucinations have been described in the late luteal phase of the menstrual cycle but are very rare. Although females with the combination of dysmenorrhea (painful menses) and premenstrual dysphoric disorder are somewhat more likely to seek treatment than females with only one of these conditions, most females with either of the conditions do not have the other condition. A wide range of general medical conditions may worsen in the premenstrual or luteal phase (e.g., migraine, asthma, allergies, and seizure disorders). There are no specific laboratory tests that are diagnostic of the disturbance. However, in several small preliminary studies, certain laboratory findings (e.g., serotonin or melatonin secretion patterns, sleep EEG findings) have been noted to be abnormal in groups of females with this proposed disorder relative t o control subjects.

It is estimated that at least 75% of women report minor or isolated premenstrual changes. Limited studies suggest an occurrence of "premenstrual syndrome" (variably defined) of 20%–50%, and that 3%–5% of women experience symptoms that may meet the criteria for this proposed disorder. There has been very little systematic study on the course and stability of this condition. Premenstrual symptoms can begin at any age after menarche, with the onset most commonly occurring during the teens to late 20s. Those who seek treatment are usually in their 30s. Symptoms usually remit with menopause. Although symptoms do not necessarily occur every cycle, they are present for the majority of the cycles. Some months the symptoms may be worse than others. Women commonly report that their symptoms worsen with age until relieved by the onset of menopause.

Research criteria for premenstrual dysphoric disorder

A.   In most menstrual cycles during the past year, five (or more) of the following symptoms were present for most of the time during the last week of the luteal phase, began to remit within a few days after the onset of the follicular phase, and were absent in the week postmenses, with at least one of the symptoms being either (1), (2), (3), or (4):
    (1)   markedly depressed mood, feelings of hopelessness, or self-deprecating thoughts
    (2)   marked anxiety, tension, feelings of being "keyed up", or "on edge"
    (3)   marked affective lability (e.g., feeling suddenly sad or tearful or increasedsensitivity to rejection)
    (4)   persistent and marked anger or irritability or increased interpersonal conflicts
    (5)   decreased interest in usual activities (e.g., work, school, friends, hobbies)
    (6)   subjective sense of difficulty in concentrating
    (7)   lethargy, easy fatigability, or marked lack of energy
    (8)   marked change in appetite, overeating, or specific food cravings
    (9)   hypersomnia or insomnia
   (10)   a subjective sense of being overwhelmed or out of control
   (11)   other physical symptoms, such as breast tenderness or swelling, headaches, joint or muscle pain, a sensation of "bloating", weight gain.

    Note: In menstruating females, the luteal phase corresponds to the period between ovulation and the onset of menses, and the follicular phase begins with menses. In nonmenstruating females (e.g., those who have had a hysterectomy), the timing of luteal and follicular phases may require measurement of circulating reproductive hormones.

B.   The disturbance markedly interferes with work or school or with usual social activities and relationships with others (e.g., avoidance of social activities, decreased productivity and efficiency at work or school).

C.   The disturbance is not merely an exacerbation of the symptoms of another disorder, such as Major Depressive Disorder, Panic Disorder, Dysthymic Disorder, or a Personality Disorder (although it may be superimposed on any of these disorders).

Criteria A, B, and C must be confirmed by prospective daily ratings during at least two consecutive symptomatic cycles. (The diagnosis may be made provisionally prior to this confirmation.)

End Notes

a. The Massachusetts Institute of Technology holds the patent for this treatment.

b. The English Homicide Act of 1957 provides that "Where a person kills or is a party to the killing of another, he shall not be convicted of murder if he was suffering from such abnormality of mind ... as substantially impaired the mental responsibility for acts and omissions in doing or being a party to the killing." 5 and 6 Eliz. 2, ch. 2, § 2[1], 1957.

c. *LaFave* § 9.8(f)(4).

d. Arizona, California, Florida, Georgia, Maryland, Ohio, Oklahoma, Rhode Island, and South Carolina have abolished diminished capacity. See, e.g., *State v. Doss*, 568 P.2d 1054 (Ariz. 1977) (en banc) Cal. Penal Code § 25. Section 2.02 of the Model Penal Code abolished specific intent and diminished capacity.

e. See Alaska Stat. § 12.47.020.

f. Alaska, Colorado, Connecticut, Delaware, Idaho, Indiana, Iowa, Kentucky, Louisiana, Maine, Michigan, Mississippi, Nebraska, New Hampshire, New Mexico, North Carolina, Ohio, Oklahoma, Oregon, Rhode Island, Tennessee, Texas, West Virginia, and Wyoming. See, e.g., *State v. Coon*, 974 P.2d 386 (Alaska 1999); *People v. Shreck*, 22 P.3d 68 (Colo. 2001); *Springfield v. State*, 860 P.2d 435 (Wyo. 1993).

g. 18 U.S.C. Appendix Ch. Five Determining the Sentence, part K Departures 5K2.13. Diminished Capacity (Policy Statement).

h. See Clephane, J.O. *Trial of Mary Harris Indicted for the Murder of Adoniram Burroughs Before the Supreme Court of the District of Columbia*, 10–12 (opening statement of Joseph Bradley) (W.H. & O.H. Morrison, Washington, DC. 1865); Goldstein, A. (1997). *Nineteenth Century Gender Roles and the Murder Trial of Mary Harris*; Kaye, N.S. (1997). *Feigned Insanity*.

i. A search of Australian law databases such as LexisNexis and AUSTLII and the archives of the two major Australian newspapers *The Sydney Morning Herald* and *The Age* newspapers was conducted. No cases were reported in which PMS or PMT was used in an Australian court during that time period. Legal practitioners report its infrequent mention in sentencing.

References

[1] *British Legal Debate: Premenstrual Tension and Criminal Behavior*, New York Times, 29 Dec 1981, at http://www.nytimes.com/ (accessed 1 Jun 2007).

[2] 2001 CCA Lexis 202, (NMCM 99 00830 17 Jul 2001).

[3] No 1KO46229 (N.Y. Crim. Ct. 3 Nov 1982).

[4] (1983). Recent decisions: criminal law – premenstrual syndrome: a criminal defense, *Notre Dame Law Review* **59** 253.

[5] *United States v Pohlot*, 827 F2d 889 (3rd Cir. 1987); *cert denied*, U.S. 98 L Ed 2d 660, 108 S Ct 710 (1988) *LaFave*, § 9.1(a).

[6] North Carolina, Massachusetts, Oregon, New York, and Pennsylvania. See, e.g., *State v. p.*, 488 S.E.2d 225 (N.C. 1997). *People v. Segal*, 429 N.E.2d 107, 444 N.Y.S.2d 588 (N.Y. 1981).

[7] 471 F.2d 969 (D.C. Cir. 1972).

[8] Hawaii, Kansas, Massachusetts, Minnesota, Mississippi, Missouri, and Tennessee. See, e.g., *State v Baker*, 691 P2d 1166 (Hawaii 1984). *State v. Grose*, 982 S.W.2d 349 (Tenn. Crim. App. 1997) appeal denied (May 11, 1998).

[9] *United States v. Brown*, 326 F.3d 1143 (10th Cir. 2003); 18 U.S.C.S. § 17 (2007).

[10] 509 U.S. 579, 113 S.C.t. 2786, 125 L.Ed.2d 469 (1993).

[11] *Daubert*, 509 U.S. 593–594 (1993).

[12] *Frye v. United States*, 293 F. 1013, 34 A.L.R. 145 (App. D.C. 1923) States following this rule include Arizona, California, the District of Columbia, Florida, Illinois, Kansas, Maryland, Minnesota, Missouri, Nebraska North Dakota, Pennsylvania, and Washington. See, e.g., *People v. Superior Court*, 137 Cal. App. 4th 353, 40 Cal. Rptr. 3d 365 (2d Dist. 2006). *Com. v. Crews*, 536 Pa. 508, 640 A.2d 395 (1994).

[13] *State v. Peters*, 192 Wis. 2d 674, 534 N.W.2d 867 (Ct. App. 1995) These states include Alabama, Georgia, Hawaii, Massachusetts, Nevada, Oregon, South Carolina, Utah, Virginia, and Wisconsin. See, e.g., *Turner v. State*, 746 So. 2d 355 (Ala. 1998).

[14] Chodorow, N. (1989). *Feminism and Psychoanalytic Theory*, Yale University Press, New Haven.

[15] Riley, T.L. (1986). Premenstrual syndrome as a legal defense, *Hamline Law Review* **9**, 193–194.

[16] D'Orban, P.T. (1983). Medicolegal aspects of the premenstrual syndrome, *British Journal of Hospital Medicine*, **30**, 404–406.

[17] Spitz, A. (1987). Premenstrual syndrome: a critical review of the literature, *Indiana Medicine* **80**(4), 378–382.

[18] Meehan, E. & MacRae, K. (1986). Legal implications of premenstrual syndrome: a Canadian perspective, *Canadian Medical Association Journal* **135**, 601–608.

[19] Horney, J. (1978). Menstrual cycles and criminal responsibility, *Law and Human Behaviour* **2**(1), 25–36.

[20] Easteal, P. (1991). Women and crime: premenstrual issues, *Trends and Issues in Crime and Criminal Justice* **31**, 1–8.

[21] Dalton, K. (1980). Cyclical criminal acts in premenstrual syndrome, *Lancet* 1070–1071.

[22] Dalton, K. (1986). Premenstrual syndrome, *Hamline Law Review* **9**(1), 143–154.

[23] Sweet, M. (1996). Periods of joy, *Sydney Morning Herald*, 1 April, p. 11.

[24] Mc Sherry, B. (1993). The return of the raging hormones theory, *Sydney Law Review* **15**, 309–310.

[25] Scutt, J. (1982). Premenstrual tension as an extenuating factor in female crime, *The Australian Law Journal* **56**, 99–100.

[26] American Psychiatric Association, (1994) Diagnostic and Statistical manual of Mental Disorders 4th ed., (Text Revision). Washington, DC.

Related Articles

Temporary Insanity

PATRICIA EASTEAL, NEIL S. KAYE AND TOM REED

Preventative Law *see* Therapeutic Jurisprudence

Primer Discharge Residue: Cartridge Discharge Residue *see* Firearm Discharge Residue: Analysis of

Printing Devices in Document Examination *see* Writing Instruments and Printing Devices

Privilege *see* Duty to Warn

Product Standard of Insanity *see* Insanity: Defense

Professional Judgment: Structured *see* Risk Assessment: Patient and Detainee

Professional Responsibility Codes for Forensic Scientists *see* Ethics: Codes of Conduct for Expert Witnesses

Profiles: Psychological and Behavioral

Profiles are most closely associated with psychological models developed by the Federal Bureau of Investigation (FBI) in their early searches for serial murderers [1] (*See* **Serial Homicide**). The term has since been applied to a great many diverse compilations of information, as well as to what are little more than stereotypes. Over the past decade or so, "profilers" have been a favorite topic of crime dramas and novels and in the process have been glamorized and misrepresented to the point where the facts have often been obscured. Of particular concern for the justice system, however, has been the introduction of "profiles" as a component of psychological syndromes that have suggested new categories of "victims" and alleged profiles of the perpetrators responsible for their victimization (*see* **Syndromes: Psychological**; **Deception: Truth Serum**).

Profiles as an Aid in Law Enforcement

In 1987, Judge Charles Becton published a law review article that drew attention to a seemingly chameleon-like way in which drug courier profiles adapted to any particular set of observations [2]. Within months, the Court of Appeals for the Ninth Circuit incorporate Judge Becton's arguments into *United States v. Sokolow* [3]; a case which it had debated for over 2 years. By the late 1980s, however, criminal profiles had become a staple of law enforcement. Even the US Supreme Court could not stand by and watch them wiped out in a single sweep of a judicial pen.

The High Court went back to basics, and they found their foundation in *Terry v. Ohio* [4]. Officer McFadden, and his detention of two men casing Zucker's clothing store on an Ohio day in 1963, had given rise to the Terry Stop "stop and frisk" exception to the Fourth Amendment and the reasonable suspicion test, which provided justification, short of probable cause, under which police officers could initiate limited investigatory action. The Supreme Court knew that it could not allow any decision that it could make in *Sokolow* to turn profiles into unrestricted hunting licenses for overenthusiastic enforcement officials, nor was it willing to set up an entirely new bureaucracy to review the constitutionality of each and every profile. The Court also recognized that profiles changed over time, and that their effectiveness would evaporate if they became frozen and subject to public scrutiny.

This solution requires that every law enforcement intervention, regardless of whether or not it was set in motion by a profile, must be justifiable through the same articulation of facts – the "totality of the circumstances" – required for a *Terry* stop. Searches made under *Sokolow* are reviewed on a case-by-case basis and have been overturned if they fail to meet appropriate standards [5]. In this single decision, the Court recognized the validity of the probabilistic assumptions underlying the application of behavioral science techniques in justice administration, yet made it impossible to elevate criminal profiles into a license for Fourth Amendment abuse.

Criminal profiles continue to serve as a tool in law enforcement, but more importantly, profiles are a means of leveraging investigative expertise, training investigative and enforcement officials, and applying systematic methodologies to the fast-changing and highly mobile environment that characterizes contemporary criminal operations. Once the intervention has been initiated, however, the profile is of no further probative relevance. Arrest and even the issuance of a search warrant require probable cause, and prosecution of any resulting charges must be based upon substantive evidence of guilt. The original profile is inadmissible in support of guilt, and is presumed to be inherently prejudicial [6].

The temptation to push these limits was brought home to the British public in a highly publicized 1995 case. Three years earlier, 23-year-old Rachel Nickell took her 2-year-old son and dog for a walk. She selected Wimbledon Common as her south London destination because of its reputation for safety, but, less than an hour later, she was found soaked in the blood of some 49 stab wounds, her child clinging to her lifeless body crying "get up mummy". Police responded with the biggest murder investigation in London history – and one of the nation's early attempts at using the new science of psychological profiling.

England's first encounter with the behavioral sciences in criminal investigation came in the 1985 "Railway Rapist" case. Although profiling had become well established in the United States through the work of the FBI Behavioral Science Unit, both serial killers and the methods for catching them were only just then taking hold in Britain. David Canter, professor of investigative psychology at Liverpool University, had a background in the psychology of building design, human behavior during fires, and the psycholinguistics of hoax fire calls; but the rigor of his science prepared him well to become that nation's leading criminal profiler. His methodical work led to the conviction of John Duffy, and inspired the Robbie Coltrane character in the hit television detective series *Cracker* [7].

By the time of the Nickell murder, however, the publicity surrounding criminal profiling had attracted a host of psychologists who had been bitten by the detective bug. It was one of these who claimed the case, produced a profile, and eventually took over much of the day-to-day police operations directed toward conviction of the suspect, Colin Stagg, targeted by the profile. Through an attractive blond undercover policewoman, the psychologist initiated an 8-month liaison with the 31-year-old Stagg in which she shared violent sexual fantasies, confessed to the ritual sexual murder of a baby and a young woman, and egged him on to match her stories; even telling him that she wished he were Nickell's murderer because "That's the kind of man I want."

Stagg never claimed credit for the killing, but from 700 pages of letters and transcribed telephone conversations and public meetings, the psychologist concluded that Stagg's fantasies, modeled upon information fed to him by those familiar with the details of the crime, revealed unique knowledge of the crime scene that could be known only by the murderer. Dragged before a judge in open court at the Old Bailey, defense quickly pointed out that Stagg had not even made good guesses – he did not know the location of the crime and had wrongly asserted that the victim had been raped.

Up until that point, Great Britain had never felt the need for an entrapment statute, but the judge recognized a "honey trap" when he saw one. Clearing the accused and acknowledging the understandable pressure on the police, the judge was, nevertheless, forced to conclude that the operation betrayed "not merely an excess of zeal, but a blatant attempt to incriminate a suspect by positive and deceptive conduct of the grossest kind". Stagg left the chaotic courtroom vowing to sue everyone involved, the police were the butt of press ridicule, and David Canter observed with typical English understatement that pulling in some "media recognized expert" can undermine "more effective, longer term development of a professional discipline" [8].

It is not just the newcomers who can make mistakes. The 1996 Summer Olympics began in the wake of the first case of suspected air terrorism on American soil, and as the investigation of the TWA flight 800 crash off New York moved ahead with commendable precision, a bomb blast rocked the Olympic festivities in Atlanta. Unwilling to stand by in the face of two national assaults, an inexperienced FBI

agent allowed the press to get word that a psychological profile had identified the private security guard who first spotted the bomb as the likely perpetrator. In moments, Richard Jewell went from hero to the object of media scrutiny and scorn.

After a week of publicized investigation, in which the entire world got to see Jewell live on CNN sitting forlorn on his own front steps as the FBI picked through his apartment, the investigation yielded nothing more than a few pathetic souvenirs of a man's only moment of glory. Pressed for an explanation, an FBI spokesperson on the scene curtly informed the press that "We don't make apologies". FBI director Louis Freeh, called before a congressional investigating committee, tried to put a better face on the public relations disaster but confided privately that "We wish we never heard of Richard Jewell". [9, 10].

This is not to say that mention of a profile, or court testimony that overlaps in any way with a profile, is necessarily prohibited. Testimony can mention a profile in the context of background as to how and why a defendant was stopped and searched, if such testimony is confined to the preliminary stop and not the actual investigation, and the fact that the individual satisfied the profile is not used to impugn the defendant [11]. Moreover, the expertise reflected in profiles *can* be the subject of expert testimony to refute assertions by the defendant [12], to supply factual information helpful to the trier of fact in placing the case in context [13], or to establish motive, intent, absence of mistake or accident, or identity of a common scheme or plan [14].

Profiles as Evidence at Trial

By their tentative and proximal nature, profiles pose serious issues of both scientific and probabilistic validity [15]. Their use, and the term itself, are therefore most appropriately restricted to investigative tools. As evidence, profiles easily become little more than a means to either link a defendant to undesirable traits or stereotypes; or for the defense to attribute by association positive or sympathetic attributes to a defendant.

Behavioral science is relevant to justice because it can assist the trier of fact to understand a party in litigation as an individual (*see* **Risk Assessment**), while profiles are a tactic to attribute the qualities of a grouping to an individual. There are circumstances in which this tactic can be attractive to either side of a case, and the law has established guidelines to restrict potential abuse.

Entrapment, the affirmative defense that alleged crimes were in reality induced by government persuasion or trickery, is a good example. An entrapment defense, as with defenses to most serious criminal charges, turns on the defendant's mental state: was the defendant an active participant or simply a passive bystander to conduct actually carried out by a government operative? Although early cases tended to hold that a defendant asserting the affirmative defense of entrapment could not establish their state of mind through expert testimony, the courts now generally consider such testimony an appropriate aid to the triers of fact [16, 17].

Most other attempts to enlist expert testimony regarding a defendant's personality profile to help disprove a criminal charge have been less successful. Introduction of psychiatric testimony regarding the "dependent personality disorder" of a defendant was excluded, for example, as support of her assertion that she was unaware that computer equipment that she sold was, in fact, stolen. Here, the court felt that imprimatur of such an official-sounding label was neither necessary nor helpful to the jury in making its assessment of the defendant's mental state [18].

Similarly, the psychological profile of a murder and robbery defendant was excluded as possible support that his crime could not have been deliberate and premeditated, holding that the profile appeared to be simply a narration of the defendant's social history with little or no rational bearing on issues of premeditation and intent [19]. Such personality testimony has also been excluded as a defense to armed robbery and assault [20], and manslaughter [21], where the defendants sought to establish that they were simply not the "type" to use a weapon.

In many instances, the testimony is simply a way in which to introduce character evidence. Testimony in support of good character is generally permissible [22], but the courts are leery of according it scientific stature [23]. Nevertheless, in two controversial decisions, lay character witness testimony has been upheld in a child molestation case [24], and a psychologist's opinion was upheld as appropriate testimony concerning a defendant charged with lewd

and lascivious acts upon a child, noting that the testimony was based, at least in part, upon standardized testing [25].

Most frequently, however, courts have excluded expert testimony aimed simply at ruling out a defendant as the guilty party. This has been the case in proposed testimony as to "peaceableness" [26], psychiatrist testimony as to lack of characteristics "likely to result in abuse of infant victim" [27], psychiatrist testimony that defendant had made previous false confessions and may therefore be mentally ill and his confession untrustworthy [28], expert testimony as to defendant's remorse or lack of remorse [29], and that the defendant had undergone a religious conversion and therefore could be rehabilitated [30]. Expert testimony is also typically not allowed as to mitigation of an offense [31]. Often, such expert testimony is proffered in place of the defendant taking the stand on his or her own behalf, thus becoming subject to cross-examination. The jury system quite correctly assumes that a defendant is his own most revealing character witness, and that if character is to be made an issue it is best presented by the defendant himself [32].

Expert behavioral testimony on behalf of a defendant can also end up working against that defendant. For example, in *State v. Hunt* [33], the defendant claimed that a borderline personality prevented him from being able to form the necessary intent to be guilty of a shooting charge. The court ruled that this assertion opened the door for broad inquiry into his mental condition, and allowed the prosecution to counter the claim with expert testimony that the defendant was actually suffering from nothing more than "antisocial personality disorder". To explain how this conclusion was reached, the expert was further permitted to recount for the jury defendant's difficulties in interpersonal relationships, including his prior "bad acts".

If profile evidence has had little impact upon the ability of the accused to fashion a defense, it *has* provided a potentially devastating weapon in the hands of the prosecution. The case of Sgt. Russell Banks illustrates just how powerful and insidious prosecution profile testimony can become, even when the "expert" does not testify as to a personal conclusion about the guilt or innocence of the defendant. In this instance, a pinpoint profile that could only describe the defendant – a stepfather living with his wife and her young daughter – combined with the known limitations of a child witness, and an aggressive child "therapist" able to lead that witness and allowed to testify as to her own conclusions, created a direct path to the defendant, which a jury would be hard pressed to ignore.

In its *Banks* holding [34], the Court of Military Appeals noted that its reversal of Sgt. Banks conviction for child rape and sodomy was consistent with the case law in both federal and state courts that has severely criticized attempts to introduce "profile" evidence to establish either guilt or innocence. As the Supreme Court of Kansas noted in the 1989 case of *State v. Clements*, "Evidence which only describes the characteristics of a typical offender has no relevance in determining whether the defendant committed a crime in question, and the only inference which can be drawn from such evidence, namely that the defendant who matches the profile must be guilty, is an impermissible one" [35]. This conclusion has been reached in cases as diverse as child molestation [36], child abuse [37], murder [38], rape [39], and shoplifting [40].

This is not to say that expert profile testimony may never be used by the prosecution. If the defendant places his own personality and character at issue, the prosecution can call experts to help rebut defense assertions [41]. In a Washington state case, a defendant who stuttered pointed to the fact that the person he allegedly assaulted was unable to identify his assailant as a stutterer. The prosecution was permitted to introduce to the jury expert scientific testimony as to the statistical percentage of probability that a stutterer would not exhibit that particular speech anomaly in certain situations [42].

Expert profile testimony as to a lack of profile can also be admissible when a defendant deviates significantly from the expectation that a lay jury may hold about people who commit particular types of crimes [24]. Finally, background testimony that does not specifically address guilt or innocence of a defendant but instead enables the jury to understand evidence that does go to guilt or innocence has been held to be permissible profile evidence.

Conclusions

The often misused term *profile* is best restricted to investigative tools used to narrow down likely suspects and establish reasonable suspicion necessary to justify an action in the field. Reasonable suspicion is reviewed on a case-by-case basis to assure protection of suspect rights. As evidence at trial, profiles easily become little more than a means to either link a defendant to undesirable traits or stereotypes; or for the defense to attribute by association positive or sympathetic attributes to a defendant. Although behavioral science evidence may be proffered for use at trial, including statistical compilations, such evidence should have relevance to the applicable party as an individual, and the term *profile* avoided when possible.

Expert testimony concerning a trait of an accused may only be used as evidence that the accused possesses such a trait. It must be left to the jury to determine whether and how such a trait may influence the facts of the case [43]. While the term *profile* may appear to give behavioral evidence an aura of scientific respectability, such labels themselves do nothing to enhance the stature of the substantive underlying observations. In fact, if anything, good science and credible observation are more readily accepted without them [44].

References

[1]   For a critique of FBI profiles and a plea that behavioral evidence is admissible by the defense, see George, J.A. (2008). Offender profiling and expert testimony: scientifically valid or glorified results? *Vanderbilt Law Review* **61**, 221–260.

[2]   Becton, C.L. (1987). The drug courier profile, *North Carolina Law Review* **65**, 417–480.

[3]   United States v. Sokolow, 490 U.S. 1 (1989).

[4]   Terry v. Ohio, 392 U.S. 1 (1968).

[5]   An interesting look at the kind of reasoning used by the appellate courts in overturning a *Sokolow* search is provided in People v. Pullman, (Not Reported in Cal.Rptr.2d, 2002) WL 31230831 Cal.App. 1 Dist., (2002).

[6]   People v. Hubbard, 530 N.W.2d 130 (Mich. Ct. App. 1995); United States v. Williams, 957 F.2d 1238 (5th Cir., 1992); United States v. Wilson, 930 F.2d 616 (Minn. 1991); United States v. Beltran-Rios, 878 F.2d 1208 (Cal. 1989); United States v. Hernandez-Cuartas, 717 F.2d 552 (Fla. 1983).

[7]   Crace, J. (Feb 17, 1995) Inside the criminal mind, *New Statesman & Society*, 29; (1995 WL 14340484).

[8]   *Guardian* (London) (1995). Sept 15 (1995 WL 9944184, 9944234, 9944240, 9944195 and 9944268).

[9]   Yoder Jr., E.M. (Aug 2, 1996) Olympic park bombing, *San Diego Union Tribune*, B8.

[10] Sack, K. (Oct 29, 1996) Jewell lambastes FBI, media for 88-day ordeal as suspect, *Austin American-Statesman* A1.

[11] United States v. Hernandez-Cuartas, 717 F.2d 552 (Fla. 1983).

[12] People v. Lopez, 26 Cal. Rptr. 2d 741 (Ct. App. 1994); United States v. Robinson, 978 F.2d 1554 (N.M. 1992); United States v. Wilson, 930 F.2d 616 (Minn. 1991); United States v. Beltran-Rios, 878 F.2d 1206 (Cal. 1989).

[13] United States v. Khan, 787 F.2d 28 (N.Y. 1986).

[14] Wilson v. State, 871 P.2d 46 (Okl. 1994).

[15] An analysis of issues of probability as they relate to criminal profiles appears in Risinger, M. (2002). Three card monte, Monty hall, modus operandi and 'offender profiling': some lessons of modern cognitive science for the laws of evidence, *Cardozo Law Review* **238**, 193–284.

[16] State v. Woods, 484 N.E.2d 773 (Ohio Com. Pl. 1984);United States v. Hill, 655 F.2d 512 (Pa. 1981).

[17] Moore, C.D. (1995). The elusive foundation of the entrapment defense, *Northwestern University Law Review* **89**, 1151–1188.

[18] United States v. DiDomenico, 985 F.2d 1159 (Conn. 1993).

[19] Hartless v. State, 611 A.2d 581 (Md. 1992).

[20] People v. Watkins, 440 N.W.2d 36 (Mich. App. 1989).

[21] State v. Hensley, 655 S.W.2d 810 (Mo. App. 1983).

[22] Green, E.D. & Nesson, C.R. (eds) (1966). *Federal Rules of Evidence*, Little, Brown, Boston, pp. 51–58.

[23] Mendez, M.A. (1996). The law of evidence and the search for a stable personality, *Emory Law Journal* **45**, 221–238.

[24] People v. McAlpin, 812 P.2d 563 (Cal. 1991).

[25] People v. Stoll, 783 P.2d 698 (Cal. 1989).

[26] State v. Arnold, 421 A.2d 932 (Me. 1980).

[27] State v. Screpesi, 611 A.2d 34 (Del. Super 1991).

[28] Stano v. Dugger, 883 F.2d 900 (Fla. 1989).

[29] Clenney v. State, 344 S.E.2d 216 (Ga. 1986).

[30] People v. Moya, 350 P.2d 112 (Cal. 1960).

[31] People v. Masor, 578 N.E.2d 1176 (Ill. Ct. App. 1991).

[32] Mueller, C.B. & Kirkpatrick, L.C. (1996). *Evidence Under the Rules*, 3rd Edition, Little, Brown, Boston, pp. 677–679.

[33] State v. Hunt, 555 A.2d 369 (Vt. 1988).

[34] United States v. Banks, 36 M.J. 150 (CMA, 1992).

[35] State v. Clements, 770 P.2d 447, 448 (Kan. 1989).

[36] United States v. Gillespie, 852 F.2d 475 (Cal. 1988).

[37] Sloan v. State, 522 A.2d 1364 (Md. Ct. App. 1987).

[38] Sanders v. State, 303 S.E.2d 13 (Ga. 1983).

[39] State v. Percy, 507 A.2d 955 (Vt. 1986).

[40] State v. McCoy, 294 N.E.2d 242 (Ohio Ct. App. 1973).

[41] United States v. Gillespie, 852 F.2d 475 (Cal. 1988); State v. Hunt, 555 A.2d 369 (Vt. 1988).

[42] State v. Briggs, 776 P.2d 1347 (Wash. Ct. App. 1989).

[43] State v. Hicks, 649 P.2d 267 (Ariz. 1982).

[44] Hadden v. State, 670 So.2d 77 (Fla. Ct. App. 1996).

CARL N. EDWARDS

Profiling: Drugs *see* Drug Profiling

Profiling: Mitochondrial DNA *see* Mitochondrial DNA: Profiling

Property Crime *see* Firesetting

Pseudoseizures *see* Seizures: Behavioral

Psychodynamic Diagnostic Manual (PDM) *see* Psychopathology: Terms and Trends

Psychological Autopsy

Origins

The psychological autopsy originated in approximately 1958 as a result of the Los Angeles County Medical Examiner's Office consulting the Los Angeles Suicide Prevention Center for assistance in distinguishing drug-related accidental overdoses from suicides [1]. This collaboration laid down the basic principles of the psychological autopsy procedure. Edwin Schneidman, a director of the LA Suicide

Table 1   Commonalities of suicide

- Purpose: seek a solution
- Stimulus: unbearable psychological pain
- Stressor: frustrated needs
- Emotion: hopelessness, helplessness
- Cognition: ambivalence
- Perception: constriction

Adapted from Schneidman, 1996

Prevention Center, is credited with coining the term *psychological autopsy*. Schneidman's initial definition of the psychological autopsy was "a thorough retrospective investigation of the intention of the decedent" [2]. The process was partially based on his observations that many suicides shared certain common characteristics that could help identify a suicidal individual. Table 1 lists some of Schneidman's "commonalities of suicide".

Over the past 50 years, the procedure has become familiar to most suicidologists, suicide researchers and major city homicide investigators. However, a single standard definition has yet to be formally agreed upon. This article uses the following definition for the psychological autopsy: "A postmortem investigative procedure requiring the identification and assessment of suicide risk factors present at the time of death, with the goal of enabling a determination of the manner of death to as high a degree of certainty as possible".

Thus, the psychological autopsy can be conceptualized as synonymous with a postmortem suicide risk assessment. The strength of framing the psychological autopsy in this manner lies in the fact that performing formal suicide risk assessments on patients who are at risk for suicide is endorsed by overwhelming clinical consensus [3], and will be further clarified below in the section on current controversies. Regardless of the definition or method used, the quality of the assessment will depend heavily on the training, knowledge, experience and clinical judgment of the investigator.

In the push toward standardization, the psychiatric autopsy has evolved through a number of iterations. Initially, Schneidman developed a list of 14 areas of inquiry to guide the investigator when conducting a psychological autopsy [2]. In the late 1980s, the Centers for Disease Control established a list of 22 criteria to assist forensic investigators, called the Operational Criteria for the Determination of Suicide

(OCDS) [4]. Shortly afterwards, suicide researchers developed the Empirical Criteria for the Determination of Suicide (ECDS). This instrument subsumed the OCDS, as well as other important criteria from the research literature [5].

While the Department of Defense had long employed the psychological autopsy method, in 2002 it published a sample model curriculum for conducting them, along with recommendations for training and peer review [6]. Finally, in 2006, leading suicidology experts and researchers proposed an initial standard protocol for lines of inquiry to improve reliability and validity [7]. This protocol, which has been further amended with the assistance of an expert from this research group (Berman, A. *Personal communication*, 2007), is presented toward the end of this article.

Despite progress in psychological autopsy research, some deaths (i.e., drug-related fatalities [8, 9]) continue to frustrate medical examiners (MEs). Thus, the psychological autopsy methods and protocol must continue to be vigorously pursued and tested.

Purpose

Psychological autopsies are an invaluable tool for assessing equivocal deaths. An "equivocal death" may be one in which the manner of death is questionable, or the circumstances surrounding the death are otherwise unclear [7]. Typical equivocal death scenarios are listed in Table 2.

When MEs perform autopsies, they attempt to classify the death into one of four categories or "modes": natural, accidental, suicide, or homicide (NASH) [10]. When a death cannot be immediately classified, it is often officially referred to as *undetermined*. Table 3 lists the basic elements of death classification.

Table 2   Typical equivocal death scenarios

- Drug-related deaths
- Autoerotic asphyxia
- Self-induced asphyxia (e.g., the "choking game")
- Drownings
- Vehicular deaths
- "Russian Roulette"
- "Suicide by cop"
- Staged death scenes

Table 3 Death classification

1. Cause: gunshot, poisoning, etc.
2. Mode: circumstances leading to cause
   a) Natural
   b) Accidental
   c) Suicide
   d) Homicide
3. Motive: reasons for the action
4. Lethality: probability of death as a result of method and circumstances chosen (low, medium, and high)
5. Intent: what the decedent wanted to happen at the time

Table 5 Psychological autopsy uses

- Assist medical examiners with "equivocal" deaths
- Research on suicide
- Insurance claims
- Criminal cases
- Estate issues, contested wills
- Malpractice claims
- Worker's compensation cases
- Product liability cases
- Organizational suicide prevention efforts

The goals of the psychological autopsy include obtaining an in-depth understanding of the decedent's personality, behavior patterns, and possible motives for suicide. The investigator strives to obtain an objective analysis of the decedent's suicide risk enhancing and protective factors. In certain cases, an experienced investigator can use the method to help sort out the degree of risk, intent and causal factors at the time of death [3]. Ultimately, this should allow for a well informed assessment of whether or not the deceased was a likely candidate for suicide. Table 4 lists some of the more important goals of the psychological autopsy.

The psychological autopsy has utility in a variety of settings. Table 5 gives a list of some of its more common uses. As noted, it can be an extremely helpful tool for assisting MEs and homicide investigators. It has been shown to have a significant impact on MEs determination in equivocal cases [11]. It has been used for several decades to collect valuable research data about suicide that ultimately informs prevention efforts [12–14]. The vast majority of these studies suggest that mental disorder is present in a preponderance of suicides. The first generation of

research driven by psychological autopsies found that more than 90% of completed suicides suffered from mental disorders, mostly mood disorders and substance use disorders [3, 15]. The second generation of psychological autopsy research has employed case-control designs, resulting in better estimations of the role of various risk factors for suicide [16].

The psychological autopsy method has also been used in a forensic context in both criminal and civil courts. While courts have admitted testimony based on psychological autopsies in many civil cases, criminal courts have been more hesitant [17]. The issue of the psychological autopsy's legal admissibility will be further discussed below. In criminal cases, the psychological autopsy may be used to establish whether a decedent was likely to have committed suicide, or whether the matter should be viewed as a homicide. In some criminal cases, most notably *Jackson v. State* (Fla. 4th DCA 1989), the psychological autopsy has been used to help analyze whether an abusive relationship played a role in a suicide [18]. In the criminal case *U.S. v. St. Jean* (US Ct. of Appeals for Armed Forces, 1996), the psychological autopsy was used by the prosecution to assist in determining whether or not a suspected homicide victim had been a likely candidate for suicide.

In civil cases, the psychological autopsy has been used to help determine whether benefits are owed to the decedent's beneficiaries [10]. This often involves life insurance payments, where many policies hold that a suicide precludes benefits. However, some policies permit payment if it can be proven that the decedent's death was an "insane suicide". "Insane suicide" is a legal term that was defined by the US Supreme Court in the case of *Mutual Life Insurance Company v. Terry* (US 1872; 82: 580). The Court held that a suicide was "sane" when the "assured, being in the possession of his ordinary reasoning faculties,

Table 4 Psychological autopsy goals

- Identify behavior patterns – stress reactions, adaptability, habit, or routine changes
- Establish presence or absence of mental illness
- Identify possible precipitants
- Determine presence or absence of motives
- Determine presence or absence of suicidal intent
- Determine suicide risk factors – both mitigating and aggravating
- Perform a postmortem suicide risk assessment
- Establish whether or not the deceased was a likely candidate for suicide

from anger, pride, jealousy, or a desire to escape from the ills of life, intentionally takes his own life."

In contrast, an "insane" suicide was defined as "when his reasoning faculties are so far impaired that he is not able to understand the moral character, the general nature, consequences, and effect of the act he is about to commit, or when he is impelled thereto by an insane impulse, which he has not the power to resist ..." Thus, a sane suicide implies the decedent had a rational understanding that his acts would result in his death, whereas an insane suicide implies the decedent was so emotionally disturbed that he did not have a rational appreciation of his actions [10].

Worker's compensation cases generally involve allegations that the decedent's employer was somehow legally responsible for his suicide. Similarly, product liability cases allege that the decedent's use of a particular product (e.g., medication) caused him to commit suicide. In psychiatric malpractice cases involving suicide, the plaintiff must prove that the doctor's negligence was a proximate cause of the decedent's suicide [19]. In addition to determinations regarding the standard of care, a postmortem suicide risk assessment must be conducted to determine the decedent's overall suicide risk and the foreseeability of the suicide.

Another potential use for the psychological autopsy may be its clinical utility in helping surviving family members better understand the tragedy and begin the grieving process [20]. The psychological autopsy may be used for other clinical purposes, such as informing an institution's morbidity and mortality conference after a client's suicide. For historical purposes and interest, psychological autopsies have been conducted on numerous public figures such as Ernest Hemingway [21], Vince Foster, (Berman, A. *Personal communication*, 2007), Howard Hughes and Marilyn Monroe.

Methods

The psychological autopsy method involves collecting and analyzing all relevant information on the deceased. This means that all applicable records are reviewed, including medical records, psychiatric records, police records, and autopsy findings. A visual inspection of the death scene via photographs is necessary, and occasionally a visit to the scene will be required. A thorough review of the decedent's

writings in the form of diaries, journals, e-mails and internet correspondence is vital. The suggested protocol at the end of this article provides a list of other important sources of data. In addition to reviewing records, structured interviews of family members, relatives or friends are necessary. Thus, a psychological autopsy synthesizes data from multiple informants and records. When performed in a comprehensive manner, the method may take anywhere from 20 to 50 or more hours to complete. The overriding principle is that the greater the amount of relevant data analyzed, the more accurate the investigator's conclusions are likely to be.

Suicide risk factors vary among different populations [22]. The investigator should consider any special nuances of the deceased, such as age group [23], mental health diagnosis, gender [24] and other factors that may allow for a more precise consideration of risk factors associated with that group. This requires keeping up to date with the evolving psychiatric and suicidology literature, which is steadily becoming more detailed about risk factors in distinct diagnostic categories such as depression [25], bipolar disorder [26], and persons who are outside the care of mental health services [27]. Some individuals may display unique, individualized behaviors suggestive of increased or decreased suicide risk that will be known only by close social contacts or treating mental health professionals [22]. Thus, an understanding of the decedent's individualized risk factors and past stress reaction patterns becomes important.

Suicide Notes

There is a considerable literature on suicide notes. Research suggests that suicide notes are left only by a minority, approximately 10–33% of all suicides [15]. Regarding persons who do leave notes, available research has not found any significant differences when compared to suicides who do not leave notes. A few studies have suggested that whites and women are slightly more likely to leave suicide notes. At least one study has suggested there are no significant differences in the themes of notes between male and female suicides [28]. Themes of love and relationships were found to be more common than achievement themes in both men and women [29]. Another study found that suicide notes written by young people were longer and rich in emotions, whereas notes written by the elderly were shorter, contained specific instructions, and were less emotional [30].

In a study of 42 suicide notes, the most common themes were: "apology/shame" (74%), "love for those left behind" (60%), "life too much to bear" (48%), "instructions regarding practical affairs postmortem" (36%), "hopelessness/nothing to live for" (21%), and "advice for those left behind" (21%) [31]. The common usage of computers, the Internet [32] and various electronic types of messaging have introduced another important source of data for the psychological autopsy. The investigator should not fail to inquire about these potential sources of information, as they may provide critical insight into the decedent's state of mind and intentions.

One important caveat regarding suicide notes is the possibility that they have been fraudulently prepared and left by another person attempting to disguise a homicide. While there has been some attempt to develop a method for distinguishing genuine from simulated suicide notes [33], more research in this area is required. In such cases, collaboration with a forensic handwriting analysis expert might be considered. Another important consideration for the investigator is the possibility that family members or others who find a suicide note may destroy it or remove it from the death scene for various motives.

Collateral Interviews

The importance of collateral interviews as part of the psychological autopsy method cannot be overstated. Careful interviews of the decedent's family members and other relevant social contacts distinguish a proper psychological autopsy from a mere analysis of demographic data and police reports. Most experts recommend a structured or semistructured approach to collateral interviews. At least one study has developed a semistructured interview for the psychological autopsy which has demonstrated inter-rater reliability [34]. For research purposes, there has been a trend toward using modified instruments such as the Structured Clinical Interview for Diagnostic and Statistical Manual of Mental Disorders, 4th ed.-Text Revision Disorders (SCID), as well as a life events calendar method, which helps identify and quantify the burden of events that may be associated with suicide [35].

Regardless of method used, collateral interviews often reveal critical information about the decedent

that cannot be obtained elsewhere. Recent theories about suicide have stressed that psychiatric illness alone is not enough to fully explain an individual suicide. Rather, a stress-diathesis model has been proposed, in which the risk for suicidal acts is determined by the interplay of biopsychosocial factors and situational variables [36]. According to this model, a diathesis may be reflected in an individual's tendency to have maladaptive responses to stressors, such as acting impulsively. Such information is most likely to be obtained via collateral interviews.

Ethics and Sensitivity. An important ethical and practical consideration related to gathering collateral data is the manner in which collateral sources should be contacted and interviewed. Interviewing surviving family and friends is a very sensitive matter that must consider the survivor's reactions. Ideally, the investigator should have adequate clinical experience in order to handle survivors' reactions with appropriate sensitivity [37]. For "research purposes", it has been recommended that a two to six-month time interval between the suicide and interview be used [37]. There does not appear to be a significant relationship between the timing of the interview and the quality of information obtained when this time frame is used [38].

While a concern about untoward emotional reactions to the interview is an obvious concern, some have noted that survivors appeared to have benefited from the interview experience in terms of being able to express their feelings and receive a mental health referral if needed [37]. Presently, there is no clearly agreed upon method for initiating contact with survivors. Investigators performing a psychological autopsy for forensic legal purposes will likely be supplied with relevant phone numbers and/or addresses of potential interviewees. Often, attorneys will have previously informed the interviewees that an investigator will be contacting them. Investigators seeking interviews for research purposes may consider a letter followed by a phone call, or vice versa [10].

Postmortem Suicide Risk Assessment

A comprehensive postmortem suicide risk assessment is necessary because of the fact that there is no single pathognomonic risk factor for suicide [22]. Single risk factors do not have adequate statistical power on which to base conclusions. Particularly in the context of forensic expert testimony, the postmortem suicide risk assessment approach is recommended [3]. This involves a careful identification and assessment of suicide risk factors present at the time of death.

Risk enhancing factors (both proximal and distal) should be carefully weighed along with risk reducing factors. When thoughtfully analyzed in the context of the totality of the decedent's circumstances, the investigator should be able to arrive at conclusion about the decedent's overall risk of suicide near the time of death. This ultimately informs the investigator's opinion about whether or not the decedent was a likely candidate to commit suicide at the time in question.

Testimony that focuses on whether the psychological autopsy yielded results consistent with an individual who committed suicide is more likely to be found admissible in court. In contrast, overreaching opinions that conclude the decedent did or did not commit suicide are more likely to be found inadmissible. For example, in the case of *State v. Guthrie* (2001 SD 61, 627 N.W. 2d 401), the court found that the expert's testimony became inadmissible when it "shifted from discussing typical suicide characteristics", to a "bold declaration" that the decedent did not die by suicide [39].

Limitations and Controversies

In both research and forensic legal settings, mental health professionals are legally and ethically obligated to note the limitations of their methods. In the case of the psychological autopsy, controversy over its limitations has existed for as long they have been performed [40]. Commonly cited controversies involving the psychological autopsy are listed in Table 6. The limitations largely involve the fact that there is no unanimously accepted standardized protocol for conducting a psychological autopsy. However, dedicated efforts are currently underway to resolve this issue [7]. Progress in this area may

Table 6   Current controversies [42]

- Lack of standardized protocol
- Lack of standardized suicidology nomenclature
- Methodological problems
- Reliability of assessment instruments
- Lack of homogeneity among studies
- Bias among collateral informants

be somewhat dependent on the field of suicidology developing a standard, comprehensive nomenclature. For example, even the basic term *suicide attempt* may have different meanings to different investigators [41].

Controversy surrounding admissibility and meeting Daubert standards may be best resolved by adopting the postmortem suicide risk assessment approach. The reasoning for this is as follows: (i) in clinical practice, the standard of care requires the clinician to gather relevant information and assess the patient's level of suicide risk; (ii) performing such suicide risk assessments on patients considered to be at risk for suicide is endorsed by overwhelming clinical consensus (i.e., it is "generally accepted"); and (iii) the psychological autopsy is similar in that it is the assessment of suicide risk factors present in the decedent near the time of death [3].

This approach to the psychological autopsy should meet the process-driven Daubert criteria, particularly where *Kumho Tire Co. v. Carmichael* (1999 536 U.S. 137, 141) has held that Daubert standards are not limited only to scientific evidence, but may include "technical, or other specialized knowledge" [43]. In the event that a court found that the postmortem suicide risk assessment did not meet Daubert criteria, it should at least meet the *Frye v. U.S.* (DC COA, 1923) criteria of "general acceptance" among mental health professionals. This line of reasoning was adopted by a Louisiana appeals court when it found the psychological autopsy admissible under Daubert. The case, *In re Succession of Pardue* (La Ct. App. 2005 915 So. 2d 415), involved estate issues and testamentary capacity. The court held that the methodology used in the psychological autopsy was sufficiently reliable and generally accepted in psychiatry.

In federal court where expert testimony is governed by the Federal Rules, opinions on the basis of the postmortem suicide risk assessment method would appear to comply with Federal Rules 703 and 702, which allows expert opinions if they are "of a type reasonably relied upon by experts in the particular field", and if the testimony is "the product of reliable principles and methods" [44].

An obvious criticism of the psychological autopsy is the problem of not being able to interview the decedent so as to more accurately determine intent. One response to this issue is that the comprehensive nature of the psychological autopsy, with its wide net of collateral data, may ultimately allow a reasonable approximation or inference of intent. Additionally, it has been argued that having no prior contact with the decedent removes the vagueness and subjectivity inherent in an interpersonal relationship with the decedent [18]. Therefore, one might argue that psychological autopsies may be more objective and less controversial than the analysis of living patients.

To date, only a restricted number of research studies have relied on standardized instruments, making the comparison of findings problematic [42]. Current studies are increasingly using the SCID, but this approach has yet to be conclusively validated for administration to proxies. However, at least two studies (of psychiatric inpatients admitted following a suicide attempt) have suggested that proxies are good judges of past history of suicide attempts, level of suicidal intent and data leading to a psychiatric diagnosis [45, 46].

The issue of bias in collateral informants requires a cautious approach by investigators. Informants' reports may be biased by many factors such as their own personal attitudes toward suicide and their emotional state at the time of the interview. Further, their recollection of circumstances may be impacted by the emotional trauma of the death of their loved one [42]. The demeanor and interpersonal style of the investigator may also become a factor. It is possible that informants may react to the investigator's personal characteristics, which may then influence the amount and type of information they are willing to divulge.

In summary, there is a considerable need for further research efforts aimed at improving the validity and reliability of the psychological autopsy [17]. There is concern that testimony based on a faulty or inadequate psychological autopsy may result in a "miscarriage of justice" [47]. Forensic experts who give testimony in court on the basis of psychological autopsy findings must be prepared to concede any relevant limitations.

Toward a Standard Protocol

In the interest of improving validity and reliability, forensic suicidology must continue to work toward an accepted, standardized protocol for the psychological autopsy [7]. Below is a recommended template that

was developed by expert consensus [7], (Berman, A. *Personal communication*, 2007) and further enhanced according to relevant research and clinical findings [5–7, 10, 20, 48–50]. The protocol may be used to guide areas of investigation and lines of inquiry for collateral interviews. Use of a standardized protocol can serve as a framework for conducting a psychological autopsy. Ultimately, a standard protocol will enhance admissibility, and aid in the testability of the method [7].

The psychological autopsy method allows for a "polyperspective" that can help illuminate key aspects of an equivocal death [51]. However, the light that it shines may also be distorted by the perspective of the investigator. Therefore, it is critical that the individual performing the psychological autopsy possess adequate training. This includes having sufficient knowledge in the fields of suicidology, related mental health concepts, and basic death scene investigation. Data obtained from the death scene and physical autopsy are often highly determinative, and meticulous inspection of the death scene and related items may be necessary in certain forensic legal cases. For example, in cases of suspected "simulated suicidal hanging", there may be important evidence suggesting a homicide that was staged to appear as though it was a suicide [52]. Detailed investigation of body position, ligature placement and knot formation may be required to distinguish a suicide from a homicidal hanging [53]. Further, in cases of suspected autoerotic asphyxiation, researchers have noted characteristic death scene findings (see Appendix 1) [54].

Finally, the problems inherent in assessments of suicidal intention require that the investigator be cognizant of the limits of the data and corresponding conclusions. This is primarily because of clinical observations that suicidal individuals are often ambivalent, and may even have multiple intentions at the same time [55]. In certain cases, the presence and degree of suicidal intent may be difficult to determine because of ambivalence, denial, minimization or confusion. In contrast, the nuances of other cases may present a rather straightforward inference that the decedent's intent was to die. In difficult cases, the investigator may choose to simply report on the results of the postmortem suicide risk assessment, or provide reliable evidence that "Natural", "Accidental" and "Homicidal" causes of death can be excluded [56].

Psychological Autopsy Protocol

Records and documents
- Medical records
- Mental health records
- Police records and related witness statements
- Legal records
- Criminal records
- School records
- Financial records
- Military records
- Suicide note(s), communication or video
- Decedent's journals, diary
- Electronic data: E-mails, text messages, instant messages, and websites
- Forensic computer analysis report if available
- Autopsy report
- Toxicology report

Death scene
- Photos of death scene and site visit if necessary
- Presence of atypical wounds (see Appendix 1)
- Decedent's relationship to site
- Evidence of rescuability versus precautions taken against
- Evidence of planning and/or rehearsal
- Evidence of staged manner of death (see Appendix 1)

Demographics
- Socioeconomic status
- Employment status
- Financial status
- Age/gender/race/height/weight
- Marital status
- Educational status
- Religion and religiosity
- Adopted vs. biological family status
- Immigrant status – acculturation issues
- Residence relative to recent mobility

Recent symptoms and behaviors
- Appeared depressed, sad, tearful, or moody
- High risk depressive symptoms [25]
  - Insomnia
  - Appetite loss
  - Weight loss
    - Feelings of worthlessness and/or inappropriate guilt
    - Physical agitation
    - Depression comorbid with anxiety
- Expressed suicidal ideation or preoccupation with death
- Appeared to have made a change for the better
- Appeared anxious, or complained recently of anxiety or panic attacks
- Appeared agitated
- Behaved in an impulsive manner
- Displayed uncontrolled rage or aggressive behavior
- Demonstrated constricted thinking or "tunnel vision"
- Disclosed feelings of guilt or shame
- Appeared confused, disoriented or psychotic
- Expressed feelings of hopelessness, helplessness or worthlessness
- Engaged in excessive risk-taking behaviors
- Mental Status evidence of:
  - Impaired memory
  - Poor comprehension
  - Poor judgment
  - Hallucinations or delusions
  - Inflated sense of self or signs of magical thinking

Precipitants
- Significant losses (relationships, job, finances, prestige, self-concept, family member, moving, or anything of importance)
- Significant (or perceived) disruption of a primary relationship
- Legal troubles or difficulties with police
- Traumatic events
- Significant life changes (negative or positive, birth of child, promotion, etc.)
- Completed or attempted suicide by a family member or loved one
- Anniversary of important death, loss, etc.
- Exposure to suicide of another via media or personal acquaintance
- Preparations for death (e.g., gave away prized items, settled personal accounts, updated will, and said "goodbye" to loved ones)
- Expression of wish to reunite with a deceased loved one, or to be "reborn"

Psychiatric history
- Prior suicidal behaviors

- – Total number of past attempts
- – Dates
- – Precipitants
- – Method, lethality
- – What stopped event, if anything? How found
- – Attitude and behavior after found
- Prescribed psychotropic medications
- Observed adverse reactions to psychotropic medications
- Lack of compliance with psychotropic medications
- Efficacy of treatment (e.g., subtherapeutic doses, poor or incorrect agent choice, inadequate blood level, etc.)
- Psychiatric hospitalization (reasons, dates, diagnoses, and treatment)
- Outpatient treatment (psychiatrist, psychologist, therapist, and Primary Care Physician PCP)
- Psychotherapy at time of death (duration, quality of alliance, compliance, and diagnosis)
- Expressing concerns about "going crazy" or losing cognitive function

Physical health

- Recent visit to physician (reasons)
- Chronic pain
- Chronic, fatal or debilitating disease
- Recent reduction in physical/functional capabilities
- Current medications (compliance or recent changes)

Substance abuse

- History and pattern of alcohol, drug abuse
- Recent attempts to discontinue use
- Recent increase in pattern of use
- Degree of use at time of death (binge drinking, etc.)
- History of "accidental overdose" (when and type of drug)

Family history

- Suicide or attempted suicide
- Nonnatural deaths
- Level of support or observed closeness in nuclear and extended families
- Physical, sexual, or emotional abuse
- Substance abuse
- Violent behavior
- Affective or other psychiatric disorders

Firearm history (if relevant)

- Ownership
- Recent purchasing or obtaining (stated purpose?)
- Recent movement of gun (from where to where?)
- Pattern of weapon care and cleaning
- Pattern of storage and use
- Accidental discharges

Social Supports and Attachments

- Ability to create and maintain close personal relationships
- Ability to express feelings as needed in relationships
- Recent talk about feeling unsupported, uncared for, unimportant
- Relative success in personal relationships
- Relative success in work
- Attachment to hobbies, interests, religion, etc.
- Recent change in any of the above attachments/supports

Emotional reactivity

- History of violence toward others
- Impulsive behaviors
- Excessive rage or aggression

Lifestyle/character

- Typical coping patterns, pattern of reaction to stress
- Perfectionism
- Self-destructive behaviors (self-mutilation, deliberate self-harm, driving while intoxicated, etc.)
- Frequent crises
- Victimization behaviors (bullied or abused)
- Tendency to dissembling (hiding emotions or stoicism)

Access to care

- History of help-seeking behaviors
- Barriers to healthcare (no insurance or no accessible caregiver)

Other areas of inquiry

- Occupational history
- Personal interests, hobbies
- Gambling history
- Degree and type of religiosity
- Description of activities/behaviors in last days before death

Factors associated with suicide risk reduction

- Evidence of future-oriented thinking or behaviors (doctor's appointments, job interviews, etc.)
- Responsibility for a child under 18 (stronger for women vs. men)
- Absence of suicidal ideas or intent
- Hopefulness
- Willingness to accept help and/or treatment for psychiatric conditions
- Low symptom severity
- Good therapeutic alliance with mental health professional
- Stable, supportive marriage or spouse
- Religious prohibition

Collateral interviews

For each interview, note the following:

- Relationship to deceased
- Time interval between death and interview
- Reactions to the death (surprise, acceptance, and beliefs)
- Attitudes about suicide
- Potential biases (pending lawsuits, insurance claims, denial, etc.)
- Assessment instruments used

Appendix 1

Evidence of Alternative or Staged Manner of Death

- **Presence of Autoerotic Characteristics** [57]
  - Body partially supported by ground
  - Ligature with self-rescue mechanism (slip knot, etc.)
  - Bondage items and/or sexual masochistic behavior (genitals, nipples, etc.)
  - Male wearing female attire
  - Protective padding between ligature and body
  - Sexual paraphernalia (vibrator, pornography, and mirrors)
  - Evidence of previous autoerotic practices
- **Presence of Atypical Self-Inflicted Gunshot Wounds** [58]
  - More than one gunshot injury
  - Gunshot injury without contact or near contact
  - Uncommon entrance wound sites (back of neck or head, ear, and eye)

- Uncommon bullet paths (downward and back to front)

Acknowledgment

The authors would like to acknowledge Alan L. Berman, PhD for his expertise and assistance, particularly with the Psychological Autopsy Protocol.

References

[1]   Schneidman, E. (1996). *The Suicidal Mind*, Oxford University Press, New York.

[2]   Schneidman, E. (1981). The psychological autopsy, *Suicide and Life-Threatening Behavior* **11**, 325–340.

[3]   Simon, R. (2002). Murder, suicide, accident, or natural death? Assessment of suicide risk factors at the time of death, in *Retrospective Assessment of Mental States in Litigation*, R. Simon & D. Shuman, eds, American Psychiatric Publishing, Washington, D.C, pp. 135–153.

[4]   Rosenberg, M., Davidson, L., Smith,J.C., Berman, A.L., Buzbee, H., Gantner, G., Gay, G.A., Moore-Lewis, B., Mills, D.H., Murray, D., O'Carroll, P.W. & Jobes, D. (1988). Operational criteria for the determination of suicide, *Journal of Forensic Sciences* **33**(6), 1445–1456.

[5]   Jobes, D., Casey, J. & Berman, A. *et al.* (1991). Empirical criteria for the determination of suicide manner of death, *Journal of Forensic Sciences* **36**(1), 244–256.

[6]   Ritchie, E. & Gelles, M. (2002). Psychological autopsies: the current department of defense effort to standardize training and quality assurance, *Journal of Forensic Sciences* **47**(6), 1370–1372.

[7]   Snider, J., Hane, S. & Berman, A. (2006). Standardizing the psychological autopsy: Addressing the daubert standard, *Suicide & Life-Threatening Behavior* **36**(5), 511–518.

[8]   Cone, E. *et al.* (2004). Oxycodone involvement in drug abuse deaths. II. Evidence for toxic multiple drug-drug interactions, *Journal of Analytical Toxicology* **28**(7), 616–624.

[9]   Wolf, B.C., Lavezzi, W.A., Sullivan, L.M. & Flannagan, L.M. (2005). One hundred seventy two deaths involving the use of oxycodone in palm beach County, *Journal of Forensic Sciences* **50**(1), 192–195.

[10] Scott, C., Swartz, E. & Warburton, K. (2006). The Psychological autopsy: solving the mysteries of death, *The Psychiatric Clinics of North America* **29**(3), 805–822.

[11] Jobes, D., Berman, A. & Josselson, A. (1986). The impact of psychological autopsies on medical examiners' determination of manner of death, *Journal of Forensic Sciences* **31**(1), 177–189.

[12] Conwell, Y., Duberstein, P., Cox, C., Herrmann, J., Forbes, N. & Caine, E. (1996). Relationships of age and axis I diagnoses in victims of completed suicide: a psychological autopsy study, *The American Journal of Psychiatry* **153**, 1001–1008.

[13] Andrew, T.A., Cheng, Tony, H.H., Chen, Chwen-Chen Chen & Rachel Jenkins (2000). Psychosocial and psychiatric risk factors for suicide: case – control psychological autopsy study, *The British Journal of Psychiatry* **177**, 360–365.

[14] Henriksson, M., Aro, H., Marttunen, M., Heikkinen, M., Isometsa, E., Kuoppasalmi, K. & Lonquist, J. (1993). Mental disorders and comorbidity in suicide, *The American Journal of Psychiatry* **150**, 935–940.

[15] Berman, A. (2000). *Comprehensive Textbook of Suicidology*, The Guilford Press, New York, pp. 268–270, 319–320.

[16] Isometsa, E. (2001). Psychological autopsy studies – a review, *European Psychiatry : The Journal of The Association of European Psychiatrists* **16**(7), 379–385.

[17] Ogloff, J. & Otto, R. (1993). Psychological autopsy: clinical and legal perspectives, *St. Louis University Law Journal* **37**, 607–646.

[18] Jacobs, D. & Kline-Benheim, M. (1995). The Psychological autopsy: a useful tool for determining proximate causation in suicide cases, *Bulletin of the American Academy of Psychiatry and the Law* **23**(2), 165–182.

[19] Knoll, J. & Gerbasi, J. (2006). Psychiatric malpractice case analysis: striving for objectivity, *The Journal of the American Academy of Psychiatry and the Law* **34**, 215–223.

[20] Berman, A. (2005). Psychological autopsy, in *Encyclopedia of Forensic and Legal Medicine*, J. Payne-James, R. Byard, T. Corey & C. Henderson, eds, Academic Press, pp. 364–371.

[21] Martin, C. (2006). Ernest hemingway: a psychological autopsy of a suicide, *Psychiatry* **69**(4), 351–361.

[22] Simon, R. (2004). *Assessing and Managing Suicide Risk: Guidelines for Clinically Based Risk Management*, American Psychiatric Publishing, Washington, D.C.

[23] Houston, K., Hawton, K. & Shepperd, R. (2001). Suicide in young people aged 15–24: a psychological autopsy study, *Journal of Affective Disorders* **63**(1–3), 159–170.

[24] Pirkola, S., Isometsa, E., Heikkinen, M., Henriksson, M., Marttunen, M. & Lonquist, J. (1999). Female psychoactive substance-dependent suicide victims differ from male–results from a nationwide psychological autopsy study, *Comprehensive Psychiatry* **40**(2), 101–107.

[25] McGirr, A., Renaud, J., Seguin, M., Alda, M., Benkelfat, C., Lesage, A. & Turecki, G. (2007). An examination of DSM-IV depressive symptoms and risk for suicide completion in major depressive disorder: A psychological autopsy study, *Journal of Affective Disorders* **97**, 203–209.

[26] Marangell, L.B., Bauer, S.M., Dennehy, E.B., Wisniewski, S.R., Allen, M.H., Miklowitz, D.J., Oquendo, M.A., Frank, E., Perlis, R.H., Martinez, J.M., Fagiolini, A., Otto, M.W., Chessick, C.A., Zboyan, H.A., Miyahara, S., Sachs, G. & Thase, M.E. (2006). Prospective predictors of suicide and suicide attempts in 1, 556 patients with bipolar disorders followed for up to 2 years, *Bipolar Disorders* **8**, 566–575.

[27] Owens, C., Booth, N., Briscoe, M., Lawrence, C. & Lloyd, K. (2003). Suicide outside the care of mental health services: a case-controlled psychological autopsy study, *Crisis* **24**(3), 113–121.

[28] Salib, E., Cawley, S. & Healy, R. (2002). The significance of suicide notes in the elderly, *Aging and Mental Health* **6**(2), 186–190.

[29] Canetto, S. & Lester, D. (2002). Love and achievement motives in women's and men's suicide notes, *The Journal of Psychology* **136**(5), 573–576.

[30] Ho, T., Yip, P., Chiu, C. & Halliday, P. (1998). Suicide notes: what do they tell us? *Acta Psychiatrica Scandinavica* **98**(6), 467–473.

[31] Foster, T. (2003). Suicide note themes and suicide prevention, *International Journal of Psychiatry in Medicine* **33**(4), 323–331.

[32] Baume, P., Cantor, C. & Rolfe, A. (1997). Cybersuicide: the role of interactive suicide notes on the Internet, *Crisis* **18**(2), 73–79.

[33] Lester, D. & Linn, M. (1998). Joseph Richman's signs for distinguishing genuine from simulated suicide notes, *Perceptual and Motor Skills* **87**(1), 242.

[34] Werlang, B. & Botega, N. (2003). Semistructured interview for psychological autopsy: an inter-rater reliability study, *Suicide & Life-Threatening Behavior* **33**(3), 326–330.

[35] Seguin, M., Lesage, A., Turecki, G., Bouchard, M., Chawky, N., Tremblay, N., Daigle, F. & Guy, A. (2007). Life trajectories and burden of adversity: mapping the developmental profiles of suicide mortality, *Psychological Medicine* **37**(11), 1575–1583.

[36] Mann, J.J., Waternaux, C., Haas, G.L. & Malone K.M. (1999). Toward a clinical model of suicidal behavior in psychiatric patients, *The American Journal of Psychiatry* **156**, 181–189.

[37] Beskow, J., Runeson, B. & Asgard, U. (1990). Psychological autopsies: methods and ethics, *Suicide & Life-Threatening Behavior* **20**(4), 307–323.

[38] Brent, D.A., Perper, J.A., Kolko, D.J. & Zelenak, J.P. (1988). The psychological autopsy: methodological considerations for the study of adolescent suicide, *Journal of the American Academy of Child and Adolescent Psychiatry* **27**(3), 362–366.

[39] Kern, J. & Swier, S. (2004). Daubert, kuhmo, and its impact on south dakota jurisprudence: an update, *South Dakota Law Review* **49**, 217–249.

[40] Hansen, M. (2000). Suicidal Missions: psychological autopsies to uncover motivation in suspicious deaths are themselves now suspect, *ABA Journal* **86**, 28–29.

[41] Silverman, M. (2006). The language of suicidology, *Suicide and Life-Threatening Behavior* **36**(5), 519–532.

[42] Pouliot, L. & De Leo, D. (2006). Critical issues in psychological autopsy studies, *Suicide and Life-Threatening Behavior* **36**(5), 491–510.

[43] Kumho Tire Co. V. Carmichael, 536 U.S. 137, 141 (1999).

[44] Federal Rules of Evidence, Available at 2008. http://www.law.cornell.edu/rules/fre/rules.htm#Rule703.

[45] Conner, K., Conwell, Y. & Duberstein, P. (2001). The validity of proxy-based data in suicide research: a study of patients 50 years of age and older who attempted suicide. II. Life events, social support and suicidal behavior, *Acta Psychiatrica Scandinavica* **104**(6), 452–457.

[46] Conner, K., Duberstein, P. & Conwell, Y. (2001). The validity of proxy-based data in suicide research: a study of patients 50 years of age and older who attempted suicide, *I Psychiatric Diagnosis Acta Psychiatrica Scandinavica* **104**(3), 204–209.

[47] Ormerod, D. (2001). Psychological autopsies: legal applications and admissibility, *The International Journal of Evidence and Proof* **5**, 1–31.

[48] Moscicki, E. (1997). Identification of suicide risk factors using epidemiologic studies, *Psychiatric Clinics of North America* **20**(3), 499–517.

[49] American Psychiatric Association (APA) (2003). Practice guideline for the assessment and treatment of patients with suicidal behaviors. *The American Journal of Psychiatry* Available at http://www.psych.org/psych_pract/treatg/pg/SuicidalBehavior_05-15-06.pdf.

[50] Shea, S. (2002). *The Practical Art of Suicide Assessment: A Guide for Mental Health Professionals and Substance Abuse Counselors*, John Wiley & Sons, New Jersey.

[51] Berman, A. (1993). Forensic suicidology and the psychological autopsy, in *Suicidology: Essay in Honour of Edwin S. Schneidman*, A. Leenaars, ed, Aronson, New York.

[52] Hazelwood, R. & Napier, M. (2005). Crime scene staging and its detection, *International Journal of Offender Therapy and Comparative Criminology* **48**(6), 744–759.

[53] Vanezis, P. & Busuttil, A. (1996). *Suspicious Death Scene Investigation*, Arnold, London, p. 153.

[54] Byrard, R., Hucker, S. & Hazelwood, R. (1990). A comparison of typical death scene features in cases of fatal male and autoerotic asphyxia with a review of the literature, *Forensic Science International* **48**(2), 113–121.

[55] Andriessen, K. (2006). On "Intention" in the definition of suicide, *Suicide and Life-Threatening Behavior* **36**(5), 533–538.

[56] O'Carrol, P., Berman, A., Maris, M., Moscicki, E., Tanney, B. & Silverman, M. (1996). Beyond the tower of babel: a nomenclature for suicidology, *Suicide and Life-Threatening Behavior* **26**, 237–252.

[57] Hazelwood, R., Dietz, P. & Burgess, A. (1983). *Auto-erotic fatalities*, Lexington Books, Lexington, MA.

[58] Karger, B., Billeb, E., Koops, B. & Brinkman, B.(2002). Autopsy features relevant for discrimination between suicidal and homicidal gunshot injuries, *International Journal of Legal Medicine* **116**, 273–278.

Further Reading

Legal Citations

Campbell v. Young Motor Co, 211 Mont. 68, 684 P.2d 1101 (1984).

Daubert v. Merrell Dow (USSC., 1993).

Frye v. United States (D.C. COA., 1923).

In re Succession of Pardue (La Ct. App. 915 So. 2d 415 2005).

Jackson v. State, 553 So. 2d 719 (Fla. 4th DCA., 1989).

Kumho Tire Co. v. Carmichael 536 U.S. 137, 141 (1999).

Mutual Life Insurance Company v. Terry (U.S. 82, 580 1872).

State v. Guthrie (SD 61, 627 N.W. 2d 4012001).

United States v. St. Jean (U.S. Ct. of Appeals for Armed Forces, 1996).

Additional References

Cavanagh, J., Carson, A., Sharpe, M. & Lawrie, S. (2003). Psychological autopsy studies of suicide: a systematic review, *Psychological Medicine* **33**(3), 395–405.

Conner, K., Cox, C., Duberstein, P., Tian, L., Nisbet, P. & Conwell, Y. (2001). Violence, alcohol, and completed suicide: a case-control study, *The American Journal of Psychiatry* **158**, 1701–1705.

Conwell, Y., Duberstein, P., Cox, C., Herrmann, J., Forbes, N. & Caine, E. (1996). Relationships of age and axis I diagnoses in victims of completed suicide: a psychological autopsy study, *The American Journal of Psychiatry* **153**, 1001–1008.

Fruehwald, S., Matschnig, T., Koeni, F., Bauer, P. & Frottier, P. (2004). Suicide In custody: case-control study, *The British Journal of Psychiatry* **185**, 494–498.

He, X.Y., Felthouse, A.R., Holzer, C.E., Nathan, P. & Veasey, S. (2001). Factors in prison suicide: one year study in Texas, *Journal of Forensic Sience* **46**(4), 896–901.

Kovasznay, B., Miraglia, R., Beer, R. & Way, B. (2004). Reducing suicides in New York State correctional facilities, *Psychiatric Quarterly* **75**(1), 61–70.

Litman, R. (1989). 500 psychological autopsies, *Journal of Forensic Sciences* **34**(3), 638–646.

Malone, K.M., Oquendo, M.A., Haas, G.L., Ellis, SP., Li, S. & Mann, J.J. (2000). Protective factors against suicidal acts in major depression: reasons for living, *The American Journal of Psychiatry* **157**, 1084–1088.

Marttunen, M., Henriksson, M., Isometsa, E., Heikkinen, M., Aro, H. & Lonnqvist, J. (1998). Completed suicide among adolescents with no diagnosable psychiatric disorder, *Adolescence* **33**(131), 669–681.

Ohberg, A. & Lonquist, J. (1998). Suicides hidden among undetermined deaths, *Acta Psychiatrica Scandinavica* **98**(3), 214–218.

Owens, C., Booth, N., Briscoe, M., Lawrence, C. & Lloyd, K. (2003). Suicide outside the care of mental health services: a case-controlled psychological autopsy study, *Crisis* **24**(3), 113–121.

Shaw, J., Baker, D., Hunt, I.M., Moloney, A. & Appleby, L. (2004). Suicide by prisoners: National clinical survey, *British Journal of Psychiatry* **184**, 263–267.

Spellman, A. & Heyne, B. (1989). Suicide? Accident? Predictable? Avoidable? The psychological autopsy in jail suicides, *The Psychiatric Quarterly* **60**(2), 173–183.

Weinberger, L.E., Sreenivasan, S., Sathyavagiswaran, L. & Markowitz, E. (2001). Child and adolescent suicide in a large, urban area: Psychological, demographic, and situational factors, *Journal of Forensic Science* **46**(4), 902–907.

Related Articles

Autoerotic Deaths

Accident Reconstruction

Crime Scene Investigation

Mass Grave Investigation

Suicide (Behavior)

JAMES L. KNOLL, IV AND
ROBERT R. HAZELWOOD

Psychological First Aid *see*
Disaster Mental Health

Psychological Profiles *see* Profiles:
Psychological and Behavioral

Psychological Syndromes *see*
Syndromes: Psychological

Psychological Testing

Introduction

Psychological testing is best understood within the larger context of psychological evaluation or assessment that, in turn, is seen as one discipline's approach to a more general and shared task of information collection. The *APA Dictionary of Psychology* [1] defines psychological assessment as "the gathering and integration of data in order to make a psychological evaluation, decision, or recommendation" (p. 751). Multiple tools of assessment are listed including interview, behavioral observations, tests, and other specialized instruments. A psychological test is a "standardized instrument (i.e., a test, inventory, or scale)" used for the purpose of measuring any of a variety of abilities, aptitudes, or attributes (p. 753).

This article includes discussion of psychological testing and differentiates it from other types of assessment and focuses on one area of personality testing (*see*, in contrast, **Neuropsychological Assessment**; **Neuropsychological Assessment: Child**; **Head Injury: Neuropsychological Assessment**). While general information is applicable to examinees of all ages, most of the tests that are discussed here were developed for use with adults.

Clinical Assessment and Formal Testing

Evaluation or assessment is used in all clinical disciplines and may involve elaborate, sophisticated technology, such as magnetic resonance imagery (MRI) to look for the presence of a brain lesion, or may depend on more informal, intuitive ways of combining personal observations to form hypotheses or conclusions, such as surmising a person acts depressed. Different clinicians within mental health "work up" a client or patient using common as well as unique tools and methods associated with the specialized training and expertise of the particular discipline. For example, almost all mental health clinicians assessing someone not only interview the person by asking common questions about mood, sleep, appetite, and daily functioning but also probe other areas more selectively.

Psychiatrists are more likely to consider medical or biological factors potentially contributing to emotional problems, whereas social workers may spend more time exploring the person's interchanges with social systems. Family therapists may look more acutely at the history of family relationships and alliances, and psychologists are more likely to use inventories and psychological testing. Each discipline's approach is a blend of commonly shared tools, literature, and research arising from several disciplines as well as unique resources based on clinical specialization and scope of practice for that particular discipline.

Differences between Psychiatric and Psychological Testing

Clinical psychologists and psychiatrists both provide assessment and treatment services in the field of mental health, but the differing educational and clinical training routes shape distinct elements that each group uses for these services (*see* **Behavioral Science Evidence**). Psychiatrists, like other physicians, attend medical school for four years during which time they focus on studying chemistry, anatomy, and physiology as well as work in a wide variety of medical speciality placements before getting the MD (medical doctor) degree. They also may take courses in research, statistics, and learning theories. During psychiatric rotations in medical school and later in residency specialization (3 or 4 years), they learn about medical tests and clinical diagnostic techniques for mental health problems, study personality theories and human development, and acquire skills for treating mental illness.

For most psychiatrists, treatment is heavily based on biological and chemical factors that medicines affect (*see* **Psychopharmacology**; **Psychopharmacology: Child and Adolescent**). Assessment is therefore oriented toward finding biological factors or markers for which medical or somatic intervention is well matched. Psychiatric assessment relies heavily on clinical observation (something physicians are well trained to do) and the use of mental status evaluation (*see* **Mental Status: Examination**). A mental status evaluation involves assessing a person's orientation (knowledge of place, time, and self); ability to attend to environment and to communicate; mood and expression of feelings; and congruence or incongruence within the situation (appearing to hallucinate or act delirious). Depending on the nature of the hypothesized mental health problem, the psychiatrist may use brief tests or inventories to support or exclude

certain diagnoses. These instruments may include behavioral inventories designed to collect information about classroom behavior of children; self-reported symptoms on a depression checklist; or a brief cognitive status exam looking for signs of dementia. More elaborate psychiatric testing is usually medically or biologically oriented as the psychiatrist reaches into his/her medical training to refine diagnosis (e.g., radiological tests looking for brain tumor; electroencephalogram (EEG) to document seizures or to find unusual electrical patterns in the brain; and blood tests to measure hormone levels or to check for problems such as anemia).

Psychologists, on the other hand, begin their training by attending a university graduate school for four or more years taking courses in personality theory and human development, measurement theory and test development, research statistics, learning theories, methods of mental health interventions, and principles of social contexts and human interactions. To a lesser degree, course work includes anatomy and physiology of the nervous system, human biochemistry, and genetics. Students in a psychology Ph.D. (doctor of philosophy) program complete both a masters level research project and a doctoral dissertation.

Clinical training involves multiple placements in clinical sites during graduate school followed by a 12-month internship in a mental health setting prior to graduation. Some states require an additional year of postgraduate supervised clinical work before licensure, and several areas of professional specialization offer residency training for one or two years. Some areas of specialization are clinical psychology (dealing with application of psychological knowledge and principles to address mental health problems), neuropsychology (study of brain–behavior relationships), experimental psychology (basic physiological or social factor research), and forensic psychology (application of psychological knowledge and principles to address legal issues). Each of these areas makes heavy use of assessment and testing.

When psychologists conduct an evaluation, they also rely on the common tools of observation and interview with the person and collateral sources (family members, teachers, institutional staff who have information about the person's behavior). As do psychiatrists, they conduct mental status evaluations and may also use brief inventories, checklists, or simple tests to support or dismiss diagnostic hunches. However, when psychologists proceed to more elaborate testing, they rely most heavily upon the tools their discipline has developed. For the most part, these tests involve either measurement of cognitive abilities (e.g., intelligence, memory, and academic skills) or personality factors (e.g., traits and emotional states).

Cognitive Testing. Cognitive testing may be thought of as a way to measure how well the brain is functioning. Neuropsychology, a speciality with its own postgraduate training and certification, has developed a vast array of tests that measure not only basic intelligence but also learning and memory, sensory perception and sensory-muscle integration, reasoning and problem solving skills, language and communication abilities, and basic academic skills such as reading (*see* **Neuropsychological Assessment**; **Neuropsychological Assessment: Child**). Cognitive testing is able to identify and to document the level of skill or the degree of impaired functioning of a person. It is often used in conjunction with neurological or radiological testing that documents impaired structure of the brain or nervous system. Findings from cognitive testing may be used for such tasks as assisting with decisions about academic placement or need for special education resources (*see* **Mental Retardation**); rehabilitation treatment planning after head injury or neurosurgery (*see* **Head Injury: Neuropsychological Assessment**); diagnosis of conditions having subtle onset such as early stage dementia; measurement of progress or lack of response to remediation efforts after head injury or stroke; or documentation of progression of effects of diseases such as Parkinson's or Multiple Sclerosis. Neuropsychologists are often called upon in forensic cases involving head injury, toxic exposure, or questions of competency or capacity (*see* **Capacity to Stand Trial**; **Capacity Assessment**; **Guardianships of Adults**).

Personality Testing. If cognitive testing is thought of as a way to measure the brain's work, personality testing may be thought of as a way to assess the mind of the person. Whereas one deals with neurophysiology and often uses physical measures, the other deals with psyche and uses measures of emotion, attitude, and traits. Personality testing explores intrapsychic (internal aspects of self, value conflicts and ambivalence, moods, motivation) and interpersonal issues (social behavioral clusters, styles of interaction, orientation toward others).

Personality testing is often used to gather information to allow psychologists to describe what a person is like; how a person is different from others and to what degree; how the person functions or is likely to function with others; whether there is significant psychopathology; extent to which a person is open and transparent in self-presentation or guarded or even deceptive (*see* **Deception: Detection of and Brain Imaging**; **Deception: Detection of**); **Malingering: Forensic Evaluations**) and prognosis for improvement with treatment for mental health problems. Psychologists are often called upon in forensic cases to use personality testing to address questions involving risk assessment (*see* **Dangerousness: Risk of**); mental illness diagnosis and treatment recommendations; competency and capacity; tort cases where emotional distress claims are made (*see* **Posttraumatic Stress Disorder**); and criminal cases where mental illness factors are being presented (*see* for example **Insanity: Defense**; **Temporary Insanity**).

Properties of Formal Testing

Testing, which is a relatively circumscribed activity involving use of tests to obtain specific scores, is one part of an overall assessment that collects information from multiple sources using multiple methods. Information usually includes records that place a person's current performance in historical context, referral information that places a person in a situational context, behavioral observations, interviews, and consideration of the person's test taking attitudinal factors (fatigue, rapport, motivation, exaggeration, or defensiveness). The person–context information can be as important as the test result information, for instance when the person is observed to be disengaged from the task or hostile toward the examiner. As a result of such situational data, the psychologist interprets data cautiously or may even disregard the scores as being invalid measures. This person–situation information, whether obtained from direct observation or from validity scales embedded within tests, helps determine if test results are considered valid for interpretation.

Together with information from these other sources, test results are then used to assist in diagnosis, to identify areas for intervention, or to provide information about current functioning.

These results are integrated into a cohesive and comprehensive understanding of the person to communicate it to others including the person being tested. Indeed, providing feedback to the person often serves as an intervention itself and can be a very important part of treatment.

Formal testing refers to an assessment process using standardized instruments that have rules for administration and for scoring responses, normative information for comparing scores, and guidelines for interpretation of results. Holding these test factors constant means there should be minimal "noise" produced so that it may be logically assumed that most of the variability of scores between examinees is a result of something associated with differences between the individual test takers. Just as the use of an accurately calibrated thermometer allows a physician to verify or rule out the presence of fever to help refine diagnostic hunches, the use of psychological testing allows psychologist to verify or rule out abnormalities and to refine diagnostic hunches on the basis of test score patterns and known psychological conditions.

Reliability

Reliability is the term used to indicate the concept of score consistency on a test. It is a measure of how closely clustered or how far apart a person's scores would be with repeated administrations of the same test or with alternate versions of the test. Reliability is a measure of how much error (or "noise" as compared to "signal") is present in test scores [2, 3].

Validity

Validity is the term used to designate the concept of score accuracy of a test. It tells how well a test works in measuring what it purports to assess. Validity may be determined by comparing a test with a "gold standard" in the field, by seeing how well test scores discriminate between known groups on a particular factor, or by how well a test covers relevant aspects of a construct but avoids tapping other constructs. Just as a rifle must shoot true before a marksman can attain target accuracy, a test must have reliability (consistency of measured scores) before its validity (accuracy of measured scores) can be established [2, 3].

Standardization

Standardization refers to the process whereby a test and its components are made standard or routine in details of administration. Test items, the order of administration of items, ways of recording and scoring responses, and ways of instructing examinees about how to take the test must become standard or fixed. Standardization and adherence to instructions regarding the test should decrease the "noise" associated with a person's scores so that differences between examinees (or the same person tested at different times) should be related to actual differences rather than to errors involved in the process of obtaining the scores [2, 3].

Norms

Norms refer to the collection of scores that represent a sample group's responses on a test. Norms can be obtained when many people take the test under the same standard conditions. The mean (average) and standard deviation (SD) (measure of variability of scores) can be calculated and used to evaluate a particular person's obtained score in relation to the cluster and range of scores produced by the norm group. Raw scores are often transformed to standard scores (mean $= 100$, $SD = 15$), T-scores (mean $=50$, $SD = 10$), or scale scores (mean $= 10$, $SD = 3$) to create a shorthand way of conveying a person's score in relation to the sample group's norms. A well-developed test has a heterogeneous (mixed gender, ethnicity, and socioeconomic status) group of individuals whose scores are used to calculate the norms. As a result, the sample group norms should be more representative of the entire population of interest than if only a homogenous group was tested and scores calculated.

By having good normative data, it is possible to determine to what degree the examinee is similar to or different from the average person taking the test. By having test data from differing groups of people with a known condition or factor, it is possible to use a person's test results to refine diagnostic hypotheses about the examinee. By using information about a person's score in relation to the norms, the psychologist can then analyze and interpret test score data. Analysis of test data can occur at three levels: specific details about skills, deficits, or symptoms based on actual scores; level of performance or information about severity of problem or level of skill based on relationship of score to group norms; and syndrome or pattern of scores, which generalizes to life context, based on research literature and clinical knowledge [3, 4].

Testing offers advantages over interview or observation alone by providing empirically quantified information that is usually more precise than interview impressions. Testing may cover a variety of constructs, and, in the case of personality testing, it covers a large array of traits in an efficient manner. Standardized administration and scoring means a common yardstick is used for measuring a person, and behavior is observed in a uniform context. Test norms allow scores to be compared to known groups, and research with such known groups provides the psychologist with a stimulating backdrop from which to generate and evaluate hypotheses related to test scores [5].

History of Psychological Testing

A brief history of psychological testing can provide a useful context for understanding its current state. A very influential English figure was Sir Francis Galton who in 1869 published "Classification of Men According to Their Natural Gifts" [6]. Galton pioneered use of questionnaires and rating scales, developed statistical methods for analysis of individual differences, and popularized forms of psychological testing. At the International Health Exhibition in London (1884), he and his assistants tested individuals willing to pay to learn about their vision and hearing sensitivity, muscle strength, reaction time, and memory. This focus of attention on individual abilities was in contrast to the emphasis on group data being collected by others. Wilhelm Wundt, a German psychologist who had established the first psychology lab in Leipzig five years before, considered individual differences to be errors and was far more interested in measures of perception that portrayed information about the species as a whole [7].

In the same tradition as Galton, James M. Cattell established a testing lab at the University of Pennsylvania (1888) and used tests to measure sensitivity to pain, perceptual discrimination, memory, and other cognitive skills as ways to study individual differences in intelligence. Cattell was the first to use the term *mental test* to describe his techniques [7]. In general, testing in clinical psychology testing has continued to focus more on individual distinctives, whereas measurement in physiological or experimental psychology has focused more on data that add to knowledge about collective or group characteristics of humans and other animals.

Psychological testing took a major leap forward in 1905 when Alfred Binet, a French psychologist, and Theodore Simon, a psychiatrist, collected 30 brief cognitive tests to use as an intelligence scale for the purpose of determining school entry for Parisian children. They later revised their collection of tests and developed the concept of mental age (the age at which an average child could pass a particular test). In the United States, Lewis Terman added some other tasks and developed the concept of intelligence quotient (IQ) that was found by dividing the attained mental age by the person's chronological age. Eventually, IQ came to be calculated in a different manner on the basis of comparison to group information and how far from the group mean a person's scores were [8].

Another major advancement in psychological testing occurred in 1917 when the US Army had to classify World War I (WWI) recruits for their suitability for military service as well as for possible officer training. In a period of two years, 1.7 million inductees were given group administered intelligence tests based on alterations of the Binet and Terman tests. For those literate in English, the Alpha version (verbal tests) was used; for illiterate or non-English speaking recruits, the Beta version (nonverbal tests) was used. Nonverbal or language free tests had been used in the United States at Ellis Island for screening immigrants for mental defects and had also been used in Chicago with unschooled juvenile delinquents.

David Wechsler, a psychology graduate student, enlisted in the Army and was trained to conduct individual intelligence tests for the 5% of recruits who failed one of the group-administered versions. Many years later as psychologist at Bellevue Psychiatric Hospital in New York City, he developed a different approach to intelligence testing that combined verbal and nonverbal tasks to result in a single score. He also collected normative data on a large group from the general population and compared each person's score to the group average (mean). This deviation derived IQ score (relationship of person's score to group average) provided information about how far a person's score was above or below the mean score for the group. In 1939, he contracted with Psychological Corporation for production and sale of his test [8].

Psychological Corporation, formed in 1921, had already been marketing intelligence tests (termed *scholastic aptitude tests*) and other specialized aptitude tests to schools and industries after the war, but the number of psychological tests had been rather limited until the mid-1930s.

Oscar Buros' first edition of *Educational, Psychological, and Personality Tests of 1933 & 1934* had been only 44 pages, but his 1938 edition of what became *Mental Measurements Yearbook* was more than 400 pages long and covered 4000 tests. The current edition is multivolume and covers thousands of tests [9]. The entry of the US military into World War II brought with it the need for testing four million recruits for military assignments. Once again, a national crisis produced a surge of testing emphasis which propelled psychological testing from academic or clinical environments into the larger culture. A similar peacetime surge occurred in the Cold War with a strong focus on achievement and aptitude testing when the space race was initiated with the launch of the Russian satellite Sputnik. These intelligence, aptitude, and achievement tests fall into the general category of cognitive testing [10].

Objective Tests

In a different line of development, another contribution out of the WWI era was the self-report inventory that formed the basis for objective personality testing. Robert Woodworth's personal data sheet was developed too late for military use in the war but was used afterwards in civilian life to screen for seriously disturbed individuals. The inventory was basically a self-report of recognized symptoms associated with psychiatric problems. This approach culminated in the 1943 publication of the Minnesota Multiphasic Personality Inventory (MMPI). Starke Hathaway, a psychologist, and Charnley McKinley, a psychiatrist, had developed the set of test items empirically by selecting those items that successfully differentiated known patient groups from a general population sample (both genders but all Caucasian samples comprised mostly of hospital visitors, some airline workers, and civilian conservation corps workers in Minnesota). The inventory was remarkable for this use of empirical research that served as a basis for item selection and for its use of three validity scales

designed to measure test taking attitude (defensiveness, exaggeration of symptoms, and subtle defensiveness) [7, 11].

From this line of development has come a wide range of objective tests that provide information about personality traits (e.g., introversion, dominance, and self-constraint); emotional states (anger, anxiety, and depression); behaviors (substance abuse, risk-taking, and antisocial acts); and interpersonal orientation (psychopathy, altruism, and cooperativeness). Often these tests are pencil and paper or computer administered self-report measures that have validity scales to assess manner of self-presentation. As the tests are usually in written form, it is important to assess the examinee's reading level to assure it is sufficient for the task. The results of the tests are thought to be explicit self-representations of the test taker. Test items are seen as stimuli, and self-report statements of endorsement or denial of particular items are seen as responses that define and describe the person. Some tests are also designed to be completed by collateral sources who know the person, and this information can be quite useful in assessment of children or when the examiner wants to know how others perceive the person [3].

Projective Tests

A different approach to personality assessment is the use of projective tests, best typified by the inkblots used by Hermann Rorschach, a Swiss psychiatrist. Others had previously used vague or ambiguous stimuli to elicit a person's responses, which then were interpreted on the basis of the assumption that the subject's internal struggles, fantasies, and needs were being projected onto this ambiguous but neutral stimulus material. Rorschach began experimenting with inkblots around 1910 and established a system for eliciting and scoring responses, which he published along with 10 inkblots in *Psychodiagnostik* (1921).

This line of assessment was further elaborated by the work of Henry Murray in the development of the Thematic Apperception Test (TAT) (picture cards used to elicit short stories from the subject), Goodenough's draw a person test (originally used as an intelligence measure), and various sentence completion or word association tests. Often projective tests are administered directly by the examiner who records responses of the examinee, but some projective tests are also self-administered (house–tree–person drawings and sentence completion tasks). Regardless of the manner of administration, the stimuli are used to evoke behavior that is thought to contain implicit information that must be discovered and interpreted by the trained examiner [12].

Personality Testing

The study of the nature of personality has a long lineage dating back at least to early Greek philosophers and playwrights. In the mid-nineteenth and early twentieth centuries, scientists such as Galton, Wundt, and James moved psychology away from being a philosophical exercise to the study of actual human behavior, many times trading erudite speculation for humble inquiry. Much of the physiological and cognitive research work of the European psychologists was laboratory based study of normal behavior but lacked a theory of person. In contrast was the work of Freud, a psychiatrist who was a seminal figure in the history of personality theory who worked with disturbed patients and searched for a model of the psyche combining understanding of normal and abnormal personality that would fit neurological evolution. His treatment approach and psychoanalytic theory came from his clinical model of inquiry and observation, and his major contributions were related to abnormal personality.

Issues in Personality Test Theory

There remains a basic division in personality research regarding whether personality is known by studying normal or abnormal behavior. In the United States, Gordon Allport studied the individual and the unique combination of the individual's normal traits. Henry Murray (who developed the TAT) studied individual differences seen in normal drives or traits and how they were integrated in the person. Both assumed personality is defined by traits that are independent of psychopathology, but both taught that the individual cannot be understood by fragmenting these traits. Eysenck, who proposed a two factor theory of neuroticism/emotional stability and extroversion/introversion, and Cattell, who developed the 16 Personality Factor (16 PF) test, carried on this line of work that now has given rise to the five factor model of Costa and McCrae [13]. This model is the

basis for the NEO-Personality Inventory (NEO-PI) [14]. In contrast, developers of inventories such as the MMPI [11] or the Personality Assessment Inventory (PAI) [15] have paid more attention to clinical groups and abnormal personality.

Those who attempt to reconcile normal and abnormal personality research must address the question articulated by Paul Meehl as to whether personality traits (enduring characteristics in contrast to temporary states) occur in a dimensional spectrum that ranges from normal to abnormal extremes or occur in categorical divisions (taxons or uniquely different groups). The thinking behind the *Diagnostic and Statistical Manual of Mental Disorders* (DSM) approach to diagnosis assumes distinct categorization. Some trait theorists such as Millon posit a dimensional approach where either extreme of a trait may be pathological [16, 17].

Those who study personality are also divided as to whether traits actually exist independent of models of thought (constructive-realist) and are largely determined by physiology or whether traits are only psychological explanations of behavior, actually determined by social domains affecting expression of biological needs (socioanalytic). The debate comes out in discussion about nature versus nurture causing behavior but goes beyond to attempt to answer whether there are really inherent basic trait domains (such as hardwired extroversion/introversion or even psychopathy) or only differences evident in the way people respond to or cope with biological needs based on social factors [18].

Atheoretical Approaches to Personality Testing

In addition to the trait research, other American work has significantly influenced personality testing from an atheoretical model. Coming out of the medical exam/psychiatric interview methodology, Hathaway (psychologist) and McKinley (psychiatrist) in the 1930s and early 1940s developed the MMPI in an attempt to find an empirically derived test that would differentiate medical patients with psychopathology from normal individuals. Even though self-report methodology, which had been developed by Woodworth in World War I with the Personal Data Sheet, had come to be criticized as too easily manipulated, Hathaway and McKinley used the technique anyway. They collected a large pool of items that were associated with psychiatric and medical symptoms and asked individuals to respond to each by endorsing or denying its occurrence in their own lives. The MMPI authors, aware that responses might be affected by efforts to distort self-presentation, created validity scales to be used in interpretation of scores. They disregarded theoretical constructs and attempted to use only empirical means to identify those particular items that produced scores able to distinguish between specific diagnostic groups of patients and nonpatients. The original hope and early emphasis with the work at the University of Minnesota and later at Menniger Clinic in Kansas was to develop a tool capable of providing psychiatric diagnosis using a practical, empirically derived approach [19, 20].

The work on the MMPI was part of a post-World War II interest in testing. Similar to the demands of WWI, the military during wartime had responded to the task of classifying millions of recruits. After the war, in the United States there was a large number of nonmedically trained mental health providers, mainly clinical psychologists, who were equipped and ready to apply science, which had been optimistically embraced by the nation, to the study and treatment of mental health problems. Testing was valued in clinical, educational, industrial, and correctional settings and was seen as a way to bring efficiency, empiricism, and objectivity to tasks in these fields.

During the rise and reign of behaviorism (1960s and early 1970s), there was strong challenge to the concept of "personality", something that was intangible and considered an unnecessary and useless myth in explaining behavior. There was no need for the concept of "self" as there was exclusive focus on what an organism did in response to particular stimuli. Testing did not go away, but there was a much stronger emphasis on behavioral assessment – identifying particular behaviors of interest and recording the circumstances and frequency of their occurrence. In the past few decades, there has been modification of this model that now includes cognitive as well as behavioral aspects of assessment and treatment [21]. With this cognitive-behavioral approach there is focus on specific assessment using specialized instruments (Beck Depression Inventory and Beck Anxiety Inventory) that make no effort to describe the person as an integrated personality or even to provide a comprehensive clinical picture. Some have suggested that these brief rating scales and inventories, which are limited in scope, represent a third type

of personality assessment: rapid personality assessment instruments [3].

Currently, in many settings outside the teaching or research environments, comprehensive personality assessment is often not seen as important or is not viewed as essential even if important. In addition, managed care of mental health services has often taken a restrictive stance toward more comprehensive testing. A survey of psychologists assumed to be in private practice found that 25% did not do personality testing at all. Of the ones who did such testing at least sometimes, about half used one or both of the two widely recognized tests (MMPI and Rorschach Inkblots) although the most utilized personality test reported was sentence completion [21].

Current Psychological Test Usage

Other surveys of psychologists have likewise documented a decided trend toward less testing in recent years. Psychologists in 1959 said 44% of their time was spent in assessment, but that figure was down to 22% in 1982. In 1971, 5 of the top 10 most often used psychological tests were projective personality tests; 1 was an objective personality test (MMPI), and 3 others were IQ tests. The core of the most popular tests remained stable through the early 1990s, but the amount of time devoted to assessment declined markedly. By the end of the decade, a study on test usage conducted for the American Psychological Association (APA) found fewer than 20% of clinical psychologists spent as much as 5 hours a week doing testing although about three-quarters of neuropsychologists spent at least that much time testing. Of those clinical psychologists with at least 5 hours a week devoted to testing, approximately 40% of their service was devoted to IQ or achievement testing and one-third to personality testing.

Neuropsychological testing was the next highest category of time spent (about 20%) but was (as expected) the major use of time for neuropsychologists who also spent about 20% of their time doing personality assessment. The MMPI/MMPI-2 was the most widely used test in the combined two groups with an IQ test (Wechsler Adult Intelligence Scale-Revised (WAIS-R)) placing second overall. Clinical psychologists also tended to use the Rorschach Inkblots (ranked fourth), but neuropsychologists did not (ranked eighteenth). No other personality tests were popular with neuropsychologists, but at least half of clinical psychologists in the survey used the TAT (ranked sixth in frequency of use) [22].

Psychological Testing in Forensic Context

In addition to neuropsychology, another area of psychology that relies heavily on assessment and testing is forensic psychology. A survey of state directors of mental health resulted in information for 41 state corrections departments. Of those responding, 40 used testing at intake while 25 used it also for pre-parole work-ups. Of those testing at intake, 26 (65%) used MMPI/MMPI-2, 18 (45%) used intelligence tests, and five (12.5%) used Rorschach Inkblots in their department protocols. Of the 25 using testing for preparole evaluations, 24 (96%) used MMPI/MMPI-2, eight (32%) used intelligence tests, and nine (36%) used Rorschach Inkblots [23].

Results of a survey of 152 forensic psychologists who were members of American Psychology-Law Society (AP-LS) or diplomates of the American Board of Forensic Psychology (ABFP) indicated they averaged 56% of their time doing forensic work, presumably largely assessment, with almost a third (29%) being spent in actual testing. When asked about most frequently used tests in particular types of adult assessments, the top five in order of weighted frequency of usage across referral questions were: MMPI-2, one of the Wechsler intelligence or memory, one of the Hare Psychopathy Checklist versions (*see* **Psychopathy Checklists**) Structured Interview of Reported Symptoms (SIRS), and PAI [24].

Another survey of 64 diplomates of ABFP asked which tests were considered acceptable for use in six areas of forensic assessment. Across areas, both the MMPI-2 and the Wechsler Adult Intelligence Scale, Third Edition (WAIS III) showed strong acceptance as did the PAI to a lesser but still major degree. The Millon Clinical Multiaxial Inventory, Third Edition (MCMI-III) was rated as acceptable in only one area (mental status at time of offense). The Rorschach *inkblots* was rated as unacceptable by the majority (52–60%) of the respondents in five of the six areas (equivocal for use in exploration of mental status at time of offense) while other projective tests were deemed unacceptable in all areas by a significant majority (60–95%). Two neuropsychological batteries (Halstead-Reitan and Luria-Nebraska) were reported to be acceptable in half of the areas as was another IQ test (Standford-Binet) [25].

Forensic Assessment: Psychology and Law

Historical Developments

Hugo Munsterberg, considered the founder of applied psychology, was the first director of the psychology lab at Harvard after leaving the University of Leipzig where he had been a student of Wilhelm Wundt. He was an early pioneer of the study of eyewitness testimony and a strong advocate of application of psychology to law. In his book *On the Witness Stand* (1908), he chastised attorneys and judges for not embracing the research findings of psychology and using them in the courtroom. He was strongly criticized and his ideas mocked, but in the 1920s law schools began hiring psychologists to teach courses. Psychology was involved in courts largely in relation to treatment and disposition of children, and psychiatrists were more involved with competency and sanity questions. But psychologists and other social scientists were involved in Brandeis briefs, the most famous being the work of Kenneth Clark and colleagues in *Brown v. Board of Education* (1954) [26]. Only after *Jenkins v. United States* (1962) [27] was the way open for psychologists to provide expert testimony on mental health issues.

Other more recent legal rulings that have significantly impacted the practice of forensic psychology have been *Daubert v. Merrell Dow Pharmaceuticals, Inc.* (1993) [28], which replaced *Frye* (1923) criteria and defined the standards for consideration of scientific expert testimony; *General Electric v. Joiner* (1997) [29], which established the authority for the trial judge to determine what proffered testimony met *Daubert* standards; and *Kumho Tire Co., LTD v. Carmichael* (1999) [30], which expanded *Daubert* criteria to other fields of technical and specialized knowledge. Although these rulings only apply to federal courts, states have their own case law decisions in these areas [31].

Prevalence of Forensic Psychological Assessment

No data were found that indicate the current extent of psychological assessment utilization by US courts, but a conservative estimate of Competency to Stand

Trial evaluations in 1993 was 50 000 [32]. A more recent work cited research indicating 4–7% of criminal cases involved referral for these competency evaluations, the most prevalent mental health evaluation for criminal courts [33]. Civil courts often refer custody case participants for psychological evaluations, and personal injury cases frequently involve mental health expert testimony. Although the data are not available, it is obvious that a significant number of legal cases involve psychological or other mental health assessment. This reliance on psychology appears to be growing as evident with the publication of this volume that verifies Munsterberg's foresight.

The practice of forensic psychology, which is heavily dependent on psychological research and assessment tools, is one of the speciality areas in which the American Board of Professional Psychology (ABPP) offers board certification or diplomate status. The APA Division 41 (AP-LS) is devoted to exploration of the interface of psychology and law. Several well respected, refereed journals (including *Law and Human Behavior; Behavioral Sciences and the Law; Psychology, Public Policy, and Law*) are devoted exclusively to publication of research in this area of disciplinary overlap.

Tensions between Clinical and Forensic Assessment Perspectives

Forensic assessment in some important ways differs from traditional clinical assessment as discussed by Melton *et al.* [34], Heilbrun [35], and Archer *et al.* [31]. Some of the major ways include purpose, scope, and understanding of who is being served (broad understanding of purpose and scope in mental health evaluation where examinee is also the client being served versus forensic assessment addressing specific legal or quasilegal question(s) regarding the examinee to assist the decision maker who is considered the client). In addition, forensic examinees are frequently mandated for an evaluation and often assumed to have significant reasons to be purposefully selective in self-disclosure so that a much stronger focus must be placed on examiner objectivity and assessment of examinee's response style (pattern of self-presentation). Because of the threats of conscious deception or selective self-presentation in forensic evaluations, there is more emphasis on use of multiple sources of data to create hypotheses or to verify information as well as strong reliance on external

sources (collateral observations, historical records, and reports of others) apart from the formal assessment interactions with the examinee.

While there are some instruments specifically developed for forensic use, these tend to be structured interviews, rating scales, or tests designed for use with a particular legal application in mind (e.g., Competence Assessment Instrument for Standing Trial (CAI), Psychopathy Checklist-Revised (PCL-R), and Competence Assessment for Standing Trial for Defendants with Mental Retardation (CAST/MR)). Quite frequently other instruments, developed for nonforensic purposes, are used in a forensic assessment because of the vast research on the instruments, validity indicators built into some of the instruments, or ability for these tests to contribute to a broad understanding of the person to develop hypotheses related to factors bearing on the legal question(s). Obvious examples would include well researched personality tests, tests of malingering, and cognitive tests including IQ measures. When any test is considered for forensic evaluation, these factors are important to consider: sufficient research and norms with a population similar to that of the examinee, adequate test development and psychometric properties, and ability to link test results to conclusions regarding the referral question [35].

A major risk inherent with use of clinical tests is overinterpretation of results where adequate validity research (relating test scores to real world conditions or outcomes) does not demonstrate clear connections between the test data and specific legal question(s) [34]. This problem was pointed out in a marked way by Jay Ziskin and David Faust, two psychologists, in the 1970s and 1980s (*Coping with Psychiatric and Psychological Testimony; The Limits of Scientific Reasoning*). They criticized mental health providers for going beyond the data and research by offering forensic opinions based on personal impressions rather than scientific conclusions. As a more recent writer noted, the task should be to provide "the best that psychology has to offer but also to be candid about the limits of our science and our expertise" (p. 131) [36].

Tensions between Psychological and Legal Perspectives

Even though psychologists are often used to conduct assessments and to provide relevant information to the courts about psychological factors having a bearing on legal issues, there remains basic tension between psychology (which is experimental, descriptive, and probabilistic in its orientation to pursue scientific truth) and law (which is adversarial, prescriptive, and decisive in its orientation to pursue social and individual justice) [34, 37]. Psychology operates from a perspective of determinism (i.e., behavior can be predicted by some combination of genetic, biological, social, interpersonal, and environmental factors) whereas law operates on an assumption of free will (i.e., behavior is the result of personal choice and responsibility as each person is a free moral agent).

Other differences are evident as law applies broad terminology to specific cases, and psychology seeks to define and operationalize terminology into quantifiable form. Questions arise about legal terms for which there are no operational definitions either in law or psychology (e.g., reasonable degree of certainty pertaining to professional opinions, best interest of the child, reasonable degree of rational understanding for competency, unable to appreciate the nature and quality or wrongfulness of acts for criminal responsibility) or where the meaning of words or use of concepts differ (insanity as a legal construct and psychosis as a mental health concept). Despite the sometimes ill-fit of the two systems of thought, courts continue to rely on psychologists for help; and psychologists continue to explore better ways to respond to the task by developing methods to tie psychological data to legal constructs in a rational manner that can be logically followed [38].

Brief Overview of Major Personality Tests

Minnesota Multiphasic Personality Inventory (MMPI and MMPI-2)

The original 550 items and norms were developed by Hathaway and McKinley in the 1930s, mostly with patients and visitors at the University of Minnesota Hospital. The instrument was developed to aid in psychiatric and medical screening [7]. A revision (MMPI-2) was published in 1989 with updated items (66 modified, 90 omitted, and 107 newly created) and contemporary norms (2600 subjects of which 5% were current psychiatric patients). Individuals in the new norm group were from seven states representing a geographic diversity and were roughly balanced for gender (56% female).

Although ethnic and socioeconomic diversity was sought, Hispanic and Asian American groups are underrepresented in the norms. The normative sample is also skewed with college graduates comprising a larger percentage than is present in the US population [20]. The current 567 item true/false inventory requires an eighth grade reading level according to the 1989 version of the manual or a sixth grade reading level according to the revised edition of the test manual published in 2001 [11]. In addition to the original three validity scales (L, F, K), there are now several others measuring tendency to acquiesce, marking responses randomly, or subtly presenting self in a consciously distorted manner. Although well respected and popularly used, the inventory is criticized for its scales being too highly intercorrelated and therefore not distinct because many items are used simultaneously for scoring on different scales.

The MMPI was originally constructed for diagnostic classification purposes, but it proved to be disappointing in that regard when used in replication studies. Meehl was influential in adapting interpretation to a larger context by focusing on patterns of scores (profiles) and code types (based on scores of highest scales in a person's profile). These profiles and code types were researched to provide psychiatric descriptions for the major groups. While code type or group profile descriptions came to be widely used, research revealed problems with temporal instability of the code types when individuals were retested [19].

Another way of using test results from the MMPI has grown through the development and use of content scales, which are comprised of items that seem to be consistently related to a similar construct. This approach led to content scales providing descriptive rather than diagnostic information about a person and has more recently led to innovations such as Restructured Clinical (RC) scales (basic clinical scales with a general demoralization factor removed) and Restructured Form (MMPI-2-RF) with RC scales and newly developed specific problem (content) scales in a shorter version. These innovations also removed the use of K-corrections in calculating scores and removed item overlap within the basic scales [19].

Personality Assessment Inventory (PAI)

The PAI, a self-report inventory comprised of 344 items to which a person marks one of four choices about how well each item applies to self, produces scores on 22 scales and 31 conceptually derived sub-scales. Scales were devised based on content and internal consistency and no item is scored on more than one major scale. Raw scores are transformed to T-scores using norms from a group of 1000 community dwelling subjects matching 1995 US census projections. Comparison clinical norms are also available based on a group of 1246 patients. Construction of the PAI was based on the assumption that normal personality constructs are distributed for both patients and nonpatients according to a bell-shaped (normal) curve. However, abnormal symptoms and constructs differ markedly within the two populations and occur very infrequently in the general population. The PAI requires a fourth grade reading level. It has four validity scales measuring positive and negative self-presentation, random responding, and overendorsement of unusual items [15, 39].

NEO-Personality Inventory-Revised (NEO-PI-R)

A third objective personality measure is the NEO-Personality Inventory-Revised (NEO-PI-R) that measures five basic stable dimensions of personality based on the work of Tupes and Christal who analyzed data that had been collected by Cattell in his work on normal personality traits. These personality domains are neuroticism, extroversion, openness to ideas, agreeableness, and conscientiousness. These five scales each have six subscales that have been developed by logical and factor analytic strategies utilizing known research on normal personality traits. This inventory is comprised of 240 items marked with one of five possible responses (strongly disagree to strongly agree). It contains no validity scales. Norms were developed using 500 males and 500 females selected to match 1995 US census projections. Forms are available for both self-rating and ratings by collateral persons who know the examinee [13, 14].

Rorschach Inkblots

This projective test, a standard set of 10 inkblots, was published by Swiss psychiatrist Hermann Rorschach in 1921 and is based on the assumption that personality can best be assessed through analysis of responses to ambiguous stimuli. Such implicit knowledge is less confounded by conscious distortion than is explicit information obtained by self-report. The assumption

is that self-report only describes behavior, but this projective task actually produces behavior that can be observed, recorded, scored, and analyzed. Over the next five decades after Rorschach's publication, several different systems for scoring and interpretation emerged in both Europe and the United States. John Exner, influenced by Meehl's writings about actuarial rather than intuitive approaches to test interpretation, set out to standardize rules for scoring responses so that empirical data could be developed and used in interpretation. His comprehensive system of coding caught on and has largely shaped the use of this instrument since its introduction in the mid-1970s. Use of Exner's system [40] leads to specific data that can be related to norms and empirical research to provide information about a person's ability to control stress; ways to process information or make sense of the world; patterns of thinking about self and the world; emotional state; and ways of perceiving events and relationships.

Despite criticisms and disfavor of projective tests in general, the Rorschach Inkblots, especially when scored and interpreted using the Exner system, has remained a respected instrument for personality assessment and has passed *Daubert* scrutiny enabling expert testimony based on its findings. It provides limited information about diagnosis with the notable exception of thought disorder but provides a wealth of information to enable an understanding a person as an individual [41].

Other Resources

Clinical and forensic uses of these and other personality tests are discussed at length in Butcher [42, 43], Goldstein [44], Meyer and Deitsch [45], Maruish [46], Strack [47], and Archer [48].

References

[1]   Vanden Bos, G.R. (ed) (2007). *APA Dictionary of Psychology*, American Psychological Association, Washington, DC.

[2]   American Psychological Association (1999). *Standards for Educational and Psychological Testing*, American Psychological Association, Washington, DC.

[3]   Adams, R.L. & Culbertson, J.L. (2000). Personality assessment: Adults and children, in *Kaplan & Sadock's Comprehensive Textbook of Psychiatry*, 4th Edition, B.J. Sadock & V.A. Sadock, eds, Lippincott, Williams, & Wilkins, Philadelphia, pp. 702–722.

[4] King, R.A., Schwab-Stone, M.E., Peterson, B.S. & Theis, A.P. (2000). Psychiatric examination of the infant, child, and adolescent, in *Kaplan & Sadock's Comprehensive Textbook of Psychiatry*, 4th Edition, B.J. Sadock & V.A. Sadock, eds, Lippincott, Williams, & Wilkins, Philadelphia, pp. 2558–2586.

[5] Meyer, G.J., Finn, S.E., Eyde, L.D., Kay, G.G., Kubiszyn, T.W., Moreland, K.L., Eisman, E.J. & Dies, R.R. (1998). *Benefits and Costs of Psychological Assessment in Healthcare Delivery: Report of the Board of Professional Affairs Psychological Assessment Work Group, Part I*, American Psychological Association, Washington, DC.

[6] Sattler, J.M. (2001). *Assessment of Children, Cognitive Applications*, 4th Edition, Author, Jerome M. Sattler, San Diego.

[7] Anastasi, A. (1988). *Psychological Testing*, 6th Edition, Macmillan, New York.

[8] Boake, C. (2002). From the Binet-Simon to the Wechsler-Bellevue: Tracing the history of intelligence testing, *Journal of Clinical and Experimental Neuropsychology* **24**, 383–405.

[9] Geisinger, K.F., Spies, R.A., Carlson, J.F. & Blake, B.S. (eds) (2007). *The Seventeenth Mental Measurements Yearbook*, Buros Institute of Mental Measurements, Lincoln. Also accessible online at http://www.unl.edu/buros/.

[10] Haney, W. (1981). Validity, vaudeville, and values: A short history of social concerns over standardized testing, *The American Psychologist* **36**, 1021–1034.

[11] Butcher, J., Graham, J., Ben-Porath, Y., Tellegen, A., Dahlstrom, G. & Kaemer, B. (2001). *MMPI-2 (Minnesota Multiphasic Personality Inventory-2) Manual for Administration, Scoring, and Interpretation*, (Revised Edition), University Press, Minneapolis.

[12] Carr, A. (1980). Psychological testing of personality, in *Comprehensive Textbook of Psychiatry, III*, H. Kaplan, A. Freedman & B. Sadock, eds, Williams & Wilkins, Baltimore, pp. 940–966.

[13] Costa Jr, P.T. & McCrae, R.R. (2000). Approaches derived from philosophy and psychology, in *Kaplan & Sadock's Comprehensive Textbook of Psychiatry*, 4th Edition, B.J. Sadock & V.A. Sadock, eds, Lippincott, Williams, & Wilkins, Philadelphia, pp. 638–651.

[14] Costa Jr, P.T. & McCrae, R.R. (1992). *Revised NEO Personality Inventory (NEO-PI-R) and NEO Five Factor Inventory (NEO-FFI) Professional Manual*, Psychological Assessment Resources, Odessa.

[15] Morey, L.C. (1991). *The Personality Assessment Inventory Professional Manual*, Psychological Assessment Resources, Odessa.

[16] Strack, S. (2006). Introduction, in *Differentiating Normal and Abnormal Personality*, S. Strack, ed, Springer, New York, pp. xvii–xxviii.

[17] Halsam, N. & Williams, B. (2006). Taxometrics, in *Differentiating Normal and Abnormal Personality*, S. Strack, ed, Springer, New York, pp. 283–310.

[18] Harkness, A.R. & Hogan, R. (1995). The theory and measurement of traits: Two views, in *Clinical Personality Assessment*, J.N. Butcher, ed, Oxford University Press, New York, pp. 28–41.

[19] Ben-Porath, Y. (2006). Differentiating normal from abnormal personality with the MMPI-2, in *Differentiating Normal and Abnormal Personality*, S. Strack, ed, Springer, New York, pp. 337–382.

[20] Pope, K., Butcher, J. & Seelen, J. (1993). *The MMPI, MMPI-2, and MMPI-A in Court*, American Psychological Association, Washington, DC.

[21] Exner Jr, J.E. (1995). Why use personality tests? A brief historical view, in *Clinical Personality Assessment*, J.N. Butcher, ed, Oxford University Press, New York, pp. 10–18.

[22] Camara, W., Nathan, J. & Puente, A. (2000). Psychological test usage: Implications for professional psychology, *Professional Psychology: Research and Practice* **31**, 141–154.

[23] Gallagher, R.W., Somwaru, D.P. & Ben-Porath, Y. (1999). Current usage of psychological tests in state correctional settings, *Corrections Compendium* **24**, 1–3, 20.

[24] Archer, R.P., Buffington-Vollum, T.K., Stredny, R.V. & Handel, R.W. (2006). A survey of psychological test use patterns among forensic psychologists, *Journal of Personality Assessment* **87**, 84–94.

[25] Lally, S.J. (2003). What tests are acceptable for use in forensic evaluations? A survey of experts, *Professional Psychology: Research and Practice* **34**, 491–498.

[26] Brown v. Board of Education, 347 U.S. 483 (1954).

[27] Jenkins v. United States, 307 F.2d 637 (1962).

[28] Daubert v. Merrell Dow Pharmaceuticals, Inc., 509 U.S. 579 (1993).

[29] General Electric v. Joiner, 522 U.S. 136 (1997).

[30] Kumho Tire Co. Ltd. v. Carmichael, 526 U.S. 137 (1999).

[31] Archer, R.P., Stredny, R.V. & Zoby, M. (2006). Introduction, in *Forensic Uses of Clinical Assessment Instruments*, R.P. Archer, ed, Lawrence Erlbaum, Mahwah, pp. 1–18.

[32] Skeem, J., Golding, S., Cohn, N. & Berge, G. (1998). Logic and reliability of evaluations of competence to stand trial, *Law and Human Behavior* **22**, 529–547.

[33] Stafford, K. (2003). Assessment of competence to stand trial, in *Handbook of Psychology: Vol. 11, Forensic Psychology*, I. Weiner, (Series Editor) A. Goldstein, (Volume Editor), John Wiley, Hoboken, pp. 359–380.

[34] Melton, G.B., Petrila, J., Poythress, N.G. & Slobogin, C. (2007). *Psychological Evaluations for the Courts: A Handbook for Mental Health Professionals and Lawyers*, 3rd Edition, Guilford, New York.

[35] Heilbrun, K. (2001). *Principles of Forensic Mental Health Assessment*, Kluwer Academic, New York.

[36] Nicholson, R.A. (1999). Forensic assessment, in *Psychology and Law: The State of the Discipline*, R. Roesch, S.D. Hart & J.R.P. Ogloff, eds, Kluwer Academic, New York, pp. 121–173.

[37] Ogloff, J.R.P. & Finkelman, D. (1999). Psychology and law: an overview, in *Psychology and Law: The State of the Discipline*, R. Roesch, S.D. Hart & J.R.P. Ogloff, eds, Kluwer Academic, New York, pp. 1–20.

[38] Grisso, T. (2003). *Evaluating Competencies: Forensic Assessments and Instruments*, 2nd Edition, Kluwer Academic, New York.

[39] Morey, L.C. & Hopwood, C.J. (2006). The Personality Assessment Inventory and the measurement of normal and abnormal personality constructs, in *Differentiating Normal and Abnormal Personality*, S. Strack, ed, Springer, New York, pp. 451–471.

[40] Exner Jr, J.E. (2003). *The Rorschach: A Comprehensive System*, 4th Edition, John Wiley, Hoboken.

[41] Ganellen, R.J. (2006). Rorschach assessment of Normal and Abnormal Personality, in *Differentiating normal and abnormal personality*, S. Strack, ed, Springer, New York, pp. 473–500.

[42] Butcher, J.N. (ed) (1995). *Clinical Personality Assessment*, Oxford University Press, New York.

[43] Butcher, J.N. & Miller, K.B. (2006). Personality assessment in personal injury litigation, in *The Handbook of Forensic Psychology*, 3rd Edition, A.K. Hess & I.B. Weiner, eds, John Wiley, New York, pp. 140–166.

[44] Goldstein, A. (ed) (2007). *Forensic Psychology: Emerging Topics and Expanding Roles*, John Wiley, Hoboken.

[45] Meyer, R.G. & Deitsch, S.E. (1996). *The Clinician's Handbook: Integrated Diagnostics, Assessment, and Intervention in Adult and Adolescent Psychopathology*, 4th Edition, Allyn and Bacon, Boston.

[46] Maruish, M.E. (ed) (2004). *The Use of Psychological Testing for Treatment Planning and Outcomes Assessment*, 3rd Edition, Lawrence Erlbaum, Mahwah.

[47] Strack, S. (ed) (2006). *Differentiating Normal and Abnormal Personality*, Springer, New York.

[48] Archer, R.P. (ed) (2006). *Forensic Uses of Clinical Assessment Instruments*, Lawrence Erlbaum, Mahwah.

PAUL ANDREWS

Psychological Trauma *see* Posttraumatic Stress Disorder

Psychopathology *see* Compulsion, Firesetting

Psychopathology: Terms and Trends

Introductoin

Society cannot exist without norms, and yet the definition of what is normal proves to be a thorny task for both social science and the field of mental health. In particular, at the interface of behavioral sciences and the law, forensic assessment requires clarity regarding threshold issues in the determination of the presence or absence of pathology and psychical suffering. Whether societal norms are identical to norms of psychical functioning or whether these two norms diverge from one another in specific and definable ways, the line between mental health and mental illness always necessarily implies an appreciation of the individual's ability to function effectively within his environment.

This environment, however, is not a biological one but rather is societal. An individual's ability to function in the social environment is mediated through his subjective interpretation of its laws and imposed constraints, that is, his perception of and ability to integrate norms. A forensic evaluator's role is precisely to introduce and assess this subjective point of view within the parameters of legal proceedings; parameters are designed to apply to all cases equally while providing for individual differences.

Norms and Normality

Psychopathology refers to the description, explanation, and logical formulation of the individual's mental state and mental processes, with the aim of characterizing abnormalities or guiding interventions in the context of treatment. Psychoanalysis has traditionally played an important role in psychopathology, along with cognitive science, neurobiology, and epidemiology (the study of diseases within populations). The overarching aim of psychopathology is the task of demarcating mental health and mental illness, two concepts whose meanings are inextricably bound up with one another, in reference to a norm.

In an article in the September 1967 issue of *Archives of General Psychiatry*, Sabshin outlines four perspectives on normality: (i) normality as health or adequate functioning; (ii) normality as utopia or optimal functioning; (iii) normality as average or statistically common behavior; and (iv) normality as process or constant redefinition of the human condition relative to advances in civilization [1]. Canguilhem offers an additional viewpoint, defining normality as the individual's capacity to adjust his relationship to the environment toward the restitution of a norm, when confronted with "error" or deviation due to an anomaly or defect [2].

As cited by Sabshin, Freud's work, *Civilization and its Discontents* [3], describes civilization's impact on human nature as an intrinsic potential source of pathology. The imposition of culture upon the biological organism necessarily induces discomfort, though not always illness. To the extent that society's norms are evolving and imperfect, absolute conformity to such norms would entirely efface the individual's initiative. Normality, thus involves the negotiation of desires within social parameters and the law.

Values, Theory, and the Problem of Stigma

In the previously cited issue of *Archives of General Psychiatry*, medical sociologist Strauss argued that deviant behavior becomes pathological through "visibility," through public attention [4]. Deviant behavior is assigned significance through societal attribution of harm or potential harm – a judgment of value. The process of distinguishing between deviant behaviors that are due to mental health problems and behaviors that are not due to mental pathology has been subject to complex debate.

Wakefield [5, 6] is a key contemporary author in this debate, who introduced the concept of *harmful dysfunction* as a criterion for disorder. Although a detailed summary of the debate is beyond the scope of this article, the concept of harmful dysfunction has gained credence and acceptance and requires elaboration. Among other topics, Wakefield has addressed the advantages of an approach to diagnosis that emphasizes the development of a common vocabulary for improved communication between clinicians and for research purposes, and which thereby allows for the clarification of causation of symptoms using multiple explanatory theories.

Wakefield developed the concept of harmful dysfunction in response to a lack of clarity regarding the definition of a "disorder." Although clinicians utilize the concept of disorder and are able to reach a consensus about what is and is not a disorder, the formulation of an operational definition of disorder remains problematic. The concept of harmful dysfunction involves two separate elements, both of which must be present in order for there to be a mental disorder. First, there must be *harm* of some kind to the individual or others. This is a value judgment, in reference to societal norms. However, harm alone would not define a mental disorder, since many forms of harmful behavior are simply social evaluative judgments. The second element *dysfunction* implies a cause that is in some way internal to the functioning of the individual – in other words, a disturbance of an evolutionary capacity from which the resulting harmful behavior flows. If there is dysfunction but no harm, then there is no disorder. Similarly, if there is harm but no dysfunction, there is no mental disorder.

Klein agrees with Wakefield and adds the "involuntary" nature of the dysfunction [7]. In a disorder, harm arises from a process that occurs without the individual choosing it. Spitzer remarks that the current diagnostic criteria may be overly inclusive of nonpathological syndromes, and that the testing of diagnostic criteria according to the harmful dysfunction analysis would result in more precise definitions of disorders. With regards to adjustment disorder (symptoms which arise in the context of life stressors) he writes, "the degree of distress … is a poor marker for discriminating disorder from nondisorder. What would be more helpful would be the issue of whether the individual's response to the stressor helped or hindered the individual in dealing with the stressor. … If the reaction, even if associated with marked distress, facilitated dealing appropriately with the stressor, then a judgment of nondisorder would be appropriate." [8].

Separation of harm from dysfunction as components of mental disorder allows for clarification of the nature of psychopathology, as defined by norms that are not entirely determined by judgments of social value. The definition of disorder as a combination of harmful manifestations and underlying dysfunction may reduce the tendency toward stigmatization of the mentally disordered person, since disorder is, thus, attributed neither to social norms nor to causes that are beyond the individual's control [9].

Diagnostic and Statistical Manual of Mental Disorders, 4th Edition, Text Revision (DSM-IV-TR)

In the United States, there is consensus by mental health forensic experts on the use of the American Psychiatric Association's *Diagnostic and Statistical Manual of Mental Disorders* (DSM) for attribution of diagnoses in legal proceedings, despite the fact that the DSM explicitly indicates that it is not designed for this purpose [10]. The first edition was issued in 1952, and involved narrative, descriptive paragraphs according to categories from the psychoanalytic orientation of psychopathology at that time. The second edition, with some revisions, was issued in 1968 and continued the previous edition's characterization of disorders through narrative paragraphs. A major conceptual shift occurred in 1980 with the release of the third edition, shaped in parallel with the research diagnostic criteria (RDC), which identified disorders according to specific criteria, which were required in order to assign the diagnosis. This was a significant step in the international standardization of diagnosis for the purposes of biomedical research, and the DSM was also applied in clinical and public mental health settings [11]. The strict set of criteria present for establishing a diagnosis were designed to focus on the phenomenology, or symptom description, rather than the underlying theory or causal explanation of the symptoms.

The same conceptual basis was retained in subsequent revisions, the DSM-III-R (R for revised), the DSM-IV and the DSM-IV-TR (TR for text revision, indicating that the accompanying text was updated without changing the criteria). However, the two editions of the DSM-IV emphasized empirical evidence, including field trials of the diagnostic criteria and classification, as well as data from published research [12]. A dramatically different system of classification, with a new conceptual basis, is likely in the forthcoming fifth edition of the DSM (see below).

The DSM-IV-TR divides mental disorders into broad categories and defines within each grouping a set of specific disorders with symptom lists and other criteria that must be met in order to assign the diagnosis. While some diagnoses are excluded or superseded by the presence of symptoms meeting criteria for another disorder, other diagnoses allow for the presence of multiple other disorders, sometimes with overlapping symptoms. Although the definitions require clinical judgment in assigning diagnosis, the method of arriving at a diagnosis specifies that if the clinical manifestations do not meet all of the necessary criteria for a given diagnosis, the diagnosis cannot be assigned.

For this reason, many clinically significant syndromes do not fit into specific DSM disorders, and the DSM provides for these through "not otherwise specified" diagnoses within each large category. The "not otherwise specified" diagnoses generally focus on a predominant symptom, such as anxiety or depressed mood, and indicate that such symptoms are present, without the individual meeting full criteria for a specific disorder. Diagnoses with the suffix "not otherwise specified" should not be taken to be less meaningful than specific diagnoses, since the individual's level of impairment may be as significant as that of a person who meets the criteria for a specific diagnosis. The reality of clinical practice suggests that disorders arise on a continuum with gradations from subtle to more severe and marked manifestations; the existence of "not otherwise specified" diagnoses reflects the reality that some symptomatic individuals with clinically significant distress or impairment do not fit neatly into the criteria which define research categories, but nevertheless closely resemble them.

The International Classification of Diseases, 10th Edition (ICD-10)

The International Classification of Diseases (ICD) includes diagnostic codes and criteria for all medical disorders, including mental health disorders [13]. The ninth version of the ICD was finalized 1 year after the task force for DSM-III was formed, without coordination of the criteria or nomenclature [14]. The preparation for a 10th edition of the ICD began well in advance of the work of the DSM-IV task force, making it impossible for the two systems to become identical [15]. During the subsequent development of the ICD-10 and the DSM-IV, international groups worked to improve the concordance between the two [15]. When both systems of classification are present in legal proceedings (e.g., where expert opinions are expressed in terms of DSM-IV-TR criteria and medical records contain ICD-10 coding), possible differences in specific criteria used to assign diagnoses should be clarified.

Beyond the Clinical Interview

Although the clinical interview and the mental status examination (*see* **Mental Status: Examination**) form the basis of diagnostic assessment, the examiner often has recourse to additional information, including documents, such as prior hospital records. Some of the criteria required for assigning a DSM diagnosis are difficult to confirm or disaffirm through the evaluee's self-report of symptoms or past behavior alone.

Parallel History

Some disorders are characterized by a lack of awareness of symptoms. Individuals with disorders such as schizophrenia or a personality disorder often manifest symptoms that they themselves are unable to perceive. Their symptoms are more readily perceived by others in their entourage. For this reason, information obtained from sources other than the evaluee (family members, employers, or the individual's treating physician) may be of value in determining the nature of the psychopathology. In addition, diagnostic criteria for some disorders include the time course of symptoms, and parallel history obtained from family members or others may be useful, for example, in confirming whether or not the symptoms of schizophrenia have been present for six months or longer, or whether elements suggestive of a personality disorder do in fact represent a life-long pattern, present from the time of childhood or adolescence.

Psychometric Validation

Although a large number of rating scales and standardized diagnostic instruments are available for the assessment of psychopathology (*see* **Psychological Testing**), the use of such techniques is not obligatory in forensic clinical practice for the determination of the presence of a mental disorder. Some examiners routinely administer psychometric tests, whereas others have recourse to them only in cases where there is ambiguity in the examination or where findings in the clinical interview suggest the presence of malingering (*see* **Malingering: Forensic Evaluations**). Caution must be exercised in relying too heavily upon the results of standardized testing, because the results are calibrated upon findings within a defined population as statistical probabilities and not as probabilities

in an individual case. Even reporting of a highly validated and reliable examination such as the Minnesota Multiphasic Personality Inventory-2 (MMPI-2) is usually expressed in terms such as "Individuals with this profile tend to …, " suggesting that the result indicates a trend that is relevant to the particular case only after appreciation in the context of findings upon clinical examination.

However, the diagnosis of a mental defect (*see* **Mental Retardation**) such as mental retardation or dementia (disturbance of memory and either language, motor activity, or complex task completion) (*see* **Neuropsychological Assessment**) does require testing beyond the clinical examination. By definition, these mental defects involve deficits in cognitive function that are sometimes subtle and require detailed evaluation with psychometrically validated techniques. In some cases, dementia may be so evident upon clinical examination that confirmation through specialized testing is unnecessary.

Genetics

Efforts in the field of neurobiology to determine the genetic basis of mental disease (*see* **Genomics and Behavioral Evidence**) have yielded results that are as yet unreliable, though some researchers propose classification of psychopathology on a genetic basis in the future [16–18]. Owing to variability in the expression of genes and environmental factors in disease causation, it appears unlikely that genetic typing will supplant clinical examination as a basis for diagnosis at any time in the near future. Even a disease with strong genetic underpinnings such as schizophrenia is present in both identical twins only approximately 50% of the time [19, 20]. Should genetic evidence in support of a diagnosis become admissible in courts, it will likely have a status similar to that of psychological testing, as data that supplements the clinical impression and not as definitive proof of diagnosis.

Neuroimaging

Recent developments in structural and functional magnetic resonance imaging (MRI) have led some jurisdictions to permit testimony from experts in brain imaging (*see* **Deception: Detection of and Brain Imaging**) as an aid in the assessment of psychopathology, though the future use of such techniques in legal proceedings remains uncertain at the time of writing of this article.

Structural Approaches

The concept of *structure* refers to the underlying organization of internal psychical functioning, at a level beyond what is manifest. Structure is interpreted in different ways by various schools of thought, particularly within psychodynamic psychiatry and psychoanalysis. The notion refers, in general, to latent relationships between different elements of the psyche, viewed as a set [21]. Recent articles utilize the concept of structure to describe the underlying organization of psychopathology, including the integration of temperament, personality, and symptoms [22–24].

Although the various conceptualizations of structure are valuable in clinical practice, they pertain to enduring patterns relating to personality diagnosis and are seldom relevant to specific legal adjudications such as insanity at the time of the criminal act. Structural assessment of a forensic evaluee is challenging under evaluation conditions, since accurate formulation may require serial interviews over a significant period of time. Hypotheses regarding structural diagnosis may lead the forensic examiner to identify traits or historical features that he may then integrate into formulations that are pertinent to criminal mitigation or the assessment of civil damages. In addition, preliminary hypotheses regarding structural diagnosis may lead to further exploration of an individual's points of vulnerability in the setting of assesment of fitness for duty or of risk for future violence.

Psychodynamic Diagnostic Manual (PDM)

In 2006, a task force representing six psychoanalytic organizations published the result of their collaborative effort to develop a system of diagnostic classification to "complement the DSM and ICD efforts of the past 30 years in cataloguing symptoms by explicating the broad range of mental functioning," and with a wider appreciation of the patient as a "whole person" with a complex and rich life history [25]. Prior to the Psychodynamic Diagnostic Manual (PDM), some authors provided cogent psychoanalytic perspectives on DSM-IV diagnoses, reflecting the perceived need for enhanced formulations of the processes underlying descriptive diagnostic categories

[26, 27]. Although the PDM includes syndromes that are recognizable to readers of the DSM-IV, it also describes other syndromes and classifies them in a manner that allows the clinician to find a basis to link diagnoses that are commonly co-occurring. In other words, in the PDM disorders are not considered as separate categories but as identifiable manifestations of the individual's underlying internal functioning.

The PDM is likely to be useful to treating clinicians, but is unlikely to supplant the DSM as a basis for expert opinion, a use for which it is not explicitly intended. The authors state quite clearly that it is not their intention to displace the DSM as a scientific classification necessary for research studies. Only time will determine whether forensic experts will refer to the PDM in supplementing their case formulations when arriving at an opinion or testifying in court. The PDM represents a consensus statement that supports what careful forensic mental health professionals already do – that is to say, to seek in detail the case-specific factors that are at issue in explaining past behavior and the likely future evolution of an individual within his personal history and in terms of idiosyncratic subjective experience.

Dimensional Approaches: the DSM-V and Beyond

Planning for the DSM-V began in 1999 and resulted in the publication in 2002 of *A Research Agenda for DSM-V* [28]. After a review of the existing literature, DSM-V workgroups were formed in 2007, with an aim to publish DSM-V by as early as 2011 [29]. A major conceptual revision of the DSM is anticipated, in light of numerous observations regarding the DSM-IV, which utilizes a *categorical* system of classification of disorders, in which the particular disorder is either present or absent. Clinicians have noted that disorders do not easily conform to such a system, since symptoms that partly meet criteria may result in significant impairments that are susceptible to treatment. Researchers have noted that categorical diagnosis may exclude individuals from studies, resulting in a skewed picture of underlying pathological processes [30].

In order to remedy such difficulties, the DSM-V workgroups began to consider the feasibility of a *dimensional* approach to diagnosis, which would retain the categorical diagnoses currently in use, with modifiers to indicate the milder versions or partial syndromes, which are nonetheless related to the primary diagnosis. This approach is based on the assumption that psychopathology exists on a continuum, although there are characteristics which define a "prototype" of the disorder [31, 32]. Previously, the terms "categorical" and "dimensional" were most widely used in the diagnosis of personality disorders, where a wide range of assessment instruments were developed, alternately defining disorders using strict criteria for determining the presence or absence of a specific entity ("borderline personality disorder" or "antisocial personality disorder") *versus* defining disorder according to the predominance of traits that were deemed to be more or less characteristic of the individual's life pattern. The clarification of relevant dimensions in disorders other than personality disorders is likely to require the development of consensus through empirical study of the types of dimensions most characteristic of the "prototype" for each specific disorder [33, 34].

The DSM-V may also include a reorganization of disorders into *spectra*, of related disorders. Beyond the identification of relevant dimensions for specific disorders, the spectrum approach seeks to group together disorders that share similar underlying processes [35, 36]. For example, pathological gambling, eating disorders, and substance abuse could be conceptualized as disturbances arising from an underlying process of compulsion (*see* **Compulsion**), and these might therefore be more likely to occur together in the same individual.

Although the process of DSM revision is lengthy and careful, including field testing of the criteria prior to finalization, commentators observe that the major conceptual change will likely require further refinement after the DSM-V is published [12, 37]. After extensive discussion, the final published criteria for DSM disorders summarize only the essential findings of the committees. For this reason, the *DSM-IV Sourcebook* [38] – a summary of debates prior to arriving at final criteria – is a useful reference when clarification is needed, and provides further information for assessment of the intended meaning of DSM diagnoses. Hopefully, the DSM-V will also be accompanied by such a companion sourcebook to aid the reader.

Relevance to Legal Proceedings

At first blush, a dimensional approach to the diagnosis of mental disease would appear to be contraindicated in the context of legal proceedings. Case law has defined, for example, what diagnoses are eligible for consideration as a "severe mental disease" leading to criminal nonresponsibility, implying that adjudications require clear thresholds provided by categorical diagnosis. However, closer scrutiny reveals that a dimensional approach is compatible with the process of expert evaluation in cases involving mental disorders, to the extent that forensic opinions do not rely solely upon diagnosis, but rather present the relationship between particular symptoms and specific behavior or distress, along a continuum of severity. A term such as "severe mental disease" is, thus, a legal term of art that can accommodate evolution in the professional standards regarding mental pathology, in accordance with contemporary scientific definitions.

Conclusion

Psychopathology is a complex and evolving field of study, with a long historical tradition that merits a closer examination than is possible in this article. Systems of classification of mental disorders have been constructed in accordance with changing needs and new findings in research. Although manuals such as the DSM and the PDM are commercially available for purchase, works such as these should be viewed as guides for use by mental health professionals in light of their education, experience, and intuition based on clinical reasoning and the specifics of each case. Through research and consensus, it has been possible to define categories of psychopathology using standardized criteria that serve as a common language, across theoretical orientations. However, debate continues as to the adequacy of these categories, particularly given the wide variety of clinical manifestations and underlying mental processes involved in the experience of each person, and efforts are under way to revise the existing classifications in light of new findings.

References

[1]   Sabshin, M. (1967). Psychiatric perspectives on normality, *Archives of General Psychiatry* **17**, 258–264.

[2] Canguilhem, G. (1989). A new concept in pathology: error (1963–1966), *The Normal and the Pathological*, Zone Books, New York.

[3] Freud, S. (1930, 1953). *Civilization and its Discontents* in J. Strachey, ed, *The Standard Edition of the Complete Psychological works of Sigmund Freud*, Hogarth Press and The Institute of Psycho-Analysis, London, Vol. 21.

[4] Strauss, A. (1967). A sociological view of normality, *Archives of General Psychiatry* **17**, 265–270.

[5] Wakefield, J.C. (1997). Diagnosing DSM-IV – Part I: DSM-IV and the concept of disorder, *Behaviour Research and Therapy* **35**(7), 633–649.

[6] Wakefield, J.C. (1999). The concept of disorder as a foundation for the DSM's theory-neutral nosology: response to Follette and Houts, part 2, *Behaviour Research and Therapy* **37**, 1001–1027.

[7] Klein, D.F. (1999). Harmful dysfunction, disorder, disease, illness, and evolution, *Journal of Abnormal Psychology* **108**(3), 421–429.

[8] Spitzer, R.L. (1999). Harmful dysfunction and the DSM definition of mental disorder, *Journal of Abnormal Psychology* **108**(3), 430–432.

[9] Dain, N. (1994). Reflections on antipsychiatry and stigma in the history of American Psychiatry, *Hospital and Community Psychiatry* **45**(10), 1010–1014.

[10] American Psychiatric Association (2000). *Diagnostic and Statistical Manual of Mental Disorders*, 4th Edition, Text Revision, APA Press, Washington, DC, pp. 32–33, 37.

[11] First, M.B. (2002). The DSM series and experience with DSM-IV, *Psychopathology* **35**, 67–71.

[12] Regier, D.A., Narrow, W.E., First, M.B. & Marshall, T. (2002). The APA classification of mental disorders: future perspectives, *Psychopathology* **35**, 166–170.

[13] World Health Organization (1990). *International Classification of Diseases and Related Health Problems*, 10th Revision, Geneva.

[14] Widiger, T.A., Frances, A.J., Pincus, H.A., Davis, W.W. & First, M.B. (1991). Toward an empirical classification for the DSM-IV, *Journal of Abnormal and Social Psychology* **100**(3), 280–288.

[15] Kendell, R.E. (1991). Relationship between the DSM-IV and the ICD-10, *Journal of Abnormal Psychology* **100**(3), 297–301.

[16] Gottesman, I.I. & Gould, T.D. (2003). The endophenotype concept in psychiatry: etymology and strategic intentions, *The American Journal of Psychiatry* **160**, 636–645.

[17] Cannon, T.D. & Keller, M.C. (2006). Endophenotypes in the genetic analyses of mental disorders, *Annual Review of Clinical Psychology* **2**, 267–290.

[18] Bearden, C.E. & Freimer, N.B. (2006). Endophenotypes for psychiatric disorders: ready for primetime? *Trends in Genetics* **22**, 306–313.

[19] Cardno, A.G. & Gottesman, I.I. (2000). Twin studies of schizophrenia: from bow-and-arrow concordances to Star Wars Mx and functional genomics, *The American Journal of Medical Genetics* **97**, 12–17.

[20] Kendler, K.S. (2001). Twin studies of psychiatric illness, *Archives of General Psychiatry* **58**, 1005–1014.

[21] Vandermersch B. (1998). *Structure du Dictionnaire de la Psychanalyse*, R. Chemama & B. Vandermersch, eds, 2nd Edition, Larousse Paris, pp. 407–408.

[22] Clark, L.A. (2005). Temperament as a unifying basis for personality and psychopathology, *Journal of Abnormal Psychology* **114**(4), 505–521.

[23] Cuthbert B.N. (2005). Dimensional models of psychopathology: research agenda and clinical utility, *Journal of Abnormal Psychology* **114**(4), 565–569.

[24] Krueger, R.F., Watson, D. & Barlow, D.H. (2005). Introduction to the special section: toward a dimensionally based taxonomy of psychopathology, *Journal of Abnormal Psychology* **114**(4), 491–493.

[25] PDM Task Force (2006). *Psychodynamic Diagnostic Manual*, Alliance of Psychanalytic Organizations, Silver Spring.

[26] Gabbard, G.O. (2000). *Psychodynamic Psychiatry in Clinical Practice*, 3rd Edition, American Psychiatric Press, Washington, DC.

[27] McWilliams, N. (1994). *Psychoanalytic Diagnosis: Understanding Personality Structure in the Clinical Process*, The Guilford Press, New York.

[28] Kupfer, D.J., First, M.B. & Regier, D.A. (2002). *A Research Agenda for DSM-V*, American Psychiatric Publishing, Washington, DC.

[29] DSM-V website at http://dsm5.org (accessed Nov 4, 2007).

[30] Kraemer, H.C. (2007). DSM categories and dimensions in clinical and research contexts, *International Journal of Methods in Psychiatric Research* **16**(S1), S8–S15.

[31] Jablensky, A. (2005). Categories, dimensions and prototypes: critical issues for psychiatric classification, *Psychopathology* **38**, 201–205.

[32] Widiger, T.A. & Samuel, D.B. (2005). Diagnostic categories or dimensions? A question for the Diagnostic and Statistical Manual of Mental Disorders – Fifth Edition, *Journal of Abnormal Psychology* **114**(4), 494–504.

[33] First, M.B. (2005). Clinical utility: a prerequisite for the adoption of a dimensional approach in DSM, *Journal of Abnormal Psychology* **114**(4), 560–564.

[34] Jablensky A. (2005). Categories, dimensions and prototypes: critical issues for psychiatric classification, *Psychopathology* **38**, 201–205.

[35] Cuthbert, B.N. (2005). Dimensional models of psychopathology: research agenda and clinical utility, *Journal of Abnormal Psychology* **114**(4), 565–569.

[36] Krueger, R.F., Markon, K.E., Patrick, C.J. & Iacono, W.G. (2005). Externalizing psychopathology in adulthood: a dimensional-spectrum conceptualization and its implications for DSM-V, *Journal of Abnormal Psychology* **114**(4), 537–550.

[37] Brown, R.A. & Barlow, D.H. (2005). Dimensional versus categorical classification of mental disorders in the fifth edition of the *Diagnostic and Statistical Manual of Mental Disorders* and beyond: comment on the

special section, *Journal of Abnormal Psychology* **114**(4), 551–556.

[38] Widiger, T.A., Frances, A.J., Pincus, H.A., First, M.B., Ross, R. & Davis, W. (1994). *DSM-IV Sourcebook*, American Psychiatric Association, Washington, DC, 3 Vols.

Suzanne Yang and François Sauvagnat

Psychopathy

Psychopathy or psychopathic personality disorder is referred to as *antisocial personality disorder* in the fourth edition of the *Diagnostic and Statistical Manual of Mental Disorders* or *DSM-IV* [1] and as dissocial personality disorder in the tenth edition of the *International Statistical Classification of Diseases and Related Health Problems* or *ICD-10* [2]. Previously, it was referred to as *sociopathy* or *sociopathic personality disorder*.

Clinical Description

According to clinical descriptions over the past 200 years [3, 4], psychopathy is characterized by a broad range of symptoms in several major domains of personality functioning. In the domain of *behavioral organization*, they include lack of perseverance, unreliability, recklessness, restlessness, disruptiveness, and aggressiveness. The *emotionality* domain includes lack of anxiety, lack of remorse, lack of emotional depth, and lack of emotional stability. The domain of *interpersonal attachment* includes detachment, lack of commitment, and lack of empathy or concern for others. The domain *interpersonal dominance* includes antagonism, arrogance, deceitfulness, manipulativeness, insincerity, and glibness or garrulousness. The *cognitive* domain includes suspiciousness, inflexibility, intolerance, lack of planfulness, and lack of concentration. Finally, the *self* domain includes self-centeredness, self-aggrandizement, self-justification, and a sense of entitlement, uniqueness, and invulnerability.

Assessment and Diagnosis

In the *DSM-IV* and *ICD-10*, the diagnostic criteria for psychopathy focus primarily on symptoms from the behavioral organization domain, especially those related to violation of explicit social norms. In many civil psychiatric settings, these diagnostic criteria have adequate reliability (e.g., stability or consistency across evaluators and time) and validity (e.g., prognostic value with respect to poor treatment response, institutional misbehavior, or community violence) [1, 5]. In forensic settings, however, the *DSM-IV* and *ICD-10* criteria are less useful. Their heavy focus on criminality leads to extremely high prevalence rate – typically 50–75% or higher – in correctional offenders and forensic psychiatric patients [1, 5]. For this reason, many forensic mental health professionals prefer more comprehensive diagnostic criteria, such as the *Hare Psychopathy Checklist Revised* or *PCL-R* [6] and its progeny, such as the *Screening Version* or *PCL:SV* [7] and the *Youth Version* or *PCL:YV* [8]. These latter tests yield a lifetime prevalence rates of ~15 to 25% – about one-third the rate observed using the *DSM* criteria for antisocial personality disorder [5, 6] – and also have superior reliability and validity (*see* **Psychopathy Checklists**).

Course

Symptoms of psychopathy may emerge as early as age 6–10 [9], and it is common for adults with psychopathy to have been diagnosed in childhood or adolescence as suffering from one of the disruptive behavior disorders. Indeed, the *DSM-IV* diagnostic criteria for antisocial personality disorder require that the person met the criteria for a conduct disorder before age 15 [1]. Unfortunately, the majority of children or adolescents so diagnosed – 50 to 75% or more – spontaneously desist antisocial behavior and do not go on to develop psychopathy as adults [9, 10]. Consequently, it is recommended not to diagnose psychopathy before the beginning of early adulthood, at least 18 years old or possibly even 25 years old [1, 2].

The course of the disorder during adulthood is characterized by relative stability. For example, there is evidence of moderate diagnostic stability across periods of several months to several years [6], persistence of symptoms across adulthood [11, 12], and long-term risk for negative health outcomes such as morbidity and mortality [13]. But there is also evidence that symptom severity may fluctuate substantially over time [14].

Prevalence

Epidemiological research in the United States indicates that the lifetime prevalence of psychopathy in the general population, according to *DSM-IV* or similar criteria, is ~1.5 to 3.5% [15, 16]; in correctional offenders, the rate is 50–75% [6].

When more comprehensive diagnostic criteria are used, the prevalence rate is considerably lower. For example, research using the *PCL-R* with correctional offenders and forensic psychiatric patients in the United States has reported lifetime prevalence rates of ~15 to 25% – about one-third the rate observed using the *DSM* criteria [6].

Gender, Age, and Sociocultural Factors

Lifetime prevalence rates of psychopathy vary across three major group factors: gender, age, and culture. First, with respect to gender, the male : female sex ratio in diagnosis is typically about 3 : 1 [15, 16]. This gender difference is not limited to a few clinical features, but is evident across the full range of symptomatology. Second, with respect to age, some epidemiological research in the United States using *DSM-III* and *DSM-III-R* criteria has reported a cohort effect, with higher lifetime prevalence rates in younger generations than in older generations [17]. Third, with respect to culture, anthropological and epidemiological research indicates that psychopathy is found across cultures [18], but there is evidence of cross-cultural differences in prevalence. For example, according to general population studies, the lifetime prevalence of psychopathy in Taiwan is much lower than that reported in the United States [19], and according to studies of correctional offenders and forensic psychiatric patients, the prevalence of psychopathy is higher in the United States than in Europe [20.]

These group differences may be due to *cultural facilitation* [20, 21]. In highly individualistic cultures such as the United States, norms and values that emphasize the importance of distinctiveness, status, self-confidence, honor, competition, and freedom from obligations to others may also foster the development of extreme manifestations of the same characteristics – for example, conceit, manipulativeness, irresponsibility, pathological dominance, and aggressiveness. Similarly, within a dominant culture, the expression of symptoms of psychopathy may be facilitated in certain subgroups, such as males or younger generations, that subscribe to more individualistic norms and values.

The group differences may also be due to inadequacies in diagnostic criteria. The current diagnostic criteria for psychopathy may be biased to reflect its prototypical manifestation in young males from individualistic cultures; if this is true, any differences due to gender, age, and culture may be smaller than suggested by research to date [20].

Comorbidity

Psychopathy has a high rate of comorbidity with substance use disorders [15, 22, 23]. This comorbidity may reflect a common etiological mechanism, or it may be that in some cases substance use disorders are a consequence or complication of psychopathy.

Psychopathy also has a high rate of comorbidity with other personality disorders, specifically, borderline, the Cluster B narcissistic, and histrionic personality disorders in *DSM-IV* or emotionally unstable and histrionic personality disorders in *ICD-10* [24, 25]. The high rate of comorbidity among them almost certainly reflects inadequacies in their diagnostic criteria (i.e., a failure to "carve nature at its joints"), as well as common etiological factors.

Low rates of comorbidity are observed between psychopathy and certain other personality disorders, specifically the Cluster C avoidant, dependent, and obsessive–compulsive personality disorders or anxious/avoidant, dependent, and anankastic personality disorder in *ICD-10* [24, 25]. The low rates of comorbidity among the disorders suggest they have independent or even competing etiologies.

The rates of comorbidity between psychopathy and most other disorders are inconsistent, unclear, or unremarkable [15, 24, 25].

Etiology

The etiology of psychopathy is unknown. Theoretical models of etiology can be divided into two main categories based on whether they view psychopathy as a true disorder, that is, a *bona fide* form of mental abnormality.

Theoretical models of psychopathy as mental abnormality have focused on the potential causal influence of social and biological factors. Overall, the research literature supports the relative importance of biological over social factors. With respect to social factors, there are no child-rearing experiences, familial dysfunctions, or adverse life experiences that are found both frequently and specifically in people with psychopathy compared with people with other personality disorders. As noted previously, however, sociocultural factors certainly appear to play a role in the expression of the disorder [20, 21]. With respect to biological factors, researchers have reported elevated rates of prenatal trauma, neurotransmitter abnormalities, and structural abnormalities of the brain associated with symptoms of psychopathy [26–28], but none of these factors is clearly pathognomonic. Also, some adoption research has reported that the heritability of psychopathy is substantial [11, 29], but molecular genetic research has not identified genetic markers. A common theme underlying many etiological theories that focus on biological factors is that psychopathy is associated with impaired ability to experience emotions and integrate them in executive functions; this core emotional deficit results in a failure of attachment to others, inattention to cues of impending punishment, and insensitivity to reward or punishment.

Other theoretical models reject the notion that psychopathy is a mental abnormality at all. First, some interpersonal and behavioral genetic theories view psychopathy as an extreme variant of the same personality traits found in all people [30, 31]. According to these theories, psychopathy is not associated with any unique or specific causal influences and any differences between people with *versus* without the disorder are quantitative rather than qualitative in nature – that is, the differences are a matter of degree rather than of kind. Second, some sociobiological and evolutionary theories view psychopathy as an adaptation [32]. According to these theories, the human species has the genetic capacity to express traits associated with psychopathy. In sociobiological theories, the genetic capacity exists in only a minority of humans and its manifestation is only partially dependent on environmental circumstances; in evolutionary theories, the genetic capacity exists in all humans, but is manifested in only a minority of

humans who are exposed to specific environmental circumstances. In both the theories, people with psychopathy have an evolutionary advantage in terms of an increased likelihood of producing offspring.

Treatment

There is no methodologically sound research on the treatment of psychopathy, and so there no good evidence that it can be successfully treated [33]. Notwithstanding methodological limitations, there is evidence that psychopathy is associated with increased risk for disruptive behavior during treatment, treatment dropout, and posttreatment recidivism [34].

Forensic Relevance

Psychopathy does not appear to impair cognitive abilities to the extent that it is relevant in the assessment of psycholegal competencies or capacities. With respect to civil-forensic evaluations, psychopathy generally is not considered by either research or law to be relevant to issues such as competence to consent to treatment, enter into contracts, or testify. With respect to criminal forensic evaluations, it is generally not considered relevant to issues such as competence to confess or stand trial, or to ability to form criminal intent.

In contrast, psychopathy does appear to impair volitional abilities to the extent that it is relevant to the assessment of risk for serious crime, and, in particular, for violence. A large body of research indicates that psychopathy is a major risk factor for disruptive behavior while institutionalized and for recidivism upon release to or while under supervision in the community [35, 36]. Explanations include the following [35]:

1. Psychopathy increases the perceived benefits of serious crime. For example, interpersonal symptoms may make demeaning, controlling, and hurting other people rewarding; and behavioral symptoms may make exciting, risk activities rewarding.
2. Psychopathy decreases the perceived costs of serious crime. For example, attachment symptoms, emotional deficit, and self symptoms may

result in failure to be deterred by anxiety, empathy, remorse, or self-punishment.

3. Psychopathy destabilizes general psychosocial adjustment. For example, all symptoms of psychopathy may increase problems in daily living, decrease social integration or cohesion, or otherwise increase interpersonal conflict.

Given the association between psychopathy and serious crime, as well as the lack of demonstrably effective treatment for psychopathy, it is understandable that psychopathy is potentially relevant in a wide range of psycholegal evaluations involving risk for serious crime. With respect to civil-forensic evaluations, psychopathy is relevant to issues such as parental capacity (i.e., risk for child abuse), employee discipline and dismissal (i.e., risk for workplace violence), and civil commitment as a sexually violent predator (i.e., risk for sexual violence). With respect to criminal forensic evaluations, it is relevant to issues such as pretrial release, sentencing, correctional classification, and community registration, notification, and supervision.

References

[1] American Psychiatric Association (1994). *Diagnostic and Statistical Manual of Mental Disorders*, 4th Edition, American Psychiatric Press, Washington, DC.

[2] World Health Organization (1992). *ICD-10: International Statistical Classification of Diseases and Related Health Problems*, 10th Revision, World Health Organization, Geneva.

[3] Arrigo, B. & Shipley, S. (2001). The confusion over psychopathy (I): historical considerations, *International Journal of Offender Therapy and Comparative Criminology* **45**, 325–344.

[4] Berrios, G. (1996). *The History of Mental Symptoms: Descriptive Psychopathology Since the Nineteenth Century*, Cambridge University Press, Cambridge.

[5] Widiger, T.A., Cadoret, R., Hare, R.D., Robins, L.N., Rutherford, M. Zanarini, M., Alterman, A., Apple, M., Corbitt, E., Forth, A.E., Hart, S.D., Kultermann, J., Woody, G. & Frances, A. (1996). DSM-IV antisocial personality disorder field trial, *Journal of Abnormal Psychology* **105**, 3–16.

[6] Hare, R.D. (2003). *Manual for the Hare Psychopathy Checklist – Revised*, 2nd Edition, Multi-Health Systems, Toronto.

[7] Hart, S.D., Cox, D.N. & Hare, R.D. (1995). *Manual for the Hare Psychopathy Checklist: Screening Version (PCL:SV)*, Multi-Health Systems, Toronto.

[8] Forth, A.E., Kosson, D.S. & Hare, R.D. (2003). *Hare Psychopathy Checklist Revised: Youth Version (PCL:YV)*, Multi-Health Systems, Toronto.

[9] Goldstein, R.B., Grant, B.F., Ruan, W.J., Smith, S.M. & Saha, T.D. (2006). Antisocial personality disorder with childhood – vs adolescence-onset conduct disorder: results from the national epidemiologic survey on alcohol and related conditions, *The Journal of Nervous and Mental Disease* **194**, 667–675.

[10] Simonoff, E., Elander, J., Holmshaw, J., Pickles, A., Murray, R. & Rutter, M. (2004). Predictors of antisocial personality: continuities from childhood to adult life, *The British Journal of Psychiatry* **184**, 118–127.

[11] Burt, S.A., McGue, M., Carter, L.A. & Iacono, W.G. (2007). The different origins of stability and change in antisocial personality disorder symptoms, *Psychological Medicine* **37**, 27–38.

[12] Hare, R.D., McPherson, L.E. & Forth, A.E. (1988). Male psychopaths and their criminal careers, *Journal of Consulting and Clinical Psychology* **56**, 710–714.

[13] Repo-Tiihonen, E., Virkkunen, M. & Tiihonen, J. (2001). Mortality of antisocial male criminals, *Journal of Forensic Psychiatry* **12**, 677–683.

[14] Lenzenweger, M.F., Johnson, M.D. & Willett, J.B. (2004). Individual growth curve analysis illuminates stability and change in personality disorder features: the longitudinal study of personality disorders, *Archives of General Psychiatry* **61**, 1015–1024.

[15] Compton, W.M., Conway, K.P., Stinson, F.S., Colliver, J.D. & Grant, B.F. (2005). Prevalence, correlates, and comorbidity of DSM-IV antisocial personality syndromes and alcohol and specific drug use disorders in the United States: results from the national epidemiologic survey on alcohol and related conditions, *Journal of Clinical Psychiatry* **66**, 677–685.

[16] Narrow, W.E., Rae, D.S., Robins, L.N. & Regier, D.A. (2002). Revised prevalence estimates of mental disorders in the United States using a clinical significance criterion to reconcile 2 surveys' estimates, *Archives of General Psychiatry* **59**, 115–123.

[17] Robins, L.N., Tipp, J. & Przybeck, T. (1991). Antisocial personality, in L.N. Robins & D.A. Reiger, eds, *Psychiatric disorders in America: The epidemiological catchment area study*, Free Press, New York, USA, pp. 258–290.

[18] Cooke, D.J. (1996). Psychopathic personality in different cultures: What do we know? What do we need to find out? *Journal of Personality Disorders* **10**, 23–40.

[19] Compton, W.M., Helzer, J.E., Hwu, H.G., Yeh, E.K., McEvoy, L., Tipp, J.E. & Spitznagel, E.L. (1991). New methods in cross-cultural psychiatry: psychiatric illness in Taiwan and the United States, *American Journal of Psychiatry* **148**, 1697–1704.

[20] Cooke, D.J., Michie, C., Hart, S.D. & Clark, D.A. (2005). Searching for the pan-cultural core of psychopathic personality disorder: Continental Europe and North America compared, *Personality and Individual Differences* **39**, 283–295.

[21] Paris, J. (1998). Personality disorders in sociocultural perspective, *Journal of Personality Disorders* **12**, 289–301.

[22] Grant, B.F., Stinson, F.S., Dawson, D.A., Chou, P.S., Ruan, W.J. & Pickering, R.P. (2004). Co-occurrence of 12-month alcohol and drug use disorders and personality disorders in the United States: results from the national epidemiologic survey on alcohol and related conditions, *Archives of General Psychiatry* **61**, 361–368.

[23] Hemphill, J., Hart, S.D. & Hare, R.D. (1994). Psychopathy and substance use, *Journal of Personality Disorders* **8**, 32–40.

[24] Hart, S.D. & Hare, R.D. (1989). Discriminant validity of the psychopathy checklist in a forensic psychiatric population, *Psychological Assessment* **1**, 211–218.

[25] Hildebrand, M. & de Ruiter, C. (2004). PCL-R psychopathy and its relation to DSM-IV Axis I and II disorders in a sample of male forensic psychiatric patients in the Netherlands, *International Journal of Law and Psychiatry* **27**, 233–248.

[26] Coccaro, E.F. (2001). Biological and treatment correlates, in *Handbook of Personality Disorders: Theory, Research and Treatment*, W.J. Livesley, ed, Guilford, New York, pp. 124–135.

[27] Neugebauer, R., Hoek, H.W. & Susser, E. (1999). Prenatal exposure to wartime famine and development of antisocial personality disorder in early adulthood, *Journal of the American Medical Association* **282**, 455–462.

[28] Rainze, A., Lencz, T., Bihrle, S., LaCasse, L. & Colletti, P. (2000). Reduced prefrontal gray matter volume and reduced autonomic activity in antisocial personality disorder, *Archives of General Psychiatry* **57**, 119–127.

[29] Cadoret, R., Troughton, E., Bagford, J. & Woodworth, G. (1990). Genetic and environmental factors in adoptee antisocial personality, *European Archives of Psychiatry and Neurological Sciences* **239**, 231–240.

[30] Livesley, W.J. (1998). The phenotypic and genotypic structure of psychopathic traits, in *Psychopathy: Theory, Research, and Implications for Society*, D.J. Cooke, A.E. Forth & R.D. Hare, eds, Kluwer Academic Publisher, Dordrecht, pp. 69–79.

[31] Miller, J.D., Lynam, D.R., Widiger, T.A. & Leukefeld, C. (2001). Personality disorders as extreme variants of common personality dimensions: can the five-factor model adequately represent psychopathy? *Journal of Personality* **69**, 253–276.

[32] Mealey, L. (1995). The sociobiology of sociopathy: an integrated evolutionary model, *The Behavioral and Brain Sciences* **18**, 523–599.

[33] Dolan, B. & Coid, J. (1993). *Psychopathic and Antisocial Personality Disorders: Treatment and Research Issues*, Gaskell, London.

[34] Hemphill, J.F. & Hart, S.D. (2002). Motivating the unmotivated: psychopathy, treatment, and change, in *Motivating Offenders to Change*, M. Mc Murran, ed, John Wiley & Sons, Chichester, pp. 193–219.

[35] Hart, S.D. (1998). The role of psychopathy in assessing risk for violence: conceptual and methodological issues, *Legal and Criminological Psychology* **3**, 121–137.

[36] Douglas, K.S., Vincent, G.M. & Edens, J.F. (2006). Risk for criminal recidivism: the role of psychopathy, in *Handbook of Psychopathy*, C.J. Patrick, ed, Guilford, New York, pp. 533–554.

Related Articles

Dangerousness: Risk of

Psychopathy Checklists

Risk Assessment: Patient and Detainee

STEPHEN D. HART

Psychopathy Checklists

Psychopathy is a specific form of personality disorder (*see* **Psychopathy**). The *Hare Psychopathy Checklist-Revised (PCL-R)* [1, 2] and the *Screening Version of the Hare Psychopathy Checklist-Revised (PCL:SV)* [3] are standardized psychological tests of lifetime psychopathic symptoms in adults. They have proven to be particularly useful forensic mental health evaluations and are in wide use, both in the original English and in numerous foreign language translations.

History

In the mid-1970s, Robert Hare was dissatisfied with the assessment procedures for psychopathy then in use, as they focused primarily on impulsive, irresponsible, and antisocial behavior and had only low-to-moderate correlations with each other [4]. Hare began work on the development of measures that were more comprehensive and reliable. His first attempt, the *Psychopathy Checklist* (PCL), was distributed informally starting in about 1980 [5] and stimulated considerable interest among researchers and forensic mental health professionals. The manual for the revised PCL, or PCL-R, was published in 1991 [1] and updated in 2004 [2].

Several derivations of PCL-R were developed by Hare and colleagues. One of these was PCL:SV, which is shorter and easier to administer than PCL-R, as well as being appropriate for use in general community and civil psychiatric settings [3]. Development of PCL:SV began in the mid-1980s, concurrent with the revision of the PCL, and a test manual was published in 1995.

Format

PCL-R and PCL:SV are multi-item observer rating scales designed to assess the lifetime presence and severity of psychopathic symptoms. Ratings are based on personal interviews and third-party information (e.g., collateral interviews and official records). Each item reflects a different symptom or characteristic of psychopathy, defined in the test manual, and is rated on a 3-point scale (0 = absent, 1 = present to a limited extent, 2 = present and severe). A small number of items can be omitted if insufficient information is available to rate them. Items are summed (and prorated, if necessary) to yield total scores. Total scores can be interpreted dimensionally, relative to norms from various comparison groups, or cut-off scores can be used to make categorical diagnoses. Items can also be summed to yield factor scores, although these are used primarily for research purposes.

PCL-R is intended for use with adult correctional offenders and forensic psychiatric patients, male or female. It comprises 20 items, some of which reflect pathological personality traits and others that reflect specific forms of antisocial conduct. Item definitions average about 200 words or so in length. Total scores range from 0 to 40; a cut-off score of 30 and higher is used to diagnose psychopathy. Norms are available for a variety of reference groups. Scores can be calculated for two superordinate factors or four subordinate factors.

PCL:SV is intended for use with adults in general community and civil psychiatric settings, in addition to adult correctional offenders and forensic psychiatric patients, male or female. It comprises 12 items, all of which tap relatively broad pathological personality traits. Each item is either a simplified version of a PCL-R item or a combination and simplification of two PCL-R items. Item definitions are shorter than in PCL-R, averaging about 50 words. Total scores

range from 0 to 24, with scores of 18 and higher used to diagnose psychopathy. Norms are available for reference groups of male or female correctional offenders, forensic psychiatric patients, civil psychiatric patients, and community residents. Scores can be calculated for two factors, isomorphic to the superordinate factors of PCL-R.

In forensic settings, PCL:SV can be used in conjunction with PCL-R as a screening test for psychopathy; most evaluators, however, tend to use PCL-R if the person being evaluated has a history of serious criminality (e.g., chronic or long-sentence offenders), and PCL:SV when the person does not (e.g., first-time, short-sentence, or less serious offenders; mentally disordered offenders; and forensic psychiatric patients).

Administration

PCL-R and PCL:SV are usually administered as part of a comprehensive psychodiagnostic evaluation. It takes about 20–30 min to score and interpret PCL-R, and about 10–15 min to score and interpret PCL:SV in these circumstances. Single-use assessment guides are available for both PCL-R and PCL:SV, which include a semistructured interview and space for recording relevant third-party information.

It is possible to administer the tests solely on the basis of third-party information if a person refuses or is otherwise unable to be interviewed, provided the quantity and quality of this information is sufficient. This procedure may, however, result in a score that is substantially lower than would have been obtained if the person had been interviewed.

It is not possible to administer PCL-R or PCL:SV without access to third-party information, except for certain research purposes.

Test User Qualifications

PCL-R and PCL:SV are controlled psychological tests. Independent use of the tests for clinical purposes is limited to people who are legally entitled to use psychological tests to assess and diagnose mental disorder. Test users also should have advanced education and training in individual assessment and psychological testing that would qualify them to practice as a mental health professional (e.g., graduate or medical degree). PCL-R manual also recommends that test users should have at least 2 years experience working in forensic settings. Completion of training workshops and supervised practice in the use of PCL-R and PCL:SV is recommended, but not required. Similarly, the manuals recommend completion of 5–10 practice cases prior to clinical use of the tests.

Psychometric Properties

The psychometric properties of PCL-R and PCL:SV have been evaluated extensively within the framework of classical test theory [2, 3, 6]. The most relevant forms of reliability for the tests are structural, inter-rater, and test–retest reliabilities. Structural reliabilities are good to excellent: Item adequacy, as indexed by corrected item-total correlation, is typically 0.40–0.50; item homogeneity, as indexed by mean inter-item correlation, is typically 0.20–0.30; and internal consistency, as indexed by Cronbach's α, is typically 0.85–0.90. Inter-rater reliabilities also are good to excellent: For items, the intraclass correlation coefficient (ICC1) is typically between 0.60 and 0.80; for total scores, ICC1 is typically 0.80–0.90; and for categorical diagnoses, inter-rater agreement, as indexed by κ, is typically 0.50–0.75. Test–retest reliability of total scores and diagnoses has been examined infrequently, but appears to be good to excellent over periods of 1 week to 1 month and at least fair over periods of 6 months to 2 years.

More recently, the tests have been evaluated within the framework of item response theory (IRT) by Cooke, Hare, and colleagues [2, 7, 8]. The interpersonal, affective, and behavioral symptoms have good discriminating power; in contrast, the discriminating power of antisocial behavioral items is weaker. The interpersonal symptoms discriminate the latent trait at high levels (i.e., psychopathy), affective symptoms at moderate levels, and behavioral symptoms, at low levels.

IRT is also being used to examine potential metric bias in PCL-R and PCL : SV scores. Some researchers have reported evidence of a small but statistically significant metric bias across dominant cultures, with offenders and patients in the United Kingdom and other European countries scoring lower on PCL-R than those in Canada and the United States, given equivalent standing on the latent trait [9, 10]. This may be due to the effects of cultural facilitation, with symptoms of psychopathy being expressed more often in highly individualistic societies. There is no evidence, however, of metric bias between ethnic majority versus minority groups within a dominant culture [11]. Only recently have researchers started to investigate metric bias across gender and age.

Association Between PCL-R and PCL:SV

Cooke and colleagues have evaluated the derivation of PCL:SV using IRT methods [8]. They found a strong association between corresponding PCL-R and PCL:SV items or item pairs. They also found that PCL:SV items had a discriminating power as good as or better than the corresponding PCL-R items or item pairs.

Total scores on PCL-R and PCL:SV are also strongly associated. Cooke and colleagues [8] reported a high correlation ($r = 0.94$) between scores on the latent trait underlying both tests according to IRT analyses, and Guy and Douglas [6] reported similar high correlations ($r = 0.94$–0.95) between (raw) total scores on the tests in forensic samples. Guy and Douglas [6] also found that PCL:SV had good validity as a screening test for high-PCL-R scores in the same two forensic samples, with large areas under the curve (AUC = 0.98) according to receiver operating characteristic (ROC) analyses.

Factor Structure

Initial investigations of the dimensionality of PCL-R and PCL:SV used exploratory factor analysis (EFA) methods. The only consistent finding was the absence of a simple, unidimensional latent variable underlying the tests. Hare and colleagues proposed a structure comprising two orthogonal (i.e., correlated) factors: one reflecting interpersonal and affective symptoms, and the other reflecting behavioral symptoms and antisocial conduct [1].

Cooke and Michie [12] overcame the limitations of EFA by using confirmatory factor analysis (CFA) methods. After omitting PCL-R and PCL:SV items tapping antisocial conduct, they found strong evidence of a hierarchical three-factor structure, comprising a superordinate general factor (psychopathy) underpinned by three correlated subordinate factors (interpersonal, affective, and behavioral symptoms).

The hierarchical three-factor structure was replicable across diverse samples of offenders and forensic psychiatric patients from different nations. Importantly, it was even found when factor-analyzing diagnostic criteria for psychopathy other than PCL-R and PCL:SV.

Subsequent to Cooke and Michie's article, several researches have found support for the three-factor hierarchical structure. But others, including Hare and his colleagues, have argued that the entire item pools of PCL-R and PCL:SV should be included in factor analyses, which they say results in the addition of a fourth subordinate factor, reflecting antisocial conduct; this view was reflected in the updated PCL-R test manual [3]. Debate continues on whether antisocial conduct should be considered a primary symptom of psychopathy versus a secondary symptom, sequela, or consequence of the disorder [13].

Validity

As PCL-R and PCL:SV have been used in virtually hundreds of published studies, only a general review of research is presented here; and as the tests are strongly associated, they are reviewed together.

One important line of research has evaluated the *concurrent validity* of PCL-R and PCL:SV, that is, their association with other procedures for assessing psychopathy. Total scores on the tests have moderate to large correlations with clinical diagnoses made using other criteria, and moderate correlations with self-report measures of psychopathy [2, 3]. Both clinical diagnoses made using other criteria and self-report measures tend to correlate more highly with PCL-R and PCL:SV items reflecting behavioral symptoms and antisocial conduct than with items reflecting the interpersonal and affective features [2, 3].

With respect to *predictive validity*, total scores on PCL-R and PCL:SV are reliably associated with serious antisocial behavior, including violence, in both institutional and community settings. Summarizing a number of reviews in recent years [14, 15], several general conclusions may be drawn. First, the predictive validity of PCL-R or PCL:SV with respect to serious antisocial behavior is typically moderate in magnitude, $r = 0.20 – 0.30$. Second, the predictive validity tends to be larger in community settings than institutional settings. Third, the predictive validity tends to be larger when the outcome reflects

general but serious antisocial conduct (e.g., "any violence"), rather than more specific or less serious antisocial conduct (e.g., "sexual violence" or "any misconduct"). Fourth, the predictive validity of psychopathy, as measured by PCL-R and PCL:SV, typically is higher than that of other established demographic, criminal history, and clinical risk factors (e.g., age, prior antisocial conduct, substance use); indeed, PCL-R and PCL:SV predict antisocial conduct about as well as do multifactor risk assessment procedures constructed theoretically or statistically. Fifth, the predictive validity of PCL-R and PCL:SV is not attributable solely or even primarily to the inclusion of items reflecting past antisocial conduct.

With respect to other aspects of *construct validity*, PCL-R and PCL:SV have been used to study the course, comorbidity, etiology, and treatment of psychopathy [16]. (*See also* **Psychopathy**.)

Forensic Applications

In the practice of forensic mental health, PCL-R and PCL:SV are used most often as part of comprehensive assessments of risk and treatability for sentencing, civil commitment, institutional classification, and release decision making. This application is supported by research on the prediction of serious antisocial conduct and on treatment response. Indeed, PCL-R and PCL:SV are incorporated explicitly into several procedures for assessing violence risk (*see* **Dangerousness: Risk of** and **Risk Assessment: Patient and Detainee**).

Forensic mental health professionals should be aware of some important limitations of PCL-R and PCL:SV [17, 18]. First, as observer ratings scales, the tests may be susceptible to distortion – unconscious or deliberate – by evaluators. To safeguard against this, evaluators should closely follow the administration instructions in the test manuals; training and supervised practice in the use of the tests may also be helpful. Second, although the tests have good psychometric properties in adult male offenders and forensic psychiatric patients in the United States and Canada, the possibility of bias due to culture and gender has not yet been ruled out. Third, the tests reflect the lifetime presence of psychopathic symptoms; this means they cannot be used to measure changes in the presence or severity of symptoms over time, or used to determine whether the person currently suffers from psychopathy. Fourth, although comprehensive, PCL-R and PCL:SV are not exhaustive in content and relatively heavily saturated with items reflecting antisocial conduct. Evaluators should consider using PCL:SV instead of PCL-R in cases where the person being assessed does not have a serious history of criminality. Fifth, although psychopathy is a robust risk factor for antisocial behavior, PCL-R and PCL:SV scores cannot be used – either on their own or in combination with other factors – to estimate the specific probability or absolute likelihood that a given person will commit a criminal or violent act with any reasonable degree of scientific certainty.

References

[1] Hare, R.D. (1991). *Manual for the Hare Psychopathy Checklist – Revised*, Multi Health Systems, Toronto.

[2] Hare, R.D. (2003). *Manual for the Hare Psychopathy Checklist – Revised*, 2nd Edition, Multi Health Systems, Toronto.

[3] Hart, S.D., Cox, D.N. & Hare, R.D. (1995). *Manual for the Hare Psychopathy Checklist: Screening Version (PCL:SV)*, Multi-Health Systems, Toronto.

[4] Hare, R.D. (1996). Psychopathy: a clinical construct whose time has come, *Criminal Justice and Behavior* **23**, 25–54.

[5] Hare, R.D. (1980). A research scale for the assessment of psychopathy in criminal populations, *Personality and Individual Differences* **1**, 111–119.

[6] Guy, L.S. & Douglas, K.S. (2006). Examining the utility of the PCL:SV as a screening measure using competing factor models of psychopathy, *Psychological Assessment* **18**, 225–230.

[7] Cooke, D.J. & Michie, C. (1997). An item response theory analysis of the Hare psychopathy checklist-revised, *Psychological Assessment* **9**, 3–14.

[8] Cooke, D.J., Michie, C., Hart, S.D. & Hare, R.D. (1999). Evaluating the screening version of the Hare psychopathy checklist-revised (PCL:SV): an item response theory analysis, *Psychological Assessment* **11**, 3–13.

[9] Cooke, D.J., Michie, C., Hart, S.D. & Clark, D.A. (2005). Assessing psychopathy in the United Kingdom: Concerns about cross-cultural generalisability, *British Journal of Psychiatry* **186**, 339–345.

[10] Cooke, D.J., Michie, C., Hart, S.D. & Clark, D.A. (2005). Searching for the pan-cultural core of psychopathic personality disorder: Continental Europe and North America compared, *Personality and Individual Differences* **39**, 283–295.

[11] Cooke, D.J., Kosson, D.S. & Michie, C. (2001). Psychopathy and ethnicity: structural, item and test generalizability of the psychopathy checklist revised (PCL–R) in Caucasian and African-American participants, *Psychological Assessment* **13**, 531–542.

[12] Cooke, D.J. & Michie, C. (2001). Refining the construct of psychopathy: Towards a hierarchical model, *Psychological Assessment* **13**, 171–188.

[13] Cooke, D.J., Michie, C., Hart, S.D. & Clark, D.A. (2004). Reconstructing psychopathy: clarifying the significance of antisocial and socially deviant behavior in the diagnosis of psychopathic personality disorder, *Journal of Personality Disorders* **18**, 337–357.

[14] Hart, S.D. (1998). The role of psychopathy in assessing risk for violence: conceptual and methodological issues, *Legal and Criminological Psychology* **3**, 121–137.

[15] Douglas, K.S., Vincent, G.M. & Edens, J.F. (2006). Risk for criminal recidivism: the role of psychopathy, in *Handbook of Psychopathy*, C.J. Patrick, (ed), Guilford, New York, pp. 533–554.

[16] Patrick, C.J. (ed) (2006). *Handbook of Psychopathy*, Guilford, New York.

[17] Hare, R.D. (1998). The Hare PCL-R: some issues concerning its use and misuse, *Legal and Criminological Psychology* **3**, 99–119.

[18] Hemphill, J.F. & Hart, S.D. (2003). Forensic and clinical issues in the assessment of psychopathy, in *Comprehensive Handbook of Psychology: Vol. 11. Forensic Psychology*, I. Weiner (series editor) & A.M. Goldstein (volume editor), eds, John Wiley & Sons, New York, pp. 87–107.

Further Reading

Patrick, C.J. (ed) (2006). *Handbook of Psychopathy*, Guilford, New York.

Related Articles

Dangerousness: Risk of

Psychopathy

Risk Assessment: Patient and Detainee

STEPHEN D. HART

Psychopharmacology

Psychopharmacology is the study of the effects of drugs on psychological function. It is a branch of pharmacology, which focuses on the nervous system. Clinical psychopharmacology is the portion of psychiatric practice, which pertains to the use of medication as a tool to treat mental disorders [1, 2].

Clinical psychopharmacology involves an assessment process, development of a treatment plan, and subsequent assessment of the effects of treatment [3].

Psychopharmacologic testimony is often relevant in both civil and criminal cases. Establishing standard of care, and causation of damages in cases alleging negligent prescription, evaluating complex disability claims, and testamentary competency are some areas for psychopharmacological consultation. Cases of suspected poisoning or suicide may also warrant psychopharmacological consultation.

Since many crimes are committed under the influence of substances (*see* **Substance Abuse**), the effect of those substances on the defendant's mental state may be relevant (*see* **Insanity: Defense**; **Temporary Insanity**; **Mitigation Testimony**). Even though voluntary intoxication may not negate a mental state in many jurisdictions, the distinction between intoxication, mental illness, and "settled insanity" [4] requires psychiatric evaluation.

Defendants who are incompetent as a result of mental disorder (*see* **Capacity to Stand Trial**) may often be restored to competence through treatment. If the defendant refuses treatment, psychopharmacological evaluation is necessary to inform the court that medication is substantially likely to render the defendant competent to stand trial and substantially unlikely to have side effects that will interfere significantly with the defendant's ability to assist counsel in conducting a defense [5].

Basic principles of psychopharmacology are outlined in this article, along with an overview of psychotherapeutic agents, and some clinical and medical legal issues related to them. Substance abuse and dependence are reviewed in **Substance Abuse**; **Addictions**.

The study of pharmacology includes an understanding of pharmacokinetics, pharmacodynamics, and drug mechanisms. Pharmacokinetics describes what happens to a drug when it enters the body. How a drug is absorbed, metabolized, activated or inactivated, and excreted, influences how much of a drug is available at the site of action. Pharmacodynamics explains the effect of drugs on the sites of action [6].

Drug effects may vary as a result of the route of administration. For example, intravenous benzodiazepines can reliably cause short-term amnesia, which is useful to anesthesiologists. The same dose of drug ingested orally will usually not have the same effect.

Once a drug is absorbed, it enters the bloodstream to be carried through the body. Most psychoactive drugs are lipid (fat) soluble. They do not dissolve well in water. Thus, they are carried through the bloodstream bound to protein.

Many drugs are metabolized through interactions with enzymes in the liver (many are metabolized throughout the body). When a drug is metabolized, it is altered, often to an inactive or water soluble form. Sometimes the metabolites are themselves active drugs. If the drug is ingested by mouth, after it is absorbed in the intestines, it goes through the portal system to the liver for first pass metabolism, and then to the general circulation, where it can effect other organs.

Drugs that are inactivated to an efficient degree by the liver are not effective when administered orally. First pass inactivation can be bypassed through alternative routes of administration: intravenous, sublingual, or intranasal.

Drugs and their metabolites are excreted through urine, feces, and perspiration. The time required for the plasma concentration of a drug to fall by one half is the half-life of the drug ($t_{1/2}$). When the amount of drug administered in a given time equals the amount eliminated, the drug has reached steady state.

In order for a drug to act on the brain, it must cross the blood–brain barrier. Factors that affect a drug's ability to enter the brain include size and charge of the drug molecule, and its lipid solubility. For example, L-Dopa will cross the blood–brain barrier, while Dopamine (DA) will not.

A drug may have a nonspecific effect on the nervous system when it affects energy metabolism, or membrane stability. Specific drug effects arise from interaction with identifiable molecular mechanisms unique to target cells, which bear receptors for that drug. Sometimes a drug with specific effects at a low dose has general effects at a higher dose. Alcohol and general anesthetics are general depressants of the central nervous system, while drugs such as caffeine can be general stimulants [6].

Psychoactive drugs generally affect psychological function through interaction with the normal function of the nervous system [1, 6–8]. The brain contains billions of neurons supported by glia. Glia are considered supporting tissue for the nerve cells. Some form myelin, which facilitates axon function. Others are involved in metabolic activity, and the formation of the blood-brain barrier. Ongoing research suggests that glia may, in fact, serve a more active role in brain function than previously believed [3].

The cell body contains the nucleus of the neuron. It is the center of metabolic activity. Dendrites extend and branch from it, and connect to the terminal processes of other neurons to form synapses. The axon is a single, often long, process, which arises out of the cell body to connect to other neurons.

The concentration of ions, like potassium, sodium, chloride, and calcium within the cell is not equal to the concentration outside the cell. As a result, the cell membrane carries a charge across it, like a microscopic battery. When a nerve fires, the membrane allows ions to cross, depolarizing it briefly. The depolarization travels down the length of the axon (an action potential). At the terminal process, packets of chemicals – neurotransmitters – are released across the membrane into the synapse, where the terminal process connects to the dendrite of another neuron.

The surface of the dendrite contains special proteins called a *postsynaptic receptor*. The axon may contain presynaptic receptors as well. Each receptor is specialized to react to a specific neurotransmitter. The effect may be to excite the neuron or to make excitation more difficult – to inhibit it (depending on the neurotransmitter and receptor). When the sum of excitatory minus inhibitory stimulation exceeds a threshold, the nerve will fire.

The system is regulated through feedback mechanisms mediated by (presynaptic) autoreceptors and secondary messengers. When stimulated, autoreceptors on the presynaptic neuron signal the cell to stop release of neurotransmitter. Secondary messengers within the postsynaptic neuron modulate metabolic processes in the cell, including protein production. This controls neural plasticity, including long-term potentiation, long-term depression, down regulation and up regulation of receptors.

Neurotransmitter molecules are removed from the synapse by the presynaptic neuron (which released them) through a reuptake process. Once removed, the neurotransmitter does not interact with the receptor, until it is released again. Some neurotransmitter is inactivated through enzyme-assisted metabolic degradation.

The synapse is the site of action of most psychoactive drugs.

Neurons are organized in circuits, with specialized function. The systems that are most interesting to the psychiatrist are the limbic system, the basal ganglia, and the thalamocortical system.

The limbic system is involved with the experience and expression of emotion. Basal ganglia are involved in both motor and cognitive function. The thalamocortical system is involved in sensation, movement, and cognition.

Drugs of abuse affect DA circuits in the nucleus acumbens, an area of the brain involved in learning and motivation. The reinforcing effect of such stimulation is difficult to overcome, as reflected in the rates of lapses and relapses in recovering addicts (*see* **Addictions**).

A non-comprehensive list of neurotransmitters follows:

- Dopamine (DA);
- serotonin (5-HT);
- acetylcholine (ACh);
- norepinephrine (NE);
- gamma aminobutyric acid (GABA);
- glutamate (Glu);
- endorphins;
- enkephalins;
- histamine; and
- aspartate.

Therapeutic Classes of Drugs

Drugs are often classified in terms that identify the target syndrome or symptoms for which the particular drug was first marketed. Thus, we have antipsychotic drugs, antidepressants, sedative hypnotics, stimulants, mood stabilizers, and cognitive enhancers. Over the course of time, however, drugs are often used effectively for purposes other than those for which they were initially marketed. Some antipsychotic drugs can be used for anxiety, depression, and mood stabilization. Some antidepressants are used for first line treatment of anxiety disorders. Other classification schemes based upon chemical structure or target chemical systems are sometimes employed by practitioners. Thus, various drugs may be described as benzodiazepine, or tricyclic, or selective serotonin reuptake inhibitor (SSRI).

Antipsychotic Medication

The practice of psychiatry was revolutionized in the 1950s with the introduction of chlorpromazine, the first effective antipsychotic drug. Its use reduced the need for restraints, seclusion, and locked psychiatric facilities [6]. As the only effective treatment for psychosis at the time, it was accepted rapidly, despite its side effects.

The success of chlorpromazine stimulated the development of other phenothiazine drugs: thioridazine, fluphenazine, perphenazine, and trifluoperazine. In attempts to increase potency while reducing side effects, the pharmaceutical industry developed butyrophenones (haloperidol), thioxanthenes (thiothixene), dihydroindolones (molindone), and dibenzoxazepines (loxapine). By the 1980s, clozapine was recognized as an effective treatment for psychotic illness, which had not responded to other medications. Its significant toxicity (agranulocytosis) necessitated weekly blood counts, and precluded its use as a first line treatment in the United States. However, its atypical neurochemical profile, its lack of movement side effects, and its affect on negative symptoms of schizophrenia, suggested significant advantages over older line medications. Olanzapine, risperidone, quetiapine, ziprasidone, and aripiprazole were developed in attempts to provide clozapine's therapeutic advantages without potentiating agranulocytosis. These second-generation antipsychotics, also known as *atypical antipsychotics* are now used more frequently than neuroleptics for treatment of chronic psychosis, as their side effects are generally milder and more easily tolerated by patients.

Antipsychotic medication is indicated for treatment of schizophrenia, schizoaffective disorder, schizophreniform disorder, or psychotic symptomatology caused by medical disorders.

Symptoms of schizophrenia can be divided into positive and negative symptoms. Atypical antipsychotics are more effective than first-generation drugs for negative symptoms, which include flat or blunted affect, inactivity, diminished pleasure in activities, and poverty of thought. First-generation drugs primarily affect positive symptoms, including delusions, hallucinations, confusion, and anxiety [9–12].

Blockade of some DA receptors (D_2) is associated with both the antipsychotic effect and movement side effects of these drugs. (In fact, the first psychiatrists to use chlorpromazine did not expect to see antipsychotic effects without an extrapyramidal syndrome.) The blockade of some serotonin receptors ($5\text{-}HT_2$) is associated with relief of negative

symptoms, as well as mitigation of movement side effects [1, 6, 7].

Side effects of antipsychotic medication include sedation, orthostatic hypotension, dry mouth, constipation, blurry vision, urinary hesitancy, extrapyramidal effects, weight gain, and metabolic effects.

First-generation antipsychotics were differentiated from each other on the basis of their side effect profiles, rather than their efficacy. These side effects, related to the drugs' effects on cholinergic, adrenergic, and histamine receptors [1] were understood in relation to differences in the structures of the side chains of these molecules.

Anticholinergic effects include dry mouth, constipation, blurry vision, confusion, and urinary hesitancy.

Adrenergic blockade may cause changes in blood pressure, and cardiac rhythm, as well as symptoms of dizziness.

Histamine blockade is associated with sedation, drowsiness, and weight gain.

Extrapyramidal side effects are caused by DA blockade. DA and ACh are neurotransmitters of the extrapyramidal motor system, involved in posture and coordinated movement. Excessive blockade of DA receptors in this system may lead to an imbalance, and one of four extrapyramidal syndromes: Akathisia, dystonia, Parkinson's syndrome, or tardive dyskinesia.

Akathisia is an uncontrolled sense of inner restlessness, which must be distinguished from anxiety. If it is mistaken for anxiety, and treated with increased dose of medication, it will be worsened.

Dystonia is spasm of the muscles, usually of the head and neck.

Parkinson's syndrome includes muscular rigidity, tremor, slowed motor responses, and diminished facial expression.

Tardive dyskinesia is an often irreversible effect of antipsychotic medication characterized by involuntary movements of the mouth and tongue, as well as of the trunk and extremities.

Akathisia, dystonia, and Parkinson's syndrome may be treated as they emerge through the use of anticholinergic agents, minor tranquilizers, or adjustment in dose of antipsychotic medication.

While various drugs have been used to diminish symptoms of tardive dyskinesia, there is no cure. Discontinuation of the antipsychotic medication will lead to initial worsening of dyskinesia. Over time, symptoms often will remit.

Atypical antipsychotic drugs are less frequently associated with tardive dyskinesia, or other extrapyramidal side effects, than older first-generation antipsychotics.

Significant weight gain is a common problem with antipsychotic drugs, and appears to be associated with an increased risk of diabetes. Aripiprazole and ziprasidone are less likely than other agents to be implicated in weight gain.

Neuroleptic malignant syndrome is a rare complication of antipsychotic drug use. It is characterized by severe muscular rigidity, fever, increased blood pressure, increased heart and respiratory rate, and changing levels of consciousness. Laboratory testing show elevations in creatine phosphokinase (CPK), sometimes along with altered liver functions, and myoglobin (a muscle protein) in the blood or urine. Immediate treatment with supportive symptomatic measures and discontinuation of antipsychotic medication is necessary when this diagnosis is made. Treatment with DA agonists as well as benzodiazepines should be considered with high fevers.

Antidepressants

Iproniazid was an antituberculous agent developed after World War II. After its mood-elevating qualities were noticed, it was investigated, and then marketed as an antidepressant in the late 1950s. The therapeutic action was a result of inhibition of monoamine oxidase (MAO) enzymes, which break down serotonin and NE.

Iproniazid was withdrawn because of toxic effects on the liver. Other MAO Inhibitors were developed, but their use was limited because of the need for dietary restrictions to avoid potentially fatal hypertensive reactions. Recently a transdermal form of selegiline was developed, allowing fewer dietary restrictions.

Around the same time that iproniazid was developed, phenothiazine-like drugs were being tested for antipsychotic effects, with the hope that new drugs could be found without the side effects of chlorpromazine. One, imipramine, was relatively ineffective in calming psychotic patients. However, it did have a therapeutic effect on depressed patients, especially those characterized by regression and inactivity. It was marketed as the first tricyclic antidepressant.

Over the following years, several other tricyclic antidepressants were developed: desipramine, amitriptyline, nortriptyline, clomipramine, trimipramine, doxepin, protriptyline, amoxapine, and maprotiline (a tetracyclic). All block the reuptake of NE into nerve terminals. Imipramine, amitriptyline, doxepin, nortriptyline, and especially clomipramine, also block reuptake of serotonin (5-HT).

These drugs are all pharmacologically "dirty". In addition to their desired effects, they bind to a host of other receptors, with resultant unwanted side effects, including faintness, cardiac arrhythmias, constipation, dry mouth, sedation, and weight gain.

SSRIs or SRIs represent an important pharmacological advance in the treatment of depression, as pharmacologically cleaner drugs, their safety, and tolerability have led to their becoming the predominant class of prescribed antidepressants.

Venlafaxine and duloxetine, serotonin and norepinephrine reuptake inhibitors (SNRIs) may be more useful than SSRIs in treating chronic pain.

Bupropion effects DA and NE reuptake. Trazodone and nefazodone block a portion of the serotonin receptors. Mirtazapine blocks some alpha-adrenergic and serotonergic receptors. These drugs are less likely to cause sexual side effects than other antidepressants.

All antidepressants are indicated for treatment of major depression, including vegetative symptoms of appetite and sleep disturbance, fatigue, diminished sex drive, anhedonia (loss of the ability to experience pleasure), agitation, restlessness, or psychomotor retardation.

In addition, many are effective for generalized anxiety disorder, panic disorder, posttraumatic stress disorder, insomnia, and enuresis.

Tricyclic antidepressants and SNRIs are effective in chronic pain conditions. SSRIs and clomipramine are effective in obsessive compulsive disorder [13–15].

Bupropion can reduce craving for cigarettes, probably as a result of its dopaminergic effect on the nucleus accumbens.

The mechanism of action of antidepressants is not fully understood. While antidepressant drugs exert immediate effects on brain receptors, the therapeutic effect is delayed, usually 2–6 weeks. This suggests that the therapeutic effects arise from a cascade of adaptive processes to repeated administration of the drug. Increased availability of serotonin and/or NE in the synapse evokes negative feedback mechanisms to restore homeostasis. This includes downregulation and desensitization of receptors, and alterations in tonic inhibition and stimulation mediated through secondary messengers in the neuron, which signal formation of new protein.

Newer antidepressants present fewer, less toxic side effects than older tricyclics and MAO Inhibitors. As a result, patients are more likely to comply with treatment long enough to obtain a therapeutic effect than those prescribed tricyclic antidepressants. Patient acceptability and relative safety in overdose have contributed to the popularity of these drugs.

Tricyclic antidepressants cause side effects related to their effects on the autonomic nervous system. These include dry mouth, dizziness, palpitations, blurry vision, constipation, tachycardia, orthostatic hypotension, and cardiac arrhythmias.

MAO Inhibitors may cause postural hypotension. Drug and diet interactions may precipitate hypertensive crisis or serotonin syndrome, which includes restlessness, muscle twitching, sweating, shivering, and tremor [16].

SRI and SNRI side effects include nausea, headache, delayed ejaculation, and impaired orgasm. Bupropion can cause anorexia, insomnia, and agitation. Trazodone can cause priapism. Mirtazapine is sedating and can cause weight gain.

Patients with bipolar disorder treated with antidepressants may be at risk of switching from depression to a hypomanic or manic state [17–19].

Mood Stabilizers

Cade first described the therapeutic effects of lithium on mania in 1949. It was first approved by the US FDA for treatment of acute mania in 1970s, and for prophylaxis of bipolar disorder in 1974.

While lithium is quite toxic, it is very effective for treatment of both manic and depressive phases of bipolar disorder. Several large-scale studies have demonstrated significant reduction in suicide risk associated with lithium therapy [20, 21]. There is an increase in suicide risk after discontinuation of lithium [22].

Adverse effects include acne, leucocytosis, hypothyroidism, hypoparathyroidism, nephrogenic diabetes insipidus, and kidney damage. Signs of toxicity include tremor, weakness, fatigue, nausea,

vomiting, cardiac arrhythmias, hypotension, shock, stupor, coma, and even death.

Safe use of lithium requires monitoring of blood levels, since the therapeutic dose is close to the toxic dose. Evaluation of serum electrolytes, thyroid, parathyroid, renal, and hematological function is necessary at the commencement of treatment and periodically during the course of therapy.

Valproate was approved by the FDA for treatment of acute mania in 1994. It is less toxic, and easier to prescribe than lithium. It consequently has been prescribed more frequently than lithium, even though the evidence of its effectiveness for prophylaxis is not robust.

In 2003, the FDA approved the use of lamotrigine for long-term treatment of bipolar disorder. This anticonvulsant demonstrates little effect on acute mania. However, it shows antidepressant effect and prophylactic effects in bipolar patients. Other anticonvulsants, which are used as mood stabilizers, include carbamazepine, gabapentin, pregabalin, topiramate, tiagabine, oxcarbazepine, and zonisamide.

Antipsychotic drugs such as olanzapine, aripiprazole, and quetiapine are also termed *mood stabilizers* because of their demonstrated roles in treatment of bipolar disorder [23].

Anxiolytics

Chlordiazepoxide and diazepam were the first benzodiazepines, introduced in the early 1960s. They were soon widely prescribed by physicians for pathological anxiety, because they were effective and safer than meprobamate and barbiturates. Other benzodiazepines were subsequently developed and marketed, including clorazepate, alprazolam, oxazepam, and clonazepam.

All benzodiazepines exhibit anxiolytic, sedative hypnotic, muscle relaxant, and anticonvulsant effects. The primary differences among them are a result of pharmacokinetic properties, including rates of absorption and elimination.

Benzodiazepines bind to specific receptors in the brain – the GABA – BZ complex. GABA is a primary inhibitory neurotransmitter in the brain. When it is bound to its receptor, a chloride channel on the membrane is opened a little, making depolarization of the nerve more difficult. GABA works more effectively in the presence of a benzodiazepine.

Sedation and drowsiness are common side effects of benzodiazepines. Motor impairment may occur, as may memory impairment. Tolerance may occur, and physical dependence is common with prolonged treatment. Abuse and dependence (*see* **Substance Abuse**; **Addictions**), as defined by Diagnostic and Statistical Manual of Mental Disorders-IV (DSM-IV) [24], are less common, but may still be problematic.

Buspirone is a unique nonsedating nonbenzodiazepine anxiolytic drug, which appears to exert its effect through actions on a subset of serotonergic receptors (5-HT$_{1A}$). It is effective for generalized anxiety disorder, but not for panic attacks. Its effect builds up slowly, over several weeks. Side effects may include dizziness, headaches, and nausea.

Addition of buspirone to an antidepressant can be beneficial for patients with inadequate or poor responses to an initial trial of antidepressant treatment [25–28].

Stimulants

Amphetamines and methylphenidate stimulate the release of DA and NE at the synapse. They are useful for the treatment of attention deficit disorder [29–32] (*see* **Psychopharmacology: Child and Adolescent**), and have been used for appetite suppression, fatigue, and treatment of poststroke depression.

Side effects include nervousness, insomnia, and agitation. Arrhythmias and seizures may occur. Hallucinations and delusions are uncommon with stimulants administered orally at usually prescribed doses. They are a frequent complication of inhaled or injected amphetamines.

Stimulant psychosis, including visual hallucinations, disorientation, agitation, pacing, and thought disorder, may persist for months after cessation of amphetamine use.

Modafinil is similar to stimulants, in that it increases wakefulness. It does not increase reinforcement, like other stimulants. Thus it is, in a class by itself, a "wakefulness promoting agent". It is indicated for narcolepsy, and the fatigue associated with shift work and sleep apnea.

Drug Interactions

Concurrent use of more than one drug, or a drug with other substances, may lead to altered pharmacological effect – a drug interaction. Pharmacokinetic interactions occur when an agent alters the absorption, distribution, or metabolism of a drug. Pharmacodynamic interaction involves changes at the receptor, or the biologically active site.

The absorption of buspirone and ziprasidone are enhanced in the presence of food. Antacids may decrease absorption of some antibiotics. Drugs that are bound strongly to protein, like fluoxetine, will displace other protein-bound drugs, possibly enhancing their action or leading to toxic effects. Excretion of lithium is diminished with certain diuretic drugs, leading to increased serum concentration. Grapefruit juice may inhibit Cytochrome P450 enzymes, which break down imipramine, leading to increased serum concentration. These are all pharmacokinetic interactions.

Many drugs are metabolized by the Cytochrome P450 family of enzymes, predominantly found in the liver, the gut, and the brain. The activity of these enzymes, in turn, is enhanced or inhibited by many drugs. Many significant pharmacokinetic drug interactions are mediated by changes in these enzymes [33]. Much variability in individual sensitivity to therapeutic agents can be explained by variations in the concentrations and activities of these enzymes.

Pharmacodynamic interactions can cause increased or decreased pharmacological effect. For example, alcohol can potentiate the sedative effect of hypnotic drugs. Lithium can potentiate the effect of antidepressant drugs. MAO Inhibitors can provoke a serotonin syndrome when administered with an SSRI.

Attention to the potential for drug interactions allows a psychopharmacologist to safely and effectively provide rational treatment.

Drug Testing

For most psychotherapeutic drugs, the relationship between serum concentration and clinical effect has not been established. Lithium, valproate, carbamazepine, and nortriptyline are important exceptions. The difference between the therapeutic dose and a toxic dose of lithium is small. Periodic measurement of serum concentration is necessary to safely prescribe it. The interactions of carbamazepine and valproate with the Cytochrome P450 enzymes necessitate blood testing to establish an appropriate therapeutic dose. Sometimes physicians will check on the concentration of other prescribed drugs when toxicity is suspected. Sometimes less expensive qualitative testing can confirm or refute suspicions of noncompliance. Generally, however, adjustment of doses of psychotropic medication is made on clinical grounds.

Qualitative testing for the presence of drugs in blood, urine, saliva, or hair samples is often part of a treatment program for patients with substance use disorders (*see* **Drug Testing: Urine**; **Amphetamine**; **Benzodiazepines**; **Cannabis**; **Cocaine**; **Opioids**). Serum concentration is often presented to the forensic psychopharmacology consultant for interpretation (**Toxicology: Forensic Applications of**).

Substances associated with dependence tend to evoke tolerance over time. Thus, without additional data, one cannot usually determine from a single sample of body fluid, the level of intoxication experienced by a user. Was the blood level the result of one use or many over time? How was the drug ingested? How long ago? Were blood levels on their way up, or down? Or was this steady state?

Concentrations of drugs obtained during necropsy are often quite different than those obtained during life (Postmortem blood has been described as a fluid resembling blood that is obtained from the vasculature after death [34]). A drug that has been concentrated in solid organs and tissues will diffuse into the blood after death, increasing its concentration. This was demonstrated in the case of a man who committed suicide by ingesting an overdose of imipramine. Concentrations of imipramine and its active metabolite, desipramine, obtained during postmortem examination 7 h after death were compared with concentrations in blood samples obtained in the emergency room 2 h prior to death. Postmortem imipramine concentrations ranged from 1.8 to 7.9 times the concentration of the emergency room sample (depending on the site in the body from which the blood was drawn), while desipramine ratios ranged from 1.6 to 6 [35].

The Volume of distribution (V_d) is a hypothetical volume of body fluid that would be necessary if the total amount of drug in the body were distributed uniformly in the same concentration as in the plasma. In general, lipophilic drugs have a high volume of distribution. Caffeine, which dissolves equally in water and in fat, has a V_d of $1 \, \text{l kg}^{-1}$. For imipramine, it is $11–16 \, \text{l kg}^{-1}$. For sertraline, it is in the range of $50–80$. Drugs with a high volume of distribution

will show the greatest change in concentration postmortem (*see* **Toxicology: Analysis**).

References

[1]   Schatzberg, A.F. & Nemeroff, C.B. (2004). *The American Psychiatric Press Textbook of Psychopharmacology*, 3rd Edition, American Psychiatric Press, Washington, DC.

[2]   Nemeroff, C.B., Heim, C.M., Thase, M.E., Klein, D.N., Rush, A.J., Schatzberg, A.F., Ninan, P.T., McCullough, J.P., Weiss Jr, P.M., Dunner, D.L., Rothbaum, B.O., Kornstein, S., Keitner, G & Keller M.B (2003). Differential responses to psychotherapy versus pharmacotherapy in patients with chronic forms of major depression and childhood trauma, *Proceedings of the National Academy of Sciences of the United States of America* **100**(24), 14293–14296.

[3]   Sadock, B.J. & Sadock, V.A. (2004). *Kaplan and Sadock's Comprehensive Textbook of Psychiatry*, 8th Edition, Lippincott Williams & Wilkins.

[4]   Feix, J. & Wolber, G. (2007). Intoxication and settled insanity: a finding of not guilty by reason of insanity, *The Journal of the American Academy of Psychiatry and the Law* **35**(2), 172–182.

[5]   Sell v. United States, 539 U.S. 166 (2003).

[6]   Brunton, L., Lazo, J. (2005). *Goodman and Gilman's the Pharmacological Basis of Therapeutics*, 11th Edition, McGraw Hill.

[7]   Seeman, P. (2004). Atypical antipsychotics: mechanism of action, *Focus* **2**(1), 48–58.

[8]   Nemeroff, C.B. (1998). Psychopharmacology of affective disorders in the 21st century, *Biological Psychiatry* **44**(7), 517–525.

[9]   Keefe, R.S.E., Silva, S.G., Perkins, D.O. & Lieberman, J.A. (1999). The effects of atypical antipsychotic drugs on neurocognitive impairment in schizophrenia: a review and meta-analysis, *Schizophrenia Bulletin* **25**(2), 201–222.

[10] Lieberman, J.A., Stroup, T.S., McEvoy, J.P., Swartz, M.S., Rosenheck, R.A., Perkins, D.O., Keefe, R.S.E., Davis, S.M., Davis, C.E., Lebowitz, B.D., Severe, J & Hsiao, J.K. The Clinical Antipsychotic Trials of Intervention Effectiveness (CATIE) Investigators, (2005). Effectiveness of antipsychotic drugs in patients with chronic schizophrenia, *New England Journal of Medicine* **353**(12), 1209–1223.

[11] Rosenheck, R., Cramer, J., Xu, W., Thomas, J., Henderson, W., Frisman, L., Fye, C. & Charney, D. The Department of Veterans Affairs Cooperative Study Group on Clozapine in Refractory Schizophrenia (1997). A comparison of clozapine and haloperidol in hospitalized patients with refractory schizophrenia, *New England Journal of Medicine* **337**(12), 809–815.

[12] Volavka, J., Czobor, P., Sheitman, B., Lindenmayer, J.-P., Citrome, L., McEvoy, J.P., Cooper, T.B., Chakos,

M. & Lieberman, J.A., (2004). Clozapine, olanzapine, risperidone, and haloperidol in the treatment of patients with chronic schizophrenia and schizoaffective disorder, *Focus* **2**(1), 59–67.

[13] Greist, J.H., Jefferson, J.W., Kobak, K.A., Katzelnick, D.J. & Serlin, R.C. (1995). Efficacy and tolerability of serotonin transport inhibitors in obsessive-compulsive disorder. A meta-analysis, *Archives of General Psychiatry* **52**(1), 53–60.

[14] Kaplan, A. & Hollander, E. (2004). A review of pharmacologic treatments for obsessive-compulsive disorder, *Focus* **2**(3), 454–461.

[15] Kobak, K.A., Greist, J.H., Jefferson, J.W., Katzelnick, D.J. & Henk, H.J. (2004). Behavioral versus pharmacological treatments of obsessive compulsive disorder: a meta-analysis, *Focus* **2**(3), 462–474.

[16] Looper, K.J. (2007). Potential medical and surgical complications of serotonergic antidepressant medications, *Psychosomatics* **48**(1), 1–9.

[17] Altshuler, L.L., Suppes, T., Black, D.O., Nolen, W.A., Leverich, G., Keck Jr, P.E., Frye, M.A., Kupka, R, McElroy, S.L., Grunze, H., Kitchen, C.M.R. & Post, R. (2007). Lower switch rate in depressed patients with bipolar II than bipolar I disorder treated adjunctively with second-generation antidepressants. *Focus* **5**(1), 107–110.

[18] Judd, L.L., Akiskal, H.S., Schettler, P.J., Endicott, J., Maser, J., Solomon, D.A., Leon, A.C., Rice, J.A. & Keller, M.B. (2002). The long-term natural history of the weekly symptomatic status of bipolar I disorder, *Archives of General Psychiatry* **59**(6), 530–537.

[19] Leverich, G.S., Altshuler, L.L., Frye, M.A., Suppes, T., McElroy, S.L., Keck Jr, P.E., Kupka, R.W., Denicoff, K.D., Nolen, W.A., Grunze, H., Martinez, M.I. & Post, R.M. (2006). Risk of switch in mood polarity to hypomania or mania in patients with bipolar depression during acute and continuation trials of venlafaxine, sertraline, and bupropion as adjuncts to mood stabilizers. *American Journal of Psychiatry* **163**(2), 232–239.

[20] Tondo, L., Jamison, K. & Baldessarini, R. (1997). Effect of lithium maintenance on suicidal behavior in major mood disorders, *Annals of the New York Academy of Sciences* **836**, 339–351.

[21] Tondo, L., Hennen, J. & Baldessarini, R. (2001). Lower suicide risk with long-term lithium treatment in major affective illness: a meta-analysis, *Acta Psychiatrica Scandinavica* **104**, 163–172.

[22] Baldessarini, R., Tondo, L. & Viguera, A. (1999). Discontinuing lithium maintenance treatment in bipolar disorders: risks and implications, *Bipolar Disorders* **1**, 17–24.

[23] Bauer, M.S. & Mitchner, L. (2004). What Is a "mood stabilizer"? an evidence-based response, *American Journal of Psychiatry* **161**(1), 3–18.

[24] American Psychiatric Association (1994). *The Diagnostic and Statistical Manual of Mental Disorders, (DSM IV)*, 4th Edition, American Psychiatric Association, Washington, DC.

[25] Thase, M.E., Friedman, E.S., Biggs, M.M., Wisniewski, S.R., Trivedi, M.H., Luther, J.F., Fava, M., Nierenberg, A.A., McGrath, P.J., Warden, D., Niederehe, G., Hollon, S.D. & Rush, A.J. (2007). Cognitive therapy versus medication in augmentation and switch strategies as second-step treatments: a STAR*D report, *The American Journal of Psychiatry* **164**(5), 739–752.

[26] Fava, M., Rush, A.J., Wisniewski, S.R., Nierenberg, A.A., Alpert, J.E., McGrath, P.J., Thase, M.E., Warden, D., Biggs, M., Luther, J.F., Niederehe, G., Ritz, L. & Trivedi, M.H. STAR*D StudyTeam, (2006). A comparison of mirtazapine and nortriptyline following two consecutive failed medication treatments for depressed outpatients: a STAR*D report, *The American Journal of Psychiatry* **163**(7), 1161–1172.

[27] Nierenberg, A.A., Fava, M., Trivedi, M.H., Wisniewski, S.R., Thase, M.E., McGrath, P.J., Alpert, J.E., Warden, D., Luther, J.F., Niederehe, G., Lebowitz, B., Shores-Wilson, K. & Rush, A.J. STAR*D Study Team, (2006). A comparison of lithium and T3 augmentation following two failed medication treatments for depression: a STAR*D report, *The American Journal of Psychiatry* **163**(9), 1519–1530.

[28] Rush, A.J., Trivedi, M.H., Wisniewski, S.R., Nierenberg, A.A., Stewart, J.W., Warden, D., Niederehe, G., Thase, M.E., Lavori, P.W., Lebowitz, B.D., McGrath, P.J., Rosenbaum, J.F., Sackeim, H.A., Kupfer, D.J., Luther, J. & Fava, M. (2006). Acute and longer-term outcomes in depressed outpatients requiring one or several treatment steps: a STAR*D report, *The American Journal of Psychiatry* **163**(11), 1905–1917.

[29] The MTA Cooperative Group (1999). Moderators and mediators of treatment response for children with attention-deficit/ hyperactivity disorder: the Multimodal Treatment Study of Children with attention-deficit/hyperactivity disorder, *Archives of General Psychiatry* **56**(12), 1088–1096.

[30] The MTA Cooperative Group (1999). A 14-month randomized clinical trial of treatment strategies for attention-deficit/hyperactivity disorder, *Archives of General Psychiatry* **56**(12), 1073–1086.

[31] Spencer, T., Wilens, T., Biederman, J., Faraone, S.V., Ablon, J.S. & Lapey, K. (1995). A double-blind, crossover comparison of methylphenidate and placebo in adults with childhood-onset attention-deficit hyperactivity disorder, *Archives of General Psychiatry* **52**(6), 434–443.

[32] Goldman L.S., Genel M., Bezman R.J., Slanetz P.J., for the Council on Scientific Affairs AMA (1998). Diagnosis and treatment of attention-deficit/hyperactivity disorder in children and adolescents, *The Journal of the American Medical Association* **279**(14), 1100–1107.

[33] Nemeroff, C., DeVane, C. & Pollock, B. (1996). Newer antidepressants and the cytochrome P450 system, *The American Journal of Psychiatry* **153**(3), 311–320.

[34] Klaasen, C.D. (2001). *Casarett & Doull's Toxicology: The Basic Science of Poisons*, 6th Edition, McGraw-Hill, New York.

[35] Pounder, D. & Jones, G. (1990). Postmortem drug redistribution – A toxicological nightmare, *Forensic Science International* **45**, 253–263.

SAMUEL I. MILES

Psychopharmacology: Child and Adolescent

Psychopharmacology's Role in Treatment of Child and Adolescent Mental and Behavioral Disorders

Psychopharmacology is the study of drug–behavior relationships and the use of medications to influence affective and emotional states and thoughts. In children and adolescents, psychotherapeutic medications are best used in conjunction with a holistic bio-psycho-social approach to identify youth's problems and at times in combination with specific nonmedication-based therapies [1]. Transactions between individual genetics, environmental, family and social stresses, and protective factors are currently considered integral to the development of or protection from psychiatric illness. The use of psychotherapeutic medication, when based on scientific evidence, has an important role in fostering improved adaptation in the face of an individual's lowered threshold toward disease. Psychotherapeutic medications are not intended to affect a cure but rather to help by reducing problematic behaviors or relieving mentally painful symptoms.

If a biologic predisposition to a mental disorder lowers the threshold at which a disease becomes evident, then understanding the nature of the risk exposure, while not always immediately evident in the chain of causality, is important. Examples include how the toxic effects of lead and mercury on the development of human nervous system lead to disease states, learning disabilities, and behavioral disorders. Likewise, fetal alcohol effects are discussed as public policy issues, while families, pediatricians, child and adolescent psychiatrists, teachers and the juvenile, and adult justice system attempt to mitigate the damage at a more individual level.

Our knowledge of the pernicious effects of multigenerational cycles of physical and mental maltreatment in childhood, leading to states of affective dyscontrol beginning in childhood and continuing throughout the life span, has expanded to include neuroanatomical and biochemical proof of the disordered states. Addictions are diseases compounded by genetic predispositions that affect motivational circuitry in the brain. Interrupting the cascading effects of untreated disease on the individual, families, and larger society is an important goal. Medication is a component in treatment. There are multiple textbooks on this subject and this article addresses only a few of the issues [2–4].

The Prescriber, Privacy, and the Court

Subpoenas to courts do not provide the authority to release confidential health information that is protected by privacy laws. The prescriber needs to assure that the person who controls protected information has consented to its release or that there has been a judicial determination that privilege does not apply. If uncertain and questioned in court, the prescriber should indicate that the information is privileged and follow the direction of the judge.

Tort Law and the Standard of Care

The use of the word prescriber rather than physician is intended to reflect the fact that many jurisdictions allow nonphysicians such as nurse practitioners to prescribe medications. The tort of negligence has been described as "conduct that falls below the standard regarded as normal or desirable in a given community for those who are perceived to be competent in carrying out their profession within the standards of reasonable skill and proficiency" [5].

In prescribing the medications for psychiatric illness, liability for malpractice does not ensue necessarily from a bad outcome but rather from deviation from the accepted use of the medication. In most jurisdictions, the standard of care in assessing negligence is a matter of medical judgment. In making this decision, rarely does the law provide an answer but rather testimony of experts, articles in learned journals and textbooks, guidelines from professional organizations, etc. will be used to advise the decision maker.

Lawsuits against prescribers of psychotherapeutic medicine often make claims of negligence in either failing to obtain an informed consent for or in the prescribing, administering, and/or monitoring of medications.

Informed Consent for Psychotheraputic Medications in Children and Adolescents

Treatment with psychotherapeutic medication requires informed consent. Applebaum and Gautheil state "Treatment without any consent or over a patient's objections may constitute a battery, but treatment after an inadequate consent is properly considered as a form of malpractice" [6].

A free person is considered to have a right to control what happens to his or her body. Most jurisdictions give the individual patient and not the prescriber of treatment the right to balance risk *versus* benefit of the procedure and to consent to it or refuse it.

Informed consent involves two essential parts: a document and a process. It is important to document it in the medical record but it is more than a signed piece of paper. Ongoing explanations help the patient make wise decisions about whether it is essential to begin or continue taking a particular treatment or medication.

The three elements of informed consent are as follows:

1. the mental *competency* to make a rational decision;
2. the *voluntary* nature of the decision; and
3. *sufficient information* to make a decision.

In children and adolescents, the issue of competence and substitute decision making are especially involved.

Competency

Statutory rules determine when the age of competence to seek or refuse psychiatric treatment occurs. This often occurs before the age of majority. Emancipated minors have full competence. Statutes and age of consent vary from one jurisdiction to another. Informed assent of the older child or adolescent helps the therapeutic relationship and improves compliance. Research trials are governed by more stringent guidelines in this regard. In the United States, the National

Commission for Protection of Human Subjects of Biomedical and Behavioral Research has established age 7 as a reasonable minimum age for children involving in some kind of assent or dissent process and "parental permission" rather than "proxy consent" is considered the norm [7].

Sometimes clarification from a court as to who has authority for decision making for a child may be necessary. Divorced or separated parents with shared decision-making powers might disagree with one another's opinion. Substitute nonparent decision makers who are actively raising the child (grandparents, foster parents, social service agency workers, etc.) may not have the medical decision-making authority to consent.

Voluntary Decision Making

Regarding the issue of substitute decision making, one should consider the agency of the prescriber. Children and adolescents rarely seek psychiatric treatment on their own and are usually dependant upon their parents who act as decision makers. Because the parents are so much a part of the child's decision to be in treatment to some extent, the prescriber should be aware when he or she is acting in their agency as well as the child's. Other situations of potential for dual agency exist when clinicians are contracted to or are employed by schools or social agencies or treatment facilities. The prescriber should assure that school authorities or others are not coercing decision maker to medicate the child.

Information to Make the Decision

To make a submissible case based on negligence in obtaining informed consent, a plaintiff must show nondisclosure, causation, and injury.[a] To show nondisclosure, a plaintiff must include evidence of the risks involved and what disclosures were made by the prescriber.[b] Some jurisdictions have a professional standard of disclosure that the sufficiency of information disclosed should be what a "reasonable clinician" would reveal to his or her patient. Expert testimony of what risks a reasonable medical practitioner would disclose under the same or similar circumstances is required.[c,d] A plaintiff must also establish causation between the inadequate disclosure and the injury.[e] The issue is whether a reasonable person in the plaintiff's position would have consented to the procedure had the proper disclosure been made.[f] The plaintiff has the burden of producing evidence from which a jury or other decision maker could determine whether a reasonable person would have consented to the procedure.[g]

Other jurisdictions use a "reasonable person" standard. This would involve disclosing the information sufficient for a reasonable patient or legal decision maker acting on that patient's behalf to make a rational decision. In those jurisdictions, the clinician should discuss the following matters with the patient and or authorized decision makers:

1. The nature of the condition for which medication is being proposed.
2. The likely outcome of nontreatment.
3. The proposed medication treatment and how and to what extent that will benefit the patient and condition.
4. The risks and side effects associated with the medication. Risks of medications or other treatments proposed that should be disclosed should include those that a reasonable person would be likely to consider significant. The standard in malpractice case law is that the information not disclosed would have been considered substantial in evaluating the risk. Exceptions to this exist when severe harm could result if disclosure were made (principle of therapeutic privilege). Transparency in self-disclosure is important. The clinician's biases and skill level should be disclosed as that might also effect a patient's decision about the risk involved. If a clinician has never treated a certain condition before or never used a certain treatment before, it may be later be judged important to have informed the decision maker of this. Disclosure of potential conflict of interests or even the appearance of such conflict is recommended.
5. Alternative treatments available with their attendant benefits and risks.

Documentation

In the defense against a claim of negligence, legible and timely documentation of prescriptions and orders along with details of the informed consent process, and instructions given to patient and caregivers support the assertion that proper care was given. Prescriptions that are difficult to read pose a hazard to the patient. The prescriber should assure patient and caregivers understand instructions about dosages and interval between doses and potential side effects is important. Warning as to the importance of parental oversight and responsibility to safeguard potentially dangerous medicines should be given.

Documentation of all other medications the patient is currently taking and consideration of drug–drug interactions is a part of clinical care.

Refills, frequency of follow-up intervals to monitor for effectiveness, appropriate compliance with therapy and side effects is important, particularly in children and adolescents with medicines that have a potential for lethality in overdose, irreversible side effects, or abuse potential.

It is important to have permission to communicate with the other individuals involved with the child or adolescent's care about all medications that are being prescribed and about signs, symptoms of side effects, and positive responses to the medications. When a patient or their decision maker will not allow this, then the prescriber's ability to treat the patient is compromised.

Law of Agency/Vicarious Liability

Multiple professional disciplines interact with individual children and families. Pediatric psychopharmacology is practiced within this greater framework. Given the multidisciplinary nature of the treatment of a child or adolescent with interactions with family, school, and larger society, there might be tensions or disagreement at times of critical decision making regarding issues such as dangerousness to self or others, diagnostic labeling, as well as treatment choice recommendations. The prescriber often does not have input on important treatment decisions. The concept of *respondeat superior* is affected by these facts. Most others interacting with the child or adolescent are not acting as agents for the prescriber. The prescriber, even a physician, collaborating with a therapist is not responsible for the actions of that therapist unless he or she is directing these activities in a supervisory manner. The nonsupervisory nature of the relationship should be made clear so that false assumptions are not made.

Medication Practices

Psychotherapeutic medications for the treatment of mental illness are considered one of the most useful and important forms of treatment available for mental illness in both adults and youth. Millions of prescriptions are written annually. Prescribing medications has become so routine and commonplace; it is easy for prescribers and patients to lose sight of the risks involved.

Multiple factors have led to the increased recognition of mental illness in children and adolescents as well as the increase in medication use including the following:

1. The nature *versus* nurture controversy of the last century yielded an increased emphasis and understanding of the biology of mental illness. Biological psychiatry with primary emphasis on the individual's biological vulnerabilities interplaying with psychosocial stressors led to popularization of the simplistic concept of "chemical imbalance". A corollary to this concept was the idea that psychotherapeutic medications righted the imbalance. This notion was applied to youth as well as adults.
2. Large epidemiologic studies such as the 1999 Methodology for Epidemiology of Mental Disorders in Children and Adolescents (MECA) showed significant functional impairment due to mental or addictive disorders in approximately 1 in 10 of the pediatric population, for a total of four million in the United States alone [8].
4. Successful marketing by the pharmaceutical industry of psychotherapeutic medications had significant impact on both prescribers and the general public in terms of *increased expectations* of relief from distressing symptoms. Given the awareness of the availability of medications helpful in treating adults, there has been a willingness to treat youth without awaiting regulatory approvals.

Pediatric Psychohamacology in Practice

It is a statement of fact that most of the medications, psychiatric or not, used in children and adolescents, with the exception of stimulants, were not extensively studied or approved for use in this population. Manufacturers regularly put in disclaimers to that effect in their labeling. Therefore, the use of "off label" (i.e., not regulatory agency approved) prescribing remains the norm rather than the exception.

Pharmacodynamics is the branch of pharmacology that studies how medicines work. In general, psychoactive medications alter the biochemical environment in the synaptic space through either the blockade or activation and enhancement (antagonism, partial agonism, and agonism) of nerve cell membrane receptors. This in turn alters the way the nerve cells communicate.

In children and adolescents, more than in the midadult period in which most new medications are studied, the brain is developing by growing, and pairing down dopaminergic, serotononergic, and noradrenergic cell networks in areas of the brain, which are important to functions of attention, mood, anxiety, and perceptions. In adult populations these brain systems are relatively stable and the medications have been studied more extensively prior to approval and widespread use. Younger, developing brain systems may be permanently affected by mechanisms that are not well understood. Because of this, children and adolescents have differential risks when administered psychotherapeutic medicines. Examples include different risks of side effects such as extrapyramidal motor side effects and dyskinesias from antipsychotics as well as possibilities of overactivation of mood and attentional systems due to increased sensitivities to antidepressants.

Pharmacokinetics studies and informs us as to the absorption, distribution, metabolism, and excretion of medicines. It is important to understand that various people and subpopulations do this differently. In children and adolescents, the phamacokinetic properties of medicines need to be studied thoroughly for the safest administration of medicines that benefit them.

Children have a higher gastric and intestinal motility than adults thus favoring more rapid absorption. Prepubescent children and adolescents usually have fewer fat stores compared with adults, which may lead to higher plasma concentration of medicines in part distributed among fat stores. The metabolic breakdown of medications and toxins in the body differs. Excretion of medicines or the metabolites of medicines, usually by the kidneys might also be affected.

Treatment

Because standard of care is determined on all clinical data available for an individual child or adolescent, the following information is intended as informational only and not intended to imply adherence or deviance from the standard. Side effects are fairly common and so management should include regular periodic monitoring and routine reassessment as to the need to continue with the medication.

History

Review of history is very important for diagnosis and treatment planning. It is not unusual for psychiatrically ill children to have comorbid medical conditions that can influence their psychiatric symptoms. Developmental history should be reviewed with specific attention to development of gross and fine motor skills, speech and language development, affective relatedness, and attachments. A medical history (allergies, adverse drug reactions, acute and chronic illnesses, hospitalizations, injuries, loss of consciousness and traumatic brain injuries, and treatments) should be obtained. Previous laboratory findings and brain imaging if available should be reviewed.

Psychosocial history should include the family of origin, adoption, foster care, exposure to influences of alleged maltreatment, abuse, trauma, and losses.

Past psychiatric treatments and results should be reviewed.

A recent physical examination by the child or adolescent's primary care provider should be reviewed. Many psychiatric medications can be teratogenic and most teen pregnancies are unplanned. Sexually active postpubertal girls should have a pregnancy test along with counseling regarding the use of appropriate methods of birth control and methods of preventing sexually transmittable disease.

Documentation of the above and appropriate laboratory tests ordered prior to initiation of medication therapies and during ongoing monitoring is important.

Diagnosis

Accurate diagnosis in children and adolescents requires clinical assessment often using multiple sources of information including interactions with, observation of, and interview of the child or adolescent, parents, caregivers, and teachers if possible. Guidelines for assessment and treatment are available from the American Academy of Child and Adolescent Psychiatry, American Academy of Pediatrics and other organizations [9, 10].

Substance Abuse. Drug and alcohol screening with clinical questions augmented by urine toxicology for substances of abuse when indicated should be routine among adolescents and preadolescents. Substance-induced behavioral effects can mimic psychiatric illness and cause or aggravate other mental illnesses. Substance use disorders and tobacco addiction need treatment along with other mental illnesses. Making appropriate referrals for treatment of addiction and dependence and identification of patients or caregivers who might be misusing medications, altering prescriptions or getting multiple prescriptions from multiple sources (doctor shopping) is important.

Examples of Therapeutic Medications. *ADHD and the Use of Stimulants and Nonstimulants in its Treatment.* Attention deficit hyperactivity disorder (ADHD) is characterized by early childhood onset of an enduring pattern of inattention and/or hyperactivity and impulsive behavior. In total, 4–12% of children are affected by the disorder [11].

Many children can contain their behaviors during office visits and so collecting information about the child's behavior in multiple settings is most useful. Well-validated and normed behavior rating scales are available and useful in assessing and measuring treatment effects. These would include the Conners' Rating Scales-Revised; Brown Attention-Deficit Scales; and Swanson, Nolan, and Pelham (SNAP-IV) [12].

Stimulant Medications. In 1937, Bradley reported on the positive effects of amphetamine on children institutionalized for neurobehavioral reasons [13]. Since then, opposing social forces have exerted pressures for either wider acceptance of these medications or for more restrictions on their use. The existence of these pressures has led scientists to explore the issue and, for the most part, demonstrate the efficacy of these medicines [14]. Concerns regarding associations with sudden cardiac death have brought these medications into greater controversy in the recent years.

Nonstimulant Medications. Atomoxetine is a selective norepinephrine reuptake inhibitor that is superior to placebo in the treatment of ADHD at appropriate doses [15]. Although the manufacturer recommends once a day dosing, avoiding adverse effects while maintaining adequate therapeutic doses often requires twice a day dosing. Because it shares features with the antidepressants it is associated with an increased risk of suicidality.

Guanfacine and clonidine are antihypertensive medications that have found usefulness. They are generally used in children who cannot tolerate or as adjuncts to the other medications.

Antidepressant Medications, Mood Disorders, and Suicide. Major depression and bipolar mood disorders are enduring and disabling conditions. Suicide is among the most feared of outcomes in the field of mental health. Ninety percent of suicides occur in the context of psychiatric illness and mood disorders are the most likely illnesses to be associated with the act [16]. Suicide is a major cause of preventable death among youth [17].

The prevalence of mood disorders is relatively low before the onset of puberty and equally distributed among the two sexes. After puberty, however, the prevalence increases to adult levels. Various epidemiologic studies point to a prevalence of 5–10% of teens and young adults suffer from major depression or other disabling depressive disorders such as dysthymia and depressive disorder not otherwise specified [18].

Pharmacotherapy with selective serotonin reuptake inhibitor (SSRI) antidepressants either with cognitive behavioral or interpersonal psychotherapy for children and adolescents with major depressive disorder had been the first line and standard of treatment until 2003 and 2004 [1] when regulators in the United Kingdom, the United States, and the European Common Market, became concerned about possible or even causal links between youth suicidality and antidepressants of all classes. UK regulators went on to advise against the use of almost all antidepressants in persons below 18 years. Black box labeling and letters of warning from manufacturers to prescribers were issued in the United States. These expressed warnings and concerns were based on collective data comparing placebo to active medication in multiple different trials, which showed increased rates of suicidality on the active medications and have been extensively reviewed [19].

The stance of regulators was contrary to the opinion of many prescribers who felt the medicines to be very helpful in the real world of clinically complex populations. The warnings had both intended and unintended consequences. Internationally, warnings had the effect of reducing prescriptions to youth by some 20% in 2004 [20]. Coincidental to this decrease in prescribing of antidepressants was a marked increase in actual suicide rates among youth. There exists epidemiologic data showing an inverse correlation between the SSRI prescriptions and suicide rates in multiple population groups in several countries [21, 22]. Antidepressant prescriptions seem to have a protective effect by reducing suicide rates such that strong arguments exist regarding the potential harm resulting from a reduction of SSRI antidepressant use [23]. Indeed, according to the United States Center for Disease Control, after having dropped some 28% from 1990 until 2004, suicide rates for youth in the United States surged 8% leading to 4599 deaths in 2004 following the issuance regulatory letters and black box warning [17]. Prescribers have been left in a conundrum of needing to treat their patients with these medicines despite alarming warnings from regulatory authorities. The best practice to follow is to assure that the diagnosis is correct, the patient makes a full informed consent and to monitor for the development of new onset of suicidal ideations or agitation.

The results of the above-noted reviews [19], which used meta-analytic methods, suggest that there is no benefit to the use of tricyclic antidepressants in children and adolescents with depressive disorders and that the risks, given their toxicity in overdose, generally outweigh the benefits of their use in this population.

SSRI antidepressant medications remain helpful in the treatment of mood and anxiety disorders [24].

Antipsychotics. Antipsychotics are used in treating hallucinations, delusions, hostility, aggression, and disorganized thinking associated with major mental illness such as bipolar disorder, major depression with psychotic features, and schizophrenia. These diseases often manifest in late adolescence or young adulthood and often go undiagnosed for several years. Antipsychotics are also used in the treatment of children with autism and mental retardation who exhibit prominent irritability, aggression, and self-injurious behavior.

It is thought that blockade of D_2 receptors in the mesocortical and prefrontal systems is responsible for the antipsychotic effects. With older antipsychotics, the degree of D_2 receptor blockade is predictive of the potency of antipsychotic effect on hallucinations, delusions, agitation, hostility, and disorganization. Many side effects are also a function of the medication's D_2 binding properties to receptors in the basal ganglia. Drug-induced Parkinson symptoms such as feeling stiff, shuffling gait, tremor, drooling, and masked facial expression led to the mislabeled term *chemical restraint* for this group of medicines that helped many people with mental illness to return to more normal lives.

The newer second generation antipsychotics (SGAs) (olanzapine, risperidone, paliperidone, ziprasidone, quetiapine, aripirazole, and clozapine) were promoted as having fewer side effects on movement and positive effects on motivational circuitry in the prefrontal cortex. The SGAs seemed to balance out many of the untoward effects of D_2 blockade through effects on serotonin 2A receptors, making them agents of first choice. Clozapine, however, because of its potential for causing dangerous agranulocytosis, is reserved for treatment refractory disease.

The number of studies supporting their efficacy and safety in children and adolescents is limited. Children, adolescents, and young adults are particularly susceptible to antipsychotic drug-induced movement disorders (Extra-Pyramidal Symptoms (EPS), akithesia, and diskinetic side effects). The newer medicines have proven to have fewer with drug-induced movement disorders in adults but have problematic effects related to weight gain, glucose regulation, lipid regulation, sedation, prolactin levels, and cardiac conduction. It is hypothesized that because of varying proportions of blockage and, in the case of aripiprazole, the partial agonism of the dopamine receptors, as well as the above noted blockade of serotonin receptors, the effectiveness and sensitivities to side effects in children and adolescents varies markedly between one medicine and another. This means caution should be exercised in their use, careful review of improvement of targeted symptoms and monitoring for side effects. Of note, risperidone received approval from the Food and Drug Administration (FDA) for an indication in the treatment of

children with autism and severe problem behaviors [25, 26].

Children and adolescents are generally treated with the lowest possible effective dose of these medications with periodic monitoring for side effects including baseline and follow-up weight measures and laboratory testing for glucose and lipid abnormalities and abnormal involuntary movements all the while examining the benefits and the need for ongoing use. Because of the potential for significant and sometimes irreversible side effects, documentation of the consideration of the risk benefit ratio prior to initiation and while continuing with these medications is important.

Mood Stabilizers. Mood stabilizers are used in the treatment of bipolar disorder and schizoaffective disorders. The term *mood stabilizer* gathered wide use after publication of reports in the late 1980s demonstrating the efficacy of carbamazepine and divalproex in adult patients with bipolar disorder giving more choices than lithium and adjunctive agents [27]. Oxcarbazapine and lamotragine are now also widely used. Use of these medications has migrated into pediatric use. These medicines are associated with potentially serious side effects; some side effects are more prominent in children and adolescents, including hirsuitism and polycystic ovary syndrome in adolescent girls associated with divalproex and increased incidences of severe rashes with lamotragine in children and adolescents. Oxcarbazapine is metabolized more rapidly in preadolescents. Patient, parent, and caregiver education as to side effects is important.

Routine laboratory evaluations include complete blood-cell count with differential and platelet counts, metabolic profile including liver function tests, pregnancy tests, thyroid function monitoring, as well as plasma drug levels of lithium, valproate, and carbamazepine.

End Notes

[a.] Wilkerson, 908 S.W.2d at p. 696.

[b.] Aiken, 396 S.W.2d at p. 673.

[c.] Aiken, 396 S.W.2d at p. 674–675.

[d.] Wilkerson, 908 S.W.2d at p. 696.

[e.] Aiken, 396 S.W.2d at p. 676.

[f.] Wilkerson, 908 S.W.2d at pp. 696–697

g. Wilkerson, at p. 697 (citing Aiken, 396 S.W.2d at p. 676).

References

[1]   March, J., Silva, S., Petrycki, S., Curry, J., Wells, K., Fairbank, J., Burns, B., Domino, M., McNulty, S., Vitiello, B. & Severe, J. (2004). Fluoxetine, cognitive-behavioral therapy, and their combination for adolescents with depression: treatment for adolescents with depression study (TADS). Randomized controlled trial, *The Journal of the American Medical Association* **292**(7), 807–820.

[2]   Martin, A. & Volkmar, F. (eds) (2007). *Lewis's Child and Adolescent Psychiatry*, 4th Edition, Lippincott, Williams & Wilkins, Philadelphia.

[3]   Coffey, C. & Brumback, R. (eds) (2006). *Pediatric Neuropsychiatry*, Lippincott, Williams & Wilkins, Philadelphia.

[4]   Conner, D. & Meltzer, B. (eds) (2006). *Pediatric Psychopharmacology Fast Facts*, W.W. Norton, New York.

[5]   Fleming, J. (1992). *The Law of Torts*, 8th Edition, Law Book, Sidney, p. 102.

[6]   Applebaum, P. & Gutheil, T. *Clinical Handbook of Psychiatry and the Law*, 4th Edition, Williams & Wilkins, Baltimore, p. 126.

[7]   Broome, M.E. (1999). Consent (Assent) for research with pediatric patients, *Seminars in Oncological Nursing* **15**(2), 96–103.

[8]   (1999). *Mental Health: A Report of the Surgeon General*, Department of Health and Human Services, Substance Abuse and Mental Health Services Administration, Center for Mental Health Services, National Institute of Mental Health, Rockville.

[9]   Kowatch, R. *et al.* (2005). Treatment guidelines for children and adolescents with bipolar disorder: child psychiatric workgroup on bipolar disorder, *Journal of the American Academy of Child and Adolescent Psychiatry* **44**, 213–235.

[10] American Academy of Pediatrics. Subcommittee on Attention-Deficit/Hyperactivity Disorder and Committee on Quality Improvement (2001). Clinical practice guideline: treatment of the school-aged child with attention-deficit/hyperactivity disorder, *Pediatrics* **108**(4), 1033–1044.

[11] Brown, R.T., Freeman, W.S., Perrin, J.M., Stein, M.T., Amler, R.W., Feldman, H.M., Pierce, K. & Wolraich, M.L. (2001). Prevalence and assessment of attention-deficit/hyperactivity disorder in primary care settings, *Pediatrics* **107**, E43.

[12] Swanson, J., Lerner, M., March, J. & Gresham, F.M. (1999). Assessment and intervention for attention-deficit/hyperactivity disorder in the schools: lessons from the MTA study, *Pediatric Clinics of North America* **46**, 993–1009.

[13] Bradley, C. (1937). The behavior of children receiving benzedrine, *The American Journal of Psychiatry* **94**, 577–585.

[14] Zametkin, A.J. & Rappaport, J.L. (1987). Neurobiology of attention deficit disorder with hyperactivity: where have we come in 50 years? *Journal of the American Academy of Child and Adolescent Psychiatry* **26**, 676–686.

[15] Michelson, D., Allen, A.J., Busner, J., Casat, C., Dunn, D., Kratochvil, C., Newcorn, J., Sallee, F.R., Sangal, R.B., Saylor, K., West, S., Kelsey, D., Wernicke, J., Trapp N.J., & Harder, D. (2002). Once-daily atomoxetine treatment for children and adolescents with attention deficit hyperactivity disorder: a randomized, placebo-controlled study, *The American Journal of Psychiatry* **159**(11), 1896–1901.

[16] Beautrais A.L., Jopyce P.R., Mulder R.T., Ferguson, D.M., Deavoll, B.J. & Nightingale, S.K. (1996). Prevalence and comorbidity of mental disorders in persons making serious suicide attempts: a case–control study, *The American Journal of Psychiatry* **153**, 1009–1014.

[17] Centers for Disease Control and Prevention WISQARS (Web-based Injury Statistics Query and Reporting System).

[18] Birmaher, B., Ryan, N.D. & Williamson, D.E., Brent, D.A., Kaufman, J., Dahl, R.E., Perel, J. & Nelson, B. (1996). Childhood and adolescent depression: a review of the past 10 years Part I, *Journal of the American Academy of Child and Adolescent Psychiatry* **35**(11), 1427–1439.

[19] U.S. Food and Drug Administration (2006). *Clinical Review: Relationship between Antidepressant Drugs and Suicidality in Adults*, Food and Drug Administration, Center for drug Evaluation and Research, Rockville.

[20] Gibbons, R.D., Brown, C.H., Hur, K., Marcus, S.M., Bhaumik, D.K., Erkens, J.A., Herings, R.M. & Mann, J.J. (2007). Early evidence on the effects of regulators' suicidality warnings on SSRI prescriptions and suicide in children and adolescents, *The American Journal of Psychiatry* **164**, 1356–1363.

[21] Ludwig, J. & Marcotte, D.D. (2005). Anti-depressants, suicide, and drug regulation, *Journal of Policy Analysis and Management* **24**, 249–272.

[22] Gibbons, R.D., Hur, K., Bhaumik, D.K. & Mann, J.J. (2006). The relationship between antidepressant prescription rates and rate of early adolescent suicide, *The American Journal of Psychiatry* **163**, 1898–1904.

[23] Gibbons, R.D., Hur, K., Bhaumik, D.K. & Mann, J.J. (2006). The relationship between antidepressant prescription rates and rate of early adolescent suicide, *The American Journal of Psychiatry* **163**(11), 1989–10904.

[24] Walkup, J. *et al.* (2002). Treatment of pediatric anxiety disorders: an open-label extension of the research units on pediatric psychopharmacology anxiety study, *Journal of Child and Adolescent Psychopharmacology* **12**(3), 175–188.

[25] McCracken, J.T., McGough, J., Shah, B., Cronin, P., Hong, D., Aman, M.G., Arnold, L.E., Lindsay, R., Nash,

P., Hollway, J., McDougle, C.J., Posey, D., Swiezy, N., Kohn, A., Scahill, L., Martin, A., Koenig, K., Volkmar, F., Carroll, D., Lancor, A., Tierney, E., Ghuman, J., Gonzalez, N.M., Grados, M., Vitiello, B., Ritz, L., Davies, M., Robinson, J. & McMahon D. Research Units on Pediatric Psychopharmacology Autism Network (2002). Risperidone in children with autism and serious behavioral problems, *The New England Journal of Medicine* **347**(5), 314–321.

[26]   Research Units on Pediatric Psychopharmacology Autism Network (2005). Risperidone treatment of autistic disorder: longer-term benefits and blinded discontinuation after 6 months, *The American Journal of Psychiatry* **162**(7), 1361–1369.

[27]   Emrich, H.M., Dose, M. & von Zerssen, D. (1985). The use of sodium valproate, carbamazepine and oxcarbazepine in patients with affective disorders, *Journal of Affective Disorders* **8**, 243–250.

ROBERT W. LOVELL

Psychosis *see* Delusions

Psychosis: Puerperal *see* Postpartum Psychosis

Psychotic Disorder: Shared *see* Temporary Insanity

Publishing in Forensics and Peer Review *see* Peer Review as Affecting Opinion Evidence

Pyromania *see* Firesetting

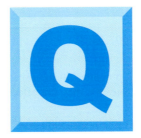

QiaAmp

The *QIAamp® DNA Micro Kit* DNA extraction method utilizes a silica-based spin column to separate DNA from other cellular components that are released after cell lysis. DNA binds, specifically, to the silica-gel membrane embedded within the microcentrifuge tube while other cellular components pass through. This process isolates a purified DNA extract as the washing steps remove inhibitory proteins and divalent cations, which are the cofactors for harmful nucleases. DNA is released from the silica column by the addition of an elution buffer. The entire procedure takes approximately 30 min. Lyophilized carrier RNA can be added to the lyzed sample at the beginning of the process to facilitate membrane binding. This is recommended for forensic samples; however, care must be taken to ensure that downstream quantitation methods are DNA specific. QiaAmp microextraction methods have the advantage of being a simple, reliable, flexible, single-tube technique that is highly amenable to automated liquid handling platforms. In many laboratories, QiaAmp is used as a postextraction purification step, particularly for degraded or severely compromised tissue.

Related Articles

DNA
Extraction

Simon J. Walsh

Quality Systems: Toxicology

Introduction

Quality management (QM) aims to ensure that the activities necessary to design, develop, and provide a product or service are effective and "fit for purpose". QM including laboratory accreditation, i.e., inspection and independent certification of laboratories to ensure, as far as possible, the quality and reliability of the work produced, is becoming increasingly important [1]. A prerequisite for laboratory accreditation is to have a documented QM system. It was thought that the likelihood of examination in court was sufficient to ensure the accuracy and reliability of forensic toxicology results, but implementation of QM systems and accreditation of laboratories by regional or national accreditation bodies provide a far more robust method of ensuring quality. Obviously, all this has to be paid for and inspectors themselves have to be trained and accredited.

The ISO 9000 family (ISO 9000:2000 and 9001: 2001) form a basis for many QM systems (Box 1) and are maintained by the International Organization for Standardization (ISO, http://www.iso.ch/iso/en/iso9000-14000/index.html, accessed 27f August 2007). A related set of standards, ISO 14000, is concerned with environmental management. ISO

Box 1. Some of the requirements in ISO 9001:2001

- A set of procedures that cover all key processes in the organization being managed
- Active monitoring of processes to ensure that they are effective
- Adequate record keeping
- Monitoring the quality of output, with implementation of appropriate corrective action if necessary
- Regular review of individual processes and the QM system itself for efficacy
- Implementation of a culture of continual improvement

---

works in collaboration with the International Electrotechnical Commission (IEC) and other metrological organizations.

ISO/IEC 17025:2005 is the main standard used by testing and reference laboratories to implement a QM system. It replaces ISO/IEC 17025:1999 (formally ISO Guide 25 and EN 45001). There is much in common with ISO 9000/9001, but ISO/IEC 17025 adds the concept of competence. There are two main sections: (i) management requirements that are primarily related to the operation and effectiveness of the laboratory QM system and (ii) technical requirements that address the competence of staff, methodology, and test/calibration equipment. ISO 15189:2007 defines standards for the operation of a medical laboratory, and is consistent with ISO 9000/9001.

Laboratory accreditation procedures and conformity assessment bodies (CABs) are assessed against ISO/IEC 17011:2004 (previously ISO/IEC Guide 58). CABs are defined as organizations providing assessment services such as testing, inspection, management system certification, personnel certification, product certification, and calibration.

Laboratory Accreditation

The International Laboratory Accreditation Cooperation (ILAC) website (http://www.ilac.org/, accessed 27 August 2007) gives details of accreditation bodies in many countries. Key elements are the Quality Policy, a statement of the quality aims of the organization, and the Quality Manual, which defines the organization's QM system. The layout of the Quality Manual should follow the outline of ISO 17025:2005.

Laboratory operations can be divided into preanalytical, analytical, and postanalytical phases (Box 2). Written procedures, usually known as *standard operating procedures (SOPs)*, should describe all aspects

---

Box 2. Stages in analytical toxicology laboratory operation

- **Preanalytical**
  Procedures must be in place to advise on appropriate sample collection (including sample tubes) and to ensure the safe transport, receipt, and storage of biological samples once in the laboratory, and for arranging the priority for the analysis
- **Analytical**
  Validated (i.e., tried and tested) procedures must be used to perform the requested or appropriate analyses to the required degree of accuracy and reliability in an appropriate timescale
- **Postanalytical**
  A mechanism for reporting results and maintaining confidentiality by telephone, fax, or other electronic means and in writing must be in place. Proper interpretation of results, especially for less-common analytes, must be provided. Full records of the analysis must be kept for at least 5 years (10 or more years in forensic work) unless otherwise determined by statute. Residues of samples must be stored appropriately until disposed of safely in an agreed timeframe

of laboratory operation, including management and health and safety aspects. The Society of Forensic Toxicologists (SOFT) and American Academy of Forensic Sciences (AAFS) have published detailed guidelines for the operation of forensic toxicology laboratories, much of which is also applicable to clinical toxicology laboratories [2].

Implementation and documentation of internal audits, both vertical (when, for example, the documentation concerning the analysis of a particular sample is examined) and horizontal (such as examining operating or quality procedures for internal consistency), are important parts of laboratory accreditation. Clinical or operational audit, i.e., examining the results generated in the light of the purpose for which they were requested, although much more difficult to undertake, is also important in the accreditation process. The results of such audits provide valuable training material.

Documentation of "quality queries", i.e., instances when mistakes or failures in processing have occurred, even if the error or failure was detected and corrected before a result was issued, and implementation and monitoring of corrective action, are also important in the accreditation process.

Method Implementation and Validation

Whatever method is used for a given analysis it must be validated, i.e., it must be shown to be "fit for purpose" [3]. Assay validation should conform, as far as possible, with the US Food and Drug Administration (FDA) Center for Drug Evaluation and Research (CDER) guidance for bioanalytical method validation [4]. Data for within-day (repeatability), between-day, and total precision should be calculated according to the protocol proposed by the Clinical and Laboratory Standards Institute [5]. A number of terms important in understanding method validation are given in Table 1.

Quantitative methods must have good precision and accuracy. Selectivity (freedom from interference, specificity) is important when a single species is to be measured, but broad specificity may be useful when screening for the presence of a particular class of compounds. The recovery of the analyte, i.e., how much of the compound of interest is recovered from the sample matrix during an extraction, for example, is important if sensitivity is limiting, but need not

be an issue if the lower limit of quantification (LLoQ), accuracy, and precision of the assay are acceptable.

Any quantitative analysis has associated errors, both random and systematic. In chromatographic and other separation methods, the "internal standard" method is often used to reduce the impact of systematic errors such as variations in injection volume, evaporation of extraction solvent, or mass spectrometry (MS) response during the analysis. Thus, a known amount of a second compound that behaves similarly to the analyte during the analysis, but elutes at a different place on the chromatogram or is otherwise detected independently of the analyte (the internal standard) is added at an appropriate stage in the analysis. Subsequently, the detector response of the analyte relative to the response of the internal standard is plotted against analyte concentration when constructing a calibration graph. Requirements for an internal standard for chromatographic assays are summarized in Box 3.

Stable isotope-labelled analogues are widely used as internal standards in MS (isotope dilution MS). Isotopic internal standards have virtually identical chemical and physical properties to the analyte and thus extraction, derivatization if needed, chromatography, and fragmentation are often virtually identical. However, the site of isotopic labeling should be chosen such that the bonds linking the isotope are not broken during fragmentation, as bonds involving heavier isotopes are more stable and the fragmentation pattern of the labeled compound could thus differ from that of the analyte. The vibrational frequencies of carbon–deuterium bonds are less than those of the corresponding carbon–hydrogen bonds, for example, so that deuterated compounds tend to be more stable than their unlabeled homologs. That labeled and unlabeled compounds may be partially resolved during the chromatographic analysis (deuterated analogs may elute slightly before the unlabeled analyte in GC-MS, for example) must be borne in mind not only with regard to choosing the correct integration parameters, but also because any ion suppression due to cochromatographed components may differ between the internal standard and the analyte(s). The internal standard may add to the degree of ion suppression in LC-MS, but generally both internal standard and analyte are affected equally by such phenomena [6].

Table 1 Terms used when reporting method validation

Term	Notes
Accuracy	The difference between the measured value and the accepted ("true") value
Calibration range	The range of concentrations between the highest and lowest calibration standards. This should encompass the range of concentrations found in the test samples
Coefficient of variation (CV)	An obsolete term for RSD
Higher limit of quantitation (HLoQ)	The highest concentration that can be quantified. Not always quoted, but important in assays with a clear upper "cutoff", for example, immunoassays and fluorescence assays
Internal standard	A second compound, not the analyte, added at an appropriate stage in the assay to correct for systematic errors in the analysis
Limit of detection (LoD)	The smallest amount of analyte that can be detected. Usually defined as some multiple (5, for example) of the baseline noise (signal-to-noise ratio = 5) or multiple of the SD of the blank signal
Linearity	A definable and reproducible relationship between a physicochemical measurement (e.g., UV absorption) and the concentration of the analyte, but not necessarily a straight line
Lower limit of quantification (LLoQ)	The lowest concentration that can be measured within defined limits. Usually a concentration for which the precision and accuracy have been set arbitrarily, e.g., RSD <20%
Precision	The scatter of measured values about a mean value. Usually quoted as RSD – within-assay (repeatability) and between-assay precision (reproducibility) is commonly given
Relative standard deviation (RSD)	The standard deviation of replicate measurements expressed as a percentage of the mean value: RSD = SD/Mean ×100% Useful when comparing precision at different concentrations
Selectivity	The ability to distinguish between the analyte and some other compound
Signal-to-noise (S/N) ratio	Strictly, the response to the analyte divided by the amplitude of the random electronic noise of the detection system. In practice, the background signal due to interfering compounds is often greater than the electronic noise

---

Box 3. Requirements for an internal standard

An internal standard must:

- Be completely resolved from the known and unknown substances in the chromatogram, or detected selectively as in MS for stable isotopes
- Elute near to (preferably just after the last) peak(s) of interest
- Have a similar detector response (peak height or area) to the analyte(s)
- Have similar chemical and physical properties to the analyte(s)
- Undergo any derivatization reaction in the same way as the analyte(s)
- Be chemically and physically stable on storage in solution and during the analysis
- Be easily available with adequate purity

Deuterium is the most commonly used stable isotope label. This is because of not only cost, but also the availability of high purity reagents. The presence of each deuterium atom in the molecule increases the M_r of the molecule by 1 atomic mass unit (u). For high-sensitivity analyses, it is recommended that the mass of the internal standard is at least 3 u greater than the analyte to reduce interference from naturally occurring isotopes. When stable isotope-labeled analogs are not available or the procedure can be used to quantify a large number of analytes simultaneously, internal standards that have chemical properties close enough to the analyte(s) to yield reliable quantitative data are used.

Reference Compounds

A fundamental starting point in any assay is obtaining certified pure reference material, or at least the best approximation to such material that can be attained. When preparing primary standards, particular attention should be paid to the M_r of salts and their degree of hydration (water of crystallization). Analytical results are normally reported in terms of free acid or base and not of a salt. The supplier, batch or lot number, purity, expiry date, and any other relevant information supplied with a compound should be recorded. Compounds should be stored in the dark under conditions recommended by the supplier. Every effort should be made to obtain a certificate of analysis or other appropriate documentation, but supply of such documentation is at the discretion of the manufacturer.

Preparation and Storage of Calibration Solutions

Assay calibration is normally done by analyzing standard solutions containing each analyte over an appropriate range of concentrations prepared in analyte-free plasma, urine, or other appropriate fluid. The chosen medium should be analyzed prior to the addition of the analyte(s) to ensure the absence of interferences.

Balances for weighing reagents or calibration standards, and automatic and semiautomatic pipettes, must be kept clean and checked for accuracy on a regular basis. Weighing of balance check weights should be recorded. Pipette accuracy should be documented by dispensing purified water and recording the weight dispensed. Weighing of reference compounds should

normally be performed by one analyst and witnessed by a second analyst, as should other steps, in preparing calibration standards and internal quality control (IQC) solutions such as calculating and performing dilutions.

The range of the calibration curve should cover the range of concentrations expected in the samples. The calibration curve should not normally be extrapolated beyond the lowest or highest standard solution. If the concentrations of some of the samples being analyzed are below the lowest calibration standard, then the assay may be repeated with the inclusion of lower concentration standards, if that is possible, or the result reported as less than the lowest standard. High concentration samples may be diluted to fit within the calibration range, provided the validity of doing so has been demonstrated during method development and if sufficient sample is available. Dilutions should be made with the same (e.g., blank plasma from the subject), or very similar (e.g., the matrix used for the calibration standards) matrix as the sample.

Neonatal calf serum is often used in the preparation of calibration solutions for plasma or serum assays. Newly prepared calibration solutions should be validated before use by comparison either with existing calibration solutions, or with IQC solutions prepared in human plasma or serum, and the results recorded. If, for any reason, neonatal calf serum proves unsuitable, human plasma or serum from an appropriate source should be used.

Blood-bank whole blood (transfusion blood) is sometimes used to prepare calibration standards. However, such blood and "plasma" derived from it (i) will usually be diluted with citrate solution, which has a high buffering capacity; (ii) may contain lidocaine and sometimes lidocaine metabolites; and (iii) may well contain plasticizers and other contaminants that may interfere in chromatographic and possibly other assays, and may alter the distribution of drugs between red cells and plasma by altering protein binding. Commercially available equine or bovine blood may suffer some of these same problems.

The question of "matrix matching" for preparation of calibration or IQC solutions is a vexed issue. Clearly true "matrix-matched" standards cannot be prepared for solid tissues such as liver or hair. Use of "blank" homogenized tissue samples or hair digests, for example, as the matrix for standard preparation is one way forward here. Analyte(s) may also be adsorbed onto hair prior to digestion.

Similarly, it is rarely possible to prepare standards in analyte-free sample from a patient or victim such that the standard has exactly the same composition as the sample submitted for analysis. The method of "standard additions" (adding known amounts of analyte to portions of the sample) is very difficult and inaccurate if only a limited sample volume is available, does not allow validation against existing calibrators, and does not permit the preparation of IQCs. Finally, "blank" human blood or urine can be used, as discussed above, but the volume of blood available is usually limited.

If newly prepared calibration standards and the IQCs meet the criteria for acceptance, portions may be transferred to labeled 3-ml plastic tubes and stored ($-20\,^{\circ}$C) until used. Cleaning records and lists of contents should be posted on all refrigerators and freezers including those used to store biological samples to meet Health and Safety requirements. Refrigerators and freezers should be fitted with failure alarms and temperature-monitoring devices and temperature records kept. Computerized temperature-monitoring devices (e.g., Tinytalk, http://www.tinytag.info/products/index.asp, accessed 10 October 2007) are available.

Calibration Graphs

Normally, a calibration graph of analyte response *versus* concentration in the calibration standards is constructed. In chromatographic assays, the response may be peak height or area, or peak height or area ratios to an internal standard. The relationship may be a straight line or a curve.

Blank samples, usually the drug-free matrix, should be prepared and analyzed along with the calibrators and unknown samples. The blank is an important part of quality control (QC). In a chromatographic assay, for example, there should be no interfering peaks in the region of the analyte(s) or internal standard(s). The response of the blank should not be so high as to limit the working range of the assay. The blank is not a zero calibrator, and normally must not be included in the calibration data. Replicate analyses of "blank" signal are necessary to define the limit of detection (LoD) and so it is important when using electronic data capture to ensure that the calibration curve is not being forced though zero.

An important criterion for an analytical method is the LoD, i.e., the minimum concentration (amount) of analyte that can be detected reliably and differentiated from any background signals measured in analyte-free samples. Defining the LoD is not as simple as it might at first seem to be, as there are random errors associated with both the blank sample and samples at or near the LoD. For chromatographic assays, the LoD might be quoted as some arbitrary multiple of the signal-to-noise ratio (S/N) such as 3, 5, or 10 times. This, of course, presupposes that the S/N can be measured and, with biological samples, the limiting factor is rarely instrument noise, but rather signals due (usually) to endogenous interfering species, in which case some multiple of the standard deviation (SD) of the blank signal may be used.

For quantitative analyses, it is usual to quote the lowest concentration or amount that can be measured with defined values of precision and accuracy; this is the lowest limit of quantitation (LLoQ). Again the criteria are arbitrary, and the relative standard deviations (RSDs) for precision and accuracy typically range from 10–15%, depending on the requirement of the assay. For trace analyses and pharmacokinetic experiments, it may be necessary to accept values as high as 20%, although the RSDs for concentrations above the LLoQ would normally be considerably lower. The concentration of the lowest calibrator may be set to the LLoQ, although for some applications it may not be necessary to measure such low concentrations. In any event, concentrations below the lowest standard should not be reported.

Reports do not always quote a higher limit of quantitation (HLoQ), particularly when the assay has a wide linear range. However, for some techniques, such as immunoassay and fluorescence detection in HPLC, the working range of the assay should be defined by both LLoQ and HLoQ. In some immunoassays, the presence of very high concentrations of an analyte can give a result suggesting the presence of a very low concentration ("hook effect").

Batch Analyses

Batch-assay calibration should normally be by analysis of standard solutions of each analyte (six to eight concentrations across the calibration range) prepared in the appropriate matrix (e.g., analyte-free neonatal calf or human serum). IQC procedures should be instituted. This involves the analysis of independently prepared solutions of known compositions that are not used in assay calibration; normally low, medium, and high concentrations of each analyte are prepared in analyte-free human serum, for example. Calibration standards are normally analyzed in duplicate, once at the beginning and once at the end of the batch. IQC samples are analyzed at the beginning and end of the batch and also after every 5–10 test samples as appropriate. External quality assessment (EQA) samples are analyzed as appropriate to conform to the requirements of particular EQA schemes. Single-point calibration methods for emergency work must be validated and the results compared with those from multipoint calibration [7].

The performance of batch analyses (analysis of a number of samples in the same analytical sequence) and analysis acceptance criteria should be as set out in the method validation guidance [4]. Typical assay-acceptance criteria are (i) chromatography (reproducible peak shape and retention time, stable baseline) and (ii) calibration graph ($r = 0.98$ or greater, intercept not markedly different from zero), and mean IQC results within acceptable limits (generally within 10% of nominal value). Acceptance criteria for patient samples are (i) "clean" chromatogram, i.e., absence as far as can be ascertained of interferences; (ii) duplicate values (peak height ratio to the internal standard) within 10% except when approaching the limit of sensitivity of the assay when duplicates within 20% may be acceptable; and (iii) results within the calibration range of the assay. Sample analyses falling outside acceptance limits may be repeated if sufficient sample is available.

While immunoassays may be performed as batch analyses, they may, depending on the instrument used, be subjected to random access analysis. IQC in such circumstance is best performed at timed intervals at low, medium, and high concentration. Some immunoassays are used as screens for the presence of drugs or metabolites, and "cutoff" concentration values are used to define positives. It is particularly important to ensure that the analytical performance at this cutoff point is properly investigated ($\pm 25\%$ of cutoff value) to minimize the risk of false positives and negatives arising from poor assay performance.

If a result above the calibration range is obtained, then, if possible, a portion of the sample should be diluted with "blank" plasma/serum and reanalyzed. If a sample is from a suspected overdose patient, then sample dilutions ($1 + 1, 1 + 3, 1 + 9$) should be made using "blank" serum at the time of the initial analysis (if the available sample volume permits) and

analyzed at the same time as the normal sample analysis. Postmortem whole-blood samples or tissue digests from suspected overdose cases, for example, may be diluted $1 + 3$ and $1 + 9$ with "blank" human serum prior to analysis using standard methods. If the information available suggests a massive overdose, further dilutions may be made as appropriate prior to the analysis.

Quality Control and Proficiency Testing

Once an analytical method has been validated and implemented, it is important to be able to show that the method continues to perform as intended. In qualitative work, known positive and negative specimens should normally be analyzed at the same time as the test sample. A negative control ("blank") helps to ensure that false positives (owing to, for example, contaminated reagents or glassware) are not obtained. Equally, inclusion of a true positive serves to check that the reagents have been prepared properly and remained stable.

In quantitative work, assay performance is monitored by the systematic analysis of IQC samples. Plotting the results for the IQC samples on a chart allows the day-to-day performance of the assay to be monitored and gives warning of any problems as they arise. When new batches of calibration and IQC samples are prepared, it is prudent to ensure comparability of the results obtained with those given by an earlier batch, or with the results obtained using external QC material.

FDA guidelines (for batch processing) require duplicate IQCs at three concentrations (high, medium, and low) to ensure that the assay is performing satisfactorily across the calibration range. The assay batch is deemed acceptable, provided four of the six controls (with at least one at each concentration) are within specification.

Quality Control Charts

QC charts are valuable in that they (i) produce evidence of satisfactory assay performance and (ii) give visual warning if assay performance begins to deteriorate. As with any QC method, it is important that reliable estimates of the parameters defining the control material are established. The mean value, μ, should be obtained from a minimum of 10 observations and the SD, σ, should be the between-assay value (interassay value). Obviously, these parameters must be measured when the analysis is performing satisfactorily.

Analytical laboratories commonly use Westgard rules to establish that assay performance is adequate [8]. Five different control rules are used to assess the acceptability of an analytical sequence. Further details and a multirule worksheet can be obtained from http://www.westgard.com/mltirule.htm (accessed 27 August 2007).

External Quality Assurance

Participation in EQA or proficiency testing (PT) schemes is an important part of QM [9]. In such schemes, portions of (sometimes lyophilized) homogenized plasma, serum, whole blood, or urine specimens are sent to a number of participating laboratories. After reconstitution in deionized water, if appropriate, the specimens are analyzed as if they were real samples and the results are reported before the true or target concentrations are made known.

EQA schemes measure interlaboratory performance and allow individual laboratories to detect and correct systematic errors. The laboratories do not have to use the same analytical method, as is usually the case with collaborative trials that are designed to test the reproducibility of a particular method. The results of EQA schemes are usually given as the z-score:

$$z = \frac{x - x_a}{\sigma_p} \qquad (1)$$

where x is an individual result, x_a is the accepted, "true" value and σ_p is known as the *target value of SD*, which should be decided on the basis of what is required of the test, and should be circulated in advance. If the result needs to be measured with high precision, then a low value of σ_p would be used. Thus, z is a measure of a laboratory's accuracy and the organizer's judgment as to what is "fit for purpose". If the results of an EQA scheme are normally distributed with a mean of x_a and variance of 1, then z-scores <2 would be deemed acceptable, whereas those >3 would not.

Toxicology EQA Schemes

Quantitative EQA schemes are available for a wide range of therapeutic drug monitoring (TDM) analytes

and some other poisons in many countries. The European Network of Forensic Science Institutes (ENFSI) website (http://www.enfsi.eu/page.php?uid=93, accessed 1 October 2008) and European Proficiency Testing Information System (http://www.eptis.bam.de/, accessed 1 October 2008) list EQA schemes for a range of analytes including drugs that are available in Europe, America, and Australia. The United Kingdom National External Quality Assessment Scheme (UKNEQAS) for therapeutic drug assays and the Dutch KKGT (Association for Quality Assessment in TDM and Clinical Toxicology) schemes, for example, have been operating for over 25 years.

There are, of course sometimes, concerns such as the possible effects of freeze-drying on analyte stability, and issues concerning the matrix used to prepare material for circulation (due to the cost of analyte-free human plasma or serum, neonatal calf serum may be used for some analytes). Nevertheless, from the datasets generated, scheme organizers can ascertain the methods that give the best performance, investigate sources of interference or bias, and, in extreme cases, report poorly performing methods to regulatory authorities. In the 30 years since the inception of these schemes, poorly performing assays have been identified and participants advised accordingly. The mean values reported have moved nearer to the intended value and the spread of results about the mean has been reduced [9].

EQA of qualitative work is also invaluable, as in drugs of abuse screening. Here, poor selectivity due to immunoassay cross-reactivity or gas chromatography (GC) injection port artifacts, as well as to manipulation of the sample by the patient, are real problems. Even with the ongoing educative role of EQA, errors (such as failure to detect morphine at $1\,\mathrm{mg}\,\mathrm{l}^{-1}$ in urine using LC-MS-MS) still occur. Often human error is the cause of such mistakes.

Well-run qualitative EQA schemes not only assess routine performance, but also add in hard-to-detect compounds or "spike" at concentrations around nationally agreed "cutoff" values. Good screening and confirmatory analytical performance from laboratories is required to ensure that the correct result is reported. Scoring of performance for a set of commonly encountered drugs such as morphine, 6-monoacetylmorphine for heroin, and 2-ethylidene-1,5-dimethyl-3,3-diphenylpyrrolidine (EDDP) for methadone, for example, helps laboratories address any problems in their procedures.

Urine is the matrix used most commonly, but schemes to support analyses in oral fluid and indeed in other matrices, such as hair, are emerging (e.g., that organized by the Society of Hair Testing, http://www.soht.org/, accessed 15 October 2007). For urine testing, scheme cutoffs are quite generous, but laboratories may also be scored against agreed workplace cutoffs (see http://www.wdtforum.org.uk/, accessed 27 August 2007). A breakdown of the performance of each recognized method type should be given to help laboratories understand why false-positive or false-negative reports have occurred in a given distribution. Meetings with users and scheme organizers are helpful to both groups. Regular clinical/forensic toxicology case schemes have also been instituted.

User Support and Staff Training

Training is an important part of QM. Clinicians, especially Accident and Emergency staff, forensic physicians, pathologists, and police need guidance not only as to what toxicological assays are useful in a given set of circumstances but also on sample collection, transport, and storage, local assay availability and turn-around time, and the interpretation of results. Especially important is guidance on blood and tissue sampling postmortem since the homogeneity of such samples cannot be taken for granted [10] and the possibility of changes in composition having occurred since death must be borne in mind when reporting results [11].

Not only do laboratory staff providing analytical toxicology services need training in providing these services and in the interpretation of results, they will also need some training in dealing with requests for tests that will need to be referred to other analytical centers. Staff in regional or national analytical centers will require extensive training in the more complicated analytical methods that they will be called upon to use. This training must encompass not only the techniques themselves (TLC, HPLC, etc.), but also their application in analytical toxicology and related areas. Knowledge of the role of local hospital laboratories, coroners, police, and the local poisons center is important [12].

There are no internationally recognized training programs in analytical toxicology. However, a training scheme for a graduate clinical scientist specializing in analytical toxicology has been developed in the UK. The training program comprises 4 years full-time study, followed by a period of higher specialist training, in some cases, leading to the award of a research degree such as Doctor of Philosophy. The American Board of Clinical Chemistry hosts an examination in Toxicological Chemistry (http://www.abclinchem.org/tox_chem/Pages/default. aspx, accessed 30 September 2008).

Participation in continuing education (CE), continuing professional development (CPD), or revalidation programs is important when staff attain career grades, i.e., when initial and higher specialist training has been completed, and may be necessary for continued specialist registration in countries where such registration is mandatory. Compliance with CPD programs may require maintenance and external audit of personal records listing educational activities, such as scientific meetings attended, papers published, lectures given, etc. Details of such a scheme maintained by the UK Royal College of Pathologists are available (http://www.rcpath.org/index.asp?PageID=620, accessed 27 August 2007). Many other countries run similar schemes.

Nongraduate scientific staff will be normally trained in-house in specific aspects of laboratory operation, although training in the operation of newer specialized instruments may sometimes be provided by manufacturers. Proper recording of training is important.

Recording and Reporting Results

It is usually advisable to contact the laboratory by telephone in advance to discuss urgent or complicated cases. A request form must accompany the samples to the laboratory. Most clinical specimens, particularly blood and urine, may be sent by post if securely packaged in compliance with current regulations. Filter-paper adsorbed dried blood may be acceptable in certain circumstances and does not require refrigeration [11].

In forensic work, it is important to be able to guarantee the identity and integrity of the specimen. Thus, such samples should be protected during transport by the use of tamper-evident seals and should, ideally,

---

Box 4. Chain of custody documents

- Name of the individual collecting the specimen
- Name of each person or entity subsequently having custody of it, and details of how it has been stored
- Date(s) the specimen was collected or transferred
- Specimen or case number
- Name of the subject or deceased
- Brief description of the specimen
- Record of the condition of tamper-evident seals

---

be submitted in person to the laboratory by the Coroner's officer or other investigating personnel. *Chain of custody* is a term used to refer to the process used to maintain and document the history of the specimen (Box 4).

Fully validated assays must include data on the stability of the analyte in the appropriate matrix under specified storage conditions. In the absence of other information, biological specimens should be stored at $2-8\,^{\circ}C$ prior to analysis, if possible, and ideally any specimen remaining after the analysis should be kept at $2-8\,^{\circ}C$ for 3–4 weeks in case further analyses are required. In forensic work, any specimen remaining must be kept (preferably at $-20\,^{\circ}C$) until destruction is authorized by the investigating authority.

All results should be recorded in laboratory notebooks or on worksheets together with information such as the date, the name of the analyst, the name of the patient, and other relevant information, the number and nature of the specimens received for analysis, and the tests performed. All specimens received in laboratories are normally allocated a unique identifying number. This number is used when referring to the tests performed on the specimen.

UV spectra, chromatograms, calibration graphs, and other documents generated during an analysis should always be kept for a time after the results have been reported. Recording the results of color tests and TLC analyses is more difficult unless a digital camera is used. Electronic data storage is dependent on the availability of hardware and software to read the data.

Reporting the results of tests in which no compounds were detected in plasma/serum or in urine, the limit of sensitivity of the test (LoD) should always be known, at least to the laboratory, and the scope of generic tests (benzodiazepines and opioids) should be defined.

The results of urgent (emergency) analyses must be communicated directly to the client without delay, and should be followed by a written report as soon as possible. Ideally, confirmation from a second independent method, or failing this, an independent duplicate, should be obtained before reporting positive findings. However, this may not always be practicable, especially if only simple methods are available or if sample amount is limiting. In such cases, it is vital that the appropriate positive and negative controls have been analyzed together with the specimen.

When reporting quantitative results, it is important to clearly state the units of measurement used. In addition, any information necessary to ensure that the clinical implications of the result are fully understood must be available and should also be noted on the written report.

Although it may be easy to interpret the results of analyses in which no compounds are detected, such results are sometimes difficult to convey to others, especially in writing. This is because it is important to give information as to the poisons excluded by the tests performed with all the attendant complications of the scope, sensitivity, and selectivity of the analyses and other factors such as sampling variations. Because of the potential medicolegal and other implications of any toxicological analysis, it is important not to use laboratory jargon such as "negative" or "not confirmed", or sweeping statements such as "absent" or "not present". The phrase "not detected" should precisely convey the laboratory result, especially when accompanied by a statement of the specimen analyzed and the LLoQ.

While chain-of-custody procedures for sample submission are widely implemented, secure systems for reporting results are also needed – it is not unknown for a report to be altered by laboratory staff in order to subvert an investigation.

Summary

Implementation of QM principles and associated laboratory accreditation procedures helps ensure that reliable results are obtained and can be defended in court. With the increasing use of point-of-care testing (POCT) devices, the principles of QM also have to be applied to such procedures in order to ensure the reliability of results. Although QM principles are more difficult to apply to the clinical interpretation of analytical results, it is vital that this aspect of the laboratory's work is not neglected.

References

[1] Burnett, D. (2002). *A Practical Guide To Accreditation In Laboratory Medicine*, ACB Venture Publications, London.

[2] SOFT/AAFS (Society of Forensic Toxicologists/ American Academy of Forensic Sciences) (2002). *Forensic Toxicology Laboratory Guidelines*, http://www. soft-tox.org/docs/Guidelines%202006%20Final.pdf (accessed 27 August 2007).

[3] Peters, F.T., Drummer, O.H. & Musshoff, F. (2007). Validation of new methods, *Forensic Science International* **165**, 216–224.

[4] FDA/CDER (Food and Drug Administration/Center for Drug Evaluation and Research) Guidance for industry (2001). *Bioanalytical Method Validation*, http://www. fda.gov/cder/guidance/4252fnl.htm (accessed 27 August 2007).

[5] Clinical and Laboratory Standards Institute (2004). *Evaluation of Precision Performance of Quantitative Measurement Methods: Approved Guideline*, 2nd Edition, Document EP05-A~ 2, http://webstore.ansi.org/ansi-docstore/product.asp?sku=EP05%2DA2 (accessed 27 August 2007).

[6] Sojo, L.E., Lum, G. & Chee, P. (2003). Internal standard signal suppression by co-eluting analyte in isotope dilution LC-ESI-MS, *The Analyst* **128**, 51–54.

[7] Peters, F.T., Jung, J., Kraemer, T. & Maurer, H.H. (2005). Fast, simple, and validated gas chromatographic-mass spectrometric assay for quantification of drugs relevant to diagnosis of brain death in human blood plasma samples, *Therapeutic Drug Monitoring* **27**, 334–344.

[8] Westgard, J.O., Barry, P.L., Hunt, M.R. & Groth, T. (1981). A multi-rule Shewhart chart for quality control in clinical chemistry, *Clinical Chemistry* **27**, 493–501.

[9] Wilson, J.F. (2002). External quality assessment schemes for toxicology, *Forensic Science International* **128**, 98–103.

[10] Flanagan, R.J. & Connally, G. (2005). Interpretation of analytical toxicology results in life and at post mortem, *Toxicological Reviews* **24**, 51–62.

[11] Flanagan, R.J., Connally, G. & Evans, J.M. (2005). Analytical toxicology: guidelines for sample collection post mortem, *Toxicological Reviews* **24**, 63–71.

[12] Flanagan, R.J. (2004). Developing an analytical toxicology service: Principles and guidance, *Toxicological Reviews* **23**, 251–263.

ROBERT J. FLANAGAN AND ROBIN WHELPTON